A Practical Approach to Cardiac Anesthesia

Fifth Edition

Editors

Frederick A. Hensley, Jr., MD
Benjamin Monroe Carraway Professor
Vice Chair of Clinical Anesthesiology, Department of Anesthesiology
University of Alabama at Birmingham
School of Medicine
Medical Director of Anesthesia Services for UAB Health System
Birmingham, Alabama

Donald E. Martin, MD
Professor of Anesthesiology
Associate Dean for Administration
Penn State University College of Medicine
Penn State Hershey Medical Center
Hershey, Pennsylvania

Glenn P. Gravlee, MD
Professor
Department of Anesthesiology
University of Colorado at Denver
and Health Sciences Center
Denver, Colorado

Wolters Kluwer Health | Lippincott Williams & Wilkins
Philadelphia • Baltimore • New York • London
Buenos Aires • Hong Kong • Sydney • Tokyo

Acquisitions Editor: Brian Brown
Product Manager: Nicole Dernoski
Vendor Manager: Alicia Jackson
Senior Manufacturing Manager: Benjamin Rivera
Marketing Manager: Lisa Lawrence
Design Coordinator: Doug Smock
Production Service: Aptara, Inc.

Two Commerce Square
2001 Market Street
Philadelphia, PA 19103 USA
LWW.com

Printed in China

Library of Congress Cataloging-in-Publication Data
A practical approach to cardiac anesthesia / editors, Frederick A. Hensley Jr., Donald E. Martin, Glenn P. Gravlee.—5th ed.
p. ; cm.
Includes bibliographical references and index.
ISBN 978-1-4511-3744-6 (alk. paper)
I. Hensley, Frederick A. II. Martin, Donald E. (Donald Eugene)
III. Gravlee, Glenn P.
[DNLM: 1. Anesthesia—methods. 2. Cardiac Surgical Procedures.
3. Heart—drug effects. WG 460]
617.9'67412—dc23

2012011794

To purchase additional copies of this book, call our customer service department at (800) 638-3030 or fax orders to (301) 223-2320. International customers should call (301) 223-2300.

Visit Lippincott Williams & Wilkins on the Internet: at LWW.com. Lippincott Williams & Wilkins customer service representatives are available from 8:30 am to 6 pm, EST.

10 9 8 7 6 5 4 3 2 1

CCS0812

❖

I dedicate this book to my children; Frederick Allen III, now in Heaven; but his spirit will always be in his parents' hearts, Theresa Jeannette, and Jennifer Elizabeth. A father could not be prouder of his children.—Frederick A. Hensley, Jr., MD

❖

I'm proud to dedicate this book to our three wonderful children, Susan, Seth, and Marc, and wish them all of the love and joy that they have brought to us.—Donald E. Martin, MD

❖

I dedicate this book to my children, Brent and Sarah, who have inspired and amazed me from infancy to adulthood.—Glenn P. Gravlee, MD

Contributors

Percy Boateng, MD
Assistant Professor
Department of CT Surgery
Drexel University College of Medicine
Attending Surgeon
Department of CT Surgery
Hahnemann Hospital
Philadelphia, Pennsylvania

John F. Butterworth, IV, MD
Professor and Chairman
Department of Anesthesiology
Virginia Commonwealth University
Virginia Commonwealth University Health System
Richmond, Virginia

Charles E. Chambers, MD
Professor of Medicine & Radiology
Penn State University
Director
Cardiac Catheterization Laboratory
Heart & Vascular Institute
Hershey Medical Center
Hershey, Pennsylvania

Joseph C. Cleveland, Jr., MD
Professor of Surgery
Surgical Director, Cardiac Transplantation and MCS
University of Colorado Anschutz Medical Center
Aurora, Colorado

Charles D. Collard, MD, MS
Professor and Vice Chairman
Department of Anesthesiology
Baylor College of Medicine
Anesthesiologist in Chief
Department of Anesthesiology
Texas Heart Institute
St. Luke's Episcopal Hospital
Houston, Texas

John R. Cooper, Jr., MD
Professor
Department of Anesthesiology
Baylor College of Medicine
Attending Anesthesiologist
Department of Cardiovascular Anesthesia
Texas Heart Institute
St. Luke's Episcopal Hospital
Houston, Texas

Jack H. Crawford MD, PhD
Assistant Professor
Department of Anesthesiology
University of Alabama at Birmingham
Birmingham, Alabama

Laurie K. Davies, MD
Associate Professor
Department of Anesthesiology & Surgery
University of Florida
Gainesville, Florida

Kishan Dwarakanath, MD
Assistant Professor
Department of Anesthesiology
Baylor College of Medicine
Attending Anesthesiologist
Cardiovascular Anesthesia
Texas Heart Institute
St. Luke's Episcopal Hospital
Houston, Texas

John W.C. Entwistle, III, MD, PhD
Associate Professor
Department of Cardiothoracic Surgery
Drexel University College of Medicine
Director of Heart Transplantation
Department of Cardiothoracic Surgery
Hahnemann University Hospital
Philadelphia, Pennsylvania

Amanda A. Fox, MD, MPH
Assistant Professor
Department of Anesthesiology
Harvard Medical School
Attending Anesthesiologist
Department of Anesthesiology
Perioperative & Pain Medicine
Brigham and Women's Hospital
Boston, Massachusetts

Thomas E.J. Gayeski, MD, PhD
Professor of Anesthesiology
Director of Cardiac Anesthesiology
Department of Anesthesiology
University of Alabama at Birmingham
Birmingham, Alabama

Mark A. Gerhardt, MD, PhD
Associate Professor
Department of Anesthesiology
The Ohio State University
The Ohio State University Medical Center
Columbus, Ohio

Joseph N. Ghansah

Neville M. Gibbs, MD, FANZCA
Clinical Professor
School of Medicine and Pharmacology
University of Western Australia
Head
Department of Anaesthesia
Sir Charles Gairdner Hospital
Nedlands, Australia

Glenn P. Gravlee, MD
Professor
Department of Anesthesiology
University of Colorado at Denver
and Health Sciences Center
Denver, Colorado

Michael S. Green, DO
Assistant Professor
Department of Anesthesiology
Drexel University College of Medicine
Program Director
Department of Anesthesiology
Hahnemann University Hospital
Philadelphia, Pennsylvania

Robert C. Groom, MS, CCP
Associate Vice President
Cardiac Services
Maine Medical Center
Portland, Maine

Ronald L. Harter, MD
Professor and Chair
Department of Anesthesiology
Wexner Medical Center at The Ohio State University
Columbus, Ohio

Eugene A. Hessel, II, MD
Professor
Department of Anesthesiology
University of Kentucky College of Medicine
Staff Anesthesiologist
Department of Anesthesiology
A.B. Chandler/University of Kentucky Medical Center
Lexington, Kentucky

Jay C. Horrow, MD, MS
Professor
Department of Anesthesiology & Perioperative Medicine
Drexel University College of Medicine
Hahnemann University Hospital
Philadelphia, Pennsylvania

Michael B. Howie, MD
Professor
Department of Anesthesiology
The Ohio State University
Columbus, Ohio

S. Adil Husain, MD
Associate Professor
Department of CT Surgery
Chief
Division of Pediatric CT Surgery
The University of Texas Health Sciences Center
Chairman
Department of Surgery
Christus Santa Rosa Children's Hospital
San Antonio, Texas

James Y. Kim, MD
Chief Fellow
Department of Anesthesiology
Emory University School of Medicine
Emory University Hospital
Atlanta, Georgia

Colleen G. Koch, MD, MS, MBA
Professor of Anesthesiology
Cleveland Clinic Lerner College of Medicine
Case Western Reserve University
Vice Chair
Research and Education
Department of Cardiothoracic Anesthesia
Cardiothoracic Anesthesia and Quality and Patient Safety Institute
Cleveland Clinic
Cleveland, Ohio

David R. Larach, MD, PhD
Chief (Retired)
Division of Cardiac Anesthesiology
The Heart Institute
St. Joseph Medical Center
Towson, Maryland

Michael G. Licina, MD
Vice Chair of Operations
Department of Cardiothoracic Anesthesia
Cleveland Clinic
Cleveland, Ohio

Jerry C. Luck, Jr., MD
Clinical Professor of Medicine
Penn State Hershey Medical Center
Cardiologist Cardiac Consultants, P.C.
Lancaster, Pennsylvania

S. Nini Malayaman, MD
Assistant Professor
Department of Anesthesiology
Drexel University College of Medicine
Attending Anesthesiologist
Department of Anesthesiology
Hahnemann University Hospital
Philadelphia, Pennsylvania

Donald E. Martin, MD
Professor of Anesthesiology
Associate Dean for Administration
Penn State University College of Medicine
Penn State Hershey Medical Center
Hershey, Pennsylvania

Thomas M. McLoughlin, Jr., MD
Professor of Surgery
Division of Surgical Anesthesiology
University of South Florida College of Medicine
Tampa, Florida
Chair
Department of Anesthesiology
Lehigh Valley Health Network
Allentown, Pennsylvania

Anand R. Mehta, MBBS
Medical College of Georgia
Department of Anesthesiology & Perioperative Medicine
Augusta, Georgia

Benjamin N. Morris, MD
Assistant Professor
Department of Anesthesiology
Wake Forest University
Winston-Salem, North Carolina

John M. Murkin, MD, FRCPC
Senate Professor of Anesthesiology
Department of Anesthesiology and Perioperative Medicine
Schulich School of Medicine
The University of Western Ontario
Director
Cardiac Anesthesiology Research
Department of Anesthesiology and Perioperative Medicine
University Hospital
London Health Sciences Center, London
Ontario, Canada

Glenn S. Murphy, MD
Clinical Associate Professor
Department of Anesthesiology
Pritzker School of Medicine
University of Chicago
Chicago, Illinois
Director
Cardiac Anesthesia
Department of Anesthesiology
North Shore University Health System
Evanston, Illinois

Gary S. Okum, MD
Associate Professor
Department of Anesthesiology and Surgery
Drexel University College of Medicine
Attending Physician
Department of Anesthesiology
Hahnemann University Hospital
Philadelphia, Pennsylvania

Ferenc Puskas, MD, PhD
Associate Professor
Department of Anesthesiology
University of Colorado Denver
Aurora, Colorado

James G. Ramsay, MD
Professor
Department of Anesthesiology
Emory University School of Medicine
Medical Director, CV ICU
Emory University Hospital
Atlanta, Georgia

Mark E. Romanoff, MD
Staff Anesthesiologist
American Anesthesiology
Carolinas Medical Center
Charlotte, North Carolina

Anne L. Rother, MBBS, FANZCA
Staff Anesthesiologist
Department of Anesthesia
Monash Medical Centre
Clayton, Australia

Roger L. Royster, MD
Professor
Department of Anesthesiology
Wake Forest University
Executive Vice Chair
Department of Anesthesiology
Wake Forest Baptist Medical Center
Winston-Salem, North Carolina

Soraya M. Samii, MD
Associate Professor
Department of Medicine
Clinical Electrophysiology
Department of Cardiology
Penn State Hershey
Hershey, Pennsylvania

Jack S. Shanewise, MD
Professor of Clinical Anesthesiology
Department of Anesthesiology
Columbia University
Director
Division of Cardiothoracic Anesthesiology
Department of Anesthesiology
Columbia University Medical Center
New York, New York

Michael L. Shelton, MD
Cardiothoracic Anesthesiology Fellow
Department of Anesthesiology
University of Alabama
Birmingham, Alabama

Linda Shore-Lesserson, MD
Division of Anesthesiology
Montefiore Medical Center
Bronx, New York

Peter Slinger, MD, FRCPC
Professor
Department of Anesthesia
University of Toronto
Staff Anesthesiologist
Department of Anesthesia
Toronto General Hospital
Toronto, Ontario

Mark Stafford-Smith, MD
Professor
Department of Anesthesiology
Duke University
Attending Anesthesiologist
Department of Anesthesiology
Duke University Medical Center
Durham, North Carolina

Brad L. Steenwyk, MD
Associate Professor of Anesthesiology
University of Alabama at Birmingham School of Medicine
Birmingham, Alabama

Erin A. Sullivan, MD
Associate Professor of Anesthesiology, Director
Division of Cardiothoracic Anesthesiology
University of Pittsburgh
Physician
Department of Anesthesiology
University of Pittsburgh Medical Center
Pittsburgh, Pennsylvania

Breandan Sullivan, MD
Assistant Professor
Department of Anesthesiology
Section on Critical Care Medicine
University of Colorado School of Medicine
Aurora, Colorado

Benjamin C. Sun, MD
Chair, Cardiac, Thoracic and Transplant Surgery
Minneapolis Heart Institute
Allina Health Systems
Minneapolis, Minnesota

Matthew M. Townsley, MD
Assistant Professor
Department of Anesthesiology
University of Alabama
Birmingham School of Medicine
Attending Anesthesiologist
Department of Anesthesiology
UAB Hospital
Birmingham, Alabama

Michael H. Wall, MD, FCCM
Professor of Anesthesiology and Cardiothoracic Surgery
Department of Anesthesiology
Washington University in St. Louis
Clinical Chief of Anesthesiology
Department of Anesthesiology
Barnes-Jewish Hospital
St. Louis, Missouri

Katarzyna M. Walosik-Arenall, MD
Cardiothoracic Anesthesia Fellow
Department of Anesthesiology
University of Alabama
Birmingham, Alabama

Andrew S. Wechsler, MD, BA
Stanley K. Brockman Professor and Chairman
Department of Cardiothoracic Surgery
Drexel University College of Medicine
Philadelphia, Pennsylvania

Nathaen S. Weitzel, MD
Assistant Professor
Department of Anesthesiology
University of Colorado
Denver, Colorado
Anesthesiologist
University of Colorado Hospital
Aurora, Colorado

Preface

We are happy to introduce you to the 2012 edition of *A Practical Approach to Cardiac Anesthesia*, the latest of five editions published over almost 25 years. During this time, the subspecialty of cardiac anesthesiology has grown and matured. Cardiac anesthesiologists' skills in echocardiography, pain management, life support, and critical care have expanded their role in the management of cardiothoracic patients.

This edition remains true to its original purpose to provide "an easily accessible, practical reference designed to help the practitioner prepare for and manage cardiac anesthetics." At the same time, it has been updated and expanded to keep pace with the rapidly changing practice of cardiothoracic anesthesia. Several new chapters have been added. "Cardiovascular Physiology: A Primer" provides an important introduction to the basics of cardiovascular physiology and monitoring. Unique aspects of the management of adult patients with congenital heart disease are now recognized with separate chapters regarding adult and pediatric patients with congenital heart disease. A chapter has been added discussing "Blood Transfusion", recognizing the expanding importance of blood management to cardiac procedures, and a chapter has been dedicated to the unique "Anesthetic Considerations for Patients with Pericardial Disease". In addition to new chapters, the discussions of echocardiography and other applications of ultrasound have been expanded and enhanced by a large number of high-quality color images. The recent technologic advances in non-invasive monitoring techniques and the most recent recommendations for perioperative glucose and implantable electronic device management are included.

The fifth edition draws on the experience of 55 authors from 29 different institutions. It is organized into five sections–Cardiovascular Physiology and Pharmacology, Anesthetic Management for Cardiac Surgery, Anesthetic Management of Specific Cardiac Disorders, Circulatory Support, and Thoracic Anesthesia and Pain Management. The book is published in full color, in an up-to-date and easily readable format. The key points in each chapter are summarized at the beginning of the chapter, with references (and hyperlinks in electronic versions) to the appropriate section of the text.

The editors would like to take this chance to thank each of the authors for sharing their knowledge and experience in the pages of this book, and also to express our appreciation for the work of Brian Brown and Nicole Dernoski, the book's editors from Wolters Kluwer, for their skillful management of the publication process.

Contents

I CARDIOVASCULAR PHYSIOLOGY AND PHARMACOLOGY

1 Cardiovascular Physiology: A Primer

Thomas E. J. Gayeski, Brad L. Steenwyk, and Jack H. Crawford

KEY POINTS

1. The heart has a fibrous skeleton that provides an insertion site at each valvular ring. This fibrous structure also connects cardiac myocytes so that "stretch" or preload results in sarcomeres lengthening and not intercellular sliding.
2. Contractility changes as a result of myoplasmic Ca^{2+} concentration change during systole.
3. Relaxation following contraction is an active process requiring ATP consumption to pump Ca^{2+} into the sarcoplasmic reticulum as well across the sarcolemma.
4. The fundamental unit of tension development is the sarcomere.
5. The endocardium receives perfusion during systole while the epicardium receives blood flow throughout the cardiac cycle. The ventricular wall is more susceptible to endocardial infarction.
6. The external stroke volume work the ventricle does is to raise the pressure of a stroke volume from VEDP (right or left) to mean arterial pressure (pulmonary or systemic, respectively).
7. Oxygen or ATP consumption occurs during release of actin–myosin bonds during relaxation of this bond. The main determinants of myocardial oxygen consumption are heart rate, contractility, and wall tension.

(*continued*)

8. The cardiovascular system regulates blood pressure and it is an example of a negative feedback loop control system. Sensors throughout the cardiovascular system all sense stretch.
9. Physiologic reserves are expansion factors allowing the cardiovascular system to maintain blood pressure. These reserves are heart rate (3-fold range), contractility, systemic vascular resistance (15-fold range), and venous capacitance (~1.5-fold range).
10. Utilizing the reserve of venous capacitance does not affect myocardial oxygen consumption.

AS A PHYSIOLOGIC PRIMER FOR CARDIAC ANESTHESIOLOGY, this chapter requires brevity and choices (or opinions)! Cardiac anatomy, physiology, pathology, and genomics are decades old, continue to evolve, and have a vast literature. Our focus is on presenting physiologic principles important to clinical management in the operating room. A detailed description and discussion of cardiac physiology can be found in 1. If these physiologic concepts are memorized and applied correctly, your patients will benefit from risk modification under your care. If they are understood, you will be able to apply them to the dynamic pathology present in the operating room and have a physiologic basis for being a consultant in cardiac anesthesiology.

I. Embryologic development of the heart.

A. The cardiovascular system begins to develop during week 3 as the primitive vascular system is formed from mesodermally derived endothelial tubes. Eventually at week 4, bilateral cardiogenic cords from paired endocardial heart tubes fuse into a single heart tube (primitive heart). This fusion initiates forward flow and is the start of the heart's transport function.

B. The primitive heart evolves into four chambers: Bulbus cordis, ventricle, primordial atrium, and sinus venosus, eventually forming bulboventricular loop with the initial contraction occurs at 21 to 22 days. These contractions result in unidirectional blood flow in week 4.

C. From weeks 4 to 7 heart development enters a critical period as it divides into the four chambers of the adult heart, the basis of the fetal circulation.

D. The framework of the heart is a fibrous skeleton, composed of fibrin and elastin, forming four rings encircling the four valves of the heart as well as intermyocyte connections.

E. The fibrous skeleton:

1 1. Serves as an anchor for the insertion of the valve cusps
2. Resists overdistention of the annuli of the valves (resisting incompetence)
3. Provides a fixed insertion point for the muscular bundles of the ventricles
4. Minimizes intermyocyte sliding during ventricular filling and contraction

II. Electrical conduction

A. By breaking the atrial intermyocyte conduction of impulses, the fibrous skeleton blocks the direct spread of electrical conduction from the atria to the ventricles.

B. Because of this separation of the atrial myocyte conduction from ventricular myocytes, the AV nodal/purkinje system creates coordinated contraction between atria and ventricles.

C. Excitation–contraction coupling

1. A purkinje fiber action potential results in the coordinated contraction of a cardiac myocyte. There are five phases of an action potential and an integrated and complex change in Na+, K+, and Ca^{2+} conductances and ion fluxes within these phases.
2. Excitation–contraction coupling starts when an action potential triggers the diffusion of Ca^{2+} ions across the sarcolemma through the Ca^{2+} release channels (ryanodine receptor channel). To shorten the time constant of this transmembrane flux, the T-tubule system markedly increases the surface area through which this flux of external Ca^{2+} occurs. In addition, the sarcoplasmic reticulum cisternae ensure rapid myoplasmic Ca^{2+} increase (Fig. 1.1).
3. The amount of Ca^{2+} transported across the sarcolemma is only about 1% of Ca^{2+} needed for contraction. However, this Ca^{2+} serves as a trigger for sarcoplasmic reticulum release of Ca^{2+} to create the Ca^{2+} concentration needed for tension development.
4. The sarcoplasmic reticulum is a complex organelle responsible for the efficient cycling of calcium concentration during each heartbeat. The external Ca^{2+} crossing the sarcolemma

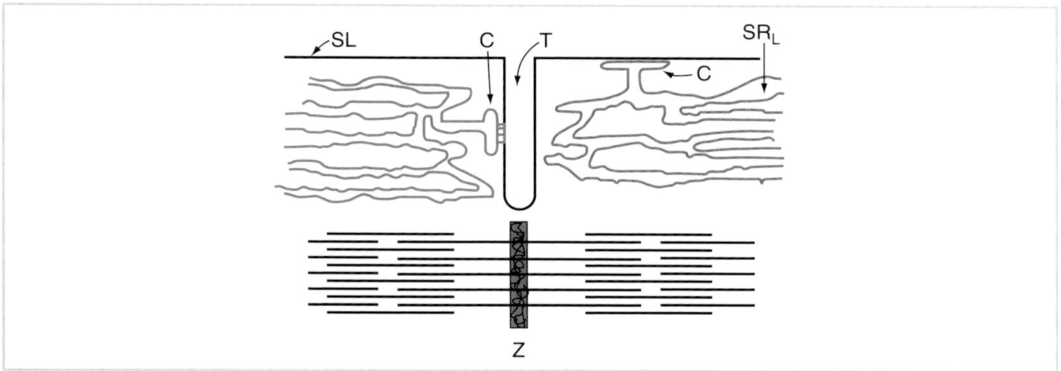

FIGURE 1.1 Relation of cardiac sarcoplasmic reticulum to surface membrane and myofibrils. The SR_L and C overlie the myofilaments; they are shown separately for illustrative purposes. SL, sarcolemma; C, cisterna; T, transverse tubule; SR_L, longitudinal sarcoplasmic reticulum; Z, Z disc.

triggers a graded release of internal Ca^{2+} from the sarcoplasmic reticulum. From relaxation to contraction, cytosolic Ca^{2+} concentration varies approximately 100-fold.

2 **5.** Three very important proteins within the sarcoplasmic reticulum are responsible for controlling calcium flux: The Ca^{2+} release channel, the sarco-endoplasmic reticulum ATP-ase (SERCA-2), and the regulatory protein of SERCA-2 (phospholamban). Alterations within phospholamban are currently an active area of interest and may play a role in the development of heart failure and other cardiomyopathies (Maclennan, Nature Reviews Molecular Cell Biology 4, 566–577 [July 2003]).

6. The graded release of Ca^{2+}, signaled by the trans-sarcolemmal Ca^{2+} flux and enhanced due to sarcoplasmic reticulum cisternae, is dependent on the amount of Ca^{2+} stored in the sarcoplasmic reticulum, the sympathetic tone (sarcolemma Ca^{2+} conductance), and the external Ca^{2+}. Increased stores lead to increased release, resulting in increased tension development for a given sarcomere length = increased contractility.

7. Any increase in contractility via any drug is a consequence of increased myoplasmic Ca^{2+} concentration during systole! Ca^{2+} binds to troponin and results in a conformational change involving tropomyosin. This change allows actin and myosin to interact, resulting in shortening of a sarcomere (Fig. 1.2).

8. Similarly, a decrease in contractility is a result of decreased Ca^{2+} binding to troponin during systole. Its cause is attributable to decreased myoplasmic Ca^{2+} during systole or decreased Ca^{2+} binding to troponin. Myoplasmic Ca^{2+} is affected by inhalational agents, induction drugs, etc. A common clinical reason for decreased Ca^{2+}–troponin affinity is intracellular acidosis.

3 **9.** Finally, for contraction to cease, Ca^{2+} must be removed from the myoplasm. Ca^{2+} is actively pumped into the sarcoplasmic reticulum as well as pumped across the sarcolemma. Depending on Ca^{2+} ion conductances in each of the sites, sarcoplasmic Ca^{2+} may be increased or decreased in the sarcoplasmic reticulum during this removal.

III. Cardiac myocyte

A. Sarcomere

1. The fundamental unit of tension development is the sarcomere. The sarcomere is composed of myosin, the tropomyosin–actin–troponin complex, and a z-disc.

2. Each actin molecule contains a myosin-binding site as well as the site for tropomyosin–troponin chain to bind. Two actin molecule chains are intertwined and form an actin polymer. Combined with a tropomyosin–troponin complex bound within the grooves to the actin polymer chains, this complex is known as a thin filament. The thin filament spans a distance of approximately 2 μm.

3. The z-disc anchors the thin filaments in place in a regular pattern as schematized below. It is a strong meshwork of filaments forming a band that anchors the interdigitated thin filaments.

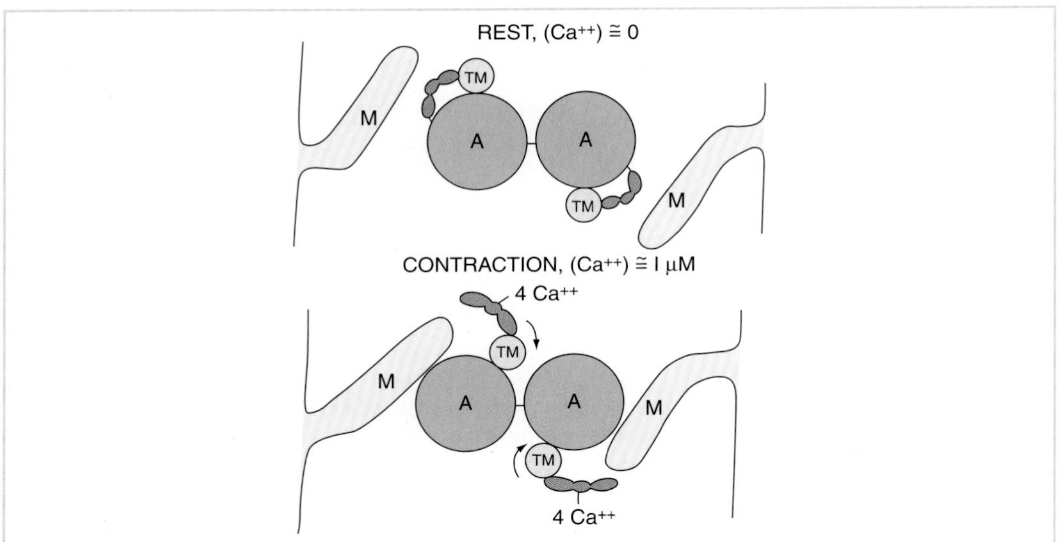

FIGURE 1.2 Schematic representation of actin–myosin dependence on Ca^{2+}–troponin binding for tension development to occur. (From Honig C. *Modern Cardiovascular Physiology*. Boston/Toronto: Little, Brown and Company; 1981.)

4. Myosin molecules aggregate spontaneously forming the thick filaments. These filaments are approximately 1.6 μm. These thick filaments are held in place by M filaments and are interdigitated amongst the thin filaments. At the center of each thick filament is a zone that has no myosin "heads." This absence explains the decrease in tension development if overstretching of the sarcomere were to occur. Each myosin head contains an ATP-ase and actin-binding site.

4 5. Together, troponin and tropomyosin and Ca^{2+} binding serve as regulatory proteins that allow actin and myosin to interact to result in shortening of the sarcomere length.

6. Each exposure of actin to myosin results in a shortening of sarcomere length. To allow for multiple shortenings to occur, actin–myosin binding is uncoupled. This ATP-consuming step, the relaxation phase, occurs because of the ATP-ase bound to myosin. This energy-dependent step, requiring oxygen consumption, occurs multiple times during a cardiac cycle.

7. Depending on preload, the sarcomere length, or the distance between z-discs, ranges from 1.8 to 2.2 μm.

IV. Organization of myocytes

A. A cardiac myocyte is approximately 12 μm long. Hence, each myocyte only has several (~6) sarcomeres in series from end to end of a myocyte.

B. As mentioned under embryology, collagen fibers link cardiac myocytes together. These collagen fiber links connect adjacent myocytes that hold all myocytes together allowing for a summation of the shortening of each myocyte into a concerted shortening of the ventricle.

C. This collagen structure also limits the cardiac myocyte from being overstretched, minimizing the risk of destroying a cell or limiting actin–myosin exposure through overstretching [1, p. 9].

D. Additional complexity is that from epicardium to endocardium, longitudinal alignment of the cardiac myocytes occurs in layers. Hence, shortening in each layer results in distortion between the layers.

5 E. This distortion results in partial occlusion of penetrating arteries arising from the surface vessels supplying blood to the inner layers of the myocardium.

F. Consequently, the endocardium is more vulnerable to ischemia than the epicardium because blood flow to the endocardium occurs primarily during systole while that to the epicardium occurs during the entire cardiac cycle.

V. Length–tension relationship

A. Consider this thought experiment. There is an idealized, single cardiac myocyte that is 12 μm long with 6 sarcomeres in series. All distances between Z-discs (sarcomere lengths) are equal for each of the 6 sarcomeres (12 μm = 6 * 2 μm). As the cardiac myocyte length changes, the length of each sarcomere changes proportionately. This single myocyte is suspended so that a strain gauge measures the tension that the myocyte generates at rest and during contraction.
   1. The idealized myocyte is stretched between two fixed points.
   2. The tension caused by the force of stretching the muscle at rest and created by the muscle during contraction is measured.
   3. The muscle is stretched at rest over a range of 10.8 to 16.2 μm. Consequently, the sarcomere lengths vary between 1.8 and 2.7 μm as this myocyte contracts.
   4. At each sarcomere length, two fixed myoplasmic Ca^{2+} concentrations are set within the cell: Zero concentration (rest) and a known value (contraction).
   5. Myocyte tension is measured for both Ca^{2+} concentrations.
   6. Plotting resting tension as a function of length results in a resting length–tension plot.
   7. Recording peak tension as a function of myocyte length, a length–tension curve can be plotted for the given Ca^{2+} concentration as depicted in Figure 1.3.

B. Compliance
   1. In our idealized myocyte model, a measured amount of tension was required to stretch the sarcomere to a value between 1.9 and 2.6 μm. If we were to plot this passive tension resulting from passive stretch of the sarcomeres, there would be very little passive tension required to stretch the sarcomeres until around 2.2 μm. As the sarcomeres become stretched beyond 2.2 μm in intact cardiac muscle, the fibrous skeleton restricts further stretching resulting in a rapid change in pressure with very little change in volume (very low compliance).
   2. This resting relationship between length and tension is the equivalent of ventricular compliance as will be discussed below.

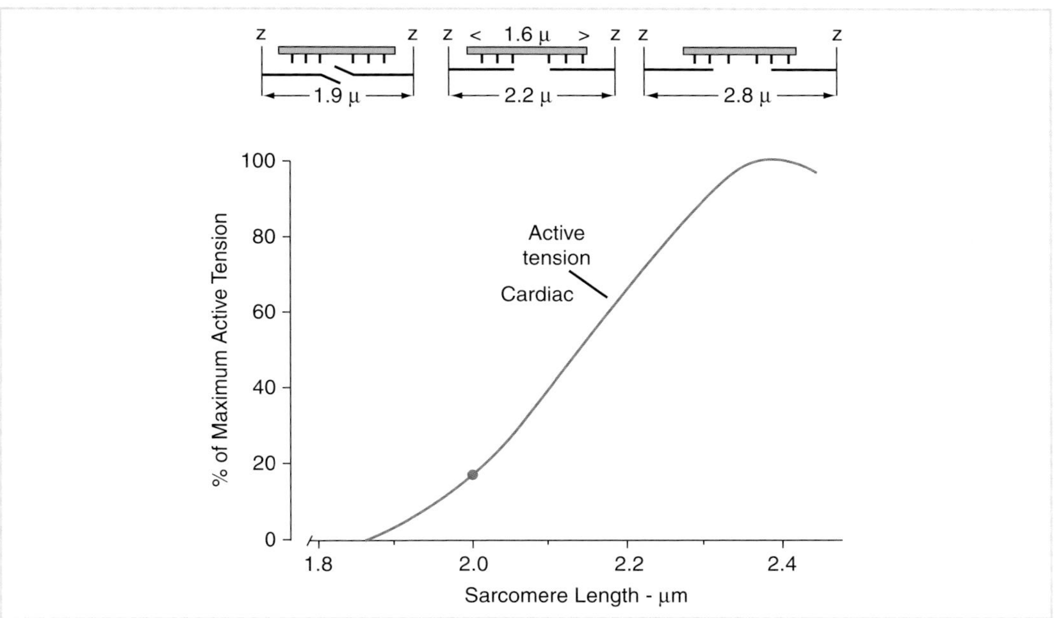

FIGURE 1.3 Top three schematic diagrams represent actin (thick filaments penetrating Z disc) and myosin (thin filaments forming sheaf between Z disc) filaments at three sarcomere lengths 1.9, 2.2, and 2.8 μm. Bottom graph represents per cent of maximum tension development versus sarcomere length for strips of cardiac muscle. Note that fibrous cardiac skeleton inhibits sarcomere stretch from approaching a sarcomere length of 2.8 μm. (Modified from Honig C. *Modern Cardiovascular Physiology.* Boston/Toronto: Little, Brown and Company; 1981.)

C. Contractility

1. For a given Ca^{2+} concentration, a fraction of troponin molecules will bind Ca^{2+} molecules.
2. This Ca^{2+} binding to each troponin results in a conformational change in its corresponding tropomyosin that allows an actin and myosin head pair, opposing each other and regulated by these tropomyosin molecules, to interact.
3. In addition to this conformational change, the percentage of the actin and myocytes heads opposed to each other is dependent on sarcomere length.
4. If one repeats the above mental experiment with a different known Ca^{2+} concentration, a new contracting length–tension curve is plotted.
5. For a range of Ca^{2+} concentrations in cardiac myocytes, a family of length–tension curves results.
6. Only through a change in myoplasmic Ca^{2+} concentration during contraction can contractility change.

D. Intracellular Ca^{2+} concentration

1. The range of myoplasmic Ca^{2+} concentrations during contraction varies depending upon Ca^{2+} fluxes across the sarcolemma at the initiation of contraction and the Ca^{2+} released from the sarcoplasmic reticulum.
2. The flux of Ca^{2+} across the sarcolemma is only ~1% of Ca^{2+} present during contraction. However, changes in this 1% result in changes in the amount of Ca^{2+} released from the sarcoplasmic reticulum.
3. The sarcoplasmic reticulum response is graded. The more the Ca^{2+} crossing the sarcolemma, the more the Ca^{2+} released from the sarcoplasmic reticulum.
4. Examples of increasing sarcolemmal Ca^{2+} flux include increasing epinephrine levels and increasing external Ca^{2+} concentration (a $CaCl_2$ bolus).
5. Increased sarcoplasmic reticulum Ca^{2+} stores result from increased Ca^{2+} flux across the sarcolemma and increased heart rate (HR).

E. Oxygen consumption

1. Each interaction of actin and myosin results in a submicron shortening of the sarcomere. For the sarcomere to shorten 15%, many actin–myosin interactions take place.
2. Therefore, shortening requires a repetitive interaction of actin–myosin complexes.
3. Each interaction requires ATP for release of the actin–myosin head. It is relaxation of the actin–myosin interaction that requires energy and consumes oxygen.
4. Remember that the more actin–myosin cycles in a unit of time, the more the oxygen consumption!

VI. A heart chamber and external work

A. The chamber wall

1. To form a ventricular chamber, individual myocytes are joined together via collagen fibrin strands. This joining of myocytes, along a particular direction but not end to end, results in a sheet of muscle with myocytes oriented along a similar axis.
2. Several such layers form the ventricular wall. These layers insert on the valvular annuli.
3. Because of the electrical distribution of the signal through the purkinje system, the layers contract synchronously resulting in shortening of the muscle layers and a reduction in the volume of the chamber itself.

B. Atria

1. Atrial contraction contributes approximately 20% of the ventricular filling volume in a normal heart and may contribute even more when left-ventricular end-diastolic pressure (LVEDP) is increased. In addition to the volume itself, the rapid rate of ventricular volume addition resulting from atrial contraction may play a role in ventricular sarcomere lengthening.

C. Ventricle

1. For a given state of contractility (myoplasmic Ca^{2+} concentration), sarcomere length determines the wall tension the ventricle can achieve as discussed above. The aggregate shortening of the sarcomeres in the layers of cardiac myocytes results in wall tension that leads to ejection of blood into the aorta and pulmonary artery (PA).

2. The active range of sarcomere length is only 1.9 to 2.2 μm or ~15% of its length. Falling below 1.8 μm results from an empty ventricle and an empty heart cannot pump blood. The collagen fiber network inhibits the stretching of sarcomeres much above 2.2 μm. This integration of structure and function is important in permitting survival. If there were no skeleton, overstretch would lead to reduced emptying that would lead to more overstretch and no cardiac output (CO).

D. Preload and compliance
   1. Preload
      a. Where clinicians speak of preload, muscle physiologists think of sarcomere length. Clinician's surrogate for initial sarcomere length is end-diastolic ventricular volume, and not ventricular pressure.
      b. As discussed above, the sarcomere length determines how many actin–myosin heads interact for a given myoplasmic Ca^{2+} concentration at any instant.
      c. Measuring sarcomere length is essentially impossible clinically. As a surrogate indirect estimate of sarcomere length, clinicians measure a chamber pressure during chamber diastole. This pressure measurement is the equivalent of the myocyte tension measurement above.
      d. A more direct surrogate estimate of sarcomere length is chamber volume. As echocardiography is commonly available, estimates of volumes are direct estimates of preload and remove assumptions about chamber compliance that are necessary from the estimate when chamber pressure is used.
      e. A plot of the relationship between chamber pressure and chamber volume results in a curve similar to the resting length tension curve for the myocyte.
      f. The slope of this curve at any point (change in volume over the change in pressure at that point) is the compliance of the chamber at that point. The pressure–volume curve is nonlinear, and this slope varies depending on ventricular volume. Ventricles become much less compliant as sarcomere length surpasses 2.2 μm because of the collagen fiber skeleton.
      g. Non-ischemic changes in compliance generally occur over long time periods. However, ischemia can change ventricular compliance very quickly. Thick ventricles, ventricles with scar formation, or ischemic ventricles have a lower compliance than normal ventricles. Less compliant ventricles require a higher pressure within them to have equal volume within them compared to a more compliant ventricle.
      h. While preload is most commonly considered in the left ventricle, it is important in all four chambers. Congenital heart disease and cardiac tamponade can make that very apparent.

E. Ventricular work
   1. For a sarcomere length between 1.9 and ~2.2 μm (preload) with a given systolic myoplasmic Ca^{2+} concentration (contractility), the cardiac myocyte will shorten, develop tension that increases with increased sarcomere length, and eject blood from the ventricle—a stroke volume (SV).
   2. In ejecting this SV the ventricle performs external work. This external work is the raising of SV from LVEDP to the ventricular pressure in systole. In the absence of valvular heart disease, the systolic pressure and ventricular pressure in systole are closely matched by those in the aorta or PA for the respective ventricles.
   3. Normal blood pressures (BPs) in the aorta and PA are not dependent on subject size and vary little amongst normal subjects. Normalizing SV to stroke volume index (SVI), SV divided by body surface area (BSA), the variability amongst subjects is small.
   4. Formally, the external work of a ventricle is the area within the pressure volume loop seen in Figure 1.4. The definition of various points and intervals is defined in the legend. We estimate this indexed work for the left ventricle (LVSWI) by multiplying the SVI in milliliter times the difference in arterial mean pressure and ventricular pressure at the end of diastole (commonly estimated as atrial pressure or PA wedge pressure) times a constant (0.0136) to convert to clinical units:

6

$$\text{LVSWI} = \text{SVI} * (\text{SBP mean} - \text{LVEDP}) * 0.0136 \ (\text{g m/m}^2)$$

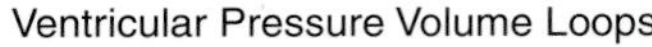

Breakdown of a Pressure-Volume Loop

- P-V loop depicts IV volume and pressure relationship
- A=MV opening & LVESV
- B=MV closure & LVEDV/LVEDP
- C=AV opening & systemic aortic diastolic pressure
- D=AV closure & LVESV/LVESP & dicrotic notch in Ao pressure tracing
- AB → LV Filling
- BC → Isovolumetric contraction
- CD → LV ejection
- DA → Isovolumetric relaxation
- LV compliance is ΔP/ΔV during filling of LV (slope of AB)
- Stroke volume = EDV − ESV
- Ejection fraction = SV/EDV

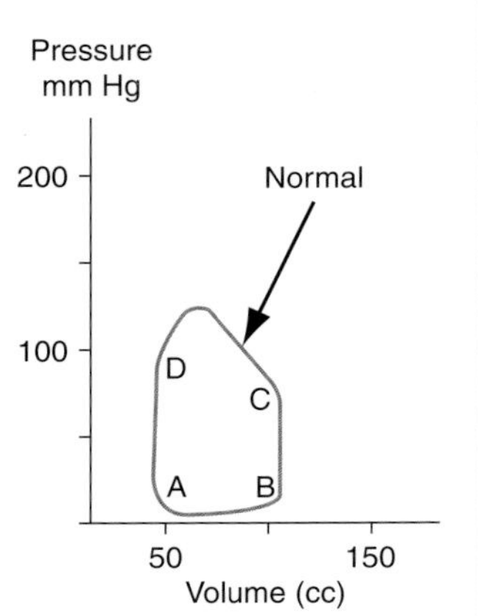

FIGURE 1.4 Idealized pressure–volume loop. Area within the loop represents LVSW. Dividing SV (Point B minus Point A volumes) by BSA results in SVI. The area within this indexed loop is the LVSWI.

5. The normal resting values for SVI and LVSWI are ~50 mL/m^2 and 50 g m/m^2.
6. In performing this work, the efficiency of the ventricle, the ratio of external work done to energy consumed to do it, approaches that of a gasoline engine—only 10%. An astonishingly inefficient process given that our lives depend on it (and we cannot improve it)!
7. Since external work includes the product of pressure difference and SV, the amount of work does not distinguish between these two variables. Evidence suggests that the ventricles can do volume work somewhat more efficiently (require less oxygen) than pressure work. The reasoning relates to how many actin–myosin cycles are required to shorten a sarcomere to a given distance! The hypothesis is that it takes fewer actin–myosin cycles to shorten the same distance for volume work compared to pressure work. This principle may explain an underlying reason for success using vasodilators to treat heart failure.

F. Starling curve

1. For a given myoplasmic Ca^{2+} concentration (contractile state), varying the sarcomere length between 1.9 μm and less than 2.2 μm increases the amount of external work changes. For a ventricle with a normal compliance, a sarcomere length of 2.2 μm corresponds to one with an LVEDP of 10 mm Hg.
2. By plotting the relationship of ventricular pressure with left ventricular work index, a Starling curve is generated.
3. By changing the contractile state and replotting the same relationship, a new curve develops resulting in a family of Starling curves idealized in Figure 1.5.

G. Myocardial oxygen consumption

1. Except for very unusual circumstances, substrate for ATP and phosphocreatine (PCr) production is readily available. At any given moment the intracellular oxygen content is
7 capable of keeping the heart contracting for seconds but the carbohydrate and lipid store can fuel the heart for almost an hour. Hence, capillary blood flow is crucial to maintain oxidative metabolism.
2. Myoglobin is an intracellular oxygen store. Its affinity for oxygen is between hemoglobin and cytochrome aa3. The maximum oxygen concentration required in mitochondria for maximal ATP production is 0.1 Torr! Myoglobin concentration is high enough to buffer interruptions in capillary flow only for seconds. Compared to high-energy phosphate buffers, this time buffer is small relative to ATP consumption rates. However, its intermediate oxygen affinity enhances unloading from the red cell into the myocyte and also serves to distribute oxygen within the cell.
3. Commonly, blood flow to regions of the heart limits oxygen delivery resulting in decreased. ATP production will result in reduced wall motion in that region—regional ischemic heart disease.

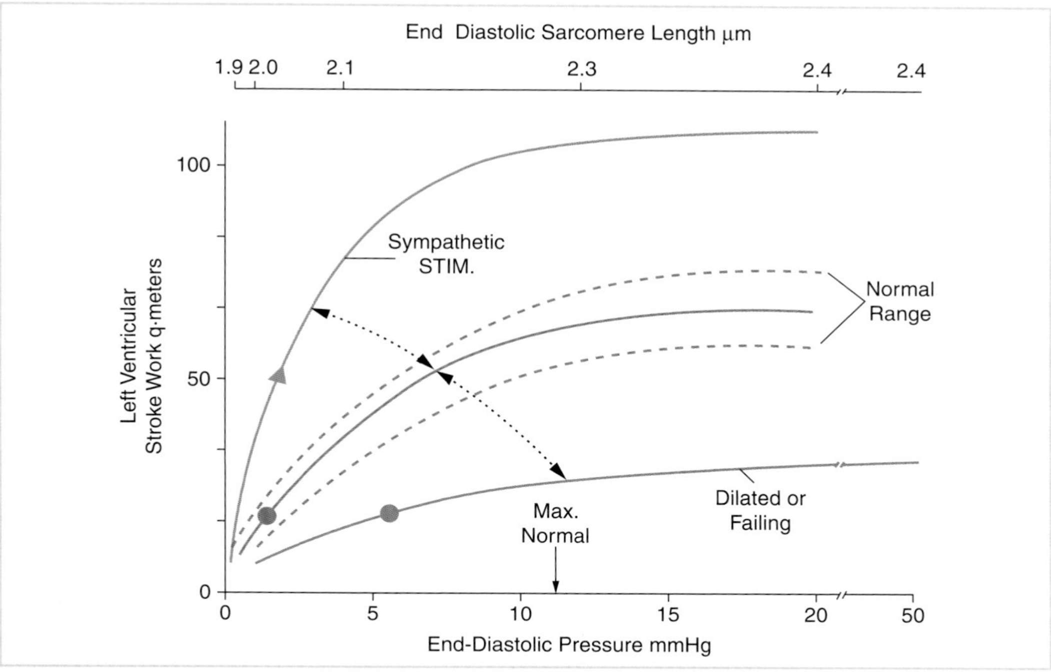

FIGURE 1.5 The Starling curve.

4. Capillaries are approximately 1 mm in length, so each capillary supplies multiple cardiac myocytes (12 μm in length) along its length. In contrast, skeletal muscle fiber is perhaps 15 cm long. Capillary length is the same—1 mm. Hence, each fiber has 150 capillaries in series to supply its entire length.
5. Capillary perfusion is organized into several capillaries supplied from a single higher-order arteriole. There are multiple levels of arteriolar structure. The lower-order, or initial, arterioles contribute to systemic vascular resistance (SVR) and the higher-order arterioles regulate regional blood flow distribution (at the local level). The intricacies are beyond the scope of this chapter.
6. This structure yields regions of perfusion on the scale of mm^3 for the regional blood flow unit. Hence, the smallest volumes for "small vessel infarcts" should be of this order of magnitude. As the vessel occlusions become more proximal, the infarct size grows.
7. Because of the size of cardiac myocytes being small relative to the capillary and unit of importance of blood flow from ischemia, infarction only affects local zones. If the cardiac myocyte had a similar structure as skeletal muscle myocyte, the consequences of a local infarct would be more global.
8. Adequate production of ATP is dependent on mitochondrial function. Approximately 30% of cell volume is occupied by mitochondria. Given the substrate store and the ability to produce ATP within this volume, oxygen availability is the limiting factor for maintaining ATP availability. Mitochondria can maximally produce ATP when their cell PO_2 is 0.1 Torr!
9. PCr is an intracellular buffer for ATP concentration. The cell readily converts ATP into PCr and vice versa. PCr is an important energy source and also serves to transport ATP between mitochondria and myosin ATP-ase.
10. Myosin ATP-ase activity is responsible for 75% of myocardial ATP consumption. The remaining 25% is being consumed by Ca^{2+} transport into the sarcoplasmic reticulum and across the sarcolemma.
11. Mitochondria play an evolving role in determining the response to ischemia. Intracellular signaling pathways in response to hypoxia may direct the cell to necrosis or even apoptosis.

VII. Control systems

A. The space program put man in space. As importantly, it brought many technical advances. In the world of systems development, control systems were an essential part. These systems allowed us to perform tasks in unexplored environments under unimagined conditions. To perform many tasks we required control systems. These systems in simplest concept permitted real-time sensing and adjustment of system outcomes through adjustment of system input and performance based on system outcome. This closed loop of an output affecting an input is referred to as a **feedback loop**.

B. Circulating levels of Ca^{2+}, thyroid hormones, and antidiuretic hormone are only a few of the systems that utilize a negative feedback loop to maintain a "normal blood level." A feedback loop is referred to as a **negative feedback loop** if a deviation from the desired level, called set point, is returned toward that level through the system response. Blood levels of all of the above protein moieties are controlled through negative feedback loop systems. In contrast, **positive feedback loops** increase the deviation from the normal level in response to a change. Outside of the physiology of the immune system, physiologic systems with positive feedback loops are generally pathologic. As considered below, perhaps the most studied biologic negative feedback loop is the cardiovascular system.

C. A simple example

1. A simple, manual system consists of a voltage source, a wall switch, and a light bulb. The system turns electrical energy into light through manually turning a light switch. A more complex system includes a light detector (**sensor**) that senses light level. If the ambient light level gets below a defined level, the controller turns the light bulb on and vice versa. This system automates light on and light off. A refinement of this automated system is one that keeps the light level constant below a defined light level (set point). In this system, light level is referred to as a **regulated variable**. If the light level is above the set point, the constant-light-level-system (CLLS) does not turn on the light. However, when the light level gets below this set point, the CLLS **controls** the amount of light coming from a light bulb such that the light level at the light sensor remains constant. This control requires that the output from the light bulb must vary. One way to vary the light output is to **control** the voltage (input) to the light bulb. This new variable output light bulb is referred to as an **effector** because it changes in response to system requirements. We will refer to the component of the system that regulates the voltage as the regulator. This CLLS system has a negative feedback loop because CLLS increases light output if natural (or artificial) light decreases and vice versa.
2. If regulating the light level becomes essential, the CLLS may become more complex. **Outside disturbances** such as snow and sleet will interfere with the sensing of ambient light. If system regulation requires adaptation to adjust for this disturbance, the system will require alteration.
3. The components of this CLLS consists of **inputs** to a light source (voltage), an **effector** that can vary light levels (light bulb), a **sensor** that detects the amount of light (a light detector), and a **comparator** that compares the signal from the sensor to a set point (the light level at which the system turns on or off). Finally, a **controller** varies the voltage to the light source in response to the signal from the sensor. The **controller** is the combination of the comparator and the regulator. Finally, the disturbances to the regulated variable as well as other systems impacting that variable are schematized (Fig. 1.6).
4. To be complete there are **positive feedback systems** as well. In a positive feedback system, the response of the system increases the difference between the regulated variable and a set point. When positive feedback occurs, the system frequently becomes unstable and usually leads to system failure. In physiology, typically pathology causes positive feedback. An example of this pathology is the response of the cardiovascular system to hypotension in the presence of coronary artery disease. Hypotension leads to an increase in HR and contractility that lead to more ischemia and more hypotension.

VIII. The cardiovascular system components

A. The simple control system model can be used to develop a model of the cardiovascular system. This model is useful if it predicts the system response to system disturbances. Modified from

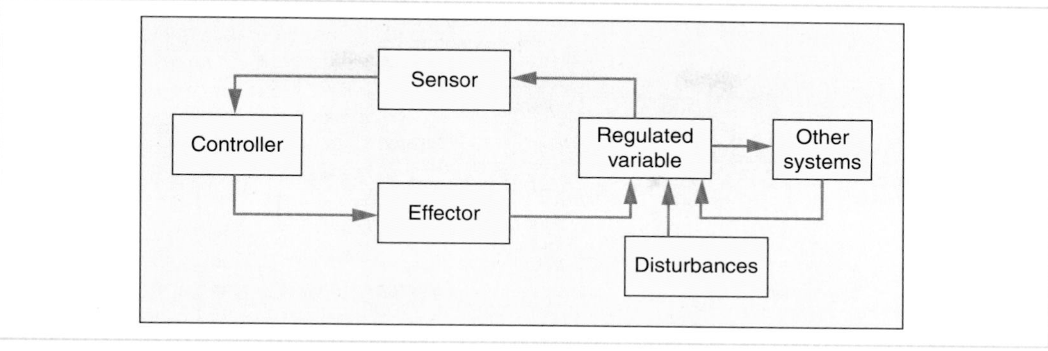

FIGURE 1.6 Diagram of a control system with a feedback loop. If the system response to a disturbance is to return the regulated variable back to the original set point, the system is a negative feedback system. Many physiologic systems are negative feedback systems.

[1, p.249], components in Figure 1.6 can be broken down into sensor, controller, and effector functions. The following discussion will summarize concepts for each function.

B. For the sensor functions, the two best characterized sensors—the baroreceptors in the carotid sinus and the volume and HR sensors in the right atrium—will be outlined in detail.

8 C. **Regulation** of a variable is defined as the variable remaining fixed despite changes in its determinants. The regulated variable in the cardiovascular system is primarily BP and occurs via a negative feedback loop.

D. Our survival requires a wide range of CO and SVR. Since BP changes only by perhaps ± 25% from our being asleep to maximal exercising, CO increasing is offset by SVR decreasing. The range for each is approximately 4 to 6-fold.

E. Individual organ survival is preserved as a consequence of system integration. It is noted from above that a well-conditioned subject can increase CO 4-fold while a sedentary person can only increase 2-fold. However, while running, his blood flow to skeletal muscle must be 100-fold greater than its minimum value. This apparent disparity—4-fold increase in CO but 100-fold increase to skeletal muscle—because blood flow to other organs is reduced.

F. The **brain** is the site of the comparator and integrator. Together the comparator and the regulator make up the **controller**. While anatomic sites for individual comparator and regulator functions are known, the specifics of interaction of these sites and regulation of control balance (what effector is utilized and how much) are largely unknown.

G. For this review, details of the sympathetic and parasympathetic outputs will not receive focus. As outputs from the controller, the nervous system signals recruit and derecruit the effectors in a predictable fashion through release of norepinephrine and acetylcholine as indicated in Figure 1.7.

H. The **effectors of the cardiovascular system—heart, venous system, and arterial system—** respond to changes in system demand. Fundamentally, the cardiovascular system must maintain BP in a normal range despite a wide range of demand, e.g., exercise or limitations of effector reserves such as dehydration and ischemic and valvular heart disease. To adapt, the effectors have a range over which they can expand their capacities. Each effector has an expandable range known as its **physiologic reserve**.

I. Effective feedback control requires functioning sensors, comparators, and effectors to have the desired effect—in this case regulation of BP. The understanding of complexities and capacities of the sensors, comparators, and effectors as well as system integration provides a clinical basis for reducing surgical and anesthetic risk.

IX. Stretch receptors: BP sensors

A. The simplified view of BP regulation presented herein is useful for organizing priorities in maintaining BP. Integration of BP regulation is more complex and requires meeting demands of competing organs.

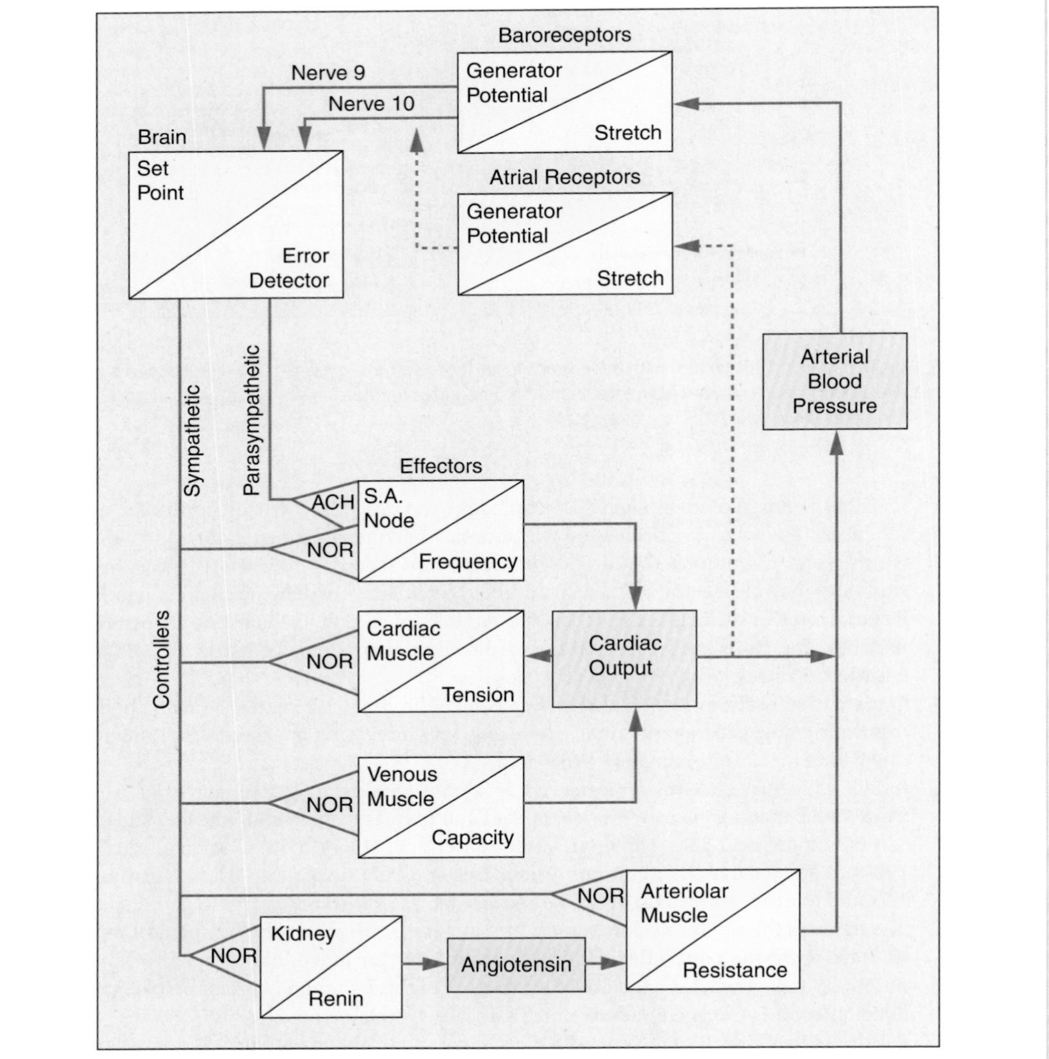

FIGURE 1.7 This simplified representation omits input to the brain from sensors throughout the vascular tree and the ventricular chambers. As discussed in the text, there are multiple inputs to the brain not represented in this simplified view. Input to the brain includes signals from sensors (receptors) that monitor blood volume, CO, SVR, and HR. Input to the effectors occurs through the sympathetic and parasympathetic systems with neural transmitters indicated. NOR, norepinephrine; ACH, acetylcholine; S.A., sinoatrial.

B. Excepting the splanchnic circulation, organs are organized in parallel with either the aorta or PA as their source of BP.

C. As a consequence, blood flow to the individual organs can be locally adjusted or centrally integrated. This organization allows for individual independent organ perfusion as long as aortic or PA BP is maintained.

D. Additional sensor sites include systemic and pulmonary venous volumes, HR, SVR, and ventricular volumes. Experiments looking at cardiovascular system responses to isolated disturbance in these locations have demonstrated their existence.

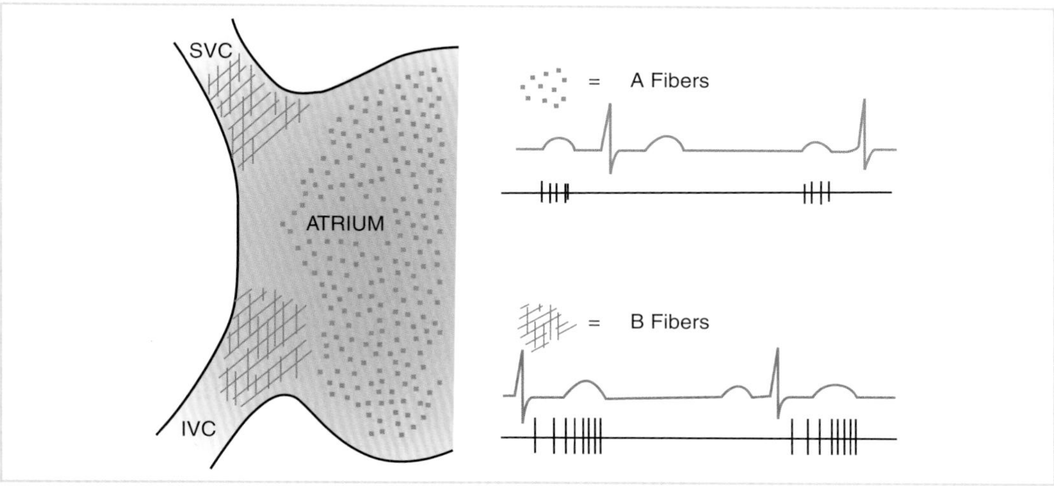

FIGURE 1.8 The A fibers (stretch receptors) are located in the body of the atrium and fire during atrial contraction and sense atrial contraction rate or HR. The B fibers (stretch receptors) are located at the intersection of the inferior vena cava (IVC) and superior vena cava (SVC). Their neural signals occur during ventricular systole when the atria are filling. Hence, they sense atrial volume.

E. All known pressure-sensitive sensors in the cardiovascular system are stretch receptors. They respond to wall stretch and not container pressure. Hence, compliance of the receptor site impacts receptor response.

F. In addition to the volume of a chamber, the rate of change of that volume may be sensed and afferent signals are sent to the brain.

G. Consequently, depending on the sensor location, sensor signals provide data that reflect BP, venous capacitance, SVR, ventricular contractility, SV, HR, and other parameters. Most of the knowledge of these sensor sites is inferred from indirect experiments.

X. Atrial baroreceptors

A. Within the right atrium, there are receptors at the junction of the superior and inferior venae cavae with the atrium (B fibers) and in the body of this atrium (A fibers, Fig. 1.8). The corresponding impulses from the respective nerves are seen on the left. **A fibers**, seen in both atria, generate impulses during atrial contraction, indicating that they **detect** HR.

B. B fibers are located only in the right atrium and impulses occur during systole when the atrium is filling. Maximum frequency of B fiber impulses occurs just prior to AV valve opening and this frequency is linearly proportional to right atrial volume. **Hence, B fibers detect atrial volume.** Hence, information necessary to infer CO is therefore available.

C. The B receptor impulse rates (volume receptor) have adrenal, pituitary, and renal effects. These effects form another negative feedback loop control system that regulates volume in the long term through the adrenal–pituitary–renal axis.

D. In addition to these B fiber signals, results from system-oriented whole animal experiments indicate that there are additional volume receptors throughout the cardiovascular system. Not surprisingly, large systemic veins, pulmonary veins, as well as right and left ventricles all have effects on the cardiovascular system that are volume dependent. The observed effects on CO, SVR, and BP clearly indicate that there is a predictable impact of these additional receptors on overall homeostasis.

XI. Arterial baroreceptors

A. The baroreceptors in the carotid sinus are the first described sensors of BP. Additional arterial baroreceptors have been discovered in the pulmonary and systemic arterial trees including a site in the proximal aorta!

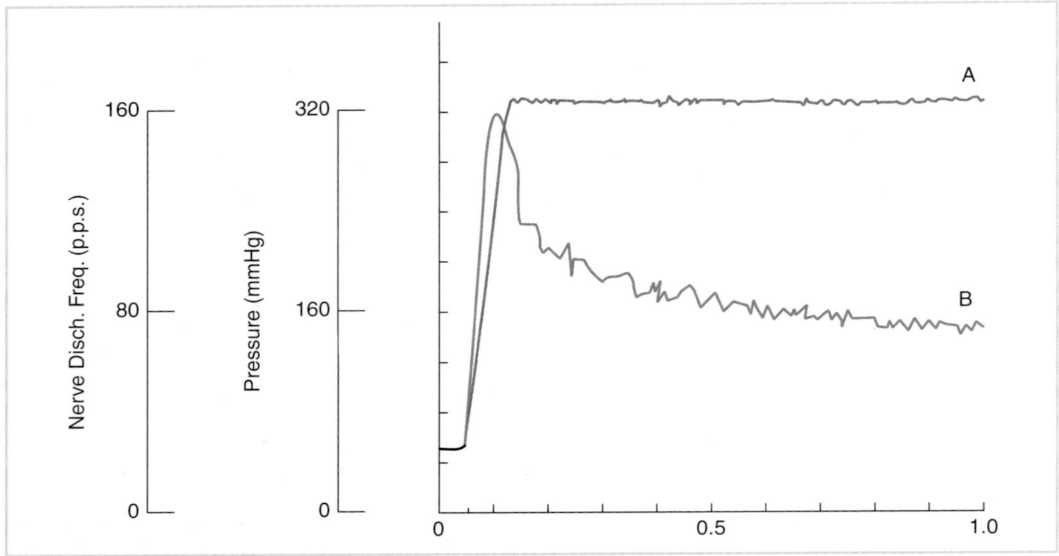

FIGURE 1.9 The nerve discharge frequency from the baroreceptor recording change from ~30 pulses/s to 80 pulses/s after the response reached a steady state. Note that there was a transient change during the rapid response phase as well.

B. "The carotid sinus baroreceptor monitors BP" is a rapid response to the common question of where BP is sensed. However, the details of what is sensed in this location are less frequently known [1, p. 246].

C. In Figure 1.9 a step change in mean BP from 50 to 330 mm Hg is plotted along with the neural discharge of the carotid sinus fiber. There is a change in the neural frequency reflecting the step change in BP and then a leveling to a steady-state discharge rate, indicating a signal correlating with mean BP.

D. In Figure 1.10, the relationship between neural impulses in a single neural fiber emanating from a carotid sinus nerve can be seen relative to the pulsatile "BP waveform" in the carotid body.

E. Signals related to contractility (upstroke of BP), SVR (the dichrotic notch in the peripheral circulation), and downstroke emanate from the carotid sinus nerve. Hence, the oscillatory shape of the BP waveform is detected and a signal sent to the brain controller.

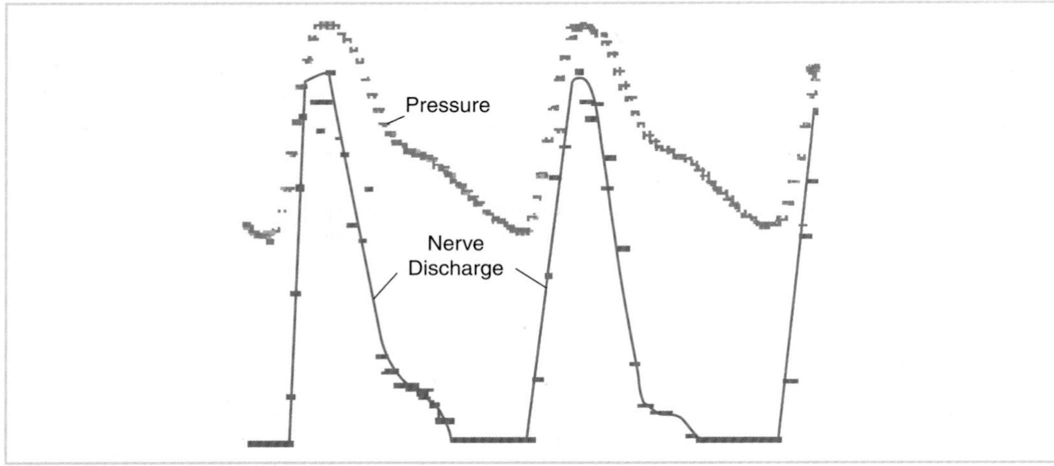

FIGURE 1.10 Note that the upslope of arterial pressure (dP/dt), the downslope (SVR), and the notch (SVR) are reflected in the action potential frequency.

F. The aortic baroreceptor is located near or in the aortic arch. Infrequently, cardiac anesthesiologists can become acutely aware of its presence. When distorted secondary to the placement of any aortic clamp, the resulting aortic baroreceptor signal results in an acute and dramatic increase in BP. The presumed mechanism is that the clamp distorts the aortic baroreceptor. This distortion results in a signal that BP has precipitously fallen. Despite the fact that the carotid baroreceptor has no such indication, hypertension ensues—imperfect system integration. Immediately releasing the cross-clamp (when possible) promptly returns the BP to a more normal level (usually). When release is not feasible, short, rapid-acting intervention—pharmacologic or reverse Trendelenburg—is required. How does reverse Trendelenburg affect the pressure?

G. Cardiovascular effectors

1. BP is the product of CO, or HR times SV times SVR plus right atrial pressure (RA):

$$BP = (CO * SVR) + RA = (SV * HR * SVR) + RA \qquad (1)$$

2. Organ perfusion is dependent on the difference between arterial pressure and RA and organ resistance. For homeostasis, a focus on perfusion is important in our view of BP.
3. The organs in the body are in parallel and the SVR is dependent on the individual resistance in a simple but more complex way than I will cover here!
4. SV is dependent upon contractility, preload, and afterload [Eq. (1)]. Sympathetic tone sets contractility, preload, and SVR. The myoplasmic Ca^{2+} concentration, fraction of blood in the thorax versus total blood volume, and the SVR are all functions of sympathetic tone.
5. HR is dependent on the sympathetic tone as well.

XII. Effectors and physiologic reserves

A. The range that each of the effectors can contribute to maintaining BP through increasing CO or changing SVR in the face of everyday life requirements (sleeping to climbing a mountain) is referred to as physiologic reserve.

B. Knowing this range for each effector gives a framework to consider which reserves can be utilized to further increase CO or perhaps increase SVR.

9 C. This concept provides a framework for considering which effector is available to lower or raise BP. To have a clinical situation where additional physiologic reserve cannot be recruited (because of pathology or exceeding a range) will increase risk and jeopardize outcome.

D. HR

1. A normal resting HR range is perhaps 60 beats per minute (bpm). A maximum attainable HR in a 25-yr old would be 220 as compared to 170 in a 55-yr old. Hence, an average expansion factor is ~2.5- to 3.5-fold.
2. The clinician must keep in mind that of the three main determinants of oxygen demand—HR, contractility, and wall tension—only HR correlated with ischemia in patients under anesthesia. Hence, this correlation tempers the use of this expansion factor.

E. Systemic vascular resistance

1. Within the systemic vascular tree, the organs in our body, recognizing the lung and liver as more complex circulations, emanate from the aorta or the PA. This arrangement is referred to as be parallel.
2. Because of the large diameters of the aorta and pulmonary artery, there is no physiologically important decrease in mean BP along either of their lengths. Consequently, each organ experiences the same mean BP. Through its own resistance, the organ determines the blood flow to it.
3. In normal life, organ blood flow requirement are met without compromising BP. Metabolic requirements (substrate supply, oxygen supply, and demand) are met despite the variability amongst organs for blood flow. The cardiovascular system maintains pressure through its effectors via central nervous system (CNS) control responding to local organ control of its resistance.
4. Looking at Equation (1), if BP is regulated, when SVR is high then CO must be proportionately lower and vice versa. What is the observed range of SVR? For a severely dehydrated person or one with a bad left ventricle, the cardiac index might be 33% of normal (1.2 LPM/M^2

[Eq. (1)]). The corresponding SVR would be three times the normal value (3,600 dyne s/cm^5 [Eq. (1)]). For a well-trained athlete who, during maximal exercise, would increase CO 7-fold, the SVR would be ~15% of normal (~200 dyne s/cm^5 [Eq. (1)]).

F. Contractility

1. Contractility is not a commonly measured clinical variable because of the difficulty in direct measurement and the impact of afterload and preload on its estimate. The clinician is left to estimate any changes. A consequence of an increase in contractility is the ability to increase wall tension in the left ventricle. This increased ability will lead to an increase in ejection rate and fraction under normal conditions. While there are differences in how trained and untrained healthy subjects achieve the increase, both increase ejection fraction (EF) from 60% to 80%. This 33% increase in EF contributes to a modest but important increase in CO.

G. Intravascular volume: Venous capacitance

1. Total blood volume can be estimated from body weight. In the ideal 70 kg person, an estimate of blood volume is 70 mL/kg or ~5 L. This blood volume is considered **euvolemia**.
2. The distribution of that volume between intrathoracic and extrathoracic (or systemic) volumes is roughly 30% and 70%, respectively.

10 3. In each of these two compartments, approximately one-third of the blood is in the arteries and capillaries and two-thirds are in the venous system.

4. The pulmonary veins hold 1,100 mL and the systemic veins hold 2,400 cc (almost half of the blood volume).
5. Relaxation of venous tone results in an increase in venous capacity for blood. If there is no change in blood volume, this results in a decrease in atrial filling pressures.
6. Returning those atrial filling pressures to their original values requires infusion of volume. The amount of intravascular volume added to return these pressures to their original values is referred to as the venous capacitance reserve.
7. In addition to the blood volume defined as euvolemia, the intrathoracic and extrathoracic compartments can expand their respective volumes by approximately 300 and 1,200 mL!
8. Thus, quantitatively, 1,500 mL of intravascular volume is an estimate of this venous capacitance reserve.
9. This reserve intravascular volume is added to a euvolemic blood volume (5 L in a 70 kg subject), and the total intravascular volume would be 6.5 L or a 30% increase.
10. Functionally, maintaining intrathoracic blood volume in the face of hemorrhage is an important task of the cardiovascular system. Maintenance of this blood volume results in maintenance of CO through shifting blood into the thorax and recruitment of HR and contractility.
11. In pathologic states resulting in chronically elevated right- or left-sided atrial pressures, venous dilation results in an increase in "euvolemic" blood volume.
12. Particularly in the systemic venous system, this increase in capacity can be large. While there is no experimental data, anecdotal observations of patients going on cardiopulmonary bypass clearly demonstrate this fact. However, the extent that the increased volumes can be recruited to maintain intrathoracic volume, the key to maintaining preload, is unknown.
13. Like hemorrhage, chronic diuresis leads to a contracted venous bed. Hence, caring for patients who are chronically or acutely made hypovolemic secondary to this management approach must include understanding the state of their venous volume status and its capacitance.
14. Worthy of note, chronic diuretic administration leads to venoconstriction. However, an acute dose of lasix will venodilate the patient with heart failure and actually lower intrathoracic blood volume due to the shift of blood into the dilated systemic veins.

H. Lymphatic circulation: A final reserve?

1. Lymphatic circulation occurs in interstitial space between the blood vessels and intracellular space. Clinically this system is rarely discussed but physiologically plays a vital role. For our purposes, its role in protection of organs from edema and recruitment of volume in times of high sympathetic tone—severe hemorrhage—will be discussed.
2. The characteristics of this space help prevent fluid accumulation in two ways—transport of fluid through the lymphatic conduits and its low compliance [2].

3. In interstitial space, the lymphatics are tented open by a collagen matrix. Because of this tenting, they are not compressed when the interstitium is edematous. Lymphatics increase their flow during edematous states.
4. Consequently, more fluid leaves the interstitium via lymphatic drainage when more fluid enters the lymphatics across the capillary.
5. The collagen matrix is a gel and this structure results in interstitial space having a low compliance. Consequently, fluid entering interstitial space raises interstitial pressure rapidly (low compliance) and the increase in interstitial pressure opposes further transudation of fluid across capillaries.
6. This increased interstitial pressure also increases lymphatic drainage.
7. This system does not only have water passing through it, but also proteins traverse this space with total proteins moving through it in ~24 hrs daily.
8. It is also dynamic during the convective transport of blood down a capillary. Exchange occurs as fluid leaves the capillary at the arteriole end and returns at the venous end. The expansion factor for this exchange is ~8-fold. Hence, crystalloid administration equilibrates across the vascular and interstitial volumes rapidly.
9. With **severe hemorrhage** with maximal sympathetic stimulation, interstitial and intracellular fluid may contribute up to 2.5 L of fluid to ***intravascular volume*** [3]. While this recruitment of intracellular and interstitial fluid compensates for intravascular depletion acutely, this depletion, particularly of intracellular volume, does so at the expense of cell function, eventually leading to acidosis and compromise of cell function.
10. All three of these compartments—intracellular, interstitial, and intravascular—have a dynamic relationship with at least equilibrium being reached in minutes after volume administration, change in sympathetic tone, or administration of vasoactive drugs.
11. In summary, for major hemorrhage, consideration of volume resuscitation requirements must include intracellular, interstitial, and intravascular compartments. Particularly when sympathetic tone is abruptly altered (induction of anesthesia), the extent of circulatory collapse may be greater than anticipated as fluid within these compartments equilibrates at the new level of sympathetic tone.

I. Brain: The controller
1. It is beyond the scope of this chapter, and to an extent our knowledge, to detail the neural pathways, interactive signaling, and psychological influence to the cardiovascular system response. Hence, the controller, our brain, is considered a black box. In this view, this controller is designed to maintain BP assuming that all the effectors are recruitable.
2. Making the controller a black box may be justifiable on another level. After we describe the system integration, we must recognize that the pharmacology we utilize affects the integration of this system in direct and indirect effects on effectors and perhaps the controller and sensors as well. Other medications affect the ability of the CNS to stimulate responses through receptor or ganglion blockade. **For anesthesiologists, in many situations, our clinical management must replace system integration.** By understanding the pharmacology present and its effect on the cardiovascular system, clinical judgment dictates a plan to control BP regulation. This control responsibility must include temporizing and maintaining BP variability. Unable to rely on the cardiovascular system alone, the clinician manipulates the effector responses to maintain BP always cognizant of the need for physiologic reserves in the face of upcoming disturbances.
3. Understanding the comorbidities anticipates the limitations in physiologic reserves and their availability for recruitment during stress. Recognition of necessary compromises for adjustment of anesthetic approach reduces the risk of morbidity.

XIII. The cardiovascular system integration

A. The cardiovascular system response to physiologic stress is predictable and reproducible. In its simplest form, if BP is altered, the integrated system response—sensors, controller, and effectors—senses the alteration and returns BP toward the original set point. This negative feedback permits us to lead our lives without considering the consequences or preparing for the disturbances to this system. As each effector is recruited to regulate BP, it can contribute less to compensating for an additional stress. We take for granted the range and automaticity of this system response.

B. In healthy subjects, the utilization of their reserves to respond to recruitment is dependent on training levels, hydration status, and psychological state amongst others. In healthy subjects, their limits are set through a complex physio-psycho state that ends with not being able to go on—hitting the wall.

C. For patients, the response of effectors may be limited by effector pathology. The most common of these is ischemic heart disease.

D. To maintain blood in the face of hypotension the cardiovascular system responses are predictable.

1. Oxygen demand. HR and contractility will be increased. Each increases myocardial oxygen consumption. Wall tension will be decreased. Since HR is a primary determinant of the onset of ischemia under anesthesia, its elevation is a reason for concern and intervention.
2. Oxygen supply. Assuming no blood loss or alteration of oxygenation, increased HR leads to reduced diastolic time. Hence, endocardial perfusion time will be reduced. Reduced diastolic systemic pressure will most likely be greater than LVEDP reduction. Consequently perfusion pressure is reduced.
3. Intervention: The anesthesiologist will most likely administer neosynepherine in response. SVR will increase, and blood volume will shift from the systemic veins into the thoracic veins, increasing preload and leading to an increase in SV. BP will rise, HR will fall, contractility will be reduced, diastolic time lengthened, and perhaps coronary perfusion pressure will rise as well.
   a. Response time required
      (1) Responding to hypotension is an everyday occurrence for an anesthesia provider. Defining hypotension is somewhat difficult. Physiologists would arrive at a value of around a mean BP of 50 mm Hg for organ function. Hypotensive anesthesia challenges that value and data indicate that a sitting position is different from a supine one. A prevalent clinical definition is "±25% of the preoperative value." Given anxiety, determining that preoperative value is not always easy. Clinicians face this dilemma and almost individually resolve it.
      (2) As an aside, cardiac anesthesiologists in the post-bypass period are confronted with BP management in the patient who frequently has hypertension, renal insufficiency, peripheral vascular disease, and an aorta that has been (minimally) cannulated. Systolic pressures, frequently under 100 mm Hg, are the norm in this setting.
      (3) If it is low, how long at the pressure will cause damage. If a neuron is without oxygen, the neuron has a lifespan of minutes. Given that reality, sacrificing all other organ functions to maintain BP is essential on the time scale of minutes.
      (4) For the kidney, even renal insufficiency created during surgery can recover. Consequently, sacrificing renal perfusion is acceptable to protect the neuron.
      (5) For a cardiac myocyte, the time constant is several minutes. The exact time constant is unclear for an individual cell but is certainly approaching an hour. After 4 hrs, the magic window for thrombolysis to be effective, 50% of myocytes will survive. Therefore, compromising myocardial oxygen supply and demand to preserve neurons is acceptable as a temporizing measure.
4. Neosynepherine administration elicits a very positive physiologic impact **if we do not stop there**. As the new controller, the anesthesia provider needs to consider why the hypotension occurred, if that reason is going to continue or get worse and how soon the remaining physiologic reserves can maintain homeostasis.
5. These considerations are crucial in determining the likelihood of long-term—the course of the operation and the early postoperative period—hemodynamic stability of the patient.
6. Frequently, volume management is key in this decision. Consider that if instead of administering neosynephrine above, a volume challenge was administered and the BP response was to increase, the oxygen demand and supply benefits would remain. However, instead

of consuming physiologic reserves through neosynephrine use, the controller would be providing physiologic reserves through increased venous capacitance and decreased SVR.

a. Achieving the balance between the need for short-term intervention and long-term stability is the responsibility of the controller, the patient's or the provider's brain.

XIV. Effect of anesthesia providers and our pharmacology on the cardiovascular system

A. The surgical patient

1. White-coat hypertension is common. Some attribute this hypertension to the flight response necessary for survival! The perioperative period is certainly a time of increased anxiety for many patients. In the context of our cardiovascular system, the anxiety represents an input that most likely alters the response at the controller level—the brain. Since non–white-pant hypertension may contribute to cardiac-related complications perioperatively, a patient who is hypertensive in the preoperative area will be given an anxiolytic as the first step to determine if it is chronic or not.
2. If the anxiolysis reduces the BP to the normal range, we attribute the hypertension to anxiety and proceed. If it does not, we attribute it to an altered set point for BP and must consider the risks and benefits, as ill-defined as they are, before proceeding.

B. The anesthetic choice

1. For a healthy patient for low-risk surgery, our closed claims data conclude that anesthetic choice has little to no bearing on outcome. Low surgical risk in the setting of normal physiologic reserves protects homeostasis to the extent that the margin for error is great. Provocative statement—perhaps but the closed claims data base would support this view.
2. For the high-risk patient with comorbidities related to diabetes, ischemic or valvular heart disease for high-risk surgery, consideration of the status of their physiologic cardiac reserves becomes extremely important. The entire perioperative period subjects the patient to increased risk. Understanding the consequences of the patient's pathology on their physiologic reserves and use of clinical management approaches to reduce the risk should influence the anesthetic choice.
3. In this chapter, we discussed physiologic reserves in the context of normal physiology. The principles related to ventricular function, determinants of myocardial oxygen consumption, and physiologic reserves apply in the pathologic situation as well.
4. Of all the physiologic reserves discussed, the physiologic reserve that is minimally affected by pathology during surgery and is not shown to affect outcomes adversely, except perhaps for gastrointestinal (GI) surgery and major trauma, is volume management to replenish or expand venous capacitance reserves. The principle that "An empty heart cannot pump blood!!!" is true. The number of patients resuscitated from hypovolemia is far greater than those who have incurred congestive heart failure due to too much fluid.

C. Treating the cause

1. When clinical signs and symptoms do not agree with clinical judgment and conclusions, more data are necessary. The two most useful monitors in the setting of unresponsive hypotension under general anesthesia are the PA catheter and the transesophageal echocardiography (TEE) examination.
2. The PA catheter has been touted and maligned as a monitoring tool. Rao et al. [4] demonstrated an improved outcome in patients undergoing surgery in the setting of a recent myocardial infarction. Using physiologic principles to guide management, Rao et al. demonstrated improved outcome in this high-risk group. A national survey demonstrated that clinicians did not understand the physiologic principles underlying the interventions in Rao's study. The mere presence of a PA catheter has not been shown to improve outcome or "The yellow snake does no good when inserted [5]." While anecdotal experience does not refute data, using the data from the PA catheter to optimize the physiologic reserves available for perioperative optimization would be the parallel to Rao's results for the high-risk setting of a recent acute myocardial infarction.
3. The TEE probe is the optimal tool for assessing ventricular volume status and regional wall motion abnormalities. An experienced echocardiographer can assess the volume status of the ventricle (intrathoracic blood volume) within a minute and almost as quickly assess

ventricular systolic function. These two data elements provide immediate help in clinical management of the unresponsive hypotension. Particularly in a setting where ventricular compliance can change (ischemia, acidosis, and sepsis) so that filling pressures may not reflect volume status of the ventricles, TEE is an essential tool. As a tool, it can be used to assess the state of venous capacitance through Trendelenburg and reverse Trendelenburg manipulation during observation. Clearly with three-dimensional echocardiographic capabilities, CO becomes measurable. The available physiologic reserves are then known.

XV. Clinical examples to discuss

A. GI surgery: A special case?

1. In GI surgery, conservative fluid management is reported to improve surgical outcomes. While the studies are limited, the outcome improvement appears real [6] but controversial [7]. Important to note when considering these data are that a bowel preparation and hydration the night before and the morning of surgery preoperatively are important parameters that may have led to reduced fluid administration intraoperatively.
2. When extrapolating these results to another operation, all interstitial spaces are not the same—specifically, the gut interstitial space is different from all other. GI function involves absorption from the GI tract. Interstitial fluid fluxes and a lymphatic system function are different from those in other organs. Globalizing fluid management from GI surgery and inferring that if the outcome improves for GI surgery due to fluid management is unsound.
3. Balancing the benefits and risks of surgery, fluid shifts, cardiac system perturbations with the risk of fluid administration, and its other benefits should be the focus.

XVI. Two examples emphasizing fluid management

A. A patient NPO for 12 hrs on a diuretic.

1. The patient is undergoing a 30-min herniorrhaphy.
2. The patient is on a diuretic for chronic hypertension.
3. In correcting volume deficit, the goal is to achieve euvolemia.
4. This 70 kg patient on a diuretic for hypertension is NPO overnight. The diuretic results in volume constriction—a guesstimate of 500 mL. Twelve hours of NPO results in sensible and insensible losses—guesstimate 1,250 mL.
5. The type and duration of surgery will result in insignificant fluid shifts.
6. The goal is euvolemia.
7. Insensible and sensible loss replacement—1,250 mL of crystalloid
   - **a.** Considerations: Nuance of the lactated ringer's versus normal saline controversy, actual ionic content of losses. Both deemed inconsequential in this patient.
8. Chronic intravascular volume contraction—500 mL of the following:
   - **a.** Crystalloid administration of 1,500 mL infusion
     - **(1)** In the intraoperative period the presence of the chronic volume depletion will not be compensated for by the CNS controller and will have to be accommodated for by the anesthesia provider.
     - **(2)** While neosynephrine could be used,
       - **(a)** The postoperative pain medications will affect BP regulation and result in hypotension more likely.
       - **(b)** Nausea and vomiting are reduced in the hydrated patient.
9. Total fluid 2,750 mL—rounded to 3 L.
   - **a.** If recruiting the venous capacitance reserve of 1,500 mL were the goal, 4,500 mL of additional crystalloid would have been infused with a hypervolemic patient but with no change in atrial filling pressure.
   - **b.** Hence, an overinfusion of 500 mL of crystalloid would not be noticed in the cardiovascular system.
10. In this setting, how do we respond to "You gave too much fluid!!!!"
    - **a.** A proposed rationale response is "The patient had an insensible deficit of 1,250 mL based on NPO status, I guesstimated that he was volume constricted because of his diuretic for hypertension—~500 mL as he was well compensated when awake—and he became hypotensive on induction, consistent with that. Given that, and that the perioperative period will have less effective cardiovascular BP regulation, hypotension

more likely, I estimated approximately 2,750 mL to get him euvolemic. If I erred, his physiologic reserve of 1,500 mL of intravascular volume would have accommodated ~5,000 more mL. He is not nauseated at the moment and I expect him to have a stable BP until his ambulatory discharge. Would you like me to order pain meds for the Phase 2 recovery." Concise, factual, and true. Have fun with your knowledge and profession!

B. This same Patient, NPO for 12 hrs on a diuretic; involved in a motor vehicle accident outside the hospital entrance

1. Same 70 kg hypertensive patient on a diuretic is involved in an MVA on his way to the hospital.
2. Vital signs in the emergency room (ER) minutes after the accident
   a. HR 180
   b. BP 60/40
3. Conscious, Foley catheter in place, large-bore access available, monitored, no head or chest trauma
4. Hematocrit (HCT) 24
5. Clearly, this clinical operating room course will be difficult. Induction, further monitors, maintenance, etc. are important considerations. But in the ER, while other decisions and actions are going on, consider volume management alone.
6. Volume management
   a. The goal of fluid replacement:
      (1) From the above patient considerations, prior to accident, returning to euvolemia required 3 L.
      (2) Ongoing and potential worsening of blood loss suggests that a goal of recruiting venous capacitance reserve (1,750 mL) through volume expansion is preferable—1,500 mL of additional venous capacity beyond euvolemia.
   b. Estimating extent of hypovolemia and crystalloid replacement for achieving the goal:
      (1) NPO times 12 hrs plus volume depletion from diuretic—3 L (from the above patient)
      (2) Recruiting venous capacitance reserve of 1,500 mL—4.5 L of crystalloid
      (3) Vital signs indicate at least a greater than 25% reduction in intrathoracic blood volume. The extrathoracic blood volume is reduced to maintain intrathoracic blood volume, and an estimate of overall intravascular volume approaching 40% is within reason (2 L of blood loss) requiring 6 L of crystalloid replacement.
      (4) Interstitial and intracellular volume recruitment (up to 25%) into intravascular space compensates for blood loss in this situation as well—1.2 L of crystalloid.
      (5) Total crystalloid administration for achieving the goal of euvolemia plus adding venous capacitance reserve assuming no ongoing blood loss is as follows:

$$\text{Total crystalloid: } 3 + 4.5 + 6 + 1.2 = \sim 15 \text{ L!!}$$

      (6) Concerning the **actual volume resuscitation**, various protocols advocate different combinations of colloid, crystalloid, fresh frozen plasma, platelets, packed red cell units as well as antifibrinolytics, platelet function enhancers, etc. Consideration of the fluids loss estimates from the individual compartments above combined with the intravascular volume, coagulation and oxygen carrying capacity issues in this case will drive ultimate fluids administered. Consideration of requirements of each of the compartments is necessary to restore intravascular volume and cell function ultimately.
   c. **Red** cell mass and coagulation
      (1) Clearly, red cell mass, commonly thought of in terms of HCT, and coagulation factors will also require consideration. There are protocols for RBC to fresh frozen plasma (FFP) ratios in trauma and this consideration is beyond the scope of this chapter.
      (2) However, an estimate of RBC requirements based on red cell mass reveals the following:
         (a) Initial HCT 24%
         (b) Initial intravascular volume of 60% of normal (contraction of 40% volume)
         (c) Desired goal of volume expansion to include euvolemia plus venous capacitance reserve: 5 5 L + ~1.5 L.

(d) This represents a 30% increase in intravascular volume or 130% of euvolemia.
(e) Your estimate without reading on of his HCT after 15 L of crystalloid
(f) The final HCT estimate calculation is as follows:

$$\text{Final HCT} = \text{Initial HCT (24)} * [\text{Initial volume (0.6)/Final volume (1.3)}]$$

(g) That value would be 11%.
(h) That HCT is too low. Setting a desired HCT, transfusing RBCs to reach it with the recognition of ongoing blood loss, and infusing FFP and platelets to correct coagulation deficiencies are dynamic considerations in trauma. Using physiologic principles outlined for volume managment, the anesthesiologist can guesstimate endpoints for product component requirements. In the face of continued bleeding, recalculating guesstimates and retesting hypotheses are essential to achieving hemodynamic and hemostatic stability.

The remainder of this book is focused on cardiac anesthesiology. The patients to whom it applies have significant pathology as it relates to the cardiovascular system. In this chapter, we reviewed patients with a normal, intact cardiovascular system. This model provides the building blocks for putting pathology into the context of the normal cardiovascular system. From the effect of hypertension on the sensors, to the effect of increased intra cranial pressure on the brain or the effect of HR and contractility in the presence of coronary artery disease, pathology impacts the desired response of the cardiovascular system. Consider the system effects as you apply your management of the anesthetic as the controller of this system. This individualization will provide a foundation for your choices and responses. In acting on principles, a reduction in morbidity and mortality may (can) be achieved (Rao).

REFERENCES

1. Honig C. *Modern Cardiovascular Physiology.* Boston/Toronto: Little, Brown and Company; 1981.
2. Mellander S, Johansson B. Control of resistance, exchange, and capacitance functions in the peripheral circulation. *Pharmacol Rev.* 1968;20:117–196.
3. Mellander S. Comparative studies on the adrenergic neuro-hormonal control of resistance and capacitance blood vessels in the cat. *Acta Physiol Scand Suppl.* 1960;50(176):1–86.
4. Rao TL, Jacobs KH, El-Etr AA. Reinfarction following anesthesia in patients with myocardial infarction. *Anesthesiology.* 1983;59(6):499–505.
5. Iberti TJ, Fischer EP, Leibowitz AB, et al. A multicenter study of physicians' knowledge of the pulmonary artery catheter. Pulmonary Artery Catheter Study Group. *JAMA.* 1990;264(22):2928–2932.
6. Walsh SR, Tang TY, Farooq N, et al. Perioperative fluid restriction reduces complications after major gastrointestinal surgery. *Surgery.* 2008;143(4):466–468.
7. Hamilton MA, Mythen MG, Ackland GL. Less is not more: A lack of evidence for intraoperative fluid restriction improving outcome after major elective gastrointestinal surgery. *Anesth Analg.* 2006;102(3):970–971.

2 Cardiovascular Drugs

John F. Butterworth, IV

KEY POINTS

1. Drug errors are a common cause of accidental injury to patients. The author suggests referring to drug package inserts or the Physician Desk Reference to check any unfamiliar drug before it is prescribed or administered.
2. Phenylephrine can be used for hypotension related to low systemic vascular resistance states or as a temporizing therapy for hypovolemia.
3. Epinephrine is a direct α_1 and α_2 and β_1 and β_2 agonist not dependent on release of endogenous norepinephrine. In the setting of a dilated left ventricle and myocardial ischemia, epinephrine may increase coronary perfusion pressure and reduce ischemia.
4. Milrinone increases intracellular concentration of cAMP. Milrinone used as a single inotropic agent has favorable effects on myocardial supply/demand balance reducing preload and afterload and has a low tendency to produce tachycardia.
5. Nitroglycerine is a direct vasodilator producing greater venous pooling than arterial dilation. Venous pooling caused by dilation decreases heart size and preload reducing MV02 and usually lessens ongoing ischemia.

NUMEROUS POTENT DRUGS ARE USED to control heart rate (HR) and rhythm, blood pressure (BP), and cardiac output before, during, and after surgery. Patients undergoing cardiovascular and thoracic operations are particularly likely to receive one of these agents. This chapter reviews the indications, mechanisms, dosing,
1 drug interactions, and common adverse events for these drugs. Drug errors are common causes of accidental injury to patients, particularly in hospitalized, critically ill patients. Therefore, we suggest that the package insert or *Physicians' Desk Reference* [1] (which contains the package insert information) be consulted before any unfamiliar drug is prescribed or administered [2]. Fortunately, it has never been easier to obtain drug information. Convenient sources of drug information include numerous books and web sites, some of which are provided at the end of this chapter [2–5]. Using a "smart" mobile telephone or tablet computer, many physicians now maintain a readily updated library of drug information in their hand or pocket at all times.

I. Drug dosage calculations

A. Conversions to milligram or microgram per milliliter

1. Drugs are administered in increments of weight or units. Unfortunately, drugs are not labeled in a uniform manner. Dilution of drugs and calculations are often necessary.

Fortunately, most modern infusion pumps do these calculations for the operator, limiting the opportunity for mistakes.

2. A drug labeled z% contains z g/dL; $10 \times z$ equals the number of grams per liter, numerically equivalent to the number of milligrams per milliliter.
   a. Example: Mannitol 25% solution contains 25 g/dL, which equals 250 g/L or 250 mg/mL.
   b. Example: Lidocaine 2% contains 2 g/dL, or 20 g/L, or 20 mg/mL.
3. Concentrations given as ratios are converted to milligrams or micrograms per milliliter as follows:

$$1{:}1{,}000 = 1 \text{ g}/1{,}000 \text{ mL} = 1 \text{ mg/mL}$$
$$1{:}1{,}000{,}000 = 1 \text{ g}/1 \text{ million mL} = 1\ \mu\text{g/mL}$$

   a. Example: Epinephrine is packaged for resuscitation in 1:10,000 dilution. Thus, it is one-tenth as concentrated as 1:1,000; therefore, 1:10,000 is 0.1 mg/mL (or 100 μg/mL).
   b. Example: A brachial plexus block is to be performed with 0.5% bupivacaine to which epinephrine 1:200,000 must be added. Because the desired concentration is five times greater than 1:1,000,000, 5 μg of epinephrine should be added for each milliliter of bupivacaine.

B. Calculating infusion rates using standard drip concentrations (adults)

1. Step 1. Dose rate (μg/min): Calculate the desired per-minute dose. Example: A 70 kg patient who is to receive dopamine at 5 μg/kg/min needs a 350 μg/min dose rate.
2. Step 2. Concentration (μg/mL): Calculate how many micrograms of drug are in each milliliter of solution. To calculate concentration (μg/mL), simply multiply the number of milligrams in 250 mL by 4. Example: When nitroglycerin is diluted 100 mg/250 mL, there are $100 \times 4 = 400$ μg/mL. Example: Dopamine, 200 mg, added to 250 mL fluid = 200/250 mg/mL = 800 mg/L = 800 μg/mL concentration.
3. Step 3. Volume infusion rate (mL/min): Divide the dose rate by the concentration (μg/min ÷ μg/mL = mL/min). The infusion pump should be set for this volume infusion rate. Example: 350 μg/min ÷ 800 μg/mL = 0.44 mL/min. Conversion of volume rate from milliliters per minute to milliliters per hour simply involves multiplying by 60 min/h (0.44 mL/min $\times$ 60 = 26 mL/h).
4. Table 2.1 can be consulted as an alternative means for determining vasoactive drug infusion rates for patients of different weights.
5. Finally, and perhaps most importantly, the wide availability of micropressor-controlled, programmable infusion pumps has largely eliminated the need for complex calculations at the bedside.

C. Preparation of drug infusions for pediatric patients

1. Most pediatric anesthesia departments, critical care units, and pharmacies have specific preferences as to how drugs should be mixed prior to infusion. We strongly recommend that practitioners adhere to the predominant practice in their unit, **whether or not the practitioner may perceive it to be optimal**. In general, patient safety is maximized when variation is minimized. We discuss two of the more common ways in which drugs are diluted for pediatric patients in the succeeding sections.
2. **Technique A: Standard, single drug concentration for all patients**
   a. **Advantages** are that it is simple (no arithmetic calculations are required) and the fluid volume administered scales upward appropriately with weight.
   b. **Disadvantages** are that the standard dilution for each drug must be remembered, and volume infusion rates may be excessive in critically ill infants.
3. **Technique B: Custom drug dilution based on patient weight.** This method permits infusion of a single fluid volume rate to patients of any weight. Our opinion is that this technique maximizes the possibility for drug dilution mistakes.

TABLE 2.1 Vasoactive drug infusion rates

Drug	Add (mg) (to 50 mL)	Dilution (μg/mL)	Starting dose (μg/kg/min)	Patient weight (kg)														
				5	10	15	20	25	30	40	50	60	70	80	90	100	120	140
Epinephrine or NE	3	60	0.1	0.5	0	1.5	2	2.5	3	4	5	6	7	8	9	10	12	14
Dopamine	400	8,000	5	0.2	0.4	0.6	0.8	1	1.2	1.6	1.8	2.2	2.6	3	3.4	3.8	4.6	5.2
Dobutamine	250	5,000	5	0.3	0.6	0.9	1.2	1.5	1.8	2.4	3	3.6	4.2	4.8	5.4	6	7.2	8.4
Inamrinone[a]	250	5,000	5	0.3	0.6	0.9	1.2	1.5	1.8	2.4	3	3.6	4.2	4.8	5.4	6	7.2	8.4
Milrinone[a]	50	1,000	0.5	0.2	0.3	0.5	0.6	0.8	0.9	1.2	1.5	1.8	2.1	2.4	2.7	3	3.6	4.2
Nitroprusside	50	1,000	0.5	0.2	0.3	0.5	0.6	0.8	0.9	1.2	1.5	1.8	2.1	2.4	2.7	3	3.6	4.2
Nitroglycerin	100	2,000	0.5	0.1	0.2	0.3	0.3	0.4	0.5	0.6	0.8	0.9	1.1	1.2	1.4	1.5	1.8	2.1

Values in the table under patient weight heading show the drug infusion rate in mL/h.
[a]Both inamrinone and milrinone are not diluted except in very small infants.

a. Step 1. Decide on a starting dose per kilogram for the drug. Some standard values are as follows:

Drug	Dose
Dopamine Dobutamine	5 μg/kg/min
Nitroprusside	0.5 μg/kg/min
Epinephrine NE Isoproterenol	0.04 μg/kg/min

b. Step 2. Multiply **starting dose** (in μg/kg/min) by **weight** (in kg) to give starting dose rate in μg/min.

c. Step 3. Decide on **volume rate** of fluid that should carry this starting dose of drug into the patient:

For most children >5 kg	0.1 mL/min (6 mL/h)
For babies	0.05 mL/min (3 mL/h)

These volumes may be decreased substantially if a continuous carrier infusion is utilized.

d. Step 4. Divide starting dose rate (step 2) by volume rate (step 3) to give desired **concentration** of drug. Units cancel: (μg/min)/(mL/min) = μg/mL.
Example: In a 6.3 kg baby

(1) Select standard starting dosages of dopamine and isoproterenol.

(2) Calculate starting dose rate:

(a) Dopamine: 5 μg/kg/min × 6 kg = 30 μg/min.

(b) Isoproterenol: 0.1 μg/kg/min × 6 kg = 0.6 μg/min.

(3) Choose volume rate: 0.05 mL/min.

(4) Calculate concentration:

(a) Dopamine: 30 μg/min ÷ 0.05 mL/min = 600 μg/mL.

(b) Isoproterenol: 0.6 μg/min ÷ 0.05 mL/min = 12 μg/mL.

(5) Dilute drugs:

(a) Dopamine: 600 mg/L (or 150 mg/250 mL).

(b) Isoproterenol: 12 mg/L (or 3 mg/250 mL).

D. **Pediatric resuscitation doses.** We find it convenient to prepare syringes of certain drugs (e.g., epinephrine and atropine) so that they contain a standard emergency dose for the patient.

II. Drug receptor interactions

A. **Receptor activation.** Can responses to a given drug dose be predicted? The short answer is: *Partially.* The more accurate answer is: *Not with complete certainty.* Many factors determine the magnitude of response produced by a given drug at a given dose.

1. **Pharmacokinetics** relates the dose to the concentrations that are achieved in plasma or at the effect site. In brief, these concentrations are affected by the drug's volume of distribution and clearance, and for drugs administered orally, by the fractional absorption [6,7].

2. **Pharmacodynamics** relates drug concentrations in plasma or at the effect site to the drug effect.

a. **Concentration of drug at the effect site (receptor)** is influenced by the concentration of drug in plasma, tissue perfusion, lipid solubility, and protein binding; diffusion characteristics, including state of ionization (electrical charge); and local metabolism.

b. **Number of receptors** per gram of end-organ tissue varies.

(1) **Upregulation** (increased density of receptors) is seen with a chronic **decrease** in receptor stimulation. Example: Chronic administration of β-adrenergic receptor antagonists increases the number of β-adrenergic receptors.

(2) **Downregulation** (decreased density of receptors) is caused by a chronic **increase** in receptor stimulation. Example: Chronic treatment of asthma with β-adrenergic receptor agonists reduces the number of β-adrenergic receptors.

c. **Drug receptor affinity and efficacy may vary.**

(1) Receptor binding and activation by an agonist produces a biochemical change in the cell. Example: α-Adrenergic receptor agonists increase protein kinase C concentrations within smooth-muscle cells. β-Adrenergic receptor agonists increase intracellular concentrations of cAMP.

(2) The biochemical change may produce a cellular response. Example: Increased intracellular protein kinase C produces an increase in intracellular [Ca^{2+}], which results in smooth-muscle contraction. Conversely, increased intracellular concentrations of cAMP relax vascular smooth muscle but increase the inotropic state of cardiac muscle.

(3) The maximal effect of a partial agonist is less than the maximal effect of a full agonist.

(4) **Receptor desensitization** may occur when prolonged agonist exposure to receptor leads to loss of cellular responses with agonist–receptor binding. An example of this is the reduced response to β_1-adrenergic receptor agonists that occurs in patients with chronic heart failure (CHF), as a result of the increased intracellular concentrations of β-adrenergic receptor kinase, an enzyme which uncouples the receptor from its effector enzyme adenylyl cyclase.

(5) Other factors including acidosis, hypoxia, and drug interactions can reduce cellular response to receptor activation.

III. Pharmacogenetics and genomics

In the future, pharmacogenetics, or how drug actions or toxicities are influenced by an individual's genetic make-up, may become a tool in helping anesthesiologists select among therapeutic options. We are learning, for example, that the genetic profile of the individual may impact the degree to which patients respond to adrenergic therapies, including vasopressors. Life-threatening arrhythmias, such as Long QT syndrome, may result from therapy with a number of commonly prescribed agents, and relatively common genetic sequence variations are now known to be an underlying predisposing factor. Droperidol, which is highly effective and safe at small doses for preventing or treating postoperative nausea, has been shown (at larger doses) to cause QT-interval lengthening and increase risk of *Torsades de Pointes* in a small cohort of susceptible patients. Therefore, a larger number of patients will be deprived of this useful medication because of our inability to identify the small number of patients who have the genetic markers associated with this rare but disastrous complication. Industry and academia are rapidly progressing toward simple assay-based genetic screens capable of identifying patients with these and other risks for adverse or inadequate drug responses, including heparin or warfarin resistance. Unfortunately, at the present time, commercially available screens are rare and have not been sufficiently evaluated to be considered the standard care. As such, detailed family history is the only practical means through which we can identify such genetic risks. At the same time, genetic variations may occur spontaneously or be present in a family but not be manifested with symptoms (phenotypically silent). Hence, continuous monitoring for adverse or highly variable drug responses, particularly those related to arrhythmias or BP instability, is the cornerstone of cardiovascular management in the perioperative period.

IV. Guidelines for prevention and treatment of cardiovascular disease

Drug treatment and drug prevention for several common cardiovascular diseases have been described in clinical practice guidelines published by national and international organizations. We provide references for the convenience of our readers. Because these recommendations evolve from year to year, we strongly recommend that readers check whether these guidelines may have been updated since publication of this volume.

A. **CAD**

1. Primary prevention (see Ref. 7)
2. Established disease (see Refs. 8,9)
3. Preoperative cardiac evaluation and prophylaxis during major surgery (see Refs. 10,11)

B. **CHF** (see Refs. 12,13)

C. **Hypertension** (see Refs. 14,15)

D. **Atrial fibrillation prophylaxis** (see Ref. 11)

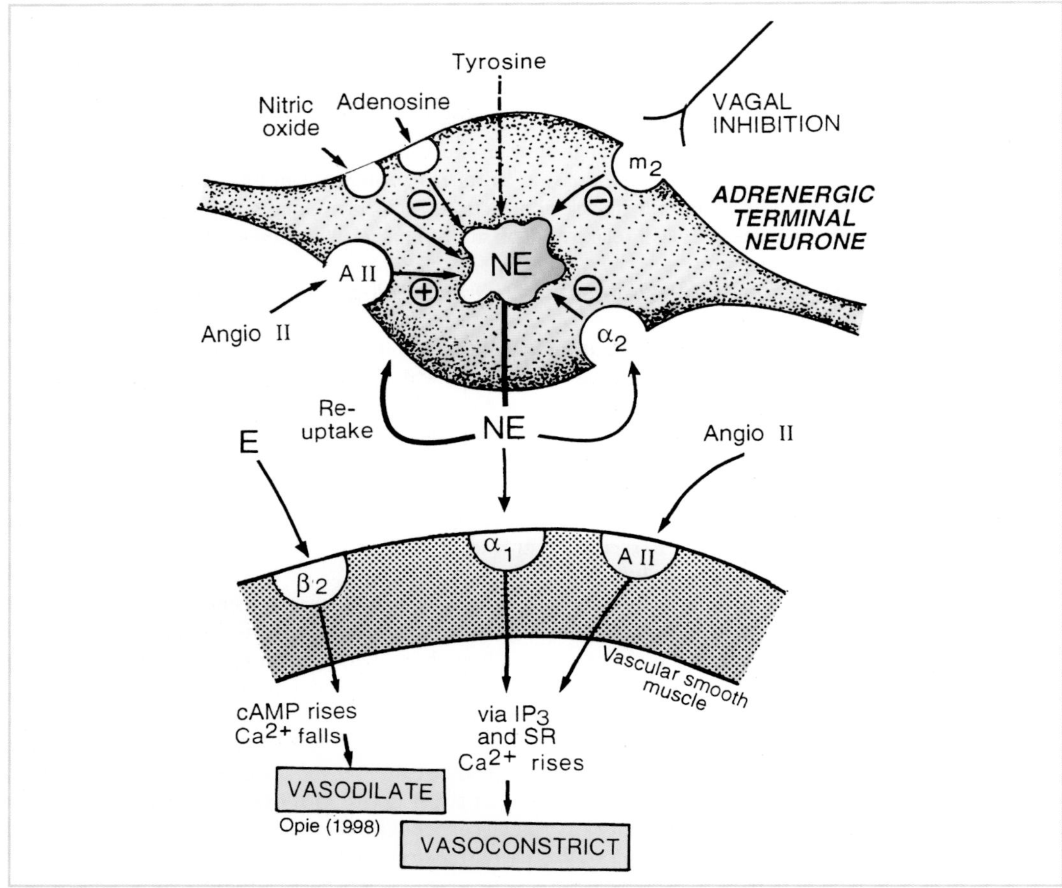

FIGURE 2.1 Schematic representation of the adrenergic receptors present on the sympathetic nerve terminal and vascular smooth-muscle cell. NE is released by electrical depolarization of the nerve terminal; however, the quantity of NE release is *increased* by neuronal (presynaptic) β_2-receptor or muscarinic-cholinergic stimulation and is *decreased* by activation of presynaptic α_2-receptors. On the *postsynaptic* membrane, stimulation of α_1- or α_2-adrenergic receptors causes vasoconstriction, whereas β_2-receptor activation causes vasodilation. Prazosin is a selective α_1-antagonist drug. Note that NE at clinical concentrations does not stimulate β_2-receptors, but epinephrine (E) does. (From Opie LH. *The Heart: Physiology from the Cell to the Circulation.* Philadelphia, PA: Lippincott Williams & Wilkins; 1998:17–41, with permission.)

V. Vasopressors

A. α-Adrenergic receptor pharmacology (Fig. 2.1)

1. Postsynaptic α-adrenergic receptors mediate peripheral vasoconstriction (both arterial and venous), especially with neurally released norepinephrine (NE). Selective activation of cardiac α-adrenergic receptors increases inotropy while **decreasing** the HR. (Positive inotropy from α-adrenergic agonists can only be demonstrated in vitro or by selective drug administration in coronary arteries to avoid peripheral effects that normally overwhelm the cardiac actions.)
2. α-Adrenergic receptors on presynaptic nerve terminals decrease NE release through negative feedback. Activation of brain α-adrenergic receptors (e.g., with clonidine) lowers BP by decreasing sympathetic nervous system activity and causes sedation (e.g., with dexmedetomidine). Postsynaptic α_2-adrenergic receptors mediate constriction of vascular smooth muscle.

3. **Drug interactions**
   a. **Reserpine interactions.** Reserpine depletes intraneuronal NE and chronic use induces a "denervation hypersensitivity" state. Indirect-acting sympathomimetic drugs show diminished effect because of depleted NE stores, whereas direct-acting or mixed-action drugs may produce exaggerated responses because of receptor upregulation. This is of greater laboratory than clinical interest because of the rarity with which reserpine is now prescribed to patients. For the rare patient receiving reserpine, we recommend titrated dosages of direct-acting drugs and careful monitoring of BP.
   b. **Tricyclic (and tetracyclic) antidepressant or cocaine interactions.** These drugs block the reuptake of catecholamines by prejunctional neurons and increase the catecholamine concentration at receptors. Interactions between these drugs and sympathomimetic agents can be very severe and of comparable or greater danger than the widely feared monoamine oxidase (MAO) inhibitor reactions. In general, if sympathomimetic drugs are required, small dosages of direct-acting agents represent the best choice.
4. **Specific agents**
   a. **Selective agonists**
      (1) **Methoxamine (Vasoxyl)**
         (a) **Methoxamine is a synthetic drug and is not a catecholamine. It is of mostly historic interest.**
         (b) **Actions.** The drug is a selective, direct, α_1 agonist that produces vasoconstriction.
         (c) **Offset.** A longer duration of action (1 to 1.5 h intramuscularly [IM]) than phenylephrine or NE; not metabolized by either MAO or catechol-O-methyl transferase (COMT).
         (d) **Indications for use**—similar to phenylephrine
         (e) **Clinical use**
            (i) Methoxamine dose (adult): 1 to 5 mg intravenous (IV) bolus; 10 to 20 mg IM.
            (ii) The long duration of action of methoxamine makes it more difficult to titrate the dosage to rapidly changing hemodynamic conditions than with phenylephrine, vasopressin, or NE.
      (2) **Phenylephrine (Neo-Synephrine)** [16]
         (a) **Phenylephrine is a synthetic noncatecholamine.**
         (b) **Actions.** The drug is a selective α_1-adrenergic agonist with minimal β-adrenergic effects. It causes vasoconstriction, primarily in arterioles.

	Phenylephrine
HR	Decreased (reflexresponse to BP elevation)
Contractility	No direct effect with systemic administration
Cardiac output (CO)	No change or decreased
BP	Increased
Systemic vascular resistance (SVR)	Increased
Preload	Minimal

         (c) **Offset** occurs by redistribution and rapid metabolism by MAO; there is no COMT metabolism.
         (d) **Advantages.** A direct agonist with short duration (less than 5 min), it increases perfusion pressure for the brain, kidney, and heart in the presence of low SVR states. When used during hypotension, phenylephrine will increase coronary perfusion pressure without altering myocardial contractility. If *hyper*tension is avoided, myocardial oxygen consumption (MvO_2) does not increase substantially. If contractility is depressed because of ischemia, phenylephrine will sometimes produce an increased CO from an increase in coronary perfusion

pressure. It is useful for correcting hypotension in patients with CAD, hypertrophic subaortic stenosis, tetralogy of Fallot, or valvular aortic stenosis.

(e) **Disadvantages.** It may decrease stroke volume (SV) and CO secondary to increased afterload; it may increase pulmonary vascular resistance (PVR); it may decrease renal, mesenteric, and extremity perfusion. Reflex bradycardia, usually not severe, may occur but will usually respond to atropine. Phenylephrine rarely may be associated with coronary artery spasm or spasm of an internal mammary, radial, or gastroepiploic artery bypass graft.

(f) **Indications for use**

(i) Hypotension due to peripheral vasodilation, low SVR states (e.g., septic shock, or to counteract effects of nitroglycerine)

(ii) For patients with supraventricular tachycardia (SVT), reflex vagal stimulation in response to increased BP may terminate the arrhythmia; phenylephrine treats both the hypotension and the arrhythmia.

2

(iii) It can oppose right-to-left shunting during acute cyanotic spells in tetralogy of Fallot.

(iv) Temporary therapy of hypovolemia until blood volume is restored, although a drug with positive inotropic action (e.g., ephedrine) usually is a better choice in patients without CAD (or hypertrophic obstructive cardiomyopathy), and in general, vasoconstrictors should not be viewed as effective treatments for hypovolemia.

(g) **Administration.** IV infusion (central line preferable) or IV bolus

(h) **Clinical use**

(i) Phenylephrine dose

(a) IV infusion: 0.5 to 10 μg/kg/min.

(b) IV bolus: 1 to 10 μg/kg, increased as needed (some patients with peripheral vascular collapse may require larger bolus injections to raise SVR).

(c) For tetralogy of Fallot spells in children: 5 to 50 μg/kg IV as a bolus dose.

(ii) **Mixing:**

(a) IV infusion: Often mix 10 or 15 mg in 250 mL IV fluid (40 or 60 μg/mL).

(b) IV bolus: Dilute to 40 to 100 μg/mL.

(iii) Nitroglycerin may be administered while maintaining or increasing arterial BP with phenylephrine. This combination may serve to increase myocardial oxygen supply while minimizing increases in $M\dot{V}O_2$.

(iv) Phenylephrine is the vasopressor of choice for short-term correction of excessive vasodilation in most patients with CAD or aortic stenosis.

b. Mixed agonists

(1) Dopamine (Intropin) [16]

See subsequent Section VI: Positive inotropic drugs.

(2) Ephedrine

(a) Ephedrine is a plant-derived alkaloid with sympathomimetic effects.

(b) Actions

(i) Mild direct α-, β_1-, and β_2-adrenergic agonist

(ii) Indirect NE release from neurons

	Ephedrine
HR	Slightly increased
Contractility	Increased
CO	Increased
BP	Increased
SVR	Slightly increased
Preload	Increased (mobilization of blood from viscera and extremities)

(c) **Offset.** 5 to 10 min IV; no metabolism by MAO or COMT; renal elimination

(d) **Advantages**

(i) Easily titrated pressor and inotrope that rarely produces unexpected excessive responses

(ii) Short duration of action with IV administration (3 to 10 min); lasts up to 1 h with IM administration

(iii) Limited tendency to produce tachycardia

(iv) Does not reduce blood flow to placenta; safe in pregnancy

(v) Good agent to correct sympathectomy-induced relative hypovolemia and decreased SVR after spinal or epidural anesthesia

(e) **Disadvantages**

(i) Efficacy is reduced when NE stores are depleted.

(ii) Risk of malignant hypertension with MAO inhibitors or cocaine

(iii) Tachyphylaxis with repeated doses (thus rarely administered by continuous infusion)

(f) **Indications**

(i) Hypotension due to low SVR or low CO, especially if HR is low, and particularly with spinal or epidural anesthesia

(ii) Temporary therapy of hypovolemia until circulating blood volume is restored, although, as previously noted, in general vasoconstrictors should not substitute for definitive treatment of hypovolemia

(g) **Administration.** IV, IM, subcutaneous (SC), by mouth (PO)

(h) **Clinical use**

(i) Ephedrine dose: 5 to 10 mg IV bolus, repeated or increased as needed; 25 to 50 mg IM.

(ii) Ephedrine is conveniently mixed in a syringe (5 to 10 mg/mL) and can be given as an IV bolus into a freely running IV line.

(iii) Ephedrine is a useful, quick-acting, titratable IV pressor that can be administered via a peripheral vein during anesthesia.

(3) **Epinephrine (Adrenaline)**

See subsequent Section IV: Positive inotropic drugs.

(4) **NE (noradrenaline, Levophed)** [16]

(a) **NE is the primary physiologic postganglionic sympathetic neurotransmitter;** NE also is released by adrenal medulla and central nervous system (CNS) neurons.

(b) **Actions**

(i) Direct α_1- and α_2-adrenergic actions and β_1-adrenergic agonist action

(ii) Limited β_2-adrenergic effect in vivo, despite NE being a more powerful β_2-adrenergic agonist than dobutamine in vitro

	NE
HR	Variable; unchanged or may decrease if BP rises (reflex); increases if BP remains low
Contractility	Increased
CO	Increased or decreased (depends on SVR)
BP	Increased
SVR	Increased
Pulmonary vascular resistance (PVR)	Increased

(c) **Offset** is by redistribution, neural uptake, and metabolism by MAO and COMT.

(d) Advantages
- **(i)** Direct adrenergic agonist. Equipotent to epinephrine at β_1-adrenergic receptors
- **(ii)** Redistributes blood flow to brain and heart because all other vascular beds are constricted.
- **(iii)** Elicits intense α_1- and α_2-adrenergic agonism; may be effective as vasoconstrictor when phenylephrine (α_1 only) lacks efficacy

(e) Disadvantages
- **(i)** Reduced organ perfusion: Risk of ischemia of kidney, skin, liver, bowel, and extremities
- **(ii)** Myocardial ischemia possible; increased afterload, HR. Contractility may increase, be unchanged, or even decrease. Coronary spasm may be precipitated.
- **(iii)** Pulmonary vasoconstriction
- **(iv)** Arrhythmias
- **(v)** Risk of skin necrosis with SC extravasation

(f) Indications for use
- **(i)** Peripheral vascular collapse when it is necessary to increase SVR (e.g., septic shock or "vasoplegia" after cardiopulmonary bypass [CPB])
- **(ii)** Conditions in which increased SVR is desired together with cardiac stimulation
- **(iii)** Need for increased SVR in which phenylephrine has proved ineffective

(g) Administration. IV only, by central line only

(h) Clinical use
- **(i)** Usual NE starting infusion doses: 15 to 30 ng/kg/min IV (adult); usual range, 30 to 300 ng/kg/min.
- **(ii)** Minimize duration of use; monitor patient for oliguria and metabolic acidosis.
- **(iii)** NE can be used with vasodilator (e.g., nitroprusside or phentolamine) to counteract α stimulation while leaving β_1-adrenergic stimulation intact; however, if intense vasoconstriction is not required, we recommend that a different drug be used.
- **(iv)** For treating severe right ventricular (RV) failure associated with cardiac surgery, the simultaneous infusion of NE into the *left atrium* (through a left atrial catheter placed intraoperatively) plus inhaled NO and/or nitroglycerine by IV infusion is useful. The left atrial NE reaches the systemic vascular bed first and it is largely metabolized peripherally before it reaches the lung where it might increase PVR (had the NE been infused through a venous line) (Table 2.2).

(5) Interactions with MAO inhibitors

(a) MAO is an enzyme that deaminates NE, dopamine, and serotonin. Thus, the MAO inhibitors treat severe depression by increasing catecholamine concentrations in the brain by inhibiting catecholamine breakdown. Administration of indirectly acting adrenergic agonists or meperidine to patients taking MAO inhibitors can produce a life-threatening hypertensive crisis. Ideally, 2 to 3 wks should elapse between discontinuing the hydrazine MAO inhibitor phenelzine and elective surgery. Nonhydrazine MAO inhibitors (isocarboxazid, tranylcypromine) require 3 to 10 days for offset of effect. Selegiline at doses 10 mg or less per day should present fewer adverse drug interactions than other MAO inhibitors.

(b) The greatest risk of inducing a hyperadrenergic state occurs with indirect-acting sympathomimetic drugs (such as ephedrine), because such agents release the intraneuronal stores of NE that were increased by the MAO

TABLE 2.2 Acute treatment of pulmonary hypertension and RV failure

Pulmonary hypertension	
Hyperventilation	Maintain P_aCO_2 at 25–28 mm Hg
Oxygen	Prevents hypoxic vasoconstriction
NO	Inspired, 0.05–80 ppm
Nitroprusside	0.1–4 μg/kg/min
Nitroglycerin	0.1–7 μg/kg/min
Alprostadil	0.05–0.4 μg/kg/min
Epoprostenol	9 ng/kg/min[a]
Tolazoline	Bolus 0.5–2 mg/kg, then 0.5–10 mg/kg/h
Phentolamine	1–20 μg/kg/min
Isoproterenol	0.02–20 μg/kg/min
Diltiazem	Effective orally; no data on IV use
Right ventricular failure	
Use therapies listed above to reduce PA pressure; in addition, the following may be utilized:	
Dobutamine	2–20 μg/kg/min
Dopamine	≤5 μg/kg/min
Epinephrine[b]	0.05–0.2 μg/kg/min
Inamrinone	5–20 μg/kg/min (maintenance)
Milrinone	0.5–0.75 μg/kg/min (maintenance)
Norepinephrine[b]	0.05–0.2 μg/kg/min (maintain coronary perfusion pressure)
Right-sided mechanical assist device	Rest, unload right heart
Intra-aortic balloon counterpulsation	Unload left heart, improve coronary perfusion to left and right heart

[a]Used mainly for chronic management of primary pulmonary hypertension.
[b]May be administered via left atrial line to reduce actions on pulmonary vasculature.

inhibitor. Because dopamine releases NE, it should be initiated with caution in the MAO-inhibited patient.

(c) In MAO-inhibited patients, preferred drugs are those with purely direct activity: epinephrine, NE, isoproterenol, phenylephrine, vasopressin, and dobutamine. All pressor drugs should be used cautiously, in small dosages with BP monitoring and observation of the electrocardiogram (ECG) for arrhythmias.

B. Vasopressin pharmacology and agonists [17]

1. Actions

a. Vasopressin is an endogenous antidiuretic hormone that in high concentrations produces a direct peripheral vasoconstriction through activation of smooth-muscle V1 receptors. Vasopressin has no actions on β-adrenergic receptors, so it may produce less tachycardia than epinephrine when used for resuscitation after cardiac arrest. Vasopressin has been administered intra-arterially in a selective fashion to control gastrointestinal bleeding.

b. Vasopressin produces relatively more vasoconstriction of skin, skeletal muscle, intestine, and adipose tissue than of coronary or renal beds. Vasopressin causes cerebrovascular dilation.

2. Advantages

a. Vasopressin is a very potent agent which acts independently of adrenergic receptors.

b. Some studies suggest that vasopressin may be effective at maintaining adequate SVR in severe acidosis, sepsis, or after CPB, even when agents such as phenylephrine or NE have proven ineffective.

c. Vasopressin may restore coronary perfusion pressure after cardiac arrest without also producing tachycardia and arrhythmias, as is common when epinephrine is used for this purpose.

3. **Disadvantages**
   a. Vasopressin produces a variety of unpleasant signs and symptoms in awake patients, including pallor of skin, nausea, abdominal cramping, bronchoconstriction, and uterine contractions.
   b. Decreases in splanchnic blood flow may be of concern in patients receiving vasopressin for more than a few hours, particularly when vasopressin is coadministered with agents such as α-adrenergic agonists and positive inotropic drugs. Increases in serum concentrations of bilirubin and of "liver" enzymes are common.
   c. Vasopressin may be associated with a decrease in platelet concentration.
   d. Lactic acidosis is common in patients receiving vasopressin infusion (but these patients are generally critically ill and already receiving other vasoactive agents).
4. **Clinical use**
   a. Vasopressin has been used as an alternative to epinephrine in treating countershock-refractory ventricular fibrillation (VF) in adults. The 2010 American Heart Association Guidelines for Cardiopulmonary Resuscitation and Emergency Cardiovascular Care Science suggest that vasopressin may be substituted either for the first or second dose of epinephrine during resuscitation, but that there is no convincing evidence that inclusion of vasopressin in resuscitation will improve outcomes relative to outcomes obtained with epinephrine alone. The typical vasopressin resuscitation dose is 40 units as an IV bolus.
   b. Vasopressin has been used in a variety of conditions associated with vasodilatory shock, including sepsis, the "vasoplegic" syndrome after CPB, and for hypotension occurring in patients receiving ACE inhibitors (or angtiotensin receptor blockers) and general anesthesia. Typical adult doses range from 4 to 6 units/h. We have found this drug to be effective and useful, but sometimes associated with troublesome metabolic acidosis. We speculate that the latter may be the result of inadequate visceral perfusion.

VI. Positive inotropic drugs

A. Treatment of low CO [16]

1. **Goals.** Increase organ perfusion and oxygen delivery to tissues
   a. Increase CO by increasing SV, HR (when appropriate) or both
   b. Maximize myocardial oxygen supply (increase diastolic arterial pressure, diastolic perfusion time, and blood O_2 content; decrease left ventricular end-diastolic pressure [LVEDP])
   c. Provide an adequate mean arterial pressure (MAP) for perfusion of other organs
   d. Minimize increases in myocardial oxygen demand by avoiding tachycardia and left ventricular (LV) dilation
   e. Metabolic disturbances, arrhythmias, or cardiac ischemia, if present, should be treated concurrently.
   f. Drug treatment of critically ill patients with intrinsic myocardial failure may include the following cardiac stimulants:
      (1) β_1-Adrenergic stimulation
      (2) Phosphodiesterase (PDE) inhibition
      (3) Dopaminergic stimulants
      (4) Calcium sensitizers (increase calcium sensitivity of contractile proteins)
      (5) Digoxin
2. **Monitoring.** Positive inotropic drug dosing is most effectively regulated using data from the arterial line, a monitor of cardiac output, and/or echocardiography. In addition, monitoring of mixed venous oxygen saturation can be extremely valuable. The inotropic drug dosage can be titrated to CO and BP endpoints, together with assessment of organ perfusion, e.g., urine output and concentration.

B. cAMP-dependent agents

1. **β-Adrenergic and dopaminergic receptor agonists**
   a. **Similarities among sympathomimetic drugs**

(1) β_1-agonist effects are primarily stimulatory.

β_1 agonists	
HR	Increased
Contractility	Increased
Conduction velocity	Increased
Atrioventricular (AV) block	Decreased
Automaticity	Increased
Risk of arrhythmias	Increased

(2) **β_2 agonists** cause vasodilation and bronchodilation, and they also increase HR and contractility (albeit with less potency than β_1 agonists).

(3) **Postsynaptic dopaminergic receptors** mediate renal and mesenteric vasodilation, increase renal salt excretion, and reduce gastrointestinal motility. Presynaptic dopaminergic receptors inhibit NE release.

(4) **Diastolic ventricular dysfunction.** Cardiac β-receptor activation enhances diastolic ventricular relaxation by facilitating the active, energy-consuming process that pumps free intracellular Ca^{2+} into storage sites. Abnormal relaxation occurring in ischemia and other myocardial disorders leads to increased diastolic stiffness. By augmenting diastolic relaxation, β-adrenergic receptor agonists reduce LVEDP and heart size (LV end-diastolic volume [LVEDV]), improve diastolic filling, reduce left atrial pressure (LAP), and improve the myocardial oxygen supply–demand ratio.

(5) **Systolic ventricular dysfunction.** More complete ventricular ejection during systole will reduce the LV end-systolic volume. This reduces heart size, LV systolic wall tension (by Laplace's law), and myocardial oxygen consumption (Mvo_2).

(6) **Myocardial ischemia.** The net effects of β-receptor stimulation on myocardial O_2 supply and demand are multifactorial and may be difficult to predict. Mvo_2 tends to increase as HR and contractility rise, but Mvo_2 is reduced by lowering LVEDV. β Agonists improve O_2 supply when LVEDP is decreased, but can worsen the supply–demand ratio particularly if HR rises or diastolic BP is lowered.

(7) **Hypovolemia** is deleterious to the patient with heart failure just as it is for the patient with normal ventricular function; however, volume overload may lead to myocardial ischemia by restricting subendocardial perfusion.

(8) **There is a risk of tissue damage or sloughing when vasoactive drugs extravasate outside of a vein.** In general, catecholamine vasoconstrictors should not be infused for long periods of time through a peripheral IV line because of the risk of extravasation or infiltration. These drugs may be given through peripheral IV lines provided that

- **(a)** No central venous catheter is available.
- **(b)** The drug is injected only into a free-flowing IV line.
- **(c)** The IV site is observed during and after the injection for signs of infiltration or extravasation.

b. Dobutamine (Dobutrex) [16]

(1) **Dobutamine is a synthetic catecholamine formulated as a racemic mixture.**

(2) **Actions**

- **(a)** Direct β_1 agonist, with limited β_2 and α_1 effects. Dobutamine has no α_2 or dopaminergic activity.
- **(b)** Dobutamine increases cardiac inotropy principally via its β_1 (and perhaps also by α_1) agonism, but HR is increased only by the β_1 effect.
- **(c)** On blood vessels, dobutamine is predominantly a vasodilator drug. Mechanisms for vasodilation include the following:
  - **(i)** β_2-mediated vasodilation that is only partially counteracted by (–) dobutamine's α_1 constrictor effects

(ii) The (+) dobutamine enantiomer and its metabolite, (+)-3-O-methyldobutamine, are α_1 *antagonists.* Thus, as dobutamine is metabolized, any α_1 agonist actions of the drug should diminish over time.

	Dobutamine
HR	Increased
Contractility	Increased
CO	Increased
BP	Usually increases, may remain unchanged
LVEDP	Decreased
LAP	Decreased
SVR	Decreased by dilating all vascular beds; slight increase may be seen in β-blocked patients
PVR	Decreased

(3) Offset. Offset of action is achieved by redistribution, metabolism by COMT, and conjugation by glucuronide in liver; an active metabolite is generated. Plasma half-life is 2 min.

(4) Advantages

(a) At low doses there is generally less tachycardia than with "equivalently inotropic" doses of isoproterenol or dopamine, whereas some studies show that "equivalently inotropic" doses of epinephrine produce LESS tachycardia than dobutamine.

(b) Afterload reduction (SVR and PVR) may improve LV and RV systolic function, which can benefit the heart with right and/or LV failure.

(c) Renal blood flow may increase (due to a β_2 effect), but not as much as with comparable (but low) doses of dopamine or dopexamine.

(5) Disadvantages

(a) Tachycardia and arrhythmias are dose-related and can be severe.

(b) Hypotension may occur if the reduction in SVR is not fully offset by an increase in CO; dobutamine is an inotrope but is not a pressor.

(c) Coronary steal is possible.

(d) The drug is a nonselective vasodilator: Blood flow may be shunted from kidney and splanchnic bed to skeletal muscle.

(e) Tachyphylaxis has been reported when infused for more than 72 h.

(f) Mild hypokalemia may occur.

(g) As a partial agonist, dobutamine can inhibit actions of full agonists (e.g., epinephrine) under certain circumstances.

(6) Indications. Low CO states, especially with increased SVR or PVR

(7) Administration. IV only (central line is preferable, but dobutamine has little vasoconstrictor activity, minimizing risk of extravasation).

(8) Clinical use

(a) Dobutamine dose: IV infusion, 2 to 20 μg/kg/min. Some patients may respond to initial doses as low as 0.5 μg/kg/min and, at such low doses, HR usually does not increase.

(b) Dobutamine increases $M\dot{V}O_2$ to a lesser degree than CO. Dobutamine increases coronary blood flow to a greater degree than dopamine when either agent is given as a single drug. However, addition of nitroglycerin to dopamine may be equally effective.

(c) Dobutamine acts similar to a fixed-ratio combination of an inotropic drug and a vasodilator drug. These two components cannot be titrated separately.

(d) In patients undergoing coronary surgery, dobutamine produces more tachycardia than epinephrine when administered to produce the same increase in SV [11].

(e) When dobutamine is given to β-blocked patients, SVR may increase.

(f) Routine administration of dobutamine (or any other positive inotrope) is not recommended. [18]

c. **Dopamine (Intropin)** [16]

(1) Dopamine is a catecholamine precursor to NE and epinephrine found in nerve terminals and the adrenal medulla.

(2) **Actions**

(a) Direct action: α_1-, β_1-, β_2-adrenergic, and dopaminergic (DA_1) agonist

(b) Indirect action: Induces release of stored neuronal NE

(c) The dose versus response relationship is often described as if "carved in stone"; however, the relationship between dose and concentration and between dose and response is highly variable from patient to patient.

	Dopamine (as commonly described)	
Dose (μg/kg/min)	**Receptor activated**	**Effect**
1–3	Dopaminergic (DA_1)	Increased renal and mesenteric blood flow
3–10	$\beta_1 + \beta_2$ (plus DA_1)	Increased HR, contractility, and CO
>10	α (plus β plus DA_1)	Increased SVR, PVR; decreased renal blood flow; increased HR, arrhythmias. Increased afterload may decrease CO

(3) **Offset** is achieved by redistribution, uptake by nerve terminals plus metabolism by MAO and COMT.

(4) **Advantages**

(a) Increased renal perfusion and urine output at low to moderate dosages (partially due to a specific DA_1 agonist effect)

(b) Blood flow shifts from skeletal muscle to kidney and splanchnic beds.

(c) BP response is easy to titrate because of its mixed inotropic and vasoconstrictor properties.

(5) **Disadvantages**

(a) There is a significant indirect-acting component; response can diminish when neuronal NE is depleted (e.g., in patients with CHF).

(b) Sinus, atrial, or ventricular tachycardia (VT) and arrhythmias may occur.

(c) Maximal inotropic effect less than that of epinephrine.

(d) Skin necrosis may result from extravasation.

(e) Renal vasodilating effects are over-ridden by α-mediated vasoconstriction at dosages greater than 10 μg/kg/min with risk of renal, splanchnic, and skin necrosis. Urine output should be monitored.

(f) Pulmonary vasoconstriction is possible.

(g) $M\text{VO}_2$ increases, and myocardial ischemia may occur if coronary flow does not increase commensurately.

(h) In some patients with severe HF, the increased BP at increased doses may be detrimental. Such patients benefit from adding a vasodilator.

(6) **Indications**

(a) Hypotension due to low CO or low SVR (although other agents are superior for the latter indication)

(b) Temporary therapy of hypovolemia until circulating blood volume is restored (but vasoconstrictors should not substitute or delay primary treatment of hypovolemia)

(c) "Recruiting renal blood flow" for renal failure or insufficiency (widely used for this purpose, but limited evidence basis)

(7) **Administration:** IV only (preferably by central venous line)

(8) **Clinical use**

(a) Dopamine dose: 1 to 20 μg/kg/min IV.

(b) Often mix 200 mg in 250 mL IV solution (800 μg/mL).

(c) Good first choice for temporary treatment of hypotension until intravascular volume can be expanded or until a specific diagnosis can be made.

(d) Correct hypovolemia if possible before use (as with all pressors)

(e) After cardiac surgery if inotropic response is not adequate at dopamine doses of 5 to 10 μg/kg/min, we recommend a switch to a more powerful agonist such as epinephrine, or a switch to or addition of milrinone.

(f) Consider adding a vasodilator (e.g., nitroprusside) when BP is adequate and afterload reduction would be beneficial (or better still, reduce the dose of dopamine).

d. Dopexamine [16]

(1) **Actions**

(a) Dopexamine is a synthetic analog of dobutamine with vasodilator action. Its cardiac inotropic and chronotropic activity is caused by direct β_2-agonist effects and by NE actions (due to baroreceptor reflex activation and neuronal uptake-1 inhibition) that *indirectly* activate β_1-receptors. In CHF, there is selective β_1 downregulation, with relative preservation of β_2-receptor number and coupling. The latter assume greater than normal physiologic importance, making dopexamine of *theoretically* greater utility than agents with primary β_1-receptor activity. Although dopexamine has been used in Europe for roughly a decade, the drug will likely never be available in the United States.

(b) Receptor activity

α_1 and α_2: Minimal

β_1: Little *direct* effect, some *indirect;* β_2: Direct agonist

DA_1: Potent agonist (activation increases renal blood flow)

(c) Inhibits neuronal catecholamine uptake-1, increasing NE actions

(d) Hemodynamic actions

	Dopexamine
HR	Increased
CO	Increased
SVR	Decreased
MAP	Little change or decrease
Preload	No change or slight decrease
PAP	No change or slight decrease

(2) **Offset.** Half-life: 6 to 11 min. Clearance is by uptake into tissues (catecholamine uptake mechanisms) and by hepatic metabolism.

(3) **Advantages**

(a) Lack of vasoconstrictor activity avoids α-mediated complications.

(b) Decreased renovascular resistance might *theoretically* help preserve renal function after ischemic insults.

(4) **Disadvantages**

(a) Less effective positive inotrope than other agents (e.g., epinephrine, milrinone)

(b) Dose-dependent tachycardia may limit therapy.

(c) Tachyphylaxis

(d) Not approved by the U.S. Food and Drug administration for release in the United States.

(5) **Indications.** Treatment of low CO states

(6) **Administration.** IV

(7) **Clinical use**

(a) Dopexamine dose: 0.5 to 4 μg/kg/min IV (maximum 6 μg/kg/min).

(b) Hemodynamic and renal effects similar to the combination of variable doses of dobutamine with dopamine 1 μg/kg/min (renal dose) or fenoldopam 0.05 μg/kg/min.

e. **Epinephrine (Adrenaline)** [16]

(1) **Epinephrine is a catecholamine produced by the adrenal medulla.**

(2) **Actions**

(a) Direct agonist at α_1-, α_2-, β_1-, and β_2-receptors

(b) Dose response (adult, approximate)

	Epinephrine	
Dose (ng/kg/min)	**Receptors activated**	**SVR**
10–30	β	Usually decreased
30–150	β and α	Variable
>150	α and β	Increased

(c) Increased contractility with all dosages, but SVR may decrease, remain unchanged, or increase dramatically depending on the dosage. CO usually increased but, at extreme resuscitation dosages, α-receptor–mediated vasoconstriction may cause a lowered SV due to high afterload.

(3) **Offset** occurs by uptake by neurons and tissue and by metabolism by MAO and COMT (rapid).

(4) **Advantages**

(a) This drug is direct-acting; its effects are not dependent on release of endogenous NE.

(b) Potent α- and β-adrenergic stimulation results in greater maximal effects and produce equivalent increases in SV with tachycardia after heart surgery than dopamine or dobutamine.

(c) It is a powerful inotrope with variable (and dose-dependent) α-adrenergic effect. Lusitropic effect (β_1) enhances the rate of ventricular relaxation.

(d) BP increases may blunt tachycardia due to reflex vagal stimulation.

(e) It is an effective bronchodilator and mast cell stabilizer, useful for primary therapy of severe bronchospasm, anaphylactoid, or anaphylactic reactions.

3

(f) With a dilated LV and myocardial ischemia, epinephrine may increase diastolic BP and decrease heart size, reducing myocardial ischemia. However, as with any inotropic drug, epinephrine may induce or worsen myocardial ischemia.

(5) **Disadvantages**

(a) Tachycardia and arrhythmias at higher doses.

(b) Organ ischemia, especially kidney, secondary to vasoconstriction, may result. Renal function must be closely monitored.

(c) Pulmonary vasoconstriction may occur, which can produce pulmonary hypertension and possibly RV failure; addition of a vasodilator may counteract this.

(d) Epinephrine may produce myocardial ischemia. Positive inotropy and tachycardia increase myocardial oxygen demand and reduce oxygen supply.

(e) Extravasation from a peripheral IV cannula can cause necrosis; thus, administration via a central venous line is preferable.

(f) As with most adrenergic agonists, increases of plasma glucose and lactate occur. This may be accentuated in diabetics.

(g) Initial increases in plasma K^+ occur due to hepatic release, followed by decreased K^+ due to skeletal muscle uptake.

(6) **Indications**

(a) Cardiac arrest (especially asystole or VF); electromechanical dissociation. Epinephrine's efficacy is believed to result from increased coronary perfusion pressure during cardiopulmonary resuscitation (CPR). Recently, the utility of high-dose (0.2 mg/kg) epinephrine was debated, the consensus is that there is no outcome benefit to "high-dose" epinephrine.

(b) Anaphylaxis and other systemic allergic reactions; epinephrine is the agent of choice.
(c) Cardiogenic shock, especially if a vasodilator is added
(d) Bronchospasm
(e) Reduced CO after CPB
(f) Hypotension with spinal or epidural anesthesia can be treated with low-dose (1 to 4 μg/min) epinephrine infusions as conveniently and effectively as with ephedrine boluses [12].

(7) Administration. IV (preferably by central line); via endotracheal tube (rapidly absorbed by tracheal mucosa); SC

(8) Clinical use

(a) Epinephrine dose
(i) SC: 10 μg/kg (maximum of 400 μg or 0.4 mL, 1:1,000) for treatment of mild-to-moderate allergic reactions or bronchospasm.
(ii) IV: Low-to-moderate dose (for shock, hypotension): 0.03 to 0.2 μg/kg bolus (IV), then infusion at 0.01 to 0.30 μg/kg/min.
High dose (for cardiac arrest, resuscitation): 0.5 to 1.0 mg IV bolus; pediatric, 5 to 15 μg/kg (may be given intratracheally in 1 to 10 mL volume). Larger doses are used when response to initial dose is inadequate. **Resuscitation** doses of epinephrine may produce extreme hypertension, stroke, or myocardial infarction. A starting dose of epinephrine exceeding a 150 ng/kg (10 μg in an adult) IV bolus should be given only to a patient in extremis! **Moderate doses** (.03–.06 μg/kg/min) of epinephrine are commonly used to stimulate cardiac function an facilitate separation from cardiopulmonary bypass.

(b) Watch for signs of excessive vasoconstriction. Monitor SVR, renal function, extremity perfusion.
(c) Addition of a vasodilator (e.g., nicardipine, nitroprusside, or phentolamine) to epinephrine can counteract the α-mediated vasoconstriction, leaving positive cardiac inotropic effects undiminished. Alternatively, addition of milrinone or inamrinone may permit lower doses of epinephrine to be used. We find combinations of epinephrine and milrinone particularly useful in cardiac surgical patients.

f. NE (noradrenaline, Levophed)

See the preceding Section V: Vasopressors.

g. Isoproterenol (Isuprel)

(1) Isoproterenol is a synthetic catecholamine.

(2) Actions

(a) Direct β_1- plus β_2-adrenergic agonist
(b) No α-adrenergic effects

	Isoproterenol
HR	Increased
Contractility	Increased
CO	Increased
BP	Variable
SVR	Decreased; dose-related dilation of all vascular beds
PVR	Decreased

(3) Offset. Rapid (half-life, 2 min); uptake by liver, conjugated, 60% excreted unchanged; metabolized by MAO, COMT

(4) Advantages

(a) Isoproterenol is a potent direct β-adrenergic receptor agonist.
(b) It increases CO by three mechanisms:
(i) Increased HR

(ii) Increased contractility → increased SV
(iii) Reduced afterload (SVR) → increased SV
(c) It is a bronchodilator (IV or inhaled).

(5) **Disadvantages**
(a) It is not a pressor! BP often falls (β_2-adrenergic effect) while CO rises.
(b) Hypotension may produce organ hypoperfusion, hypotension, and ischemia.
(c) Tachycardia limits diastolic filling time.
(d) Proarrhythmic
(e) Dilates all vascular beds and is capable of shunting blood away from critical organs toward muscle and skin.
(f) Coronary vasodilation can reduce blood flow to ischemic myocardium while increasing flow to nonischemic areas producing coronary "steal" in patients with "steal-prone" coronary anatomy.
(g) May unmask pre-excitation in patients with an accessory AV conduction pathway (e.g., Wolff—Parkinson–White [WPW] syndrome).

(6) **Indications**
(a) Bradycardia unresponsive to atropine when electrical pacing is not available
(b) Low CO, especially for situations in which increased inotropy is needed and tachycardia is not detrimental, such as the following:
(i) Pediatric patients with fixed SV
(ii) After resection of ventricular aneurysm (small fixed SV)
(iii) Denervated heart (after cardiac transplantation)
(c) Pulmonary hypertension or right heart failure
(d) AV block: Use as temporary therapy to decrease block or increase rate of idioventricular foci. Use with caution in second-degree Mobitz type II heart block—may intensify heart block.
(e) Status asthmaticus: Intravenous use mandates continuous ECG and BP monitoring.
(f) β-Blocker overdose
(g) Isoproterenol should not be used for cardiac asystole. CPR with epinephrine or pacing is the therapy of choice because isoproterenol-induced vasodilation results in reduced carotid and coronary blood flow during CPR.

(7) **Administration.** IV (safe through peripheral line, will not necrose skin); PO

(8) **Clinical use and isoproterenol dose.** IV infusion is 20 to 500 ng/kg/min.

2. **PDE inhibitors**

a. **Inamrinone (Inocor)** [16]

(1) **Inamrinone is a bipyridine derivative that inhibits the cyclic guanosine monophosphate (cGMP)-inhibited cAMP-specific PDE III, increasing cAMP concentrations in cardiac muscle (positive inotropy) and in vascular smooth muscle (vasodilation).**

	Inamrinone
HR	Generally little change (tachycardia at higher doses)
MAP	Variable (the decrease in SVR may be offset by increase in CO)
CO	Increased
LAP	Decreased
SVR	Decreased
PVR	Decreased
Mvo_2	Generally little change (increase in oxygen consumption from increased CO is offset by decrease in wall tension)

(2) **Offset**
(a) The elimination half-life is 2.5 to 4 h, increasing to 6 h in patients with CHF.
(b) Offset occurs by hepatic conjugation, with 30% to 35% excreted unchanged in urine.

(3) Advantages

(a) As a vasodilating inotrope, inamrinone increases CO by augmenting contractility *and* decreasing cardiac afterload.

(b) Favorable effects on Mvo_2 (little increase in HR; decreases afterload, LVEDP, and wall tension)

(c) It does not depend on activation of β-receptors and therefore retains effectiveness despite β-receptor downregulation or uncoupling (e.g., CHF) and in the presence of β-adrenergic blockade.

(d) Low risk of tachycardia or arrhythmias

(e) Inamrinone may act synergistically with β-adrenergic receptor agonists and dopaminergic receptor agonists.

(f) Pulmonary vasodilator

(g) Positive lusitropic properties (ventricular relaxation) at even very low dosages

(4) Disadvantages

(a) Thrombocytopenia after chronic (more than 24 h) administration

(b) Will nearly always cause hypotension from vasodilation if given by rapid bolus administration. Hypotension is easily treated with IV fluid and α agonists.

(c) Increased dosages may result in tachycardia (and therefore increased Mvo_2).

(d) Less convenient than milrinone because of photosensitivity and reduced potency

(5) Administration. IV infusion only. Do not mix in dextrose-containing solutions.

(6) Clinical use

(a) Inamrinone loading dose is 0.75 to 1.5 mg/kg. When given during or after CPB, usual dosage is 1.5 mg/kg.

(b) IV infusion dose range is 5 to 20 μg/kg/min (usual dosage is 10 μg/kg/min).

(c) Used in cardiac surgical patients in a manner similar to milrinone

(d) The popularity of this agent has steadily declined since the introduction of milrinone, largely due to milrinone's lack of an adverse action on platelet function. Inamrinone is included here mostly for completeness.

b. Milrinone (Primacor) [16]

(1) Actions

(a) Milrinone has powerful cardiac inotropic and vasodilator properties. Milrinone increases intracellular concentrations of cAMP by inhibiting its breakdown. Milrinone inhibits the cGMP-inhibited, cAMP-specific PDE (commonly known by clinicians as "type III") in cardiac and vascular smooth-muscle cells. In cardiac myocytes, increased cAMP causes positive inotropy, lusitropy (enhanced diastolic myocardial relaxation), chronotropy, and dromotropy (AV conduction), as well as increased automaticity. In vascular smooth-muscle cells, increased cAMP causes vasodilation.

(b) Hemodynamic actions

	Milrinone
HR	Usually no change or slight increase
CO	Increased
BP	Variable
SVR and PVR	Decreased
Preload	Decreased
Mvo_2	Often unchanged or slight increase

(2) Onset and offset. When administered as an IV bolus, milrinone rapidly achieves its maximal effect. The elimination half-life of milrinone is considerably shorter than that of inamrinone.

4

(3) **Advantages**
   (a) Used as a single agent, milrinone has favorable effects on the myocardial oxygen supply–demand balance, due to reduction of preload and afterload, and minimal tendency for tachycardia.
   (b) Milrinone does not act via β-adrenergic receptors and it retains efficacy when β-adrenergic receptor coupling is impaired, as in CHF.
   (c) It induces no tachyphylaxis.
   (d) Milrinone has less proarrhythmic effects than β-adrenergic receptor agonists.
   (e) When compared to dobutamine at equipotent doses, milrinone is associated with a greater decrease in PVR, greater augmentation of RV ejection fraction, less tachycardia, fewer arrhythmias, and lower $M\text{VO}_2$.
   (f) This drug may act synergistically with drugs that stimulate cAMP production, such as β-adrenergic receptor agonists.
   (g) Even with chronic use, milrinone (unlike inamrinone) does not cause thrombocytopenia.

(4) **Disadvantages**
   (a) Vasodilation and hypotension are predictable with rapid IV bolus doses.
   (b) As with all other positive inotropic drugs, including epinephrine and dobutamine, independent manipulation of cardiac inotropy and SVR cannot be achieved using only milrinone.
   (c) Arrhythmias may occur.

(5) **Clinical use**
   (a) Milrinone loading dose: 25 to 75 (usual dose is 50) μg/kg given over 1 to 10 min. Often it is desirable to administer the loading dose before separating the patient from CPB so that hypotension can be managed more easily [13].
   (b) Maintenance infusion: 0.375 to 0.75 μg/kg/min (usual maintenance is 0.5 μg/kg/min). Dosage should be reduced in renal failure.

(6) **Indications**
   (a) Low CO syndrome, especially in the setting of increased LVEDP, pulmonary hypertension, RV failure
   (b) To supplement/potentiate β-adrenergic receptor agonists
   (c) Outpatient milrinone infusion has been used as a bridge to cardiac transplantation.

3. **Glucagon**
   a. **Glucagon is a peptide hormone produced by the pancreas.**
   b. **Actions.** Glucagon increases intracellular cAMP, acting via a specific receptor.

	Glucagon
Contractility	Increased
AV conduction	Increased
HR	Increased
CO	Increased, with a variable effect on SVR

   c. **Offset** of action of glucagon occurs by redistribution and proteolysis by the liver, kidney, and plasma. Duration of action is 20 to 30 min.
   d. **Advantages.** Glucagon has a positive inotropic effect even in the presence of β-blockade.
   e. **Disadvantages**
      (1) Consistently produces nausea and vomiting
      (2) Tachycardia
      (3) Hyperglycemia and hypokalemia
      (4) Catecholamine release from pheochromocytomas
      (5) Anaphylaxis (possible)

f. **Indications for glucagon include the following:**
   (1) Severe hypoglycemia (especially if no IV access) from insulin overdosage
   (2) Spasm of sphincter of Oddi
   (3) Heart failure from β-blocker overdosage

g. **Administration.** IV, IM, SC

h. **Clinical use**
   (1) Glucagon dose: 1 to 5 mg IV slowly; 0.5 to 2 mg IM or SC.
   (2) Infusion: 25 to 75 μg/min.
   (3) Rarely used (other than for hypoglycemia) because of gastrointestinal side effects and severe tachycardia.

C. cAMP-independent agents

1. **Calcium** [16]

a. **Calcium is physiologically active only as the free (unbound) calcium ion (Ca_i).**
   (1) Normally, approximately 50% of the total plasma calcium is bound to proteins and anions and the rest remains as free calcium ions.
   (2) Factors affecting ionized calcium concentration:
      (a) Alkalosis (metabolic or respiratory) decreases Ca_i.
      (b) Acidosis increases Ca_i.
      (c) Citrate binds (chelates) Ca_i.
      (d) Albumin binds Ca_i.
   (3) Normal plasma concentration: $[Ca_i] = 1$ to 1.3 mmol/L.

b. **Actions of calcium salts**

	Calcium
HR	No change or decrease (vagal effect)
Contractility	Increase (in response to Ca bolus during hypocalcemia)
BP	Increase
SVR	Usually increase
Preload	Little change
CO	Variable

c. **Offset.** Calcium is incorporated into muscle and bone and binds to protein, free fatty acids released by heparin, and citrate.

d. **Advantages**
   (1) It has rapid action with duration of approximately 10 to 15 min (7 mg/kg dose).
   (2) It reverses hypotension caused by the following conditions:
      (a) Halogenated anesthetic overdosage
      (b) Calcium-blocking drugs (CCBs)
      (c) Hypocalcemia
      (d) CPB, especially with dilutional or citrate-induced hypocalcemia, or when cardioplegia-induced hyperkalemia remains present (administer calcium salts only after heart has been well reperfused to avoid augmenting reperfusion injury)
      (e) β-blockers (watch for bradycardia!)
   (3) It reverses cardiac toxicity from hyperkalemia (e.g., arrhythmias, heart block, and negative inotropy).

e. **Disadvantages**
   (1) Minimal evidence that calcium salts administered to patients produce even a transient increase in CO.
   (2) Calcium can provoke digitalis toxicity which can present as ventricular arrhythmias, AV block, or asystole.
   (3) Calcium potentiates the effects of hypokalemia on the heart (arrhythmias).
   (4) Severe bradycardia or heart block occurs rarely.
   (5) When extracellular calcium concentration is increased while the surrounding myocardium is being reperfused or is undergoing ongoing ischemia, increased cellular damage or cell death occurs.

(6) Post-CPB coronary spasm may occur rarely.

(7) Associated with pancreatitis when given in large doses to patients recovering from CPB.

(8) Calcium may inhibit clinical responses to epinephrine and dobutamine [14].

f. Indications for use

(1) Hypocalcemia

(2) Hyperkalemia (to reverse AV block or myocardial depression)

(3) Intraoperative hypotension due to decreased myocardial contractility from hypocalcemia or calcium channel blockers

(4) Inhaled general anesthetic overdose

(5) Toxic hypermagnesemia

g. Administration

(1) Calcium chloride: IV, preferably by central line (causes peripheral vein inflammation and sclerosis).

(2) Calcium gluconate: IV, preferably by central line.

h. Clinical use

(1) Calcium dose

(a) 10% calcium chloride 10 mL (contains 272 mg of elemental calcium or 13.6 mEq): adult, 200 to 1,000 mg slow IV; pediatric, 10 to 20 mg/kg slow IV

(b) 10% calcium gluconate 10 mL (contains 93 mg of elemental calcium or 4.6 mEq): adult, 600 to 3,000 mg slow IV; pediatric, 30 to 100 mg/kg slow IV

(2) During massive blood transfusion (more than 1 blood volume replaced with citrate-preserved blood), a patient may receive citrate, which binds calcium. In normal situations, hepatic metabolism quickly eliminates citrate from plasma, and hypocalcemia does not occur. However, hypothermia and shock may decrease citrate clearance with resultant severe hypocalcemia. Rapid infusion of albumin will transiently reduce ionized calcium levels.

(3) Ionized calcium levels should be measured frequently to guide calcium salt therapy. Adults with an intact parathyroid gland quickly recover from mild hypocalcemia without treatment.

(4) Calcium is not recommended during resuscitation unless hypocalcemia, hyperkalemia, or hypermagnesemia are present.

(5) Calcium should be used with care in situations in which ongoing myocardial ischemia may be occurring or during reperfusion of ischemic tissue. "Routine" administration of large doses of calcium to all adult patients at the end of CPB is unnecessary and may be deleterious if the heart has been reperfused only minutes earlier.

(6) Hypocalcemia is frequent in children emerging from CPB.

2. Digoxin (Lanoxin)

a. Digoxin is a glycoside derived from the foxglove plant.

b. Actions

(1) Digoxin inhibits the integral membrane protein Na-K ATPase, causing Na^+ accumulation in cells and increased intracellular Ca_i, which leads to increased Ca^{2+} release from the sarcoplasmic reticulum into the cytoplasm with each heartbeat, ultimately causing a mildly increased myocardial contractility.

(2) Hemodynamic effects

(a) Digoxin

	Calcium
Contractility	Increased
AV conduction	Decreased
Ventricular automaticity	Increased rate of phase 4 depolarization
Refractory period	Decreased (in atria and ventricles); increased in AV node

(b) Hemodynamics in CHF

	Calcium
HR	Decreased
SV	Increased
SVR	Decreased
$M\dot{V}O_2$	Decreased

c. Offset. Digoxin elimination half-life is 1.7 days (renal elimination). In anephric patients, half-life is more than 4 days.

d. Advantages

(1) Supraventricular antiarrhythmic action

(2) Reduced ventricular rate in atrial fibrillation or flutter

(3) An orally active positive inotrope which is not associated with increased mortality in CHF

e. Disadvantages

(1) Digoxin has an extremely low therapeutic index; 20% of patients show toxicity at some time.

(2) Increased $M\dot{V}O_2$ and SVR occur in patients without CHF (angina may be precipitated).

(3) The drug has a long half-life, and it is difficult to titrate.

(4) There is large interindividual variation in therapeutic and toxic serum levels and dosages. The dose response is nonlinear; near-toxic levels may be needed to achieve a change in AV conduction.

(5) Toxic manifestations may be life-threatening and difficult to diagnose. Digoxin can produce virtually any arrhythmia. For example, digitalis is useful in treating SVT, but digitalis toxicity can trigger SVT.

(6) Digoxin may be contraindicated in patients with accessory pathway SVT. Please refer to Digoxin use for SVT in Section VIII.E.

f. Indications for use

(1) Supraventricular tachyarrhythmias (see Section VIII.E)

(2) CHF (mostly of historical interest for this condition)

g. Administration. IV, PO, IM

h. Clinical use (general guidelines only)

(1) Digoxin dose (assuming normal renal function; decrease maintenance dosages with renal insufficiency)

(a) Adult: Loading dose IV and IM, 0.25 to 0.50 mg increments (total 1 to 1.25 mg or 10 to 15 μg/kg); maintenance dose, 0.125 to 0.250 mg/day based on clinical effect and drug levels

(b) Pediatric digoxin (IV administration)

Age	Total digitalizing dose (DD) (μg/kg)	Daily maintenance dose (divided doses, normal renal function)
Neonates	15–30	20%–35% of DD
2 mos–2 yrs	30–50	25%–35% of DD
2–10 yrs	15–35	25%–35% of DD
>10 yrs	8–12	25%–35% of DD

(2) Digoxin has a gradual onset of action over 15 to 30 min or more; peak effect occurs 1 to 5 h after IV administration.

(3) Use with caution in the presence of β-blockers, calcium channel blockers, or calcium.

(4) Always consider the possibility of toxic side effects.

(a) Signs of toxicity include arrhythmias, especially with features of both increased automaticity and conduction block (e.g., junctional tachycardia with a 2:1 AV block). Premature atrial or ventricular depolarizations, AV block, accelerated junctional tachycardia, VT or VF (may be unresponsive to countershock), or gastrointestinal or neurologic toxicity may also be apparent.

(5) Factors potentiating toxicity

(a) Hypokalemia, hypomagnesemia, hypercalcemia, alkalosis, acidosis, renal insufficiency, quinidine therapy, and hypothyroidism may potentiate toxicity.

(b) Beware of administering calcium salts to digitalized patients! Malignant ventricular arrhythmias (including VF) may occur, even if the patient has received no digoxin for more than 24 h. Follow ionized calcium levels to permit use of smallest possible doses of calcium.

(6) Therapy for digitalis toxicity

(a) Increase serum [K^+] to upper limits of normal (unless AV block is present).

(b) Treat ventricular arrhythmias with phenytoin, lidocaine, or amiodarone.

(c) Treat atrial arrhythmias with phenytoin or amiodarone.

(d) β-Blockers are effective for digoxin-induced arrhythmias, but ventricular pacing may be required if AV block develops.

(e) Beware of cardioversion. VF refractory to countershock may be induced. Use low-energy synchronized cardioversion and slowly increase energy as needed.

(7) Serum digoxin levels

(a) Therapeutic: Approximately 0.5 to 2.5 ng/mL. Values of less than 0.5 ng/mL rule out toxicity. Values exceeding 3 ng/mL are definitely toxic.

(b) Increased serum concentrations may not produce clinical toxicity in children or hyperkalemic patients, or when digitalis is used as an atrial antiarrhythmic agent.

(c) "Therapeutic" serum concentrations may produce clinical toxicity in patients with hypokalemia, hypomagnesemia, hypercalcemia, myocardial ischemia, hypothyroidism, or those recovering from CPB.

(8) Because of its long duration of action, long latency of onset, and increased risk of toxicity, digoxin is not used to treat acute heart failure.

(9) For all indications, digoxin is much less widely used in recent years.

3. **Triiodothyronine (T_3, liothyronine IV)** [16]. T_3 is the active form of thyroid hormone. It has multiple cellular actions on the nucleus and on mitochondria, affecting gene transcription and oxidative phosphorylation. There is evidence that CPB induces a state of low plasma thyrotropin (T_3), termed the "euthyroid sick" syndrome. Laboratory studies demonstrate that T_3 stimulates cardiac inotropy and lusitropy even in the face of overwhelming β-adrenergic receptor blockade and without increasing intracellular concentrations of cAMP. Despite reports that liothyronine would facilitate the separation from CPB of patients who could not be weaned using conventional therapies, larger clinical trials failed to identify efficacy of T_3. Doses that have been suggested include a bolus of 0.4 μg/kg IV followed by 0.4 μg/kg infused over 6 h. T_3 is advocated over thyroxine because of the very slow onset time of the latter hormone and the reduced ability of critically ill patients to convert T_4 to T_3. In treatment of myxedema coma, corticosteroids should be given with liothyronine.

4. **Levosimendan** [19]

a. Actions

(1) Binds in Ca-dependent manner to cardiac troponin C, shifting the Ca^{2+} tension curve to the left. Levosimendan may stabilize Ca^{2+}-induced confirmational changes in troponin C.

(2) Its effects are maximized during early systole when intracellular Ca^{2+} concentration is greatest and least during diastolic relaxation when Ca^{2+} concentration is low.

(3) Levosimendan also inhibits PDE III activity.

(4) Hemodynamic actions

Levosimendan	
HR	Increased
CO	Increased
SVR	Decreased
MAP	Unchanged
PCWP	Unchanged
$M\dot{V}O_2$	Unchanged

b. **Advantages**
(1) Does not increase intracellular Ca^{2+}
(2) Does not work via cAMP so should not interact with β agonists or PDE inhibitors

c. **Disadvantages**
(1) Unknown potency relative to other agents
(2) Has not received regulatory approval in major North American or Western European countries

d. **Indications**
Where approved, drug's indications include acute heart failure and acute exacerbations of CHF.

e. **Administration**
(1) IV

f. **Clinical use**
(1) 8 to 24 μg/kg/min
(2) Despite its biochemical actions on PDE, levosimendan is not associated with increased cAMP, so it may have reduced tendency for arrhythmias relative to sympathomimetics.

VII. β-Adrenergic receptor–blocking drugs [3,5]

A. **Actions.** These drugs bind and antagonize β-adrenergic receptors typically producing the following cardiovascular effects:

Levosimendam	
HR	Decreased
Contractility	Decreased
BP	Decreased
SVR	Increased (unless drug has intrinsic sympathetic activity [ISA])
AV conduction	Decreased
Atrial refractory period	Increased
Automaticity	Decreased

B. **Advantages of β-adrenergic-blocking drugs**
1. Reduce $M\dot{V}O_2$ and decrease HR and contractility
2. Increase the duration of diastole, during which majority of blood flow and oxygen are delivered to the left ventricle.
3. Synergistic with nitroglycerin for treating myocardial ischemia; blunt reflex tachycardia and increased contractility secondary to nitroglycerin, nitroprusside, or other vasodilator drugs
4. Have an antiarrhythmic action, especially against atrial arrhythmias
5. Decrease LV ejection velocity (useful in patients with aortic dissection)
6. Antihypertensive, but should not be first-line agents for essential hypertension
7. Reduce dynamic ventricular outflow tract obstruction (e.g., tetralogy of Fallot, hypertrophic cardiomyopathy)
8. Use of these agents is associated with reduced mortality after myocardial infarction, chronic angina, CHF, and hypertension.

C. **Disadvantages**
1. Severe bradyarrhythmias are possible.

2. Heart block (first, second, or third degree) may occur, especially if prior cardiac conduction abnormalities are present, or when IV β-blockers and certain IV calcium channel blockers are coadministered.
3. May trigger bronchospasm in patients with reactive airways
4. CHF can occur in patients with low ejection fraction newly receiving large doses. Elevated LVEDP may induce myocardial ischemia because of elevated systolic wall tension.
5. Signs and symptoms of hypoglycemia (except sweating) are masked in diabetics.
6. SVR may increase because of inhibition of β_2 vasodilation; use with care in patients with severe peripheral vascular disease or in patients with pheochromocytoma without α-blockade treatment.
7. Risk of coronary artery spasm is present in rare susceptible patients.
8. Acute perioperative withdrawal of β-blockers can lead to hyperdynamic circulation and myocardial ischemia.

D. **Distinguishing features of β-blockers** (Table 2.3)

1. **Selectivity.** Selective β-blockers possess a greater potency for β_1- than for β_2-receptors. They are less likely to cause bronchospasm or to increase SVR than a nonselective drug. However, β_1 selectivity is dose-dependent (drugs lose selectivity at higher dosages). Caution must be exercised when an asthmatic patient receives any β-blocker.
2. **Intrinsic sympathomimetic activity (ISA).** These drugs possess "partial agonist" activity. Thus, drugs with ISA will block β-receptors (preventing catecholamines from binding to a receptor) but also will cause mild stimulation of the same receptors. A patient receiving a drug with ISA would be expected to have a greater resting HR and CO (which shows no change with exercise) but a lower SVR compared to a drug without ISA.
3. **Duration of action.** In general, the β-blockers with longer durations of action are eliminated by the kidneys, whereas the drugs of 4 to 6 h duration undergo hepatic elimination. Esmolol, the ultrashort–acting β-blocker (plasma half-life, 9 min), is eliminated within the blood by a red blood cell esterase. After abrupt discontinuation of esmolol infusion (which under most circumstances we **do not recommend**), most drug effects are eliminated within 5 min. The duration of esmolol does not change when plasma pseudocholinesterase is inhibited by echothiophate or physostigmine.

E. **Clinical use**

1. **β-Blocker dosage**
   a. See Table 2.3.
   b. Begin with a low dose and slowly increase until desired effect is produced.
   c. For metoprolol IV dosage use 1 to 5 mg increments (for adults) as tolerated while monitoring the ECG, BP, and lung sounds. Intravenous dosage is much smaller than oral dosage because first-pass hepatic extraction is bypassed. The usual acute IV metoprolol dose is 0.02 to 0.1 mg/kg.
2. If β-blockers must be given to a patient with bronchospastic disease, choose a selective β_1 blocker such as metoprolol or esmolol and consider concomitant administration of an inhalation β_2 agonist (such as albuterol).
3. **Treatment of toxicity.** β-agonists (e.g., isoproterenol, possibly in large doses) and cardiac pacing are the mainstays. Calcium, milrinone, inamrinone, glucagon, or liothyronine may be effective because these agents do not act via β-receptors.
4. **Assessment of β-blockade.** When β-blockade is adequate, a patient should not demonstrate an increase in HR with exercise.
5. **Use of α agonists in β-blocked patients.** When agonist drugs with α or both α and β actions are administered to patients who are β-blocked, e.g., with an epinephrine-containing IV local anesthetic test dose, a greater elevation of BP can be expected owing to α vasoconstriction unopposed by β_2 vasodilation. This may produce deleterious hemodynamic results (increased afterload with little increased CO).
6. Esmolol is given by IV injection (loading dose), often followed by continuous infusion. (For details on esmolol dosing for SVT, see Section VIII.E.) It is of greatest utility when the required duration of β-blockade is short (i.e., to attenuate a short-lived stimulus). Esmolol's

TABLE 2.3 β-Adrenergic–blocking drugs

	Acebutolol (Sectral)	**Atenolol (Tenormin)**	**Carvedilol (Coreg)**	**Esmolol (Brevibloc)**	**Labetalol (Trandate)**
β Half-life[a] (h)	3–4	6–9	7–10	9 min	3–8
Elimination	H (60%–70%)	R (85%)	H (98%)	Blood	H
Active metabolites	Yes	No	Yes	No	No
β_1 Selectivity	Yes	Yes	No	Yes	No
ISA	Yes	No	No	No	No
α Antagonist	No	No	Yes	No	Yes
IV use	No	No	No	Yes	Yes
Initial PO dose[b] (mg)	200/day	25/day	6.25 bid	—	100 bid
Maximum PO dose[b] (mg)	600 bid[c]	50 mg bid[c]	25 mg bid	—	600 mg bid
Maximum usual IV[d] dose		—		0.25–0.5 mg/kg load, then 50–200 μg/kg/min	20 mg load, then 40–80 q10min to max 300

	Metoprolol (Lopressor)	**Nadolol (Corgard)**	**Nebivolol (Bystolic)**	**Pindolol (Visken)**	**Propranolol (Inderal)**	**Sotalol[e] (Betapace)**	**Timolol[f] (Blocadren)**
β Half-life[a] (h)	3–4	14–24	12–19 hrs	3–4	3.5–6	7–15	3–4
Elimination	H	R (75%)		H (60%) R (40%)	H	R	H (80%) R (20%)
Active metabolites	No	No	Yes	No	Yes	No	No
β_1 Selectivity	Yes	No	Yes (at lower doses)	No	No	No	No
ISA	No	No	No	Yes	No	No	No
α Antagonist	No	No	No (but vasodilates via NO	No	No	No	No
IV use	Yes	No	No	No	Yes	No	No
Initial PO dose[b] (mg)	50/day	20/day	5 mg once daily	5 bid	20 bid	80 bid[c]	5 bid
Maximum PO dose[b] (mg)	100 bid[c]	320/day[c]	40 mg once daily	30 bid[c]	40 bid	320/day	30 bid[c]
Maximum usual IV[d] dose	15 in 5 mg increments	—	—	—	4–8 in 120 mg bid 0.5–1-mg increments	—	

[a]Half-life may not be predictive of clinical duration of action.
[b]Usual dosages for adults.
[c]Decrease dosage in renal failure.
[d]IV doses must be given in small, divided doses with careful monitoring. Adult dosages are given.
[e]Sotalol also has class III antidysrhythmic activity.
[f]Timolol eye drops can produce systemic β blockade.
[g]In percentage after oral dose.
ISA, Intrinsic sympathomimetic activity; IV, intravenous; H, Hepatic elimination; R, renal elimination.

ultrashort duration of action plus its β_1 selectivity and lack of ISA make it a logical choice when it is necessary to initiate a β-blocker in patients with asthma or another relative contraindication. It is also useful in critically ill patients with changing hemodynamic status.

7. Labetalol is a combined α and β antagonist (α/β ratio = 1:7), which produces vasodilation without reflex tachycardia. Labetalol is useful for preoperative or postoperative control of hypertension. During anesthesia, its relatively long duration of action makes it less useful than other agents for minute-to-minute control of HR and BP. However, treatment with labetalol or another β-adrenergic receptor antagonist will reduce the needed dosage of short-acting vasodilators.
8. β-Adrenergic receptor antagonist withdrawal. Abrupt withdrawal of chronic β-blocker therapy may produce a withdrawal syndrome including tachycardia and hypertension. Myocardial ischemia or infarction may result. Thus, chronic β-blocker therapy should not be abruptly discontinued perioperatively. The authors have seen this syndrome complete with myocardial ischemia after abrupt discontinuation of esmolol when it had been infused for only 48 h!
9. Certain β-adrenergic receptor blockers are now part of the standard therapy of patients with Class B through Class D CHF. The drugs most often used are carvedilol and metoprolol-XL, and these agents have been shown to prolong survival in heart failure. β-adrenergic receptor blocker therapy is associated with improved LV function and improved exercise tolerance over time. These agents counteract the sympathetic nervous system activation that is present with CHF. In animal studies, β-adrenergic receptor blocker therapy reduces “remodeling,” which is the process by which functional myocardium is replaced by connective tissue. Importantly, not all β-adrenergic receptor blockers have been shown to improve outcome in CHF, so reduced mortality should not be considered a “class effect” of β-adrenergic receptor blockers.

F. Specific agents

1. See Table 2.3.

VIII. Vasodilator drugs [16]

A. Comparison

1. Sites of action

Arterial (decreased SVR)	Both arterial and venous
Calcium channel blockers	Angiotensin-converting enzyme (ACE) inhibitors
Hydralazine	Angiotensin receptor blockers (ARBs)
Phentolamine	Nitroglycerin Nitroprusside Prazosin Alprostadil Trimethaphan Nesiritide

2. **Mechanisms of action**
   - a. Direct vasodilators: Calcium channel blockers, hydralazine, minoxidil, nitroglycerin, nitroprusside.
   - b. α-adrenergic blockers: Labetalol, phentolamine, prazosin, terazosin, tolazoline.
   - c. Ganglionic blocker: Trimethaphan.
   - d. ACE inhibitor: Enalaprilat, captopril, enalapril, lisinopril.
   - e. ARBs: Candesartan, irbesartan, losartan, olmesartan, valsartan, telmisartan.
   - f. Central α_2 agonists (reduce sympathetic tone): Clonidine, guanabenz, guanfacine.
   - g. Calcium channel blockers (see Section VII)
   - h. Nesiritide: Binds to natriuretic factor receptors.
3. **Indications for use**
   - a. **Hypertension, increased SVR states.** Use arterial or mixed drugs. First-line agent for long-term treatment of essential hypertension should be thiazide diuretic with ACE inhibitors, ARBs, calcium channel blockers, β-blockers, as secondary choices. Other oral agents are not associated with outcome benefit.

b. **Controlled hypotension.** Short-acting drugs are most useful (e.g., nitroprusside, nitroglycerine, nicardipine, clevidipine, nesiritide, and volatile inhalational anesthetics).
c. **Aortic valvular regurgitation.** Reducing SVR will tend to improve oxygen delivery to tissues.
d. **CHF.** Vasodilation reduces $M\dot{V}O_2$ by lowering preload and afterload (systolic wall stress, due to reduced LV size and pressure). Vasodilation also improves ejection and compliance. More importantly, ACE inhibitors and ARBs inhibit "remodeling" and increase longevity in patients with heart failure.
e. **Thermoregulation.** Vasodilators are often used during the cooling and rewarming phases of CPB to facilitate tissue perfusion and accelerate temperature equilibration. This is especially important during pediatric CPB procedures and others involving total circulatory arrest where an increased CBF promotes brain cooling and brain protection during circulatory arrest.
f. **Pulmonary hypertension.** Vasodilators can improve pulmonary hypertension that is not anatomically fixed. Presently, inhaled NO is the only truly selective pulmonary vasodilator.
g. **Myocardial ischemia.** Vasodilator therapy can improve myocardial O_2 balance by reducing $M\dot{V}O_2$ (decreased preload and afterload), and nitrates and calcium channel blockers can dilate conducting coronary arteries to improve the distribution of myocardial blood flow. ACE inhibitors prolong lifespan in patients who have had a myocardial infarction.
h. **Intracardiac shunts.** Vasodilators are used in the setting of nonrestrictive cardiac shunts, especially ventricular septal defects and aortopulmonary connections, to manipulate the ratio of pulmonary artery to aortic pressures. This allows control of the direction and magnitude of shunt flow.

4. **Cautions**
a. **Hyperdynamic reflexes.** All vasodilator drugs decrease SVR and BP and may activate baroreceptor reflexes. This cardiac sympathetic stimulation produces tachycardia and increased contractility. Myocardial ischemia resulting from increased myocardial O_2 demands can be additive to ischemia produced by reduced BP. Addition of a β-blocker can attenuate these reflexes.
b. **Ventricular ejection rate.** Reflex sympathetic stimulation will also increase the rate of ventricular ejection of blood (dP/dt) and raise the systolic aortic wall stress. This may be detrimental with aortic dissection. Thus, addition of β-blocker (or a ganglionic blocker) is of theoretical benefit for patients with aortic dissection, aortic aneurysm, or recent aortic surgery.
c. Stimulation of the renin–angiotensin system is implicated in the "rebound" increased SVR and PVR when some vasodilators are discontinued abruptly. Renin release can be attenuated by concomitant β-blockade, and renin's actions are attenuated by ACE inhibitors and ARBs.
d. **Intracranial pressure (ICP).** Most vasodilators will increase ICP, except for trimethaphan and fenoldopam.
e. Use of nesiritide for decompensated CHF was associated with increased mortality.

B. **Specific agents**
1. **Direct vasodilators**
a. **Hydralazine (Apresoline)**
(1) **Actions**
(a) This drug is a direct vasodilator.
(b) It primarily produces an arteriolar dilatation, with little venous (preload) effect.

Hydralazine	
HR	Increased (reflex)
Contractility	Increased (reflex)
CO	May increase (reflex)
BP	Decreased
SVR and PVR	Decreased
Preload	Little change

(2) **Offset** occurs by acetylation in the liver. Patients who are slow acetylators (up to 50% of the population) may have higher plasma hydralazine levels and may show a longer effect, especially with oral use.

(3) **Advantages**

(a) Selective vasodilation. Hydralazine produces more dilation of coronary, cerebral, renal, and splanchnic beds than of vessels in the muscle and skin.

(b) Maintenance of uterine blood flow (if hypotension is avoided).

(4) **Disadvantages**

(a) Slow onset (5 to 15 min) after IV dosing; peak effect should occur by 20 min. Thus, at least 10 to 15 min should separate doses.

(b) Reflex tachycardia or coronary steal can precipitate myocardial ischemia.

(c) A lupus-like reaction, usually seen only with chronic PO use, may occur with chronic high doses (more than 400 mg/day) and in slow acetylators.

(5) **Clinical use**

(a) Hydralazine dose

(i) IV: 2.5 to 5 mg bolus every 15 min (maximum 20 to 40 mg)

(ii) IM: 20 to 40 mg every 4 to 6 h

(iii) PO: 10 to 50 mg every 6 h

(iv) Pediatric dose: 0.2 to 0.5 mg/kg IV every 4 to 6 h, slowly

(b) Slow onset limits use in acute hypertensive crises.

(c) Doses of vasodilators can be reduced by the addition of hydralazine, decreasing the risk of cyanide toxicity from nitroprusside or prolonged ganglionic blockade from trimethaphan.

(d) Addition of a β-blocker attenuates reflex tachycardia.

(e) Patients with CAD should be monitored for myocardial ischemia.

(f) Enalaprilat, nicardipine, and labetalol are replacing hydralazine for many perioperative applications.

b. Nitroglycerin (glyceryl trinitrate) [16]

(1) **Actions**

(a) Nitroglycerin is a direct vasodilator, producing greater venous than arterial dilation. A nitric acid-containing metabolite activates vascular cGMP production.

	Nitroglycerin
HR	Increased (reflex)
Contractility	Increased (reflex)
CO	Variable; often decreased, due to decreased preload (CO may increase when NTG treats ischemia)
BP	Decreased (high dosages)
Preload	Marked decrease
SVR	Decreased (high dosages)
PVR	Decreased

5

(b) Peripheral venous effects. Venodilation and peripheral pooling reduce effective blood volume, decreasing heart size and preload. This effect usually reduces $M\dot{V}O_2$ and increases diastolic coronary blood flow.

(c) Coronary artery

(i) Relieves coronary spasm.

(ii) Flow redistribution provides more flow to ischemic myocardium and increases endocardial-to-epicardial flow ratio.

(iii) There is increased flow to ischemic regions through collateral vessels.

(d) Myocardial effects

(i) Improved inotropy due to reduced ischemia

(ii) Indirect antiarrhythmic action (VF threshold increases in ischemic myocardium because the drug makes the effective refractory period more uniform throughout the heart)

- **(e)** Arteriolar effects (higher dosages only)
  - **(i)** Arteriolar dilatation decreases SVR. With reduced systolic myocardial wall stress, $M\dot{V}O_2$ decreases, and ejection fraction and SV may improve.
  - **(ii)** Arteriolar dilation often requires large doses, exceeding 10 μg/kg/min in some patients, whereas much lower doses give effective venous and coronary arterial dilating effects. When reliable peripheral arteriolar dilation is needed to control a hypertensive emergency, nicardipine, nitroprusside, or clevidipine are often better choices (and can be used together with nitroglycerin).

(2) **Offset** occurs by redistribution, metabolism in smooth muscle and liver. Half-life in humans is 1 to 3 min.

(3) **Advantages**
- **(a)** Preload reduction (lowers LV and RV end-diastolic and LA and RA pressures)
- **(b)** Unlike nitroprusside, virtually no metabolic toxicity
- **(c)** Effective for myocardial ischemia
  - **(i)** Decreases infarct size after coronary occlusion
  - **(ii)** Maintains arteriolar autoregulation, so coronary steal unlikely
- **(d)** Useful in acute exacerbations of CHF to decrease preload and reduce pulmonary vascular congestion
- **(e)** Increases vascular capacity; may permit infusion of residual pump blood after CPB is terminated
- **(f)** Not as photosensitive as nitroprusside
- **(g)** Dilates the pulmonary vascular bed and can be useful in treating acute pulmonary hypertension and right heart failure
- **(h)** Attenuates biliary colic and esophageal spasm

(4) **Disadvantages**
- **(a)** It decreases BP as preload and SVR decrease at higher dosages. This may result in decreased coronary perfusion pressure.
- **(b)** Reflex tachycardia and reflex increase in myocardial contractility are dose-related. Consider reducing dose or administering a β-blocker (if BP is satisfactory).
- **(c)** It inhibits hypoxic pulmonary vasoconstriction (but to a lesser extent than nitroprusside). Monitor PO_2 or supplement inspired gas with oxygen.
- **(d)** It may increase ICP.
- **(e)** It is adsorbed by polyvinyl chloride IV tubing. Titrate dosage to effect; increased effect may occur when tubing becomes saturated. Special infusion sets that do not adsorb drug are expensive and unnecessary.
- **(f)** Tolerance. Chronic continuous therapy (for longer than 24 h) can blunt hemodynamic and antianginal effects. Tolerance during chronic therapy may be avoided by discontinuing the drug (if appropriate) for several hours daily.
- **(g)** Dependence. Coronary spasm and myocardial infarction have been reported after abrupt cessation of chronic industrial exposure.
- **(h)** Methemoglobinemia. Avoid administering doses greater than 7 to 10 μg/kg/min for prolonged periods.

(5) **Clinical use**
- **(a)** Nitroglycerin dose
  - **(i)** IV bolus: A bolus dose of 50 to 100 μg may be superior to infusion for acute ischemia. Rapidly changing levels in blood may cause more vasodilation than a constant infusion (and thus may be more likely to produce hypotension).
  - **(ii)** Infusion: Dose range, 0.1 to 7 μg/kg/min.
  - **(iii)** Sublingual: 0.15 to 0.60 mg.
  - **(iv)** Topical: 2% ointment (Nitropaste), 0.5 to 2 in. every 4 to 8 h; or controlled-release transdermal preparation (Transderm-Nitro, Nitrodisc), 5 to 10 mg (or more) every 24 h or as needed.

(b) Unless non-polyvinyl chloride tubing is used, infusion requirements may decrease after the initial 30 to 60 min.
(c) Nitroglycerin is better stored in bottles than in bags if storage for more than 6 to 12 h is anticipated.
(d) When administered during CPB, venous pooling may cause decreases in pump reservoir volume.

c. Nitroprusside (Nipride) [16,20]

(1) Actions

(a) Nitroprusside (SNP) is a direct-acting vasodilator. The nitrate group is converted into NO in vascular smooth muscle, which causes increased cGMP levels in cells.
(b) It has balanced arteriolar and venous dilating effects.

	Nitroprusside
HR	Increased (reflex)
Contractility	Increased (reflex)
CO	Variable
BP	Decreased (dose-dependent)
SVR	Decreased (dose-dependent)
PVR	Decreased (dose-dependent)

(2) Advantages

(a) SNP has a very short duration of action (1 to 2 min) permitting precise titration of dose.
(b) It has pulmonary vasodilator in addition to systemic vasodilator effects.
(c) SNP is highly effective for virtually all causes of hypertension except high CO states.
(d) A greater decrease in SVR (afterload) than preload is produced at low dosages.

(3) Disadvantages

(a) Cyanide and thiocyanate toxicity may occur.
(b) SNP solution is unstable in light and so must be protected from light. Photodecomposition inactivates nitroprusside over many hours but does not release cyanide ion.
(c) Reflex tachycardia and increased inotropy (undesirable with aortic dissection because of increased shearing forces) respond to β-blockade.
(d) Hypoxic pulmonary vasoconstriction is blunted and may produce arterial hypoxemia from increased venous admixture.
(e) Vascular steal. All vascular regions are dilated equally. Although total organ blood flow may increase, flow may be diverted from ischemic regions (previously maximally vasodilated) to nonischemic areas that, prior to SNP exposure, were appropriately vasoconstricted. Thus, myocardial ischemia may be worsened. However, severe hypertension is clearly dangerous in ischemia, and the net effect often is beneficial. ECG monitoring is important.
(f) Patients with chronic hypertension may experience myocardial, cerebral, or renal ischemia with abrupt lowering of BP to "normal" range.
(g) Rebound systemic or pulmonary hypertension may occur if SNP is stopped abruptly (especially in patients with CHF). SNP should be tapered.
(h) Mild preload reduction due to venodilation occurs; fluids often must be infused if CO falls.
(i) Risk of increased ICP (although ICP often decreases with control of hypertension)
(j) Platelet function is inhibited (no known clinical consequences).

(4) Toxicity

(a) Chemical formula of SNP is $Fe(CN)_5NO$. SNP reacts with hemoglobin to release highly toxic free cyanide ion (CN^-).
(b) SNP + oxyhemoglobin → four free cyanide ions + cyanomethemoglobin (nontoxic).

(c) Cyanide ion produces inhibition of cytochrome oxidase, preventing mitochondrial oxidative phosphorylation. This produces tissue hypoxia despite adequate PO_2.

(d) Cyanide detoxification

(i) Cyanide + thiosulfate (and rhodanase) → thiocyanate. Thiocyanate is much less toxic than cyanide ion. Availability of thiosulfate is the rate-limiting step in cyanide metabolism. Adults can typically detoxify 50 mg of SNP using existing thiosulfate stores. Thiosulfate administration is of critical importance in treating cyanide toxicity. Rhodanase is an enzyme found in liver and kidney that promotes cyanide detoxification.

(ii) Cyanide + hydroxocobalamin → cyanocobalamin (vitamin B_{12}).

(e) Patients at increased risk of toxicity:

(i) Those resistant to vasodilating effects at low SNP dosages (requiring dose greater than 3 μg/kg/min is necessary for effect)

(ii) Those receiving a high-dose SNP infusion (greater than 8 μg/kg/min) for any period of time. In this setting, frequent blood gas measurements must be performed, and consideration must be given to the following:

(a) First and foremost, decrease dosage by adding another vasodilator or a β-blocker.

(b) Consider monitoring mixed venous oxygenation (see Section f.2).

(iii) Those receiving a large total dose (greater than 1 mg/kg) over 12 to 24 h

(iv) Those with either severe renal or hepatic dysfunction

(f) Signs of SNP toxicity

(i) Tachyphylaxis occurs in response to vasodilating effects of SNP.

(ii) Elevated mixed venous PO_2 (due to decreased cellular O_2 utilization) occurs in the absence of a rise in CO.

(iii) There is metabolic acidosis.

(iv) No cyanosis is seen with cyanide toxicity (cells cannot utilize O_2; therefore, blood O_2 saturation remains high).

(v) Chronic SNP toxicity is due to elevated thiocyanate levels and is a consequence of long-term therapy or thiocyanate accumulation in renal failure. Thiocyanate is excreted unchanged by the kidney (elimination half-life, 1 wk). Elevated thiocyanate levels (greater than 5 mg/dL) can cause fatigue, nausea, anorexia, miosis, psychosis, hyperreflexia, and seizures.

(g) Therapy of cyanide toxicity

(i) Cyanide toxicity should be suspected when a metabolic acidosis or unexplained rise in mixed venous PO_2 appears in any patient receiving SNP.

(ii) As soon as toxicity is suspected, SNP must be discontinued and substituted with another agent; lowering the dosage is not sufficient because clinically evident toxicity implies a marked reduction in cytochrome oxidase activity.

(iii) Ventilate with 100% O_2.

(iv) Treat severe metabolic acidosis with bicarbonate.

(v) Mild toxicity (base deficit less than 10, stable hemodynamics when SNP stopped) can be treated by sodium thiosulfate, 150 mg/kg IV bolus (hemodynamically benign).

(vi) Severe toxicity (base deficit greater than 10, or worsening hemodynamics despite discontinuation of nitroprusside:

(a) Create methemoglobin that can combine with cyanide to produce nontoxic cyanomethemoglobin, removing cyanide from cytochrome oxidase:

(1) Give 3% sodium nitrite, 4 to 6 mg/kg by slow IV infusion. (repeat one-half dose 2 to 48 h later as needed), *or*

(2) Give amyl nitrite: Break 1 ampule into breathing bag. (Flammable!)

(b) Sodium thiosulfate, 150 to 200 mg/kg IV over 15 min, should also be administered to facilitate metabolic disposal of the cyanide. Note that thiocyanate clearance is renal dependent.

(c) Consider hydroxocobalamin (vitamin B_{12}) 25 mg/h.

Note: These treatments should be administered even during CPR; otherwise, O_2 cannot be utilized by body tissues.

(5) Clinical use

(a) SNP dose: 0.1 to 2 μg/kg/min IV infusion. Titrate dose to BP and CO. Avoid doses greater than 2 μg/kg/min: Doses as high as 10 μg/kg/min should be infused for no more than 10 min.

(b) Monitor oxygenation.

(c) Solution in a bottle or bag must be protected from light by wrapping in metal foil. Solution stored in the dark retains significant potency for 12 to 24 h. It is not necessary to cover the administration tubing with foil.

(d) Because of the potency of SNP, it is best administered by itself into a central line using an infusion pump. If other drugs are being infused through the same line, use sufficient "carrier" flow so that changes in one drug's infusion rate does not change the quantity of other drugs entering the patient per minute.

(e) Infusions should be tapered gradually to avoid rebound increases in systemic and PA pressures.

(f) Use this drug cautiously in patients with concomitant untreated hypothyroidism or severe liver or kidney dysfunction.

(g) Continuous BP monitoring with an arterial catheter is recommended.

d. NO

(1) Actions

(a) NO is a vasoactive gas naturally produced from L-arginine primarily in endothelial cells. Before its molecular identity was determined it was known as *endothelium-derived relaxing factor.* NO diffuses from endothelial cells to vascular smooth muscle, where it increases cGMP and affects vasodilation, in part by decreasing cytosolic calcium. It is an important physiologic intercellular signaling substance and NO or its absence is implicated in pathologic conditions such as reperfusion injury and coronary vasospasm.

(b) It is inhaled to treat pulmonary hypertension, particularly in respiratory distress syndrome in infancy.

	NO
PVR	Decreased
SVR	No change
RVSWI*	Decreased

*RVSWI, right ventricular stroke work index.

(2) Offset. NO rapidly and avidly binds to the heme moiety of hemoglobin, forming the inactive compound nitrosylhemoglobin, which in turn degrades to methemoglobin. NO's biologic half-life in blood is approximately 6 s.

(3) Advantages

(a) Inhaled NO appears to be the long-sought "selective" pulmonary vasodilator. It is devoid of systemic actions.

(b) Unlike parenterally administered pulmonary vasodilators, inhaled NO favorably affects lung *V*/*Q* relationships, because it vasodilates primarily those lung regions that are well ventilated.

(c) There is low toxicity, provided safety precautions are taken.

(4) **Disadvantages**

(a) Stringent safety precautions are required to prevent potentially severe toxicity, such as overdose or catastrophic nitrogen dioxide-induced pulmonary edema.

(b) Methemoglobin concentrations may reach clinically important values, and blood levels must be monitored daily.

(c) Chronic administration may cause ciliary depletion and epithelial hyperplasia in terminal bronchioles.

(d) NO is corrosive to metal.

(5) **Clinical use**

(a) NO is inhaled by blending dilute NO gas into the ventilator inlet gas. Therapeutic concentrations range from 0.05 to 80 parts per million (ppm). The lowest effective concentration should be used, and responses should be carefully monitored. The onset of action for reducing PVR and RVSWI is typically 1 to 2 min.

(b) NO must be purchased prediluted in nitrogen in assayed tanks, and an analyzer must be used intermittently to assay the gas stream entering the patient for NO and nitrogen dioxide. NO usually is not injected between the ventilator and the patient (to avoid overdose), and it must never be allowed to contact air or oxygen until it is used (to prevent formation of toxic nitrogen dioxide).

(c) NO has been used to treat persistent pulmonary hypertension of the newborn, other forms of pulmonary hypertension, and the adult respiratory distress syndrome with variable success and to date no effect on outcomes.

e. **Nesiritide [21]**

(1) **Actions**

(a) Nesiritide binds to A and B natriuretic peptide receptors on endothelium and vascular smooth muscle, producing dilation of both arterial and venous systems from increased production of cGMP. It also has indirect vasodilating actions by suppressing the sympathetic nervous system, the renin–angiontensin–aldosterone system, and endothelin.

	Nesiritide
HR	No direct effect
Contractility	No direct effect (reflex increase)
CO	No direct effect (reflex increase)
BP	Decreased
Preload	Decreased
Afterload	Decreased
SVR	Decreased
PVR	Decreased

(b) Diuretic and natriuretic effects. Although nesiritide as a "cardiac natriuretic peptide" would be expected to have major diuretic and natriuretic effects, the agent seems most effective at this in healthy patients.

(c) Nisertide may be hydrolyzed by neutral endopeptidase. A small amount of administered drug may be eliminated via the kidneys.

(2) **Current clinical use.** Initial studies suggested that use of nesiritide was associated with reduced mortality in HF patients compared to the use of standard positive inotropic agents. The most recent data from a large clinical trial demonstrated that nesiritide offered no advantage over standard agents for acute decompensated HF.

(a) Typical doses are as follows:

(i) 2 μg/kg loading dose

(ii) 0.01 μg/kg/min maintenance infusion

2. ***α*-Adrenergic blockers** [3,5]

a. **Labetalol (Normodyne, Trandate)**

See preceding *β*-adrenergic receptor blocker section in which this agent was presented.

b. Phentolamine (Regitine)

(1) Actions

(a) Competitive antagonist at α_1, α_2, and 5-hydroxytryptamine (5-HT, serotonin) receptors

(b) Primarily arterial vasodilation with little venodilation

Phentolamine	
HR	Increased (reflex)
Contractility	Increased (reflex)
BP	Decreased
SVR	Decreased
PVR	Decreased
Preload	Little change

(2) Offset occurs by hepatic metabolism, in part by renal excretion. Offset after IV bolus occurs after 10 to 30 min.

(3) Advantages

(a) Good for high NE states such as pheochromocytoma.

(b) Antagonizes undesirable α stimulation. For example, reversal of deleterious effects of NE extravasated into skin is achieved by local infiltration with phentolamine, 5 to 10 mg in 10 mL saline.

(c) Has been combined with NE for positive inotropic support with reduced vasoconstriction after CPB.

(4) Disadvantages

(a) Tachycardia arises from two mechanisms:

(i) Reflex via baroreceptors

(ii) Direct effect of α_2 blockade. Blockade of presynaptic receptors eliminates the normal feedback system controlling NE release by presynaptic nerve terminals. As α_2 stimulation decreases NE release, blockade of these receptors allows increased presynaptic release. This results in increased β_1 sympathetic effects only, as the α-receptors mediating postsynaptic α effects are blocked by phentolamine. Myocardial ischemia or arrhythmias may result. Thus, the tachycardia and positive inotropy are β effects that will respond to β-blockers.

(b) Gastrointestinal motility is stimulated and gastric acid secretion increased.

(c) Hypoglycemia may occur.

(d) Epinephrine may cause hypotension in α-blocked patients ("epinephrine reversal") via a β_2 mechanism.

(e) Arrhythmias occur.

(f) There is histamine release.

(5) Clinical use

(a) Phentolamine dose

(i) IV bolus: 1 to 5 mg (adult) or 0.1 mg/kg IV (pediatric)

(ii) IV infusion: 1 to 20 μg/kg/min

(b) When administered for pheochromocytoma, β blockade may also be instituted.

(c) β-Blockade will attenuate tachycardia.

(d) Phentolamine has been used to promote uniform cooling of infants during CPB prior to DHCA (dose, 0.1 to 0.5 mg/kg).

c. Phenoxybenzamine (Dibenzyline)

(1) Actions

(a) Noncompetitive antagonist at α_1 and α_2-receptors

(b) Primarily arterial vasodilation with little venodilation

Phentolamine	
HR	Increased (reflex)
Contractility	Increased (reflex)
BP	Decreased
SVR	Decreased
PVR	Decreased
Preload	Decreased

(2) **Offset** occurs by hepatic metabolism, in part by renal excretion. Offset after IV bolus occurs after 10 to 30 min.

(3) **Advantages**

(a) Used for high NE states such as pheochromocytoma

(b) Given PO to prepare patients for excision of pheochromocytoma

(c) Slow onset and prolonged duration of action (half-life of roughly 24 h)

(4) **Disadvantages**

(a) Tachycardia arises from two mechanisms:

(i) Reflex via baroreceptors

(ii) Direct effect of α_2 blockade. Blockade of presynaptic receptors eliminates the normal feedback system controlling NE release by presynaptic nerve terminals. As α_2 stimulation decreases NE release, blockade of these receptors allows increased presynaptic release. This results in increased β_1 sympathetic effects only, as the α-receptors mediating postsynaptic α effects are blocked by phentolamine. Myocardial ischemia or arrhythmias may result. Thus, the tachycardia and positive inotropy are β effects that will respond to β-blockers.

(b) "Stuffy" nose and headache are common.

(c) Creates marked apparent hypovolemia; adequate preoperative rehydration may result in marked postoperative edema.

(d) No IV form

(5) **Clinical use**

(a) Phenoxybenzamine dose

(i) PO dose: 10 mg (adult) bid.

(ii) Increase dose gradually up to 30 mg tid—limited by onset of side effects or by elimination of hypertension.

(b) When administered for pheochromocytoma, β-blockade should not be added until phenoxybenzamine dose has reached a steady state, unless there is exaggerated tachycardia or myocardial ischemia.

(c) Some authors advocate doxazosin or calcium channel blockers rather than phenoxybenzamine for preoperative preparation of pheochromocytoma, arguing that there are fewer side effects (preoperatively and postoperatively) with these agents.

d. Prazosin, doxazosin, and terazosin

(1) **Actions.** A selective α_1 competitive antagonist, prazosin's main cardiovascular action is vasodilation (arterial and venous) with decreased SVR and decreased preload. Reflex tachycardia is minimal.

(2) **Offset** occurs by hepatic metabolism. The half-life is 4 to 6 h.

(3) **Advantages**

(a) Virtual absence of tachycardia

(b) The only important cardiovascular action is vasodilation.

(4) **Disadvantages.** Postural hypotension with syncope may occur, especially after the initial dose.

(5) **Indications.** Oral treatment of chronic hypertension (but is not a first-line agent).

(6) **Administration.** PO

(7) **Clinical use**

(a) Prazosin dose: Initially 0.5 to 1 mg bid (maximum 40 mg/day).

(b) Prazosin is closely related to two other α_1-blockers with which it shares a common mechanism of action:

(i) Doxazosin (Cardura). Half-life: 9 to 13 h. Dose: 1 to 4 mg/day (maximum 16 mg/day).

(ii) Terazosin (Hytrin). Half-life: 8 to 12 h. Dose: 1 to 5 mg/day (maximum 20 mg/day).

e. **Tolazoline (Priscoline)**

(1) **Actions**

(a) Tolazoline, an imidazoline derivative, is a competitive α-adrenergic antagonist belonging to the same family as phentolamine.

(b) In addition to blocking α_1- and α_2-receptors, tolazoline also stimulates muscarinic cholinergic receptors (enhancing gastrointestinal motility and salivary secretions), causes histamine release from mast cells, and displays a sympathomimetic effect.

	Tolazoline
HR	Increased, often marked
CO	Increased
BP	Decreased
SVR	Decreased
PVR	Decreased
PVR/SVR ratio	Variable

(2) **Offset** occurs by hepatic metabolism and renal excretion, with a half-life in neonates of 3 to 10 h.

(3) **Disadvantages**

(a) Tolazoline is *not* a selective pulmonary vasodilator. Generally, substantial systemic vasodilation occurs also, with hypotension. If PVR is fixed and SVR decreases, then the PVR/SVR ratio actually may increase.

(b) Sympathomimetic effect (possibly due to enhanced neuronal NE release) plus reflex sympathetic activation lead to marked tachycardia and arrhythmias. Pulmonary vasoconstriction may occur in some patients.

(c) Peptic ulceration, abdominal pain, and nausea may occur.

(d) Hypotension may occur.

(e) Thrombocytopenia may occur.

(4) **Clinical use**

(a) Tolazoline is used primarily as a pulmonary vasodilator in neonates with persistent pulmonary hypertension.

(b) Tolazoline dose: Bolus 0.5 to 2 mg/kg; infusion 0.5 to 10 mg/kg/h.

3. **Angiotensin converting enzyme (ACE) inhibitors**

a. **Benazepril (Lotensin)**

(1) An oral ACE inhibitor used primarily to treat hypertension; it is largely similar to captopril (see Section b: Captopril). **Benazepril** must first be converted to an active metabolite in the liver.

(2) Benazepril dose: 10 to 40 mg PO in 1 or 2 daily doses.

b. **Captopril (Capoten)**

(1) **Actions**

(a) In common with all ACE inhibitors, captopril blocks the conversion of angiotensin I (inactive) to angiotensin II in the lung. This decrease in plasma angiotensin II levels causes vasodilation, generally without reflex increases in HR or CO.

(b) Many tissues contain ACE (including heart, blood vessels, and kidney), and inhibition of the local production of angiotensin II may be important in the mechanism of action of ACE inhibitors.
(c) Plasma and tissue concentrations of kinins (e.g., bradykinin) and prostaglandins increase with ACE inhibition and may be responsible for some side effects.
(d) Captopril, enalaprilat, and lisinopril inhibit ACE directly, but benazepril, enalapril, fosinopril, quinapril, and ramipril are inactive "prodrugs" and must undergo hepatic metabolism into the active metabolites.

(2) **Offset** occurs primarily by renal elimination with a half-life of 1.5 to 2 h. Dosages of all ACE inhibitors (except fosinopril) should be reduced with renal dysfunction.

(3) **Advantages** (in common with all ACE inhibitors)
(a) Oral vasodilator with efficacy in chronic hypertension
(b) No tachyphylaxis or reflex hemodynamic changes
(c) Improved symptoms and prolonged survival in CHF, hypertension, and after MI
(d) May retard progression of renal disease in diabetics
(e) Antagonizes LV remodeling after myocardial infarction

(4) **Disadvantages** (in common with all ACE inhibitors)
(a) Reversibly decreased renal function, due to reduced renal perfusion pressure. Patients with renal artery stenosis bilaterally (or in a single functioning kidney) are at particular risk of renal failure.
(b) Increased plasma K^+ and hyperkalemia may occur, due to reduced aldosterone secretion.
(c) Not all angiotensin arises through the ACE pathway ("angiotensin escape").
(d) ACE inhibition also leads to accumulation of bradykinin (which may underlie side effects of ACE inhibitors).
(e) Allergic phenomena (including angioedema and hematologic disorders) occur rarely. Captopril may induce severe dermatologic reactions.
(f) Many patients develop a chronic nonproductive cough.
(g) Chronic use of ACE inhibitors (and ARBs) appears associated with exaggerated hypotension with induction of general anesthesia.
(h) Severe fetal abnormalities and oligohydramnios may occur during second- and third-trimester exposure.

(5) **Indications**
(a) Hypertension
(b) CHF
(c) Myocardial infarction (secondary prevention)
(d) For all indications, outcome benefits appear to be a drug class effect; any ACE inhibitor will provide them.
(e) Prevention of renal insufficiency (in the absence of renal artery stenosis), especially in at-risk population (diabetics)

(6) **Administration.** PO

(7) **Clinical use**
(a) Captopril dose
(i) Adults: 12.5 to 150 mg PO in 2 or 3 daily doses, with the lower doses being used for treatment of heart failure
(ii) Infants: 50 to 500 μg/kg daily in three doses
(iii) Children older than 6 mos: 0.5 to 2 mg/kg/day divided into three doses
(b) Interactions. ACE inhibitors interact with digoxin (reduced digoxin clearance) and with lithium (Li intoxication). May predispose to exaggerated hypotension with anesthesia. Captopril interacts with allopurinol (hypersensitivity reactions), cimetidine (CNS changes), and insulin or oral hypoglycemic drugs (hypoglycemia).

c. Enalapril (Vasotec)

(1) Actions. An oral ACE inhibitor used to treat hypertension and CHF, enalapril is very similar to captopril (see Section b). The drug must first be converted to an active metabolite in the liver.

(2) Clinical use. Enalapril dose: 2.5 to 40 mg/day PO in one or two divided doses.

d. Enalaprilat (Vasotec-IV)

(1) Actions. Enalaprilat is an IV ACE inhibitor that is the active metabolite of enalapril. It is used primarily to treat severe or acute hypertension and is very similar to captopril (see Section b).

(2) Offset is by renal elimination, with a half-life of 11 h.

(3) Advantages

(a) This drug has a longer duration of action than nitrates, thereby avoiding the need for continuous infusion. It can help extend BP control into the postoperative period.

(b) Unlike hydralazine, reflex increases in HR, CO, and MvO_2 are absent.

(4) Disadvantages

(a) There is a longer onset time (15 min) than with IV nitroprusside. Peak action may not occur until 1 to 4 h after the initial dose.

(b) Pregnancy. Oligohydramnios and fetal abnormalities may be induced. Use during pregnancy should be limited to life-threatening maternal conditions.

(5) Enalaprilat IV dose

(a) Adults: 1.25 mg IV slowly every 6 h (maximum 5 mg IV every 6 h). In renal insufficiency (creatinine clearance less than 30 mL/min), initial dose is 0.625 mg, which may be repeated after 1 h; then 1.25 mg.

(b) Pediatrics: A dosage of 250 μg/kg IV every 6 h has been reported to be effective in neonates with renovascular hypertension.

e. Fosinopril (monopril)

(1) An oral ACE inhibitor most often used for hypertension, fosinopril is very similar to captopril (see Section b). The drug must first be converted to an active metabolite in the gastrointestinal tract and liver.

(2) Unlike other ACE inhibitors, substantial biliary excretion occurs, so that doses do not need to be altered with renal insufficiency.

(3) Fosinopril dose: 10 to 80 mg PO in 1 or 2 daily dose.

f. Lisinopril (prinivil, zestril)

(1) Lisinopril is an oral ACE inhibitor most often used for hypertension. It is very similar to captopril (see Section b). The drug must first be converted to an active metabolite in the liver.

(2) Lisinopril dose: 5.40 mg PO once daily.

g. Quinapril (accupril)

(1) An oral ACE inhibitor used primarily to treat hypertension, quinapril is very similar to captopril (see Section b). The drug must first be converted to an active metabolite in the liver.

(2) Quinapril dose: 5 to 80 mg PO daily in one or two divided doses.

h. Ramipril (altace)

(1) An oral ACE inhibitor used primarily to treat hypertension, ramipril is very similar to captopril (see Section b). The drug must first be converted to an active metabolite in the liver.

(2) Ramipril dose: 1.25 to 10 mg PO once daily.

i. Aceon (perindopril)

(1) An oral ACE inhibitor used primarily to treat hypertension or HF-LV dysfunction after MI. It is very similar to captopril (see Section b). This prodrug must be hydrolyzed to an active metabolite in the liver.

(2) Perindopril dose: 2 to 8 mg daily (most often given as a single dose).

j. **Mavik (trandolopril)**

(1) An oral ACE inhibitor used primarily to treat hypertension or HF-LV dysfunction after MI. It is very similar to captopril (see Section b). This prodrug must be hydrolyzed to an active metabolite in the liver.

(2) Trandolopril dose: 1 to 8 mg daily in patients not already receiving a diuretic. Usual starting dose is 1 mg daily (2 mg daily for control of hypertension in blacks).

k. **Univasc (moexipril)**

(1) An oral ACE inhibitor used primarily to treat hypertension or HF-LV dysfunction after MI. It is very similar to captopril (see Section b.). This prodrug must be hydrolyzed to an active metabolite in the liver.

(2) Moexipril dose: 7.5 mg to 30 mg daily (most often as a single dose).

4. **Angiotensin receptor blockers (ARBs)**

a. **Actions**

(1) Plasma concentrations of angiotensin II and aldosterone may increase despite treatment with ACE inhibitors because of accumulation of angiotensin or because of production catalyzed via non-ACE–dependent pathways (e.g., chymase).

(2) Selective Angiotensin type-1 receptor (AT1) blockers prevent angiotensin II from directly causing the following:

(a) Vasoconstriction

(b) Sodium retention

(c) Release of NE

(d) LV hypertrophy and fibrosis

(3) Angiotensin type-2 receptors (AT-2) are not blocked: Their actions including NO release and vasodilation remain intact.

b. **Advantages**

(1) Oral vasodilator

(2) No tachyphylaxis or reflex hemodynamic changes

(3) ARBs have minimal interaction with CYP system, so few drug interactions.

(4) Improved symptoms and survival in CHF, hypertension, and after MI

(5) Stroke prevention in hypertension and LV dysfunction

(6) May retard progression of renal disease (particularly in diabetics)

(7) Antagonizes LV remodeling after myocardial infarction

(8) Lacks common side effects of ACE inhibitors (cough, angioedema)

c. **Disadvantages**

(1) There is the potential for decreased renal function, due to reduced renal perfusion pressure. Patients with renal artery stenosis bilaterally (or in a single functioning kidney) are at particular risk.

(2) Increased plasma K^+ and hyperkalemia may occur, especially when clinicians fail to recognize the consequences of reduced aldosterone secretion.

d. **Indications**

(1) Intolerance of ACE inhibitors—outcome benefits of ACE inhibitors appear to be largely shared by ARBs

(2) Hypertension

(3) CHF

(4) Prevention of renal insufficiency (in the absence of renal artery stenosis) in at-risk population (diabetics)

(5) **Data are inconclusive as to whether there is an outcome benefit to adding ARBs to an ACE inhibitor.**

e. **Specific agents**

(1) **Losartan (Cozaar)**

(a) Both drug and first metabolite antagonize angiotensin

(b) Requires dosage adjustment in both renal and hepatic disease

(c) Peak concentration about 1 h after oral administration

(d) Dosing 25–100 mg/day in 1 or 2 daily doses

(e) Takes 4 to 6 wks to see peak effect

(2) **Irbesartan (Avapro)**
   (a) Once-daily dosing
   (b) Primarily hepatic metabolism
   (c) Usual dose 150–300 mg daily in 1 dose

(3) **Candesartan (Atacand)**
   (a) Taken as a prodrug (candesartan cilexetil is hydrolyzed to candesartan during absorption from GI tract)
   (b) Only ARB that is totally dependent on metabolism for clinical effect
   (c) Prodrug is not detectable in blood after oral dosing (assumed to be completely metabolized to candesartan).
   (d) Usual dose 8–32 mg once daily
   (e) Most of the drug is eliminated unchanged in urine (30%) and feces (70%, 25% of this as inactive metabolite).
   (f) Dose adjustment required with renal disease; no adjustment required in mild to moderate hepatic disease

(4) **Eprosartan (Teveten)**
   (a) Approximately two-thirds of oral dose eliminated unchanged in bile; remainder eliminated unchanged in urine
   (b) Usual dose 400–800 mg in 1 or 2 daily)
   (c) Peak blood concentration 1 to 3 h after oral dose
   (d) Most of the drug eliminated unchanged in feces with remainder eliminated unchanged in urine (small fraction of conjugated drug)
   (e) No need to routinely adjust dosage in patients with mild to moderate renal or hepatic disease

(5) **Telmisartan (Micardis)**
   (a) Typical dose 40 to 80 mg/day in 1 daily dose
   (b) No dosage adjustment required for renal disease; manufacturer urges "caution" in hepatic disease.
   (c) Steady-state concentrations were achieved after 5 to 7 days of dosing.
   (d) Almost all of the administered drug is eliminated unchanged in bile.

(6) **Valsartan (Diovan)**
   (a) Typical dose 80 mg to 320 mg in 1 daily dose
   (b) Extensively studied in both hypertension and heart failure
   (c) Maximum concentration reached within 3 h of oral dosing
   (d) Most of the administered drug eliminated unchanged in bile
   (e) Should be given 40 mg twice daily in heart failure; once-daily dosing is approved in hypertension.

(7) **Olmesartan (Benicar)**
   (a) Omesartan medoxomil is a prodrug (de-esterified in GI tract much like candesartan)
   (b) Peak blood concentrations after oral dosing within 3 h
   (c) 60% administered dose eliminated unchanged in bile, remainder eliminated unchanged in urine
   (d) Once-daily dosing in hypertension
   (e) Usual doses 20 to 40 mg daily
   (f) No dosage adjustment recommended in patients with mild to moderate renal or hepatic disease

5. **Direct renin inhibitor.** Aliskiren is the single member of this class. It is used for treatment of hypertension and has the same side effects and contraindications as the ARBs. It is dosed at 150–300 mg in a single daily dose.

6. **Central α_2 agonists**

   a. **Clonidine (Catapres)**

   (1) **Actions**
      (a) Clonidine reduces sympathetic outflow by activating central α_2 receptors thereby reducing NE release by peripheral sympathetic nerve terminals.

(b) Clonidine is a partial agonist (activates receptor submaximally but also antagonizes effects of other α_2 agonists).

(c) There is some direct vasoconstrictor action at α_2-receptors on vascular smooth muscle, but this effect is outweighed by the vasodilation induced by these receptors.

(d) Has "local anesthetic" effect on peripheral nerve and produces analgesia by actions on spinal cord when administered via epidural or caudal route

(e) **Has been added to intermediate-duration local anesthetics (e.g., mepivacaine) to nearly double the duration of analgesia after peripheral nerve blocks**

(2) **Offset**

(a) Long duration (β half-life; 12 h)

(b) Peak effect 1.5 to 2 h after an oral dose

(3) **Advantages**

(a) α_2 Agonists potentiate general anesthetics and narcotics through a central mechanism. This effect can reduce substantially doses of anesthetics and narcotics required during anesthesia.

(b) There are no reflex increases in HR or contractility.

(c) Clonidine reduces sympathetic coronary artery tone.

(d) It attenuates hemodynamic responses to stress.

(e) Prolongs duration of regional anesthesia

(4) **Disadvantages**

(a) Rebound hypertension prominent after abrupt withdrawal

(b) Clonidine may potentiate opiate drug effects on CNS.

(c) Sedation is dose-dependent.

(5) **Clinical use**

(a) Clonidine dose

(i) Adult: 0.2 to 0.8 mg PO daily (maximum 2.4 mg/day). When used as anesthetic premedication, the usual dose is 5 μg/kg PO.

(ii) Pediatrics: 3 to 5 μg/kg every 6 to 8 h.

(b) Rebound hypertension frequently follows abrupt withdrawal. Clonidine should be continued until immediately before the operation, and either it should be resumed soon postoperatively (by transdermal skin patch, nasogastric tube, or PO) or another type of antihypertensive drug should be substituted. Alternatively, clonidine can be replaced by another drug 1 to 2 wks preoperatively.

(c) Intraoperative hypotension may occur.

(d) Transdermal clonidine patches require 2 to 3 days to achieve therapeutic plasma drug levels.

(e) Guanabenz and guanfacine are related drugs with similar effects and hazards.

(f) Use of clonidine may improve hemodynamic stability during major cardiovascular surgery.

(g) Clonidine attenuates sympathetic responses during withdrawal from alcohol or opioids in addicts.

(h) It may reduce postoperative shivering.

(i) It may be added to intermediate-duration local anesthetic solutions prior to peripheral nerve blocks to prolong the duration of action.

b. **Guanabenz (Wytensin)**

(1) Oral α_2 agonist is similar to clonidine.

(2) Guanabenz dose: 4 mg PO bid (maximum 32 mg PO bid).

c. **Guanfacine (Tenex)**

(1) Oral α_2 agonist is similar to clonidine.

(2) Actions. Guanfacine has a longer duration of action than clonidine due to renal elimination (half-life: 15 to 20 h).

(3) Guanfacine dose: 1 mg PO daily (maximum 3 mg daily).

7. **Other vasodilators**
   a. **Fenoldopam**
      (1) **Actions**
         (a) Fenoldopam is a short-acting DA-1 receptor agonist which causes peripheral vasodilation. The mechanism appears to be through stimulation of cAMP.
         (b) Unlike dopamine, fenoldopam has no α- or β-adrenergic receptor activity at clinical doses and thus no direct actions on HR or cardiac contractility.
         (c) Fenoldopam stimulates diuresis and natriuresis.
      (2) **Advantages**
         (a) Relative to other short-acting IV vasodilators, fenoldopam has almost no systemic toxic effects.
         (b) Fenoldopam alone among vasodilators stimulates diuresis and natriuresis comparable to "renal dose" (0.5 to 2 μg/kg/min) dopamine.
         (c) Fenoldopam, unlike dopamine, reduces global and regional cerebral blood flow.
      (3) **Disadvantages**
         (a) As is true for other dopaminergic agonists, fenoldopam may induce nausea in awake patients.
      (4) **Clinical use**
         (a) Fenoldopam is an appropriate single agent to use whenever a combination of a vasodilator and "renal dose" dopamine is employed; for example, for hypertensive patients recovering after CPB.
         (b) Fenoldopam carries no risk of cyanide or of methemoglobinemia and may have theoretical advantages over both nitroprusside and nitroglycerin for control of acute hypertension.
         (c) For treatment of urgent or emergent hypertension in adults we initiate fenoldopam at 0.05 μg/kg/min and double the dose at 5- to 10-min intervals until it achieves BP control. Doses of up to 1 μg/kg/min may be required.
         (d) The limited data available in pediatrics suggest that weight-adjusted doses at least as great as those used in adults are necessary.
         (e) For inducing diuresis and natriuresis, we have found that doses of 0.05 μg/kg/min are effective in adults.
   b. **Alprostadil (Prostaglandin$_1$, PGE$_1$, Prostin VR)**
      (1) **Actions.** This drug is a direct vasodilator acting through specific prostaglandin receptors on vascular smooth-muscle cells.
      (2) **Offset** occurs by rapid metabolism by enzymes located in most body tissues, especially the lung.
      (3) **Advantages**
         (a) Alprostadil selectively dilates the ductus arteriosus (DA) in neonates and infants. It may maintain patency of an open DA for as long as 60 days of age and may open a closed DA for as long as 10 to 14 days of age.
         (b) Metabolism by lung endothelium reduces systemic vasodilation compared with its potent pulmonary vascular dilating effect.
      (4) **Disadvantages**
         (a) Systemic vasodilation and hypotension
         (b) May produce apnea in infants (10% to 12%), especially if birth weight is less than 2 kg. Fever and seizures are also possible.
         (c) Expensive agent
         (d) Reversible platelet inhibition
      (5) **Administration.** Infused IV or through umbilical arterial catheter
      (6) **Indications for use**
         (a) Cyanotic congenital heart disease with reduced pulmonary blood flow
         (b) Severe pulmonary hypertension with right heart failure

(7) **Clinical use**

(a) Alprostadil dose: Usual IV infusion starting dose is 0.05 μg/kg/min. The dose should be titrated up or down to the lowest effective value. Doses as great as 0.4 μg/kg/min may be required.

(b) Intravenous alprostadil is sometimes used in combination with left atrial NE infusion for treatment of severe pulmonary hypertension with right heart failure.

c. **Epoprostenol (PGI_2)** is used for the long-term treatment of primary pulmonary hypertension and pulmonary hypertension associated with scleroderma. The acute treatment of pulmonary hypertension and RV failure is summarized in Table 2.2.

IX. Calcium channel blockers [3,5]

A. General considerations

1. **Tissues utilizing calcium.** Calcium is required for cardiac contraction and conduction, smooth-muscle contraction, synaptic transmission, and hormone secretion.
2. **How calcium enters cells.** Calcium ions (Ca^{2+}) reach intracellular sites of action in two ways, by entering the cell from outside or by being released from intracellular storage sites. These two mechanisms are related because Ca^{2+} crossing the sarcolemma acts as a trigger (Ca-induced Ca release), releasing sequestered Ca^{2+} from the sarcoplasmic reticulum into the cytoplasm. These processes can raise intracellular free Ca^{2+} concentrations 100-fold.
3. **Myocardial effects of calcium.** The force of myocardial contraction relates to the free ionized calcium concentration in cytoplasm. Increased [Ca^{2+}] causes contraction and decreased [Ca^{2+}] permits relaxation. At the end of systole, energy-consuming pumps transfer Ca^{2+} from the cytoplasm back into the sarcoplasmic reticulum, decreasing free cytoplasmic [Ca^{2+}]. If ischemia prevents sequestration of cytoplasmic Ca^{2+}, diastolic relaxation of myocardium is incomplete. This abnormal diastolic stiffness of the heart raises LVEDP.
4. **Myocardial effects of CCBs.** CCBs owe much of their usefulness to their ability to reduce the entry of the "trigger" current of Ca^{2+}. This reduces the amount of Ca^{2+} released from intracellular stores with each heartbeat. Therefore, all CCBs in large enough doses reduce the force of cardiac contraction, although this effect often is counterbalanced by reflex actions in patients. Clinical dosages of some CCBs, such as nifedipine and nicardipine, do not produce myocardial depression in humans.
5. **Vascular smooth muscle and the cardiac conduction system are particularly sensitive to Ca^{2+} channel blockade.** All CCBs cause vasodilation.
6. **Site selectivity.** CCBs affect certain tissues more than others. Thus, verapamil in clinical dosages depresses cardiac conduction, whereas nifedipine does not.
7. **Direct versus indirect effects.** Selection of a particular CCB is based primarily on its relative potency for direct cellular effects in the target organ versus its relative potency for inducing cardiovascular reflexes.

B. Clinical effects common to all CCBs

1. **Peripheral vasodilation**

a. **Arterial vasodilation reduces LV afterload,** and this helps offset any direct negative cardiac inotropic action.

b. **Venous effects.** Preload usually changes little because venodilation is minimal, and negative inotropy often is offset by reduced afterload. However, if CCBs reduce myocardial ischemia and diastolic stiffness, filling pressures may decrease.

c. **Regional effects.** Most vascular beds are dilated, including the cerebral, hepatic, pulmonary, splanchnic, and musculoskeletal beds. Renal blood flow autoregulation is abolished by nifedipine, making it pressure-dependent.

d. **Coronary vasodilation is induced by all CCBs.** These drugs are all highly effective for coronary vasospasm.

e. **CCBs versus nitrates**

(1) Unlike nitrates, CCBs do not incite tachyphylaxis.

(2) Unlike nitrates, several CCBs are associated with increased bleeding.

f. **Reversal of vasodilation.** α Agonists such as phenylephrine often restore BP during CCB-induced hypotension, but usual doses of calcium salts are often ineffective.

2. **Depression of myocardial contractility.** The degree of myocardial depression that occurs following administration of a CCB is highly variable, depending on the following factors:
   a. **Selectivity.** The relative potency of the drug for myocardial depression compared with its other actions is an important factor. Nifedipine and other dihydropyridines are much more potent as vasodilators than as myocardial depressants; clinical dosages that cause profound vasodilation have minimal direct myocardial effects. Conversely, vasodilating dosages of verapamil may be associated with significant myocardial depression in some patients.
   b. **Health of the heart.** A failing ventricle will respond to afterload reduction with improved ejection. An ischemic ventricle will pump more effectively if ischemia is reversed. As CCBs reduce afterload and ischemia, CO may rise with CCB therapy in certain situations. Direct negative inotropic effects may not be apparent.
   c. **Sympathetic reflexes** can counteract direct myocardial depression and vasodilation due to CCBs.
   d. **Reversal of myocardial depression.** Calcium salts, β agonists, and PDE inotropes all can be used to help reverse excessive negative inotropy and heart block. Electrical pacing may be needed.
3. **Improving myocardial ischemia**
   a. **CCBs may improve oxygen supply** by the following actions:
      (1) Reversing coronary artery spasm
      (2) Vasodilating the coronary artery, increasing flow to both normal and poststenotic regions. Diltiazem and verapamil appear to preserve coronary autoregulation, but nifedipine may cause a coronary steal.
      (3) Increasing flow through coronary collateral channels
      (4) Decreasing HR (prolonging diastolic duration during which subendocardium is perfused) with verapamil and diltiazem
   b. **CCBs may improve oxygen consumption** by
      (1) Diminishing contractility
      (2) Decreasing peak LV wall stress (afterload reduction)
      (3) Decreasing HR (by verapamil and diltiazem)
4. **Electrophysiologic depression**
   a. **Spectrum of impairment of AV conduction**
      (1) **Verapamil.** Clinical doses usually produce significant electrophysiologic effects. Thus, verapamil has a high relative potency for prolonging AV refractoriness compared with its vasodilating potency.
      (2) **Dihydropyridines.** On the other hand, nifedipine and other drugs of this class in dosages that produce profound vasodilation have no effect on AV conduction.
      (3) **Diltiazem** is intermediate between nifedipine and verapamil.
   b. **AV node effects.** The depression of AV nodal conduction by CCBs may be beneficial for its antiarrhythmic effect.
   c. **Sinoatrial (SA) node effects.** Diltiazem and verapamil decrease sinus rate, whereas nifedipine and nicardipine often increase HR slightly.
   d. **Ventricular ectopy** due to mitral valve prolapse, atrial or AV nodal disease, and some forms of digitalis toxicity may respond to CCBs.
5. **Clinical uses**
   a. **Myocardial ischemia** mainly for symptom reduction; note that outcome benefit is not well established for CCBs.
   b. **Hypertension** (outcome benefits are better established for thiazide diuretics and ACE inhibitors; short-acting CCBs have been associated with *worsened* outcomes)
   c. **Hypertrophic cardiomyopathy** by relieving LV outflow obstruction
   d. **Cerebral vasospasm following subarachnoid hemorrhage** (nimodipine)
   e. **Possible reduction of cyclosporine nephrotoxicity with concomitant CCB therapy in transplant recipients.** Also, CCBs may potentiate the immunosuppressive action of cyclosporine.
   f. **Migraine prophylaxis**

C. Specific agents

1. **Amlodipine (Norvasc)**
   a. **Actions.** A dihydropyridine CCB with actions closely resembling those of nifedipine (see Section 7), amlodipine is primarily a vasodilator without important negative cardiac inotropy. It is used most commonly for oral treatment of hypertension.
   b. **Amlodipine dose:** 2.5 to 10 mg PO once daily; decrease with hepatic dysfunction
2. **Bepridil (Vascor)**
   a. **Actions.** In addition to inhibiting Ca channels, bepridil also inhibits voltage-gated Na channels, prolongs cardiac repolarization, and causes additional negative cardiac inotropy by a non-calcium channel mechanism. Its vasodilator actions are selective for the coronary circulation; nevertheless, hypotension may be induced.
   b. **Offset** is by hepatic metabolism (with active metabolites). The elimination half-life is 33 h.
   c. **Advantages**
      (1) Oral treatment of angina pectoris that is not controlled by other medical therapies
      (2) Does not cause clinical myocardial depression but not recommended for use with severe LV dysfunction
   d. **Disadvantages**
      (1) Proarrhythmic action. Bepridil can increase QT intervals, which may cause ventricular arrhythmias; *Torsades de Pointes* occurs rarely. For this reason, bepridil is contraindicated in patients with a prolonged QT interval, conduction abnormalities, or elevated K^+.
      (2) T-wave abnormalities may be induced.
   e. **Bepridil dose:** 200 to 400 mg PO once daily
3. **Diltiazem (Cardizem)**
   a. **Diltiazem is a benzothiazepine calcium blocker.**
   b. **Actions.** Diltiazem has a selective coronary vasodilating action, causing a greater increase in coronary flow than in other vascular beds.

	Diltiazem
HR	Slight decrease
Contractility	No change or small decrease
BP	Decreased
Preload	No change
SVR	Decreased
AV conduction	Slowed

   c. **Offset** occurs by hepatic metabolism (60%) and renal excretion (35%). Plasma elimination half-life is 3 to 5 h. The active metabolite is desacetyldiltiazem.
   d. **Advantages**
      (1) Diltiazem often decreases HR of patients in sinus rhythm.
      (2) It is effective in treating and preventing symptoms of classic or vasospastic myocardial ischemia. Diltiazem does *not* improve outcome in these conditions.
      (3) Used for rate control of SVT (see Section VIII.E).
      (4) Perioperative hypertension can be controlled with IV diltiazem.
   e. **Disadvantages**
      (1) Sinus bradycardia and conduction system depression are possible.
      (2) No evidence for outcome benefit in hypertension or CAD relative to other agents
   f. **Indications**
      (1) Myocardial ischemia, both classic angina and coronary artery spasm
      (2) Hypertension
      (3) Supraventricular tachycardia, including atrial fibrillation or flutter (see Section VIII.E).
      (4) Sinus tachycardia, especially intraoperative or postoperative
   g. Diltiazem dose (adult) (see Section VIII.E)

4. **Felodipine (Plendil)**
   a. **Actions.** A dihydropyridine CCB with actions closely resembling those of nifedipine (see Section 7). Felodipine is primarily a vasodilator without clinically important negative cardiac inotropy. It is used most commonly for oral treatment of hypertension.
   b. **Felodipine dose:** 2.5 to 10 mg PO once daily.
5. **Isradipine (DynaCirc)**
   a. **Actions.** A dihydropyridine CCB with actions closely resembling those of nifedipine (see Section 7), isradipine is primarily a vasodilator without clinically important negative cardiac inotropy. It is used most commonly for oral treatment of hypertension.
   b. **Isradipine dose:** 5 to 10 mg PO in 2 daily doses
6. **Nicardipine (Cardene)**
   a. **Actions.** A dihydropyridine calcium blocker with actions closely resembling those of nifedipine (see Section 7), nicardipine is primarily a vasodilator without clinically important negative cardiac inotropy. It is used most commonly for treatment of hypertension.
   b. IV nicardipine
      (1) The IV preparation is a highly effective vasodilator that is widely used in surgical patients, causing only minimal HR increase and no increase in ICP. Nicardipine lacks the rebound hypertension that can follow nitroprusside withdrawal. Nicardipine causes less venodilation than nitroglycerin.
      (2) **Offset.** Metabolism occurs in the liver, with plasma α and β half-lives of 3 and 14 min, respectively. When IV administration is stopped, 50% offset vasodilation occurs in approximately 30 min.
      (3) **Clinical use.** Nicardipine IV is effective for control of perioperative hypertension; it also improves diastolic LV function during ischemia by acceleration of myocardial relaxation (lusitropy). Nicardipine can elevate plasma cyclosporine levels.
   c. **Nicardipine dose:** PO: 60–120 mg in 3 daily doses; IV: 1 to 4 μg/kg/min in adults, titrated to BP. The drug causes phlebitis when infused for more than 12 h through a peripheral IV catheter.
7. **Nifedipine (Adalat, Procardia)**
   a. **Nifedipine is a dihydropyridine calcium channel blocker.**
   b. **Actions**

	Nifedipine
HR	Increased (reflex)
Contractility	Increased (reflex)
BP	Decreased
Preload	No change, or slightly decreased
SVR	Markedly decreased
AV conduction	Increased (reflex)

   c. **Offset** occurs by hepatic metabolism. Plasma elimination half-life is 1.5 to 5 h, and there are no active metabolites.
   d. **Advantages**
      (1) Profound vasodilation is the predominant effect.
         (a) Coronary vasodilation and relief of coronary vasospasm reduce myocardial ischemia.
         (b) Peripheral vasodilation can improve CO via LV unloading.
      (2) Virtually no myocardial depression occurs in clinical dosages. Therefore, nifedipine can be used in patients with poor ventricular function.
      (3) Generally this drug is devoid of conducting system toxicity.
      (4) It may be combined with β-blockers without increased risk of AV block, or with nitrates provided that the patient is monitored for excessive vasodilation.
   e. **Disadvantages**
      (1) It is extremely light-sensitive; thus, no IV preparation is available.

(2) Administration must be PO or via mucosa of the nose or mouth.
(3) Severe hypotension is possible due to peripheral vasodilation.
(4) No significant antiarrhythmic effect occurs unless relief of myocardial ischemia decreases ischemia-induced arrhythmias.
(5) Peripheral edema is possible (not due to heart failure).
(6) The drug must be avoided in hypertrophic cardiomyopathy due to increased aortic outflow tract obstruction.
(7) Short-acting versions of this drug have been associated with *worsened* outcome when used for chronic treatment of essential hypertension.

f. Clinical use

(1) Nifedipine dose: PO, 10 to 40 mg tid; sublingual, 10 to 20 mg liquid (extracted from capsule). In hypertension, use extended-release formation at 30–90 mg in 1 daily dose
(2) Nifedipine generally is selected for its vasodilator and antianginal properties.
(3) The sublingual (or intranasal) route is useful in treatment of hypertensive emergencies when no IV is present.
(4) If excessive vasodilation with hypotension occurs, phenylephrine may be used (high dosages may be required).
(5) In rare patients, angina is exacerbated with nifedipine. This may be related to hypotension or to a coronary steal phenomenon.

8. Nimodipine (Nimotop)

a. Actions. A dihydropyridine CCB with actions closely resembling those of nifedipine (see Section I), nimodipine lacks clinically important negative cardiac inotropy. It is a more effective dilator of cerebral arteries compared with other CCBs. Its primary use is in patients with subarachnoid hemorrhage for oral treatment and prophylaxis of cerebral vasospasm and neurologic deficits.

b. Nimodipine dose: 60 mg PO (or by nasogastric tube) every 4 h.

9. Verapamil (Calan, Isoptin) (see Section VIII.E).

10. Flunarizine (a vasodilating CCB indicated for prophylaxis against migraine headaches in countries other than the United States, where it has not received regulatory approval)

X. Pharmacologic control of HR and rhythm

A. Overview of arrhythmias [5,22,23]

1. Conduction pathway. Drug effects on the cardiac rhythm depend upon the anatomy and physiology of the cardiac conduction pathway. The cardiac impulse normally arises in the SA node and passes through the atria to enter the AV node. Impulses then transit the conduction system (including the His bundle, the major bundle branches, and the Purkinje fiber network) before spreading into the ventricular myocardium. Agents that inhibit conduction from the sinus node to (or through) the AV node prolong the interval from the P wave (which represents atrial systole) to the QRS complex (which represents ventricular systole), manifest as the "PR" interval on the ECG (Fig. 2.1). Conversely, agents that prolong conduction through the specialized conduction system or the ventricle lengthen the QRS complex.

2. The role of the conduction system in arrhythmias. Drugs that suppress AV nodal conduction (β-blockers, calcium channel blockers, adenosine) terminate SVTs that originate in the AV node, or involve the AV node in a re-entrant pathway (Table 2.4). Conversely, rhythms that originate in atrial tissue above the AV node, including atrial flutter or fibrillation, as well as paroxysmal rhythms stimulated by catecholamines (common in perioperative patients), respond to AV nodal blockade with slowing of the ventricular response rate, since the passage of impulses from the atrium to the ventricle through the AV node is slowed. Junctional tachycardias, common in surgical patients, arise in the conduction system, and may convert to sinus rhythm in response to AV nodal blockers only if they originate very close to the AV node, but are otherwise unresponsive to drugs acting on the AV node. Ventricular arrhythmias usually exhibit no beneficial response to AV nodal blockade, since these rhythms originate in tissues distal to the AV node.

3. Initiating the cardiac action potential (AP). The effects of drugs on the surface ECG can be predicted from their effects on the ion channel currents that compose the cardiac

TABLE 2.4 The response of common supraventricular tachyarrhythmias to IV adenosine

SVT	Mechanism	Adenosine response
AV nodal re-entry	Re-entry within AV node	Termination
AV reciprocating tachycardias (orthodromic and antidromic)	Re-entry involving AV node and accessory pathway (WPW)	Termination
Intra-atrial re-entry	Re-entry in the atrium	Transiently slows ventricular response
Atrial flutter/fibrillation	Re-entry in the atrium	Transiently slows ventricular response
Other atrial tachycardias	Abnormal automaticity cAMP-mediated triggered activity	Transient suppression of the tachycardia termination
AV junctional rhythms	Variable	Variable

AV, Atrioventricular.
Adapted from ref 24 Balser JR. Perioperative management of arrhythmias. In: Barash PG, Fleisher LA, Prough DS, eds. *Problems in Anesthesia*. Vol. 10. Philadelphia, PA: Lippincott-Raven; 1998:201.

AP (Fig. 2.2). The cardiac AP represents the time-varying transmembrane potential of the cardiac myocyte before, during, and after a depolarization. The AP is divided into five distinct phases; the channels responsible for "Phase 0" initiate the AP and underlie impulse propagation. In the atria and the ventricles, the phase 0 current is generated by sodium channels, and is inhibited by the local anesthetic-type drugs (lidocaine, procainamide, etc.) that prolong the QRS complex. In AV and SA nodal cells (not shown in Fig. 2.2), phase 0 is produced by L-type calcium channels, so drugs that suppress calcium channels (β-blockers and calcium channel blockers) slow the HR by acting on the SA node, and prolong the PR interval by slowing conduction through the AV node. The latter effect renders the AV node a more efficient "filter" for preventing rapid trains of atrial beats from passing into the ventricle, and hence the rationale for AV nodal blockade during SVT.

4. **The later phases of the AP** [17–19] reflect repolarization, and are modulated by a number of outward (mainly potassium) and inward (mainly calcium) currents. In general, the long plateau (phase 2) is maintained by L-type calcium current, and is terminated (phase 3) by potassium currents (Fig. 2.2) and inactivation of the calcium currents. Hence, the QT interval on the ECG reflects the length of the AP, and is determined by a delicate balance between these currents. Drugs that reduce or shorten calcium current tend to abbreviate the AP plateau, shorten the QT, and reduce the inward movement of calcium ions into the cardiac cell (hence, the negative inotropic effect). Conversely, agents that block outward potassium current prolong the AP and the QT interval on the ECG. An example is shown in Figure 2.2.
5. **Re-entry** underlies a wide variety of supraventricular and ventricular arrhythmias, and implies the existence of a pathological circus movement of electrical impulses around an anatomic loop (accessory pathway or infarct scar) or a "functional" loop (ischemia or drug-induced dispersion of AP duration). Fibrillation, in either the atrium or ventricle, is believed to involve multiple coexistent re-entrant circuits of the functional type. Drugs may terminate re-entry through at least two mechanisms. Agents that suppress currents responsible for initiation of the AP, the Na current in ventricle (Fig. 2.2) or the calcium current in the AV node, may slow or block conduction in a re-entrant pathway, and thus terminate an arrhythmia. Interventions that prolong the AP, such as potassium channel blockade (Fig. 2.2), in turn prolong the refractory period of cells in a re-entrant circuit, and thus "block" impulse propagation through the circuit. Agents operating through the latter mechanism are more effective in suppressing fibrillation in the atrium and ventricle.
6. **Triggered automaticity** may occur during phase 2 or 3 (early afterdepolarization, or "EAD") or phase 4 (delayed afterdepolarization, or "DAD"). Drugs that block potassium channels prolong the duration of the AP, lengthening the QT interval on the ECG (Fig. 2.2), and thereby stimulate EADs. In addition, low serum potassium, hypomagnesemia, and slow HR synergistically prolong the QT and precipitate EADs. EADs in turn elicit a polymorphic VT known as *Torsades de Pointes.* At the same time, inherited mutations that suppress potassium channel function provoke the congenital long QT syndrome, an inherited condition where the QT interval is prolonged and the risk for *Torsades de*

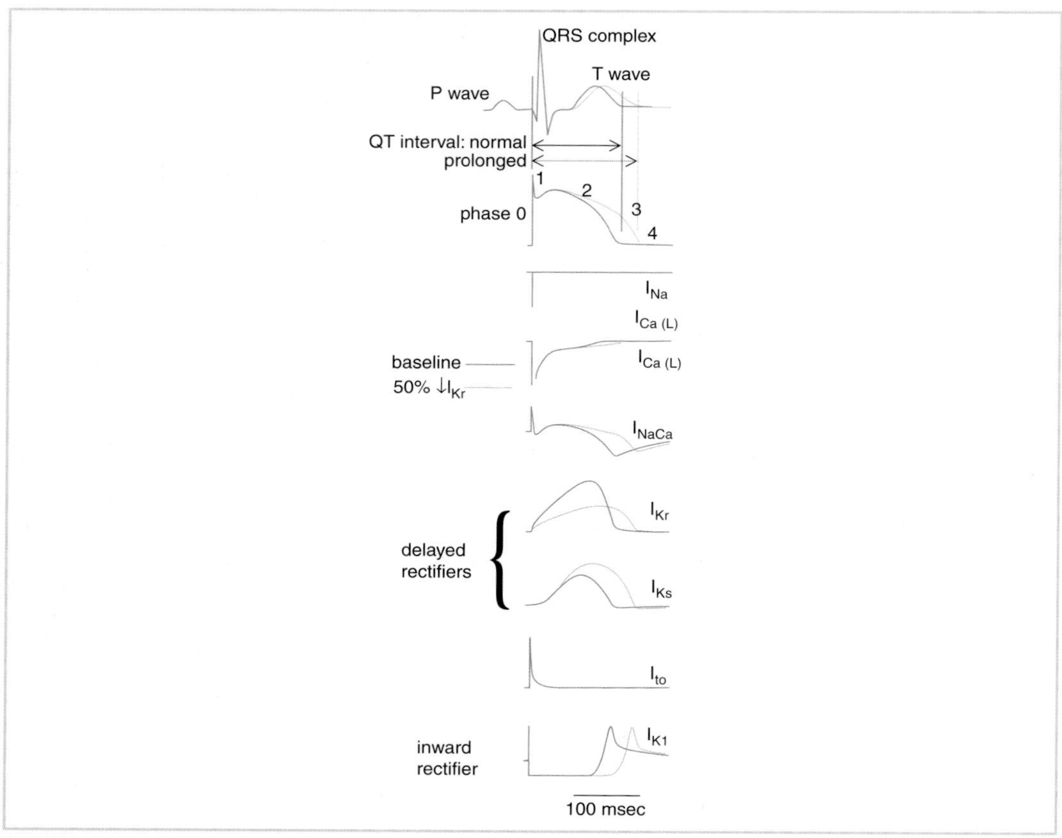

FIGURE 2.2 Relationship between the ECG **(top)**, the AP in the ventricle **(second panel)**, and individual ion currents. The amplitudes of the currents are not on the same scales. The *solid lines* represent the baseline; the *dotted lines* the computation when I_{Kr} is reduced by 50%. Note that this change not only prolongs the action potential duration (APD) (as expected), but also generates changes in the time course of $I_{Ca\text{-}L}$, I_{Ks}, and the sodium–calcium exchange current, each of which thus also modulates the effect of reduced I_{Kr} on the APD. (From Roden DM, Balser JR, George AL Jr, et al. Cardiac ion channels. *Annu Rev Physiol.* 2002;64:431–475, with permission. 2002 by Annual Reviews www.annualreviews.org.)

Pointes is increased. Moreover, "silent" mutations in potassium channels may provoke QT prolongation and torsades only during exposure to potassium-channel–blocking drugs; hence, the "acquired" and congenital long QT syndromes are mechanistically related and represent distinct points on a continuum of ion channel dysfunction. Drugs commonly used in the perioperative period that may prolong the QT and provoke torsades are listed in Table 2.5. More comprehensive listings are available on-line (see, for example, http://www.arizonacert.org/medical-pros/drug-lists/drug-lists.htm).

DADs are most common during conditions of intracellular calcium ion (Ca^{2+}) overload. Common clinical entities are digitalis toxicity, excess catecholamine states (exercise, acute myocardial infarction, perioperative stress), and heart failure. Arrhythmias provoked by DADs are responsive to maneuvers aimed at lowering intracellular Ca^{2+}, such as calcium channel blockade.

B. Nonsustained ventricular tachycardia (NSVT) [5,17,22]

1. **Definition and etiology.** NSVT is three or more premature ventricular contractions (PVCs) occurring at a rate exceeding 100 beats/min, and lasting 30 s or less without hemodynamic compromise. These arrhythmias occur up to 50% of patients during or after thoracic and major vascular surgeries, often in the absence of cardiac disease.

TABLE 2.5 QT-prolonging drugs (partial listing emphasizing agents used perioperatively)

Antiarrhythmics	Quinidine, procainamide, disopyramide, sotalol, amiodarone, ibutilide, dofetilide
Antipsychotics	Haloperidol, risperidone, isoperidene, Chlorpromazine, thioridazine
Antihistamines	Terfenadine, astemizole
Antifungals	Ketoconazole, fluconazole, itraconazole
Antibiotics	Trimethoprim–sulfamethoxazole, erythromycin, clarithromycin
Antidepressants	Amitriptyline, imipramine, doxepin
Opioid	Methadone
GI	Cisapride, droperidol, ondansetron

2. **Management.** The rhythms do not influence early or late mortality in patients with preserved LV function, and do not require suppressive drug therapy in most circumstances. However, NSVT with normal LV function may be the first sign of a reversible, life-threatening condition, such as hypoxemia or cardiac ischemia, and therefore should always trigger a thorough evaluation. Among patients with low CO following CABG (requiring pressor support), NSVT is an independent predictor of more serious, life-threatening arrhythmias. Similarly, patients who undergo aortic valve replacement and have NSVT are at increased risk for sustained ventricular arrhythmias. There are no studies available to guide therapy in these circumstances, so clinical management is empiric. Hemodynamically unstable patients with marginal perfusion may deteriorate with recurrent episodes of NSVT (problematic ventricular pacing or intra-aortic balloon counterpulsation) and may benefit from suppression with IV amiodarone, lidocaine, or β blockade if hemodynamically tolerated. Repletion of postbypass hypomagnesemia (2 g $MgCl_2$ IV) reduces the incidence of NSVT after cardiac surgery.

C. **Sustained ventricular arrhythmias** [5,17,22]

1. **Monomorphic VT.** The mechanism for monomorphic VT is a re-entrant pathway around scar tissue from a healed myocardial infarction, producing a constant QRS morphology. Patients may have a stable (perfusing) BP with this rhythm, and procainamide or amiodarone are often preferred over lidocaine for chemical cardioversion. In cases of hemodynamic instability, DC countershocks should be utilized for cardioversion and antiarrhythmic drug therapy considered as a means to maintain sinus rhythm. Monomorphic VT is less common during surgery than the polymorphic VTs (discussed later).
2. **Long QT polymorphic VT (*Torsades de Pointes*).** As discussed earlier, this rhythm is usually an acquired complication of therapy with drugs that prolong the QT interval (Table 2.5). The management of *Torsades* is distinctive. Following DC countershocks to achieve conversion, additional maneuvers are aimed at shortening the QT interval in order to maintain sinus rhythm. This includes IV magnesium sulfate and maneuvers to increase the HR (atropine, isoproterenol, or ventricular pacing). Antiarrhythmic drug therapy is considered when the rhythm is refractory to these measures, and agents producing minimal potassium channel blockade, such as lidocaine or phenytoin, should be chosen to avoid further prolongation of the QT interval. Among the antiarrhythmic agents that prolong the QT interval, the incidence of *Torsades de Pointes* is lowest with amiodarone; hence, IV amiodarone is a rational alternative therapy for polymorphic VT of unclear etiology that is refractory to other therapies.
3. **Normal QT polymorphic VT and VF** are the most common, life-threatening ventricular arrhythmias in perioperative patients, and may occur in patients with ischemic or structural heart disease. IV antiarrhythmic agents are common adjuncts to DC countershocks, and the agents recommended include procainamide and amiodarone. There are no prospective clinical data evaluating the efficacy of antiarrhythmic agents during cardiac arrest in perioperative patients, but in blinded, randomized, prospective trials, IV amiodarone is superior to placebo or lidocaine in producing a short-term survival benefit when treating

out-of-hospital cardiac arrest refractory to DC cardioversion [22]. There are no convincing human clinical trials to support lidocaine as an effective therapy for treating shock-resistant VT/VF, and the agent now carries an "indeterminate" recommendation in published guidelines. Bretylium was removed from the ACLS treatment guidelines because of a high occurrence of side effects (postganglionic adrenergic blockade, orthostatic hypotension with continuous infusion), limited availability from the manufacturer, and the availability of safer agents. In all cases, defibrillation is the means to achieve conversion to sinus rhythm, and these antiarrhythmic agents should be viewed as supplements to help maintain sinus rhythm.

4. **Specific agents available in IV form** [5,17,22]
   a. **Procainamide (Pronestyl, Procan-SR)**
      (1) **Dosing**
         (a) **Loading dose**
            (i) IV: 10 to 50 mg/min (or 100 mg every 2 to 5 min) up to 17 mg/kg.
            (ii) Pediatric IV: 3 to 6 mg/kg given slowly.
         (b) **Maintenance dose**
            (i) Adult: IV infusion, 2 mg/kg/h; PO, 250 to 1,000 mg every 3 h
            (ii) Children: IV infusion, 20 to 50 μg/kg/min; PO, 30 to 50 mg/kg/day divided into four to six doses.
      (2) **Pharmacokinetics**
      Therapeutic plasma level is usually 4 to 10 μg/mL. With bolus administration, the duration of action is 2 to 4 h. Metabolism is both hepatic (50%, *N*-acetylprocainamide) and renal. Slow acetylators are more dependent on renal elimination. Patients with reduced renal function require lower maintenance doses, and need close monitoring of serum levels and the ECG QT intervals.
      (3) **Adverse effects**
         (a) High serum levels or rapid loading may cause negative inotropic and chronotropic effects, leading to hypotension and hypoperfusion. Overdose may require pacing and/or β-agonist therapy.
         (b) High serum levels of procainamide and/or its principal active metabolite (*N*-acetylprocainamide) induce QT prolongation and *Torsades de Pointes.* Discontinuation of therapy should be considered if the corrected QT interval exceeds 450 ms.
         (c) CNS excitability may occur with confusion and seizures.
         (d) A lupus-like syndrome may be seen with long-term therapy.
   b. **Amiodarone (Cordarone)**
      (1) **Dosing**
         (a) PO: 800 to 1,600 mg/day for 1 to 3 wks, gradually reducing dosage to 400 to 600 mg/day for maintenance.
         (b) IV:
            (i) Loading: For patients in a perfusing rhythm, 150 mg over 10 min in repeated boluses until sustained periods of sinus rhythm occur. For patients in pulseless VT/VF, more rapid bolus administration may be warranted. Patients often require 2 to 4 or more boluses for a sustained response.
            (ii) Maintenance: 1 mg/min for 6 h, then 0.5 mg/min thereafter, with the goal of providing approximately 1 g/day.
      (2) **Pharmacokinetics.** The drug is metabolized hepatically, but has very high lipid solubility that results in marked tissue accumulation. The elimination half-life is 20 to 100 days. Hence, for patients treated chronically, it is usually unnecessary to "reload" amiodarone when doses are missed during surgery, and postoperatively patients usually resume their preoperative dosing.
      (3) **Adverse effects**
         (a) Amiodarone is an α- and β-receptor noncompetitive antagonist, and therefore has potent vasodilating effects, and can render negative inotropic effects.

Hence, vasoconstrictors, IV fluid, and occasionally β agonists are required for hemodynamic support, especially during the IV amiodarone loading phase.

(b) Amiodarone blocks potassium channels and typically prolongs the QT interval, but is only rarely associated with *Torsades de Pointes.* The risk of torsades on amiodarone therapy is poorly correlated with the QT interval, and QT prolongation on amiodarone, if not excessive, does not usually require cessation of therapy.

(c) Amiodarone use may cause sinus bradycardia or heart block due to β-receptor blockade, and patients requiring sustained IV amiodarone therapy sometimes require pacing or low doses of supplemental β agonists.

(d) The side effects of long-term oral dosing (subacute pulmonary fibrosis, hepatitis, cirrhosis, photosensitivity, corneal microdeposits, hypothyroidism, or hyperthyroidism) are of little concern during short-term (days) IV therapy.

(e) This drug may increase the effect of oral anticoagulants, phenytoin, digoxin, diltiazem, quinidine, and other drugs.

c. Lidocaine (lignocaine, Xylocaine)

(1) Dosing

(a) Loading dose: 1 mg/kg IV, a second dose may be given 10 to 30 min after first dose. Loading dose is sometimes doubled for patients on CPB who are experiencing VF prior to separation. The total dose should not exceed 3 mg/kg.

(b) Maintenance dose: 15 to 50 μg/kg/min (i.e., 1 to 4 mg/min in adults).

(2) Pharmacokinetics. Duration of action is 15 to 30 min after administration of a bolus dose. Metabolism is hepatic, and 95% of metabolites are inactive. However, for infusions lasting more than 24 h, serum levels should be monitored. Many factors that reduce hepatic metabolism will increase serum levels, including CHF, α agonists, liver disease, and advanced age.

(3) Adverse effects

(a) CNS excitation may result from mild to moderate overdose, producing confusion or seizures. At higher doses, CNS depression will ensue, producing sedation and respiratory depression. At still higher doses lidocaine will produce severe myocardial depression.

(b) Lidocaine, like other antiarrhythmics with sodium-channel–blocking properties (amiodarone, procainamide), slows ventricular excitation. Hence, patients with AV nodal block who are dependent upon an idioventricular rhythm may become asystolic during lidocaine therapy.

D. Bradyarrhythmias [5,17,22]

1. Asystole

a. CPR with cardiac compressions should be instituted immediately. As hypoxemia is a common cause of asystole, efforts to secure the airway and provide oxygenation may be critical resuscitation measures.

b. The ECG recording of VF is sometimes "fine" (low-amplitude), and may be confused with asystole. If VF cannot be excluded, DC countershocks should be applied.

c. Definitive therapy consists of ventricular pacing and/or transcutaneous pacing if immediately available (see Chapter 15).

d. For pharmacologic therapy, useful drugs include atropine (1 mg IV, repeat every 3 to 5 min) and epinephrine (1 mg IV push, repeat every 3 to 5 min). Isoproterenol infusion may be a poor choice for asystole because of reduced coronary perfusion pressure during CPR.

2. HR below 40 bpm

a. Cardiac compressions may induce VF, so if possible, pharmacologic agents or pacing should be utilized to increase the HR.

b. Certain persons (i.e., trained athletes) may tolerate HRs near 40 bpm. Patients with reduced diastolic compliance (aortic stenosis, hypertensive cardiomyopathy, ongoing ischemia, etc.) cannot increase SV in response to bradycardia, and poorly tolerate extreme bradycardia.

c. For pharmacologic therapy, useful drugs include atropine, isoproterenol, and epinephrine. *Avoid antiarrhythmics such as lidocaine, procainamide, bretylium, or amiodarone because these agents may slow a ventricular escape rhythm, worsening the bradycardia.*

3. **Drug therapies for bradyarrhythmias** [5,17,22]
   a. **Atropine**
      (1) **Dosing.** IV bolus: In adults, use 0.4 to 1 mg (may repeat); in children, use 0.02 mg/kg (minimum 0.1 mg, maximum 0.4 mg, may repeat).
      (2) **Pharmacokinetics.** The HR effects of IV atropine appear within seconds, and effects last as long as 15 to 30 min; when given IM, SC, or PO, offset occurs in approximately 4 h. There is minimal metabolism of the drug, and 77% to 94% of it undergoes renal elimination.
      (3) **Adverse effects.** Atropine is a competitive antagonist at muscarinic cholinergic receptors, and its adverse effects are largely systemic manifestations of this receptor activity.
         (a) Tachycardia (undesirable with coronary disease)
         (b) Exacerbation of bradycardia by low dosages (0.2 mg or less in an adult)
         (c) Sedation (especially in pediatric and elderly patients)
         (d) Urinary retention
         (e) Increased intraocular pressure in patients with closed-angle glaucoma. Atropine may be safely given, however, if miotic eye drops are given concurrently.
   b. **Glycopyrrolate**
      (1) **Dosing (adults).** 0.1 mg IV, repeated at 2- to 3-min intervals
      (2) **Differences from atropine.** Less likely to cause sedation, but also less likely to produce tachycardia and less likely to be effective for treatment of critical bradycardia. This agent may be chosen to manage mild intraoperative bradycardia, or as an antagonist to the HR slowing effects of neostigmine when reversing neuromuscular blockade. Atropine remains the drug of choice in severe or life-threatening sinus bradycardia.
   c. **Isoproterenol (Isuprel)**
      (1) **General features.** Isoproterenol is a synthetic catecholamine with direct β_1- and β_2-agonist effects, and thus has both positive inotropic (through β_1-mediated enhanced contractility plus β_2-mediated vasodilation) and positive chronotropic effects. Isoproterenol is the drug of choice for drug treatment of bradycardia with complete heart block.
      (2) **Dosing.** IV infusion is 0.02 to 0.50 μg/kg/min.
      (3) **Pharmacokinetics.** The agent is used as a continuous infusion, and has a short half-life (2 min) making it titratable. It is partly metabolized in the liver (MAO, COMT) and partly excreted unchanged (60%).
      (4) **Adverse effects**
         (a) The major potential adverse effect of isoproterenol is myocardial ischemia in patients with CAD, because the combination of tachycardia, positive inotropy, and hypotension may create a myocardial oxygen supply–demand mismatch.
         (b) The agent may provoke supraventricular arrhythmias, or may unmask pre-excitation in patients with an accessory AV conduction pathway (e.g., WPW syndrome).

E. **Supraventricular arrhythmias** [5,17,22,23]
   1. **Therapy-based classification**
      a. **General.** SVT often foreshadows life-threatening conditions that may be correctable in the surgical patient. Hence, the initial management of the hemodynamically stable surgical patient who suddenly develops SVT should not be on heart-directed pharmacologic therapies, but rather on potential correctable etiologies that may include hypoxemia (O_2 saturation), hypoventilation (end tidal CO_2), hypotension (absolute or relative hypovolemia due to bleeding, anaphylaxis, etc.), light anesthesia, electrolyte abnormalities (K^+ or Mg^{2+}), or cardiac ischemia (HR, nitroglycerine).

b. Hemodynamically unstable patients. Patients with low BP (e.g., systolic BP less than 80 mm Hg), cardiac ischemia, or other evidence of end-organ hypoperfusion require immediate *synchronous* DC cardioversion. While some patients may only respond transiently to cardioversion in this setting (or not at all), a brief period of sinus rhythm may provide valuable time for correcting the reversible causes of SVT (see earlier) and/or instituting pharmacologic therapies (see later). During cardiac or thoracic surgery, patients may experience SVT during dissection of the pericardium, placement of atrial sutures, or insertion of the venous cannulae required for CPB. If hemodynamically unstable SVT occurs during open thoracotomy, the surgeon should attempt open synchronous cardioversion. Patients with critical coronary lesions or severe aortic stenosis with SVT may be refractory to cardioversion, and thus enter a malignant cascade of ischemia and worsening arrhythmias that requires the institution of CPB. Hence, early preparation for CPB is recommended before inducing anesthesia in those cardiac surgery patients judged to be at exceptionally high risk for SVT and consequent hemodynamic deterioration.

c. Hemodynamically stable patients

(1) Adenosine therapy (Table 2.4)

(a) In certain patients the SVT involves a re-entrant pathway involving the AV node. These rhythms typically have a regular R–R interval, and are common in relatively healthy patients. Adenosine administered as a 6 mg IV bolus (repeated with 12 mg if no response) may terminate the SVT.

(b) Many of the rhythms commonly seen in the perioperative period do not involve the AV node in a re-entrant pathway, and AV nodal block by adenosine in such cases will produce only transient slowing of the ventricular rate. This may lead to "rebound" speeding of the tachycardia following the adenosine effect. Adenosine should be avoided in cases where the rhythm is recognizable and known to be refractory to adenosine (atrial fibrillation, atrial flutter). The hallmark of atrial fibrillation is an irregularly irregular R–R interval.

(c) Junctional tachycardias are common during the surgical period (particularly after surgery for congenital heart disease in children), and sometimes convert to sinus rhythm in response to adenosine, depending on the proximity of the site of origin to the AV node. Ventricular arrhythmias exhibit no response to adenosine since these rhythms originate.

(2) Rate control therapy

(a) Rationale for rate control. In most cases, ventricular rate control is the mainstay of therapy.

(i) Lengthening diastole serves to enhance LV filling, thus enhancing SV.

(ii) Slowing the ventricular rate reduces $M\text{VO}_2$ and lowers the risk of cardiac ischemia.

(b) Rationale for drug selection. The most common selections are IV β-blockers or calcium channel blockers because of their rapid onset.

(i) Among the IV β-blockers, esmolol has the shortest duration of action, rendering it titratable on a minute-to-minute basis, and allowing meaningful dose adjustments during periods of surgery that provoke changes in hemodynamic status (i.e., bleeding, abdominal traction). The drug has obligatory negative inotropic effects that are problematic for patients with severe LV dysfunction.

(ii) Both IV verapamil and IV diltiazem are calcium channel blockers that are less titratable than esmolol, but nonetheless rapidly slow the ventricular rate in SVT. Moreover, IV diltiazem has less negative inotropic action than verapamil or esmolol and is therefore preferable in patients with heart failure.

(iii) IV digoxin slows the ventricular response during SVT through its vagotonic effects at the AV node, but should be temporally supplemented with other IV agents because of its slow onset (approximately 6 h).

(c) **Accessory pathway rhythms.** AV nodal blockade can reduce the ventricular rate in WPW, and improve hemodynamic status. However, 10% to 35% of patients with WPW eventually develop atrial fibrillation. In this case, the rapid rate of atrial excitation (greater than 300 impulses/min), normally transmitted to the ventricle after "filtering" by the AV node, is instead be transmitted to the ventricle via the accessory bundle at a rapid rate. The danger of inducing VT/VF in this scenario is exacerbated by treatment with classic AV nodal blocking agents (digoxin, calcium channel blockers, β-blockers, and adenosine) because they reduce the accessory bundle refractory period. Hence, WPW patients who experience atrial fibrillation should not receive AV nodal blockers. IV procainamide slows conduction over the accessory bundle, and is an option for treating AF in patients with accessory pathways.

d. Specific rate control agents [5,17,22,23]

(1) Esmolol

(please also see the earlier section on β-blockers)

(a) **Dosing.** During surgery and anesthesia, the standard 0.25 to 0.5 mg/kg load (package insert) may be accompanied by marked hypotension. In practice, reduced IV bolus doses of 12.5 to 25 mg are titrated to effect, followed by an infusion of 50 to 200 μg/kg/min. Transient hypotension during the loading phase may usually be managed with IV fluid or vasoconstrictors (phenylephrine).

(b) **Pharmacokinetics.** Esmolol is rapidly eliminated by a red blood cell esterase. After discontinuation of esmolol, most drug effects are eliminated within 5 min. The duration of esmolol action is not affected when plasma pseudocholinesterase is inhibited by echothiophate or physostigmine.

(c) **Adverse effects**

(i) Esmolol is a potent, selective β_1-receptor antagonist, and may cause hypotension through both vasodilation and negative inotropic effects.

(ii) Compared to nonselective β-blockers, esmolol is less likely to elicit bronchospasm, but should still be used with caution in patients with known bronchospastic disease.

(2) Verapamil

(a) **Dosing**

(i) IV load (adults): 5 to 15 mg, consider administering in 1- to 2 mg increments during surgery and anesthesia, or in unstable patients. Dose may be repeated after 30 min.

(ii) Maintenance IV: 5 to 15 mg/h.

(iii) PO (adults): 40 to 80 mg tid to qid (maximum 480 mg/day).

(iv) Pediatric dose: 75 to 200 μg/kg IV; may be repeated.

(b) **Pharmacokinetics.** Elimination occurs by hepatic metabolism, and plasma half-life is 3 to 10 h, so lengthy intervals (hours) between dose increments for IV infusions should be utilized to avoid cumulative effects.

(c) **Adverse effects**

(i) Verapamil blocks L-type calcium channels and may cause hypotension because of both peripheral vasodilation and negative inotropic effects, especially during the IV loading phase. The vasodilatory effects may be mitigated by administration of IV fluid or vasoconstrictors (i.e., phenylephrine). Patients with severe LV dysfunction may not tolerate IV verapamil, and may be better candidates for IV diltiazem (see later).

(ii) Verapamil (given chronically) reduces digoxin elimination and can raise digoxin levels, producing toxicity.

(3) Diltiazem

(a) **Dosing (adult)**

(i) IV loading: 20 mg IV over 2 min. May repeat after 15 min with 25 mg IV if HR exceeds 110 bpm. Smaller doses or longer loading periods may be used in patients who have myocardial ischemia, hemodynamic instability, or who are anesthetized.

(ii) Maintenance: Infusion at 5 to 15 mg/h, depending on HR control.

(iii) PO dose: 120 to 360 mg/day (sustained-release preparations are available).

(b) Pharmacokinetics. Metabolism is both hepatic (60%) and renal excretion (35%). Plasma elimination half-life is 3 to 5 h, so lengthy intervals (hours) between dose increases for IV infusions should be utilized to avoid cumulative effects.

(c) Adverse effects

(i) Diltiazem, like all calcium channel blockers, elicits vasodilation and may evoke hypotension. At the same time, partly due to its afterload reducing properties, IV diltiazem is less likely to compromise CO in patients with reduced LV function (relative to other AV nodal blockers) and is the drug of choice for rate control in this circumstance.

(ii) Sinus bradycardia is possible, so diltiazem should be used with caution in patients with sinus node dysfunction or those also receiving digoxin or β-blockers.

(4) High-dose IV magnesium sulfate

(a) Dosing. Regimens including a 2 to 2.5 g initial bolus, followed by a 1.75 g/h infusion, are described.

(b) Issues with use. High-dose magnesium is used rarely for SVT, but may nonetheless successfully provide rate control for patients with SVT. In some cases, rates of conversion to sinus rhythm exceeding placebo or antiarrhythmic agents have been noted. *The use of these high magnesium doses requires close monitoring of serum levels, and should be avoided in patients with renal insufficiency.* An increased requirement for temporary pacing due to the AV nodal blockade has also been noted. Magnesium potentiates neuromuscular blockers; thus, this agent can cause life-threatening hypoventilation in spontaneously breathing patients who have residual blood levels of these agents.

e. Cardioversion of SVT

(1) Limitations of pharmacologic or "chemical" cardioversion

(a) The 24-h rate of spontaneous conversion to sinus rhythm for recent-onset perioperative SVT exceeds 50%, and many patients who develop SVT under anesthesia will remit spontaneously within hours of emergence.

(b) Most of the antiarrhythmic agents with activity against atrial arrhythmias have limited efficacy when utilized in IV form for rapid chemical conversion. Although 50% to 80% efficacy rates are cited for many IV antiarrhythmics in uncontrolled studies, these findings are an artifact of high placebo rates of conversion (approximately 60% over 24 h). Although improved rates of chemical cardioversion are seen with high doses of IV amiodarone (approximately 2 g/day), the potential for undesirable side effects in the perioperative setting requires further study.

(c) Most agents have adverse effects, including negative inotropic effects or vasodilation (amiodarone, procainamide). In addition, these agents may provoke polymorphic ventricular arrhythmias (*Torsades de Pointes*). While less common with amiodarone, newer IV agents that exhibit high efficacy for converting atrial fibrillation (i.e., ibutilide) exhibit rates of torsades as high as 8%.

(2) Rationale for cardioversion. In the operating room, chemical cardioversion should be aimed mainly at patients who cannot tolerate (or do no respond to) IV rate control therapy, or who fail DC cardioversion and remain hemodynamically unstable. Intraoperative elective DC cardioversion in an otherwise stable patient with SVT also carries inherent risks (VF, asystole, and stroke). Moreover, the underlying factors provoking SVT during or shortly after surgery are likely to persist beyond the time of cardioversion, inviting recurrence. Hence, when elective DC cardioversion is considered, it may be prudent to first establish a therapeutic level of an antiarrhythmic agent that maintains sinus rhythm (i.e., procainamide, amiodarone), with a view to preventing SVT recurrence following electrical cardioversion. Guidelines for administration of IV procainamide and amiodarone are provided in an earlier section of this chapter (see Section VIII, C4).

f. **SVT prophylaxis for postoperative patients** [17,25]
SVT may occur during the days following surgery, and occurs within the first 4 postoperative days in up to 40% of cardiac surgeries. Many postoperative prophylaxis regimens have been evaluated, and are discussed in recent reviews. Prophylactic administration of a number of drugs typically used to slow AV nodal conduction (particularly β-blockers and amiodarone) may reduce the incidence of postoperative atrial fibrillation (particularly after cardiothoracic surgery), but by no means eliminate the problem. Nonetheless, antiarrhythmic prophylaxis should be considered in selected patients at high risk for hemodynamic or ischemic complications from postoperative SVT.

XI. Diuretics [26,35]

A. **Actions.** Most IV diuretics act at the loop of Henle in the kidney to block resorption of electrolytes from the tubule. Loop diuretics block the sodium-potassium-chloride transporter. Thiazide diuretics block the electroneutral sodium-chloride transporter. Amiloride and triamterene block apical (non–voltage-gated) sodium channels. Spironolactone binds and inhibits the mineralocorticoid receptor. This action increases excretion of water and electrolytes (Na, Cl, K, Ca, and Mg) from the body.

B. **Adverse effects**

1. Effect shared by all diuretics
   a. Cross-sensitivity with sulfonamides (except ethacrynic acid)
2. Effects shared by thiazides and loop diuretics
   a. Skin reactions
   b. Interstitial nephritis
   c. Hypokalemia
   d. Hypomagnesemia (effects of thiazides and loop diuretics are diminished by potassium-sparing diuretics such as spironolactone or triameterene)
   e. Risk of hyponatremia greater with thiazides than with loop diuretics
3. Effects specific to loop diuretics
   a. Increased serum uric acid
   b. Ototoxicity. Deafness, usually temporary, may occur with large drug doses or coadministration with an aminoglycoside antibiotic. One possible mechanism for this is drug-induced changes in endolymph electrolyte composition.
4. Effects of thiazide diuretics
   a. Hypercalcemia
   b. Hyperuricemia
   c. Mild metabolic alkalosis (“contraction” alkalosis)
   d. Hyperglycemia, glucose intolerance
   e. Hyperlipidemia
   f. Rare pancreatitits
5. Effects of potassium-sparing diuretics
   a. Hyperkalemia (sometimes with metabolic acidosis)
   b. Gynecomastia (with increased doses of spironolactone)
   c. Amiloride excreted by kidneys, so duration prolonged in renal failure

C. **Specific drugs**

1. **Loop diuretics**
   a. **Furosemide (Lasix)**
      (1) **Pharmacokinetics.** Renal tubular secretion of unchanged drug and of glucuronide metabolite. Half-life of 1.5 h

(2) **Clinical use**

(a) **Dosing**

(i) Adults: The usual oral dosing is 20–320 mg in 2 daily dose. The usual IV starting dose for patients not currently receiving diuretics is 2.5 to 5 mg, increasing as necessary to a 200 mg bolus. Patients already receiving diuretics usually require 20 to 40 mg initial doses to produce a diuresis. A continuous infusion (0.5 to 1 mg/kg/h) at approximately 0.05 mg/kg/h in adults produces a more sustained diuresis with a lower total daily dose compared with intermittent bolus dosing. Patients resistant to loop diuretics (e.g., after long-term dosing in hepatic failure) may benefit from combinations of furosemide and thiazide diuretics.

(ii) Pediatric: 1 mg/kg (maximum, 6 mg/kg). The pediatric infusion rate is 0.2 to 0.4 mg/kg/h.

(b) Because furosemide is a sulfonamide, allergic reactions may occur in sulfonamide-sensitive patients (rare).

(c) Furosemide often causes transient vasodilation of veins and arterioles, with reduced cardiac preload.

b. **Bumetanide (Bumex)**

(1) **Pharmacokinetics.** Combined renal and hepatic elimination. Half-life is 1 to 1.5 h.

(2) **Clinical use**

(a) **Dosing:** The usual oral dosing is 25–100 mg in 2 or 3 daily doses. 0.5 to 1 mg IV, may be repeated every 2 to 3 h to a maximum dose of 10 mg/day.

(b) Myalgias may occur.

c. **Ethacrynic acid (Edecrin)**

(1) **Pharmacokinetics.** Combined renal and hepatic elimination

(2) **Clinical use**

(a) **Dosing:** 50 mg IV (adult dose) or 0.5 to 1 mg/kg (maximum 100 mg) titrated to effect

(b) Usually is reserved for patients who fail to respond to furosemide or bumetanide, or who are allergic to sulfonamides (thiazides and furosemide are chemically related to sulfonamides)

2. **Thiazide diuretics**

a. **Mechanism/pharmacokinetics.** The mechanism of the antihypertensive effect of thiazide diuretics remains the subject of debate. All thiazides increase the urinary excretion of sodium and chloride, acting on the sodium-chloride symporter in the distal renal tubules.

b. **Clinical use and dosing** (Table 2.6)

3. **Potassium-sparing diuretics**

a. **Amiloride (Midamor)**

(1) **Mechanism/pharmacokinetics**

Amiloride works by inhibiting sodium channels in renal epithelium of the late distal tubule and collecting duct. This mildly increases the excretion of sodium and chloride. Amiloride decreases the lumen-negative voltage across the membrane, decreasing the excretion of K^+, H^+, Ca^{2+}, and Mg^{2+}. Amiloride has 15% to 25% oral bioavailability. It has a roughly 21-h half-life and is predominantly eliminated by the renal excretion of the intact drug.

(2) **Clinical use**

Amiloride is a weak diuretic, so it is almost never used as a sole agent, but most commonly in combination with other, stronger diuretics (such as thiazides or loop diuretics) to augment their diuretic and antihypertensive effects and reduce the risk of hypokalemia.

(a) **Dosing:** Usual dose is 5–10 mg/day in 1 or 2 doses added to a loop or thiazide diuretic. Doses more than 10 mg/day have rarely been given.

TABLE 2.6 Thiazides and related diuretics: dosages

	Daily oral dose	Frequency of dosage
Bendroflumethazide	2.5–10 mg	As single dose
Chlorothalidone	12.5–50 mg	As single dose
Chlorothiazide	125–500 mg	As single dose
Hydrochlorothiazide	12.5–50 mg	As single dose
Indapamide[a]	1.25–5 mg	As single dose
Metolazone[a]	1.25–5 mg	As single dose

[a]Not a thiazide but a sulfonamide qualitatively similar to thiazides.
Adapted from reference 26 Ives HE. Diuretic agents. In: Katzung BG, Master S, Treveor A eds. Basic and Clinical Pharmacology. 12th Ed. New York, NY: McGraw-Hill, 2012 and The Medical Letter vol 10, 113, Jan 2012.

(b) This agent is also available as a combination product with hydrochlorothiazide (Moduretic).

b. Eplerenone (Inspra)

(1) Mechanism/pharmacokinetics

This agent has the same mechanism of action as spironolactone and it is used for the same indications. It is an effective antihypertensive. It has been shown to prolong life in patients with LV dysfunction following myocardial infarction.

(2) Dosing: The drug is initiated at 25 mg/day and may be increased to 100 mg/day as tolerated by the patient.

c. Spironolactone (Aldactone)

(1) Mechanism/pharmacokinetics

Spironolactone is a competitive antagonist to the mineralocorticoid receptor found in the cytoplasm of epithelial cells in the late distal tubule and collecting duct. Thus, it opposes the actions of endogenous aldosterone. After binding the receptor, the aldosterone–receptor complex migrates to the cell nucleus, regulating production of a series of "aldosterone-induced proteins." The AIPs ultimately increase transepithelial sodium-chloride transport, and the lumen-negative transepithelial membrane potential, increasing the secretion of K^+ and H^+ into the tubular lumen. Spironolactone antagonizes these effects. Spironolactone has also been shown to inhibit the cardiac remodeling process and to prolong life in patients with chronic HF. The side effects of spironolactone include hyperkalemia and gynecomastia. Spironolactone has about a 65% oral bioavailability and a very short half-life. It has active metabolites with prolonged (16-h half-life) actions.

(2) Clinical use

Spironolactone is a weak diuretic, so it is almost never used as a sole agent, but most commonly in combination with other, stronger diuretics (such as thiazides or loop diuretics) to augment their diuretic and antihypertensive effects and reduce the risk of hypokalemia. Spironolactone prolongs life in patients with heart failure and is now part of standard therapy for symptomatic patients with this condition.

(a) Dosing: The usual dose is 12.5 to 25 mg/day, but this may be increased as needed up to 100 mg/day in 1 or 2 daily doses. This agent is also available as a combination product with hydrochlorothiazide (Aldactazide).

d. Triameterene

(1) Mechanism/pharmacokinetics

This agent is believed to have the same mechanism of action as amiloride and it is used for the same indications as amiloride. It is approximately one-tenth as potent as amiloride. Triamterene has 50% oral bioavailability and a half-life of roughly 4.5 h. It is eliminated through hepatic biotransformation to an active metabolite that is excreted in the urine.

(2) This agent is usually given in doses of 50 to 150 mg/day in one or two doses in combination with thiazide or loop diuretics. It is also found in a combination product with hydrochlorothiazide (Dyazide).

4. Osmotic diuretics

a. Mannitol

(1) Mechanism/pharmacokinetics. Mannitol is an osmotic diuretic that is eliminated unchanged in urine. It is also a free-radical scavenger.

(2) Clinical use

(a) Unlike the loop diuretics (e.g., furosemide), mannitol retains its efficacy even during low glomerular filtration states (e.g., shock).

(b) Diuresis with this agent may have protective effects in some clinical scenarios (i.e., CPB, poor renal perfusion, hemoglobinuria, or nephrotoxins), possibly related to free-radical scavenging.

(c) As an osmotically active agent in the bloodstream, it is sometimes used to reduce cerebral edema and ICP. Mannitol is administered routinely (as prophylaxis) by many clinicians during anesthesia for patients with intracranial mass lesions.

(3) Dosing: Initial dose is 12.5 g IV to a maximum of 0.5 g/kg.

(4) Adverse effects

(a) It may produce hypotension if administered as a rapid IV bolus.

(b) It may induce transient pulmonary edema as intravascular volume expands before diuresis begins.

ACKNOWLEDGMENTS

The current version of this chapter is based on the one in the previous edition, and the author acknowledges with thanks the important contributions of the coauthors of that previous version: Drs Jeffrey Balser and David Larach.

REFERENCES

1. *Physician's Desk Reference.* 65th ed. Montvale, NJ: Medical Economics Company, Inc.; 2011.
2. Epocrates: http://www.epocrates.com. (accessed 21 March 2012)
3. Brunton LL, Chabner B, Knollman B. *Goodman & Gilman's: The Pharmacological Basis of Therapeutics.* 12th ed. New York, NY: McGraw-Hill; 2011.
4. Drug Facts and Comparisons (www.factsandcomparisons.com) accessed 21 March 2012.
5. *The Medical Letter.* New Rochelle, NY: The Medical Letter, Inc. (www.medicalletter.org) accessed 21 March 2012.
6. Opie LH. Heart Physiology from Cell to Circulation. 4th Ed. Philadelphia, PA: Lippincott Williams & Wilkins; 2004.
7. Smith SC Jr, Benjamin EJ, Bonow RO, et al. World Heart Federation and the Preventive Cardiovascular Nurses Association. AHA/ACCF Secondary Prevention and Risk Reduction Therapy for Patients with Coronary and other Atherosclerotic Vascular Disease: 2011 update: A guideline from the American Heart Association and American College of Cardiology Foundation. *Circulation.* 2011;124(22):2458–2473.
8. Fraker TD Jr, Fihn SD, Gibbons RJ, et al. 2007 Chronic angina focused update of the ACC/AHA 2002 guidelines for the management of patients with chronic stable angina: A report of the American College of Cardiology/American Heart Association Task Force on Practice Guidelines Writing Group to develop the focused update of the 2002 guidelines for the management of patients with chronic stable angina. *Circulation.* 2007;116(23):2762–2772.
9. Kushner FG, Hand M, Smith SC Jr, et al. 2009 Focused updates: ACC/AHA guidelines for the management of patients with ST-elevation myocardial infarction (updating the 2004 guideline and 2007 focused update) and ACC/AHA/SCAI guidelines on percutaneous coronary intervention (updating the 2005 guideline and 2007 Focused Update): A report of the American College of Cardiology Foundation/American Heart Association Task Force on Practice Guidelines. *Circulation.* 2009;120(22):2271–2306.
10. Fleischmann KE, Beckman JA, Buller CE, et al. 2009 ACCF/AHA focused update on perioperative beta blockade. *J Am Coll Cardiol.* 2009;54(22):2102–2128.
11. Fernando HC, Jaklitsch MT, Walsh GL, et al. The society of thoracic surgeons practice guideline on the prophylaxis and management of atrial fibrillation associated with general thoracic surgery: Executive summary. *Ann Thorac Surg.* 2011;92(3):1144–1152.
12. Jessup M, Abraham WT, Casey DE, et al. 2009 Focused update: ACCF/AHA guidelines for the diagnosis and management of heart failure in adults: A report of the American College of Cardiology Foundation/American Heart Association Task

Force on Practice Guidelines: Developed in collaboration with the International Society for Heart and Lung Transplantation. *Circulation.* 2009;119(14):1977–2016.

13. Task Force for Diagnosis and Treatment of Acute and Chronic Heart Failure 2008 of European Society of Cardiology. ESC guidelines for the diagnosis and treatment of acute and chronic heart failure 2008: The Task Force for the Diagnosis and Treatment of Acute and Chronic Heart Failure 2008 of the European Society of Cardiology. Developed in collaboration with the Heart Failure Association of the ESC (HFA) and endorsed by the European Society of Intensive Care Medicine (ESICM). *Eur Heart J.* 2008;29(19):2388–2442.
14. Rosendorff C, Black HR, Cannon CP, et al. Treatment of hypertension in the prevention and management of ischemic heart disease: A scientific statement from the American Heart Association Council for High Blood Pressure Research and the Councils on Clinical Cardiology and Epidemiology and Prevention. *Circulation.* 2007;115(21):2761–2788.
15. Rabi DM, Daskalopoulou SS, Padwal RS, et al. The 2011 Canadian Hypertension Education Program recommendations for the management of hypertension: Blood pressure measurement, diagnosis, assessment of risk, and therapy. *Can J Cardiol.* 2011;27(4):415–433.e1-2.
16. Butterworth JF IV, Prielipp RC, MacGregor DA, et al. Pharmacologic cardiovascular support. In: Kvetan V, Dantzker DR, eds. *The Critically Ill Cardiac Patient: Multisystem Dysfunction and Management.* Philadelphia, PA: Lippincott-Raven; 1996:167–192.
17. Hazinski MF, Nolan JP, Billi JE, et al. Part 1: Executive summary: 2010 International consensus on cardiopulmonary resuscitation and emergency cardiovascular care science with treatment recommendations. *Circulation.* 2010;122(16 suppl 2): S250–S275.
18. Fellahi JL, Parienti JJ, Hanouz JL, et al. Perioperative use of dobutamine in cardiac surgery and adverse cardiac outcome: propensity-adjusted analyses. *Anesthesiology.* 2008;108(6):979–987.
19. Mebazaa A, Pitsis AA, Rudiger A, et al. Clinical review: Practical recommendations on the management of perioperative heart failure in cardiac surgery. *Crit Care.* 2010;14(2):201.
20. van den Born BJ, Beutler JJ, Gaillard CA, et al. Dutch guideline for the management of hypertensive crisis – 2010 revision. *Neth J Med.* 2011;69(5):248–255.
21. O'Connor CM, Starling RC, Hernandez AF, et al. Effect of nesiritide in patients with acute decompensated heart failure. *N Engl J Med.* 2011;365(1):32–43.
22. Sampson KJ, Kass RS. Antiarrhythmic drugs. Chapter 29. In: Brunton LL, Chabner B, Knollman B, eds. *Goodman & Gilman's: The Pharmacological Basis of Therapeutics.* 12th ed. New York, NY: McGraw-Hill; 2011.
23. Wann LS, Curtis AB, January CT, et al. 2011 ACCF/AHA/HRS focused update on the management of patients with atrial fibrillation (updating the 2006 guideline): A report of the American College of Cardiology Foundation/American Heart Association Task Force on Practice Guidelines. *Circulation.* 2011;123(1):104–123. Aug 2;124(5):e173.
24. Balser JR. Perioperative management of arrhythmias. In: Barash PG, Fleisher LA, Prough DS, eds. *Problems in Anesthesia.* Vol. 10. Philadelphia: Lippincott Williams & Wilkins 1998:201.
25. Reilly RF, Jackson EK. Regulation of renal function and vascular volume. Chapter 25. In: Brunton LL, Chabner B, Knollman B, eds. *Goodman & Gilman's: The Pharmacological Basis of Therapeutics.* 12th ed. New York, NY: McGraw-Hill; 2011.
26. Ives He. Diuretic agents. In: Katzung BG, Masters S, Treveor A, eds. *Basic and Clinical Pharmacology.* 12th Ed. New York, NY: McGraw-Hill; 2012.

II ANESTHETIC MANAGEMENT FOR CARDIAC SURGERY

3 The Cardiac Surgical Patient

Donald E. Martin and Charles E. Chambers

KEY POINTS

1. Inability to climb two flights of stairs showed a positive predictive value of 82% for postoperative pulmonary or cardiac complications.
2. Silent ischemia is more common in the elderly and diabetic patients, with 15% to 35% of all myocardial infarctions (MIs) occurring as silent events.
3. Isolated asymptomatic ventricular arrhythmias, even nonsustained ventricular tachycardia (VT), have not been associated with complications following noncardiac surgery.
4. Patients with left bundle branch block and especially with right coronary artery disease in whom a Swan-Ganz catheter is being placed may need availability of a transcutaneous pacemaker because of the risk of inducing right bundle branch block, and thus complete heart block, during passage of the pulmonary artery catheter.

(continued)

5. Hypertension with blood pressure lower than 180/110 has not been found to be an important predictor of increased perioperative cardiac risk, but it may be a marker for chronic cardiovascular disease.
6. The presence of carotid stenosis increases the risk of postoperative stroke from approximately 2% in patients without carotid stenosis to 10% with stenosis of greater than 50%, and to 11% to 19% with stenosis of >80%.
7. Selective use of pharmacologic perfusion imaging in only patients who have at least one of two clinical risk factors for ischemic disease (age >70 yrs and congestive heart failure) can maximize the usefulness of this procedure in predicting cardiac outcome.
8. PCI is not beneficial when used solely as a means to prepare a patient with coronary artery disease for surgery.
9. Elective surgery requiring interruption of anti-platelet therapy should not be scheduled within 1 month of bare metal stent (BMS) placement or within 12 months of drug eluting stent (DES) placement.
10. Angiotensin-converting enzyme (ACE) inhibitors and angiotensin II receptor blockers appear to cause perioperative hypotension, so it is prudent to hold these agents the morning of surgery but re-start them as soon as the patient is euvolemic postoperatively.

Cardiovascular disease is our society's number 1 health problem. According to the most recent CDC data, heart disease alone affects 26.8 million Americans, or about 12% of our population [1]. Of the 34 million Americans hospitalized in 2007, 3.9 million (11.5%) had heart disease. Heart disease remains the leading cause of death in patients greater than age 65, with an age adjusted death rate of 100 per 10,000, or 1%, per year. Furthermore, of the 45 million surgical procedures performed in the United States in 2007, approximately 6.9 million procedures involved the cardiovascular system. 405,000 were coronary artery bypass procedures, which represents a 13% decrease since 2003 and is associated with an increase in the number of percutaneous angioplasties and stents [2]. In contrast, the number of valve procedures has increased, with the number of valve repair procedures growing faster than the number of valve replacements [3]. The prime goals of preoperative evaluation and therapy for cardiac surgical procedures, therefore, are to quantify and reduce the patient's risk during surgery and the postoperative period.

The factors that are important in determining perioperative morbidity and anesthetic management must be assessed carefully for each patient.

I. Patient presentation

A. Clinical perioperative risk assessment—multifactorial risk indices

Multifactorial risk indices, which identify and assign relative importance to many potential risk factors, have become increasingly sophisticated over the last three decades and are used with increasing frequency to combine multiple risk factors into a single risk estimate, to determine an individual patient's risk of morbidity and mortality following heart surgery, to guide therapy, and to "risk adjust" the surgical outcomes of populations. One of the first multifactorial risk scores was developed by Paiement, in 1983 [4], and identified eight simple clinical risk factors:

1. poor left ventricular function
2. congestive heart failure
3. unstable angina or MI within 6 mos
4. age greater than 65 yrs
5. severe obesity
6. reoperation
7. emergency surgery
8. severe or uncontrolled systemic illness.

Recent models still incorporate many of these eight factors.

The preoperative clinical factors that affect hospital survival following heart surgery have been studied by multiple authors from the 1990s until the present time [3,5–9]. The initial studies focused on coronary artery bypass grafting (CABG) surgery, but more recent indices have been validated for valvular surgery and combined valve and CABG surgery as well.

The most important risk factors in these studies are compared in Table 3.1. The earlier indices assigned "point values" to indicate the relative risk of postoperative mortality associated with each preoperative risk factor, usually based on multivariate analysis. More recent studies provide more specific odds ratios of mortality associated with each of a larger number of predictors.

In 2001, Dupuis and colleagues developed and validated the cardiac risk evaluation (CARE) score, which incorporated similar factors but viewed them more intuitively in a manner similar to American Society of Anesthesiologists (ASA) physical status (Table 3.2) [9]. In 2004, Ouattara and colleagues [11] compared the CARE score to two other multifactorial indices, the Tu score [12] and Euroscore [5]. Their analysis found no difference among these scores in predicting mortality and morbidity following cardiac surgery at that time. However, in recent years the Society of Thoracic Surgeons continues to report more specific predictors and is updated annually to provide valuable risk data on CABG, valve, and combined procedures based on increasing volumes of cumulative data, making this perhaps the most robust of the risk indices.

B. **Functional status.** For patients undergoing most general and cardiac surgical procedures, perhaps the simplest and single most useful risk index is the patient's functional status, or
1 exercise tolerance. In major noncardiac surgery, Girish and colleagues found the inability to climb two flights of stairs showed a positive predictive value of 82% for postoperative pulmonary or cardiac complications [13]. This is an easily measured and sensitive index of cardiovascular risk, which takes into account a wide range of specific cardiac and noncardiac factors.

The level of exercise producing symptoms, as described classically by the New York Heart Association and Canadian Cardiovascular Society classifications, predicts the risk of both an ischemic event and operative mortality. During coronary revascularization procedures, operative mortality for patients with class IV symptoms is 1.4 times that of patients without preoperative congestive heart failure [14].

C. **Genomic contributions to cardiac risk assessment.** Genetic variations are the known basis for more than 40 cardiovascular disorders. Some of these, including familial hypercholesteremia, hypertrophic cardiomyopathy, dilated cardiomyopathy, and "channelopathies" such as the long QT syndrome, are known as monogenetic disorders, caused by alterations in one gene. These usually follow traditional Mendelian inheritance patterns, and their genetic basis is relatively easy to identify. Genetic testing is able to identify these diseases in up to 90% of patients before they become symptomatic, allowing prophylactic treatment and early therapy. For example, genetic identification of the sub-type of long QT syndrome can determine an affected patient's risk of dysrhythmias associated with exercise, benefit from β-blockers, or need for Implantable Cardioverter Defibrillator (ICD) implantation [15].

Some of the areas of the greatest expansion of genomic medicine, however, are in its application to chronic diseases such as coronary artery and vascular disease. However, the causes of these disorders are multi-factorial, including environmental as well as genetic factors, and are at best due to complex interactions of many genes. Nevertheless, genetic information can be used to determine a patient's susceptibility to disease, and this information can guide prophylactic therapy. Commercial tests are currently available for susceptibility to atrial fibrillation (AF) and MI. Genetic variants have been found which help to determine susceptibility to preoperative complications, including 4 which help to determine susceptibility to postoperative MI and ischemia. Similarly, genetic information may be used to determine variations in patient susceptibility to drugs, as for example a single allele variation can render patients

TABLE 3.1 Multifactorial indices of cardiovascular risk for cardiac surgical procedures: summary of risk factors in recent multifactorial indices

Risk factor	Euro score (Nashef et al.) (1999[a])[16]	Bernstein et al. (2000[b])	New York State model (Hannan et al.) (2000[c])	New York State model (Hannan et al.) (2000[c])	Society of Thoracic Surg. risk model for mortality (2009[d])	Society of Thoracic Surg. risk model for mortality (2009[e])	Society of Thoracic Surg. risk model (2009[f])
Surgical procedure(s) studied	CABG/ combination	CABG/Valve/ combination	Isolated aortic valve Replacement	Multiple valve replacement plus CABG	CABG	Isolated aortic valve replacement	Valve plus CABG
Measure of risk assessment	Risk score (Points)	Risk score (Points)	Odds ratio	Odds ratio	Odds ratio	Odds ratio	Odds ratio
Age	1	2.5–11	1.06	1.05	1.36–4.7	1.43–3.34	1.29–3.95
Surgical procedure	2–3	0–6	N/A	N/A	N/A	N/A	N/A
Cardiac factors							
Previous cardiac operation	3	10–20	N/A	N/A	3.13–4.19	2.11–2.48	2.2–2.46
Urgency of surgery	2	N/A	N/A	N/A	1.16–8	1.29–7.94	1.25–4.56
Left main disease or multiple vessel disease	N/A	2.5	N/A	N/A	1.17	1.19	1.12
Structural defect—LV aneurysm, VSD, ASD, acute mitral regurgitation	4	1.5–12	N/A	N/A	1.31	N/A	N/A
Severity of angina	2	N/A	N/A	N/A	1.12	1.21	1.11
Previous MI	2	4	N/A	N/A	1.37–1.7	1.14	1.19–1.55
Cardiogenic shock	3	12	3.97–8.68	N/A	1.41–2.29	1.47–1.62	1.43–1.68
Congestive heart failure	N/A	2.5	2.26	2.18	1.21–1.39	1.29–1.83	0.91–1.48
Decreased LV EF	1–3	6.5–8	N/A	N/A	1.19–6.0	1.09–5	1.1–5.5
Supra-ventricular arrhythmias	N/A	N/A	N/A	N/A	1.36	1.2	1.2
Ventricular arrhythmias	3	1	N/A	2.62	N/A	N/A	N/A
Pulmonary hypertension	2	11	2.35	N/A	N/A	N/A	N/A
Endocarditis	3	6.5	N/A	N/A	N/A	1.95	2.04

Systemic factors							
Hypertension	N/A	3	N/A	N/A	N/A	1.12	N/A
Cerebrovascular disease	2	2	N/A	N/A	1.14–1.31	N/A	1.0–1.22
PVD	2	0.5–3.5	1.96	2.13–3.55	1.42	1.25	1.29
Chronic obstructive pulmonary disease	1	6	N/A	N/A	1.22–2.35	1.27	1.19
Diabetes mellitus	N/A	3	2.52	1.87	1.01–1.3	1.27–1.62	1.12–1.31
Hepatic disease	N/A	12.5	N/A	N/A	N/A	N/A	N/A
Renal insufficiency	2	3.5–13.5	5.51	3.55–9.37	1.66–3.84	1.55–2.85	1.57–3.20
Anemia	N/A	N/A	N/A	N/A	N/A	N/A	N/A
Albumin <4	N/A	N/A	N/A	N/A	N/A	N/A	N/A
Female gender	1	6	N/A	N/A	1.31	1.23	1.36
High or low body mass index	N/A	1	N/A	N/A	1.6–2.2	0.98–1.75	1.04–1.58
Other factors	Neurologic dysfunction 2	Preoperative Endotracheal tube 4 Idiopathic thrombocytopenic purpura 12 Prior angioplasty Failure 5.5 Substance abuse 4.5			Immunosupressive treatment 1.48	Immunosupressive treatment 1.42 Co-existing mitral stenosis 1.24	Additional valve disease 1.10–1.27 Immunosuppressive therapy 1.35
Total risk score	39	97	N/A	N/A	N/A	N/A	N/A

CABG, coronary artery bypass grafting; LV, left ventricle; VSD, ventricular septal defect; ASD, atrial septal defect; MI, myocardial infarction; LVEF, left ventricular ejection fraction; PVD, peripheral vascular disease; N/A, not applicable (either not included in this risk index or not significant); the various studies quantify severity of each risk factor in different ways, so a range of values indicates the range of relative risk for all levels of severity

[a]Nashef SA, Roques F, Michael P, et al. European system for cardiac operation risk evaluation (Euroscore). *Eur J Cardiothoracic Surgery.* 1999;16:9–13.

[b]Bernstein AD, Parsonnet V: Bedside estimation of risk as an aid for decision-making in cardiac surgery. *Ann Thorac Surg.* 2000;69:823–828.

[c]Hannan EL, Racz MJ, Jones RH: Predictors of mortality for patients undergoing cardiac valve replacements in New York state. *Ann Thorac Surg.* 2000;70:1212–1218.

[d]Shahian DM, O'Brien SM, Filardo G, et al.: The Society of Thoracic Surgeons 2008 cardiac surgery risk models: part I—coronary artery bypass grafting surgery. *Ann Thorac Surg.* 2009;88:S2–S22.

[e]O'Brien SM, Shahian DM, Filardo G, et al.: The Society of Thoracic Surgeons 2008 cardiac surgery risk models: part 2—isolated valve surgery. *Ann Thorac Surg.* 2009;88:S23–S42.

[f]Shahian DM, O'Brien SM, Filardo G, et al.: The Society of Thoracic Surgeons 2008 cardiac surgery risk models: part 3—valve plus coronary artery bypass grafting surgery. *Ann Thorac Surg.* 2009;88:S43–S62.

TABLE 3.2 Cardiac anesthesia risk evaluation (CARE)

	Risk factor present in three categories		
Risk score	**Cardiac disease**	**Systemic medical disease**	**Surgery**
1	Stable	None	Noncomplex
2	Stable	Controlled	Noncomplex
3	Unstable cardiac disease	(and/or) Uncontrolled medical problem	(or) Complex surgery[a]
4	Unstable cardiac disease	(and/or) Uncontrolled medical problem	(and) Complex surgery[a]
5	Chronic or advanced cardiac disease—surgery undertaken as last hope		
E	Emergency: surgery undertaken as soon as diagnosis made and facilities available		

[a]Complex surgery: examples include reoperation, multiple valve or combined valve/coronary artery bypass grafting (CABG) surgery, left ventricular aneurysmectomy, CABG of diffuse or calcified disease.
DuPuis J, Wang F, Nathan H, et al. The cardiac anesthesia risk evaluation score: a clinically useful predictor of mortality and morbidity after cardiac surgery. *Anesthesiology* 2001;94:194–204, with permission.

much more susceptible to warfarin. Gene therapy may also target drug delivery to specific tissues [15].

D. Risk associated with surgical problems and procedures. The complexity of the surgical procedure itself may be the most important predictor of perioperative morbidity for many patients. Most, but not all, cardiac surgical procedures include the risks associated with cardiopulmonary bypass. Any procedure requiring cardiopulmonary bypass is associated with greater morbidity, caused by a systemic inflammatory response along with the risk of microemboli and hypoperfusion and most often involving the central nervous system, kidneys, lungs, and gastrointestinal tract. The extent of morbidity increases with the increased bypass duration.

Procedures on multiple heart valves, or on both the aortic valve and coronary arteries, carry a statistical morbidity much higher than that for procedures involving only a single valve or CABG alone. The mortality rate over the last decade for each procedure, for patients in the Society of Thoracic Surgeons database, is approximately 2.3% for CABG, 3.4% for isolated valve procedures, and 6.8% for valve procedures along with CABG [3,14,16].

II. Preoperative medical management of cardiovascular disease

A. Myocardial ischemia. In patients with known CAD, the most important risk factors that need to be assessed preoperatively are: (i) the amount of myocardium at risk; (ii) the ischemic threshold, or the heart rate at which ischemia occurs; (iii) the patient's ventricular function or ejection fraction (EF); (iv) the stability of symptoms, because recent acceleration of angina may reflect a ruptured coronary plaque; and (v) adequacy of current medical therapy.

1. **Stable coronary syndrome (stable angina pectoris).** Chronic stable angina most often results from obstruction to coronary artery blood flow by a fixed atherosclerotic coronary lesion in at least one of the large epicardial arteries. In the absence of such a lesion, however, the myocardium may be rendered ischemic by coronary artery spasm, vasculitis, trauma, or hypertrophy of the ventricular muscle, as occurs in aortic valve disease.

   Neither the location, duration, or severity of angina, nor the presence of diabetes or peripheral vascular disease (PVD), indicate the extent of myocardium at risk, or the anatomic location of the coronary artery lesions. Therefore, the clinician must depend on diagnostic studies, such as myocardial perfusion imaging (MPI), stress echocardiography, and cardiac catheterization to assist in establishing risk. Though some centers use cardiac computed tomography (CT) scanning for this purpose, and though it does have a high sensitivity for detecting coronary calcification and coronary artery disease, it currently still has a low specificity, so it cannot yet be recommended as a definitive test. In patients with chronic stable angina, a reproducible amount of exercise, with its associated increases in heart rate and blood pressure, often precipitates angina. This *angina threshold,* which can be determined on preoperative exercise testing, is an important guide to perioperative hemodynamic management. Stable angina often responds to medical therapy as well as to PCI. Patients are referred for CABG surgery when refractory to medical therapy and not candidates for PCI.

a. Principles of the medical management of stable angina [17]

- **(1)** aspirin at 75 to 162 mg daily
- **(2)** β-blockade as initial therapy when not contraindicated
- **(3)** calcium antagonists or long-acting nitrates as second-line therapy, or as first-line therapy when beta blockade is contraindicated
- **(4)** use of ACE inhibitors indefinitely in patients with left ventricle (LV) EF <40%, diabetes, hypertension, or chronic renal failure
- **(5)** annual influenza vaccine
- **(6)** reducing risk by:
  - **(a)** Lipid management—reduce low density lipoproteins to <100 mg/dL using diet, exercise, and statin therapy.
  - **(b)** Blood pressure control—reduce to less than 140/90 or to less than 130/80 for patients with diabetes or kidney disease, for patients with coronary disease initially treating with β-blockers and ACE inhibitors.
  - **(c)** Smoking cessation
  - **(d)** Diabetes control
  - **(e)** Weight loss
  - **(f)** Diet and exercise

2. Acute coronary syndrome (unstable angina pectoris). Sometimes called crescendo angina, or unstable coronary syndrome, this symptom complex usually presents as:

a. Rest angina, within the first week of onset

b. New onset angina markedly limiting activity, within 2 wks of onset

c. Angina which is more frequent, of longer duration, or occurs with less exercise.

These symptoms often indicate rapid growth, rupture, or embolus of an existing plaque. Patients in this category have a higher incidence of MI and sudden death, and increased incidence of left main occlusion. The clinical factors important in determining the risk of MI or death in patients with unstable angina are shown in Table 3.3.

d. Medical management for acute coronary syndrome. Diagnostic and revascularization procedures are the central parts of the management for most patients with acute coronary syndrome. However, they are often accompanied or preceded by medical therapy. The medical management of unstable angina or of a non-ST segment elevation MI has two parts: (i) anti-ischemic therapy and (ii) antiplatelet and anticoagulant therapy. Medical anti-ischemic therapy depends largely on the presence or absence of ongoing ischemia and must be accompanied by an aggressive approach to secondary prevention or risk factor modification (Table 3.4 and Table 3.5).

3. Myocardial ischemia without angina may be manifested by fatigue, rapid onset of pulmonary edema, cardiac arrhythmias, syncope, or an "anginal equivalent," most often characterized as indigestion or jaw pain. Silent ischemia is more common in the elderly and diabetic patients, with 15% to 35% of all MIs occurring as silent events, documented only on routine electrocardiogram (ECG). Whether related to coexisting disease or delayed therapy, silent ischemia has been associated with an unfavorable prognosis.

4. Prior MI interval between prior infarction and surgery.
In the non-cardiac surgical population, the occurrence of an MI within the 30 d before surgery is a significant preoperative risk factor [10]. Bernstein [6] assigns additional risk

TABLE 3.3 Risk factors for death or MI in patients with unstable angina

	High risk	Intermediate risk	Low risk
	Any one of the following	**No high-risk factors, but any of the following**	**No high- or intermediate-risk factors, but any of the following**
History	Accelerated angina within 48 hrs	Prior MI, CVD, PVD, CABG. Aspirin use	
Angina	Prolonged rest angina (>20 min)	Prolonged (>20 min) rest pain, now resolved, with risk factors Rest angina relieved with NTG Nocturnal angina New onset or progressive class III or IV angina within 2 wks	Increased angina frequency, severity, duration Lower angina threshold New onset angina
Clinical findings	Pulmonary edema New or worsening MR murmur, S3, rales, hypotension, bradycardia, tachycardia, age > 70 yrs	Age > 70 yrs	
EKG	Angina at rest with transient >0.5 mm ST changes Bundle branch block or new sustained VT	T-wave changes Pathological Q waves or resting ST-depression less than 1 mm in multiple lead groups	Normal or unchanged EKG
Cardiac markers	Elevated cardiac TnT, TnI (>0.1 ng/ml), or CK-MB elevated	Slightly elevated cardiac TnT, TnI, (>0.01 but <0.1 ng/mL) or elevated CK-MB	Normal

CABG, coronary artery bypass grafting; CK-MB, creatine kinase-MB fraction; CVD, cerebrovascular disease, MI, myocardial infarction, MR, mitral regurgitation; NTG, nitroglycerin; PVD, peripheral vascular disease; TnI, troponin I, TnT, troponin T; VT, ventricular tachycardia.

Data from, Anderson JL, Adams CD, Antman EM, et al.: 2011 ACCF/AHA focused update incorporated into the ACC/AHA 2007 guidelines for the management of patients with unstable angina/non-ST-elevation myocardial infarction: a report of the American College of Cardiology Foundation/American Heart Association task force on practice guidelines. *Circulation* 2011; 123:e426-e579 accessed 8-2-11 at http://circ.ahajournals.org/content/123/18/e436.full.pdf with permission.

to an MI occurring 48 hrs before surgery and Eagle et al. [18] conclude that CABG has increased risk in patients with unstable angina, early postinfarction angina (within 2 days of a non-ST-Elevation Myocardial Infarction (non-STEMI) and during an acute MI), and that risk may be reduced by delaying CABG for 3 to 7 days after MI in stable patients. Coronary revascularization procedures, however, offer improved survival in patients with unstable angina and LV dysfunction.

B. Congestive heart failure

1. **Clinical assessment and medical management of heart failure.** Ventricular dysfunction can occur almost immediately in association with an ischemic event. If no infarction occurs and the myocardium is reperfused, the ventricle recovers function quickly. Short episodes of ischemia followed by reperfusion may actually precondition the heart, so when it is exposed to more severe ischemia, the size and severity of MI is reduced. A MI may be associated with "stunned" myocardium, which recovers function within days to weeks, or "hibernating" myocardium, which may recover months after infarction and revascularization. Ventricular dysfunction and heart failure have been classified into four stages, A through D, based on cardiac structural changes and symptoms of heart failure. Management depends on the stage of the disease. ACE inhibitors and angiotensin II receptor blockers are usually used as first-line therapy, with the addition of β-blockers, aldosterone antagonists, diuretics, and implanted devices for more severely affected patients (Fig. 3.1).
2. **Perioperative morbidity.** Evidence of congestive heart failure or ventricular dysfunction preoperatively is associated with an increased operative mortality. Recent series summarized

TABLE 3.4 Medical therapy for unstable angina: anti-ischemic therapy

Ongoing ischemia or high-risk factors[a]	Without ongoing ischemia or high-risk factors[a]
β-blockers in the absence of contraindications[b]	β-blockers in the absence of contraindications[b]
ACE inhibitors in any patients, especially for those with LV dysfunction (EF < 40%), heart failure, hypertension or diabetes mellitus	ACE inhibitors in any patients, especially for those with LV dysfunction (EF < 40%), heart failure, hypertension or diabetes mellitus
Angiotensin receptor blockers for those patients with LV dysfunction and heart failure intolerant to ACE inhibitors	Angiotensin receptor blockers for those patients with LV dysfunction and heart failure intolerant to ACE inhibitors
Aldosterone receptor blockers for those patients without renal dysfunction or hyperkalemia already receiving ACE inhibitors with LV dysfunction, heart failure, or diabetes mellitus	Aldosterone receptor blockers for those patients without renal dysfunction or hyperkalemia already receiving ACE inhibitors with LV dysfunction, heart failure, or diabetes mellitus
Nitrates	
Nondihydropyridine calcium antagonists (verapamil or diltiazem) when β-blockers cannot be used	

[a]EKG changes, or ischemia associated with CHF, S_3 gallop, mitral regurgitation, hemodynamic instability, EF less than 40%, malignant ventricular arrhythmias.
[b]Contraindications to β-blocker therapy:

1. Marked first-degree AV blocks (EKG PR interval >0.24 s)
2. Any second- or third-degree AV block without a pacemaker
3. Asthma
4. Severe LV dysfunction with CHF (may require slowly increasing doses)
5. COPD: β-Blockers may be used cautiously, beginning with low doses of β-1 selective agents
6. Patients should not receive β-blockers during episodes of bradycardia (HR <50) or hypotension

LV, left ventricular; EF, ejection fraction; ACE, angiotensin converting enzyme; AV, atrio-ventricular; CHF, congestive heart failure; COPD, chronic obstructive pulmonary disease.
Adapted from Anderson JL, Adams CD, Antman EM, et al.: 2011 ACCF/AHA focused update incorporated into the ACC/AHA 2007 guidelines for the management of patients with unstable angina/non-ST-elevation myocardial infarction: a report of the American College of Cardiology Foundation/American Heart Association task force on practice guidelines. *Circulation* 2011; 123:e426-e579 accessed 8-2-11 at http://circ.ahajournals.org/content/123/18/e436.full.pdf with permission.

in Table 3.1 show a 1.5- to 2.5-fold greater risk of postoperative morbidity or mortality in patients with preoperative congestive heart failure, and a 1.4- to 12-fold greater risk in patients with preoperative cardiogenic shock.

In patients undergoing aortic valve replacement (AVR) for critical aortic stenosis and depressed EF, a cardiothoracic ratio of ≥0.6 is possibly the most important predictor of operative mortality, increasing the risk in some series more than 10-fold.

TABLE 3.5 Medical therapy for unstable angina and non-ST elevation MI: antiplatelet and anticoagulation therapy

Medical management without stenting	Medical management and BMS	Medical management and DES
Aspirin—75–162 mg daily indefinitely	Aspirin—162–325 mg daily for 1 month then 75–162 mg daily indefinitely	Aspirin—162–325 mg daily for 3–6 months then 75–162 mg daily indefinitely
Clopidogrel 75 mg daily for 1 month to 1 year	Clopidogrel 75 mg daily for 1 month to 1 year	Clopidogrel 75 mg daily for at least 1 year

Warfarin to maintain an INR of 2.0–2.5 along with aspirin indicated for patients requiring anticoagulation for other reasons or for those with high coronary artery disease risk and low bleeding risk who do not tolerate clopidogrel
Adapted from Anderson JL, Adams CD, Antman EM, et al.: 2011 ACCF/AHA focused update incorporated into the ACC/AHA 2007 guidelines for the management of patients with unstable angina/non-ST-elevation myocardial infarction: a report of the American College of Cardiology Foundation/American Heart Association task force on practice guidelines. *Circulation* 2011; 123:e426-e579 accessed 8-2-11 at http://circ.ahajournals.org/content/123/18/e436.full.pdf with permission.

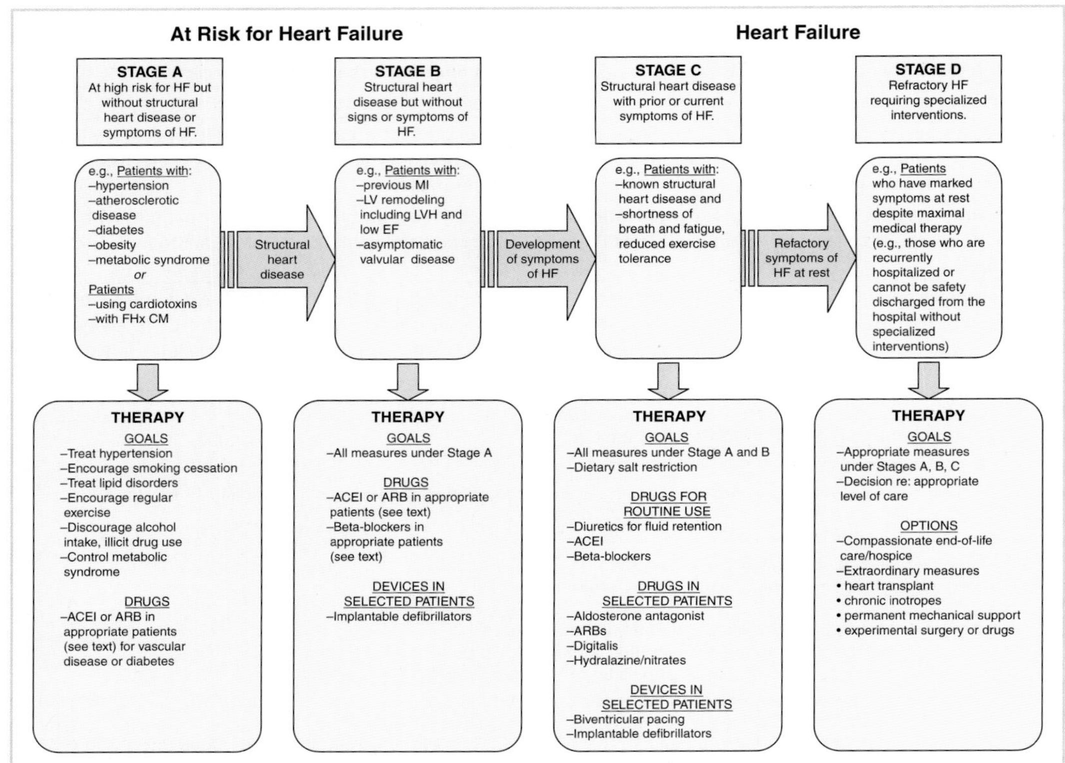

FIGURE 3.1 Functional classification and stages in the development of heart failure, and medical management of each stage. ACEI, angiotensin-converting enzyme inhibitor; ARB, angiotensin II receptor blocker; EF, ejection fraction; FHx CM, family history of cardiomyopathy; HF, heart failure; LV, left ventricular; LVH, left ventricular hypertrophy; and MI, myocardial infarction. [From Hunt SA, Abraham WT, Marshall HC, et al. 2009 Focused update incorporated into the ACC/AHA 2005 guideline update for the diagnosis and management of heart failure in adults: a report of the American College of Cardiology/American Heart Association Task Force on Practice Guidelines (Writing committee to update the 2001 guidelines for the evaluation and management of heart failure). *Circulation* 2009;119:e391–e479]

C. Dysrhythmias

1. **Incidence.** Cardiac dysrhythmias are common in patients presenting for cardiac surgery, and become increasingly common with age after 50. In the perioperative period, abnormal rhythms occur in more than 75% of patients. However, those dysrhythmias are life-threatening in less than 1%.
2. **Supraventricular tachycardia (SVT).** SVTs appear most often in the preoperative history as palpitations or near-syncope. AF and flutter, the most common SVTs, increase in frequency with age and in association with organic heart disease. Preoperative patients with SVT who are hemodynamically stable are usually managed acutely with vagal maneuvers, adenosine, verapamil, or diltiazem to reduce heart rate and potentially convert the SVT back to sinus rhythm. Those with AF are in addition managed with anticoagulation to reduce stroke risk. However, in the last two decades, either surgical or catheter-based ablation have become more common, especially in patients unresponsive to medical therapy or in whom there may be structural abnormalities.

3. **Ablation therapy**
   Catheter ablation using radiofrequency (RF) energy was first used in 1982. Medication can often control atrioventricular (AV) nodal reentrant tachycardia, However, when medications are ineffective, RF ablation can be performed. This procedure has a 97% success rate, 5% recurrence rate during the patient's lifetime, and causes heart block requiring pacer therapy in 0.5% to 1% of patients in which it is used [19].

   AF is the most frequent supraventricular arrhythmia. It can be caused by multiple reentrant circuits and also by a single focus in the SVC or pulmonary veins. Antiarrhythmic drugs can maintain sinus rhythm in one-half to two-third of patients with AF but may reduce the quality of life, decrease left ventricular function, and increase the risk of embolic complications.

   The Maze procedure is a surgical procedure which disrupts the re-entrant pathways or ablates arrhythmogenic foci in the atria, often by isolating the ostia of the pulmonary veins. Thereby it converts the fibrillation to sinus rhythm, reducing the need for anticoagulation. However, this procedure is not always successful, and therefore a second type of procedure ablates the AV node, isolating the fibrillating atria from the ventricles, without attempting to prevent the AF itself. This procedure requires a permanent pacemaker to drive the ventricles, as well as ongoing anticoagulation to prevent thrombosis in the fibrillating atria.

   The Atrial Fibrillation Follow-up Investigation of Rhythm Management (AFFIRM) investigated the relative benefits of simple AF rate control versus conversion to sinus rhythm in patients older than age 65 [20]. Though the two treatments led to no difference in major bleeding, death, stroke, or quality of life, antiarrhythmic therapy and catheter ablation were recommended in symptomatic individuals in whom the arrhythmia interferes with their regular activities. A worldwide AF ablation survey reported 4550 of 8745 patients (52%) in sinus rhythm after ablation alone. With drug therapy, they reported a 75.9% success rate [21].
4. **Ventricular arrhythmias and VT.** Ventricular dysrhythmias have been classified according to clinical presentation (stable or unstable), type of rhythm (sustained or nonsustained VT, bundle-branch re-entrant or bidirectional VT, Torsades de pointes, ventricular flutter or fibrillation), or associated disease entity. Ventricular arrhythmias may lead directly to ventricular fibrillation and sudden cardiac death, especially if they
   3 occur in the setting of acute or recent infarction. However, isolated asymptomatic ventricular arrhythmias, even nonsustained VT, have not been associated with complications following noncardiac surgery. Patients with preoperative ventricular arrhythmias associated with left ventricular dysfunction and an EF < 30% to 35% are often managed with the prophylactic implantation of an ICD. Those not controlled with or not candidates for ICD therapy are managed medically with β-blockers as the first-line therapy. Amiodarone is the second-line drug used to prevent sudden cardiac death, with studies showing some survival benefit, and sotalol can also be effective though with greater proarrhythmic effects [22].
5. **Bradycardia.** Anesthetics frequently affect sinus node automaticity but rarely cause complete heart block. Asymptomatic patients with ECG-documented AV conduction disease (PR prolongation or single or bifascicular bundle branch block) rarely require temporary pacing perioperatively. However, symptomatic patients, or patients with Mobitz II or complete heart block, require preoperative evaluation for permanent pacing. Patients with a recent MI or with both first-degree AV block and bundle branch block may need temporary transvenous or transcutaneous pacing perioperatively (See Chapter 17—"Rhythm Management Devices").

   4 Patients with left bundle branch block in whom a Swan-Ganz catheter is being placed may need availability of a transcutaneous pacemaker because of the risk of inducing right bundle branch block, and thus complete heart block, during passage of the pulmonary artery catheter. Patients with a left bundle branch block and right CAD may be at particular risk during the passage of a Swan-Ganz catheter.

Patients with an indwelling cardiac pacemaker or ICD need to have their device identified and evaluated preoperatively. Special precautions need to be considered, as outlined in Chapter 17, to prevent untoward effects of electromagnetic interference in the operating room.

D. **Hypertension**

Systemic hypertension is one of the most common diseases of adulthood and is perhaps the most treatable cause of cardiovascular morbidity, including MI, stroke, PVD, renal failure, and heart failure. The contribution of hypertension to perioperative morbidity and the implications for anesthetic management depend on (i) blood pressure level, both with stress and at rest; (ii) the etiology of hypertension; (iii) pre-existing complications of hypertension; and (iv) physiologic changes due to drug therapy.

1. **Blood pressure level.** Data summarized in the JNC VII report in 2003 indicate that cardiovascular risk begins to increase at blood pressures above 115/75 and doubles with each increment of 20/10. Patients with blood pressures of 120–139/80–89 are considered prehypertensive and require drug therapy if they have associated diabetes or renal disease. Patients with blood pressures of 140–159/90–99 are considered hypertensive and all require chronic drug therapy. Those with blood pressures greater than 160/100, classified as stage 2 hypertensive, usually require combination drug therapy. Further, for patients older than 50 yrs, systolic blood pressure >140 is a much more important cardiovascular risk factor than diastolic blood pressure [23].

   In contrast to the usual emphasis on the resting, unstimulated blood pressure in determining chronic medical management, preoperatively the patient's blood pressure under stress, as in the preoperative clinic or holding area, may be a better predictor of their perioperative morbidity. Intraoperative cardiac morbidity in the form of dysrhythmias and ischemic ECG changes may be more frequent in Stage 3 hypertensive patients with awake systolic blood pressures greater than 180 mm Hg and diastolic blood pressures of greater than 110 mm Hg, and this morbidity may be reduced by preoperative treatment. In these patients the benefits of improving hypertensive control preoperatively should be weighed
   5 against the risks of delaying surgery. Blood pressure lower than 180/110 has not been found to be an important predictor of increased perioperative cardiac risk, but it may be a marker for chronic cardiovascular disease [10].

2. **Etiology.** The most common "primary" or "essential" hypertension is likely caused by a combination of multiple genetic and environmental factors, with the genetic contribution, at least, being irreversible. However, it is important preoperatively to exclude the 5% to 15% of patients with treatable causes of secondary hypertension, especially patients shown in Table 3.6. Common causes of secondary hypertension are usually renal, endocrine, or drug related, which account for an additional 5% to 10% of hypertensive patients. Other rare disorders are found in less than 1% of patients (Table 3.7). A laboratory investigation of secondary hypertension, when indicated, should include urinalysis, creatinine, glucose, electrolytes, calcium, EKG, and chest films. More extensive testing is usually not indicated unless blood pressure cannot be controlled or a high clinical suspicion exists [23]. Pheochromocytoma, although very rare, is particularly important because of its potential morbidity in association with anesthesia. Therefore, it should be ruled out preoperatively in patients with headache, labile or paroxysmal hypertension, abnormal pallor, or perspiration, even if delay of surgery is required.

TABLE 3.6 Risk factors for secondary hypertension
• Blood pressure not controlled by two or more agents
• Increase in previously well controlled blood pressure
• Sudden onset, labile, or paroxysmal hypertension
• Hypertension with onset before age 25 or after age 50

TABLE 3.7 Causes of hypertension

Medical cause (incidence)	Drug-induced hypertension
Essential hypertension (85%–95%)	Amphetamines Caffeine
Common causes of secondary hypertension	Cocaine
Renal (2%–6%)	Chlorpromazine
Renal parenchymal disease	Cyclosporine
Renovascular disease	Erythropoietin
Endocrine (1%–2%)	Ethanol
Pheochromocytoma	Licorice
Cushing disease	MAO inhibitors
Thyroid or parathyroid disease	Nicotine
Hyperaldosteronism	NSAIDs
Aortic coarctation (2%–5%)	Oral contraceptives
Sleep apnea (1%)	Steroids
Rare causes of secondary hypertension	Sympathomimetics
Renin-producing tumors	Nasal decongestants
Adrenogenital syndrome	Weight loss regimens
Acromegaly	
Hypercalcemia	
Familial dysautonomia	
Porphyria, neuropathies	

MAO, monamine oxidase; NSAIDS, non-steroidal anti-inflammatory drugs.
Adapted from Chobanian AV, Bakris GL, Black HR, et al. The seventh report of the joint national committee on prevention, detection, evaluation, and treatment of high blood pressure. *JAMA* 2003;289:2560–2572, with permission.

3. **Sequelae of hypertension.** The hypertensive state can lead to sequelae most evident in the heart, central nervous system, and kidney. In particular, patients with established hypertension may exhibit (i) LV hypertrophy leading to decreased ventricular compliance; (ii) neurologic symptoms, such as headache, dizziness, tinnitus, and blurred vision that may progress to cerebral infarction; and (iii) renal vascular lesions leading to proteinuria, hematuria, and decreased glomerular filtration progressing to renal failure.
4. **Antihypertensive therapy.** Today antihypertensive medications are the most prescribed class of medications, and more than 75 individual or combination drugs are prescribed. The primary objective of antihypertensive therapy is to reduce cardiovascular morbidity by lowering the blood pressure. However, specific classes of antihypertensive agents are effective in preventing end organ damage, especially to the heart and the kidney, beyond that directly associated with lowering the blood pressure. The recommended antihypertensive drug classes for patients with specific comorbid conditions are shown in Table 3.8 [23]. The properties of specific medications are discussed in Chapter 2.

E. **Cerebrovascular disease**

1. **The association of preoperative cerebrovascular disease with increased perioperative neurologic dysfunction.** CNS dysfunction of at least some degree is common after cardiopulmonary bypass with temporary postoperative neurocognitive defects occurring in up to 80% of patients and stroke in 1% to 5% [24]. Arrowsmith, et al. found that aortic atherosclerosis is associated with the highest risk of adverse neurologic events (odds ratio 4.52) and that a history of neurologic disease ranked second, with an odds ratio of 3.19 [25]. Patients with a preoperative stroke are more likely to have a perioperative

TABLE 3.8 Antihypertensive therapy for patients with other systemic disease

	Recommended antihypertensive drug classes					
Coexisting condition	**Diuretic**	**β-Blocker**	**ACE inhibitor**	**Angiotensin II receptor blocker**	**Calcium channel blocker**	**Aldosterone antagonist**
Heart failure	x	x	x	xx		x
Recent MI		x	x			x
High coronary artery disease risk	x	xx	x		x	
Diabetes	x	x	xx	xx	x	
Chronic renal disease			xx	xx		
Recurrent stroke prevention	x		x			

x, indicated; xx, first-line therapy; ACE, angiotensin converting enzyme; MI, myocardial infarction.
Adapted from Chobanian AV, Bakris GL, Black HR, et al. The seventh report of the joint national committee on prevention, detection, evaluation, and treatment of high blood pressure. *JAMA* 2003;289:2560–2572, with permission.

6 stroke. Even in the absence of a prior cerebral ischemic event, the presence of carotid stenosis increases the risk of postoperative stroke from approximately 2% in patients without carotid stenosis to 10% with stenosis of greater than 50%, and to 11% to 19% with stenosis of greater than 80% [26].

2. **Genetic factors.** Genetic factors may modify the risk or severity of postoperative CNS injury. Genes related to thrombotic factors and inflammatory factors such as platelet receptors, C-reactive protein, and interleukin-6, have been associated with the risk of postoperative cognitive dysfunction.
3. **Effect of the surgical procedure.** Cardiopulmonary bypass may increase the risk of postoperative cognitive dysfunction, but neurologic deficits are still seen following off pump coronary artery bypass surgery, likely because of effects such as blood pressure lability, low cardiac output, the systemic inflammatory reaction to the procedure, or manipulation of the ascending thoracic aorta.

   As may be expected, several authors have shown increased postoperative cerebral dysfunction following open aortic or mitral valve procedures compared to CABG. However, in these series, the duration of cardiopulmonary bypass was also longer for the valve procedures, making it difficult to establish a causal relationship. Even though it is apparent that carotid artery stenosis represents a risk factor for perioperative stroke, it is not nearly as clear that simultaneous carotid endarterectomy reduces this risk. Therefore, recent texts recommend that combined carotid endarterectomy and CABG not usually be undertaken. Rather, at the present time epiaortic scanning to modify the surgical technique during the cardiac procedure, and possibly neurophysiologic monitoring, may offer more benefit [27].

III. Noninvasive cardiac imaging

A. **Echocardiography.** Transthoracic echocardiography provides specific preoperative assessment of several types of cardiac abnormalities. First, two dimensional (2D) and Doppler echocardiography together provide quantitative assessment of the severity of valvular stenosis or insufficiency (see Chapter 12) and of pulmonary hypertension. Second, assessment of regional wall motion provides a more sensitive and specific assessment of the existence and extent of MI than a surface EKG. Third, 2D echocardiography provides a quantitative assessment of global ventricular function, or ejection fraction (EF). Fourth, echocardiography can detect even small pericardial effusions. Fifth, echocardiographs can detect anatomic cardiac abnormalities, from atrial septal defects (ASD) and ventricular septal defects (VSD) to aneurysms and mural thrombi.

Perioperative transthoracic echocardiography predicts postoperative cardiac events in noncardiac surgical patients at increased clinical cardiac risk. Decreased preoperative systolic dysfunction on echo has been associated with postoperative MI, pulmonary edema, and "major cardiac events," such as ventricular fibrillation, cardiac arrest, or complete heart block. LV hypertrophy, mitral regurgitation, and increased aortic valve gradient on preoperative echo also appear to predict postoperative "major cardiac events."

B. Preoperative testing for myocardial ischemia

1. **Exercise tolerance testing.** The exercise tolerance test (ETT) is often used as a simple and inexpensive initial test to evaluate chest pain of unknown etiology. It is also used preoperatively to determine functional capacity and identify significant ischemia or dysrhythmias for prognostic stratification preoperatively. ETT is rarely useful as a screening test in asymptomatic patients. To better address the prognostic value of the ETT, the Duke risk score was developed [28]. This risk score equals the exercise time in minutes, minus five times the extent of the ST segment depression in millimeters, minus four times the level of angina with exercise (0—no angina, 1—typical angina, 2—typical angina requiring stopping the test). The score typically ranges from −25 to +15. These values correspond to low-risk (with a score of ≥+5), moderate-risk (with scores ranging from −10 to +4), and high-risk (with a score of <−11) categories.
   a. **Limitations of ETT**
      (1) Inability to exercise because of systemic disease, particularly PVD.
      (2) Abnormal resting ECG precluding ST segment analysis (left bundle branch block, LV hypertrophy, digoxin therapy).
      (3) β-blocker therapy that prevents the patient from achieving 85% of his or her maximum permissible heart rate.
2. **Stress echocardiography.** Stress echocardiography can use exercise stress or pharmacologic stress, with dobutamine, to increase myocardial work. Abnormally contracting myocardial segments seen on stress echocardiography are classified as either *ischemic,* if their reduced contraction pattern is in response to stress, or *infarcted,* if their contractility remains consistently depressed before, during, and after stress.

   Sixteen recent studies evaluated in the 2007 ACC/AHA Guidelines for Perioperation Cardiovascular Evaluation showed that 0% to 33% of vascular patients who had a positive preoperative Dobutamine Stress Echocardiogram (DSE) subsequently suffered a post operative MI or death. The negative predictive value was much higher—93% to 100% [10]. Wall motion abnormalities at low workloads were especially important predictors of short- and long-term outcomes. DSE has indications similar to pharmacologic perfusion imaging with comparable sensitivity, but possibly increased specificity.

   For patients with poor acoustic windows due to body habitus or severe lung disease, myocardial contrast agents are now available to improve imaging. Still, for some patients, a difficult echocardiographic window or global poor ventricular function may preclude its use. Further, this test cannot be used for those patients in whom a recent MI, an intracranial or abdominal aneurysm, or other vascular malformation would make tachycardia or hypertension risky.
3. **Radionuclide imaging.** Radionuclide stress imaging is used to assess the perfusion and the viability of areas of myocardium. This technique cannot provide an anatomic diagnosis of a cardiac lesion. It is a more sensitive and specific test than ETT and can provide an assessment of global LV function as well. MPI is a nuclear technique employing intravenous radioisotopes, either thallium-201 or the cardiac-specific technetium-99 perfusion agents, sestamibi (Cardiolite), or tetrofosmin (Myoview), as an indicator of the presence or absence of CAD.

   Exercise stress or pharmacologic stress is necessary to increase coronary blood flow for the test. Pharmacologic vasodilators are preferable but contraindicated in patients with severe bronchospastic lung disease, in which case dobutamine may be used. The available pharmocologic vasodilators—adenosine (Adenoscan), dipyridamole (Persantine), and regadenoson (Lexiscan)—are used to produce maximal coronary vasodilation of approximately four to five times resting values. Vessels with fixed coronary stenoses will not dilate, allowing less isotope to reach the myocardium.

Myocardium underperfused by these vessels will show up as a "defect" on stress scans when compared to surrounding myocardium supplied by nonobstructed coronaries. When compared to the images acquired at rest, any defects still present—*fixed* or *persistent defects*—are suggestive of nonviable or infarcted myocardium. Defects present on stress and not at rest, termed *reversible defects,* suggest viable myocardium at risk for ischemia when stressed.

A perfusion scan may be performed in three different ways. When thallium is chosen, only a single injection is required because the isotope redistributes; however, a repeat image should be taken 4 hrs after the stress images are taken. With the technetium agents, particularly best for larger patients due to the higher energy (KeV), separate rest and stress injections are required because no redistribution is seen. Finally, dual isotopes studies utilizing thallium for the initial rest image and technetium for the stress image allows for the fastest patient through put.

The technique used to acquire these images is single photon-emission computed tomography (SPECT). In the studies of noncardiac surgical patients reviewed by the ACC/AHA Task Force on Perioperative Cardiovascular Evaluation, reversible defects on nuclear perfusion scanning identified 2% to 20% of patients suffering postoperative MI or cardiac death. The negative predictive value of a normal scan is much better, at approximately 99%. Fixed defects did not usually predict perioperative cardiac events. The sensitivity and specificity of nuclear perfusion imaging is similar for pharmacologic and stress-based techniques [10]. The predictive value of the test can be improved by using it in high-risk
7 sub-groups. Selective use of pharmacologic perfusion imaging in only patients who have at least one of two clinical risk factors for ischemic disease (age >70 yrs and congestive heart failure) can maximize the usefulness of this procedure in predicting cardiac outcome in patients undergoing noncardiac surgery of all types.

Contraindications to pharmacologic stress with dipyridamole, adenosine or regadenoson are:

- unstable angina or MI within 48 hrs
- severe primary bronchospasm
- methylxanthine ingestion within 24 hrs
- allergy to dipyridamole or aminophylline
- For adenosine only, first-degree heart block (PR interval >0.28 seconds) and recent oral dipyridamole ingestion (<24 hrs ago).

Pharmacologic vasodilators should be used in patients who cannot exercise, or have a medical condition, such as a cerebral aneurysm, which would contraindicate exercise. Pharmacologic stress testing with vasodilators, such as adenosine or dipyridamole, is also preferable to exercise or dobutamine in patients with left bundle branch block, because of spurious septal changes with exercise or catecholamines, which lead to false positive tests.

4. **Positron emission tomography (PET) scan.** PET scanning techniques use different radioisotopes than SPECT imaging. These isotopes decay with a higher energy photon with a shorter half life and can assess both regional myocardial blood flow and myocardial metabolism on a real-time basis. PET scanning techniques can be combined with CT and magnetic resonance imaging (MRI) to provide PET metabolic and anatomic information simultaneously.
5. **Magnetic resonance imaging (MRI).** MRI has been used for some time to provide both high resolution and three-dimensional imaging of cardiac structures. It is now becoming important in perfusion imaging, atherosclerosis imaging, and coronary artery imaging. With the development of dedicated cardiovascular MRI scanning, molecular imaging techniques and biochemical markers are providing the capacity for MRI diagnosis of cardiac function. Changes in molecular composition of the myocardium can change its magnetic moment and MRI signal, allowing MRI to detect lipid accumulation, edema, fibrosis, rate of phosphate turnover, and intracellular pH in ischemic areas. Finally, MRI imaging can be gated to the cardiac cycle, allowing rapid and accurate

assessment of myocardial function. Gated images are used to detect regional myocardial abnormalities that may be caused by ischemia, infarction, stunning, hibernation, and postinfarct remodeling. MRI is the diagnostic technique of choice for arrhythmogenic right ventricular (RV) dysplagia and can differentiate myocardial infiltration and diastolic dysfunction associated with sarcoidosis, hemochromatosis, amyloidosis, and endomyocardial fibrosis. Contrast-enhanced MRI has a higher sensitivity and specificity than either CT scan or TEE in aortic dissection. Dobutamine stress MRI is an accurate and rapid test for myocardial ischemia, which may eventually replace dobutamine echocardiography.

MRI can be used to diagnose CAD involving the native major epicardial arteries with an accuracy of approximately 87% and is even better for assessing saphenous vein and internal mammary artery graft patency. However, it is still not commonly used clinically for this purpose.

6. **Computed tomography.** Since its introduction into clinical practice in 1973, CT has undergone significant advances. CT for calcium scoring has been utilized clinically to estimate cardiac risk but is not effective for defining atherosclerotic disease. With the development of a higher temporal resolution scan, in conjunction with contrast injection, coronary imaging is now possible. As these imaging techniques advance in the cardiology arena, they can be used for imaging the pericardium, cardiac chambers, and great vessels. However, imaging protocols require aggressive β-blockade to achieve heart rates of 60 bpm or less in order to decrease image blurring and improve resolution.

   Though more widely applied in recent years, less extensive clinical expertise and prognostic data preclude recommending this technique as a substitute for other more established diagnostic techniques at this time.

IV. Cardiac catheterization

A. **Overview.** Cardiac catheterization still is considered the gold standard for diagnosis of cardiac pathology before most open heart operations and for definition of lesions of the coronary vessels. More than 95% of all patients undergoing open heart operations have had catheterization prior to the procedure. The remaining 5% are assessed only by noninvasive techniques, such as echocardiography and Doppler flow studies. They have pathologic findings, such as an ASD or VSD, which are adequately defined by noninvasive means.

As an invasive procedure, serious complications occur in approximately in 0.1% of patients and include stroke, heart attack, and death. Significant access site complications occur in approximately 0.5%.

If only coronary anatomy is to be delineated, often only a systemic-arterial or left-sided catheterization will be performed. However, if any degree of LV dysfunction, valvular abnormality, pulmonary disease, or impaired RV function exists clinically, a right-sided (Swan-Ganz) catheterization will also be performed. A range of normal hemodynamic values obtained from right- and left-sided catheterization is included in Table 3.9.

Interpretation of catheterization data emphasizes the following areas.

B. **Assessment of coronary anatomy**

1. **Procedure.** Radiopaque contrast is injected through a catheter placed at the coronary ostia to delineate the anatomy of both the right and left coronary arteries. Multiple views are important to define branch lesions, decrease artifacts at points of tortuosity or vessel overlap, and determine more clearly the degree of stenosis, particularly in eccentric lesions. Two common projections of the coronary arteries are the right anterior oblique (RAO) and the left anterior oblique (LAO) views (Fig. 3.2).
2. **Interpretation.** The degree of vessel stenosis generally is assessed by the percent reduction in diameter of the vessel, which in turn correlates with the reduction in cross-sectional area of the vessel at the point of narrowing. Lesions that reduce vessel diameter by greater than 50%, reducing the cross-sectional area by greater than 70%, are considered significant. Lesions are also characterized as either focal or segmental. There is a great deal of inter-observer variability in interpretation with particular

TABLE 3.9 Normal hemodynamic values obtained at cardiac catheterization

Parameter	Measurement	Value
Peripheral arterial or aortic pressure	Systolic/diastolic Mean	≤140/90 mm Hg ≤105 mm Hg
Right atrial pressure	Mean	≤6 mm Hg
Right ventricular pressure	Systolic/end-diastolic	≤30/6 mm Hg
Pulmonary artery pressure	Systolic/diastolic Mean	≤30/15 mm Hg ≤22 mm Hg
Pulmonary artery wedge pressure	Mean	≤12 mm Hg
Left ventricular pressure	Systolic/end-diastolic	≤140/12 mm Hg
Cardiac index		2.5–4.2 L min^{-1} m^{-2}
End-diastolic volume index		<100 mL/m^{-2}
Arteriovenous O_2 content difference		≤5.0 mL/dL
Pulmonary vascular resistance		20–130 dynes sec cm^{-5} Or 0.25–1.6 Woods units
Systemic vascular resistance		700–1,600 dynes sec cm^{-5} Or 9–20 Woods units

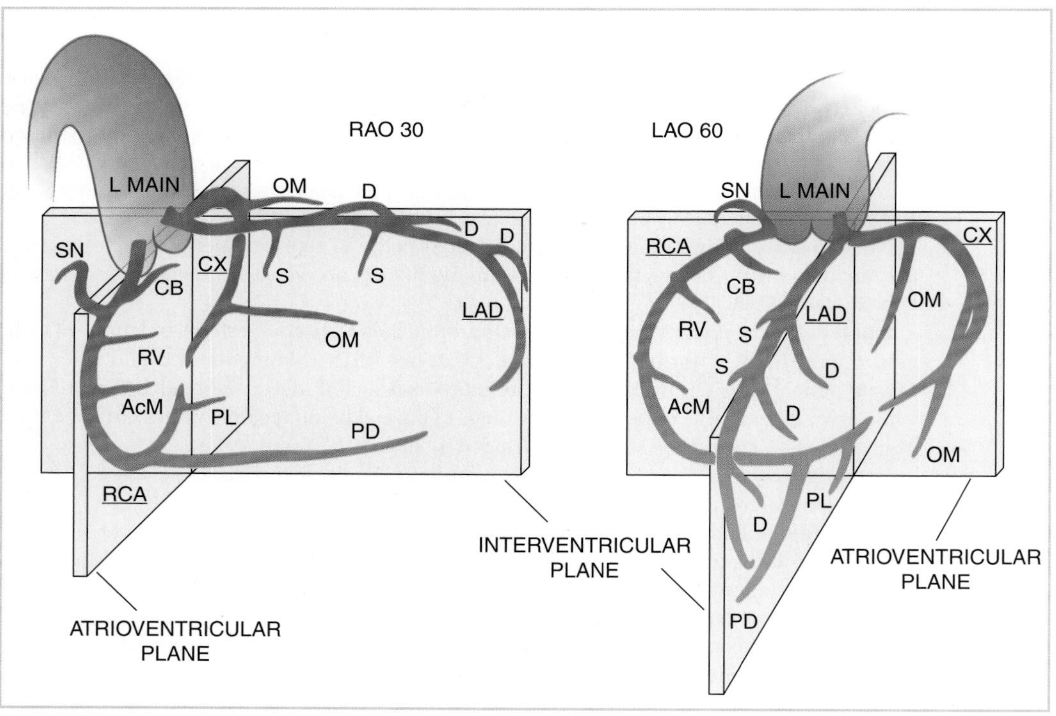

FIGURE 3.2 Representation of coronary anatomy relative to the interventricular and AV valve planes. Coronary branches are L Main, left main; LAD, left anterior descending; D, diagonal; S, septal; CX, circumflex; OM, obtuse marginal; RCA, right coronary; CB, conus branch; SN, sinus node; AcM, acute marginal; PD, posterior descending; PL, posterolateral left ventricular. RV, right ventricle. (Reproduced from Baim DS, Grossman W. Coronary angiography. In: Grossman W, ed. *Cardiac catheterization and angiography.* 3rd ed. Philadelphia: Lea & Febiger, 1986:185, with permission.)

concern regarding intermediate lesions (50% to 70%) and their physiologic significance. Adjunct imaging techniques include fractional flow reserve (FFR) and intravascular ultrasound (IVUS) that may assist in defining the need for revascularization of these vessels.

C. **Assessment of left ventricular function.** Both global and regional measures of ventricular function can be obtained from catheterization data.

1. **Global ventricular measurements**
   a. **Left ventricular end-diastolic pressure (LVEDP).** An elevated value above 15 mm Hg usually indicates some degree of ventricular dysfunction. LVEDP is an index that may reflect either systolic or diastolic dysfunction and is acutely affected by preload and afterload. Without examining other indices of function, an isolated measurement of elevated LVEDP simply indicates that something is abnormal. Associated with a normal LV contractile pattern and cardiac output, an elevated LVEDP measurement may indicate a decrease in left ventricular compliance.
   b. **Left ventricular EF**
      (1) **Calculation.** EF is defined as the volume of blood ejected (stroke volume (SV)) per beat divided by the volume in the LV before ejection The SV is equal to the EDV minus the end-systolic volume (ESV). The equation for EF determination is therefore:

$$EF = \frac{[EDV - ESV]}{EDV} = \frac{SV}{EDV}$$

      (2) **Mitral regurgitation.** An EF of greater than 50% is normal in the presence of normal valvular function. However, in the presence of significant mitral regurgitation, an EF of 50% to 55% suggests moderate LV dysfunction, because part of the volume is ejected backward into a low-resistance pathway (i.e., into the left atrium).
2. **Regional assessment of ventricular function.** LV contraction observed during ventriculography provides a qualitative assessment of overall ventricular function but is not as specific as the calculated EF. Routine ventriculography is less commonly performed when concerns for contrast volume, patient instability or prior assessment of function are present.

   Qualitative regional differences in contraction may be evident. For examination, the heart is divided into segments. The anterior, posterior, apical, basal, inferior (diaphragmatic), and septal regions of the LV are examined (Figs. 3.3 and 3.4). Motion of each one of these

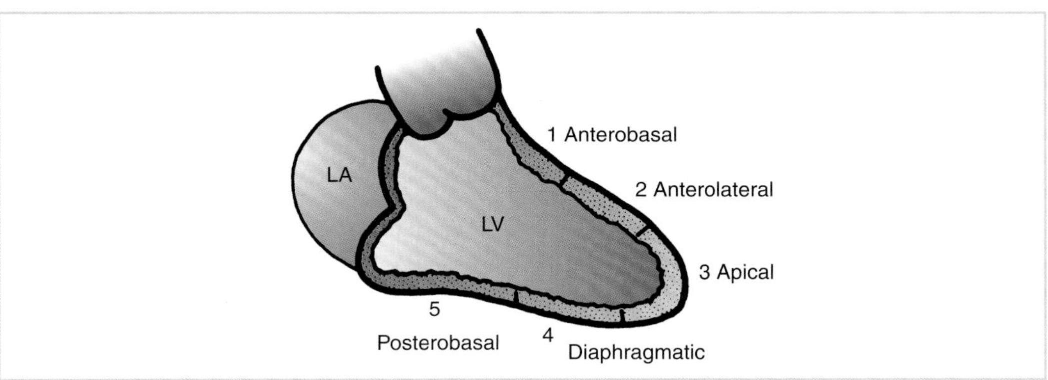

FIGURE 3.3 Terminology for left ventricular segments 1–5 analyzed from right anterior oblique ventriculogram. LV, left ventricle; LA, left atrium. (Reproduced from CASS Principal Investigators and Associates. National Heart, Lung, and Blood Institute Coronary Artery Surgery Study [Part II]. *Circulation* 1981;63[Suppl.]:1–14, Figure 2, with permission.)

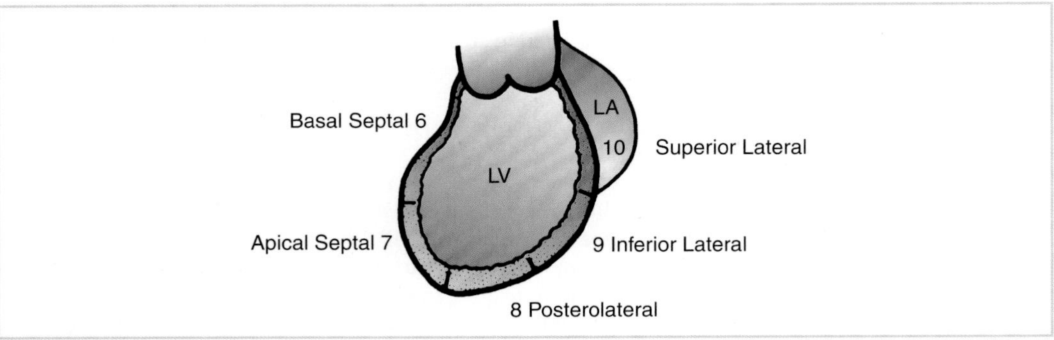

FIGURE 3.4 Terminology for left ventricular segments 6–10 analyzed from left anterior oblique ventriculogram. LV, left ventricle; LA, left atrium. (Reproduced from CASS Principal Investigators and Associates. National Heart, Lung, and Blood Institute Coronary Artery Surgery Study [Part II]. *Circulation* 1981;63[Suppl.]:1–14, Figure 3, with permission.)

particular regions is defined as normal, hypokinetic (decreased inward motion), akinetic (no motion), or dyskinetic (outward paradoxical motion) in relation to the other normally contracting segments.

Regional wall motion abnormalities are usually secondary to prior infarction or acute ischemia. However, very infrequently myocarditis as well as rare infiltrative processes by myocardial tumors may lead to regional wall motion abnormalities.

D. **Assessment of valvular function.** This section will be limited to a brief discussion of the methods utilized to study lesions of the aortic and mitral valves. The specific hemodynamic patterns of acute and chronic valvular disease will be discussed in Chapter 12.

1. **Regurgitant lesions**
   a. **Qualitative assessment.** A relative scale of 1+ to 4+ (4+ being the most severe) is used to quantify the severity of valvular incompetence during the injection of dye. Visual inspection is utilized to determine the intensity and rapidity of washout of dye from the LV after aortic root injection (aortic regurgitation) or from the left atrium after ventricular injection (mitral regurgitation).
   b. **Pathologic V waves.** In patients with mitral regurgitation, the pulmonary capillary wedge trace may manifest giant V waves. Normal or physiologic V waves are seen in the left atrium at the end of systole and are secondary to filling from the pulmonary veins against a closed mitral valve. With valvular incompetence, the regurgitant wave into the left atrium is superimposed on a physiologic V wave, producing a giant V wave (Fig. 3.5).
2. **Stenotic lesions.** The severity of valvular stenosis can be determined only by knowing the size of the pressure drop across the stenotic valve and the flow across the stenosis during either systolic ejection or diastolic filling. One cannot uniformly assess the severity of stenosis solely by examining the pressure gradient across the valve.

   Gorlin and Gorlin [29] described an equation for determining valve area based on these two factors in the *American Heart Journal* in 1951. A simplified version of this equation is:

$$\text{Valve area} = \frac{\text{cardiac output (Liters/min)}}{\sqrt{\text{mean pressure gradient}}}$$

   With the peak pressure gradient and cardiac output given on the catheterization report, a quick estimate of either aortic or mitral valve area can be made.

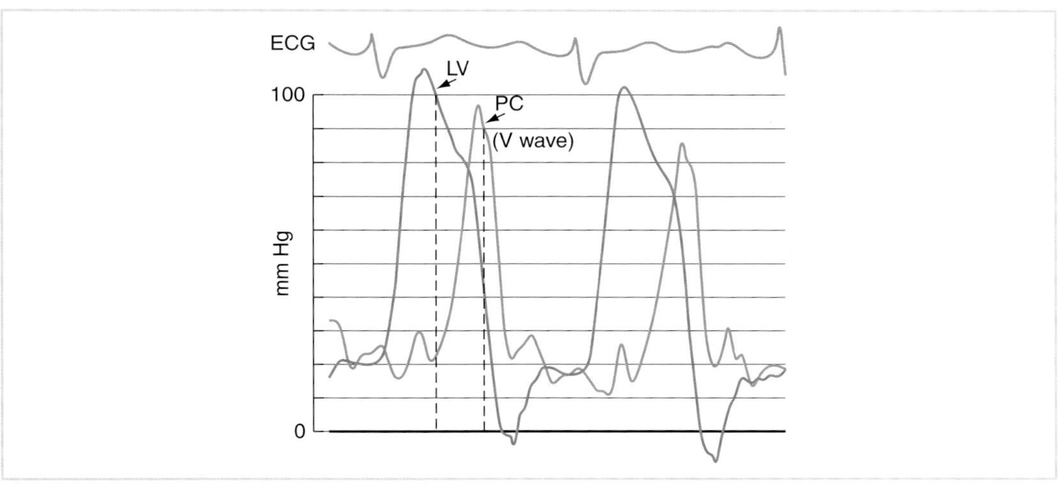

FIGURE 3.5 Left ventricular (LV) and pulmonary capillary wedge (PC) pressure tracings taken in a patient with ruptured chordae tendineae and acute mitral insufficiency. The giant V wave results from regurgitation of blood into a relatively small and noncompliant left atrium; ECG illustrates the timing of the PC V wave, whose peak follows ventricular repolarization, as manifest by the T wave of the ECG. (Reproduced from Grossman W. Profiles in valvular heart disease. In Grossman W, Baim DS, eds. *Cardiac Catheterization, Angiography, and Intervention.* 4th ed. Philadelphia: Lea & Febiger, 1991:564, with permission.)

When examining combined regurgitant and stenotic lesions of the same valve, the total or angiographic cardiac output must be used in the calculation; otherwise, the severity of stenosis will be overestimated. Values for normal and abnormal valve areas are discussed in Chapter 12.

Remember that catheterization data represent only *one* point in time, and medical management may have changed the hemodynamic pattern and catheterization results at the time of cardiac operation.

V. Interventional Cardiac Catheterization

A. Percutaneous coronary intervention (PCI). In 1977, Andreas Gruentzig brought therapeutic options to the invasive cardiology practice with the first percutaneous transluminal coronary angioplasty (PTCA). Multiple technologies have advanced since the initial balloon dilation. Current technology has evolved to include niche devices including rotational coronary atherectomy, various thrombectomy techniques, distal protection devices for saphenous vein graphs, and coronary stents [30].

However, post-PCI re-stenosis, a recurrent blockage resulting from a local vascular response to injury, occurs in one-third of balloon dilations and limits their effectiveness. Intracoronary stents were developed to provide local stabilization for PCI-induced coronary dissection and to prevent re-stenosis. Their wide-spread use has significantly reduced the need for emergent coronary bypass surgery. The original BMS reduced restenosis rates significantly, while DES, covered with polymer-based anti-inflammatory medications, have reduced re-stenosis rates an additional 46–55% [31].

The need for emergency coronary artery bypass graft surgery (CABG) has dramatically decreased with the use of coronary artery stents. Emergency CABG in patients undergoing PCI decreased from 2.9% before the use of stents to 0.3% with stents [32]. In 2009 the National Cardiovascular Data Registry (NCDR) reported the rate of emergency CABG following PCI was 0.4% [33].

Several studies have reported on the frequency of procedure-related indications for emergent CABG following PCI. These include: dissection (27%), acute vessel closure (16%), perforation (8%), and failure to cross the lesion (8%). Three-vessel disease was also present in 40% of patients requiring emergency CABG [34]. The strongest predictors of the need for emergency CABG in several studies, however, are cardiogenic shock (OR = 11.4), acute MI or emergent PCI (OR = 3.2–3.8), multivessel or three-vessel disease (OR = 2.3–2.4), and type C lesion (OR = 2.6) [34]). In-hospital mortality for emergency CABG after PCI ranges from 7.8% to 14%.

8 Though a large proportion of patients come for surgery with a history of PCI at some time in the past, it is now well established that PCI is not beneficial when used solely as a means to prepare a patient with coronary artery disease for surgery.

B. Preoperative management of patients with prior interventional procedures

1. Post-coronary stent anti-platelet therapy and stent thrombosis

a. Coronary artery stent thrombosis

Coronary artery stents are effective in preventing re-stenosis, but as foreign bodies they increase the long term, and perhaps even permanent, risk of coronary artery thrombosis. Metal stents are associated with the greatest inflammatory response, in the first 4 to 6 weeks, which then leads to re-epithelialization and a decrease in the risk of subsequent thrombosis after approximately 6 weeks. In contrast, DES are designed to inhibit inflammation and so these stents remain exposed for a much longer period of time, and so are associated with a much longer risk of stent thrombosis, extending at least to, and perhaps much longer than, 1 year. Unfortunately, there is no reliable way to determine when endothelialization actually occurs.

Because thrombosis occurs quickly, in comparison to re-stenosis, it is associated with a very high risk (greater than 50% in some series) of MI and death. Therefore, anti-platelet therapy is required to reduce the risk of thrombosis. Anti-platelet therapy may be particularly useful in the perioperative period, with its associated thrombotic risk.

b. Anti-platelet agents

Aspirin and clopidogrel have been the mainstays of anti-platelet therapy. Since they work by different mechanisms, they have at least an additive, or perhaps super-additive effect. Ticlopidine is approximately as effective as clopidogrel in reducing the risk of thrombosis, but does have increased side effects. More recently, prasugrel has been introduced and cangrelor is an investigational drug, which may provide new therapeutic options preoperatively. Table 3.10 compares the properties of these four agents.

Prasugrel has been found to be somewhat more effective than clopidogrel at reducing the risk of stent thrombosis, with its associated MIs and death. So, it may be useful for patients at extremely high risk of stent thrombosis. Cangrelor, appears to have a similar efficacy and a much more rapid onset and shorter duration, because of its reversible binding to receptors. Therefore, it is being studied as a possible purging agent, specifically used in patients with coronary artery stents in preparation for surgical procedures.

TABLE 3.10 Anti-platelet agents commonly used to prevent coronary stent thrombosis

Drug	Drug class (mechanism)	Dosage form	Commonly used dose	Duration of action
Aspirin	Salicylate (Cyclooxygenase inhibition)	Oral	325 mg loading dose 81 mg daily	7 days
Clopidogrel (Plavix)	Thienopyridine (ADP antagonist)	Oral	300 mg loading dose 75 mg daily	7 days
Ticlopidine (Ticlid)	Thienopyridine (ADP antagonist)	Oral	500 mg loading dose 250 mg b.i.d.	10 days
Prasugrel (Effient)	Thienopyridine (ADP antagonist)	Oral	600 mg loading dose 10 mg daily	7 days
Cangrelor (investigational)	(Platelet receptor P2Y12blockade)	Intravenous		1 day

TABLE 3.11 Risk factors for coronary stent thrombosis

Clinical	**Angiographic**
Advanced age	Long stents
Acute coronary syndrome	Multiple lesions
Diabetes	Overlapping stents
Low ejection fraction	Ostial or bifurcation stents
Prior brachytherapy	Small vessels
Renal failure	Suboptimal stent results

c. Prevention of coronary artery stent thrombosis
Continuous treatment with the combination of aspirin and adenosine diphosphate (ADP) antagonist after PCI reduces major adverse cardiac events (MACE). On the basis of randomized clinical trials, aspirin 162 to 325 mg daily should be given for at least 1 month after PCI, followed by daily long-term use of aspirin indefinitely at a dose of 81 to 162 mg. In patients for whom there is concern about bleeding, the lowest dose of 81 mg can be used.

Likewise, $P2Y_{12}$ inhibitors (thienopyridines) should be given for a minimum of 1 month after BMS, as the second part of dual anti-platelet therapy (DAPT), with a minimum of 2 weeks for patients at significant increased risk of bleeding, and for 12 months after DES in all patients who are not at high risk of bleeding. In the US, there are currently four approved DES: sirolimus-eluting stents (SES), paclitaxel-eluting stents (PES), zotarolimus-eluting stents (ZES), and everolimus-eluting stents (EES). Each of these stents are presumed to be associated with delayed healing and a longer period of risk for thrombosis compared with BMS, and require longer duration of DAPT. Current guidelines recommend at least 12 months of DAPT following any DES in order to avoid late (after 30 days) thrombosis.

A growing number of cardiologists, however, recommend extending DAPT beyond 1 year based on observational data analysis, and randomized trials to determine whether longer DAPT reduces stent thrombosis risk are in progress. Late stent thrombosis risk, after 1 year, is likely higher in DES than BMS and has been observed at a rate of 0.2% to 0.4% per year. The greatest risk of stent thrombosis is within the first year regardless of stent type and ranges from 0.7% to 3% depending on patient and lesion complexity [35].

Risk factors for both early and late stent thrombosis are shown in Table 3.11. In addition, of course, any subsequent surgery would result in increased thrombotic risk in the perioperative period.

d. Perioperative anti-platelet therapy in patients with coronary artery stents
9 According to current recommendations, elective surgery requiring interruption of DAPT should not be scheduled within 1 month of BMS placement or within 12 months of DES placement. Urgent or emergent surgeries require communication between the patient's cardiologist, anesthesiologist, and the surgical team. However, most guidelines recommend that, for these procedures which cannot be delayed, if the thienopyridine must be stopped it should be stopped as close to surgery as possible and re-started as soon as possible postoperatively, and aspirin should be continued if at all possible [36]. In cardiac surgery, the preoperative use of aspirin has resulted in greater blood loss and need for reoperation, but no increase in mortality, and is in fact associated with an increased saphenous vein graft patency rate [10].

If and when cangrelor is available in the US, it will also provide the option of switching from clopidogrel to cangrelor 1 week preoperatively and thereby continuing DAPT until 1 day preoperatively, because of cangrelor's rapid offset.

C. Percutaneous valvular therapy

1. Aortic valvuloplasty

Percutaneous valvuloplasty leads to at least a 50% reduction in gradient in more than 80% of cases. Complications are relatively infrequent, including femoral artery laceration in up to 10%

of patients, stroke in 1%, and a less than 1% incidence of cardiac fatality. Contraindications to aortic balloon valvuloplasty are significant PVD and moderate or greater aortic insufficiency. Aortic insufficiency usually increases during valvuloplasty. However, the acute development of severe aortic regurgitation can lead to pulmonary congestion and possibly death. Restenosis can occur as early as 6 months after the procedure and nearly all patients will have restenosis by 2 years. The most common indication for percutaneous aortic valvuloplasty is currently to temporarily improve poor left ventricular function in order to allow AVR.

2. **Mitral valvuloplasty**

Percutaneous mitral valvuloplasty (PMC) has been performed for 30 years as an alternative to surgery for patients with rheumatic mitral stenosis. The factor leading to success with mitral valvuloplasty is proper patient selection. Absolute contraindications to mitral valvuloplasty include:

a. a known left atrial (LA) thrombus, or a recent embolic event within the preceding 2 months
b. severe cardiothoracic deformity
c. bleeding abnormality.

Relative contraindications include:

a. significant mitral regurgitation
b. pregnancy
c. concomitant significant aortic valve disease
d. significant CAD

All patients must undergo transesophageal echocardiography (TEE) to exclude LA thrombus.

The procedure is reported to be successful in 85% to 99% of cases. Risks of percutaneous mitral commissurotomy include a procedural mortality of 0% to 3%, hemopericardium in 0.5% to 12% of patients, systemic embolism in 0.5% to 5%, and failure of the inter-atrial septum to close completely. Severe mitral regurgitation occurs in 2% to 10% of procedures and may require emergent surgery. Restenosis rates depend on the amount of calcium on the mitral valve commissures [37].

3. **Percutaneous valve replacement and repair**

Surgical valve replacement/repair is still the treatment of choice for stenotic aortic valves and regurgitant mitral valves when the surgical morbidity and mortality are not prohibitive. The first catheter-based alternative to surgical valve replacement was percutaneous pulmonic valve replacement. Success in this procedure led to similar procedures on the aortic and mitral valves. These percutaneous procedures are performed under general anesthesia with fluoroscopic and echocardiographic guidance. The results in high-risk patients have been promising, and the devices are now being tested in a lower risk group, as a true alternative to surgery [38]. Retrograde, antegrade, and transapical approaches to the aortic valve are used. For patients with severe vascular disease, the transapical approach using a small thoracotomy incision may be most suitable. This approach requires that general anesthesia be administered to a patient with critical aortic stenosis and may pose particular challenges for the anesthesiologist.

The percutaneous approach for MR includes techniques to replace and to repair the mitral valve [39]. Two approaches have been used. The first involves placement of a device within the coronary sinus. This device can then be shortened, decreasing the size of the mitral annulus and the amount of MR, similar to a surgically placed annuloplasty ring. The second approach uses percutaneous suturing of the mitral leaflets with the MitraClip® (Evalve, Menlo Park, CA). A report on 107 patients described procedural success in 74% with a 9% rate of major but not lethal adverse events in a high-risk cohort. Trials are currently comparing the device to surgical repair. Both temporary and permanent mitral valve implantations have been attempted experimentally.

As this field expands, the role of the cardiac anesthesiologist in the catheterization laboratory for these complex procedures will likely expand [30].

VI. Management of preoperative medications

A. β-Adrenergic blockers. β-Adrenergic blockers are used commonly for the treatment of hypertension, stable and unstable angina, as well as MI. These drugs can also be used to treat

SVT, including that due to pre-excitation syndromes, and the manifestations of systemic disease ranging from hyperthyroidism to migraine headaches. β-Blocker therapy is beneficial in the perioperative period, and the magnitude of the benefit is directly proportional to the patient's cardiac risk [40]. Further, abrupt withdrawal of β-blockers can lead to a rebound phenomenon, manifest by nervousness, tachycardia, palpitations, hypertension, and even MI, ventricular arrhythmias, and sudden death. Many authors have found that preoperative treatment with β-blocking agents reduces perioperative tachycardia and lowers the incidence of ischemic events. [10,40]. Therefore, administration of β_1 selective blockers should continue or be instituted in patients at risk for ischemic heart disease and without systolic heart failure or heart block. Continuation of β-blockade intraoperatively and postoperatively is essential to avoid rebound phenomenon.

B. **Statins (HMG-CoA inhibitors).** Statins are used chronically to reduce the levels of low-density lipoproteins. However, they have also been shown to slow coronary artery plaque formation, increase plaque stability, improve endothelial function, and exhibit antithrombogenic, anti-inflammatory, antiproliferative, and leukocyte-adhesion-limiting effects. All of these effects would be expected to reduce both short- and long-term cardiovascular morbidity. Several large recent retrospective studies, the most recent by Lindenauer et al., have shown that preoperative statin use resulted in a significant reduction in postoperative mortality from 3.05% to 2.13% [41].

Because all of these studies are retrospective and recorded only the patients taking statins during hospitalization, we have no indication of the duration of statin use needed to provide a beneficial effect or whether discontinuing statins several days preoperatively will reduce their protective effect. However, until more is known, it would be wise to continue statins preoperatively in those patients already taking the drugs, recognizing the small incremental risks of hepatotoxicity and rhabdomyolysis.

C. **Anticoagulant and antithrombotic medication**

1. Warfarin—approaches to preoperative therapy for patients taking chronic warfarin for (a) AF, (b) mechanical prosthetic heart valve, or (c) DVT/pulmonary embolus were recently reviewed by Watts and Gibbs. A simple but comprehensive approach, based on their recommendations, is shown in Tables 3.12 to 3.14.

TABLE 3.12 Preoperative anticoagulation management for chronic AF

Thromboembolism risk	Comorbid conditions	Suggested preoperative anticoagulation
High risk	TIA/CVA/systemic embolism within 30 d	Stop warfarin 5 d preoperatively Hospital admission for IV heparin 4 d until 4 hrs preop
	Mitral valve prosthesis or mitral valve disease	Stop warfarin 5 d preoperatively Enoxaparin 1–1.5 mg/kg/d 4 d until 24 hrs preop
Moderate risk	Prior TIA/CVA/PE/systemic embolus greater than 30 d ago LV failure LA enlargement Ischemic heart disease Hypertension Diabetes Age >75	Stop warfarin 5 d preoperatively Enoxaparin 40 mg SQ daily 4 d until 24 hrs before surgery
Low risk	None of the above risk factors	Stop warfarin 5 d preoperatively Enoxaparin 20 mg SQ daily 4 d until 24 hrs before surgery

Check PT/INR immediately preoperatively.
TIA, transient ischemic attack; CVA, cerebrovascular accident; d, days; hrs, hours; PE, pulmonary embolus; LV, left ventricular; LA, left atrial.
Adapted from Watts S, Gibbs N. Outpatient management of the chronically anticoagulated patient for elective surgery. *Anaesth Intensive Care* 2003;31:150, with permission.

TABLE 3.13 Management of preoperative anticoagulation for mechanical prosthetic heart valve

Thromboembolism risk	Comorbid conditions	Suggested preoperative anticoagulation
High	TIA/CVA/systemic embolism within 30 d Mural thrombus Mechanical mitral valve Prosthesis of any type Caged ball or single leaflet aortic valve prosthesis (if known) Multiple prosthetic valves	Stop warfarin 5 d preoperatively Hospital admission for IV heparin 4 d until 4 hrs preoperatively
Moderate	Bileaflet tilting disk aortic valve and any of the following risk factors: 1. Recent valve replacement <90 d 2. AF 3. Prior TIA/CVA/PE/systemic embolus greater than 30 d ago 4. LV failure 5. Hypertension 6. Diabetes 7. Age >75	Stop warfarin 5 d preoperatively Enoxaparin 1–1.5 mg/kg/d SQ from 4 d until 24 hrs preoperatively
Low	Bileaflet tilting disk aortic valve and none of the above risk factors	Stop warfarin 5 d preoperatively Enoxaparin 40 mg SQ daily from 4 d until 24 hrs before surgery

Check PT/INR immediately preoperatively.
TIA, transient ischemic attack; CVA, cerebrovascular accident; d, days; hrs, hours; PE, pulmonary embolus; LV left ventricular; AF, atrial fibrillation.
Adapted from: Watts S, Gibbs N. Outpatient management of the chronically anticoagulated patient for elective surgery. *Anaesth Intensive Care* 2003;31:151, with permission.

TABLE 3.14 Preoperative anticoagulation management for venous thromboembolism

Thromboembolism risk	Comorbid conditions	Suggested preoperative anticoagulation
High	TIA/CVA/DVT/PE/systemic embolism within 30 d	Stop warfarin 5 d preoperatively Hospital admission for IV heparin 4 d until 4 hrs preoperatively
Moderate	Prior venous thromboembolism occurring (1) within the past 1–3 mo, (2) with cessation of warfarin, or (3) with any of the following risk factors: 1. Malignancy 2. Antiphospholipid antibody 3. Factor V Leiden 4. Prothrombin gene mutation 5. Obese (BMI >40) 6. Preoperative immobility	Stop warfarin 5 d preoperatively Enoxaparin 40 mg SQ daily from 4 d until 24 hrs before surgery
Low	Thromboembolic event >3 mos ago None of the above risk factors	Stop warfarin 5 d preoperatively Enoxaparin 20 mg SQ daily from 4 d until 24 hrs before surgery

Check PT/INR immediately preoperatively.
TIA, transient ischemic attack; CVA, cerebrovascular accident; DVT, deep venous thrombosis; d, days; hrs, hours; mo, months; PE, pulmonary embolus; BMI, body mass index.
Adapted from Watts S, Gibbs N. Outpatient management of the chronically anticoagulated patient for elective surgery. *Anaesth Intensive Care* 2003;31:152, with permission.

2. Dibigatran is a potent, non-peptide small molecule that reversibly inhibits both free and clot-bound thrombin. It has been approved for stroke prevention in patients with AF. Though peak effect occurs in 2 to 4 hrs after administration, its estimated half-life is 15 hrs with normal renal function. Based on the pharmacokinetics, in patients with normal renal function (eGFR >50 cc/min) discontinuation of two doses results in a decrease in the plasma level to about 25% of baseline and discontinuation of four doses will decrease the level to about 5% to 10% [42].
3. **Antithrombotic and antiplatelet therapy** with agents such as clopidogrel (Plavix), cilostazol (Pletal), or combinations of agents should be stopped, if possible, 1 week preoperatively. Because of a concern for longer duration of action, ticlopidine (Ticlid) should be discontinued 2 wks preoperatively, and Fondaparinux (Arixtra) 1 mo preoperatively, using other agents as a bridge to surgery, if needed. Glycoprotein IIb/IIIa Inhibitors—(eptifibatide, tirofiban, abciximab) should be stopped approximately 48 hrs preoperatively.

D. Antihypertensives

Preoperatively, chronic antihypertensive medications should usually be continued until the morning of surgery, and be begun again as soon as the patient is hemodynamically stable postoperatively. Continuation of β-blockers and α-2 agonists until the morning of surgery are particularly important because of the risks of rebound hypertension with sudden withdrawal of
10 these drugs. In contrast, patients receiving ACE inhibitors and angiotensin II receptor blockers appear to be particularly prone to perioperative hypotension, so several authors recommend holding these agents the morning of surgery but re-starting them as soon as the patient is euvolemic postoperatively [43].

E. Antidysrhythmics

Preoperative patients may require any of a large number of oral antidysrhythmic agents, including amiodarone, or calcium channel blockers. Therapy for ventricular dysrhythmias should be continued perioperatively.

Complete preoperative evaluation and proper premedication, including especially the use of β-blockade in appropriate patients with good ventricular function, smooth the patient's transition into the operating room and may reduce the incidence of perioperative ischemia in susceptible patients.

REFERENCES

1. Summary Health Statistics for Adults: National Health Interview Survey 2009, http://www.cdc.gov/nchs/data/series/sr_10/sr10_249.pdf accessed 7-27-11.
2. Hall MJ, DeFrancis CJ, Williams SN, et al. National Hospital Discharge Survey: 2007 Summary. Centers for Disease Control http://www.cdc.gov/nchs/data/nhsr/nhsr029.pdf accessed 7-27-11.
3. Shahian DM, O'Brien SM, Filardo G, et al. The Society of Thoracic Surgeons 2008 cardiac surgery risk models: part 3—valve plus coronary artery bypass grafting surgery. *Ann Thorac Surg.* 2009;88:S43–S62.
4. Paiement B, Pelletier C, Dryda I, et al. A simple classification of the risk in cardiac surgery. *Can Anaesth Soc J.* 1983;30:61.
5. Nashef SA, Roques F, Michael P, et al. European system for cardiac operation risk evaluation (Euroscore). *Eur J. Cardiothoracic Surgery.* 1999;16:9–13.
6. Bernstein AD, Parsonnet V. Bedside estimation of risk as an aid for decision-making in cardiac surgery. *Ann Thorac Surg.* 2000;69:823–828.
7. Hannan EL, Racz MJ, Jones RH, et al. Predictors of mortality for patients undergoing cardiac valve replacements in New York state. *Ann Thorac Surg.* 2000;70:1212–1218.
8. Shroyer AL, Plomondon ME, Grover FL, et al. the 1996 coronary artery bypass risk model: the Society of Thoracic Surgeons Adult Cardiac National Database. *Ann Thorac Surg.* 1999;67:1205–1208.
9. Dupuis JY, Wang F, Nathan H, et al. The cardiac anesthesia risk evaluation score: a clinically useful predictor of mortality and morbidity after cardiac surgery. *Anesthesiology* 2001;94:194–204.
10. Fleisher LA, Beckman JA, Brown KA, et al. 2009 ACCF/AHA focused update on perioperative beta blockade incorporated into the ACC/AHA 2007 guidelines on perioperative cardiovascular evaluation and care for noncardiac surgery: a report of the American College of Cardiology Foundation/American heart association task force on practice guidelines. *Circulation* 2009;120:e169–e276.
11. Ouattara A, Niculescu M, Ghazouani S, et al. Predictive performance and variability of the cardiac anesthesia risk evaluation score. *Anesthesiology* 2004;100:1405–1410.

12. Tu JV, Jaglal SB, Naylor D, et al. Multicenter validation of a risk index for mortality, intensive care unit stay, and overall hospital length of stay after cardiac surgery. *Circulation* 1995;91:677–684.
13. Girish M, Trayner E, Dammann O, et al. Symptom-limited stair climbing as a predictor of postoperative cardiopulmonary complications after high-risk surgery. *Chest* 2001;120:1147–1151.
14. Shahian DM, O'Brien SM, Filardo G, et al. The Society of Thoracic Surgeons 2008 cardiac surgery risk models: part 1—coronary artery bypass grafting surgery. *Ann Thorac Surg.* 2009; 88:S2–S22.
15. Sharma S, Durieux ME. Molecular and genetic cardiovascular medicine. In: Kaplan JA, Reich DL, Savino JS, eds. *Kaplan's Cardiac Anesthesia: the Echo Era.* 6th ed. St. Louis: Saunders; 2011.
16. O'Brien SM, Shahian DM, Filardo G, et al. The Society of Thoracic Surgeons 2008 cardiac surgery risk models: part 2—isolated valve surgery. *Ann Thorac Surg.* 2009;88:S23–S42.
17. Fraker TD, Fihn SD. 2007 chronic angina: focused update of the ACC/AHA 2002 guidelines for the management of patients with chronic stable angina. *Circulation* 2007;116:2762–2772.
18. Eagle KA, Guyton RA, Davidoff R, et al. ACC/AHA 2004 guideline update for coronary artery bypass graft surgery: a report of the American College of Cardiology/American Heart Association Task Force on practice guidelines. *Circulation* 2004;110:e340–437.
19. Marine JE. Catheter ablation therapy for supraventricular arrhythmias. *JAMA* 2007;298:2768–2778.
20. Wyse DG, Waldo AL, DiMarco JP, et al. Atrial Fibrillation Follow-up Investigation of Rhythm Management (AFFIRM Investigators). A comparison of rate control and rhythm control in patients with atrial fibrillation. *N Eng J Med.* 2002;347:1825–1833.
21. Cappato R, Calkins H, Chen S-A, et al. Worldwide survey on the methods, efficacy, and safety of catheter ablation for human atrial fibrillation. *Circulation* 2005;111:1100–1105.
22. Zipes DP, Camm J, Borggrefe M, et al. ACC/AHA/ESC 2006 guidelines for management of patients with ventricular arrhythmias and the prevention of sudden cardiac death—executive summary. *Circulation* 2006;114:1088–1132.
23. Chobanian AV, Bakris GL, Black HR, et al. The seventh report of the joint national committee on prevention, detection, evaluation, and treatment of high blood pressure. *JAMA* 2003;289:2560–2572.
24. Newman MF, Kirchner JL, Phillips-Bute B, et al. Longitudinal assessment of neurocognitive function after coronary-artery bypass surgery. *N Engl J Med.* 2001;344:395–402.
25. Arrowsmith JE, Grocott HP, Reves JG, et al. Central nervous system complications of cardiac surgery. *Br J Anaesth.* 2000;84:378–393.
26. Ahonen J, Salmenpera M. Brain injury after adult cardiac surgery. *Acta Anaesthesiol Scand.* 2004;48:4–19.
27. Murkin JM. Central nervous system dysfunction after cardiopulmonary bypass. In: Kaplan JA, Reich DL, Savino JS, eds. *Kaplan's Cardiac Anesthesia: The ECHO Era.* St. Louis: Saunders; 2011.
28. Mark DB, Hlatky MA. Exercise treadmill score for predicting prognosis in coronary artery disease. *Ann Intern Med.* 1987;106:793–800.
29. Gorlin R, Gorlin SG. Hydraulic formula for calculation of the area of the stenotic mitral valve, other cardiol valves, and central circulatory shunts. *Am Heart J.* 1951;41:1–29.
30. Kozak M, Chambers CE. Cardiac catheterization laboratory: diagnostic and therapeutic procedures in the adult patient. In: Kaplan JA, Reich DL, Savino JS, eds. *Kaplan's Cardiac Anesthesia: The Echo Era.* 6th ed. Philadelphia: Elsevier; 2011:33–73.
31. Kirtane AJ, Gupta A, Iyengar S, et al: Safety and efficacy of drug-eluting and bare metal stents: comprehensive meta-analysis of randomized trials and observational studies. *Circulation* 2009;119:3198–3206.
32. Yang EH, Gumina RJ, Lennon RJ. Emergency coronary artery bypass surgery for percutaneous coronary interventions: changes in the incidence, clinical characteristics, and indications from 1979 to 2003. *J Am Coll Cardiol.* 2005;46:2004–2009.
33. Kutcher MA, Klein LW, Ou FS, et al. Percutaneous coronary interventions in facilities without cardiac surgery on site: a report from the National Cardiovascular Data Registry (NCDR). *J Am Coll Cardiol.* 2009;54:16–24.
34. Roy P, de Labriolle A, Hanna N, et al. Requirement for emergent coronary artery bypass surgery following percutaneous coronary intervention in the stent era. *Am J Cardiol.* 2009;103:950–953.
35. Levine GN, Bates ER, Blankenship JC, et al. 2011 ACCF/AHA/SCAI guidelines for percutaneous coronary intervention. *J Am Coll Cardiol.* Published online Nov 7, 2011; doi:10.1016/j.jacc.2011.08.007; http://content.onlinejacc.org/cgi/content/full/j.jacc.2011.08.007vl
36. American Society of Anesthesiologists Committee on Standards and Practice Parameters. Practice alert for the perioperative management of patients with coronary artery stents. *Anesthesiology* 2009;110:22–23.
37. Vahanian A, Palacios IF. Percutaneous approaches to valvular disease. *Circulation* 2004;109:1572–1579.
38. Momenah TS, Oakley RE, Najashi KA, et al. Extended application of percutaneous pulmonary valve implantation. *J Am Coll Cardiol.* 2009;53:1859–1863.
39. Piazza N, Asgar A, Ibrahim R. Transcatheter mitral and pulmonary valve therapy. *J Am Coll Cardiol.* 2009;53:1837–1851.
40. Lindenauer PK, Pekow P, Wang K, et al. Perioperative beta-blocker therapy and mortality after major noncardiac surgery. *N Engl J Med.* 2005;353:349–361.
41. Lindenauer PK, Pekow P, Wang K, et al. Lipid-lowering therapy and in-hospital mortality following major noncardiac surgery. *JAMA* 2004;291:2092–2099.
42. van Ryn J, Stangier J, Haertter S, et al. Dabigatran eteilate—a novel, reversible, oral direct thrombin inhibitor: interpretation of coagulation assays and reversal of anticoagulant activity. *Thromb Haemost.* 2010;103:1116–1127.
43. Comfere T, Sprung J, Kumar MM, et al. Angiotensin system inhibitors in a general surgical population. *Anesth Analg.* 2005;100:636–644.

4 Monitoring the Cardiac Surgical Patient

Mark A. Gerhardt and Katarzyna M. Walosik-Arenall

KEY POINTS

1. For cardiac anesthesia, a five-electrode surface ECG monitor should be used in the diagnostic mode, with a frequency response of 0.05 to 100 Hz.
2. After a rapid pressure change (performed by flushing the pressure line and known as the "pop test"), an underdamped system will continue to oscillate for a prolonged time. In terms of pressure monitoring, this translates to an overestimation of systolic BP and an underestimation of diastolic BP. An overdamped system will not oscillate at all but will settle to baseline slowly, thus underestimating systolic and overestimating diastolic pressures. A critically damped system will settle to baseline after only one or two oscillations and will reproduce systolic pressures accurately.
3. Air within a catheter or transducer causes most pressure monitoring errors.
4. The radial artery pressure may be significantly lower than the aortic pressure at the completion of cardiopulmonary bypass (CPB) and for 5 to 30 min following CPB.
5. Standards in the United States and the United Kingdom suggest that ultrasound guidance is the preferred technique for internal jugular catheter placement.
6. If subclavian vein cannulation is unsuccessful on one side, an attempt on the contralateral side is contraindicated without first obtaining a chest x-ray film. Bilateral pneumothoraces can be lethal.

(continued)

7. The current consensus is that pulmonary artery catheter (PAC) placement may have benefit in high-risk patients, or those with special indications. However, in routine coronary artery bypass patients, the PAC has little, if any, benefit.
8. In cardiac surgical patients with ascending aortic atheroma identified by epiaortic scanning, modification of the surgical technique and neuroprotective strategies have been reported to reduce the incidence of neurologic complications from ~60% to 0%.
9. Monitoring temperature at one core site and one shell site is recommended. Nasal temperature is recommended for core temperature, and bladder or rectal temperature for shell temperature.
10. Though low serum calcium may affect myocardial pumping function, administration of calcium during potential neural ischemia or reperfusion may likely worsen the outcome and should be avoided.

PATIENTS PRESENTING FOR CARDIAC SURGERY require extensive monitoring because of (a) severe, often unstable cardiovascular disease and hemodynamics, (b) coexisting multisystemic diseases, (c) the abnormal physiologic conditions associated with CPB, and (d) special considerations for minimally invasive cardiac surgery. Monitoring techniques have been developed to provide early warning of conditions that may lead to potentially life-threatening complications. Current trends in monitoring include size reduction, minimally invasive device development, and advanced display technology [1].

I. Cardiovascular monitors

A. Electrocardiogram. The intraoperative use of the electrocardiogram (ECG) facilitates the intraoperative diagnosis of dysrhythmias, myocardial ischemia, and cardiac electrical silence during cardioplegic arrest. A five-lead system, including a V5 lead, is preferable for cardiac surgical patients. Use of five electrodes (one lead on each extremity and one precordial lead) allows the simultaneous recording of the six standard frontal limb leads as well as one precordial unipolar lead.

1. **Indications**
   a. **Diagnosis of dysrhythmias**
   b. **Diagnosis of ischemia** (see Chapter 11 "Anesthetic Management of Myocardial Revascularization"). In the anesthetized patient, the detection of ischemia by ECG becomes more important because the usual symptom, angina, cannot be elicited.
   c. **Diagnosis of conduction defects**
   d. **Diagnosis of electrolyte disturbances**
   e. **Monitor effect of cardioplegia during aortic cross-clamp**
2. **Techniques**
   a. **The three-electrode system.** This system utilizes electrodes only on the right arm, left arm, and left leg. The potential difference between two of the electrodes is recorded, whereas the third electrode serves as a ground. Three ECG leads (I, II, III) can be examined.

      The three-lead system has been expanded to include the augmented leads. It identifies one of the three leads as the exploring electrode and couples the remaining two at a central terminal with zero potential. This creates leads in three more axes (aVR, aVL, aVF) in the frontal plane (Fig. 4.1). Leads II, III, and aVF are most useful for monitoring the inferior wall, and leads I and aVL for the lateral wall. Several additional leads have been developed for specific indications (Table 4.1).
   b. **The five-electrode system.** All limb leads act as a common ground for the precordial unipolar lead. The unipolar lead usually is placed in the V_5 position, along the anterior axillary line in the fifth intercostal space, to best monitor the left ventricle (LV). The precordial lead can also be placed on the right precordium to monitor the right ventricle (RV; V_{4R} lead).
      (1) **Advantages.** With the addition of only two electrodes to the ECG system, seven different leads can be monitored simultaneously. More important, all but the posterior wall of the myocardium can be monitored for ischemia. In patients with coronary artery disease, the unipolar V_5 lead is the best single lead in diagnosing myocardial ischemia [2]; moreover, 90% of ischemic episodes will be detected by

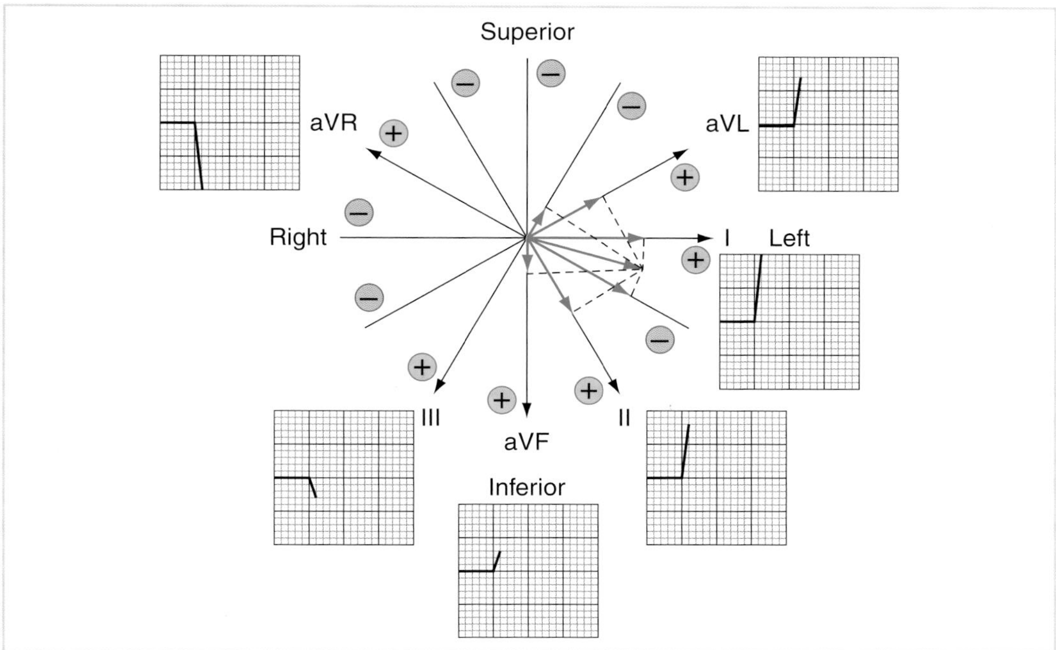

FIGURE 4.1 The six frontal plane axes that are available from three leads (right arm, left arm, and left leg) are shown. I, II, and III are bipolar leads, meaning that the potential between two electrodes (one positive, one negative) is monitored. The augmented leads (*aVR, aVL,* and *aVF*) are unipolar leads; one lead is the exploring electrode (the positive terminal), and the other two are connected and set at zero potential (indifferent, or neutral). The potential difference is then the absolute difference between the exploring and zero terminals. Connecting the two indifferent leads together produces the augmented lead axes that are between the bipolar lead axes. A sample electrical vector is shown (*heavy arrow*), with its projections to the six frontal axes. The direction of the electrical vector, then, is dictated by the direction of the deflection seen on the axis of each particular lead of the surface ECG. (From Thys DM, Kaplan JA. *The ECG in Anesthesia and Critical Care.* New York, NY: Churchill Livingstone; 1987:5, with permission.)

ECG if leads II and V_5 are analyzed simultaneously. Therefore, a correctly placed V_5 lead in conjunction with limb leads should enhance the diagnosis of the vast majority of intraoperative ischemic events. Multiple ECG leads are also useful in the diagnosis of atrial and ventricular dysrhythmias.

(2) **Disadvantage.** The V_5 electrode does not interfere with the operative field for a median sternotomy, although it will interfere with a left thoracotomy incision. All leads should be protected with waterproof tape, as surgical preparation solutions will loosen electrode patches and interfere with the electrical signal.

c. **Semi-Invasive ECG.** Semi-invasive leads are not routinely used but specific application may provide valuable information.

(1) **Esophageal.** Esophageal leads can be incorporated into the esophageal stethoscope. The esophageal lead is sensitive for the detection of posterior wall ischemia and the diagnosis of atrial dysrhythmias.

(2) **Endotracheal.** ECG leads have been incorporated into the endotracheal tube and may be useful in pediatric cardiac patients for the diagnosis of atrial dysrhythmias.

(3) **Epicardial electrodes.** Cardiac surgeons routinely place ventricular and/or atrial epicardial pacing wires at the conclusion of CPB prior to sternal closure. In addition to AV pacing, these pacing wires can be utilized to record atrial and/or ventricular epicardial ECGs. These leads are most useful in the postoperative diagnosis of complex conduction problems and dysrhythmias.

TABLE 4.1 Bipolar and augmented leads for use with three electrodes

Lead identifier	Right arm electrode: Function (location)	Left arm electrode: Function (location)	Left leg electrode: Function (location)	Lead select	Useful for diagnosing
Standard leads					
I	Negative (right arm)	Positive (left arm)	Ground (left leg)	I	Lateral ischemia
II	Negative (right arm)	Ground (left arm)	Positive (left leg)	II	Dysrhythmias (maximal P wave and QRS height); inferior ischemia
III	Ground (right arm)	Negative (left arm)	Positive (left leg)	III	Inferior ischemia
Augmented leads					
aVR	Positive (right arm)	Common ground (left arm)	Common ground (left leg)	aVR	
aVL	Common ground (right arm)	Positive (left arm)	Common ground (left leg)	aVL	Lateral ischemia
aVF	Common ground (right arm)	Common ground (left arm)	Positive (left leg)	aVF	Inferior ischemia
Special leads					
MCL_1	Ground (right arm)	Negative (Under left clavicle)	Positive (V_1 position)	III	Dysrhythmias (maximal P wave and QRS height)
CS_5	Negative (under right clavicle)	Positive (V_5 position)	Ground (left leg)	I	Anterior ischemia
CM_5	Negative (manubrium sternum)	Positive (V_5 position)	Ground (left leg)	I	Anterior ischemia
CB_5	Negative (center of right scapula)	Positive (V_5 position)	Ground (left leg)	I	Anterior ischemia; dysrhythmia (maximal P wave)
CC_5	Negative (right anterior axillary line)	Positive (V5 position)	Ground (left leg)	I	Global ischemia

Modified from Griffin RM, Kaplan JA. ECG lead systems. In: Thys D, Kaplan J, eds. *The ECG in Anesthesia and Critical Care*. New York, NY: Churchill Livingstone; 1987:20.

3. **Computer-assisted ECG interpretation.** Computer programs for online analysis of dysrhythmias and ischemia are currently widely available with a 60% to 78% sensitivity in detecting ischemia compared with the Holter monitor [3]. Typically, the current ECG signal is displayed along with a graph showing the trend (e.g., ST depression) over a recent time period, usually the past 30 min.
4. **Recommendations for ECG monitoring.** It is recommended that for cardiac anesthesia, a five-electrode surface ECG monitor be used in the diagnostic mode, with a frequency response of 0.05 to 100 Hz. Ideally, this monitor should display at least two leads simultaneously evaluating dysrhythmias and ischemia of two different areas of myocardium supplied by two different coronary arteries. Typically, leads V_5 and II are monitored. None of the standard ECG leads can detect posterior wall ischemia or RV ischemia.

1

B. Noninvasive blood pressure monitors

1. **Indications in the cardiac patient.** Noninvasive methods for measuring blood pressure (BP) are not adequate for monitoring hemodynamic parameters during a cardiac surgical procedure and should only be used until an arterial catheter is placed. Noninvasive devices will not function when pulsatile flow is absent including during cardiopulmonary bypass or when continuous-flow left ventricular assist devices (LVAD) are used.

C. Intravascular pressure measurements. Invasive monitors via intravascular catheters are required to safely administer a cardiac anesthetic. Arterial pressure can be measured by placing a catheter in a peripheral artery or femoral artery. Central venous access is obtained to measure the central venous pressure (CVP) and serve as conduit for PAC placement to measure intracardiac pressures. The components of a system of intravascular pressure measurement are the intravascular catheter, fluid-filled connector tubing, a transducer, and an electronic analyzer and display system.

1. **Characteristics of a pressure waveform.** Pressure waves in the cardiovascular system can be characterized as complex periodic sine waves. These complex waves are a summation of a series of simple sine waves of differing amplitudes and frequencies, which represent the natural harmonics of a fundamental frequency. The first harmonic, or fundamental frequency, is equal to the heart rate (Fig. 4.2), and the first 10 harmonics of the fundamental frequency will contribute significantly to the waveform.
2. **Properties of a monitoring system**
   a. **Frequency response** (or **amplitude ratio**) is the ratio of the measured amplitude versus the input amplitude of a signal at a specific frequency. The frequency response should be constant over the desired range of input frequencies—that is, the signal is not

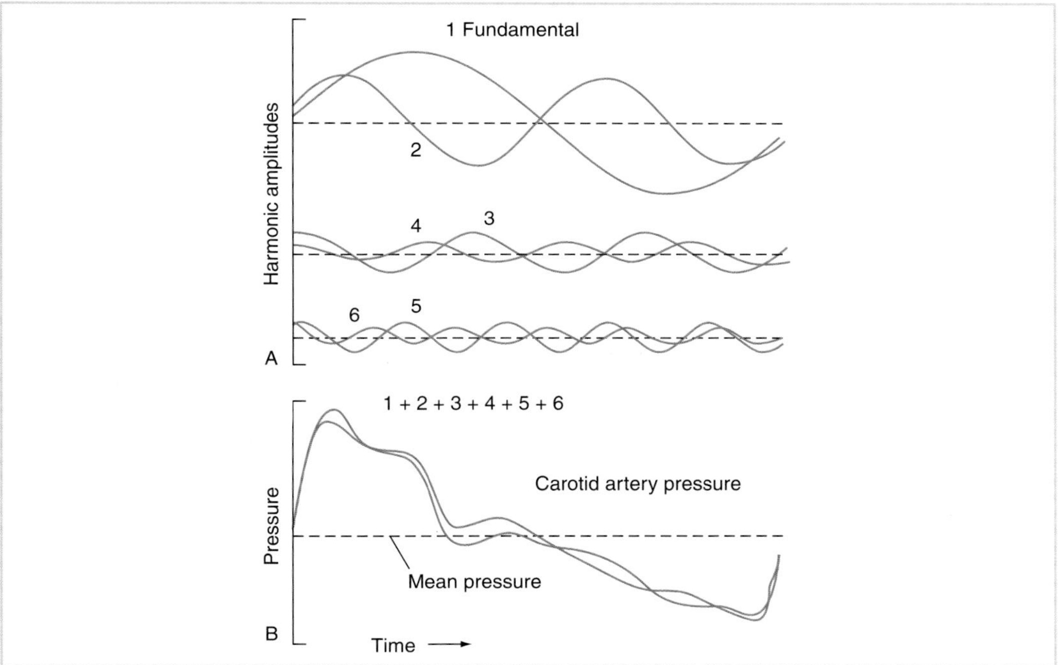

FIGURE 4.2 **A:** Generation of the harmonic waveforms from the fundamental frequency (heart rate) by Fourier analysis. **B:** The first six harmonics are shown. The addition of the six harmonics reproduces an actual BP wave. The first six harmonics are superimposed, showing a likeness to, but not a faithful reproduction of, the original wave. The first 10 harmonics of a pressure wave must be sensed by a catheter–transducer system, if that system is to provide an accurate reproduction of the wave. (From Welch JP, D'Ambra MN. Hemodynamic monitoring. In: Kofke WA, Levy JH, eds. *Postoperative Critical Care Procedures of the Massachusetts General Hospital.* Boston, MA: Little, Brown and Company; 1986:146, with permission.)

distorted (amplified or attenuated). The ideal amplitude ratio is close to 1. The signal frequency range of an intravascular pressure wave response is determined by the heart rate. For example, if a patient's heart rate is 120 beats/min, the fundamental frequency is 2 Hz. Because the first 10 harmonics contribute to the arterial waveform, frequencies up to 20 Hz will contribute to the morphology of an arterial waveform at this heart rate.

b. Natural frequency (or **resonant frequency**), a property of all matter, refers to the frequency at which a monitoring system itself resonates and amplifies the signal. The natural frequency (***f_n***) of a monitoring system is directly proportional to the catheter lumen diameter (*D*), inversely proportional to the square root of three parameters: The tubing connection length (*L*), the system compliance **($\Delta V/\Delta P$)**, and the density of fluid contained in the system (δ). This is expressed as follows:

$$f_n \alpha \mathrm{D} \cdot \mathrm{L}^{-1/2} \cdot (\Delta \mathrm{V}/\Delta \mathrm{P})^{-1/2} \cdot \delta^{-1/2}$$

To increase f_n and thereby reduce distortion, it is imperative that a pressure-sensing system be composed of short, low-compliance tubing of reasonable diameter, filled with a low-density fluid (such as normal saline).

Ideally, the natural frequency of the measuring system should be at least 10 times the fundamental frequency to reproduce the first 10 harmonics of the pressure wave without distortion. In clinical practice, the natural frequency of most measuring systems is in the range from 10 to 20 Hz. If the input frequency is close to the system's natural frequency (which is usually the case in clinical situations), the system's response will be amplified (Fig. 4.3). Therefore, these systems require the correct amount of **damping** to minimize distortion.

c. The **damping coefficient** reflects the rate of dissipation of the energy of a pressure wave. Figure 4.4 shows the relationship among frequency response, natural frequency, and damping coefficient.

When a pressure-monitoring system with a certain natural frequency duplicates a complex waveform with any one of the first 10 harmonics close to the natural frequency of the system, amplification will result if correct damping of the catheter–transducer unit is not performed. The problem is compounded when the heart rate is fast (as in

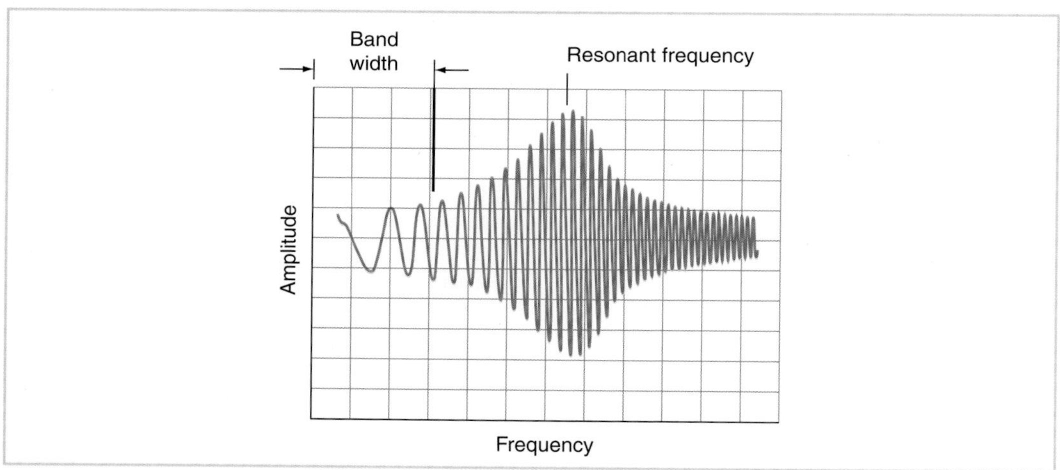

FIGURE 4.3 Pressure recording from a pressure generator simulator, which emits a sine wave at increasing frequencies (*horizontal axis*). The frequency response (ratio of signal amplitude$_{OUT}$ to signal amplitude$_{IN}$) is plotted on the vertical axis for a typical catheter–transducer system. The useful band width (range of frequency producing a "flat" response) and the amplification of the signal in the frequency range near the natural frequency of the system are shown. (From Welch JP, D'Ambra MN. Hemodynamic monitoring. In: Kofke WA, Levy JH, eds. *Postoperative Critical Care Procedures of the Massachusetts General Hospital.* Boston, MA: Little, Brown and Company; 1986:148, with permission.)

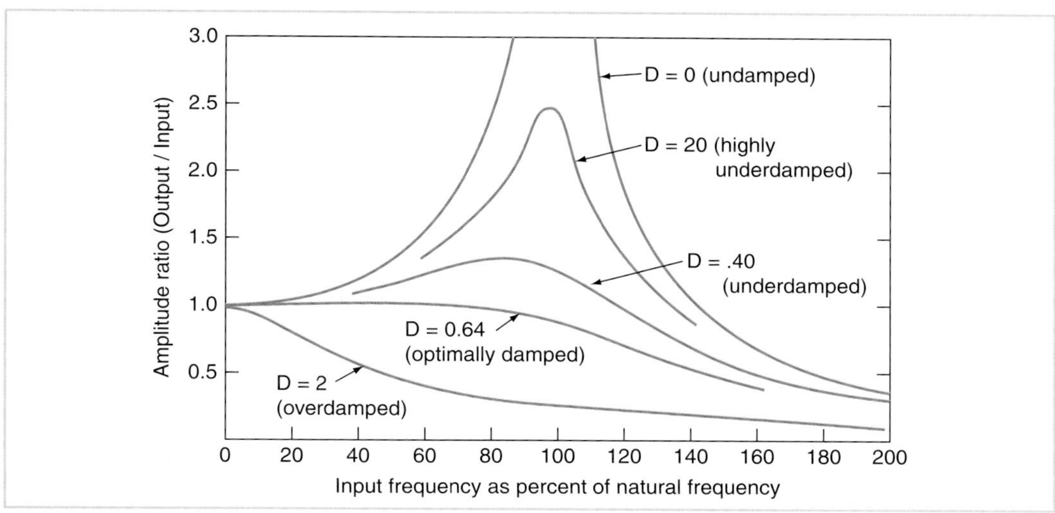

FIGURE 4.4 Amplitude ratio (or frequency response) on the vertical axis is plotted as a function of the input frequency as a percentage of the natural frequency (rather than as absolute values). In the undamped or underdamped system, the signal output is amplified in the region of the natural frequency of the transducer system; in the overdamped system, a reduction in amplitude ratio for most input frequencies is seen. This plot exhibits several important points: (i) If a catheter–transducer system has a high natural frequency, less damping will be required to produce a flat response in the clinically relevant range of input frequencies (10 to 30 Hz). (ii) For systems with a natural frequency in the clinically relevant range (usual case), a level of "critical" (optimal) damping exists that will maintain a flat frequency response. D, damping coefficient (From Grossman W. *Cardiac Catheterization.* 3rd ed. Philadelphia, PA: Lea & Febiger; 1985:122, with permission.)

a child or a patient with a rapid atrial rhythm), which increases the demands of the system by increasing the input frequency (Fig. 4.5). **Correct damping of a pressure-monitoring system should not affect the natural frequency of the system.**

Both the natural frequency and the damping coefficient of a system can be estimated using an adaptation of the square wave method known as the "pop" test. The natural

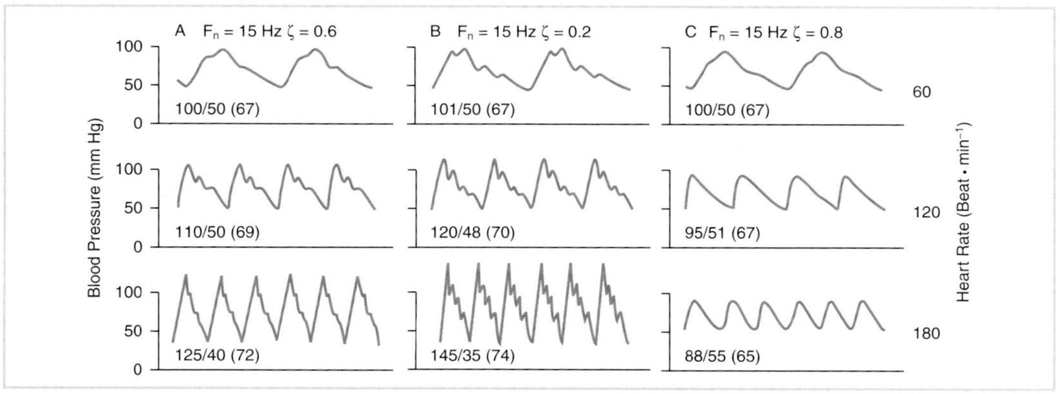

FIGURE 4.5 Comparison of three catheter–transducer systems with the same natural frequency (15 Hz) under different conditions of heart rate. Pressures are displayed as systolic–diastolic (mean). The reference BP for all panels is 100/50. **A:** A critically damped system ($\zeta = 0.6$) provides an accurate reproduction until higher heart rates (greater than 150) are reached. **B:** An underdamped system ($\zeta = 0.2$) shows distortion at lower rates, leading to overestimation of systolic and underestimation of diastolic pressures. **C:** An overdamped system ($\zeta = 0.8$) demonstrates underestimation of systolic pressure and overestimation of diastolic pressure. Also note that diastolic and mean pressures are affected less by the inadequate monitoring systems. f_n, natural frequency; ζ, damping coefficient.

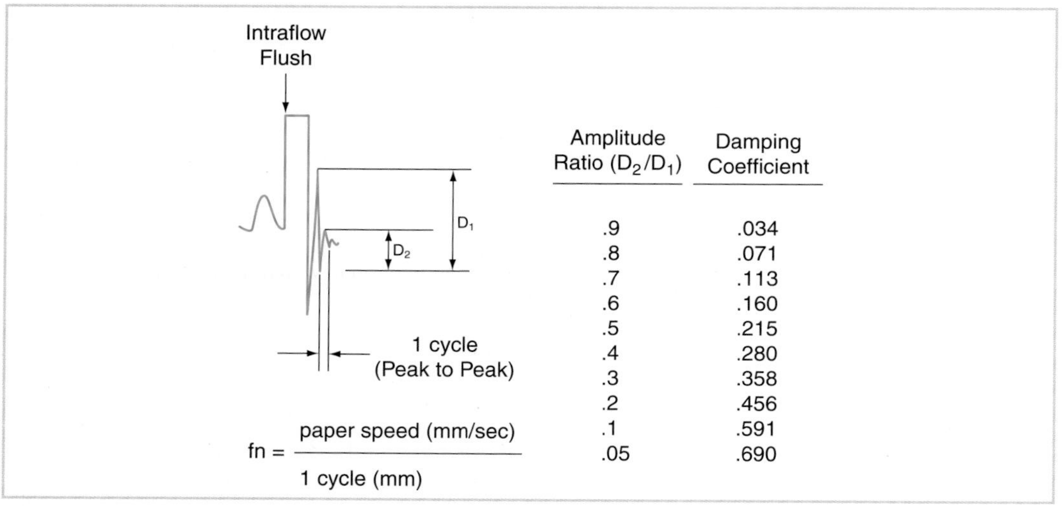

Amplitude Ratio (D_2/D_1)	Damping Coefficient
.9	.034
.8	.071
.7	.113
.6	.160
.5	.215
.4	.280
.3	.358
.2	.456
.1	.591
.05	.690

FIGURE 4.6 The "pop" test allows one to derive f_n and ζ of a catheter–transducer system. The test should be done with the catheter in the artery in order to test the system in its entirety, as all components contribute to the harmonics of the system. The test involves a rapid flush (with the high-pressure flush system used commonly), followed by a sudden release. This produces a rapid decrease from the flush bag pressure and, owing to the inertia of the system, an overshoot of the baseline. The subsequent oscillations about the baseline are used to calculate f_n and ζ. For example, the arterial pulse at the far left of the figure is followed by a fast flush and sudden release. The resulting oscillations have a definite period, or cycle, measured in millimeters. The natural frequency f_n is the paper speed divided by this period, expressed in cycles per second, or Hertz. If the period were 2 mm and the paper speed 25 mm/s, $f_n = 12.5$ Hz. For determining f_n, a faster paper speed will give better reliability. The ratio of the amplitude of one induced resonant wave to the next, D_2/D_1, is used to calculate damping coefficients **(right column).** A damping coefficient of 0.2 to 0.4 describes an underdamped system, 0.4 to 0.6 an optimally damped system, and 0.6 to 0.8 an overdamped system. (From Bedford RF. Invasive blood pressure monitoring. In: Blitt CD, ed. *Monitoring in Anesthesia and Critical Care Medicine.* New York, NY: Churchill Livingstone; 1985:59, with permission.)

frequency is estimated by measuring the time period of one oscillation as the system settles to baseline after a high-pressure flush. The damping coefficient is calculated by measuring the amplitude ratio of two successive peaks (Fig. 4.6).

2 After a rapid pressure change (performed by flushing the pressure line), an underdamped system will continue to oscillate for a prolonged time. In terms of pressure monitoring, this translates to an overestimation of systolic BP and an underestimation of diastolic BP. An overdamped system will not oscillate at all but will settle to baseline slowly, thus underestimating systolic and overestimating diastolic pressures. A critically damped system will settle to baseline after only one or two oscillations and will reproduce systolic pressures accurately. An optimally or *critically* damped system will exhibit a constant (or *flat*) frequency response in the range of frequencies up to the f_n of the system (Fig. 4.4). If a given system does not meet this criterion, components should be checked, especially for air, or the system replaced. Even an optimally damped system will begin to distort the waveform at higher heart rates because the 10th harmonic exceeds the system's natural frequency (Fig. 4.5).

3. **Strain gauges.** The pressure-monitoring transducer can be described as a variable-resistance transducer. A critical part of the transducer is the diaphragm, which acts to link the fluid wave to the electrical input. When the diaphragm of a transducer is distorted by a change in pressure, voltages are altered across the variable resistor of a Wheatstone bridge contained in the transducer. This in turn produces a change in current, which is electronically converted and displayed.
4. **Sources of error in intravascular pressure measurement**
   a. **Low-frequency transducer response.** Low-frequency response refers to a low-frequency range over which the ratio of output-to-input amplitude is constant (i.e., no

distortion). If the natural frequency of the system is low, its frequency response will also be low. Most transducer systems used in clinical anesthesia can be described as underdamped systems with a low natural frequency. Thus, any condition that further decreases f_n response should be avoided. Air within a catheter–transducer system causes most monitoring errors. Because of its compressibility, air not only decreases the response of the system but also leads to overdamping of the system. Therefore, the myth that an air bubble placed in the pressure tubing decreases artifact by increasing the damping coefficient is incorrect. A second common cause of diminution of frequency response is the formation of a partially obstructing clot in the catheter.

b. **Catheter whip.** Catheter "whip" is a phenomenon in which the motion of the catheter tip itself produces a noticeable pressure swing. This artifact usually is not observed with peripheral arterial catheters but is more common with PAC or LV catheters.

c. **Resonance in peripheral vessels.** The systolic pressure measured in a radial arterial catheter may be up to 20 to 50 mm Hg higher than the aortic pressure due to decreased peripheral arterial elastance and wave summation (Fig. 4.7).

d. **Changes in electrical properties of the transducer.** *Electrical balance,* or *electrical zero,* refers to the adjustment of the Wheatstone bridge within the transducer so that zero current flows to the detector at zero pressure. Transducers should be electronically balanced periodically during a procedure because the zero point may drift, for instance, if the room temperature changes. The pressure waveform morphology may not change with baseline drift of a transducer.

e. **Transducer position errors.** By convention, the reference position for hemodynamic monitoring during cardiac surgery is the right atrium (RA). With the patient supine, the RA lies at the level of the midaxillary line. Once its zero level has been established, the transducer must be maintained at the same level as the RA. *If the transducer position changes, falsely high or low-pressure values will result.* This can be significant especially when monitoring CVP, PA pressure, or pulmonary capillary wedge pressure (PCWP) where the observed change is a greater percentage of the measured value. For

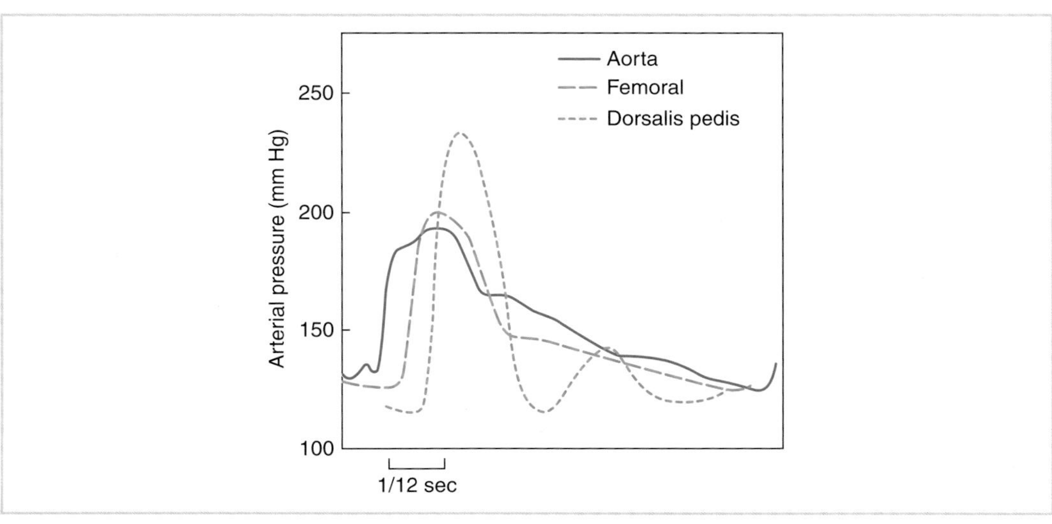

FIGURE 4.7 Change of pulse pressure in different arteries. The central aortic waveform is more rounded and has a definite dicrotic notch. The dorsalis pedis and, to a lesser extent, the femoral artery show a delay in pulse transmission, sharper initial upstrokes (and thus higher systolic pressure), and slurring (femoral) and loss (dorsalis) of the dicrotic notch. The dicrotic notch is better maintained in the upper-extremity pressure wave (not shown). The small second "hump" in the dorsalis wave probably is due to a reflected wave from the arterial–arteriolar impedance mismatching. (From Welch JP, D'Ambra MN. Hemodynamic monitoring. In: Kofke WA, Levy JH, eds. *Postoperative Critical Care Procedures of the Massachusetts General Hospital.* Boston, MA: Little, Brown and Company; 1986:144, with permission.)

example, if a patient has a mean arterial pressure of 100 mm Hg and a of 10 mm Hg, a 5 mm Hg offset due to transducer position would be displayed as a 5% or 50% change in the arterial or CVP pressures, respectively.

D. Arterial catheterization

1. **Indications.** Arterial catheterization ("art line") has become the standard in the monitoring of the cardiac surgical patient. Indications for arterial pressure monitoring are as follows:
   a. **Small or rapid changes in arterial perfusion pressure may increase patient risk requiring beat-to-beat assessment.** Cardiac surgical patients frequently have critical coronary artery disease and/or valvular heart disease. Cardiac surgical patients are at high risk of becoming hemodynamically unstable in the perioperative period.
   b. **Wide variation in BP or intravascular volume is anticipated.**
   c. **Frequent blood sampling, especially arterial blood gas (ABG) analysis, is required.**
   d. **Assessment of BP cannot be performed by other methods.** CPB and continuous flow LVAD (nonpulsatile flow), dysrhythmia, or marked obesity require arterial pressure catheters.
2. **Sites of cannulation.** Several sites can be used for cannulation of the arterial tree:
   a. **Radial artery.** The radial artery is the most commonly utilized site because catheter insertion is convenient and the radial artery provides a reasonably accurate estimation of the true aortic pressure.
      (1) **Technique.** Table 4.2 summarizes the steps used for radial arterial cannulation. One technique, transfixing the radial artery for catheter insertion, is shown in Figure 4.8. Ultrasound-guided radial artery cannulation [4] can be especially beneficial when difficulty placing the catheter via the traditional method is encountered. Table 4.3 and Figure 4.9 describe ultrasound guidance for arterial cannulation. Ultrasound guidance may be the method of choice with improved first-pass

TABLE 4.2 Steps for arterial catheter placement

Steps	Rationale and possible complications
1. Immobilize and dorsiflex at wrist	Too much dorsiflexion or tape too tight—occludes artery
2. Immobilize thumb with tape	Stabilize the artery against the radial head
3. Palpate artery 3–4 cm along its course	Increases the likelihood of a central puncture
4. a. Make small skin wheal with 0.5% lidocaine after sterile preparation **b.** Infiltrate deeper planes on either side of artery	Keep volume small for this and deeper infiltration to avoid altering anatomy Decreases the incidence of spasm
5. Make skin nick with 18-gauge needle	Facilitates maneuvering of the catheter
6. Introduce 20-gauge, 2-inch catheter-over-needle unit	Larger bore possibly associated with increased thrombogenesis
7. Advance in rapid, short, 1 mm increments until flashback is seen. Three options available: **a.** Advance unit 0.5 mm; slide catheter off needle into artery **b.** Advance unit until flashback stops, then withdraw needle (holding catheter stationary); when flashback returns, advance catheter into artery **c.** Advance unit several millimeters, remove needle completely, back catheter until good flow returns, advance catheter into artery either directly or after passing flexible wire	Rapid advance increases chance of arterial wall puncture These three methods are not mutually exclusive but describe three different depths of needle and catheter tip placement: **a.** Placement in the arterial **lumen** **b.** Placement in the **back wall** of the artery (catheter tip will remain in lumen with this method) **c.** Placement of needle and catheter **through** back wall—also termed *transfixing* the artery. Wire should be advanced through lumen of catheter only if pulsatile flow via catheter is present; forcing wire may result in arterial dissection
8. Remove air from tubing	Prevents arterial air emboli

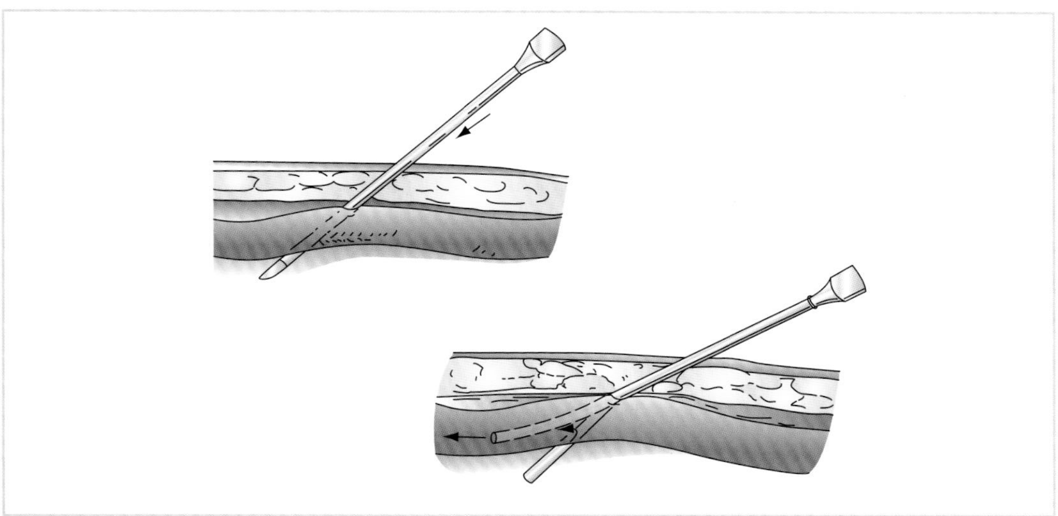

FIGURE 4.8 One technique used for radial artery cannulation. The needle–catheter unit is advanced through the artery, as shown in the **upper drawing.** The **lower drawing** shows the needle removed and the catheter withdrawn until pulsatile flow is obtained (indicating that the catheter tip is in the lumen). The catheter then is advanced into the artery. (Redrawn from Freis ES. Vascular cannulation. In: Kofke WA, Levy JH, eds. *Postoperative Critical Care Procedures of the Massachusetts General Hospital.* Boston, MA: Little, Brown and Company; 1986:137, with permission.)

success when difficulty such as low flow states (shock), or nonpulsatile flow (extracorporeal membrane oxygenation [ECMO], LVAD, cardiac arrest), or nonpalpable pulses (secondary to peripheral edema, hematoma, arterial vasospasm) are encountered.

(2) **Contraindications.** Inadequate collateral flow to the hand is a relative contraindication to the use of a radial artery catheter. Very few ischemic complications have been reported from arterial catheterization even in patients with a positive Allen's test indicating limited collateral ulnar artery flow [5].

(3) **Radial artery harvest.** If a coronary bypass that will utilize the radial artery as a free graft is planned, an alternative site must be used. Usually the radial artery to be harvested is known preoperatively, and the contralateral radial artery can be used.

b. **Femoral artery.** The femoral artery offers two advantages over the radial site: Assessment of central arterial pressure and appropriate access should placement of an intra-aortic balloon pump become necessary during the surgical procedure. Placement of a femoral artery catheter as an additional catheter site should be considered in any patient in whom difficulty in weaning from CPB is expected (e.g., those with markedly depressed ejection fraction, severe wall-motion abnormalities, or significant coronary disease).

(1) **Technique.** The femoral artery is entered most easily using a Seldinger technique after sterile preparation and draping. The femoral artery typically lies at the midpoint between the pubic tubercle and the anterior superior iliac spine. These bone landmarks can be used to guide identification of the femoral pulse in difficult cases.

(2) **Contraindications.** Cannulation of the femoral artery should be avoided in patients with prior vascular surgery involving the femoral arteries or a skin infection of the groin.

c. **Aortic root.** Aortic root cannulation is an option when the chest is open and difficulties are encountered in obtaining a reliable BP. Pressure tubing can be handed to the anesthesiologist from the sterile field after a needle or catheter is inserted in the aortic root by the surgeon.

TABLE 4.3 Steps for ultrasound-guided arterial catheterization

Steps	Rationale and possible complications
1. Prior to sterile draping of the site, the operator performs an initial scan of the intended site	Demonstrates vessel patency and any anatomical variations
2. Arterial blood flow is confirmed. **a.** Pulsibility—Partial compression of the artery improves visualization of pulsibility **b.** Compressibility—Transducer pressure typically collapses venous structures while only partially compressing arterial structures **c.** Doppler—When tilting the transducer in the direction of the heart, color flow Doppler reveals arterial flow as red and venous flow as blue. Additionally, pulse wave Doppler can be placed through the vessel for additional confirmation	Often venous structures lie in proximity to arteries
3. The location is prepped and draped sterilely. A sterile sheath is draped over the ultrasound probe and sterile gel placed on the site of interest	Site positioning should be maintained from the initial ultrasound evaluation. For example, changing wrist extension from 45° to greater than 60° can change radial artery height and impede catheterization.
4. The proceduralist stabilizes the ultrasound probe with his/her nondominant hand obtaining the desired view: **a.** Transverse Plane **b.** Longitudinal Plane—obtained by centering the artery in the transverse plane and rotating the probe 90°. (See Figure 4.9.)	**a.** Allows for easier visualization of smaller arteries **b.** Allows direct visualization of the needle entering the vascular structure, thus reducing posterior wall perforation
5. With the dominant hand, a lidocaine skin wheal is applied slightly distal to the site of the ultrasound probe **6.** The arterial needle and catheter are then inserted at the site of the skin wheal and advanced into the plane of the ultrasound until they are visualized adjacent to the artery. Once the artery is penetrated, the operator can release the ultrasound probe, freely his/her non-dominant hand to aid in catheter placement	

d. Axillary artery. The axillary artery, like the femoral artery, provides the anesthesiologist with a superficial, large artery that has good access to the central arterial tree.

(1) **Technique.** The axillary artery is most easily entered using a Seldinger technique.

(2) **Contraindications.** The increased risk of cerebral embolus of air or debris must be recognized. Flushing the arterial line must be performed with caution and low pressure.

e. Brachial artery. The brachial artery is an easily accessible artery located medially in the antecubital fossa.

(1) **Brachial artery** cannulation is similar to that described for the radial artery. The elbow must be immobilized with a long arm board for stability.

(2) **Contraindications.** Concern about compromised flow distal to catheter placement has limited its use at many institutions. Brachial catheterization is a secondary option or is not utilized in non-heparinized surgical procedures. A purported benefit has been the elimination of the pressure discrepancy seen occasionally with radial arterial lines in the immediate postbypass period (see Section I.D.4.e).

f. Ulnar artery. The ulnar artery can be used in those rare circumstances when the radial artery cannot be entered easily.

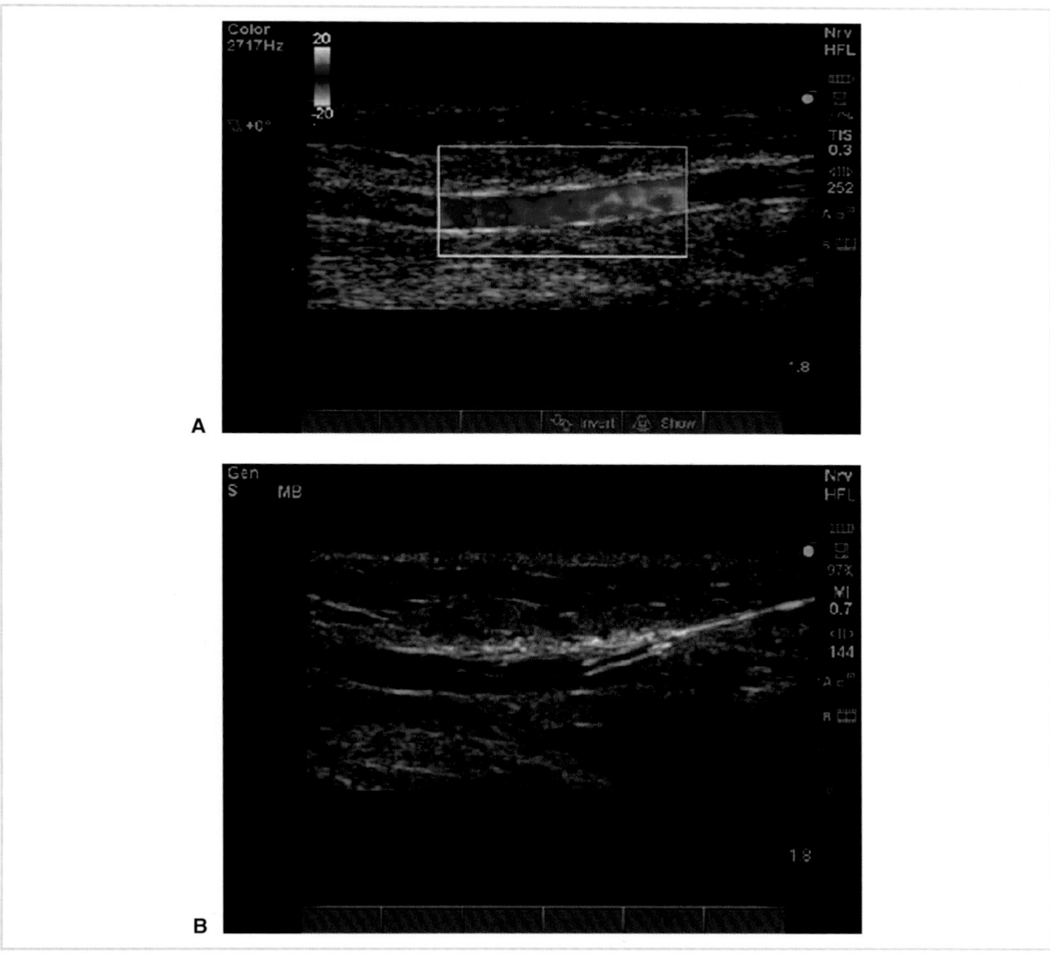

FIGURE 4.9 Ultrasound-guided radial artery cannulation. **A:** Color flow Doppler demonstrates patent flow in the radial artery. **B:** After flow is confirmed, a catheter is advanced with ultrasound guidance into the radial artery. (From Mikhael R. *Radial Artery Cannulation (In-Plane Approach)*. 2010. Graphic. MSH Obstetric Anesthesia Ultrasound Group. http://oba.mikhaels.org/currentconcepts/ultrasound/module.php?section =vascular&name =multimedia)

g. **Dorsalis pedis and posterior tibialis arteries.** In general, the distal location increases distortion of the arterial wave (Fig. 4.7). The dorsalis pedis artery is technically easier to cannulate.

3. **Interpretation of arterial tracings.** The arterial pressure waveform contains a great deal of hemodynamic information.
   a. **Heart rate and rhythm.** The heart rate can be determined from the arterial pressure wave. This is especially helpful if the patient is being paced or if electrocautery is being used. In the presence of numerous atrial or ventricular ectopic beats, the arterial trace can provide useful information on the hemodynamic consequences of these dysrhythmias (i.e., if an ectopic beat is perfusing).
   b. **Pulse pressure.** The difference between the systolic and diastolic pressures provides useful information about fluid status and valvular competence. Pericardial tamponade and hypovolemia are accompanied by a narrow pulse pressure on the arterial

waveform. An increase in pulse pressure may be a sign of worsening aortic valvular insufficiency or hypovolemia.

c. **Respiratory variation and volume status.** Hypovolemia is suggested by a decrease in arterial systolic pressure with positive-pressure ventilation (pulsus paradox). Positive intrathoracic pressure impedes venous return to the heart with a more pronounced effect in the hypovolemic patient. Because this finding is not uniformly seen in patients with hypovolemia, correlation with other findings can help make the diagnosis.

d. **Qualitative estimates of hemodynamic indices.** Inferences can be made regarding contractility, stroke volume, and vascular resistance from the arterial waveform. Contractility can be grossly judged by the rate of pressure rise during systole, keeping in mind that heart rate, preload, and afterload can affect this parameter. Stroke volume can be estimated from the area under the aortic pressure wave from the onset of systole to the dicrotic notch. Finally, the position of the dicrotic notch correlates with the systemic resistance. A notch appearing high on the downslope of the pressure trace suggests a high vascular resistance, whereas a low resistance tends to cause a dicrotic notch that is lower on the diastolic portion of the pressure trace. These elements are incorporated into the algorithms of pulse pressure analysis monitors for non-invasive cardiac output (CO).

4. **Complications of arterial catheterization**

a. **Ischemia.** The incidence of ischemic complications after radial artery cannulation is low. A classic study demonstrated that although abnormal flow patterns were present in up to 25% of patients between 1 and 7 days after radial artery catheterization, there were no adverse signs of ischemia with these findings [5].

b. **Thrombosis.** Although the incidence of thrombosis from radial artery catheterization is high, studies have not demonstrated adverse sequelae. Recanalization of the radial artery occurs in a majority of cases. Patients with increased risk include those with diabetes or severe peripheral vascular disease.

c. **Infection.** With proper sterile technique, the risk of infection from cannulation of the radial artery should be minimal. In a series of 1,700 cases, no catheter site was overtly infected [5].

d. **Bleeding.** Although transfixing the artery will put a hole in the posterior wall, the layers of the muscular media will seal the puncture. In the patient with a bleeding diathesis, however, there is a greater tendency to bleed. Unlike central venous catheters, arterial catheters are not heparin bonded and thus have increased risk of thrombus development.

e. **False lowering of radial artery pressure immediately after CPB.** The radial artery pressure may be significantly lower than the aortic pressure at the completion of CPB. Forearm vasodilation secondary to rewarming may lead to arteriovenous AV shunting, resulting in a steal phenomenon 5 to 30 min or longer in duration. Alternatively, the inaccuracy of radial pressure may be due to hypovolemia and vasoconstriction. If suspicion arises that a peripheral arterial trace is dampened following CPB, a direct pressure measurement should be obtained from a central site.

5. **Recommendations for BP monitoring.** In high-risk patients, invasive arterial pressure monitoring should commence prior to induction. Under most circumstances, the radial artery pressure measurement will be sufficient and accurate before and after CPB. In the patient with poor LV function, addition of a femoral arterial catheter before CPB may be warranted. Certain surgical procedures, for example, a thoracoabdominal aortic aneurysm repaired with left heart partial bypass, require both an upper and lower extremity arterial catheters. If an internal mammary artery (IMA) is dissected, retraction of the chest wall and compression of the subclavian artery can dampen or obliterate the radial artery traces. The surgeon should be informed for possible change in retractor position. A dampened radial pressure during IMA harvest may also be associated with a brachial plexus injury.

TABLE 4.4 Sites for internal jugular cannulation

Approaches	Landmarks	Complications
Central	Apex of triangle formed by lateral (clavicular) and medial (sternal) head of SCM. Aim needle caudally and laterally toward ipsilateral nipple	Low incidence of pneumothorax; hemothorax; medial direction has higher incidence of carotid puncture
Posterior	Intersection of lateral border of lateral (clavicular) head of SCM and line drawn laterally from cricoid ring. Aim needle caudally and ventrally (anteriorly) toward sternal notch	Higher incidence of carotid puncture; low incidence of pneumothorax; hemothorax
Anterior	Medial border of medial head, 5 cm above clavicle. Direct needle toward ipsilateral nipple	Carotid puncture more likely unless retracted medially; hemothorax
Supraclavicular	Interscalene groove 2 cm above clavicle. Direct needle caudally and medially	Higher chance of pneumothorax and subclavian artery puncture; hemothorax

SCM, sternocleidomastoid muscle.

E. **Central venous pressure.** CVP measures RA pressure and is affected by circulating blood volume, venous tone, and RV function.

1. Indications
   a. **Monitoring.** Monitoring of CVP is indicated for all cardiac surgical patients.
   b. **Fluid and drug therapy.** CVP can be used to infuse fluid or blood products; as a port for administering vasoactive drugs; and for postoperative hyperalimentation.
   c. **Special uses.** One may elect to place a CVP catheter, with delayed PAC placement in selected patients. Placement of a PAC can be difficult in patients with numerous congenital cardiac disorders, in those with anatomic distortion of the right-sided venous circulation, or in those requiring surgical procedures of the right heart or implantation of a right heart mechanical assist device.
2. **Techniques.** There are numerous routes by which a catheter can be placed in the central circulation.
   a. **Internal jugular.** The internal jugular vein (IJV) is the most common access route for the cardiac anesthesiologist.
      (1) **Techniques.** Cannulation of the IJV is relatively safe and convenient and various approaches exist for its cannulation (Table 4.4, Fig. 4.10). The process of cannulation, regardless of the approach, involves the steps outlined in Table 4.5.
      (2) **Contraindications and recommendations.** Relative contraindications for internal jugular central line placement include the following:
         (a) Presence of carotid disease.
         (b) Recent cannulation of the IJV (with the concomitant risk of thrombosis).
         (c) Contralateral diaphragmatic dysfunction.
         (d) Thyromegaly or prior neck surgery.

      In these cases, the IJV on the contralateral side should be considered. It should be remembered that the thoracic duct lies in close proximity to the left IJV and that laceration of the left brachiocephalic vein or superior vena cava by the catheter is more likely with the left-sided approach. This risk is due to the more acute angle between the left internal jugular and innominate veins.
      (3) **Sonographic guidance.** Ultrasound guidance of IJV cannulation [6] has quickly gained acceptance as several studies have suggested improved success rates and decreased complications with its use. There is debate whether ultrasound guidance should become the standard of care [7,8]. The Agency for Healthcare Research and Quality in the United States and the National Institute for Clinical Excellence in the United Kingdom suggest that the preferred method for internal jugular

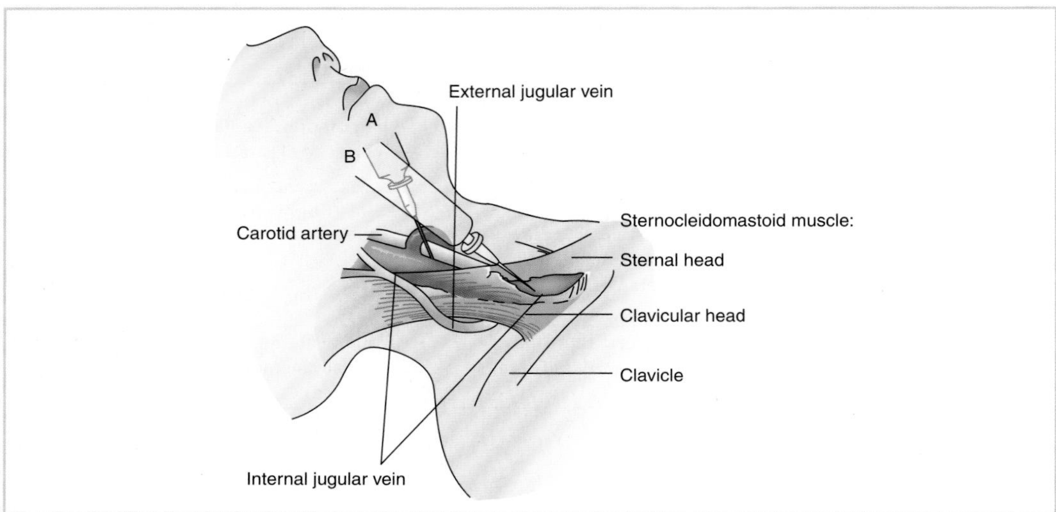

FIGURE 4.10 Two methods for internal jugular cannulation. **A:** Anterior approach. **B:** Central approach (see text for further details). (Redrawn from Freis ES. Vascular cannulation. In: Kofke WA, Levy JH, eds. *Postoperative Critical Care Procedures of the Massachusetts General Hospital.* Boston, MA: Little, Brown and Company; 1986:130, with permission.)

catheter placement is ultrasound guidance, particularly for inexperienced operators. Several commercially available hand-held ultrasound units are currently available. Alternatively, a hand-held probe from the Transesophageal echocardiography (TEE) machine can be utilized for ultrasonography. When anatomic landmark techniques prove to be difficult, ultrasound guidance becomes an invaluable tool. It can facilitate access in patients with thrombosis, hematoma formation, or vessel atrophy from multiple prior cannulations. Ultrasound-guided internal jugular cannulation (Table 4.6) requires the ability to correctly distinguish the easily compressible jugular vein from the carotid artery (CA), as shown in Figure 4.11.

b. External jugular. The external jugular vein courses superficially across the sternocleidomastoid muscle to join the subclavian vein close to the junction of the internal jugular and subclavian veins. Its course is more tortuous, and the presence of valves makes central line placement more difficult. The placement of rigid central catheters (e.g., PAC introducer) via the external jugular increases the risk of vessel trauma and is not recommended. Pliable central catheters and short catheters can be used to acquire intravenous access.

c. Subclavian. The subclavian vein is readily accessible and thus has been popular for use during cardiopulmonary resuscitation.

(1) Techniques. The patient is placed in a head-down position to distend the vein and decrease risk of air embolism. Optimal positioning can be obtained by placing a roll vertically under the patient's spine to anatomically retract the clavicle.

(2) Advantages. The main advantage to subclavian vein cannulation is its relative ease and the stability of the catheter during long-term cannulation.

(3) Disadvantages

(a) Subclavian vein cannulation carries the highest rate of pneumothorax of any approach. **If subclavian vein cannulation is unsuccessful on one side, an**
6 **attempt on the contralateral side is contraindicated without first obtaining a chest x-ray film.** Bilateral pneumothoraces can be lethal. Subclavian vein placement for cardiac surgery can be associated with compression of the central line during sternal retraction.

(b) The subclavian artery is entered easily.

TABLE 4.5 Steps for right internal jugular cannulation

Steps	Rationale and possible problems
1. Verify functioning ECG	Critical for monitoring dysrhythmias
2. Remove pillow, rotate head completely to left. Ask patient to raise head off the bed and note the position of tensed sternocleidomastoid muscle	Optimizes visualization of landmarks
3. Place patient in Trendelenburg position	Distends IJ and reduces risk of air embolism; may worsen symptoms due to congestive or right ventricular failure
4. Perform careful sterile preparation and drape	Mandatory for central venous cannulation; full glove and gown should be used
5. Recheck landmarks, skin wheal, and, in awake patients, deeper infiltration with 1% lidocaine	IJ often is superficial and may be found during infiltration; withdraw on syringe before injecting local anesthetic
6. Remove local anesthetic from syringe, replace infiltration needle with 19- or 21-gauge $1^1/_2$-inch "finder" needle	Not necessary if vein has been found previously; presence of local anesthetic will make aspirated blood appear bright red
7. Once vein has been located:	
a. Leave finder needle in place *or*	Serves as reminder of vein location
b. Remove finder, remember direction	Finder needle may interfere with subsequent cannulation
8. Insert 18-gauge $1^3/_4$-inch catheter over needle unit into IJ, following same line	Constant aspiration as unit is advanced is required to see flashback
9. When flashback is seen, advance unit ≈1 mm, then advance catheter over needle into vein	Once IV placement is established, end of catheter is capped with finger or syringe to avoid air embolism
10. If blood is not aspirated freely:	Catheter is probably through back wall
a. Remove needle	Patient may be hypovolemic, and IV fluid bolus will increase success
b. Replace syringe and aspirate	
c. Withdraw catheter until free flow of blood occurs	Increased head-down position may be needed
d. Advance catheter slowly into vein, or insert a wire through catheter	
11. Confirm IV placement by	
a. Check for lack of pulsatile flow	If arterial cannulation is diagnosed, remove catheter and hold pressure for at least 5 min to avoid hematoma formation
b. Measure pressure in the 18-gauge catheter and simultaneous arterial pressure, comparing absolute values and pressure waveforms	
c. Compare IJ and arterial blood samples, visually or by oximetry	
12. Pass flexible wire through catheter, remove catheter	ECG should be monitored because arrhythmias can result
13. Place CVP catheter over wire or dilator-introducer assembly (PAC)	Skin nick needed if larger introducer will be placed
14. Place sterile dressing	

ECG, electrocardiogram; IJ, internal jugular; IV, intravenous; CVP, central venous pressure; PAC, pulmonary artery catheter.

(c) In a left-sided cannulation, the thoracic duct may be lacerated.

(d) The right subclavian approach may make threading the PAC into the RA difficult because an acute angle must be negotiated by the catheter in order to enter the innominate vein. The left subclavian approach is recommended as the first option for PAC placement.

d. Arm vein

(1) Techniques. Central access can be obtained through the veins of the antecubital fossa ("long-arm CVP"). This has a limited role in most cardiac surgical procedures.

TABLE 4.6 Steps for ultrasound-guided cannulation of internal jugular

Steps	Rationale and possible complications
1. Steps 1–4 as described in Table 4.5	
2. Ultrasound probe is covered in a sterile sheath and sterile ultrasound gel is placed on the patient's skin	
3. Ultrasound probe is utilized to find the IJ vein. This should be distinguished from the CA	The IJ should be compressible and non-pulsatile. Additionally, color flow Doppler can be used by tilting the transducer in the direction of the heart. Arterial flow, going toward the transducer, will appear red, and venous flow, moving away from the transducer, will appear blue
4. The course of the IJ is scanned to find the best cannulation site	By scanning the course of the IJ, an area can be found where the IJ and carotid have the least amount of overlap. Additionally, the area of the largest IJ diameter can be found
5. The proceduralist stabilizes the ultrasound probe with his/her nondominant hand obtaining the desired view	
a. Transverse plane (see Figure 4.11)	Allows visualization of the carotid and IJ in same window
b. Longitudinal plane—obtained by centering the artery in the transverse plane and rotating the probe 90°	Allows visualization of the true needle tip entering the vessel. Allows visualization of posterior wall of vessel, and thus perforation of posterior wall. However, the relationship to the CA is lost
6. With the dominant hand, an 18-gauge $1^3/_4$-inch catheter over needle unit is inserted under ultrasound guidance until a flash is obtained	
7. The catheter is advanced over the needle	
8. The pressure waveform in the catheter is determined to confirm placement in the vein	
9. A flexible wire is placed through the catheter	
10. The ultrasound probe is used to confirm the placement of the wire in the vein (and lack of wire in the carotid; see Figure 4.9)	
11. Place CVP catheter over wire or dilator-introducer assembly	
12. Place sterile dressing	

IJ, internal jugular; CA, carotid artery; CVP, central venous pressure.

3. **Complications.** The site-specific complications of CVP catheter insertion are listed in Table 4.7. The most severe complications of CVP insertion usually are preventable.
4. **Interpretation**
   a. **Normal waves.** The normal CVP trace contains three positive deflections, termed the *A*, *C*, and *V* waves, and two negative deflections termed the *X* and *Y* descents (Fig. 4.12).
   b. **Abnormal waves.** A common abnormality in the CVP trace occurs in the presence of AV dissociation, when RA contraction occurs against a closed tricuspid valve. This produces a large "cannon A wave" that is virtually diagnostic. Abnormal V waves can occur with tricuspid valve insufficiency, in which retrograde flow through the incompetent valve produces an increase in RA pressure during systole.
   c. **RV function.** CVP offers direct measurement of RV filling pressure.
   d. **LV filling pressures.** The CVP can be used to estimate LV filling pressures. Parameters that distort this estimate include LV dysfunction, decreased LV compliance (i.e., ischemia), pulmonary hypertension, or mitral valvular disease. In patients with coronary

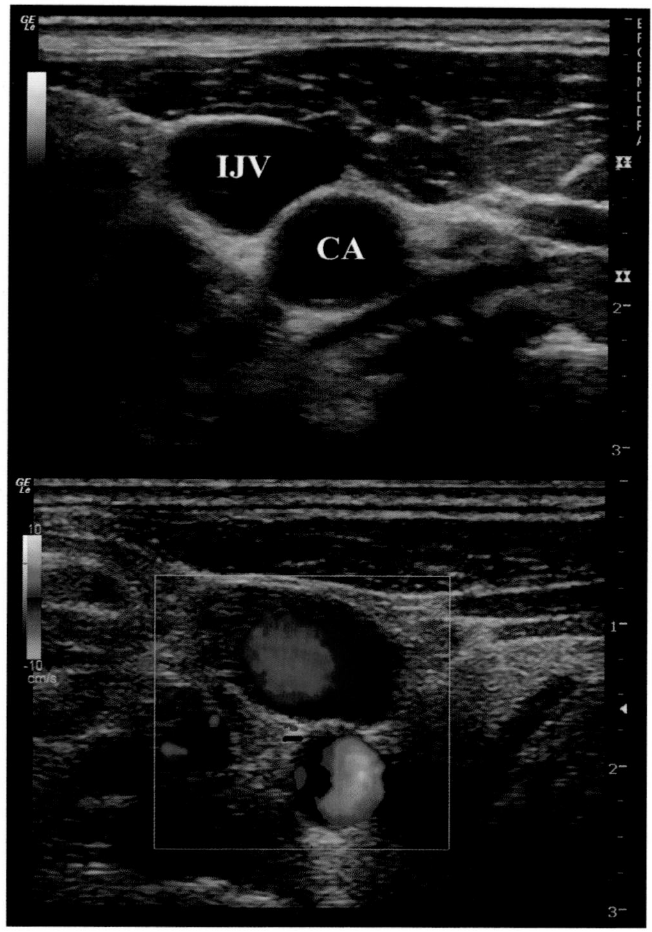

FIGURE 4.11 Ultrasound-guided internal jugular catheterization. The top picture demonstrates the two-dimensional examination showing the IJV lateral to the CA. The bottom picture with the transducer oriented caudad demonstrates the IJV with blue flow and CA with red flow. (From Barash P, Cullen B, eds. *Clinical Anesthesia*. Philadelphia, PA: Lippincott Williams & Wilkins; 2009:747.)

artery disease but good ventricular function (ejection fraction greater than 40% and no regional wall-motion abnormalities), CVP correlates well with PCWP. However, because RV is a thinner walled chamber, the compliance of RV is higher than that of LV. Therefore, for any given preload, CVP will be lower than either PA diastolic pressure or PCWP. Although the absolute number has not been shown to correlate with preload conditions and stroke volume, evaluating trends over time and cyclic changes during mechanical ventilation can help guide fluid therapy.

F. **PA catheter**

1. **Parameters measured**

a. **PA pressure** reflects RV function, pulmonary vascular resistance (PVR), and left atrial (LA) filling pressure.

b. **PCWP** is a more direct estimate of LA filling pressure. With the balloon inflated and "wedged" in a distal branch PA, a valveless hydrostatic column exists between the distal port and the LA at end-diastole (Fig. 4.13).

TABLE 4.7 Complications of central venous cannulation for each of four cannulation sites

Complication	Internal jugular	Subclavian	Femoral	External jugular
Infection	x	x	x	x
Air embolism	x	x	x	x
Catheter shearing and embolization	x	x	x	x
Thrombophlebitis	x	x	x	x
Local extravasation of fluid and drugs	x	x	x	x
Thoracic Duct Injury	x	x		
Pneumothorax	x	x		
Hemothorax	x	x		
Pericardial tamponade	x	x		
Sites of Tissue trauma				
Nerve	Brachial plexus	Brachial plexus	Femoral	
Artery	Carotid Subclavian	Subclavian	Femoral	
Vein	SVC	SVC	Inferior vena cava	SVC
Other	Thoracic duct (L) Cervical nerve roots	Thoracic duct (L)		
Sites of fluid infusion with malpositioned catheter	Mediastinum, pericardium, pleural cavity	Pleural cavity, mediastinum	Retroperitoneum, peritoneal cavity	Retrograde up ipsilateral or contralateral internal jugular

SVC, superior vena cava; L, left side.

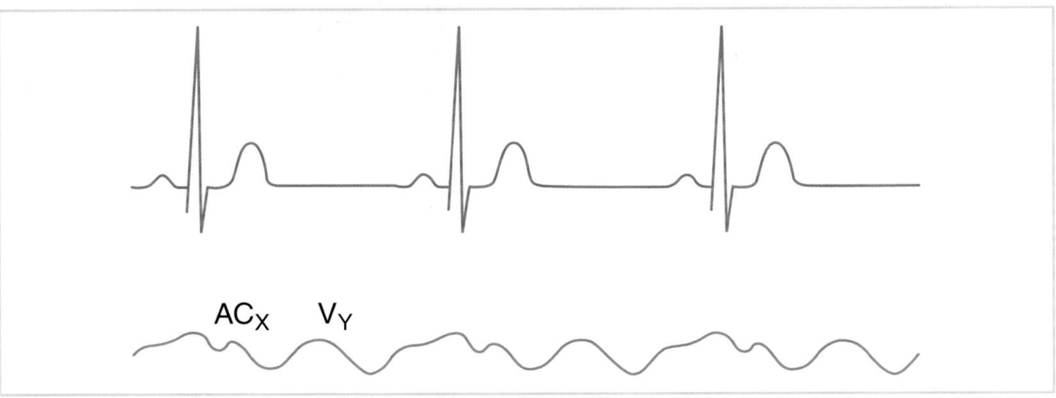

FIGURE 4.12 Relationship between ECG **(top)** and CVP **(bottom).** The normal CVP trace contains three positive deflections, known as the *A, C,* and *V waves,* and two negative deflections, the *X* and *Y* descents. The *A* wave occurs in conjunction with the P wave on the ECG and represents atrial contraction. The *C* wave occurs in conjunction with the QRS wave and represents the bulging of the tricuspid valve into the RA with right ventricular contraction. The *X* descent occurs next as the tricuspid valve is pulled downward during the latter stages of ventricular systole. The final positive wave, the *V* wave, occurs after the T wave on the ECG and represents right atrial filling before opening of the tricuspid valve. The *Y* descent occurs after the *V* wave when the tricuspid valve opens and the atrium empties into the ventricle. (Modified from Reich DL, Moskowitz DM, Kaplan JA. Hemodynamic monitoring. In: Kaplan JA, ed. *Cardiac Anesthesia.* 4th ed. Philadelphia, PA: WB Saunders; 1999:330.)

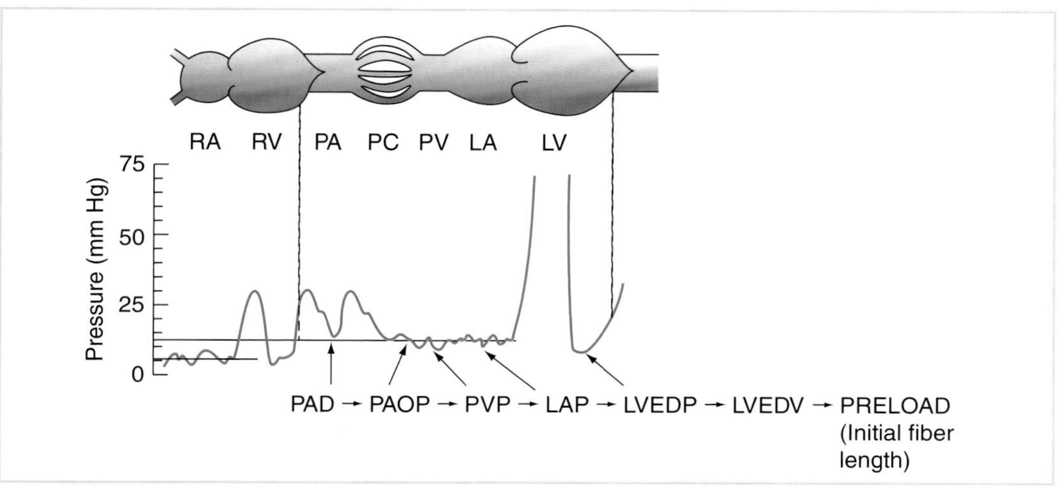

FIGURE 4.13 The cardiopulmonary circulation. **Top:** Valveless conduit from PA to LV is depicted with the mitral valve open at end-diastole. **Bottom:** Typical pressure waveforms corresponding to each chamber or vessel, with *horizontal lines* drawn at values for right ventricular and left ventricular preload. *LA,* left atrium; *LVEDP,* LV end-diastolic pressure; *LVEDV,* LV end-diastolic volume; *PC,* pulmonary capillary bed; *PV,* pulmonary vein; *RA,* right atrium; *RV,* right ventricle. Note that during diastole, the pulmonic valve is closed, which explains why the PA diastolic pressure, LA pressure, and LVEDP (equal to 12 mm Hg) are greater than the RA pressure and RV end-diastolic pressure (not labeled, but equal to 5 mm Hg). (From Tuman KJ, Carroll GC, Ivankovich AD. Pitfalls in interpretation of pulmonary artery catheter data. *J Cardiothorac Anesth.* 1989;3:626, with permission.)

c. **CVP.** A sampling port of the PAC is located in the RA and allows measurement of the CVP.

d. **CO.** A thermistor located at the tip of the PAC allows measurement of the output of the RV by the thermodilution technique. In the absence of intracardiac shunts, this measurement equals LV output.

e. **Blood temperature.** The thermistor can provide a constant measurement of blood temperature, which is an accurate reflection of core temperature.

f. **Derived parameters.** Several indices of ventricular performance and cardiovascular status can be derived from the parameters measured by PAC. Their formulas, physiologic significance, and normal values are listed in Table 4.8.

g. **Mixed venous oxygen saturation.** Oximetric PAC can measure real-time PA venous blood oxygen saturation providing information on end-organ oxygen utilization.

h. **RV performance.** New PAC technology allows for improved assessment of RV function distinct from LV dysfunction.

2. **Indications for PA catheterization.** There is no consensus among cardiac anesthesiologists regarding PAC use. PAC guidelines have been published [9]. In some institutions, cardiac surgery with CPB represents a universal indication for PA pressure monitoring in adults; other institutions rarely use PAC [10,11]. In the late 1990s several observational studies, randomized control trials, and meta-analyses did not show positive outcome benefits with the use of the PAC. Between 1994 and 2004, PAC use decreased 65% in medical intensive care units (ICUs) and 63% in surgical ICUs. Proponents of the PAC suggest that timing of catheter placement, patient selection, interpretation of PAC data, and early appropriate intervention are required for this monitor to meaningfully affect patient outcome. Decreased mortality has been reported in high-risk surgical patients in which PACs were inserted preoperatively and interventions were protocol driven. In elective cardiac surgical patients, Polanen reported in 2000 that PAC protocols reduce hospital and ICU length of stay [12]. Therefore, the current
7 consensus appears to be that PACs may have benefit in high-risk patients or those with special indications. However, in routine patients they have limited, if any, benefit.

TABLE 4.8 Derived hemodynamic indices

Parameter	Physiologic significance	Formula	Normal value
SVR	Reflects impedance of the systemic vascular tree; assumes laminar flow of homogeneous fluid	80 · (MAP–CVP)/CO	700–1,600 dyne · s · cm^{-5}
PVR	Reflects impedance of pulmonary circuit	80 · (PAM–PCWP)/CO	20–130 dyne · s · cm^{-5}
CI	Index of CO to BSA, allows for meaningful comparison between patients	CO/BSA	2.5–4.2 L · min^{-1} · m^{-2}
SVI	Reflects fluid status and ventricular performance	CI/HR · 1000	40–60 mL · $beat^{-1}$ · m^{-2}
LVSWI	Estimates work of LV, reflects contractile state	(MAP–PCWP) · SVI · 0.0136	45–60 g · m · m^{-2}
RVSWI	Estimates work done by right ventricle and RV performance	(PAM–CVP) · SVI · 0.0136	5–10 g · m · m^{-2}

MAP, mean arterial pressure; CVP, central venous pressure; CO, cardiac output; SVR, systemic vascular resistance; PVR, pulmonary vascular resistance; PAM, pulmonary artery mean pressure; PCWP, pulmonary capillary wedge pressure; CI, cardiac index; BSA, body surface area; Stroke volume index; HR, heart rate; LVSWI, left ventricular stroke work index; RVSWI, right ventricular stroke work index.

Modified from Kaplan JA. Hemodynamic monitoring. In: Kaplan JA, ed. *Cardiac Anesthesia*. 2nd ed. Philadelphia, PA: WB Saunders; 1987:203.

Particular indications for PACs are listed in Table 4.9. Differentiation of left versus right ventricular function and assessment of intracardiac filling pressures during cardioplegia administration (enhanced myocardial protection) are two indications that cannot be performed with CVP alone. Discordance in right and left heart function occurs with variable frequency where pressures measured on the right side (i.e., CVP) do not adequately reflect those on the left side [13].

a. **Assessing volume status.** In many patients with differences in RV and LV function, volume status is difficult to determine because of the large disparity between right (CVP) and left (PCWP) ventricular filling pressures. Myocardial ischemia, LV dysfunction, and positive pressure ventilation can exacerbate these differences.
b. **Diagnosing RV failure.** The RV is a thin-walled, highly compliant chamber that can fail during cardiac surgery either because of a primary disease process (inferior myocardial infarction), inadequate myocardial protection, or intracoronary air (predilection for the right coronary artery) as a result of the surgical procedure. RV failure presents as an increase in CVP, a decrease in the CVP to mean PA gradient, and a low CO.
c. **Diagnosing LV failure.** Knowledge of PA and wedge pressures can aid in the diagnosis of left-sided heart failure if other causes (ischemia, mitral valve disease) are eliminated.

TABLE 4.9 Indications for using the pulmonary artery catheter in cardiac surgery

Assessment/management of right ventricular failure
Assessment/management of pulmonary hypertension
Differentiation/treatment of various shock states, management of multiple organ failure
Management of left ventricular failure unresponsive to therapy, requiring escalating inotropes or intra-aortic balloon pump
Aortic surgery requiring suprarenal cross-clamping
Orthotopic heart transplantation

Modified from Kaplan JA. Monitoring of the heart and vascular system. In: Kaplan JA, ed. *Cardiac Anesthesia, The Echo Era*. 6th ed. St. Louis, MO: Elsevier Saunders; 2011:435.

TEE can aid in correlating the clinical paradigm to PAC measurements. Simultaneous readings of high PA pressures and wedge pressure in the presence of systemic hypotension and low CO are hallmarks of LV failure.

d. Diagnosing pulmonary hypertension. Note that with normal PVR, the PA diastolic and wedge pressure agree closely with one another. This relationship is lost with pulmonary hypertension.

e. Assessing valvular disease

(1) Tricuspid and pulmonary valve stenosis can be diagnosed by means of a PAC by measuring pressure gradients across these valves, although in adults TEE is the primary diagnostic modality for these lesions.

(2) Mitral valvular disease is reflected in the PA and wedge pressure waveform morphology. Mitral insufficiency appears as an abnormal V wave and an increase in pulmonary venous pressure from the regurgitant flow into the LA. V waves can also appear in other conditions, including myocardial ischemia, ventricular pacing, and presence of a ventricular septal defect depending on the compliance of the LA. In patients with chronic mitral valve insufficiency, the LA has a high compliance and a large regurgitant volume will not always result in a dramatic V wave.

f. Early diagnosis of ischemia. PAC, ECG, and TEE can assist detection of myocardial ischemia. Significant ischemia (transmural or subendocardial) is often associated with a decrease in ventricular compliance, which is reflected in either an increase in PA pressure or an increase in PCWP. In addition, the development of pathologic V waves may occur secondary to ischemia of the papillary muscle (Fig. 4.14).

3. Contraindications for PAC Placement

a. Significant tricuspid/pulmonary valvular pathology: Tricuspid/pulmonary stenosis, endocarditis, or mechanical prosthetic valve replacement.

b. Presence of a right-sided mass (tumor/thrombosis) that would cause a pulmonary or paradoxical embolization if dislodged.

c. Left bundle branch block (LBBB): LBBB is a relative contraindication. The incidence of transient right bundle branch block (RBBB) during PAC placement is ~5%. In a patient with LBBB, this can result in complete heart block when floating the PAC through the right ventricular outflow track. Therefore, external pacing should be immediately available for these patients.

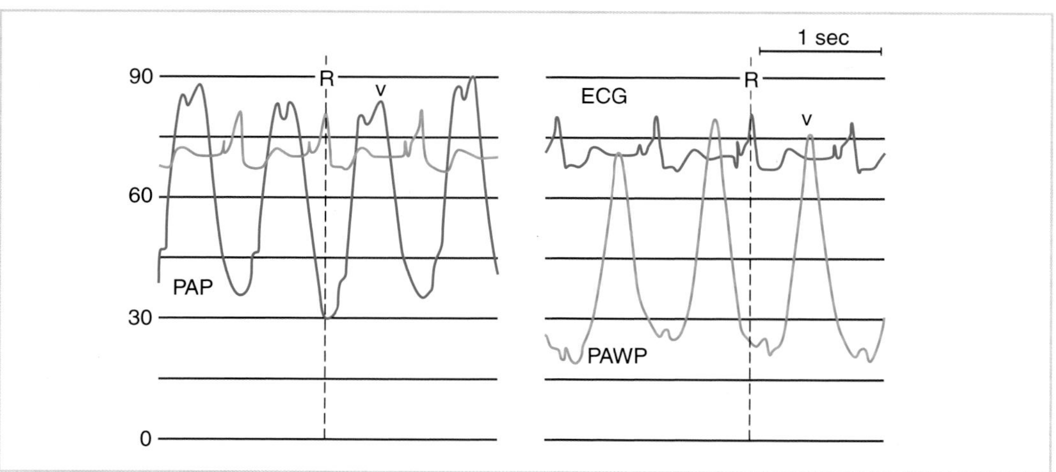

FIGURE 4.14 V waves secondary to severe mitral regurgitation. The tall systolic v wave in the PA wedge pressure (PAWP) trace also distorts the PA tracing, thereby giving it a bifid appearance. LVED pressure is best estimated by measuring PAWP at the time of the ECG R wave before the onset of the regurgitant v wave. (From Mark JB. *Atlas of Cardiovascular Monitoring.* New York, NY: Churchill Livingstone; 1998, Figure 17–11.)

4. **Interpretation of PA pressure data**
   a. **Effects of ventilation.** The effects of ventilation on PA pressure readings can be significant in the low-pressure system of the right-sided circulation because airway or transpleural pressure is transmitted to the pulmonary vasculature.
      (1) When a patient breathes spontaneously, the negative intrapleural pressure that results from inspiration can be transmitted to the intravascular pressure. Thus, low or even "negative" PA diastolic, wedge, and CVPs may occur with spontaneous ventilation.
      (2) Positive airway pressures are transmitted to the vasculature during positive-pressure ventilation, leading to elevations in pulmonary pressures. Mean airway pressure is the parameter which correlates most closely with the changes in PA and CVP pressure measurements.
      (3) The established convention is to evaluate pressures at **end-expiration**. The digital monitor numerical readout may give incorrect information because these numbers reflect the absolute highest (systolic), lowest (diastolic), and mean (area under pressure curve) values for **several seconds**, which may include one or more breaths. Damping is not accounted for by the monitor. Thus, inspection and interpretation of the waveform data is required to correctly evaluate the clinical scenario.
   b. **Location of catheter tip.** PA pressure measurements depend on where the tip of the catheter resides in the pulmonary vascular tree. In areas of the lung that are well ventilated but poorly perfused (West zone I), the readings will be more affected by the changes in airway pressure. Likewise, even when the tip is in a good location in the middle or lower lung fields, large amounts of positive end-expiratory pressure (>10 mm Hg) will affect PA values.
5. **Timing of placement.** A debate exists regarding whether PAC insertion before induction is indicated in adult patients with good LV function. The discomfort that might be associated with placement needs to be balanced with acquisition of hemodynamic data. In appropriately sedated patients, placement of a PAC is not associated with any significant hemodynamic changes. The hemodynamic data collected in the catheterization laboratory may not accurately reflect the current hemodynamic status, especially if the patient had episodes of myocardial ischemia during the catheterization or may be experiencing ischemia when entering the operating room.
6. **Types of PACs.** A variety of PACs are currently available for clinical use. The standard thermodilution catheter has a PA port for pressure monitoring and a thermistor for CO measurements at its tip, an RA port for CVP monitoring and for injection of cold saline 30 cm from the tip, and a lumen for inflation of the balloon. In addition, PACs are available that provide the following:
   a. **Venous infusion port (VIP).** VIP PACs have a third port 1 cm proximal to the CVP (31 cm from the tip) for infusion of drugs and fluids.
   b. **Pacing.** Pacing PACs have the capacity to provide intracardiac pacing. Pacing PACs are seldom used for cardiac procedures because usually patients already have a temporary pacing wire for symptomatic bradycardia prior to anesthetic care. Epicardial pacing wires are routinely placed by the surgeon intraoperatively for postoperative bradycardia.
      (1) Pacing PACs have a separate lumen terminating 19 cm from the catheter tip. When the catheter tip lies in the PA with a normal-sized heart, this port is positioned in the RV. A separate sterile, prepackaged pacing wire can be placed through this port to contact the RV endocardium for RV pacing.
      (2) PACs with thermodilution and atrial or AV pacing with two separate bipolar pacing probes have been shown to provide stable pacing before and after CPB.
   c. **Mixed venous oxygen saturation (S_vO_2).** Special fiberoptic PACs can be used to monitor S_vO_2 continuously. The normal S_vO_2 is 75%, with a 5% to 10% increase or decrease considered significant. Decreased oxygen delivery or increased oxygen

utilization result in a decreased S_vO_2. Four mechanisms can result in a significant decrease in S_vO_2:

(1) Decrease in CO
(2) Decreased hemoglobin concentration
(3) Decrease in arterial oxygen saturation (S_aO_2)
(4) Increased O_2 utilization.

Changes in S_vO_2 usually precede hemodynamic changes by a significant period of time, making this a useful clinical adjunct to other monitors. Some cardiac anesthesiologists advocate S_vO_2 monitoring for off-pump coronary artery bypass (OPCAB) procedures and any patient with severe LV dysfunction and/or valve disease.

d. Ejection fraction catheter. PACs with faster thermistor response times can be used to determine RV ejection fraction in addition to the CO. The thermistor responds rapidly enough that the exponential decay that normally results from a thermodilution CO (see Section I.H.1.b [2]) has end-diastolic "plateaus" with each cardiac cycle. From the differences in temperature of each succeeding plateau, the residual fraction of blood left in the RV after each contraction is calculated, as is RV stroke volume, end-diastolic volume, and end-systolic volume. Monitoring these parameters can be helpful in patients with RV dysfunction secondary to pulmonary hypertension, infarction, or reactive pulmonary disease.

e. Continuous CO. PACs that use low power thermal filaments to impart small temperature changes to RV blood have been developed (**Intellicath,** Baxter Edwards; and **Opti-Q,** Abbott Critical Care Systems, Mountain View, CA, USA). Fast-response thermistors in the PA allow for semicontinuous (every 30 to 60 s) CO determinations.

7. Techniques of insertion. General guidelines are outlined in Table 4.10. The introducer is placed in a manner similar to that described for CVP insertion. However, special care should be observed with PAC placement, noting especially the following points:

a. Sedation. Because the patient is under a large drape for a longer period of time, he or she should be asked questions periodically to check for oversedation. A clear drape allows visual inspection of the patient's color and may produce a less suffocating feeling.

b. ECG monitoring during placement. It is essential to monitor the ECG during placement of the catheter because dysrhythmias are the most common complication associated with PAC insertion.

c. Pulse oximetry. Pulse oximetry gives an audible signal of rhythm and may alert the physician to an abnormal rhythm.

d. Preferred approach. The right IJV approach offers the most direct route to the RA and thus results in the highest rate of successful PA catheterization. The left subclavian route is next most effective.

e. Balloon inflation. Air should be used for balloon inflation. If any suspicion exists about balloon competency, the PAC should be removed and the balloon inspected directly to avoid iatrogenic air embolism.

f. Waveform. A vast majority of cardiac anesthesiologists use waveform analysis to guide placement of the PAC tip. TEE or the use of fluoroscopy can aid placement in some situations. Representative waveforms are shown in Figure 4.15.

8. Complications. Complications [14] can be divided into vascular access, PAC placement/manipulation, and monitoring problems.

a. Vascular Access. See Table 4.7 for complications of central venous cannulation.

b. PAC placement/manipulation.

(1) Cardiac Arrhythmias: Reported incidence ranges from 12.5% to 70%. PVCs are the most common arrhythmia. Fortunately, most arrhythmia resolve with either catheter withdrawal or with advancement of the catheter tip from the RV into the PA. There appears to be a higher incidence when the patient is positioned in the Trendelenburg position versus right-tilt position.

TABLE 4.10 Steps for pulmonary artery catheter insertion

Steps	Rationale and comments
1. Establish monitoring: BP cuff, ECG, pulse oximetry	Monitor for ischemia, hypoxemia, arrhythmia
2. Place nasal cannula	Avoids hypoxemia in sedated patient in head-down position
3. Cannulate central circulation, place dilator-introducer	See Table 4.5
4. Remove catheter from package. Place sheath over catheter	Exercise care so as to not damage balloon
5. Hand off proximal end to assistant. Flush appropriate ports of catheter with heparinized saline. Monitor at least the distal port	Placing a PAC requires nonsterile assistant to connect ports to transducer tubing
6. Check balloon for competence	Should be done after sheath is placed over catheter
7. While watching monitor and holding 30-cm mark fixed, raise the distal tip from horizontal to vertical position	Ensures that the correct monitor channel is connected to the distal port. Only the pressure channel for the distal port should reflect a rise in pressure
8. Insert PAC to 20 cm with balloon down	Puts balloon past end of introducer; inflation before this point may damage balloon
9. Inflate balloon with 1.5 cc of air or CO_2	Do not force air into balloon; there is a small amount of resistance before the opening pressure is reached
10. Advance slowly, monitoring the distal port	Look for progressive pressure changes from RA to RV, PA, and PCWP (Fig. 4.15)
11. When RV reached, advance more rapidly	Avoids arrhythmia but advancing slowly may be required to reach the pulmonary outflow tract
12. If RV or PA is difficult to enter:	
a. Have patient take deep breath	Increases pulmonary blood flow
b. Place in head-up position or tilt table to left or right	Places the RV or PA outflow at highest point where balloon will float
c. Flush PA port with 1–2 mL cold sterile saline	Stiffens catheter, making threading easier
13. When PA entered, advance slowly	Look for phase shift of V wave or damping of phasic pulse, or both, indicating catheter "wedging"
14. Release balloon	PA trace should return
15. "Size" the PA by inserting gas in 0.5-cc increments, watching PA trace	If PCWP is seen before full 1.5 cc is inserted, the catheter should be pulled back 3–4 cm to reduce risk of PA rupture
16. Do not withdraw the catheter at any time with the balloon inflated	Avoids rupture of pulmonic or tricuspid valves

BP, blood pressure; ECG, electrocardiogram; PAC, pulmonary artery catheter; RA, right atrium; RV, right ventricle; PA, pulmonary artery; PCWP pulmonary capillary wedge pressure.

(2) Mechanical Damage: Catheter knotting and entanglement of cardiac structures, although rare, can occur. Damage to intracardiac structures such as valves, chordae, and even RV perforation has been reported. The presence of IVC filters, indwelling catheters, and pacemakers can increase the risk of such complications. The incidence of knotting is estimated at 0.03% and this complication can be decreased with careful attention to depth of insertion and expected waveforms. To reduce the risk of knotting, a catheter should be withdrawn if the RV waveform is still present 20 cm after its initial appearance or when the absolute depth of 60 cm is reached without a PA tracing.

(3) PA Rupture: This is a rare complication with an incidence of 0.03% to 0.2%. Risk factors include pulmonary hypertension, age greater than 60, hyperinflation of the balloon, improper (distal) catheter positioning, and coagulopathy. During CPB,

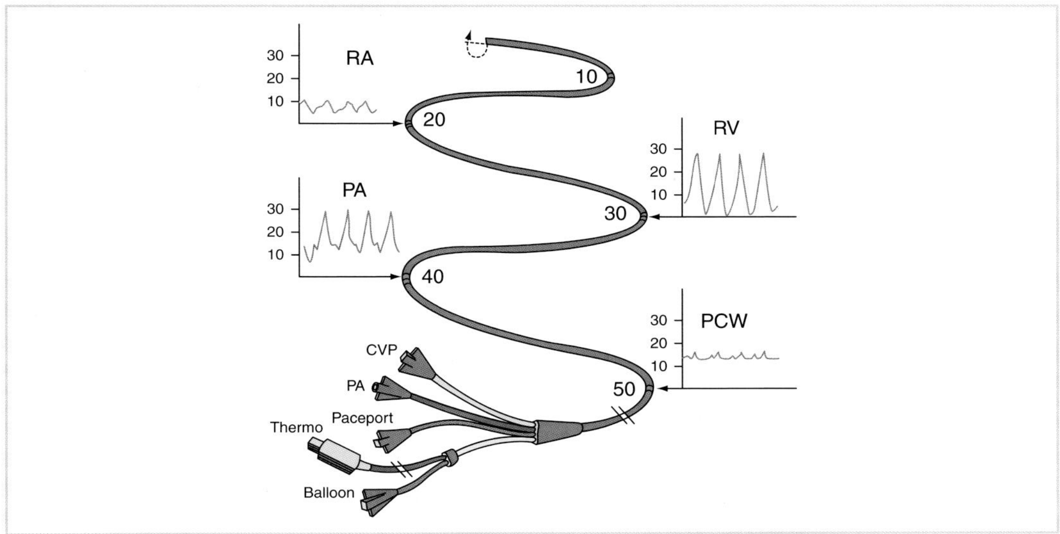

FIGURE 4.15 Pressure waves that will be encountered as a PAC is inserted into the wedged position from the right IJV. Distances on the catheter correspond to insertion distances read at the diaphragm of the introducer and are approximate. Actual distances may vary by +5 cm. PACs should not be advanced more than 60 cm from this approach because this increases the risk of PA rupture or catheter knotting. *CVP,* central venous pressure; *PCW,* pulmonary capillary wedge; *RA,* right atrium; *RV,* right ventricle; *Thermo,* thermistor connection for CO determination.

distal migration of the catheter tip may occur, thus some advocate pulling the PAC back a few centimeters prior to initiating bypass.

(4) Thrombosis: Although thrombus formation on PACs has been noted at 24 hr, the incidence of thrombogenicity substantially increases by 72 hrs.

(5) Pulmonary Infarction: It can occur as a complication of continuous distal, wedging from catheter migration, or embolization of previously formed thrombus.

(6) Infection: The incidence of bacteremia and blood stream infection related to PAC is 1.3% to 2.3%. Additionally, the PAC can contribute to endothelial damage of the tricuspid and pulmonary valves leading to endocarditis.

(7) **Other: Balloon rupture, heparin-induced thrombocytopenia (HIT) secondary to heparin-coated catheters, anaphylaxis from latex (balloon) allergy, and hepatic venous placement have all been included in PAC-related complications.**

c. Monitoring Complications.

(1) Errors in equipment and data acquisition: Examples include inappropriate pressure transducer leveling and over/underdamping of pressure system.

(2) Misinterpretation or misapplication of data: Misinterpretation can occur when not considering ventilation modes, ventricular compliance changes, or intrinsic cardiac/pulmonary pathologies.

(3) Expense.

9. Conclusions. PACs provide a wealth of information about the right and left sides of the circulation. For this reason, they are used for every cardiac surgical procedure in some institutions because their benefits are perceived to outweigh the risks. Studies that show low morbidity rates with PAC use support this viewpoint. In other institutions, however, clinicians are more selective about which patients require PACs, because use of PA monitoring has not been demonstrated to incontrovertibly improve outcomes of cardiac surgery. The widespread application of TEE may make intraoperative PAC data less useful except for S_vO_2 [15]. Additionally, non-invasive CO monitoring may also replace some uses of the PAC, although these monitors have technologic obstacles to solve prior to routine use (without invasive monitoring) during cardiac surgery.

G. **LA pressure.** In some patients (especially pediatric), direct LA pressure can be measured after surgical insertion of an LA catheter via the LA appendage in the open chest. LA catheters also are used in corrective surgery for congenital lesions when PAC insertion is not possible. The LA pressure tracing is comparable to the CVP tracing, with A, C, and V waves occurring at identical points in the cardiac cycle. LA catheters are used to monitor valvular function (after mitral valve replacement or mitral valvuloplasty) or to monitor LV filling pressures, whether or not a PAC is available. LA pressure measured directly is more accurate than that measured with a PAC because the effects of airway pressure on the pulmonary vasculature are removed. However, LA pressure does not necessarily reflect LV end-diastolic pressure (LVEDP) in the presence of mitral valvular disease. Air should be meticulously removed from LA flush systems to avoid catastrophic air emboli.

H. **Cardiac output**
   1. **Methods**
      a. **Thermodilution with cold injectate.** This method is the most commonly utilized CO technique because of its ease of use and ability to repeat measurements over time. The indicator is an aliquot of saline (typically 10 mL, which is at a lower temperature than the temperature of blood) injected into the RA. The change in temperature produced by injection of this indicator is measured in the PA by a thermistor and is integrated over time to generate a value for RV output, which is equal to systemic CO if no intracardiac shunts are present. This method requires no withdrawal of blood and no arterial line, uses an inexpensive indicator, and is not greatly affected by recirculation. The thermodilution method underestimates the CO with right-side valvular lesions. Thermodilution remains accurate for forward LV CO for mitral and aortic valve lesions.
      b. **Continuous thermodilution.** A thermal filament in the catheter heats blood ~15 to 25 cm before its tip, thus generating a PA temperature change that is measured via a distal thermistor. The input and output signals are correlated to generate CO values.
      c. **RV ejection fraction.** Improved preload estimates might be obtained with this type of PAC [16].
   2. **Assumptions and errors.** Specific errors in CO determination are mentioned below:
      a. **Thermodilution method**
         (1) **Volume of injectate.** Because the output computer will base its calculations on a specific volume, an injectate volume less than that for which the computer is set will cause a falsely high value of CO, and vice versa.
         (2) **Temperature of injectate.** If the injectate temperature parameter is incorrect, errors can occur. For example, an increase of 1°C will cause a 3% overestimation of CO. The controversy over iced versus room-temperature injectate centers around the concept that a larger difference between the injectate temperature and blood temperature should increase the accuracy of the CO determination. Studies have not supported this hypothesis, and the extra inconvenience of keeping syringes on ice, together with the increased risk of infection (nonsterile water surrounding the Luer tip), make the iced saline method a less attractive alternative.
         (3) **Shunts.** Intracardiac shunts will cause erroneous values for thermodilution CO values. This technique should not be used if a communication exists between the pulmonary and systemic circulations. A shunt should always be suspected when thermodilution CO values do not fit the clinical findings.
         (4) **Timing with the respiratory cycle.** As much as a 10% difference in CO will result, depending on when injection occurs during the respiratory cycle. These changes are most likely due to actual changes in pulmonary blood flow during respiration.
         (5) **Catheter position.** The tip of the pulmonary catheter must be in the PA and must not be "wedged"; otherwise, nonsensical curves are obtained.
   3. **Minimally Invasive CO Monitoring:** The desire to assess cardiac function and adequate tissue perfusion in critically ill patients is traditionally accomplished using the PAC. The

controversy about its invasive nature and potential harm has provoked the development of less invasive CO monitoring devices [17,18]. Just as the PAC has its nuances, these devices have their own sets of limitations that must be considered.

a. **Accuracy and precision.** Accuracy refers to the capability of a measurement to reflect the true CO. This means that a measurement is compared to a "gold standard" method. Given the wide spread use of the PAC, the thermodilution method is the practical "gold" standard to which new non-invasive CO monitors are compared. However, it is important to take into account that the inherent error for thermodilution measurements of CO are in the 10% to 20% range. *Precision* indicates the reproducibility of a measurement and refers to the variability between determinations. For the thermodilution method, studies of precision have involved probability analyses of large numbers of CO determinations. Using this approach, it was found that with two injections, there was only a 50% chance that the numbers obtained were within 5% of the true CO. If three injections yield results that are within 10% of one another, there is a 90% probability that the average value is within 10% of the true CO.

   Given that the practical gold standard carries with it some inaccuracies, new methods based on it will also hold their own similar inherent error. Table 4.11 shows the relative accuracy and precision of invasive and non-invasive techniques to measure CO.

b. **Methods:** Minimally invasive CO monitors can be classified into one of the four main groups: Pulse pressure analysis, pulsed Doppler technologies, applications of Fick's principle using partial CO_2 rebreathing, and bioimpedance/bioreactance.
   (1) **Pulse pressure analysis:** Monitors based on that principle stroke volume can be tracked continuously by analysis of the arterial waveform. These monitors require an optimal arterial waveform, thus arrhythmias, intra-aortic balloon pumps, left ventricular assist devices, and even properties of the arterial line monitoring systems (such as over/under damping) can alter accuracy of the CO measurement. Three common pulse contour analysis devices are compared in Table 4.12.
   (2) **Doppler devices:** CO can be measured using the change in frequency of an ultrasonic beam as it measures blood flow velocity. To achieve accurate measurements, at least three conditions must be met: (i) The cross-sectional area of the vessel must be known; (ii) the ultrasound beam must be directed parallel to the flow of blood; (iii) the beam direction cannot move to any great degree between measurements. Clinical use of this technique is associated with reduced accuracy and precision.

TABLE 4.11 Accuracy and precision of cardiac output measurements

Method	"Gold-standard" comparison	Accuracy	Precision
O_2 consumption (Fick method)	Rotameter or electromagnetic flow probe placed in PA	Good	Good
Thermodilution	Fick method	Overestimates output by as much as 10%	Poor; repeat measurements needed
Dye dilution	Fick method thermodilution	Yields lower values compared to both methods	Good
Doppler ultrasound	Thermodilution	Good, if initial estimate of vessel diameter is accurate	Poor; probe can move easily
TEE	Ventricular angiography	Good, if ventricular asynergy is not present	Good

PA, pulmonary artery; TEE, transesophageal echocardiography.

TABLE 4.12 CO monitors utilizing pulse wave analysis

	FloTrac System	PiCCO*plus* System	LiDCO*plus* System
Requires external calibration	No	Yes	Yes
Requires central line	No	Yes	No
Type of calibration	—	Transpulmonary thermodilution via (CVL)	Pulmonary lithium indicator
Special arterial catheter	No	Yes, thermistor-tipped catheter	No
Preferred arterial site	Any site	Femoral	Any site
Alternative sites	—	Radial/brachial (require longer catheter)	—
Method	Concept that the area under the curve of the systolic arterial waveform is proportional to stroke volume. Standard deviation of pulse pressure is correlated with "normal" stroke volume based on a database of patient demographics (age, sex, weight, height). Impedance is also derived from this demographic data	Concept that the area under the curve of the systolic arterial waveform is proportional to stroke volume. Calibration used to determine the individual aortic impedance. Recalibration recommended every 8 hrs in stable patients; increased frequency of recalibration (up to every 1 hr) needed in patients with hemodynamic instability (significant changes of vascular resistance)	Concept of conservation of mass (power). Suggests that after calibration and correction for compliance, the relationship of net power and net flow is linear. Calibration used to determine resistance of vasculature; recalibration recommended Q 8 hr. Lithium calibration negatively affected by: 1. Changes in electrolytes 2. Changes in hematocrit 3. High peak doses of muscle relaxant 4. Patient on lithium 5. Patients <40 kg
Additional assessments provided	Stoke volume variation	Global end-diastolic volume; extravascular lung volume; stroke volume variation	Stroke volume variation

CVL, central venous line.

Two methods that use ultrasound are as follows:

(a) Transtracheal. Flow in the ascending aorta is determined with a transducer bonded to the distal portion of the endotracheal tube, designed to ensure contact of the transducer with the wall of the trachea. This method is not yet fully validated in humans, and a study of cardiac patients reported poor correlation when compared to thermodilution.

(b) Transesophageal. Several esophageal Doppler probes are available which are smaller than conventional TEE probes. CO is obtained by multiplying the cross-sectional area of the aorta by the blood flow velocity. Flow in the aorta is measured using a transducer placed in the esophagus. Aortic cross-sectional area is provided from a nomogram or measured by M-mode echocardiography.

(c) TEE. In addition to the Doppler technique mentioned above, TEE utilizes Simpson's rule in which the LV is divided into a series of disks to estimate CO without the use of Doppler. End-diastolic and end-systolic dimensions measured by echocardiography are converted to volumes, allowing stroke volume and CO to be determined. Given the size of the monitor and probe, this technique can provide intermittent CO, but is not ideal for continuous CO measurement desired in ICU settings.

TABLE 4.13 Indications for intraoperative transesophageal echocardiography TEE

Indication
Judge adequacy of valvuloplasty procedures
Mitral or tricuspid valve repair
Mitral commissurotomy
Judge adequacy of valve replacement
Rule out perivalvular leak
Rule out malfunctioning prosthesis
Judge adequacy of repair of congenital heart disease
Atrial or ventricular septal defect closure
Flow through an intracardiac baffle
Flow post arterioplasty (e.g., repair of pulmonary branch stenosis)
Flow through a pulmonary-to-systemic shunt
Assessment of left or right ventricular function
Global performance
Wall-motion abnormalities
Specific systolic and diastolic functional indices
Evaluation of myotomy or myomectomy in hypertrophic obstructive cardiomyopathy
Evaluation of retained intracardiac air

Summary: The PAC still remains the practical gold standard for evaluating CO. It also provides true mixed venous saturation and pulmonary pressures that cannot be obtained from non-invasive devices. Invasive hemodynamic monitoring remains the standard in the operating theater. However, select stable cardiac patients may be candidates in the ICU or stepdown units postoperatively for minimally invasive device monitoring.

I. Echocardiography

1. **TEE.** Echocardiography, and especially **TEE,** has gained widespread use in the cardiac operating room. Indications for intraoperative TEE are listed in Table 4.13. For a complete discussion of TEE, see Chapter 5—"Transesophageal Echocardiograhy".
2. **Epiaortic scanning.** The importance of aortic atheromas, especially in the ascending aorta and/or aortic arch, in association with poor neurologic outcomes has long been recognized. Aortic atheromas with a mobile component present the greatest risk. The introduction and use of TEE to detect aortic atheroma [19] was a significant improvement over surgical palpation. However, TEE had significant limitations particularly in the detection of disease near the typical aortic cannulation site (distal ascending aorta, proximal aortic arch) because the airway structures interfere with the TEE signal. Epiaortic scanning [20,21] is a
8 highly sensitive and specific monitoring modality to detect atheroma in the thoracic aorta including regions where TEE evaluation is not possible. In cardiac surgical patients with identified atheroma, modification of the surgical technique and neuroprotective strategies has been reported to reduce neurologic complication from ~60% to 0% [22].

II. Pulmonary system

A. Pulse oximetry

1. **Indications**
   a. **Preoperative uses.** Document baseline O_2 saturation, assess the need for supplemental O_2 after premedication is administered, and provide an audible alarm for dysrhythmias.
   b. **Assessment of oxygenation intraoperatively.**
   c. **Assessment of perfusion.** The pulse oximeter utilizes plethysmography as a part of its basic operation. Thus, adequacy of perfusion is likely when the oximeter shows a saturation reading.

TABLE 4.14 Pulse oximetry in cardiac procedures

Advantages	Disadvantages
Ease of use	Poor perfusion states (shock, hypothermia) make the saturation unobtainable
Continuous monitor	Some dyes (methylene blue) interfere with the light absorbance
Noninvasive	Electrocautery causes interference
Most models have a variable pitch that correlates with the degree of saturation (obviates the need to view the screen)	Despite shielding, the oximeter cable can cause interference on other monitors if wires cross
Accuracy	Requires pulsatile flow to operate Extraneous lights (e.g., older Pilling operating room lights) cause interference

d. **Pulse rate.** In the patient with a dysrhythmia, not every beat will lead to adequate perfusion, and this will be sensed by the pulse oximeter. An audible monitor of the heart rhythm is available.

2. **Advantages and disadvantages** are listed in Table 4.14. Of note, cardiac surgery was found to be an independent predictor of pulse oximetry failure in one study that detected a better than 9% intraoperative oximetry failure rate of at least a 10-min period [23].

B. **Capnography**

1. **Indications**

a. **All patients.** End-tidal capnography offers evidence of endotracheal intubation, ventilation, and perfusion.

b. **Patients with lung disease.** Capnography assesses the severity of small airway obstruction and assists adjustment of ventilatory parameters (i.e., increasing the I:E ratio).

c. **Patients with pulmonary hypertension or reactive pulmonary vasculature.** Hypercarbia results in increased PA pressures and may worsen RV function. Factors contributing to elevated arterial CO_2 include insufflation of CO_2 during endoscopic vein harvest, hypoventilation during IMA takedown, and temporary holding ventilation for surgical manipulation.

III. **Temperature.** Cardiac anesthesia is unique in that therapeutic hypothermia is utilized frequently and aggressively in many cases. Distribution of thermal energy can be manipulated, via CPB, more rapidly and extensively than any other anesthetic case. Unique to cardiac anesthesia are circulatory arrest procedures with cooling to 17°C. Temperature monitoring for cardiac anesthesia has unique considerations. This section will introduce these topics without detailed discussion of thermal issues common to all anesthesiologists [24].

A. **Indications**

1. **Assessment of cooling and rewarming**

2. **Diagnosing hazardous hypothermia or hyperthermia.** Below 32°C, the myocardium is irritable and subject to complex arrhythmias, especially ventricular tachycardia and fibrillation. The risk of dysrhythmia is particularly high in pediatric patients. Hypothermia inhibits coagulation thus increasing bleeding/transfusion risk. Likewise, significant enzyme desaturation and cell damage can occur with temperatures greater than or equal to 41°C.

B. **Sites of measurement.** Numerous possible sites exist to measure temperature. These sites can be grouped into the core or the shell.

1. **Core temperature**

a. **General considerations.** The core temperature represents the temperature of the vital organs. The term *core temperature* used here is perhaps a misnomer because gradients exist even within this vessel-rich group during rapid changes in blood temperature.

b. **PAC thermistor.** This is the best estimate of the core temperature when pulmonary blood flow is present (i.e., before and after CPB).

c. **Nasopharyngeal temperature.** Nasopharyngeal temperature provides an accurate reflection of brain temperature during CPB. The probe should be inserted into the nasopharynx to a distance equivalent to the distance from the naris to the tip of the earlobe. Nasopharyngeal temperature should be monitored in all hypothermic circulatory arrest procedures and CPB cases with hypothermia requiring rewarming.

d. **Tympanic membrane temperature.** Temperature at this site reflects brain temperature, and may provide an alternative to nasopharyngeal temperature.

e. **Bladder temperature.** This modality has been used to measure core temperature, although it may be inaccurate in instances when renal blood flow and urine production are decreased.

f. **Esophageal temperature.** Because the esophagus is a mediastinal structure, it will be greatly affected by the temperature of the blood returning from the extracorporeal pump and should NOT be used routinely for cases involving CPB.

g. **CPB arterial line temperature.** This is the temperature of the heat exchanger (i.e., the lowest temperature during active cooling and the highest temperature during active rewarming). During either of these phases, a gradient always exists between the arterial line temperature and any other temperature.

h. **CPB venous line temperature.** This is the "return" temperature to the oxygenator and probably best reflects core temperature during CPB when no active warming or cooling is occurring.

2. **Shell**

a. **General.** The shell compartment represents the majority of the body (muscle, fat, bone), which receives a smaller proportion of the blood flow, thus acting as an energy sink that can significantly affect temperature fluxes. Shell temperature lags behind core temperature during cooling and rewarming. At the point of bypass separation, the core temperature will be significantly higher than shell temperature. The final equilibrium temperature with thermal redistribution probably will be closer to the shell temperature than the core temperature measured initially.

b. **Rectal temperature.** Although traditionally thought of as a core temperature, during CPB procedures the rectal temperature most accurately reflects muscle mass temperature. If the tip of the probe rests in stool, a significant lag will exist with changing temperatures.

c. **Skin temperature.** Skin temperature is affected by local factors (warming blanket) and is rarely utilized in cardiac surgery.

C. **Risks of temperature monitoring**

Epistaxis with nasopharyngeal temperature monitoring. Most cardiac anesthesiologists consider the benefits of neurologic protection (measured by brain temperature) to outweigh bleeding risks. If the nasal mucosa is traumatized during probe placement, epistaxis can result, especially when the patient has been given heparin.

D. **Recommendations for temperature monitoring.** Monitoring temperature at two sites is recommended: A core site and a shell site. Arterial and venous line temperatures are available directly from the CPB apparatus. Nasal temperature monitoring is recommended for core temperature because it will most rapidly reflect the changes in the arterial blood temperature.
9 Nasal temperature monitoring is recommended for circulatory arrest cases to document brain temperature. Bladder or rectal temperature monitoring is simple to establish and is recommended for monitoring shell temperature.

IV. Renal function

A. Indications for monitoring

1. **Increased incidence of renal failure after CPB.** Acute renal failure is a recognized complication of CPB, occurring in 2.5% to 31% of cases. Acute renal failure is related to the preoperative renal function as well as to the presence of coexisting disease. The nonpulsatile renal blood flow during CPB has been speculated as a contributing mechanism, although continuous-flow LVAD has not been associated with excessive renal failure.

2. **Use of diuretics in CPB prime.** Mannitol is used routinely during CPB for two reasons:
   a. **Hemolysis** occurs during CPB, and serum hemoglobin levels rise. Urine output should be maintained to avoid damage to renal tubules.
   b. **Deliberate hemodilution** is induced with the onset of hypothermic CPB. Maintenance of good urine output during and after CPB allows removal of excess free water.

B. **Urinary catheter.** This monitor is the single most important monitor of renal function during surgical cases involving CPB. Establishing a urinary catheter should be a priority in emergencies.

1. **Anuria on bypass.** It is not uncommon for oliguria or anuria while the patient is on CPB. Hypothermia and the reduction of arterial flow will cause a diminution in renal function. Therefore, anuria should not usually be treated aggressively with additional diuretic therapy, especially while the patient is hypothermic.
   a. **How much urine is adequate?** After CPB, adequacy of urine output depends on several factors, all of which should be optimized:
      (1) Volume status
      (2) CO
      (3) Hemoglobin concentration
      (4) Amount of surgical bleeding

C. **Electrolytes.** Serum electrolytes, especially potassium and magnesium, should be checked toward the end of CPB and after bypass. In the vast majority of patients with adequate renal function, potassium and magnesium concentrations will decline during CPB (secondary to mannitol and improved perfusion). Replacement of potassium has to account for cardioplegia
10 which contains potassium and hyperglycemia. A low serum ionized calcium level may be the cause of diminished pump function. The timing of the calcium therapy may affect neurologic outcome; administration during periods of neural ischemia and/or reperfusion may worsen the outcome. Many cardiac anesthesiologists will not administer calcium until at least 15 to 20 min following acceptable perfusion (e.g., after aortic cross-clamp removal).

V. Neurologic function

A. **General considerations.** The cardiac surgical patient is at increased risk of having an adverse neurologic event during surgery because of CPB (core cooling, alterations in blood flow) and because of the potential to introduce emboli (air, atheromatous material, thrombus). Neurologic risk assessment in cardiac surgical patients [25] and risk factor modification are extremely important for the anesthesiologists. Advances in processing capability have made available new devices to monitor neurologic function during surgery [26–28]. Monitoring the central nervous system is done for three primary reasons: (i) to diagnose cerebral ischemia, (ii) to assess the depth of anesthesia and prevent intraoperative awareness, and (iii) to assess the effectiveness of medications given for brain or spinal cord protection. The indications and types of neurologic monitors are outlined briefly here; for in depth applications, see Chapter 22.

B. **Indications for monitoring neurologic function**

1. Associated carotid disease
2. Diagnosis of embolic phenomenon
3. Diagnosis of aortic cannula malposition
4. Diagnosis of inadequate arterial flow on CPB
5. Confirmation of adequate cooling
6. Hypothermic circulatory arrest, in an adult or a child (see Chapters 22 and 23)

C. **Monitors of CNS electrical activity**

1. **Electroencephalogram** (see Chapter 22). The electroencephalogram (EEG) measures the electrical currents generated by the postsynaptic potentials in the pyramidal cell layer of the cerebral cortex. The basic principle of clinical EEG monitoring is that cerebral ischemia causes slowing of the electrical activity of the brain, as well as a decrease in signal amplitude. An experienced electroencephalographer can interpret raw EEG data from four or eight channels, but would be hard pressed to also administer an anesthetic and monitor other organ systems.

2. **Processed EEG.** To increase its intraoperative utility, the EEG data are processed by fast Fourier analysis into a single power versus time **spectral array** that is more easily interpreted. Examples of power spectrum analysis include **compressed spectral array, density spectral array,** and **bispectral index (BIS)**. The BIS monitor analyzes the phase relationships between different frequency components over time, and the result is reduced via a proprietary method to a single number scaled between 0 (electrical silence) and 100 (alert wakefulness). The role of BIS monitoring in cardiac surgery is in evolution [29]. The BIS may be a useful indicator of the depth of anesthesia for many procedures, but its significance in cardiac anesthesia has not been determined. Studies of BIS values as a predictor of anesthetic depth during intravenous anesthesia (narcotic plus benzodiazepine) are conflicting. One study found a positive correlation between the BIS and arousal or hemodynamic responses [30], whereas another study found no such correlation between the BIS value and plasma concentrations of fentanyl and midazolam [31]. The BIS monitor may have added benefit in the management of cardiac anesthesia. During hypothermic circulatory arrest, the BIS monitor should be isoelectric (BIS of zero). Many cardiac anesthesiologists monitor the BIS during cooling and to observe the effect of supplemental intravenous anesthetic (historically thiopental) administered for neuroprotection. Evidence supporting BIS data as a monitor of neurologic function in patients at risk for hypoxic or ischemic brain injury continues to accumulate [32]. Abnormally low BIS scores and prolonged low BIS score may be associated with poor neurologic outcomes.
3. **Evoked potentials**
   a. **Somatosensory evoked potentials (SSEPs).** SSEPs can be used to monitor the integrity of the spinal cord. It is most useful in operations such as surgery for a thoracic aneurysm, in which the blood flow to the spinal cord may be compromised. A stimulus is applied to a peripheral nerve (usually the tibial nerve), and the resultant brainstem and brain activity is quantified. Specific uses are discussed further in Chapter 23.
   b. **Visual evoked response and brainstem audio evoked responses.** These techniques do not have routine clinical application in cardiac surgical procedures and are not discussed here.
   c. **Motor evoked potentials (MEPs).** MEPs are useful to monitor the spinal cord during surgery of the descending aorta and are discussed in more detail in Chapter 23.

D. **Monitors of cerebral metabolic function**

1. **Jugular bulb venous oximetry.** Measuring the oxygen saturation of the cerebral jugular bulb with a fiberoptic catheter [33] is analogous to measuring the mixed venous oxygen saturation in the PA. Cerebral oxygen consumption is the product of cerebral blood flow **(CBF)** and the oxygen extraction by the brain. If CBF decreases, oxygen extraction would increase and the jugular O_2 saturation would decrease. Owing to a significant interpatient variability, trend monitoring yields more information than individual measurements.
2. **Near-infrared spectroscopy (NIRS).** NIRS is a noninvasive method to monitor cerebral metabolic function [33]. A near-infrared light is emitted from a scalp sensor and penetrates the scalp, skull, cerebrospinal fluid, and brain. The light is reflected by tissue but differentially absorbed by hemoglobin-containing moieties. The amount of absorption correlates with the oxygenation state of the hemoglobin in the tissue. Again, trend monitoring is possible because NIRS data are updated continuously. Currently, the role of NIRS cerebral oximetry application during cardiac surgery is controversial. Improved outcomes have not been conclusively demonstrated and the cost benefit is unclear.

E. **Monitors of CNS hemodynamics**

1. **Transcranial Doppler ultrasonography (TCD).** The Doppler technology in TCD monitoring is similar to that used in echocardiography. One difference is the signal attenuation caused by the skull, which is a source of artifact. Nonetheless, this technology is very useful in detecting emboli in the cerebral circulation.

VI. Electrical safety in the cardiac operating room

A. **Electrical hazards.** The major hazards can be classified as macroshock, microshock, and thermal burns. Some general electrical terms are listed in Table 4.15. Our discussion will focus on microshock hazard.

TABLE 4.15 Electrical terms

Term	Meaning
Ampere (amp or A)	Unit of electron flow, or current (I). One amp = 6.24×10^{18} electrons per second passing a point. Amount of current in a circuit will depend on voltage and resistance
Volt (V)	Potential difference that produces a current of 1 amp in a substance with a resistance of 1 Ω
Resistance (Ω)	Analogous to flow resistance. Related to current and voltage by: Resistance (Ω) = potential (V)/current (I)
Hertz (Hz)	For AC, it refers to the frequency with which the current changes polarity each second
Macroshock	Current >1 mA, which is the perception threshold
Microshock	Current <1 mA, which requires a means to bypass skin resistance in order to cause hazard
Electrical burn	Thermal injury resulting from the dissipation of electrical energy in the form of injurious heat

AC, alternating current.

1. **Macroshock.** *Macroshock* is an uncommon occurrence in the operating room because of (i) isolation transformers, (ii) isolation of electrical equipment, (iii) patient isolation from ground, (iv) proper grounding of equipment, and (v) line isolation monitoring.
2. **Microshock.** The term *microshock* applies to very small amounts of current (i.e., 50 to 100 mA). Significant morbidity has resulted from currents as low as 20 μA and often takes the form of cardiac dysrhythmias. Standard operating room isolation transformers provide no protection against currents of this magnitude. **Microshock cannot occur unless the skin resistance has been bypassed.** Because cardiac patients often have indwelling catheters that lead directly to the heart, as well as intracavitary or epicardial pacemaker wires, these patients are more susceptible to microshock hazard from these low-resistance pathways.
3. **Burns.** Electricity is a form of energy, and dissipation of energy takes the form of heat. *Burns* usually are a complication secondary to use of the electrocautery unit. Improper patient grounding is the usual cause.

B. Determinants of electrical hazard

1. **Current density.** The disruption of physiologic function produced by a given electrical current is inversely proportional to the area over which this current is applied. In the case of a small-bore central venous catheter in the RA, the amount of current needed to produce a significant arrhythmia is small.
2. **Current duration.** Cardiac muscle can recover quickly from a direct current (DC) that is applied for only microseconds but may become depolarized if the current is applied for 1 or more seconds.
3. **Type of current. DC** is the unidirectional, nonoscillating current that results when a constant voltage is applied across a resistor. When DC passes through skeletal or cardiac muscle, a sustained contraction can result. **Alternating** current (AC) is the current that changes polarity at a specified rate. It is the rate, or **frequency,** of the change in polarity that determines the magnitude of the hazard. Low-frequency ACs, such as the standard 60 Hz, can cause significant tetanic contraction of skeletal muscles as well as ventricular fibrillation with small currents.
4. **Skin resistance.** Resistance across intact skin can be as large as 1 million Ω when the skin is dry. This amount can drop by a factor of 1,000 when skin is wet. A centrally placed fluid-filled catheter that punctures the skin lowers resistance to 500 Ω and places the patient at a higher risk of sustaining a microshock injury.
5. **Current threshold (AC).** *Current threshold* is a term used by some to quantify that amount of current at 60 Hz needed to cause ventricular fibrillation. Several studies have determined the value to be anywhere between 50 and 1,000 μA (microshock range). One group found that as the catheter size decreases (resulting in an increased current density), the total amount of current needed to produce fibrillation also decreases.

C. **Results of microshock**

1. **Ventricular fibrillation.** In humans, the current threshold is estimated to be approximately 10 to 1,000 μA.
2. **Dysrhythmias.** Rhythm disturbances may occur before reaching currents needed to produce ventricular fibrillation. It is important to note that these rhythm disturbances can cause severe hypotension and mortality similar to that associated with ventricular fibrillation. Pump failure produced by rhythm disturbances occurs at approximately half the current threshold needed to produce ventricular fibrillation.

D. **Mechanisms of microshock.** Electrical hazard is possible when there is a path by which electrical current can flow from an electronic device through a patient to ground *and* there is some fault in the electrical grounding of the apparatus. These conditions must be present simultaneously in order for a shock hazard to exist. If the circuit includes an intracardiac monitor such as a CVP line, the leakage current can be transmitted directly to the heart, creating a microshock hazard.

E. **Prevention of electrical hazard.** Traditionally, the risk of electrical misadventure in the operating room was reduced with line isolation monitors separating the OR environment from the main power source. In most hospitals with up-to-date equipment, every device has its own safety monitor. The line isolation monitor may be obsolete. Many new or refurbished operating rooms do not even have line isolation monitors. Thus, microshock and burns are the focus of current electrical safety protocols.

1. **Macroshock.** The combined use of isolation transformers and line isolation monitors has historically provided some protection against macroshock.
2. **Microshock.** Avoidance of the conditions that lead to an AC path will prevent microshock hazard. Good equipment design and maintenance are essential. Equipment that incorporates infrared coupling between patient connections and the internal circuitry will effectively eliminate any possible current flow through a patient. Isolation of the monitoring equipment–patient connection from the internal circuitry by an isolation transformer reduces the risk of microshock hazard. In addition, any equipment that bypasses skin resistance (central fluid-filled catheters, epicardial pacemakers) should be handled with care to avoid any leakage current reaching the patient. (For example, the caregiver could touch a faulty piece of equipment and then touch a CVP catheter simultaneously.)
3. There is no substitute for vigilance in preventing electrical hazards (macroshock or microshock). The situations in which measuring or recording systems display excess noise in the form of humming or drifting in the baseline may represent a problem with the electronic circuitry. In older hospitals where the line-isolation monitor is used, an alarm should trigger immediate identification and removal of the offending piece of equipment.

VII. Point-of-care clinical testing.

Point-of-care clinical testing. Improved patient outcomes and resource utilization can be acquired via point-of-care testing. Point-of-care testing is defined as the clinical tests that are performed at the patient's bedside (i.e., in the operating room) or immediately adjacent to the patient rather than sending specimens to a central laboratory facility. Many cardiac surgical suites now utilize point-of-care testing for routine clinical tests.

A. **Coagulation.** Cardiac surgery patients, especially with CPB, are universally anticoagulated with heparin. The vast majority of patients receive protamine to ameliorate the heparin effects. CPB results in platelet dysfunction, decreased platelet number, and dilution of coagulation

TABLE 4.16 Internet simulators

PAC	http://www.pacep.org/
Transesophageal echo	http://pie.med.utoronto.ca/tee/TEE_content/TEE_virtualTEE.html
Capnography	http://www.capnography.com/
Pulse oximetry	http://vam.anest.ufl.edu/simulations/pulseoximeter.php
TEG	http://vam.anest.ufl.edu/simulations/teg.php

PAC, Pulmonary artery catheter; TEG, thromboelastography.

TABLE 4.17 Internet resources

American Heart Association (AHA)	heart.org
American Society of Anesthesiology (ASA)	asahq.org
American Society of Echocardiography (ASE)	asecho.org
ASE/SCA Guidelines	anesthesia-analgesia.org
Anesthesia Patient Safety Foundation (APSF)	apsf.org
Canadian Society of Echocardiography (CSE)	csecho.ca
Congenital Cardiac Anaesthesiologists Society	pedsanesthesia.org/ccas
European Association of Cardiothoracic Anesthesia (EACTA)	eacta.org
Foundation for Anesthesia Education and Research (FAER)	faer.org
International Anesthesia Research Society (IARS)	iars.org
Society of Cardiovascular Anesthesiologists (SCA)	scahq.org
Society of Critical Care Medicine (SCCM)	sccm.org
Society of Thoracic Surgeons (STS)	sts.org

factors. Monitoring coagulation status is critical. Detailed discussion of coagulation management during cardiac surgery is described in Chapter 19 (Coagulation/Anticoagulation).

1. **Activated clotting time (ACT).** Monitoring of adequate heparin effect is most often accomplished by measuring the ACT. For CPB, prolongation of the ACT to greater than 400 s is usually deemed adequate. OPCAB procedures sometimes use "partial heparinization" with an ACT target of about 300 s (although many cardiac anesthesiologists administer the full heparin dose in case emergent conversion to CPB is required).
2. **Thromboelastography (TEG).** TEG provides unique advantages over ACT and traditional coagulation parameters [34] because it provides functional information on platelets, clotting factors, and fibrinolytic processes. The introduction of small, reliable devices has spawned a renewed interest and utilization by cardiac anesthesiologists.

B. **Glucose.** Glucose control during cardiac surgery improves patient outcomes [30]. Many cardiac anesthesiologists treat any glucose measurement greater than 200 mg/dL. An insulin infusion is indicated for treatment. Blood glucose should be measured every 30 to 60 min and when otherwise indicated.

C. **Arterial blood gas (ABG).** Frequent ABG measurement is required for cardiac surgical procedures, especially during CPB. Point-of-care ABG analysis simultaneously measures serum electrolytes (potassium, sodium, ionized calcium) and hematocrit.

VIII. Additional Resources. The World Wide Web provides an abundance of resources to gain further knowledge about monitoring devices. Such resources not only include recently published studies and practice guidelines, but also online simulations for the less experienced (Table 4.16 and Table 4.17).

REFERENCES

1. Daniels JP, Ansermino JM. Introduction of new monitors into clinical anesthesia. *Curr Opin Anesth.* 2009;22:775–781.
2. London MJ, Hollenberg M, Wong MG, et al. Intraoperative myocardial ischemia: localization by continuous 12-lead electrocardiography. *Anesthesiology.* 1988;69:232–241.
3. Leung JM, Voskanian A, Bellows WH, et al. Automated electrocardiograph ST segment trending monitors: accuracy in detecting myocardial ischemia. *Anesth Analg.* 1998;87:4–10.
4. Shiloh AL, Eisen LA. Ultrasound-guided arterial catheterization: a narrative review. *Intensive Care Med.* 2010;36(2):214–221.
5. Slogoff S, Keats AS, Arlund C. On the safety of radial artery cannulation. *Anesthesiology.* 1983;59:42–47.
6. Karakitsos D, Labropoulos N, De Groot E, et al. Real-time ultrasound-guided catheterisation of the internal jugular vein: a prospective comparison with the landmark technique in critical care patients. *Crit Care.* 2006;10(6):R162.
7. Hessel EA. Con: we should not enforce the use of ultrasound as a standard of care for obtaining central venous access. *J Cardiothorac Vasc Anesth.* 2009;23(5):725–728.
8. Augoustides JG, Cheung AT. Pro: ultrasound should be the standard of care for central catheter insertion. *J Cardiothorac Vasc Anesth.* 2009;23(5):720–724.

9. American Society of Anesthesiologists Task Force on Pulmonary Artery Catheterization. Practice guidelines for pulmonary artery catheterization: an updated report by the American Society of Anesthesiologists Task Force on Pulmonary Artery Catheterization. *Anesthesiology.* 2003;99(4):988–1014.
10. Greenberg SB, Murphy GS, Vender JS. Current use of the pulmonary artery catheter. *Curr Opin Crit Care.* 2009;15(3):249–253.
11. Leibowitz AB, Oropello JM. The pulmonary artery catheter in anesthesia practice in 2007: an historical overview with emphasis on the past 6 years. *Semin Cardiothorac Vasc Anesth.* 2007;11(3):162–176.
12. Polonen P, Hippelainen M, Takala R, et al. A prospective randomized study of goal-oriented hemodynamic therapy in cardiac surgical patients. *Anesth Analg.* 2000;90:1052–1059.
13. Tuman KJ, Carroll GC, Ivankovich AD. Pitfalls in interpretation of pulmonary artery catheter data. *J Cardiothorac Anesth.* 1989;3:625–641.
14. Evans DC, Doraiswamy VA, Prosciak MP, et al. Complications associated with pulmonary artery catheters: a comprehensive clinical review. *Scand J Surg.* 2009;98(4):199–208.
15. Savage RM, Lytle BW, Aronson S, et al. Intraoperative echocardiography is indicated in high-risk coronary artery bypass grafting. *Ann Thorac Surg.* 1997;64:368–373.
16. Cheatham ML, Nelson LD, Chang MC, et al. Right ventricular end-diastolic volume index as a predictor of preload status in patients on positive end-expiratory pressure. *Crit Care Med.* 1998;26:1801–1806.
17. Funk DJ, Moretti EW, Gan TJ. Minimally invasive cardiac output monitoring in the perioperative setting. *Anesth Analg.* 2009;108(3):887–897.
18. Lee AJ, Cohn JH, Ranasinghe JS. Cardiac output assessed by invasive and minimally invasive techniques. *Anesthesiol Res Pract.* 2011; Epub 2011 Jul 6. Article ID 475151.
19. Konstadt SN, Reich DL, Kahn R, et al. Transesophageal echocardiography can be used to screen for ascending aortic atherosclerosis. *Anesth Analg.* 1995;81:225–228.
20. Hogue CW Jr, Palin CA, Arrowsmith JE. Cardiopulmonary bypass management and neurologic outcomes: an evidence-based appraisal of current practices. *Anesth Analg.* 2006;103:21–37.
21. Murkin JM. Applied neuromonitoring and improving CNS outcomes. *Semin Cardiothorac Vasc Anesth.* 2005;9:139–142.
22. Djaiani GN. Aortic arch atheroma: stroke reduction in cardiac surgical patients. *Semin Cardiothorac Vasc Anesth.* 2006;10:143–157.
23. Reich DK, Timcenko A, Bodian CA, et al. Predictors of pulse oximetry data failure. *Anesthesiology.* 1996;84:859–864.
24. Insler SR, Sessler DI. Perioperative thermoregulation and temperature monitoring. *Anesthesiol Clin.* 2006;24(4):823–837.
25. Newman MF, Wolman R, Kanchuger M, et al. Multicenter preoperative stroke risk index for patients undergoing coronary artery bypass graft surgery. Multicenter Study of Perioperative Ischemia (McSPI) Research Group. *Circulation.* 1996;94:II74–II80.
26. Bhatia A, Gupta AK. Neuromonitoring in the intensive care unit. I. Intracranial pressure and cerebral blood flow monitoring. *Intensive Care Med.* 2007;33(7):1263–1271.
27. Bhatia A, Gupta AK. Neuromonitoring in the intensive care unit II. Cerebral oxygenation monitoring and microdialysis. *Intensive Care Med.* 2007;33(8):1322–1328.
28. Grocott HP, Davie S, Fedorow C. Monitoring brain function in anesthesia and intensive care. *Curr Opin Anesthesiol.* 2010;23:759–764.
29. Saidi N, Murkin JM. Applied neuromonitoring in cardiac surgery: patient specific management. *Semin Cardiothorac Vasc Anesth.* 2005;9:17–23.
30. Heck M, Kumle B, Boldt J, et al. Electroencephalogram bispectral index predicts hemodynamic and arousal reactions during induction of anesthesia in patients undergoing cardiac surgery. *J Cardiothorac Vasc Anesth.* 2000;14:693–697.
31. Barr G, Anderson RE, Samuelsson S, et al. Fentanyl and midazolam anaesthesia for coronary bypass surgery: a clinical study of bispectral electroencephalogram analysis, drug concentrations and recall. *Br J Anaesth.* 2000;84:749–752.
32. Myles PS, Daly D, Silvers A, et al. Prediction of neurological outcome using bispectral index monitoring in patients with severe ischemic-hypoxic brain injury undergoing emergency surgery. *Anesthesiology.* 2009;110(5):1106–1115.
33. Tobias JD. Cerebral oxygenation monitoring: near-infrared spectroscopy. *Expert Rev Med Devices.* 2006;3:235–243.
34. Luddington RJ. Thrombelastography/thromboelastometry. *Clin Lab Haematol.* 2005;27:81–90.

5 Transesophageal Echocardiography

Jack S. Shanewise

KEY POINTS

1. The majority of cardiac surgical transesophageal echocardiography (TEE) imaging uses 2-dimensions, which is accomplished via phased array transducers consisting of 64 to 128 small crystals activated sequentially.
2. Pulsed-wave Doppler (PWD) profiles blood flow velocity at a single point along the ultrasound beam, whereas continuous-wave Doppler (CWD) detects the maximum velocity profile along the full length of the ultrasound beam. CWD permits measurement of higher-velocity blood flows (e.g., aortic stenosis) than PWD.

3. Color-flow Doppler (CFD) is a form of PWD that superimposes velocity information onto a 2D image, which assesses blood flow direction when it is predominantly moving either toward or away from the transducer.
4. Before placing a TEE probe, significant esophageal pathology should be ruled out by asking the patient about swallowing difficulty and about known esophageal dysfunction.
5. Global and regional left ventricular systolic and diastolic function can be assessed qualitatively or quantitatively using TEE, as can left ventricular preload (end-diastolic volume). Wall motion can be graded on a scale of 1 (normal) to 5 (dyskinesis).
6. A comprehensive TEE examination typically involves 20 standard views, which are shown in Figure 5.2.
7. Several TEE modalities can be used to assess mitral regurgitation, the easiest way being CFD.
8. Aortic stenosis can be assessed using a variety of TEE modalities including imaging in several planes, planimetry in a short-axis view to trace aortic valve area (AVA), and AVA assessment by continuity equation.
9. TEE is useful for interrogating the proximal ascending aorta, the aortic arch, and the descending aorta, but it has a "blind spot" for the distal ascending aorta that requires epiaortic echocardiography for diagnostic interrogation. Complete thoracic aortic interrogation is important in the presence of advanced aortic arteriosclerosis and aortic dissection.
10. TEE assessment of new left ventricular regional wall motion abnormalities is the most sensitive bedside monitor of myocardial ischemia.
11. TEE is highly sensitive for detecting intracardiac air.
12. Intraoperative TEE is indispensable during surgery for cardiac valve repair or replacement and for ventricular assist device placement.
13. Real-time 3D TEE shows promise especially in intraoperative assessment of operations for mitral valve disease and congenital heart disease.

I. Basic principles of ultrasound imaging

Medical ultrasound is produced by a piezoelectric crystal that vibrates in response to a high-frequency, alternating electrical current. The same crystal is deformed by returning echoes producing an electrical signal that is detected by the instrument. Ultrasound transmitted from the transducer into the patient interacts with the tissues in four ways: (i) Reflection, (ii) refraction, (iii) scattering, and (iv) attenuation. Ultrasound is reflected when it encounters the interface between tissues of different acoustic impedance, primarily a function of tissue density, and the timing, intensity, and phase of these echoes are processed to form the image. The velocity of transmission of ultrasound through soft tissues is relatively constant (1,540 m/s), and the time it takes the waves to travel to an object, be reflected, and return is determined by its distance from the transducer. Selecting the frequency of an ultrasound transducer is a trade-off between image resolution and depth of penetration. Higher frequencies have better resolution than lower frequencies, but they do not penetrate as far into tissue. The frequency of the ultrasound used in transesophageal echocardiography (TEE) typically ranges from 3.5 to 7 million cycles per second (MHz).

II. Basic principles of Doppler echocardiography

A. **Doppler echocardiography** uses ultrasound scattered from blood cells to measure the velocity and direction of blood flow. The Doppler effect increases the frequency of waves scattered from cells moving toward the transducer and decreases the frequency of waves from cells moving away. This change in the transmitted frequency (F_T) and the scattered frequency (F_S) is called Doppler shift ($F_S - F_T$) and is related to the velocity of blood flow (V) by the Doppler equation:

$$V = \frac{c(F_S - F_T)}{2F_T(\cos\theta)}$$

where c is the speed of sound in blood (1,540 m/s) and θ is the angle between the direction of blood flow and the ultrasound beam. The 2 in the denominator corrects for the time it takes the ultrasound to travel to and from the blood cells. In order to get a reasonably accurate (less than

6% error) measurement of blood velocity with Doppler echocardiography, the angle between the flow and the ultrasound beam (θ) should be less than 20 degrees.

B. **The Bernoulli equation** describes the relationship between the flow velocity through a stenosis and the pressure gradient across the stenosis. It is a complex relationship that includes factors for convective acceleration, flow acceleration, and viscous resistance. In certain clinical applications, such as aortic and mitral stenosis, a simplified form may be used. The **simplified Bernoulli equation** is:

$$\Delta P = 4V^2$$

where ΔP is the pressure gradient in millimeters of mercury (mm Hg) and V is the velocity in meters per second (m/s). The simplified Bernoulli equation should only be used in applications validated against another gold standard.

III. Modes of cardiac ultrasound imaging

A. **M-mode echocardiography** was the primary imaging mode for echocardiography for many years before the development of two-dimensional (2D) imaging in the late 1970s. It directs pulses of a single, linear beam of ultrasound into the tissues and displays the distance from the transducer of the returning echoes on the y-axis of a graph with signal strength indicated by brightness. The x-axis of the graph shows time, and motion of the structures is seen as curved lines. M-mode is useful for precisely timing events within the cardiac cycle. Its other advantage is very high temporal resolution, making thousands of images per second, which allows detection of high-frequency oscillating motion, such as vibrating vegetations.

B. **Two-dimensional echocardiography** is made by very rapidly moving the ultrasound beam through a plane, creating multiple scan lines that are displayed simultaneously to construct a 2D tomographic image. Mechanical transducers accomplish this by physically rotating or oscil-
1 lating the crystal. However, TEE probes usually have phased-array transducers, which consist of an array of many (64 to 128) small crystals that are electrically activated in sequence to move the beam through the imaging plane. The number of 2D images that can be formed each second is called frame rate (temporal resolution), which is determined by the width (number of scan lines per image) and depth (time for each pulse to return) of the imaging sector. Typical frame rates for 2D echocardiography are 30 to 60 frames per second, which is fast enough to accurately reflect most motion in the heart.

C. **Pulsed-wave Doppler (PWD)** measures the velocity and direction of blood flow in a specific location, called sample volume, which can be placed by the user in the area of interest of a 2D image. The velocity of flow is displayed with time on the x-axis and velocity on the y-axis. Velocities going toward the transducer are above the baseline of the y-axis and velocities away from the transducer below the baseline. PWD uses one transducer to both send and receive signals, determining the depth of the sample volume from the transducer by listening at a predetermined interval after transmission. This limits the maximum rate at which pulses can be sent (pulse repetition frequency), which in turn limits the maximum Doppler shift (**Nyquist
2 limit**) and the blood velocity that can be measured with PWD. The farther the sample volume is from the transducer, the lower the maximum velocity that can be measured. Typically, velocities more than 1.5 to 2 m/s cannot be measured with PWD.

D. **Continuous-wave Doppler (CWD)** measures the velocity and direction of blood flow along the line of sight of the ultrasound beam. The information is displayed with time on the x-axis and velocity on the y-axis, as with PWD. CWD uses two transducers: One to continuously transmit and the other to continuously receive. As a result, all returning signals are superimposed on the display, so CWD cannot determine the depth from the transducer from which a returning signal originated (range ambiguity), only its direction. But, unlike PWD, CWD has no limit on the maximum velocity measured. CWD is used to measure blood velocity too high for PWD, such as aortic stenosis (AS), and to determine the maximum velocity of a flow profile, such as with mitral stenosis.

E. **Color-flow Doppler (CFD)** is a form of PWD that superimposes the velocity information onto the simultaneously created 2D image of the heart, allowing the location and timing of flow disturbances to be easily seen. Flow toward the transducer usually is mapped as red and away as blue. Some CFD maps, called **variance maps,** add green to indicate turbulence in the
3 flow. Since it is a form of PWD, CFD cannot accurately measure higher flow velocities, such as mitral regurgitation (MR) and AS, and these flows appear as a mixture of red and blue, called

mosaic pattern. Also, as the flow velocity passes the limit of the CFD velocity scale (Nyquist limit), the color will alias, or change from red to blue or from blue to red, depending on the direction of flow. The aliasing velocity or Nyquist limit for CFD varies with the depth of the color sector, but typically is less than 100 cm/s. Since the instrument must develop both the 2D and Doppler images, the frame rate is lower with CFD than with 2D imaging alone, typically in the range from 12 to 24 frames per second. At frame rates below 15 frames per second, the image becomes noticeably jerky as the eye can discern the individual images. Decreasing the width and depth of the 2D image and the CFD sector within it will increase the frame rate.

F. **Tissue Doppler** is a form of PWD that measures the velocity of tissue motion at specific points in the myocardium. Its most common application is to measure the velocity of mitral annular motion to assess systolic function of the left ventricle (LV). More sophisticated analysis can be performed between two adjacent points in the myocardium to measure strain (tissue deformation over time) and strain rate (rate of deformation) to assess systolic and diastolic functions in different regions of the LV and the right ventricle (RV). Evaluation of synchrony of ventricular contraction is also possible with tissue Doppler.

IV. Indications for TEE during cardiac surgery

TEE can be used as a diagnostic tool during cardiac surgery to direct the surgical procedure and diagnose unanticipated problems and complications. TEE also is useful to the cardiac anesthesiologist as a monitor of cardiac function. Often, TEE is used for both purposes during heart surgery. The recently revised American Society of Anesthesiologists and the Society of Cardiovascular Anesthesiologists (ASA/SCA) Practice Guidelines for Perioperative TEE state that "For adult patients without contraindications, **TEE should be used in all open heart (e.g., valvular procedures) and thoracic aortic surgical procedures and should be considered in coronary artery bypass graft surgeries"** [1].

The ACC/AHA 2006 Practice Guidelines for the Management of Patients With Valvular Heart Disease recommend that intraoperative TEE be performed for valve repair surgery, valve replacement surgery with a stentless xenograft, homograft, or autograft valve, and for valve surgery for infective endocarditis. The guidelines also state that intraoperative TEE is reasonable for all patients undergoing cardiac valve surgery [2].

V. Safety, contraindications, and risk of TEE

A. **Preoperative screening** for esophageal disease should be completed before proceeding with TEE. The patient should be interviewed when possible and asked about a history of esophageal disease, dysphagia, and hematemesis. The medical record should be reviewed as well. Relative contraindications to TEE are listed in Table 5.1. The presence of a relative contraindication requires balancing the risk with the importance of TEE to the procedure. In patients with distal esophageal or gastric pathology, it often is possible to obtain the information needed with TEE without advancing into the distal esophagus. Preoperative esophagoscopy is another option to consider when the need for TEE is important and the risk is unclear.

4

TABLE 5.1 Relative contraindications to transesophageal echocardiography

History
Dysphagia
Odynophagia
Mediastinal radiation
Recent upper gastrointestinal surgery
Recent upper gastrointestinal bleeding
Thoracic aortic aneurysm
Esophageal pathology
Stricture
Tumor
Diverticulum
Varices
Esophagitis
Recent chest trauma

TABLE 5.2 Complications of transesophageal echocardiography
Dental and oral trauma (usually minor)
Laryngeal dysfunction
Postoperative aspiration
Endotracheal tube displacement
Bronchial compression in infants
Aortic compression in infants
Upper gastrointestinal bleeding (mucosal injury)
Pharyngeal perforation (rare)
Esophageal perforation (rare)

B. **TEE probe insertion and manipulation** should be performed gently. The probe must never be forced through a resistance, and excessive force must never be applied to the control wheels.

C. **Complications of TEE** are uncommon in properly screened patients, but they may be serious [3]. Complications of TEE are listed in Table 5.2. Serious injuries may not be apparent at the time of the procedure [4].

VI. Intraoperative TEE examination

A. **Probe insertion** is performed after the patient is anesthetized and the endotracheal tube is secured. An orogastric tube is inserted and the contents of the stomach and the esophagus are suctioned. As the mandible is displaced anteriorly, the probe is gently inserted into the posterior pharynx in the midline and advanced into the esophagus. A laryngoscope may be used to displace the mandible and better visualize the esophageal opening if necessary. As the probe is advanced into the thoracic esophagus (approximately 30 cm), the heart should come into view. On rare occasions, the probe cannot be placed in the esophagus, in which case the TEE is abandoned.

B. **Probe manipulation** is accomplished by advancing and withdrawing the probe within the esophagus, rotating the probe to the patient's left (counterclockwise) or right (clockwise). Assuming that the transducer is facing anteriorly (toward the heart), the tip flexes anteriorly and posteriorly with the large control wheel, and flexes to the patient's right and left (can be envisioned as "wagging," as in a dog's tail) with the small control wheel. With a multiplane TEE probe, the angle of the transducer is rotated axially from 0 degrees (horizontal plane), through 90 degrees (vertical plane), to 180 degrees (mirror image of 0 degree horizontal plane) (Fig. 5.1).

C. **Machine settings** are adjusted to optimize the TEE image. These settings are continuously adjusted by the user as the examination proceeds.

1. **Transducer frequency** is adjusted to the highest frequency that provides adequate depth of penetration to the structure being examined.
2. **Image depth** is adjusted to center the structure being examined in the display.
3. **Overall image gain** and **dynamic range** (compression) are adjusted so that the blood in the chambers appears nearly black and is distinct from the shades of gray representing tissue.
4. **Time gain compensation** controls are adjusted so that there is uniform brightness from the near field to the far field of the image.
5. **CFD gain** is adjusted to a threshold that just eliminates any background noise within the color sector.

D. **TEE views.** The ASE/SCA Guidelines for performing a comprehensive intraoperative multiplane TEE examination [5] define 20 views that comprise a comprehensive TEE examination (Table 5.3). These 20 views are shown in Figure 5.2. The views are named for the location of the transducer (echocardiographic window), a descriptive term of the imaging plane (e.g., short axis [SAX] or long axis [LAX]), and the major anatomic structure in the view. All of these views can be developed in most patients. Additional views may be needed to completely examine a patient with a particular form of pathology. The sequence in which these views are obtained will vary from examiner to examiner, but it is generally most efficient to develop the midesophageal (ME) views and then the transgastric (TG) views.

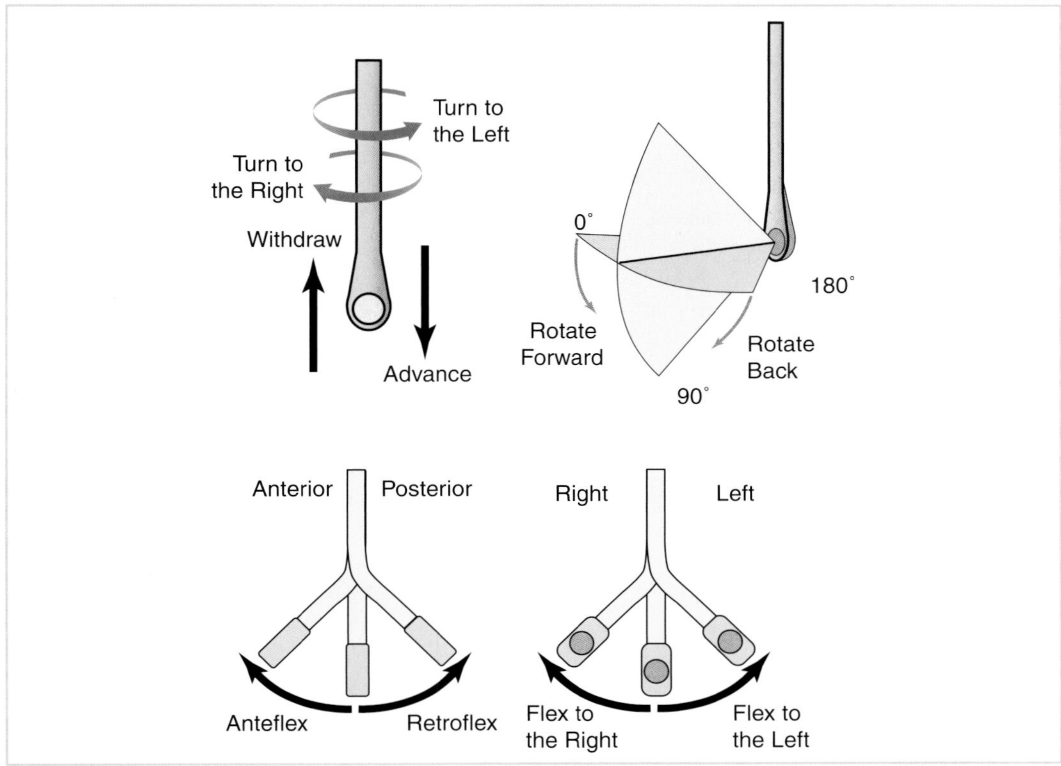

FIGURE 5.1 Terminology used to describe manipulation of the probe and transducer during image acquisition. (From Shanewise JS, Cheung AT, Aronson S, et al. ASE/SCA guidelines for performing a comprehensive intraoperative multiplane transesophageal echocardiography examination: recommendations of the American Society of Echocardiography Council for Intraoperative Echocardiography and the Society of Cardiovascular Anesthesiologists Task Force for Certification in Perioperative Transesophageal Echocardiography. *Anesth Analg.* 1999;89:870–884, with permission).

1. **ME views** are developed with the TEE transducer posterior to the left atrium (LA). With a multiplane TEE probe, detailed examinations of cardiac chambers and valves can be completed in most patients from this window alone.
2. **TG views** are obtained by passing the transducer into the stomach and directing the imaging plane superiorly through the diaphragm to the heart. Images of the LV and right ventricle (RV and the mitral valve (MV) and tricuspid valve (TV) are made from this window. Views to align the Doppler beam parallel to flow through the left ventricular outflow tract (LVOT) and aortic valve (AV) can be developed from the TG window.
3. **Upper esophageal (UE) views** are made with the transducer at the level of the aortic arch, which is examined in LAX and SAX. In many patients, images of the main pulmonary artery (PA) and pulmonic valve (PV) also may be developed, allowing alignment of the Doppler beam parallel to flow in these structures.

E. **Examination of specific structures**

1. **Left ventricle.** The LV is examined with the ME four-chamber, ME two-chamber, ME LAX, TG mid-SAX, and TG two-chamber views.
   a. **LV size** is assessed by measuring the inside diameter at the junction of the basal and mid-thirds at end diastole using the ME two-chamber or TG two-chamber view. Normal is less than 5.4 cm for women and less than 6 cm for men. Normal thickness of the LV wall is 1.2 cm or less at end diastole and is best measured with TEE from the TG mid-SAX view [6].
   b. **LV global function** may be assessed quantitatively or qualitatively. Fractional area change (FAC) is a 2D TEE equivalent of ejection fraction (EF) and is obtained by

TABLE 5.3 Recommended transesophageal echocardiographic cross section

Window (depth from incisors)	Cross section (panel in Fig. 4.2)	Multiplane angle range	Structures imaged
UE (20–25 cm)	Aortic arch LAX (s)	0°	Aortic arch, left brachiocephalic vein
	Aortic arch SAX (t)	90°	Aortic arch, PA, PV, left brachiocephalic vein
Midesophageal (30–40 cm)	Four chamber (a)	0°–20°	LV, LA, RV, RA, MV, TV, IAS
	Mitral commissural (g)	60°–70°	MV, LV, LA, LAA
	Two chamber (b)	80°–100°	LV, LA, LAA, MV
	LAX (c)	120°–160°	LV, LA, AV, LVOT, MV, asc aorta
	RV inflow–outflow (m)	60°–90°	RV, RA, TV, RVOT, PV, PA
	AV SAX (h)	30°–60°	AV, IAS, coronary ostia, LVOT, PV
	AV LAX (i)	120°–160°	AV, LVOT, prox asc aorta, right PA
	Bicaval (l)	80°–110°	RA, SVC, IVC, IAS, LA, CS
	Asc aortic SAX (o)	0°–60°	Asc aorta, SVC, PA, right PA
	Asc aortic LAX (p)	100°–150°	Asc aorta, right PA
	Desc aorta SAX (q)	0°	Desc thoracic aorta, left pleural space
	Desc aorta LAX (r)	90°–110°	Desc thoracic aorta, left pleural space
TG (40–45 cm)	Basal SAX (f)	0°–20°	LV, MV, RV, TV
	Mid-SAX (d)	0°–20°	LV, RV, papillary muscles
	Two chamber (e)	80°–100°	LV, MV, chordae, papillary muscles, CS, LA
	LAX (j)	0°–120°	LVOT, AV, MV
	RV inflow (n)	100°–120°	RV, TV, RA, TV chordae, papillary muscles
Deep TG (45–50 cm)	LAX (k)	0°–20° (anteflexion)	LVOT, AV, asc aorta, arch

UE, upperesophageal; LAX, long axis; SAX, short axis; TG, transgastric; asc, ascending; AV, aortic valve; CS, coronary sinus; desc, descending; IAS, interatrial septum; IVC, inferior vena cava; LA, left atrium; LAA, left atrial appendage; LV, left ventricle; LVOT, left ventricular outflow tract; MV, mitral valve; PA, pulmonary artery; prox, proximal; PV, pulmonic valve; RA, right atrium; RV, right ventricle; RVOT, right ventricular outflow tract; SVC, superior vena cava; TV, tricuspid valve. Lower case letters in parenthesis refer to views shown in Figure 4.2.

5

measuring the LV chamber area in the TG mid-SAX view by tracing the endocardial border to measure the end diastolic area (EDA) and the end systolic area (ESA) and using the formula: FAC = (EDA − ESA)/EDA. Normal FAC is greater than 0.50. This method is not as accurate when wall-motion abnormalities are present in the apex or the base of the LV. **Qualitative assessment of LV function is performed by considering all views of the LV and estimating the EF (estimated ejection fraction [EEF]) as normal (EEF greater than 55%), mildly decreased (EEF 45% to 54%), moderately decreased (EEF 35% to 44%), moderately severely decreased (EEF 25% to 34%), or severely decreased (EEF less than 25%). EEF by experienced echocardiographers correlates with nonechocardiographic measures of EF as well or better than quantitative echocardiographic measurements of EF** [7].

c. **Assessment of regional LV function.** The LV is divided into 17 regions or segments (Fig. 5.3). Each segment is rated qualitatively for thickening during systole using the following scale: 1 = normal (greater than 30% thickening), 2 = mild hypokinesis (10% to 30% thickening), 3 = severe hypokinesis (less than 10% thickening), 4 = akinesis (no thickening), and 5 = dyskinesis (thinning and paradoxical motion during systole). An increase in scale of 2 or more in a region should be considered significant and suggestive of myocardial ischemia [8].

d. **Assessment of diastolic LV function** can be made by examining with PWD the transmitral inflow velocity profile during diastole. The normal pattern has an E wave corresponding to early passive filling of the LV, followed by a period of diastasis,

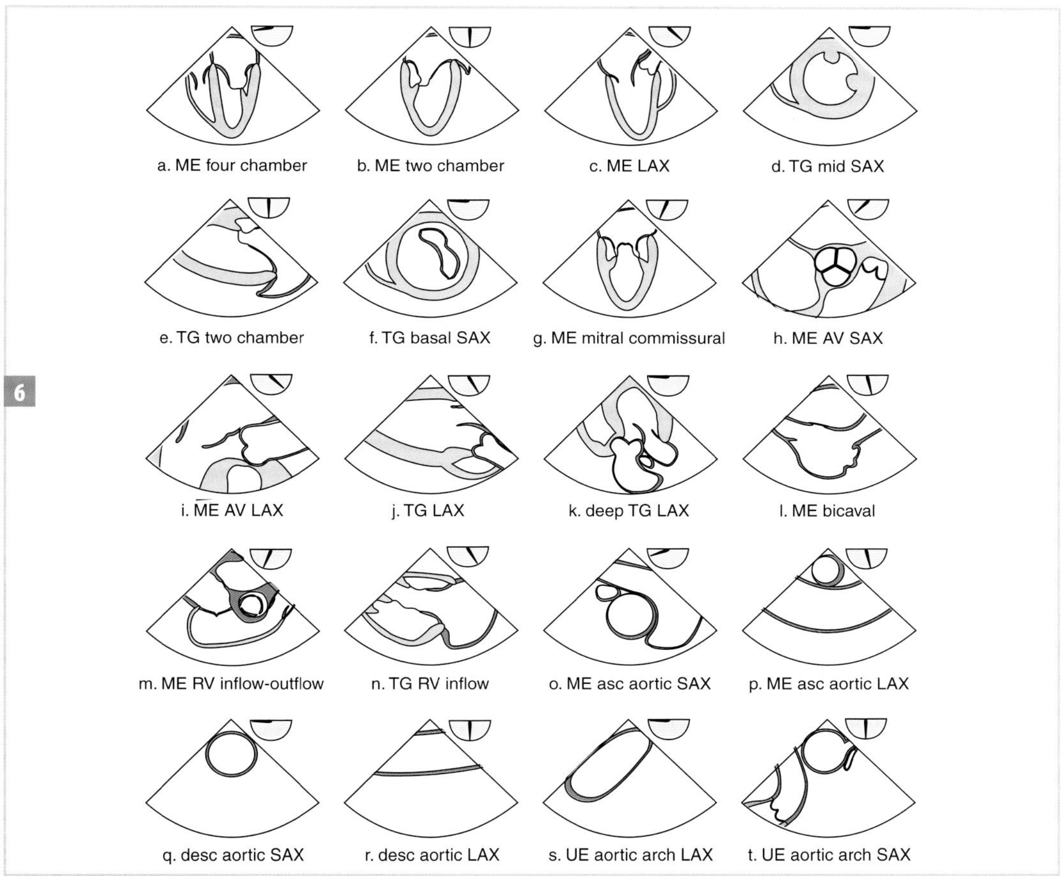

FIGURE 5.2 Twenty cross-sectional views (a. through t.) composing the recommended comprehensive transesophageal echocardiographic examination. Approximate multiplane angle is indicated by the icon adjacent to each view. asc, ascending; AV, aortic valve; desc, descending; LAX, long axis; ME, midesophageal; RV, right ventricle; SAX, short axis; TG, transgastric; UE, upper esophageal. (From Shanewise JS, Cheung AT, Aronson S, et al. ASE/SCA guidelines for performing a comprehensive intraoperative multiplane transesophageal echocardiography-examination: recommendations of the American Society of Echocardiography Council for Intraoperative Echocardiography and the Society of Cardiovascular Anesthesiologists Task Force for Certification in Perioperative Transesophageal Echocardiography. *Anesth Analg.* 1999;89:870–884, with permission.)

and finally an A wave corresponding to atrial contraction in late diastole (Fig. 5.4A). Milder forms of diastolic dysfunction result in the **impaired relaxation pattern** with decreased peak E-to-A velocity ratio and prolonged E-wave deceleration time (Fig. 5.4B). Advanced diastolic dysfunction causes the **restrictive pattern** with increased peak E-to-A velocity ratio and decreased E-wave deceleration time (Fig. 5.4C). As diastolic dysfunction progresses from mild to severe over a number of years, the transmitral flow pattern may pass through a period in which it appears normal, a condition termed **pseudonormal pattern**. Normal may be distinguished from pseudonormal by examination of the pulmonary venous inflow velocity profile, which normally has positive inflow waves during systole (S wave) and diastole (D wave) and a small, negative wave corresponding to atrial contraction (A wave) (Fig. 5.5A). The pseudonormal pattern has prolongation of the A wave and attenuation of the S wave compared to the normal pattern (Fig. 5.5B). Age and preload also affect the transmitral and pulmonary venous inflow velocity patterns.

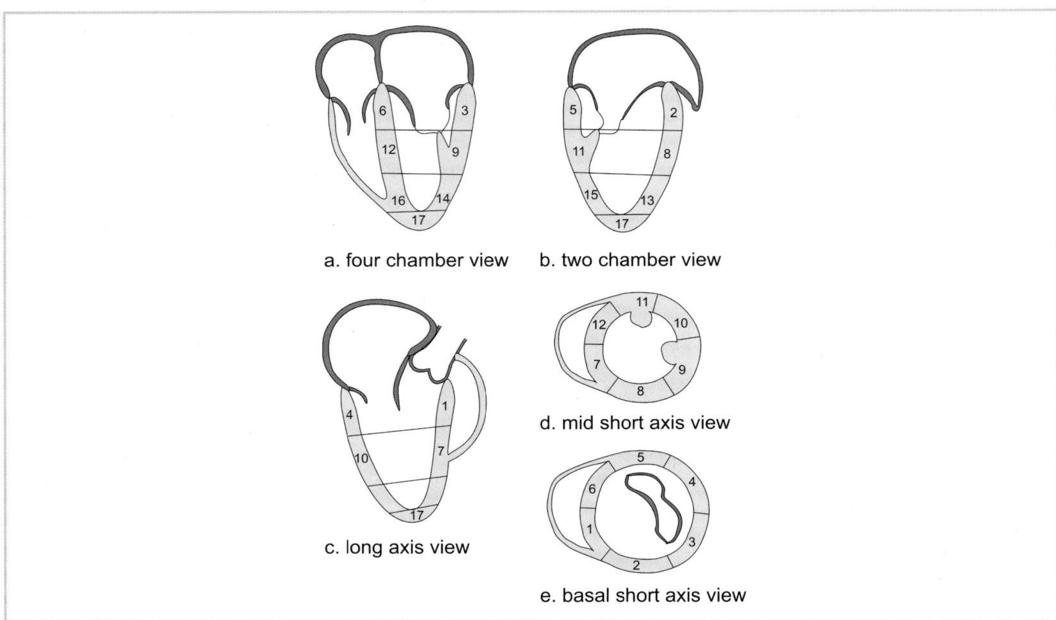

FIGURE 5.3 Seventeen-segment model of the LV. **A:** Four-chamber views show the three inferoseptal and three anterolateral segments. **B:** Two-chamber views show the three anterior and three inferior segments. **C:** Long-axis views show the two anteroseptal and two inferolateral segments. **D:** Mid–short-axis views show all six segments at the midlevel. **E:** Basal short-axis views show all six segments at the basal level. Basal segments: *1,* basal anteroseptal; *2,* basal anterior, *3,* basal anterolateral; *4,* basal inferolateral; *5,* basal inferior; *6,* basal inferoseptal. Mid-segments: *7,* mid-anteroseptal; *8,* mid-anterior; *9,* mid-anterolateral; *10,* mid-inferolateral; *11,* mid-inferior; *12,* mid-inferoseptal. Apical segments. *13,* apical anterior; *14,* apical lateral; *15,* apical inferior; *16,* apical septal; *17* apical cap or true apex. (Modified from Shanewise JS, Cheung AT, Aronson S, et al. ASE/SCA guidelines for performing a comprehensive intraoperative multiplane transesophageal echocardiography examination: recommendations of the American Society of Echocardiography Council for Intraoperative Echocardiography and the Society of Cardiovascular Anesthesiologists Task Force for Certification in Perioperative Transesophageal Echocardiography. *Anesth Analg.* 1999;89:870–884, with permission.)

2. **Mitral valve.** The MV is examined with the ME four-chamber, ME mitral commissural, ME LAX, and TG basal SAX views, with and without CFD. It consists of an anterior leaflet and a posterior leaflet joined at two commissures, the anterolateral and the posteromedial. There is a papillary muscle corresponding to each commissure. The posterior leaflet is divided into three scallops and the anterior leaflet into thirds for purposes of describing the location of lesions (Fig. 5.6). Prolapse of the MV is present when a portion of the leaflet moves to the atrial side of the annulus during systole. Flail is said to be present when a chordae tendineae is ruptured and the corresponding segment of the valve leaflet is seen oscillating in the LA during systole.

   a. **Mitral regurgitation**

   Judging severity of MR with TEE is based on several factors [9]. The structure of the valve leaflets is examined with 2D echocardiography, looking for defects of coaptation.
7 CFD is used to detect retrograde flow through the valve into the LA. The width of the jet as it passes through the valve and its size in the LA are noted. Eccentric jets of MR tend to be more severe than central jets of a similar size. CFD also can detect flow convergence proximal to the regurgitant orifice, indicating more significant MR. Pulmonary venous inflow velocity profile is examined with PWD for systolic flow reversal, a specific but not very sensitive sign of severe MR. Severity is graded on a semiquantitative scale of 1+ (mild) to 4+ (severe). Most patients have at least trace amounts of MR detected with TEE.

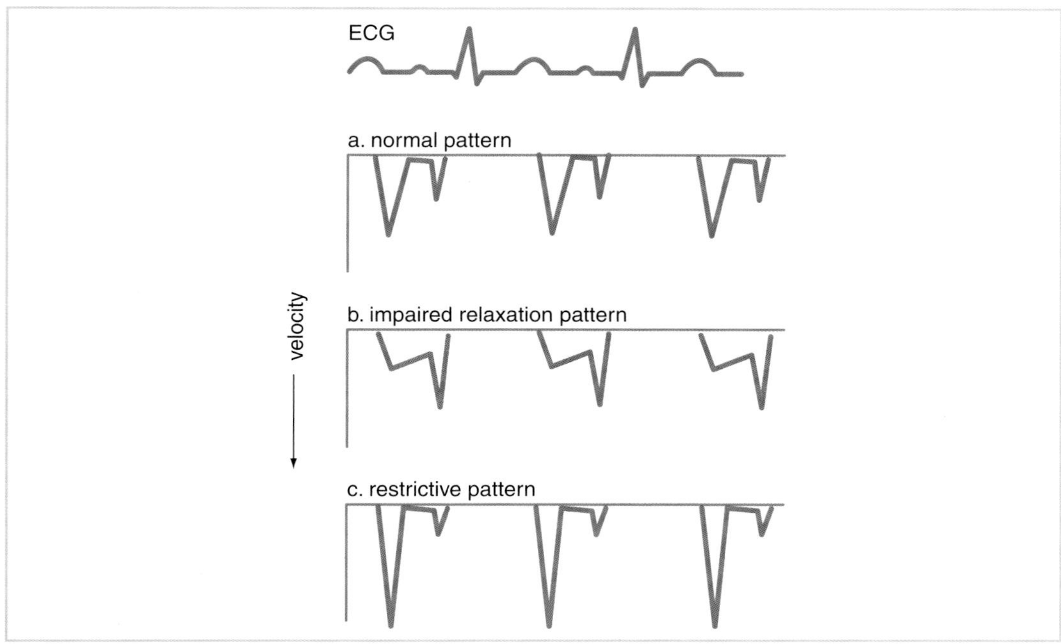

FIGURE 5.4 Transmitral inflow velocity profiles measured with PWD by placing the sample volume between the open tips of the mitral leaflets. **A:** Normal pattern. The pseudonormal pattern has a similar appearance. **B:** Impaired relaxation pattern indicative of mild diastolic dysfunction. The peak E-wave velocity is less than the A wave (E-to-A reversal) and the deceleration time of the E wave is prolonged. **C:** Restrictive pattern indicative of advanced diastolic dysfunction. The peak E-wave velocity is increased and the E-wave deceleration time is decreased. *A,* atrial filling wave; *E,* early filling wave.

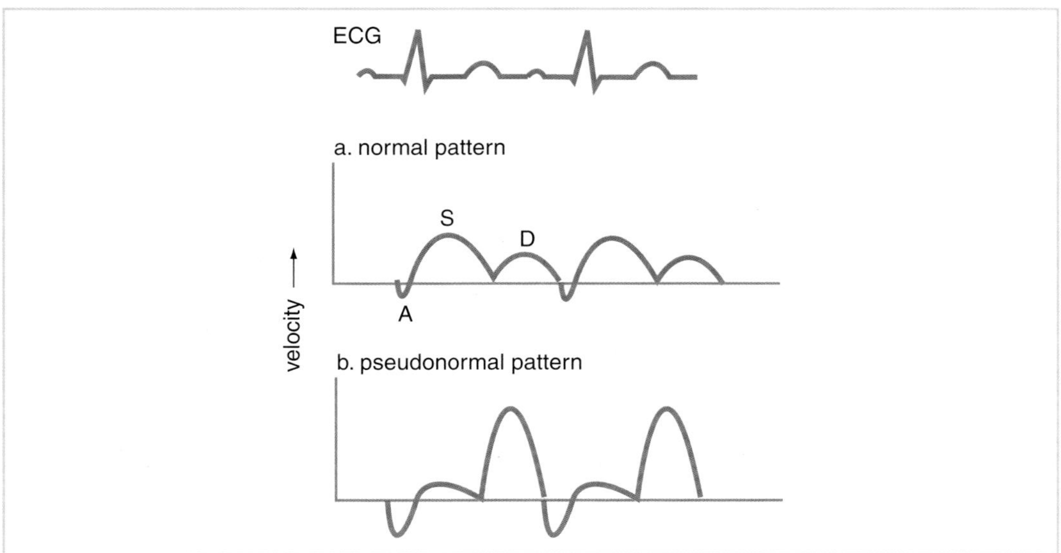

FIGURE 5.5 Pulmonary venous inflow velocity profiles measured with PWD by placing the sample volume in the left upper pulmonary vein. **A:** Profile seen with normal-diastolic function and transmitral inflow. The S wave is larger than the D wave and a small A reversal is present. **B:** Pattern seen with diastolic dysfunction and pseudonormal transmitral inflow. The S wave is attenuated and smaller than the D wave and an enlarged A wave is present. *A,* atrial reversal wave; *D,* diastolic wave, *S,* systolic wave.

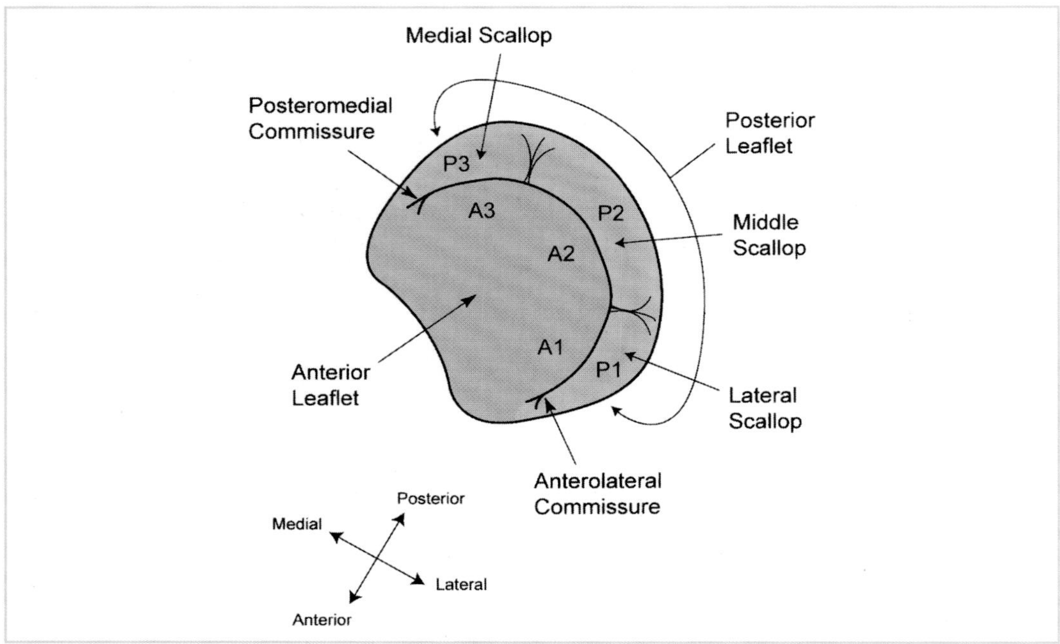

FIGURE 5.6 Anatomy of the MV. *A1,* lateral third of the anterior leaflet; *A2,* middle third of the anterior leaflet; *A3,* medial third of the anterior leaflet; *P1,* lateral scallop of the posterior leaflet; *P2,* middle scallop of the posterior leaflet; *P3,* medial scallop of the posterior leaflet. (From Shanewise JS, Cheung AT, Aronson S, et al. ASE/SCA guidelines for performing a comprehensive intraoperative multiplane transesophageal echocardiography examination: recommendations of the American Society of Echocardiography Council for Intraoperative Echocardiography and the Society of Cardiovascular Anesthesiologists Task Force for Certification in Perioperative Transesophageal Echocardiography. *Anesth Analg.* 1999;89:870–884, with permission.)

Functional MR is due to dilation of the MV annulus or displacement of the papillary muscles causing a decrease in the surface of coaptation of the MV leaflets. The structure of the valve leaflets is normal. Functional MR can be very dynamic and is markedly affected by loading conditions. The most common causes of functional MR are regional wall-motion abnormalities (RWMAs) from coronary artery disease and generalized dilation of the LV.

Myxomatous degeneration of the MV is a common cause of MR requiring surgery. The leaflets are elongated and redundant, prolapsing into the LA during systole. Rupture of a chordae is common in this condition and causes a flail segment of the involved leaflet. TEE can be used to locate the portion of the MV involved and is helpful in guiding surgical therapy. Prolapse and flail of the middle scallop of the posterior leaflet is the most common form and most amenable to repair by resection of the involved portion and reinforcement of the annulus with an annuloplasty ring.

Rheumatic MR is caused by thickening and shortening of the MV leaflets and chordae restricting motion and closure during systole. This type of MR typically is difficult to repair and usually requires prosthetic valve replacement.

Proximal isovelocity surface area (PISA) is a method to quantify MR with echocardiography using CFD and CWD. It is most commonly applied to central MR and is probably not as accurate for eccentric MR. The flow velocity of blood increases as it converges towards the regurgitant orifice and can be seen with CFD. When the velocity reaches the limit on the CFD scale, aliasing of the signal occurs and the color mapped onto the 2D image changes from red to blue on the ventricular side of the valve. This change in color represents a hemispheric shell of blood converging towards the

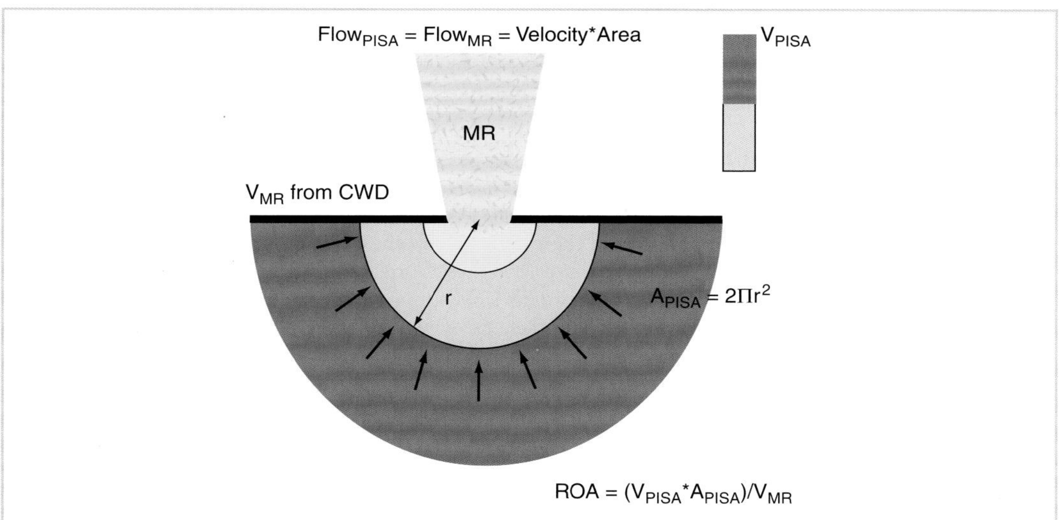

FIGURE 5.7 Diagram of the PISA method to measure ROA in central MR. The horizontal line represents the MV with a central regurgitant orifice. As the blood flow converges on the orifice, the velocity increases and causes aliasing of the CFD signal, changing the color from red to blue creating the PISA (*small arrows*) on the ventricular side of the valve. The velocity of the blood at the PISA (V_{PISA}) is taken from the CFD scale. The size of the PISA (A_{PISA}) is calculated by measuring its radius (*r, large arrow*) and using the formula for the surface area of a hemisphere: $A_{PISA} = 2\Pi r^2$. The peak velocity of the MR (V_{MR}) is measured by using CWD aimed through the orifice. Flow$_{PISA}$ = $V_{PISA} \cdot A_{PISA}$ and Flow$_{MR}$ = $V_{MR} \cdot$ ROA. By the continuity principle, Flow$_{MR}$ = Flow$_{PISA}$, so ROA = $(V_{PISA} \cdot A_{PISA})/V_{MR}$.

regurgitant orifice called PISA (Fig. 5.7). If the surface area of this hemisphere (A_{PISA}) is measured and multiplied by the aliasing velocity toward the transducer (V_{PISA}—taken from the CFD scale), the instantaneous flow at the PISA in mL/s is obtained. A_{PISA} is calculated by measuring the radius (r) of the PISA and using the formula for the area of a hemisphere: $(A_{PISA}) = 2\Pi r^2 = 6.28r^2$. By the continuity principle, the instantaneous flow (mL/s) is the same at the PISA as at the regurgitant orifice, both of which are the product of an area and a velocity: $A_{PISA} \cdot V_{PISA} = \text{ROA} \cdot V_{MR}$, where ROA is the regurgitant orifice area. The peak instantaneous velocity of the MR (V_{MR}) is measured with CWD, allowing the ROA to be calculated. Rearranging the formula,

$$\text{ROA} = \frac{(A_{PISA} \cdot V_{PISA})}{V_{MR}}$$

ROA less than 0.2 cm^2 is mild MR and greater than 0.4 cm^2 is severe MR.

If the CFD is adjusted so that the aliasing velocity toward the transducer is close to 40 cm/s, and the V_{MR} is assumed to be about 500 cm/s (most patients with reasonable hemodynamics) the formula simplifies to:

$$\text{ROA} = \frac{r^2}{2}$$

b. Mitral stenosis

Significant mitral stenosis almost always is due to rheumatic heart disease. Severe mitral annular calcification is a rare cause of significant stenosis. Two-dimensional images show thickening of the leaflets with fusion at the commissures and restricted opening during diastole. Doppler velocity measurements of the transmitral inflow shows increased peak and mean velocities, which can be used to calculate peak and mean transvalvular gradients ($\Delta P = 4V^2$).

The best gauge of severity of mitral stenosis is mitral valve area (MVA). MVA less than 1 cm^2 is considered severe, and from 1 to 1.5 cm^2 moderate.

TEE can be used to measure valve area in mitral stenosis by the following methods:

(1) Planimetry. Images of the stenotic orifice may be directly measured from the TG basal SAX view. The imaging plane is moved above and below the valve until the minimal orifice is seen, then the image is frozen in diastole and the orifice traced. Calcification of the annulus or leaflets may create acoustic shadowing limiting the ability to accurately image the orifice in many patients.

(2) Pressure half-time. The rate at which the pressure gradient decreases across a stenotic MV during diastole is directly related to the severity of the stenosis. A gauge of this rate is the pressure half-time, which can be measured from the transmitral inflow velocity profile. An empirically derived formula gives the MVA in square centimeters as:

$$\text{MVA} = \frac{220}{\text{PHT}}$$

where PHT is the pressure half-time in milliseconds. This formula has been validated only for patients with rheumatic mitral stenosis. It cannot be used if there is more than mild aortic regurgitation (AR) or immediately after a mitral commissurotomy.

(3) PISA. In mitral stenosis the flow velocity of blood increases as it converges toward the stenotic orifice and can be seen with CFD. When the velocity reaches the limit on the CFD scale going away from the transducer, aliasing of the signal occurs and the color mapped onto the 2D image changes from blue to red on the atrial side of the valve. This change in color represents a hemispheric shell of blood converging toward the stenotic orifice called PISA (Fig. 5.8). If the surface area of this

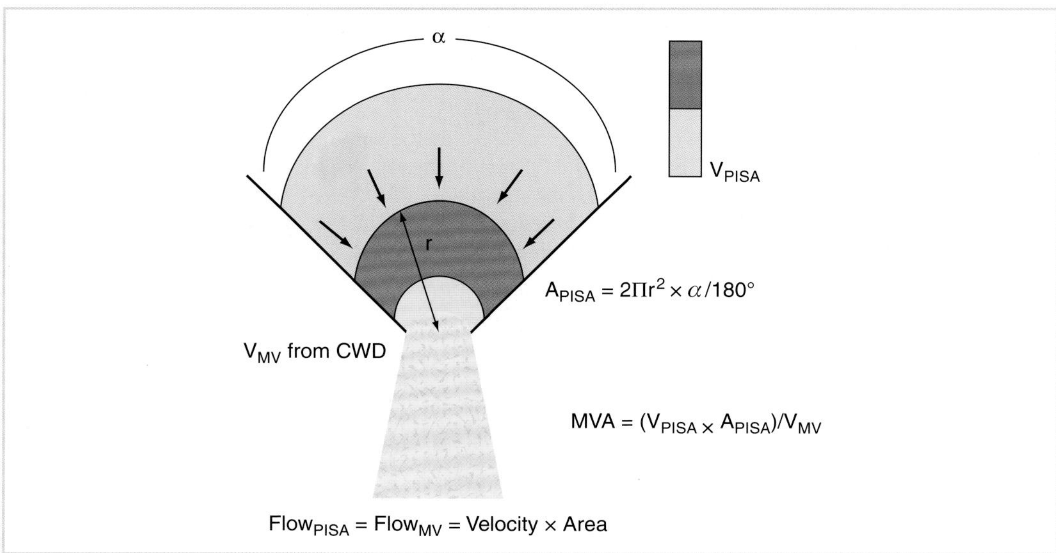

FIGURE 5.8 Diagram of the PISA method to measure MV area in mitral stenosis. The *thick lines* represent the MV with a central stenotic orifice. As the blood flow converges on the orifice, the velocity increases and causes aliasing of the CFD signal, changing the color from blue to red creating the PISA (*small arrows*) on the atrial side of the valve. The velocity of the blood at the PISA (V_{PISA}) is taken from the CFD scale. The size of the PISA (A_{PISA}) is calculated by measuring its radius (*r, large arrow*) and using the formula for the surface area of a hemisphere reduced by the ratio of the angle formed by the leaflets (α) and 180 degrees: $A_{PISA} = 2\Pi r^2 \cdot \alpha/180°$. The peak velocity of the transmitral inflow (V_{MV}) is measured by using CWD aimed through the stenotic orifice. $Flow_{PISA} = V_{PISA} \cdot A_{PISA}$ and $Flow_{MV} = V_{MV} \cdot MVA$. By the continuity principle, $Flow_{MV} = Flow_{PISA}$, so $MVA = (V_{PISA} \cdot A_{PISA})/V_{MV}$.

hemisphere (A_{PISA}) is measured and multiplied by the aliasing velocity going away from the transducer (V_{PISA}—taken from the CFD scale), the instantaneous flow at the PISA in mL/s is obtained. A_{PISA} is calculated by measuring the radius of the PISA and using the formula for the area of a hemisphere and reducing it by the ratio of the angle formed by the MV leaflets (α angle) and 180 degrees: $A_{PISA} = 2\Pi r^2 \cdot (\alpha/180°) = 6.28\, r^2 \cdot (\alpha/180°)$. The CFD scale is adjusted so that the radius of the PISA is between 1 and 1.5 cm. By the continuity principle, the instantaneous flow (mL/s) is the same at the PISA as at the stenotic orifice, both of which are the product of an area and a velocity: $A_{PISA} \cdot V_{PISA} = \text{MVA} \cdot V_{MV}$, where MVA is the MV area and V_{MV} is the peak transmitral inflow velocity measured with CWD. Rearranging,

$$\text{MVA} = \frac{(A_{PISA} \cdot V_{PISA})}{V_{MV}}$$

3. **Aortic valve.** The AV is examined in the ME AV SAX and ME AV LAX views, with and without CFD. Doppler measurements of flow velocity through the AV are made from the TG LAX and deep TG LAX views, which allow the ultrasound beam to be directed parallel to AV flow. The AV is a semilunar valve that has three cusps: (i) The right coronary cusp, which is most anterior and adjacent to the RV outflow tract, (ii) the noncoronary cusp, which is adjacent to the atrial septum, and (iii) the left coronary cusp.

   a. **Aortic regurgitation**

   The severity of AR is assessed with TEE primarily by the size of the regurgitant jet on CFD and the depth to which it extends into the LV [9]. The valve cusps also should be examined with 2D echocardiography, looking for perforations and defects in coaptation. Other signs of severe AR include holodiastolic flow reversal in the descending thoracic aorta measured with PWD, pressure half-time of AR less than 300 ms as taken from the AR velocity profile measured with CWD from the TG LAX or deep TG LAX views, presystolic closure of the MV, and presystolic MR.

   b. **Aortic stenosis**

   Evaluation of AS with TEE is based on the appearance of the valve on 2D images and Doppler velocity measurements of the flow through the stenotic valve. In AS, the valve leaflets are thickened with markedly restricted opening during systole. Calcification of the cusps and the annulus may cause acoustic shadowing. TEE may be used to quantify the severity of AS by three methods:

   (1) **Transaortic gradients** may be calculated with the simplified Bernoulli equation ($\Delta P = 4V^2$) by using CWD to measure the flow velocity in meters per second through a stenotic AV from the TG LAX or deep TG LAX views. For example, if the peak AV outflow velocity is 5 m/s, the peak instantaneous gradient would be 100 mm Hg. Peak velocities greater than 4 m/s (peak gradient greater than 64 mm Hg) are consistent with severe AS, but severe AS may be present with lower velocities if stroke volume (SV) is low due to poor ventricular function.

   (2) AV area **by planimetry**. AV area (AVA) is a better means of assessing severity of AS than gradients and may be measured by planimetry from the ME AV SAX view. The 2D image is frozen during systole at the level of the free edge of the leaflets, scrolled to identify the maximum systolic orifice, which is then traced using the caliper function. Acoustic shadowing from calcification may obscure the image in many patients and make planimetry difficult. **AVA less than 1 cm^2 is considered significant.**

   (3) **AVA by continuity equation.** AVA may be calculated using the continuity equation, which states that the same amount of flow passes through the AV and the LVOT with each stroke. Flow rate is equal to the velocity of the flow multiplied by the area through which the flow occurs (Flow = $V \cdot A$) and by the continuity equation is the same at the AV and the LVOT. Thus,

8

$$\text{Flow}_{\text{AV}} = \text{Flow}_{\text{LVOT}}$$

$$V_{\text{AV}} \cdot A_{\text{AV}} = V_{\text{LVOT}} \cdot A_{\text{LVOT}}$$

rearranging, we obtain

$$A_{\text{AV}} = \left(\frac{V_{\text{LVOT}} \cdot A_{\text{LVOT}}}{V_{\text{AV}}} \right)$$

The area of the LVOT is obtained from the ME LAX view of the AV by measuring its diameter during systole and applying the formula for the area of a circle:

$$A_{\text{CIRCLE}} = \Pi r^2 = \Pi \left(\frac{D}{2} \right)^2 = \left(\frac{\Pi}{4} \right) \cdot D^2 = 0.785 \cdot D^2$$

V_{LVOT} is measured with PWD by placing the sample volume just proximal to the AV in the LVOT and V_{AV} by directing the CWD through the stenotic valve. It is most convenient to use units of centimeters per second and centimeters in order to obtain the AVA in units per square centimeter. Common pitfalls in using the continuity equation to measure AVA are underestimation of the LVOT diameter, an error that is squared in the calculation, and underestimating the peak AV velocity due to a large angle between the direction of the flow and the Doppler beam. It is also possible to mistake the velocity profile of MR for AS because they both are systolic and in the same general direction.

4. **Right ventricle.** The RV is examined in the ME four-chamber, ME RV inflow–outflow view, and TG RV inflow view, assessing size and global function. The RV appears to be somewhat smaller than the LV in most views and does not normally share the apex with the LV. Pressure and/or volume overload will cause RV enlargement. Global function usually is based on qualitative assessment of decrease in chamber size during systole. It is rated as normal function or as mild, moderate, or severe decrease in function.
5. **Tricuspid valve.** The TV lies between the RV and the right atrium (RA) and has three leaflets: Anterior, posterior, and septal. It is examined with the ME four-chamber, ME RV inflow–outflow view, and TG RV inflow view, with and without CFD. Some tricuspid regurgitation (TR) usually is detected. Severity of TR is graded on a semiquantitative scale of 1+ (mild) to 4+ (severe) based primarily on the size of the regurgitant jet. Significant TR usually is due to annular dilation secondary to right heart failure. Tricuspid stenosis is uncommon and usually due to rheumatic heart disease. On TEE it causes high-velocity, turbulent flow across the TV detected with CFD, PWD, and CWD.
6. **Pulmonic valve.** The PV is located anterior and to the left of the AV and is examined with the ME RV inflow–outflow view and UE aortic arch SAX view with and without CFD. PWD and CWD measurements of flow across the PV are made with the UE aortic arch SAX view because the Doppler beam is parallel to the flow in this view. Trace pulmonic regurgitation usually is seen and normal. Pulmonic stenosis usually is congenital and rare in adults. It causes high-velocity, turbulent flow across the valve seen with CFD, PWD, and CWD.
7. **Left atrium.** The LA is examined in the ME four-chamber and ME two-chamber views for size and the presence of masses. It normally is less than 5 cm in its anteroposterior and mediolateral dimensions. Thrombus usually is associated with atrial fibrillation and LA enlargement and is most commonly in the LA appendage, seen at the superior lateral aspect of the body of the atrium.
8. **Right atrium.** The RA is examined in the ME four-chamber and ME bicaval views for size and masses. A variably sized fold of tissue at the junction of the inferior vena cava (IVC) and the RA, the **Eustachian valve,** is seen frequently. Fine, filamentous mobile strands may be seen in this region as well and are termed **Chiari network**. Both are normal structures.

9. **Interatrial septum.** The interatrial septum (IAS) is examined in the ME four-chamber, ME LAX, and ME bicaval views. Two portions usually are seen, the thinner fossa ovalis centrally and a thicker region anteriorly and posteriorly. Atrial septal defects are seen with 2D echocardiography and interatrial shunts with CFD. Atrial septal aneurysms cause redundancy and hypermobility of the IAS. Agitated saline contrast may be injected into the RA following release of positive airway pressure to look for the appearance of contrast in the LA. This indicates the presence of a patent foramen ovale, which may predispose patients to right-to-left interatrial shunting in the presence of right heart failure causing hypoxemia and/or paradoxical systemic embolization.
10. **Thoracic aorta.** Although most of the thoracic aorta lies close to the esophagus and can be easily seen with TEE, the trachea may come between the esophagus, the distal ascending aorta, and the proximal aortic arch, obscuring TEE images of these parts of the aorta.
    a. **Ascending aorta**
    The ascending aorta is examined with the ME ascending aortic SAX and ME ascending aortic LAX views by withdrawing the TEE probe superior to the LA from the ME AV views to the level of the right PA. The distal third may be obscured by the trachea and not well seen with TEE. The inside diameter is normally less than 3.5 cm at the midlevel (anterior to the right PA). A more complete and detailed examination of the ascending aorta may be performed after sternotomy with epiaortic echocardiography, in which an echocardiographic transducer is covered by a sterile sheath and placed directly on the aorta in the surgical field by the surgeon.
    b. **Aortic arch**
    The aortic arch is examined with the UE aortic arch LAX and UE aortic arch SAX views. The distal arch is easily seen in most patients, but the proximal arch may be obscured by the trachea. The inside diameter normally is less than 3 cm. The great vessels often are seen coursing toward the head to the right of the image in the UE aortic arch SAX view.
    c. **Descending thoracic aorta**
    The descending thoracic aorta is examined in SAX (approximately 0 degree multiplane angle) and LAX (approximately 90 degree angle) from the arch to the diaphragm. The inside diameter normally is less than 3 cm. The proximal descending thoracic aorta is lateral to the esophagus and the distal portion is posterior, so the probe must be rotated as different levels are examined to keep the aorta centered in the image. It often is possible to see the proximal abdominal aorta by advancing the probe past the diaphragm.
    d. **Aortic diseases.** Three common abnormalities of the aorta are detected with TEE:
        (1) **Atherosclerosis**
        Atherosclerosis causes thickening and irregularity of the intimal layer of the aorta that is easily seen with TEE. The normal intima is smooth and less than 2 mm thick. Severity of atherosclerosis is graded on a five-point scale: Grade 1 for normal or minimal disease (intima less than 2 mm thick), grade 2 for mild disease (intima 2 to 3 mm thick), grade 3 for moderate or sessile disease (intima 3 to 5 mm thick), grade 4 for severe or protruding disease (intima greater than 5 mm thick), and grade 5 for mobile lesions. The location and extent of the lesions also are noted.
        (2) **Aneurysm**
        Aneurysmal dilations of the aorta are classified by their location and shape as either diffuse (sometimes termed fusiform) or saccular (a sac coming out the side of the vessel, similar in concept to a bulging hernia). They often are associated with atherosclerotic changes and/or mural thrombus, which are easily seen with TEE. Aneurysms with inside diameter 4 cm or less are considered mild and those greater than 6 cm are considered severe.
        (3) **Dissection**
        An aortic dissection is the separation through the media of the intimal layer from the rest of the aorta. With TEE, a mobile membrane is seen within the aorta

dividing the vessel into a true and a false lumen. CFD is applied to the aorta to characterize the flow in the true and false lumens. Dissections are classified into type A, which involve the ascending aorta and are a surgical emergency, and type B, which do not involve the ascending aorta and usually are treated without surgery. TEE findings that may be associated with type A aortic dissections include aneurysmal dilation of the aorta, hemopericardium and tamponade, left hemothorax, AR, and RWMAs due to coronary artery ostial involvement.

VII. Monitoring applications of TEE

A. Assessing preload

The most direct measurement of preload is LV end-diastolic volume. TEE provides 2D images of the LV, so LV EDA of the TG mid-SAX view has been used as an estimation of end-diastolic volume. Studies have shown that decreases in blood volume as little as 1.5% can be detected by this technique [10] and that correlation between EDA and cardiac output is better than that between PA occlusion pressure and cardiac output [11].

B. Measuring intracardiac pressures

Measuring flow velocities with Doppler echocardiography and applying the modified Bernoulli equation allow calculation of gradients between chambers of the heart at various locations. If the absolute pressure of one of these chambers is known, the pressure of the other chamber can be calculated. Thus, by measuring the peak velocity of TR with CWD, one can estimate the peak RV systolic pressure as the RV to RA gradient ($\Delta P = 4V_{TR}^2$) plus the RA pressure. This equals the PA systolic pressure if there is no pulmonic stenosis. Similar logic can be used to measure LA, PA diastolic, and LV end-diastolic pressures by measuring the velocities of MR, pulmonic regurgitation (PR), and AR jets and knowing the LV systolic (same as systolic BP), RV diastolic (same as central venous pressure [CVP]), and aortic diastolic (same as diastolic BP) pressures.

C. Measuring cardiac output

Calculating SV with TEE requires making two measurements: (i) The velocity profile of flow with PWD or CWD and (ii) the area through which the flow occurs with 2D echocardiography. These measurements can be made with TEE in several locations: AV, LVOT, MV, and PA. The accuracy of this technique depends on both the velocity and area measurements being made **in the same location and at the same time in the cardiac cycle**. The velocity profile of the flow is traced and integrated through time to yield a value called **velocity time integral** (VTI), which is in units of length, usually centimeters. Then the area *A* through which the flow passes is measured with 2D echocardiography to give a value in units of length squared, usually square centimeters. The product of VTI and A yields the SV in units of volume, usually cubic centimeters or milliliters. SV times the heart rate gives the cardiac output. The best validated technique for intraoperative TEE uses CWD across the AV from the TG LAX or deep TG LAX views [12]. The area of the valve then is calculated from the ME AV SAX view by measuring the intercommissural distance S and applying the formula for the area of an equilateral triangle: $A_{\Delta} = 0.433\ S^2$. This technique is only applicable if the AV is normal.

D. Detecting myocardial ischemia

10 Appearance of a new RWMA on TEE during surgery has been shown to be a more sensitive indicator of myocardial ischemia than electrocardiographic changes and a better predictor of progression to myocardial infarction [13]. After complete baseline examination of all LV segments is recorded for comparison, the TG mid-SAX view is monitored because it simultaneously shows regions supplied by all three major coronary arteries. An increase in the wall-motion score of two or more grades in a segment suggests acute ischemia. Severe hypovolemia also may produce wall-motion abnormalities without ischemia [14]. TEE is not a true monitor for ischemia unless it is continuously observed during surgery and is more often checked at crucial points of the operation, such as aortic cross clamping, or when another monitor suggests ischemia, such as electrocardiographic or hemodynamic changes.

E. Intracardiac air

Air in the heart is easily seen with TEE as hyperdense or white areas within the chambers. In a supine patient, air in the LA accumulates along the IAS and adjacent to the right upper

pulmonary vein. Air in the LV accumulates along the apical septum. Tiny white spots seen floating within the chambers are microscopic bubbles and are not of great concern. Large
11 bubbles have air–fluid levels visible on TEE as straight lines perpendicular to the direction of gravity that wobble as the heart beats. They typically have a shimmering artifact extending from the air–fluid level away from the transducer. Large bubbles should be evacuated before discontinuing cardiopulmonary bypass (CPB).

VIII. TEE for specific types of surgery

A. Coronary artery bypass grafting

TEE for coronary artery bypass graft (CABG) surgery focuses on global and regional LV functions. Baseline examination of all segments of the LV is performed and recorded for later comparison. A baseline RWMA may represent previously infarcted, nonviable myocardium, chronically ischemic hibernating myocardium, or acutely ischemic myocardium. Examination of the LV is repeated after grafting. The appearance of a new RWMA before or after bypass grafting should be considered acute ischemia. A new RWMA seen immediately after CPB may indicate stunned myocardium, i.e., viable muscle that is perfused but transiently not functioning due to inadequate cardiac protection during CPB. RV infarction causes dilation and hypokinesis of the RV on TEE, often associated with significant TR. Complications of coronary artery disease, such as ischemic MR, LV thrombus, LV aneurysm, ruptured papillary muscle, and postinfarction ventricular septal defect, may be detected with TEE. TEE also is important in detecting atherosclerosis in the aorta, which may increase the risk of stroke during CABG surgery.

B. Valve repair surgery

12 Intraoperative TEE is very helpful during valve repair surgery. Detailed baseline examination of the diseased valve can provide the surgeon with information about the mechanism and etiology of the lesion, indicating the feasibility of repair and the type of repair needed. Assessment of the repair after CPB is done so that problems can be detected and immediately addressed. MV repairs are assessed with TEE for three potential problems:

1. **Residual regurgitation.** Residual MR is assessed with CFD after MV repair. Ideally there is no or only trace MR. Mild (1+) MR probably is acceptable. **Moderate (2+) or more MR should lead to consideration of revision of the repair or valve replacement.**
2. **Systolic anterior motion (SAM) of the MV.** Repair of myxomatous MVs with redundant leaflets can cause mitral SAM, which is easily diagnosed with TEE. There is abnormal anterior motion of the excessive leaflet tissue toward the ventricular septum during systole. This leads to dynamic LVOT obstruction and MR. SAM can be managed successfully in some cases by increasing intravascular volume, administering pure α-agonist drugs, and stopping positive inotropic drugs. In severe cases that do not respond to appropriate treatment, revision of the repair or valve replacement is needed.
3. **Stenosis.** Excessive narrowing of the mitral orifice by valve repair creating stenosis is possible but very uncommon. This is seen on TEE by limited opening of the leaflets and high peak transmitral inflow velocity (greater than 2 m/s).

C. Valve replacement surgery

After valve replacement surgery, the prosthesis is evaluated with TEE. CFD is used to examine the valve annulus for paravalvular leaks. Trace paravalvular leaks often are seen after CPB and are not a cause for concern. Moderate (2+) or more regurgitation may need to be addressed surgically. Different types of prosthetic valves have characteristic normal CFD patterns of regurgitation that should not be confused with pathologic regurgitation. Bileaflet mechanical valve prostheses may have a leaflet immobilized, usually in the closed position, by impinging tissue, so TEE evaluation of these valves should document that both leaflets move freely. An immobile leaflet should be corrected immediately with surgical intervention. Stentless aortic bioprostheses and aortic homograft prostheses may develop significant AR if they are not inserted properly. This can be detected with CFD. Moderate (2+) or more AR usually warrants further surgical intervention.

D. Surgery for congenital heart disease

TEE can confirm the diagnosis before CPB and occasionally finds previously undiagnosed lesions in patients with complex congenital heart disease. Septal defect closure and adequacy of flow through prosthetic conduits and intracardiac baffles are assessed intraoperatively with TEE using CFD, PWD, and CWD, allowing immediate correction of inadequate repairs.

E. Surgery for infective endocarditis

TEE is helpful in confirming the location and extent of infection and assessing the severity of associated lesions such as valvular regurgitation, abscesses, and fistulae. Intraoperative TEE often detects progression of the infection since the preoperative studies guiding the surgical intervention. TEE examination after CPB confirms the adequacy of the resection of infected tissue and repair of hemodynamic lesions.

F. Surgery for hypertrophic obstructive cardiomyopathy

TEE is used before CPB to measure the thickness of the ventricular septum and the location of contact of the MV with the septum to guide the surgeon in sizing the myectomy. The adequacy of the myectomy is assessed with TEE after CPB by looking for residual SAM, measuring residual gradients across the LVOT, and assessing severity of residual MR. Moderate (2+) or more MR and a peak LVOT gradient greater than 50 mm Hg indicates that a more extensive myectomy is needed. Complications of the repair such as ventricular septal defect and AR are assessed with TEE after CPB. CFD often reveals a small jet of diastolic flow in the region of the myectomy from the transected septal perforator artery, which is inconsequential.

G. Thoracic aortic surgery

TEE is helpful in monitoring cardiac function and providing definition of thoracic aortic pathology, but it is often difficult to image the distal ascending aorta and proximal arch with TEE. Caution should be used performing TEE in patients with thoracic aortic aneurysms, especially involving the aortic arch, as the esophagus may be deviated, increasing the risk of injury. A complete baseline examination of the LV is important to identify changes occurring during application and removal of the aortic cross clamp during surgery on the descending thoracic aorta. When left atrial to aortic or femoral artery partial left heart bypass is used, TEE LV EDA is used to assess adequacy of LV filling to balance flow between the proximal and the distal aorta.

H. Transplantation surgery

1. Heart transplantation

Pre-transplant examination of the recipient heart focuses on identifying left heart thrombus to help prevent dislodgement with surgical manipulation. Right heart pressures are estimated and aortic cannulation sites are also assessed before CPB. Adequacy of air evacuation from the donor heart is checked with TEE before coming off CPB. Evaluation of donor heart function with TEE after CPB helps direct hemodynamic support. Stenosis of the PA anastomosis is excluded by measuring the peak velocity across it with CWD. RV dysfunction after CPB is common and is manifested on TEE by a hypocontractile, dilated RV with TR secondary to annular dilatation. After CPB, the atrial transplant suture line often creates a mass visible with TEE along the lateral aspects of the LA and RA and the midportion of the atrial septum. If the vena cavae are individually anastomosed, both the superior vena cava (SVC) and IVC anastomoses should be interrogated using the bicaval view within 1 to 3 cm of the cavoatrial junction for stenosis and CFD flow acceleration (suggesting or confirming a stenotic anastomosis).

2. Lung transplantation

A comprehensive baseline examination is recorded for comparison later during the procedure. For single lung transplants and bilateral sequential lung transplants, TEE is used to monitor RV function during PA clamping. **RV failure causes increased size and decreased contractility seen with TEE, usually associated with increasing TR secondary to annular dilatation and may necessitate going on CPB.** Cardiac function is monitored as well during reperfusion, watching for changes in volume and contractility of the ventricles. Air embolism with reperfusion is also detected with TEE. After transplantation, patency of the pulmonary vein-to-left atrium anastomoses is assessed using CFD and PWD to measure pulmonary venous inflow velocity.

I. Ventricular assist device implantation

Intraoperative TEE plays a crucial role during VAD implantation surgery. For a VAD to function properly, the native valve at the outflow of the assisted ventricle must be reasonably competent (PV for right ventricular assist device, AV for left ventricular assist device [LVAD]). TEE is used to assess these valves, and if significant regurgitation is present, a prosthetic valve may be inserted or the native valve sewn shut. TEE is used to detect any intracardiac shunts with TEE such as patent foramen ovale, atrial septal defect, or VSD, because a properly functioning VAD will decompress the assisted side of the heart and can change the direction of an existing intracardiac shunt. TEE is used to detect thrombus within the left heart to avoid systemic embolization with manipulation or insertion of the VAD cannulae into the heart. The aorta is examined for atherosclerosis to avoid atheroembolism with aortic cannulation, clamping, or anastomosis of the outflow conduit. Before separating from CPB, TEE is used to check the orientation of the VAD cannulae to detect and correct obstruction of the inflow cannula against the wall of the ventricle. Intracardiac air is identified and removed. While weaning a VAD patient from CPB, TEE helps maintain stable hemodynamics with its ability to assess the assisted ventricle's decompression and the nonassisted ventricle's volume and function, including the detection of acute atrioventricular valve incompetence that can accompany acute ventricular failure. This is especially an issue with LVAD patients, where impaired RV function may limit LV preload, and hence the VAD's ability to deliver a normal cardiac output. Once off CPB but before decannulation, agitated saline contrast is injected into the RA to rule out right to left shunting not detected before CPB because of elevated left heart filling pressures. With a properly functioning LVAD, the AV typically will not open after CPB. The function of a VAD depends on an adequate filling volume, and TEE can be helpful in making decisions about fluid replacement therapy. Some LVAD patients are expected to have recovery of ventricular function and eventual explantation of the VAD. Usually, the timing of the explantation is determined by periodically decreasing the VAD flow while TEE is used to assess the function of the recovering ventricle. TEE is also very helpful in the detection of postoperative complications such as cardiac tamponade and VAD prosthetic valve dysfunction.

IX. Three-dimensional echocardiography

Three-dimensional (3D) reconstruction of echocardiographic images from a series of 2D images has been in clinical use for over 15 years. This technique has been most helpful in assessing complex congenital heart defects. TEE transducers that acquire echocardiographic data from
13 a volume of space and create a 3D image in real time are now commercially available and are being used at many centers for intraoperative applications. Reports are appearing in the literature describing how 3D echocardiography adds important information to the standard 2D examination. Three-dimensional TEE is already providing new and useful information about the anatomical relationships of complex structures close to the LA, such as the MV. As this technology continues to evolve and becomes more practical, echocardiography will be transformed in the same way as was in the 1970s with the development of 2D imaging.

A. Fundamental limitations of ultrasound imaging

The ability to use ultrasound to make medical images is based on a fundamental, physical fact: The velocity of sound transmission through soft tissue is relatively constant at about 1,540 m/s. But this fact also imposes a fundamental limitation that becomes important in 2D echocardiography and critical in 3D. Since it takes a fixed amount of time for ultrasound to leave a transducer, travel to and from the reflector in the tissues, and be detected by the transducer, there is an absolute limit to the pulses per second of ultrasound (pulse repetition frequency) a system can transmit without one pulse interfering with the reflection of the previously sent pulse. Thus, the absolute maximum pulse repetition frequency when imaging at 15 cm depth (30 cm travel distance) is about 5,000 pulses/s. An ultrasound system constructs the image by synthesizing information from many pulses, rapidly scanning the ultrasound beam through a plane for 2D or a volume of space in real-time 3D, and is limited in either the width and depth of the image or the speed with which it can generate a coherent image (frame rate).

There are two methods of producing 3D images with ultrasound: (i) Off-line computed rendering of a series of 2D images acquired separately within a short period of time and (ii) real-time insonation of a volume of tissue.

B. Computed rendering of 2D images into 3D

Off-line rendering has been available for over 15 years and uses the same computing algorithms developed in radiology for 3D renderings of CT and MRI images. In the past, these techniques had been limited to the radiology suite, but as the cost and size of computers dramatically fell, the technology was applied to portable ultrasound systems and currently is capable of producing a high-quality 3D image with a TEE transducer in about 2 min. The process begins with the positioning of the TEE probe and development of a 2D image of the structure to be examined. Then, as the probe is held perfectly still, a series of 2D images are acquired by automatically advancing the multiplane angle through 180 degrees step-wise in 3 to 5 degree increments. Image acquisition is triggered by the ECG so that each 2D image starts and ends at the same point in the cardiac cycle, and translation of the heart (changing of the heart's position within the thorax) minimized, usually by gating acquisition to end expiration or by pausing ventilation, which is easily accomplished in anesthetized patients. With TEE, acquisition takes about 1 min. Once image acquisition is completed, the system then combines the series of 2D images into a 3D image in about 20 or 30 s. The main advantages of the off-line rendering are the ability to create 3D images of larger volumes at higher frame rates than real-time 3D and images that include CFD in much greater detail. Off-line rendering can be done with a conventional 2D multiplane TEE probe. The disadvantages are the time it takes to create the image and the requirement to keep the heart from translating during acquisition. Also, 3D rendering is less accurate in patients with irregular rhythms.

C. Real-time insonation of a volume of tissue

TEE probes capable of real-time 3D image acquisition have been commercially available since 2009. The 3D TEE transducer has a rectangular array of over 2,000 elements that systematically scans an ultrasound beam through a pyramidal volume of tissue with the apex at the probe. This creates a 3D image that responds to real-time probe manipulation and heart translation and requires no extended time to acquire or render. But real-time 3D is much more limited than off-line rendering in its frame rate and its displayed image width and depth, and real-time CFD is much more limited as well. Newer versions of real-time 3D systems can increase the size of the volume acquired or the quality of CFD by acquiring five to seven real-time beats and "stitching" them into a more detailed or larger image. This requires ECG and respiratory gating, but over a shorter period than conventional off-line rendering systems. The real-time 3D TEE probe is a little larger than a 2D multiplane probe, and considerably more expensive.

D. 3D image display and manipulation

Once a 3D echo image (dataset) has been acquired, it can be displayed in a number of ways. It is typically shown as a pyramidal shaped volume that may be manipulated using the system software (Fig. 5.9). The volume can be rotated on each of three axes, allowing it to be seen from any point of view; top or bottom, front or back, left or right. The volume of data may also be cropped from any side by using an editing function that removes part of the image with an erasure plane that is gradually brought into the pyramid until the desired structure is exposed. Some systems can create a 2D image by orienting a plane through the 3D volume. Another display mode shows two or more 2D images of the structures simultaneously in synchronized motion (Fig. 5.10). The 3D volumetric displays are highly processed images that require smoothing and interpolation by computer algorithms and are thus prone to artifacts, especially drop out. It takes some time and practice to learn how to properly fine tune the settings of the system to optimize 3D image quality. While 3D echo will provide us with new insights into the structure and function of complex structures such as the MV, for now significant findings should be confirmed and refined with 2D imaging.

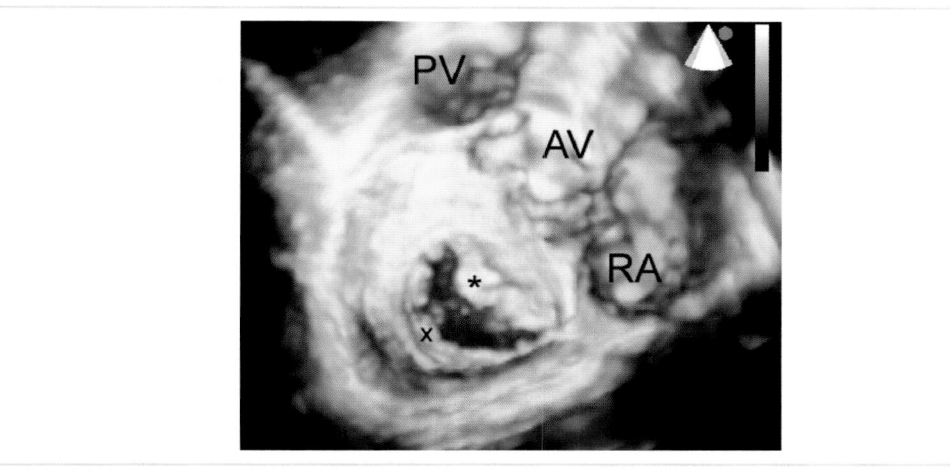

FIGURE 5.9 The MV in mid-diastole viewed from the atrial side. * indicates the anterior leaflet and × the posterior leaflet. An oblique view of the AV is seen, as well. PV, pulmonic valve; AV, aortic valve; RA, right atrium.

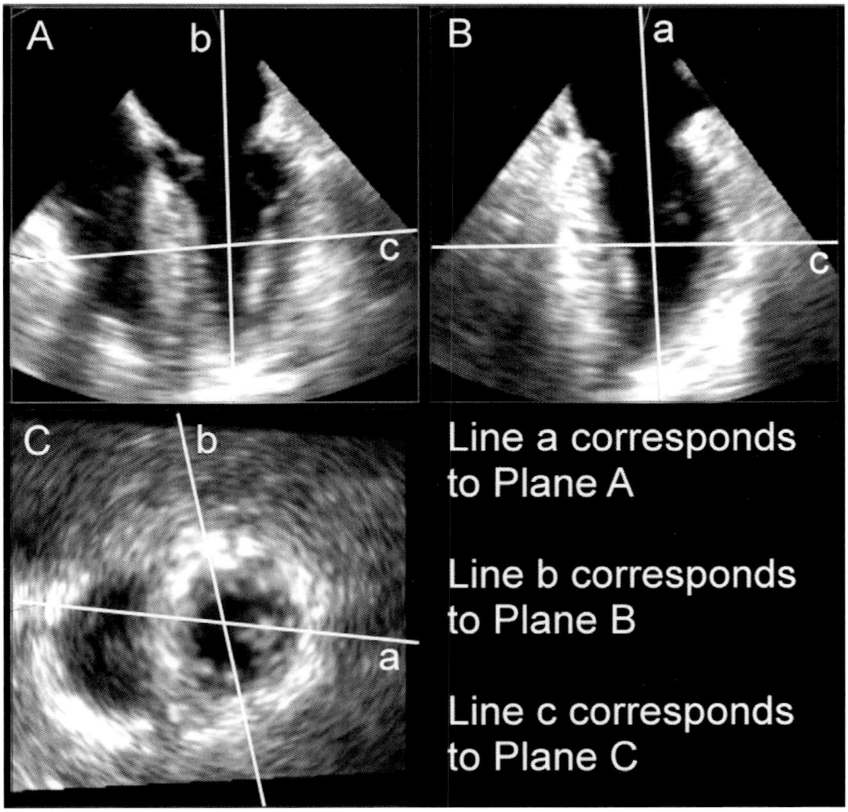

FIGURE 5.10 2D views of the heart derived from a 3D volume of data. Plane A is a four-chamber view, Plane B is a two chamber view, and Plane C is an SAX view. The lines show how the 2D planes are aligned within the 3D volume and can be manipulated with the software to modify the 2D images displayed.

REFERENCES

1. Practice guidelines for perioperative transesophageal echocardiography. A report by the American Society of Anesthesiologists and the Society of Cardiovascular Anesthesiologists Task Force on Transesophageal Echocardiography. *Anesthesiology.* 2010;112:1–13.
2. Bonow RO, Carabello BA, Chatterjee K, et al. ACC/AHA 2006 guidelines for the management of patients with valvular heart disease: a report of the American College of Cardiology/American Heart Association Task Force on Practice Guidelines (Writing Committee to Develop Guidelines for the Management of Patients with Valvular Heart Disease). *American Heart Association Web Site.* http://www.americanheart.org. *Circulation.* 2006;114:e84–e231.
3. Kallmeyer IJ, Collard CD, Fox JA, et al. The safety of intraoperative transesophageal echocardiography: a case series of 7200 cardiac surgical patients. *Anesth Analg.* 2001;92:1126–1130.
4. Brinkman WT, Shanewise JS, Clements SD, et al. Transesophageal echocardiography: not an innocuous procedure. *Ann Thorac Surg.* 2001;72:1725–1726.
5. Shanewise JS, Cheung AT, Aronson S, et al. ASE/SCA guidelines for performing a comprehensive intraoperative multiplane transesophageal echocardiography examination: recommendations of the American Society of Echocardiography Council for Intraoperative Echocardiography and the Society of Cardiovascular Anesthesiologists Task Force for Certification in Perioperative Transesophageal Echocardiography. *Anesth Analg.* 1999;89:870–884.
6. Lang RM, Bierig M, Devereux RB, et al. Chamber Quantification Writing Group. American Society of Echocardiography's Guidelines and Standards Committee. European Association of Echocardiography. Recommendations for chamber quantification: a report from the American Society of Echocardiography's Guidelines and Standards Committee and the Chamber Quantification Writing Group, developed in conjunction with the European Association of Echocardiography, a branch of the European Society of Cardiology. *J Am Soc Echocardiography.* 2005;18:1440–1463.
7. Stamm RB, Carabello BA, Mayers DL, et al. Two-dimensional echocardiographic measurement of left ventricular ejection fraction: prospective analysis of what constitutes an adequate determination. *Am Heart J.* 1982;104:136–144.
8. Smith JS, Cahalan MK, Benefiel DJ, et al. Intraoperative detection of myocardial ischemia in high-risk patients: electrocardiography versus two-dimensional transesophageal echocardiography. *Circulation.* 1985;72:1015–1021.
9. Zoghbi WA, Enriquez-Sarano M, Foster E, et al. American Society of Echocardiography. Recommendations for evaluation of the severity of native valvular regurgitation with two-dimensional and Doppler echocardiography. *J Am Soc Echocardiography.* 2003;16:777–802.
10. Cheung AT, Savino JS, Weiss SJ, et al. Echocardiographic and hemodynamic indexes of left ventricular preload in patients with normal and abnormal ventricular function. *Anesthesiology.* 1994;81:376–387.
11. Thys DM, Hillel Z, Goldman ME, et al. A comparison of hemodynamic indices derived by invasive monitoring and two-dimensional echocardiography. *Anesthesiology.* 1987;67:630–634.
12. Darmon PL, Hillel Z, Mogtader A, et al. Cardiac output by transesophageal echocardiography using continuous-wave Doppler across the aortic valve. *Anesthesiology.* 1994;80:796–805.
13. Leung JM, O'Kelly B, Browner WS, et al. Prognostic importance of postbypass regional wall-motion abnormalities in patients undergoing coronary artery bypass graft surgery. SPI Research Group. *Anesthesiology.* 1989;71:16–25.
14. Seeberger MD, Cahalan MK, Rouine-Rapp K, et al. Acute hypovolemia may cause segmental wall motion abnormalities in the absence of myocardial ischemia. *Anesth Analg.* 1997;85:1252–1257.

6 Induction of Anesthesia

Ferenc Puskas, Michael B. Howie, and Glenn P. Gravlee

KEY POINTS

1. On the day of surgery, most cardiovascular medications should be administered orally, with the exceptions of angiotensin-converting enzyme (ACE) inhibitors, angiotensin receptor blockers, and (selectively) diuretic agents.
2. The presence of a large-bore intravenous (IV) catheter and an arterial catheter prior to induction of anesthesia is recommended for most cardiac surgical patients. Central venous access can typically await induction of anesthesia and endotracheal intubation.
3. Prior to induction of anesthesia, critical emergency drugs should be prepared for immediate administration. Practices vary, but these drugs should include a vasopressor, vasodilator, inotrope, β-adrenergic blocker, and heparin.
4. Induction of anesthesia can be achieved using many different approaches. The most important underlying principle is suppression of the stress response while avoiding hypotension.
5. Hemodynamically tenuous patients likely will not tolerate traditional induction doses of propofol or thiopental, but even drugs typically unassociated with hypotension can cause hypotension in cardiac surgical patients as a result of anesthetic-induced reduction in sympathetic tone, synergistic circulatory depression when some induction drugs are given in combination (e.g., midazolam and fentanyl), and/or initiation of positive pressure ventilation.
6. Opioids suppress the stress response in a dose-related manner until a maximum effect is reached at an approximate dose-equivalency of 8 μg/kg of fentanyl.

(continued)

7. With appropriate topicalization, sedation, and systemic stress response suppression (e.g., β-adrenergic blockers), awake intubation can be safely accomplished in cardiac patients with difficult airways.
8. Etomidate offers hemodynamic stability during induction, but also suppresses adrenal cortical function for approximately 24 h.
9. Muscle relaxant timing is important during induction, i.e., early enough to avert opioid-induced chest wall rigidity but late enough to avoid awake paralysis.

POTENT INHALATIONAL AGENTS INDUCE VASODILATION and some myocardial depression, but can be safely used during induction especially to complement IV agents such as etomidate and fentanyl.

Induction of anesthesia in a cardiac patient is more than a simple transition from an awake to a stable anesthetic state. Considering all aspects of the patient's cardiac condition allows selection of an anesthetic that best accommodates the patient's current cardiac status and medications. No single agent or technique can guarantee hemodynamic stability. Hemodynamic change with induction can be attributed to the patient's pathophysiology and to a reduction in sympathetic tone potentially causing vasodilation, cardiac depression, and relative hypovolemia.

I. Premedication

A. Just as the patient's chronic medications can mostly be used to advantage, so can premedication be an integral component of the anesthetic technique.

1 B. **With rare exception, chronic cardiac medications should be administered orally preoperatively on the day of surgery** with as little water as possible.

1. Some clinicians prefer to withhold diuretics on the morning of surgery, which seems reasonable.
2. ACE inhibitors and angiotensin receptor blockers have been associated with hypotension following induction of anesthesia (and perhaps during separation from cardiopulmonary bypass). Although somewhat controversial, we prefer to discontinue the patient's usual dose of these drugs 1 day (24 h) before surgery in order to reduce the risk for hypotension and for acute kidney injury, which has been associated with ACE inhibitor use in cardiac surgery [1].

II. Preinduction period.

Unstable patients (e.g., critical aortic stenosis, congestive heart failure) probably should not be premedicated before they reach a preanesthetic holding area that permits observation by an anesthesia caregiver, and we perceive that few practitioners currently administer sedatives or opioids prior to the patient's arrival in such an area. Some examples of premedication regimens are shown in Table 6.1, but monitoring catheters, such as arterial and central venous "lines," ideally should be placed under the influence of premedication, such as IV midazolam (if not after induction of anesthesia).

A. **Basic monitors** and supplemental oxygen are important to initiate before giving supplemental sedation (if needed) and placing invasive monitors.

TABLE 6.1 Anesthetic premedication for cardiac surgical patients

Poorly compensated patients	**Lorazepam or midazolam 1–2 mg intravenously (approximately 15–20 μg/kg)**
Compensated patients	I. Midazolam 1–5 mg (15–70 μg/kg) intravenously, titrated to effect with or without IV morphine 2–5 mg (0.03–0.07 mg/kg), hydromorphone 1–2 mg (15–30 μg/kg), or fentanyl 50–100 μg (0.5–1 μg/kg) intravenously after arrival in the preinduction area or the operating room
	II. Morphine 3–10 mg (0.05–0.15 mg/kg) with or without scopolamine 0.3–0.4 mg (4–5 μg/kg), both given intramuscularly 30–60 min before transport to operating room area is an effective but now seldom-used premedication technique
	III. Lorazepam 2–4 mg (30–40 μg/kg) by mouth with or without an orally (e.g., methadone 5–10 mg or 0.1 mg/kg) or intramuscularly (e.g., morphine 0.1 mg/kg) administered narcotic 30–60 min before arrival in operating room area

1. Electrocardiogram
2. Noninvasive blood pressure (BP)
3. Pulse oximeter

B. Invasive monitors can be useful during induction [2], so some clinicians choose to place central "access" catheters, such as a central venous catheter or pulmonary artery (PA) catheter, before induction of anesthesia. It appears that most anesthesiologists defer central line place-
2 ment until after anesthetic induction, which is an equally acceptable approach that does not appear to affect patient outcomes. In patients with low cardiac outputs, onset time for anesthetic induction drugs and for vasoactive drugs can be noticeably delayed when this approach is chosen. It appears that most anesthesiologists prefer to place the arterial catheter before inducing anesthesia, as do we, but some prefer to await induction of anesthesia for this intervention as well.

1. In emergency situations, it may be necessary to proceed with anesthetic induction before placing invasive monitors. Examples include:
   - **a.** Ruptured or rupturing thoracic aortic aneurysm
   - **b.** Cardiac tamponade
   - **c.** Ventricular rupture
2. In these situations, if a large-bore IV catheter is already present, opening the chest is far more important than PA or central venous pressure catheter measurements. It is highly desirable to initiate intra-arterial BP monitoring before anesthetic induction in such cases. If the anesthesiologist is busy stabilizing the patient and preparing for induction, the surgery team can be asked to assist with radial or femoral arterial line placement under local anesthesia.

C. Clinical tips in preparing for cardiac anesthesia

1. Emergency drugs that may be needed can be prepared as dilute bolus doses in syringes or as IV or syringe infusion pumps attached to a peripheral IV or to the infusion port of the PA (or some other central venous) catheter via a manifold.
2. **The drugs selected for anesthesia depend on the patient's condition and the preferences of the anesthesiologist.**
   - **a.** Commonly fentanyl or sufentanil, and less commonly remifentanil, are selected as opioids.
   - **b.** Among the potent inhalational agents, isoflurane probably should be selected for economy, desflurane for rapid titratability, and sevoflurane for inhalational induction for an airway that is suspected to be difficult (as a judgment-based alternative to awake intubation).
   - **c.** IV amnestic agents may include benzodiazepines such as midazolam, lorazepam, or diazepam, or any of the traditional induction agents described below.
   - **d.** For muscle relaxation, succinylcholine (or no muscle relaxant) is suggested for a suspect airway; pancuronium for economy and low heart rates (HRs); vecuronium, rocuronium, or cisatracurium for hemodynamic blandness; and cisatracurium in the case of liver or renal failure. Note that even moderate to severe impairment in renal or hepatic function need not contraindicate any muscle relaxant per se, but may instead simply merit adjustments in dosing frequency.
3. **Specific cardiovascular medications to have available** (asterisk indicates probable need to have the drug drawn up and ready for administration) before surgery:
   - **a.** Anticholinergic: Atropine* (preferred over glycopyrrolate for faster onset)
   - **b. Inotrope: Epinephrine*, dobutamine, or dopamine as infusions; epinephrine also in a syringe for bolus administration**

3 - **c.** Phosphodiesterase III inhibitor: Milrinone
   - **d.** Calcium chloride
   - **e.** Ephedrine* as a bolus (mixed vasopressor/inotrope)
   - **f.** Vasopressors
     - **(1) Phenylephrine as a 50- to 100-μg bolus*, or as an infusion, or norepinephrine**
     - **(2)** Vasopressin (for vascular collapse and resuscitation, especially after left ventricular assist device placement)

g. **Vasodilators: Nitroglycerin***, nicardipine, and nitroprusside
h. Antiarrhythmics and antitachycardic agents
   (1) Adenosine
   (2) Esmolol*, metoprolol, or propranolol
   (3) Diltiazem or verapamil
   (4) Lidocaine*
   (5) Amiodarone
   (6) Magnesium
i. Anticoagulation and its reversal
   (1) **Heparin***
   (2) Protamine
j. **To be most prepared, at least one inotrope, one vasopressor, and one vasodilator should be set up and connected in a pump that is preprogrammed and ready to use. Similarly, syringes should be prepared for bolus administration of at least one vasopressor, inotrope, vasodilator, and probably a β-adrenergic blocker as well.**
k. A custom-built IV pole with a built-in electrical outlet and the capability for attachment of multiple IV infusion or syringe pumps should be available. In the case of syringe pumps, battery operation is acceptable if there is a reliable mechanism for recharging the syringe pumps before each procedure.

D. **Last-minute checks:** Immediately before anesthetic induction, the following points should be considered:
1. Reassessment of the patient's overall cardiopulmonary and airway status
2. Integrity of breathing circuit and immediate availability of suction
3. Availability of blood for transfusion
4. Proximity of a surgeon or a senior resident
5. Any special endotracheal tube needs (double-lumen, bronchial blocker)
6. Immediate availability of emergency cardiac drugs

III. Induction.

The cardiac anesthesiologist must often induce a patient who under normal circumstances would not receive a general anesthetic. Objectives include:

A. **Attenuation of hemodynamic responses** to laryngoscopy and surgery without undue hypotension

4

1. Conservative drug amounts, as the anesthetic requirement rapidly becomes relatively minor during surgical skin preparation and draping (exception: high-dose opioid induction technique) (Table 6.2)
2. Use drug onset time and interactions to advantage.
3. Adapt induction drug doses to physical status of patient.

B. **Guiding principles** for anesthetic induction include:
1. Modifications of techniques as new knowledge are gained. For example, trace the history of sufentanil as used during anesthetic induction.
   a. In the 1980s, the recommended induction dose of sufentanil was as high as 25 μg/kg.
   b. In the 1990s, recommendations changed to 6 to 10 μg/kg.
   c. In the new millennium, as little as 0.1 μg/kg is used.
   d. Combinations of sufentanil or fentanyl with etomidate and muscle relaxants exemplify efficient induction techniques.
2. Physiologic issues
   a. Hypovolemia, which is often difficult to assess, is frequently caused by diuretics and prolonged nothing by mouth (NPO) status.
      (1) This is difficult to assess because of the absence of preoperative urine output documentation or left ventricular (LV) preload assessment.
      (2) Most cardiac patients do not tolerate more than 10% depletion of intravascular volume without hemodynamic compromise.
      (3) Tachycardia and vasoconstriction, which are useful compensatory mechanisms in normal individuals, may be deleterious in cardiac patients or may be

TABLE 6.2 Recommended induction doses

Drug	Induction dose
Hypnotics	
Propofol	1–2 mg/kg
Thiopental	2–4 mg/kg
Etomidate	0.15–0.3 mg/kg
Ketamine	0.5–1.5 mg/kg
Opioids	
Fentanyl	3–10 μg/kg
Sufentanil	0.1–1 μg/kg
Remifentanil	0.1–0.75 μg/kg/min or bolus 0.5–1 μg/kg
Muscle relaxants	
Cisatracurium	70–100 μg/kg
Vecuronium	70–100 μg/kg
Pancuronium	70–100 μg/kg
Rocuronium	0.3–1.2 mg/kg
Succinylcholine	1–2 mg/kg
Maintenance of anesthesia in critically ill patients	
Sedative/hypnotic agent	
Propofol infusion	20–120 μg/kg/min
Lorazepam single bolus	2–4 mg (25–50 μg/kg)
Diazepam intermittent boluses	4–8 mg (50–100 μg/kg)
Midazolam infusion	0.25–0.5 μg/kg/min
Plus	
An opioid infusion (or intermittent boluses)	
Remifentanil	0.05–0.1 μg/kg/min
Fentanyl	0.03–0.1 μg/kg/min
Sufentanil	0.1–0.5 μg/kg/h
or	
Dexmedetomidine	0.5–1 μg/kg/h

impaired or even precluded as a result of the patient's chronic cardiovascular drug regimen.

(4) Anesthetic drugs may impair appropriate hemodynamic responses [3].

- **(a)** Propofol and thiopental reduce BP by inducing venodilation with peripheral pooling of blood, decreasing sympathetic tone to decrease systemic vascular
5 resistance (SVR), and depressing myocardial contractility.
- **(b)** In decreasing order of circulatory depression, propofol is most depressant, thiopental slightly less so, midazolam is intermediate, and etomidate is the least depressant.

(5) The most physiologically efficient method of combating hypovolemia is to augment intravascular volume in the preinduction period using balanced salt solutions, being careful not to overdo this in patients with mitral valve lesions or congestive heart failure. The presence or absence of susceptibility to congestive heart failure may be subtle in patients with LV diastolic dysfunction. In general, the trend has been toward more conservative use of fluids in the precardiopulmonary bypass period in order to minimize hemodilution and the need for RBC transfusion. At times, this occurs at the expense of circulatory support with vasopressors. This philosophy is sound as long as sufficient cardiac output is maintained to perfuse the vital organs and (arguably) is most safely applied if one can measure cardiac output to ensure an adequate cardiac index (under anesthesia, probably greater than or equal to 1.8 L/min/m^2). The initiation of an inotropic infusion (low-dose epinephrine 0.01 to 0.03 mcg/kg/min or dopamine 1 to 3 mcg/kg/min) in such patients sometimes helps to maintain a stable perfusion pressure and cardiac output during the preinduction period.

3. **Pharmacodynamic issues.** With the exception of ketamine, which can stimulate the cardiovascular system, all anesthetics decrease BP by some combination of removing sympathetic tone, directly decreasing SVR, directly depressing the myocardium, increasing venous pooling (reducing venous return), or inducing bradycardia.

Important individual drug characteristics to be considered:

a. In critically ill patients, ketamine can decrease BP because depletion of catecholamines may lead to an inability of indirect central nervous system-mediated sympathomimetic effects to counterbalance its direct negative inotropic effects.

b. The conflict between the need to attenuate the hemodynamic response to intubation and other noxious stimuli without overdosing can be illustrated by propofol.

(1) Propofol may induce hypotension if used for induction, yet a small dose may not suppress the hypertensive response to laryngoscopy.

(2) In combination with other drugs: After an induction dose of propofol, systolic BP fell an average of 28 mm Hg when no fentanyl was administered, whereas it fell 53 mm Hg when 2 μg/kg of fentanyl was administered. However, the hemodynamic response to intubation was decreased in proportion to the preinduction dose of fentanyl [4].

(3) Propofol can be given in small increments (0.5 to 1 mg/kg) judging from the patient's physical status and can be used with a small well-timed dose of opioid (e.g., 1 to 3 μg/kg of fentanyl 1 to 2 min preceding propofol).

c. The principle of using the relationship between the plasma drug concentration and the bioeffector site onset (biophase or Ke_0) must be considered, such that the maximal effects of both the opioid and hypnotic are used to best advantage.

(1) The mean onset time for peak effect of propofol is 2.9 min and for fentanyl is 6.4 min. Ideally, endotracheal intubation should be performed at the peak concentration of both drugs and after optimal muscle relaxation has been achieved. This may require a second dose or a continuous infusion of ultrashort-acting induction agents such as propofol, because the muscle relaxant onset time may occur after the peak effect of the bolus dose of the induction agent has dissipated from rapid redistribution.

6 **d. Increasing the opioid dose beyond 8 μg/kg of fentanyl, 0.75 μg/kg of sufentanil, or 1.2 μg/kg/min of remifentanil does not further attenuate the stress response (increased BP and HR) to intubation.**

e. Depth of anesthesia provided by propofol or other sedative–hypnotic agents does not determine the degree of stress-response suppression; rather, the central nervous system level of opioid analgesia tends to do so.

f. Reducing the doses of anesthetic drugs is often the safest way to induce critically ill patients.

g. For a hemodynamically stable patient, one might prefer a hemodynamically bland muscle relaxant except for patients with a baseline HR less than 50 beats/min or with valvular regurgitation, where pancuronium can still be useful.

h. Induction drugs are administered most efficiently through a central venous catheter, such as the side-port introducer, or an infusion port in a PA catheter.

i. Muscle relaxants are given early in the sequence. Onset time is important to consider. This can be defined for most agents in the context of ED_{95}, or the average dose required to induce 95% suppression of the twitch response. For most nondepolarizing neuromuscular blockers, the time to achieve maximum twitch suppression at a dose of

$1 \times ED_{95}$ is 3 to 7 min. Use of $2 \times$ or $3 \times ED_{95}$ reduces onset time to 1.5 to 3 min, and to as low as 1 to 1.5 min for $3 \times ED_{95}$ with rocuronium (0.9 mg/kg).

- **(1)** Succinylcholine (1 to 2 mg/kg) can be used to reduce onset time of neuromuscular blockade to 1 to 1.5 min.

j. An example of a drug combination that combines rapid onset (intubating conditions in 1 to 2 min) and good suppression of the stress response to laryngoscopy is remifentanil 1 μg/kg, etomidate 0.2 mg/kg, and succinylcholine 1.5 mg/kg, all administered as a simultaneous bolus.

k. High-dose opioid induction techniques:

- **(1)** Achieved popularity in the 1970s with morphine (1 to 2 mg/kg) or fentanyl (50 to 100 μg/kg) because of the combination of excellent stress–response suppression and hemodynamic stability.
- **(2)** Sufentanil (10 to 25 μg/kg) rose to popularity for the same reasons in the 1980s.
- **(3)** This technique lost favor in the 1990s because of long postoperative intubation times, but it is still potentially useful for high-risk patients who will require overnight mechanical ventilation regardless of the anesthetic technique chosen.
- **(4)** Because of the marked vagotonic effects of bolus high-dose opioids, pancuronium nicely complements this technique and should be given early in the induction sequence to minimize chest wall rigidity.
- **(5)** These doses of fentanyl and sufentanil can be given as a bolus or over 3 to 5 min. Morphine must be given slowly (5 to 10 mg/min) to avoid hypotension. A recent study indicated that morphine may still have a place in cardiac anesthesia, as it reduced the degree of postoperative pain and the incidence of postoperative fever [5].
- **(6)** Beware of hypotension if hypnotics are given simultaneously and of inadequate amnesia if they are not.

7

C. Anticipated difficult intubation. The cardiac patient with a difficult airway imposes a conflict between our instincts to preserve and protect the airway and those to avoid hemodynamic stress. Concerns about loss of airway control supersede those about hemodynamic stimulation, yet both airway safety and hemodynamic stability can be achieved with awake intubation. Suggestions for accomplishing "awake" endotracheal intubation (by any of several techniques) while still preventing potentially deleterious hemodynamics follow:

1. **Adequate airway anesthesia** either greatly attenuates or prevents the hemodynamic stress of endotracheal intubation. Specific techniques that may prove helpful include:
   - **a.** Nebulized 4% lidocaine for 15 or more minutes prior to airway.
   - **b.** Topical sprays such as Cetacaine or 10% lidocaine, although toxicity can result from either of these agents if used to excess.
   - **c.** Nerve blocks: Glossopharyngeal and superior laryngeal blocks can anesthetize the pharynx down to the level of the vocal cords.
   - **d.** Transcricoid or transtracheal injection of 4% lidocaine can suppress the cough reflex, as can injection of 4% lidocaine via the suction or injection port of a fiberoptic bronchoscope upon reaching the vocal cords and trachea.
2. **Low to moderate levels of sedation** can facilitate patient cooperation and may induce amnesia:
   - **a.** Midazolam titrated to effect.
   - **b.** Opioids in low doses, but beware of the combined sedative and respiratory depressant effects of opioids combined with sedative/hypnotics, such as midazolam.
   - **c.** Conservative infusion doses of propofol (e.g., 10 to 40 μg/kg) can be helpful and may reduce the gag and cough reflex modestly, but can also result in dysphoria or airway obstruction.
   - **d.** Some practitioners select dexmedetomidine for this purpose, whereas others remain unimpressed with its efficacy or desirability. Favorable aspects include sedation (without reliable amnesia!), tendency to decrease HR and BP, and possibly modest airway

reflex suppression. Typically the dose for awake intubation would be 1 μg/kg administered intravenously over approximately 10 min.

3. **Adjuncts that may help prevent or treat hypertension or tachycardia:**
   a. **β-Adrenergic blockers (e.g., esmolol** bolus [0.25 to 1 mg/kg] or infusion [100 to 300 μg/kg/min])
   b. Vasodilators (e.g., nicardipine 500 to 750 μg or nitroglycerin 50 to 100 μg bolus, or continuous infusion titrated to effect)
   c. Mixed adrenergic blocker: IV labetalol titrated to effect (bolus dose typically 10 to 20 mg every 5 to 10 min)
4. Be prepared to proceed with a gentle IV induction once endotracheal intubation has been achieved. If the preparations above have been successful, the patient will tolerate the presence of the endotracheal tube without coughing or distress, which reduces the urgency to proceed with induction.

IV. Opioids

A. Basic structures and opioid receptors

1. Rigid interlocked molecules of the morphine group known as pentacyclides and flexible molecules of phenylpiperidine rings, such as fentanyl
2. There are three opioid receptors (μ, κ, and δ) with subgroups.
   a. Opioid receptors are γ-protein–coupled receptors.

B. Properties of opioids. Analgesia is more than the relief of pain or of the conscious perception of a nociceptive stimulus.

A noxious stimulus can affect an ostensibly unconscious (and unparalyzed) person as demonstrated by movement in the form of a withdrawal reflex. The stimulus can produce increased autonomic activity. Narcotics in general are poor hypnotics and cannot be counted upon to induce amnesia.

C. Induction pharmacokinetics:

1. Pharmacokinetics are similar among three modern synthetic opioids (fentanyl, sufentanil, and alfentanil) with a few differences [6].
   a. All have a three-compartment model.
   b. **Ninety-eight percent of fentanyl is redistributed from the plasma in the first hour.**
   c. Brain levels parallel plasma levels with a lag of 5 min.
   d. Fentanyl has a large volume of distribution, which can limit hepatic access. However, the liver will clear all the fentanyl it gets.
   e. Sufentanil is 7 to 10 times more potent than fentanyl. It has a higher pK_a and only 20% is ionized.
   f. Sufentanil is half as lipid soluble as fentanyl and is more tightly bound to receptors. It has a lower volume of distribution and a faster recovery time.
   g. Alfentanil, typically administered as a continuous infusion, is less potent than fentanyl and shorter acting than sufentanil, but has been largely superseded by remifentanil (see below).
2. Remifentanil pharmacokinetics:
   a. Remifentanil has a unique pharmacokinetic profile, as it is subject to widespread extrahepatic hydrolysis by nonspecific tissue and blood esterases.
   b. It has an onset time of 1 min and a recovery time of 9 to 20 min. These properties make it very advantageous when there is variation of surgical stimulus or a desire for early postoperative extubation. The anesthesiologist can give as much as he or she feels is needed without impeding rapid recovery.
   c. Careful provision of postoperative pain control is essential, as remifentanil-induced analgesia dissipates rapidly after the infusion is terminated.

V. Other IV anesthetic agents

A. Etomidate

1. **Etomidate, a very useful induction agent for cardiac patients, is 10 times more potent than propofol, with a recommended dose range of 0.15 to 0.3 mg/kg.**
2. It is reliable at achieving hypnosis, especially when combined with an opioid. Administering the primary dose just after giving an opioid may attenuate myoclonus, which sometimes occurs as a result of subcortical disinhibition.

3. Etomidate reaches the brain in 1 min.
4. There may be an increased incidence of epileptiform activity in patients with known epileptic seizure disorders.
5. A dose of etomidate typically produces a 10% to 15% decrease in mean arterial pressure and SVR and a 3% to 4% increase in HR and cardiac output.
6. Importantly, stroke volume, left ventricular end-diastolic volume (LVEDV), and contractility remain unchanged in normovolemic patients.
7. Etomidate can be used to anesthetize heart transplant patients, because it preserves myocardial contractility better than any induction technique other than a high-dose opioid induction.
8. Although traditional induction doses of etomidate and opioids given individually most often preserve hemodynamics, when they are given together hypotension may ensue.
9. Since even a single dose of etomidate has been shown to induce significant adrenal suppression for more than 24 h (not associated with increased vasopressor requirement), it should be used with caution in high-risk cardiac surgical patients or followed by glucocorticoid supplementation for 24 to 48 h [7].

B. Propofol

1. A normal induction dose of 2 mg/kg will drop BP 15% to 40%.
2. Because propofol resets the baroreceptor reflex, lower BP does not increase HR.
3. There are significant reductions in SVR, cardiac index, stroke volume, and LV stroke work index.
4. There is direct myocardial depression at doses above 0.75 mg/kg.
5. Propofol should be titrated according to the patient's age, weight, and individual need and ideally injected into a central vein, thereby allowing the smallest dose to be used effectively and avoiding pain on injection.
6. Propofol's metabolic clearance is 10 times faster than that of thiopental.
7. There is extensive redistribution and movement from the central compartment to a peripheral one, which enables rapid recovery.
8. Unless one wishes to decrease BP, use of propofol for induction does not have an advantage over etomidate. Because it has direct myocardial depressant effects and easily induces hypotension, propofol should be used with caution or reserved for use in hemodynamically stable cardiac patients with good ventricular function.

C. Thiopental

1. **Thiopental is currently not available in the United States.**
2. **It has a rapid onset and can be used safely in hemodynamically stable patients.**
3. Rapid redistribution to highly perfused tissues causes cessation of thiopental's effects.
4. Cardiovascular effects
   a. Predominantly venous pooling and resultant decreased cardiac preload.
   b. Myocardial depressant above 2 mg/kg.
   c. Increases HR by activating baroreceptor reflex.
   d. In patients who have low cardiac output, a greater proportion of the drug dose goes to the brain and myocardium; thus, a smaller amount of thiopental has a larger effect.
   e. Overall, there is a dose-related negative inotropic effect from a decrease in calcium influx.

D. Midazolam

1. **Midazolam is a good premedicant but is difficult to titrate to a minimum effective dose for induction because of a large variation in the required dose and a relatively slow onset time to peak CNS effect of 3 to 7 min. A typical induction dose is 0.1 to 0.2 mg/kg.**
2. It is an effective amnestic, and this constitutes its appeal.
3. The hypotensive effect from an induction dose is similar to or less than that for thiopental, and it is dose related.
4. In patients who have high cardiac filling pressures, midazolam seems to mimic low-dose nitroglycerin by reducing filling pressures.
5. The addition of opioids produces a supra-additive hypotensive effect.

E. Lorazepam and Diazepam

1. Lorazepam is a very potent benzodiazepine (approximately 1.5 times as potent as midazolam), and diazepam is approximately half as potent as midazolam.
2. Because of its potency, lorazepam produces anxiolytic, sedative, and amnestic effects in lower doses and with fewer side effects than midazolam. Diazepam's cardiovascular effects are comparable to those for midazolam, i.e., generally modest preload and afterload reduction that appears to be enhanced in the presence of potent opioids such as fentanyl, sufentanil, and remifentanil.
3. Lorazepam is useful in sick cardiac patients when only small amounts of drugs are desired. Both lorazepam and diazepam can complement high-dose opioid inductions as long as the slower onset times are understood and accommodated.
4. If rapid recovery is expected, as in minimally invasive direct coronary artery bypass surgery, lorazepam is a poor choice because of its relatively long clinical action (typically several hours). Diazepam in moderate to high doses (greater than 0.15 mg/kg for most patients) can exhibit a prolonged action as well, and it has an active metabolite. Diazepam's clinical offset is disproportionately prolonged in elderly patients when compared to lorazepam or midazolam.
5. Onset times are relatively slow (lorazepam peaks in 5 to 10 min, diazepam is slightly faster) in the context of induction of anesthesia, but are acceptable in the context of IV sedation for "line" placement before induction of anesthesia.

F. Ketamine

1. Ketamine produces a unique cataleptic trance known as dissociative anesthesia.
2. It is extensively redistributed and eliminated.
3. Bioavailability on IV injection is 97% and 2 mg/kg produces unconsciousness in 20 to 60 s.
4. **Ketamine induces significant increases in HR, mean arterial pressure, and plasma epinephrine levels.** This sympathetic nervous system stimulation is centrally mediated.
5. Ketamine may be advantageous in hypovolemia, major hemorrhage, or cardiac tamponade.
6. It allows humane obtundation of the hemodynamically unstable patient, giving the surgeon an opportunity to rapidly intervene and correct a life-threatening problem (e.g., cardiac tamponade). In these situations, skin preparation should be performed before induction.
7. **The hemodynamic stimulatory effect of ketamine depends on the presence of a robust myocardium and sympathetic reserve. In the absence of either, hypotension may ensue from myocardial depression** [8].
8. Coronary blood flow may not be sufficient to meet the increased oxygen demands induced by sympathetic stimulation.
9. Ketamine should be avoided in patients with elevated intracranial pressure.
10. The S^+ isomer produces much longer periods of hypnosis and analgesia, and less postanesthetic stimulation. This compound, currently available in some European countries, may become available in the United States.
11. Ketamine is very useful for patients who have experienced severe acute blood loss.

VI. Inhalational agents

A. Hemodynamic effects. Similar but generally modest levels of myocardial depression occur with all three popular inhalational agents, **isoflurane, desflurane,** and **sevoflurane.** Serious consequences may occur in patients with congestive heart failure, however, as a narrow range of anesthetic concentrations may be tolerated by the compromised myocardium. **The predominant hemodynamic effect of these three agents is dose-dependent vasodilation,** hence reducing BP and SVR [9]. All three agents also induce a dose-dependent reflex tachycardia that can be attenuated or prevented by β-adrenergic blockers or opioids.

B. Desflurane is uniquely titratable for induction of anesthesia because of its rapid onset and offset, which remarkably matches that of a remifentanil infusion. Because of its pungent aroma, however, desflurane is poorly tolerated unless it is preceded by an IV induction.

C. Sevoflurane has a much more pleasant aroma, suitable for inhalational induction, offers hemodynamic stability in most induction situations, and has an onset time only slightly slower than that of desflurane.

D. **Isoflurane,** like desflurane, has a pungent aroma, and it is best introduced after an IV induction.

E. **Nitrous oxide** is seldom used during anesthetic induction in cardiac surgical patients, but it is generally safe to use for induction with the probable exception of patients with markedly increased pulmonary vascular resistance.

F. **Clinical use.** Whereas clinically significant brain concentrations (greater than or equal to 1 × minimal anesthetic concentration [MAC]) can be attained with desflurane and sevoflurane in 2 to 4 min, generally lower concentrations are achieved over the same time frame with isoflurane. Consequently, **desflurane and sevoflurane are more likely to reach concentrations consistent with stress–response suppression (generally 1.3 to 1.5 times MAC) during a customary induction period than isoflurane.** One potential drawback to desflurane is sympathetic stimulation when the inspired concentration is increased rapidly, perhaps owing to its airway irritant effects. Any of these inhalation agents can be used during induction as a complement to an IV induction. Desflurane can be useful in cardiac anesthesia not as much because of its rapid offset as because of its rapid onset.

VII. Muscle relaxants

A. **A suspected difficult intubation** precludes giving the patient a neuromuscular blocker before achieving intubation unless one is highly confident that mask ventilation will succeed and that an emergency alternative airway (e.g., laryngeal mask, fiberoptic intubation) can also succeed.

B. **Succinylcholine** still has the fastest onset and offset of all muscle relaxants.

C. **Significant** β-adrenergic blockade and high-dose opioid induction are potential indications for otherwise obsolescent **pancuronium,** as its vagolytic effects tend to counter the vagotonia and bradycardia induced by higher doses of opioids.

D. **Intermediate-duration agents:** Cisatracurium, rocuronium, and vecuronium are hemodynamically bland.

   1. If hepatic or renal failure exists, cisatracurium appears to be the wisest choice.

E. **Timing of the administration** of the muscle relaxant is important.

   1. Laryngoscopy should await optimal relaxation (see Section I.B.3.i). Early administration
9 obviates opioid-induced truncal rigidity, which may impair mask ventilation and result in systemic oxygen desaturation, yet one should also ensure amnesia with a sedative-hypnotic agent before administering the muscle relaxant.

VIII. Applications of old drugs in sick patients.

One busy cardiac surgery center blends the principles of careful patient assessment, cautious dosing, and fiscal restraint by commonly choosing the following preinduction sequence:

A. Patient arrives in anesthetic preinduction area or operating room.

   1. A large-bore (16-gauge or larger) IV catheter is placed.
   2. Light premedication is administered, typically midazolam 1 to 2 mg IV.
   3. A 20-gauge radial or brachial arterial catheter is placed using local anesthesia.

B. IV induction of anesthesia proceeds using the following:

   1. Fentanyl 250 to 500 μg in consideration of the patient's size and hemodynamic stability.
   2. Etomidate 0.15 to 0.2 mg/kg with the same consideration.
   3. After ensuring that mask ventilation can be accomplished, succinylcholine 1 to 2 mg/kg is administered.
   4. Endotracheal intubation is accomplished.

C. After endotracheal intubation, the next steps are as follows:

   1. Placement of central venous access (e.g., double-lumen CVP or 9 French introducer with single-lumen IV catheter or a PA catheter placed through the introducer for hemodynamic monitoring)
   2. As hemodynamics permit, careful initiation of isoflurane is administered at 0.5 to 1 MAC with titration to BP and bispectral index.
   3. If needed, IV phenylephrine is titrated to support BP.
   4. Upon recovery from succinylcholine, transition to vecuronium (initial dose approximately 0.03 to 0.05 mg/kg, subsequent doses 0.01 to 0.02 mg/kg) for maintenance of neuromuscular blockade. For longer cases when fast tracking is not anticipated, pancuronium (30 to 50 μg/kg) is an acceptable alternative.

IX. Inhalational Induction in very sick patients. This technique is a good alternative to gently induce very sick patients with low ejection fraction undergoing LVAD placement or heart transplantation. The technique is recommended only in patients who clearly have empty stomachs in order to avoid the potential for aspiration, as the induction period is prolonged:

A. Patient is in the operating room, monitors placed.
B. Large bore (16 gauge or larger) IV catheter is placed.
C. Light premedication with midazolam 1 to 2 mg IV.
D. Twenty-gauge radial arterial catheter is placed using local anesthetic (2% lidocaine).
E. An inotropic infusion (usually epinephrine or dopamine) is connected to the peripheral IV, programmed and ready to go.
F. Start preoxygenation and 2% sevoflurane, maintain 2% during entire induction period, and decrease it only if hemodynamic instability ensues.
G. Administer fentanyl typically 150 to 500 μg in divided doses, depending on the patient size and age.
H. Consider administering additional midazolam boluses usually up to 5 mg total, or increasing the inspired concentration of sevoflurane to 3% to 4% if hemodynamics remain stable.
I. Upon loss of consciousness, after testing the airway, administer 0.6 to 0.9 mg/kg rocuronium to allow for rapid intubation.
J. When mask ventilating, hyperventilate with small tidal volumes to decrease PA pressure, and to avoid intrathoracic overinflation that may increase pulmonary vascular resistance and decrease venous return. For similar reasons, avoid positive-end-expiratory pressure and be aware of the possibility of "breath-stacking" in patients with reactive airways disease or chronic obstructive pulmonary disease (COPD). The latter patients may require prolonged expiratory time.

X. Immediate postinduction period. After induction and intubation, several different techniques may be used for maintenance of anesthesia. First priorities, however, are to assess the airway (confirm endotracheal tube location via end-tidal CO_2 and auscultation), assess hemodynamic stability, and respond appropriately to any problems identified.

A. A low-dose continuous infusion of the opioid used for induction or of remifentanil (0.1 μg/kg/min) can be implemented.
B. Consider adding an inhalational agent for maintenance of anesthesia and amnesia.
C. Continuous infusion or intermittent bolus doses of a sedative–hypnotic agent (e.g., midazolam) can be initiated if no potent inhalational agent is used.
D. A propofol infusion may be useful in hemodynamically robust patients.
E. Some clinicians prefer a dexmedetomidine infusion for its augmentation of analgesia and tendency to avoid hypertension, although its offset time is relatively long (15 min or more), it can induce hypertension at onset, and bradycardia and hypotension may occur.
F. The treatment of postinduction hypotension deserves mention. There is a tendency to administer phenylephrine boluses of 100 to 200 μg as a "knee-jerk" response to hypotension, when at times either rapid volume infusion, an alternative vasoactive drug, or both may be more appropriate.
    1. If the heart appears empty based on filling pressures, echocardiography findings, cardiac output measurement, or respiratory variation in systolic pressure, then rapid administration of crystalloid or colloid is appropriate.
    2. If the induction has used drugs most likely to reduce SVR and preload without affecting myocardial contractility (e.g., midazolam or etomidate with an opioid and a muscle relaxant), then phenylephrine is appropriate. If the need appears likely to be sustained because of a lengthy interval to surgical incision, then consider a continuous phenylephrine infusion of 0.1 to 1 μg/kg/min.
    3. If the HR is low or if there is a strong possibility of myocardial depression as well (e.g., propofol was used for induction or >0.5 MAC of a volatile agent is in use), then consider using a bolus of ephedrine (5 to 15 mg) or epinephrine (10 to 25 μg).
G. A simple technique used daily and varied in dosage according to the physical status of the patient probably provides the most consistent results for most clinicians.

REFERENCES

1. Sun J-Z, Cao L-H, Liu H. ACE inhibitors in cardiac surgery: Current studies and controversies. *Hypertension Res.* 2011;34: 15–22.
2. Reich DL, Kaplan JA. Hemodynamic monitoring. In: Kaplan JA, ed. *Cardiac Anesthesia.* 4th ed. Philadelphia, PA: WB Saunders; 1999:321–358.
3. Harrison NL, Sear JW. Barbiturates, etomidate, propofol, ketamine, and steroids. In: Evers AS, Maze M, eds. *Anesthetic Pharmacology: Physiologic Principles and Clinical Practice.* Philadelphia, PA: Churchill Livingstone; 2004:395–416.
4. Billard V, Moulla F, Bourgain JL, et al. Hemodynamic response to induction and intubation: Propofol/fentanyl interaction. *Anesthesiology.* 1994;81:1384–1393.
5. Murphy GS, Szokil JW, Marymont JH, et al. Morphine-based cardiac anesthesia provides superior early recovery compared with fentanyl in elective cardiac surgery patients. *Anesth Analg.* 2009;109:311–319.
6. Bovill JG. Opioids. In: Bovill JG, Howie MB, eds. *Clinical Pharmacology for Anaesthetists.* London: WB Saunders; 1999: 87–102.
7. Morel J, Salard M, Castelain C, et al. Hemodynamic consequences of etomidate administration in elective cardiac surgery: A randomized double blinded study. *Br J Anesth.* 2011;107(4):503–509.
8. Schuttler J, Zsigmond EK, White PF. Ketamine and its isomers. In: White PF, ed. *Textbook of Intravenous Anesthesia.* Philadelphia, PA: Williams & Wilkins; 1997:171–188.
9. Pagel PS, Warltier DC. Anesthetics and left ventricular function. In: Warltier DC, ed. *Ventricular Function, a Society of Cardiovascular Anesthesiologists Monograph.* Baltimore, MD: Williams & Wilkins; 1995:213–252.

7 Anesthetic Management in the Precardiopulmonary Bypass Period

Anand R. Mehta, Mark E. Romanoff, and Michael G. Licina

KEY POINTS

1. The incidence of ischemia during this period has been reported to be 7% to 56%.
2. The Society of Thoracic Surgeons recommends a cephalosporin as the primary prophylactic antibiotic for adult cardiac surgery. In patients considered high risk for staphylococcus infection (either presumed or known staphylococcal colonization), it would be reasonable to combine cephalosporins with vancomycin.
3. An incidence of hypertension as high as 88% is found with sternotomy during a narcotic-based anesthetic.
4. Sternotomy is the time of the highest incidence of awareness and recall during cardiac surgery, and has been reported to be associated
5. Sinus tachycardia with heart rates greater than 100 beats/min has been associated with a 40% incidence of ischemia. Heart rate greater than 110 beats/min was associated with a 32% to 63% incidence of ischemia.
6. The most likely cause of dysrhythmia in the prebypass period is surgical manipulation of the heart.

THE PERIOD OF TIME BETWEEN induction of anesthesia and institution of cardiopulmonary bypass (CPB) is characterized by widely varying surgical stimuli. Anesthetic management during this high-risk period must strive to:

1. Optimize the myocardial O_2 supply/demand ratio and monitor for myocardial ischemia. The incidence
1 of ischemia during this period has been reported to be 7% to 56% [1].
2. Hemodynamics must be optimized to maintain adequate organ perfusion. This is best achieved by optimizing the preload, afterload, contractility, heart rate, and rhythm depending on the underlying cardiac dysfunction and its associated complications.
3. Manage "fast track" patients with short-acting agents.

Adverse hemodynamic changes increase the risk of developing ischemia, heart failure, hypoxemia, or dysrhythmias. These complications may alter surgical management and lead to urgent institution of CPB with failure to perform internal mammary artery (IMA) or radial artery dissection, along with an increased risk of bleeding.

A few simple rules may assist in the management of cardiac patients before CPB:

1. **"Keep them where they live."**
   A review of the preoperative vital signs and tests of cardiac performance (echocardiography, cardiac catheterization, and other imaging modalities) helps in guiding the management of the hemodynamics during this period.
2. **"The enemy of good is better."**
   If the patient's blood pressure and heart rate are acceptable, does it matter if the cardiac index is 1.8 L/min/M^2? When a patient is anesthetized, oxygen consumption decreases, so a lower cardiac index may be adequate. Trying to increase it to "normal" may lead to other problems, such as dysrhythmias or myocardial ischemia. Additional parameters such as mixed venous oxygen saturation and presence of acidosis should be considered prior to treatment.
3. **"Do no harm."**
   These patients are frequently very ill. If you are having problems managing the patient, ask for help.

I. Management of events before CPB

A. Stages of the pre-CPB period. The pre-CPB period can be subdivided into stages based on the level of surgical stimulation.

1. **High levels of stimulation** include incision, sternal split, sternal spread, sympathetic nerve dissection, pericardiotomy, and aortic cannulation. Inadequate anesthesia or sympathetic activation at these times leads to increased catecholamine levels, possibly resulting in hypertension, dysrhythmias, tachycardia, ischemia, or heart failure (Table 7.1).
2. **Low-level stimulation** occurs during preincision, radial artery harvesting, internal mammary (thoracic) artery dissection, and CPB venous cannulation. Risks during these periods include hypotension, bradycardia, dysrhythmias, and ischemia (Table 7.1).

B. Preincision. This period includes surgical preparation and draping. Several parameters should be checked during this time:

1. **Confirm bilateral breath sounds** after final patient positioning.
2. **Check pressure points.** Ischemia, secondary to compression and compounded by decreases in temperature and perfusion pressure during CPB, may cause peripheral neuropathy or damage to soft tissues.
   a. **Brachial plexus injury** can occur if the arms are hyperextended or if chest retraction is excessive (e.g., occult rib fracture using a sternal retractor) [2]. Excessive chest retraction can occur not only with the sternal spreader but also during IMA dissection even if the arms are tucked to the sides. If the arms are placed on arm boards, obtain

TABLE 7.1 Typical hemodynamic responses to surgical stimulation before cardiopulmonary bypass

	Preincision	Incision	Sternotomy and sternal spread	Sympathetic dissection	IMA dissection	Cannulation
Surgical stimulation	↓	↑	↑↑	↑	↓	↓
Heart rate	↓↓	— or ↑	↑↑	— or ↓	— or ↓	— or ↓[a]
Blood pressure	↓↓	↑	↑↑↑	↑ or ↑↑	— or ↓	↓
Preload	— or ↓	— or ↑	— or ↑	— or ↑	— or ↓	↓
Afterload	— or ↓	↑↑	↑↑ or ↑↑↑	↑ or ↑↑	— or ↓	— or ↓
Myocardial O_2 demand	↓	— or ↑	↑↑ or ↑↑↑	↑ or ↑↑	↓	↓

All values are compared with control (preinduction) values.
[a]Dysrhythmias secondary to mechanical stimulation of the heart are likely.
IMA, internal mammary artery; ↑, slightly increased; ↑↑, moderately increased; ↑↑↑, markedly increased; ↓, slightly decreased; ↓↓, moderately decreased; —, unchanged.

the proper position by minimizing pectoralis major muscle tension. Do not extend arms more than 90 degrees from the body to avoid stretching the brachial plexus.

b. **Ulnar nerve injury** can occur from compression of the olecranon against the metal edge of the operating room table. To obtain the proper position, provide adequate padding under the olecranon. Do not allow the arm to contact the metal edge of the operating room table.

c. **Radial nerve injury** can occur from compression of the upper arm against the "ether screen" or the support post of the chest wall sternal retractors used in IMA dissection.

d. **Finger injury** can occur secondary to pressure from members of the operating team leaning against the operating table if the fingers are positioned improperly. To obtain the proper position, hands should be next to the body, with fingers in a neutral position away from the metal edge of the table. One method to prevent upper extremity injury is to have the patient position himself or herself. The patient can grasp a surgical towel in each hand to ensure that the fingers are in a comfortable and protected position.

e. **Occipital alopecia** can occur 3 wks after the operation secondary to ischemia of the scalp, particularly during hypothermia. To obtain the proper position, pad and reposition the head frequently during the operation.

f. **Heel skin ischemia and tissue necrosis** are possible. Heels should be well padded in such a way as to redistribute weight away from the heel to the lower leg.

g. **The eyes** should be closed, taped, and free from any pressure.

h. Commercial foam dressings may be applied prophylactically to various pressure points (sacrum and heels) to prevent pressure sores as these patients are bed ridden and may have compromised circulation.

3. **Adjust fresh gas flow.**

a. Use of 100% O_2 maximizes inspired O_2 tension. A lower inspired oxygen concentration may prevent absorption atelectasis and reduce the risk of O_2 toxicity. The inspired oxygen concentration can be titrated based on pulse oximeter readings and arterial blood gases (ABGs).

b. Nitrous oxide can be used during the pre-CPB period in stable patients. It will, however,

(1) Decrease the concentration of inspired oxygen (FiO_2)

(2) Increase pulmonary vascular resistance (PVR) in adults

(3) Increase catecholamine release

(4) Possibly induce ventricular dysfunction

(5) Some evidence suggests that nitrous oxide should not be used in patients with an evolving myocardial infarct or in patients with ongoing ischemia because the decrease in FiO_2 and potential catecholamine release theoretically can increase the risk of ischemia and infarct size. This point remains controversial.

4. **Check all monitors and lines after final patient position is achieved.**

a. Intravenous (IV) infusions should flow freely, and the arterial pressure waveform should be assessed for dampening or hyper-resonance.

b. IV injection ports should be accessible.

c. All IV and arterial line connections (stopcocks) should be taped or secured to prevent their movement and minimize the risk of blood loss from an open connection.

d. Confirm electrical and patient reference "zero" of all transducers (see Chapter 4).

e. Nasopharyngeal temperature probes, if required, must be placed prior to heparinization to avoid excessive nasal bleeding.

5. **Check hemodynamic status.**

a. Cardiac index, ventricular filling pressures, mixed venous oxygen saturation (S_vO_2), and cardiac work indices should be evaluated after intubation.

b. If transesophageal echocardiography (TEE) is used, check and document the position of the probe and the presence or absence of dental and oropharyngeal injury. Make sure the TEE probe is not in a locked position, as this may lead to pressure necrosis in the gastrointestinal tract.

c. A baseline TEE examination should be performed to document the ejection fraction, wall-motion abnormalities, valve function, and shunts (see Chapter 5). The TEE probe should be placed before heparinization to avoid excessive bleeding.

6. **Check blood chemistry.**
   a. Once a stable anesthetic level is achieved, and ventilation and FiO_2 have been constant for 10 min, an ABG measurement should be obtained to confirm adequate oxygenation and ventilation, and to correlate the ABG with noninvasive measurements (pulse oximetry and end-tidal CO_2 concentration). Maintain normocapnia, as hypercapnia may increase PVR. Hypocapnia may promote myocardial ischemia and cardiac dysrhythmias.
   b. Mixed venous hemoglobin O_2 saturation can be measured with a mixed venous blood gas at this time, if necessary, to calibrate a continuous mixed venous PA catheter.
   c. Electrolytes, calcium, and glucose levels should be determined as clinically indicated. High glucose levels should be treated to minimize neurologic injury and to decrease postoperative infection rates. Intraoperative hyperglycemia is an independent risk factor for other perioperative complications, including death, after cardiac surgery [3]. Perioperative glucose management of diabetic patients must be started in the prebypass period. Glucose control may be achieved by a continuous infusion of insulin with the infusion rate depending on the patient's blood sugar. Boluses of IV insulin may lead to large swings in blood sugar; thus, an IV infusion is preferred. It is imperative to treat the trends of blood glucose rather than absolute blood glucose levels to minimize intraoperative hypoglycemia. Thus, glycemic control should be based on the velocity of glucose change rather than an absolute value.
   d. A blood sample to determine a baseline activated clotting time (ACT) before heparinization may be drawn at the same time as the sample for ABG. The blood can be taken from the arterial line after withdrawal of 5 to 10 mL of blood depending on the dead space of the arterial line tubing and avoiding residual heparin, if present, in the flush solution. The perfusionist may require a blood sample to perform a heparin dose–response curve, which in some institutions is used to determine the initial heparin dosage.
   e. Before any manipulation of the arterial line (zeroing, blood sample withdrawal), it is important to announce your intentions. This avoids alarming your colleagues, who may notice the loss of the arterial waveform.

7. **Antibiotics**
   a. Antibiotics are often administered before incision and should be timed not to coincide with the administration of other medications, should an allergic reaction occur.
   b. For cardiac patients, the Surgical Care Improvement Project (SCIP) and The Society of Thoracic Surgeons (STS) Practice guidelines recommend that preoperative prophylactic antibiotics are to be administered within 1 h prior to incision with the exception of 2 h for vancomycin or fluoroquinolones and discontinued 48 h after the end of surgery for cardiac patients.
   c. The STS recommends a cephalosporin as the primary prophylactic antibiotic for adult cardiac surgery. In patients considered high risk for staphylococcus infection (either presumed or known staphylococcal colonization), it would be reasonable to combine cephalosporins with vancomycin.
   d. Exclusive vancomycin use for cardiac surgical prophylaxis should be avoided as it provides no gram-negative coverage.
   e. In patients with a history of an immunoglobulin-E–mediated reaction to penicillin, vancomycin should be administered with additional gram-negative coverage [4,5].

8. **Antifibrinolytics.** Excessive fibrinolysis is one of the causes of blood loss following cardiac surgery. Antifibrinolytic agents are commonly used to minimize bleeding and thereby reduce the exposure to blood products.
   a. **Aprotinin (serine protease inhibitor).** The FDA has suspended the use of aprotinin after the BART trial which demonstrated that aprotinin has a worse risk-benefit profile

than the lysine analogs with a trend toward increased mortality in patients receiving aprotinin [6].

   b. Epsilon-aminocaproic acid (EACA) and Tranexamic acid (lysine analogs). With the suspended use of aprotinin, EACA and tranexamic acid are the only anti-fibrinolytics available. Both are effective agents in reducing postoperative blood loss. However, EACA at equipotent doses to tranexamic acid is associated with a higher rate of temporary renal dysfunction. Tranexamic acid is associated with seizures at higher doses [7].

9. **Preparation for saphenous vein excision** involves lifting the legs above the level of the heart. Increased venous return increases the myocardial preload. This change is desirable in patients with low filling pressures and normal ventricular function but may be detrimental in patients with borderline ventricular reserve. Gradual elevation of the legs may be useful in attenuating the hemodynamic changes. The reverse occurs when the legs are returned to the neutral position.
10. **Endoscopic saphenectomy** for harvesting vein grafts for coronary artery bypass grafting is becoming common. As in a laparoscopic procedure, carbon dioxide is the insufflating gas of choice during this procedure. Mechanical ventilation may have to be adjusted depending on the rise in CO_2 as detected by an end-tidal monitor and ABG analysis. When using carbon dioxide insufflation, CO_2 embolism has been reported in two patients. These were associated with no untoward consequences because of prompt recognition and treatment. Frail, elderly patients with fragile tissue are at risk for this complication. Preventive measures include maintenance of a right atrial pressure to insufflation pressure gradient of greater than or equal to 5 mm Hg and addition of positive end-expiratory pressure (PEEP). Hemodynamic deterioration secondary to transmission of gas through a patent foramen ovale into the left heart and coronary circulation has also been reported [8].
11. **Maintenance of body temperature** is not a concern during the pre-CPB time period with the exception of off-pump coronary artery bypass grafting (OPCAB). It is preferable to allow the temperature to drift down slowly, as this allows for more homogeneous hypothermia at institution of CPB. Before CPB, increasing the room temperature, humidifying anesthetic gases, warming IV solutions, and using a warming blanket are not necessary. These measures must be available for post-CPB management. The physiologic changes associated with mild hypothermia (34 to 36°C) include the following:
    a. Decrease in O_2 consumption and CO_2 production (8% to 10% for each degree Celsius)
    b. Increase in systemic vascular resistance (SVR) and PVR
    c. Increase in blood viscosity
    d. Decrease in central nervous system (CNS) function (amnesia, decrease in cerebral metabolic rate or O_2 consumption [$CMRo_2$] and decrease in cerebral blood flow)
    e. Decrease in anesthetic requirement (minimum alveolar concentration [MAC] decreases 5% for each degree Celsius)
    f. Decrease in renal blood flow and urine output
    g. Decrease in hepatic blood flow
    h. Minimal increase in plasma catecholamine levels
12. **Maintain other organ system function**
    a. Renal system [9]
        (1) Inadequate urine output must be addressed immediately:
            (a) Rule out technical problems first (kinked urinary catheter tubing or disconnected tubing).
            (b) Optimize and maintain an adequate intravascular volume and cardiac output using central venous pressure (CVP), pulmonary artery catheter (PAC), or TEE as a measure of preload and cardiac performance.
            (c) Avoid or treat hypotension.
            (d) Maintain adequate oxygenation.
            (e) Mannitol (0.25 g/kg IV) may be used to redistribute renal blood flow to the cortex and to maintain renal tubular flow.

(f) Dopamine (2.5 to 5 μg/kg/min) infusion may be given to increase renal blood flow by renal vascular dilation. Currently, there is no evidence that "renal" dose dopamine will prevent perioperative renal dysfunction. Its use may increase the incidence of perioperative atrial dysrhythmias.

(g) Diuretics (furosemide, 10 to 40 mg; bumetanide, 0.25 to 1 mg) can be given to maintain renal tubular flow if other measures are ineffective or if the patient had taken preoperative diuretics.

(2) Patients undergoing emergent surgery may have received a large radiocontrast dye load at angiography. Avoiding dye-induced acute tubular necrosis, utilizing the techniques mentioned earlier, is crucial.

b. CNS

(1) Adequate cerebral perfusion pressure must be maintained.

(a) The patient's preoperative lowest and highest mean arterial pressures should be the limits accepted in the operating room to avoid cerebral ischemia. Remember "keep them where they live."

(b) Elderly patients have a decreased cerebral reserve and are more sensitive to changes in cerebral perfusion pressure.

(2) Patients at risk for an adverse cerebral event include those with known carotid artery disease, peripheral vascular disease, or a known embolic focus. Management considerations for these patients are discussed in Chapter 22.

c. Pulmonary system

(1) Maintain normal pH, P_aCO_2, and adequate P_aO_2.

(2) Treatment of systemic hypertension with a vasodilator may induce hypoxemia secondary to inhibition of hypoxic pulmonary vasoconstriction. FiO_2 may have to be increased.

(3) Use of an air–oxygen mixture may prevent absorption atelectasis.

13. Prepare for incision.

a. Ensure adequate depth of anesthesia using clinical signs. If available, a bispectral index (BIS) monitor may be helpful. A small dose of a narcotic or hypnotic or increased concentration of inhaled agent may be necessary.

b. Ensure adequate muscle relaxation to avoid movement with incision and sternotomy. If movement occurs, make sure the patient is anesthetized as you are paralyzing the patient.

C. Incision

1. An adequate depth of anesthesia is necessary but may not be sufficient to avoid tachycardia and hypertension in response to the stimulus of incision. If hemodynamic changes occur, they are usually short lived, so medications with a brief duration of action are recommended.

a. Treatment can include:

(1) Vasodilators

(a) Nitroglycerin (20- to 80-μg bolus) or infusion

(b) Sodium nitroprusside infusion

(2) β-blockers

(a) Esmolol (0.25 to 1 mg/kg)

2. Observe the surgical field for patient movement and blood color. Despite an abundance of monitors, the presence of bright red blood remains one of the best ways to assess oxygenation and perfusion.

3. If the patient responds clinically to the incision (tachycardia, hypertension, other signs of "light" anesthesia, or clinically significant BIS monitor value changes), then the level of anesthesia must be deepened before sternotomy. Do not allow sternal split until the patient is anesthetized adequately and hemodynamics are controlled.

D. Sternal split

3 **1.** A very high level of stimulation accompanies sternal split. The incidence of hypertension has been reported to be as high as 88% during a narcotic-based anesthetic. A cumulative

dose of fentanyl, 50 to 70 μg/kg, before sternal split should decrease the incidence of hypertension to less than 50%. However, fentanyl doses greater than 150 μg/kg are necessary for further reduction in the incidence of hypertension [10]. This high dose of fentanyl, will prevent the patient from being ready for early extubation. Hypertension and tachycardia, if they occur, should be treated as described for skin incision.

Bradycardia secondary to vagal discharge can occur. It is usually self-limiting, but if it is persistent and causes hemodynamic compromise then a dose of atropine or ephedrine may be necessary.

2. A reciprocating power saw is often used to open the sternum. The lungs should be "deflated" during opening of the internal table of the sternum to avoid damage to the lung parenchyma.
3. The patient should have adequate muscle relaxation during sternotomy to avoid an air embolism. If the patient gasps as the right atrium is cut, air can be entrained owing to the negative intrapleural pressure.

4. This is the most common time period for awareness and recall due to the intense stimulation.
   a. Awareness has been reported with fentanyl dosages as large as 150 μg/kg and with lower fentanyl doses supplemented with amnestic agents. Awareness usually, but not always, is associated with other symptoms of light anesthesia (movement, sweating, increased pupil size, hypertension, or tachycardia). A BIS monitor may be helpful, but recall has occurred in patients with an "adequate" BIS reading.
   b. If an amnestic agent has not been administered previously, it should be considered before sternotomy because these agents decrease the incidence of recall but will not produce retrograde amnesia. Amnestic supplements do not always protect against the hypertension and tachycardia associated with awareness. However, amnestic supplements may cause hypotension. The most common amnestic agents, their dosages, and side effects include:
      (1) Benzodiazepines (midazolam, 2.5 to 20 mg; diazepam, 5 to 15 mg; lorazepam, 1 to 4 mg) in divided doses usually are well tolerated but can decrease SVR and contractility in patients with poor ventricular function, especially when the drugs are added to a narcotic-based anesthetic.
      (2) Scopolamine, 0.2 to 0.4 mg IV, may cause tachycardia if it is administered rapidly. It may prolong emergence in a "fast track" patient and it will cause pupillary dilation.
      (3) Nitrous oxide may lead to catecholamine release, LV dysfunction, increased PVR, and increased risk of hypoxia. The use of nitrous oxide in noncardiac surgery (ENIGMA trial) was associated with an increased long-term risk of myocardial infarction. Nitrous oxide-induced inactivation of methionine synthetase increases plasma homocysteine levels in the postoperative period. This can lead to endothelial dysfunction and hypercoagulability. The ENIGMA-II trial is presently studying this hypothesis to ascertain the risks and benefits of using nitrous oxide [11].
      (4) Inhalation agents can cause myocardial depression, bradycardia, tachycardia, dysrhythmias, or decreases in SVR, but they are effective in low concentrations and have become a standard part of the anesthetic technique to "fast track" the patient.
      (5) Droperidol (0.0625 to 2.5 mg) may cause hypotension by blocking α_1-receptors. This effect may last several hours.
      (6) Ketamine (5 to 100 mg) can cause sympathetic stimulation unless the patient is pretreated with a narcotic or benzodiazepine.
      (7) Propofol (10 to 50 mg) can cause decreased blood pressure and cardiac output.
      (8) Sodium thiopental (25 to 150 mg) can cause decreased blood pressure and cardiac output.
5. **Concerns with cardiac reoperation ("redo heart")**
   a. The pericardium is usually not closed after heart surgery, and the aorta, RV, and bypass grafts may adhere to the underside of the sternum. At reoperation, these structures can be easily injured when the sternum is opened. A clue to this potential problem may

be provided radiologically if there is no space between the heart and the inner sternal border. Although using an oscillating saw decreases this risk, it does not eliminate it. As this takes longer than the usual sternotomy, ventilation should not be held. Knowing the proximity of mediastinal structures to the sternum is necessary, and if preoperative imaging suggests that they may be in jeopardy, extra measures before reopening the sternum, such as peripheral cannulation and CPB (with or without deep hypothermic circulatory arrest), may be necessary to avoid catastrophe [12]. Venous cannulae may be passed into the right atrium through the femoral vein. The correct positioning of these cannulae may be identified on the mid-esophageal bicaval view using TEE. Axillary or subclavian cannulation may be the preferred site for peripheral arterial inflow site as compared to the femoral artery in patients with concurrent descending, thoracoabdominal, or abdominal aortic aneurysms. A discussion with the surgeon is necessary to place the arterial line for monitoring in the contralateral superior extremity in case of either subclavian or axillary cannulation. Femoral arterial cannulation may be an alternative.

b. If a graft is cut, the patient may develop profound ischemia. Nitroglycerin may be helpful, but if significant myocardial dysfunction or hypotension occurs, the ultimate treatment is prompt institution of CPB.

c. If the right atrium, RV, or great vessels are cut, a surgeon or assistant will put a "finger in the dike" while the tear is fixed or a decision is made to go emergently on CPB. CPB can be initiated using the following:

  (1) "Sucker bypass" with a femoral artery cannula or aortic cannula and the cardiotomy suckers are used as the venous return line if the right atrium cannot be cannulated.

  (2) Complete femoral vein–femoral artery bypass

d. The prolonged surgical dissection increases the risk of dysrhythmias.

  (1) The availability of external defibrillator pads or sterile external paddles should be considered. Defibrillation may be necessary before complete exposure of the heart, rendering internal paddles ineffective.

  (2) Many institutions use a defibrillation pad that adheres to the back and is placed before induction. This allows for use of an internal paddle even if the heart is not totally exposed, as current will flow in an anteroposterior fashion through the heart.

e. Volume replacement (crystalloid, colloid, blood) may be necessary to provide adequate preload if hemorrhage is brisk during the dissection.

  (1) Adequate IV access for volume replacement must be available prior to the start of the surgical procedure. This may be accomplished by securing two large-bore peripheral IV lines or a large-bore multilumen central venous access catheter in a central vein.

  (2) Have at least 2 units of blood available in case it is necessary to transfuse the patient.

  (3) After the patient is heparinized, the surgical team should use the CPB suckers to help salvage blood.

6. Concerns with urgent or emergent cardiac operation

a. Indications include:

  (1) Cardiac catheterization complications (failed angioplasty with persistent chest pain, coronary artery dissection) [13]

  (2) Persistent ischemia with or without chest pain that is refractory to medical therapy or an intra-aortic balloon pump (IABP)

  (3) Left main coronary artery disease or left main equivalent

  (4) Acute aortic dissection

  (5) Fulminant infective endocarditis

  (6) Ruptured chordae tendineae

  (7) Acute ischemic ventricular septal defect

  (8) Multiple high-grade lesions with significant myocardium at risk

  (9) Emergent LVAD placement

b. Continue blood pressure, pulse oximeter, and electro-cardiographic (ECG) monitoring during transport and preparation.
c. Aggressively treat ischemia and dysrhythmias that may be present.
d. Continue heparin infusion until sternotomy. This will increase operative bleeding but will decrease the risk of worsening coronary thrombosis.
e. Consider heparin resistance and increase the initial heparin dose to avoid delays in starting CPB because the ACT is too low.
f. Continue antianginal therapy, particularly the nitroglycerin infusion, during an acute myocardial ischemic event.
g. Maintain coronary perfusion pressure. Phenylephrine or norepinephrine boluses and/or infusions may be necessary. An IABP may be in use or required. Maintain IABP triggers.
h. In these cases, time is of the essence. Decisions must be made regarding the risks and benefits of additional monitoring (arterial line and PA catheter) relative to the delay required for catheter insertion. Access to the central circulation and some form of direct blood pressure monitoring are required before surgery can begin.
   (1) If all lines are placed before induction at your institution, then the decision involves how to proceed while the patient is awake. If the patient has resolution of chest pain and ECG changes, then proceed cautiously with monitoring line insertion. It is often necessary to replace a femoral PA line with one that is closer to the patient's head for accessibility. Keep the femoral catheter in place for monitoring until just before floating the new PA catheter, at which time it should be pulled back to avoid complications.
   (2) If ischemia is still present while the patient is awake, proceed to the induction of anesthesia with the monitors you have. Often, after anesthesia is induced, the reduction in myocardial O_2 demand will significantly improve the ischemia and correct hemodynamic changes. In this case, insertion of further monitoring would be appropriate.
   (3) If the patient continues to have significant hemodynamic and ischemic changes, after induction, that are unresponsive to treatment, proceed to CPB urgently.
   (4) In an arrest situation, go directly to CPB. The surgeon can hand off central venous and PA lines before weaning the patient from CPB. TEE is a fast alternative to obtain much of the information derived from a PA catheter.
i. Urgency of initiating CPB does not supersede obtaining adequate heparinization documented by ACT, or adequate anesthetic levels. In a cardiac arrest situation, use double or triple the usual dose of heparin to ensure adequate heparinization. The surgeon may give the heparin directly into the heart if access is not available.
j. If a "bailout" (coronary perfusion) catheter has been placed across a coronary dissection, it should not be disturbed. It can be withdrawn from the femoral arterial sheath just before application of the aortic cross-clamp.
k. Fibrinolytic or antiplatelet agents may have been given in the catheterization laboratory. These drugs will increase bleeding before and after CPB.

E. Sternal spread

1. Very high level of stimulation can be expected
2. Visually confirm equal inflation of the lungs after the chest is open.
3. PA catheter malfunction with sternal spread has been reported. Most occurrences are with external jugular or subclavian approaches and involve kinking of the PA catheter as it exits the introducer sheath. A reinforced introducer can decrease the incidence of kinking. The surgeon could decrease the amount of sternal retraction.Sheath withdrawal may rectify the problem but can lead to the following:
   a. Loss of the IV line
   b. Bleeding
   c. Contamination of the access site
4. Innominate vein rupture, as well as brachial plexus injury, is possible after aggressive sternal spread.

F. **IMA and radial artery dissection**

1. This is a period of low-level stimulation.
2. The chest is retracted to one side using the chest wall retractor, and the table is elevated and rotated away from the surgeon. The left IMA (LIMA) is most commonly grafted to the left anterior descending artery.
   a. This procedure can cause difficulties in blood pressure measurement.
      (1) Left-sided radial arterial lines may not function during LIMA dissection owing to compression of the left subclavian artery with sternal retraction. The same may be true with a right-sided catheter and a right IMA (RIMA) dissection.
      (2) Transducers must be kept level with the right atrium.
   b. Extubation may occur with patient movement during retraction.
   c. Radial nerve injury due to compression by the support post of the Favaloro retractor is possible.
3. **Bleeding** may be extensive but hidden from view in the chest cavity (consider volume replacement to treat hypotension).
4. **Heparin,** 5,000 units, may be given during the vessel dissection process.
5. Papaverine may be injected into the IMA for dilation and to prevent spasm. Systemic effects may include hypotension or anaphylaxis.
6. IMA blood flow usually should be more than 100 mL/min (25 mL collected in 15 s) to be considered acceptable for grafting.
7. Mechanical ventilation may need to be adjusted if the motion of the lungs interferes with the surgical dissection of the IMA. This may be achieved by reducing the tidal volume and increasing the respiratory rate to achieve constant minute ventilation.
8. If the radial artery is being harvested as a conduit, the arterial line should be placed on the other side.

G. **Sympathetic nerve dissection**

1. After the pericardium is opened, the postganglionic sympathetic nerves are dissected from the aorta to allow insertion of the aortic cannula.
2. This is the most overlooked period of high-level stimulation because of sympathetic discharge. Treatment of hemodynamic changes is explained in Section I.C.

II. Perioperative stress response

A. **Afferent loop**

1. The body responds to stress with a catabolic response and an increase in substrate mobilization. This response is mediated primarily through the hypothalamic–pituitary–adrenal axis.
2. Stimuli that can trigger this response include the following:
   a. **Psychologic**
      (1) Preoperative anxiety
      (2) Light anesthesia, awareness
   b. **Physiologic**
      (1) Pain associated with invasive monitor placement
      (2) Intubation
      (3) Surgical stimulation
      (4) Changes in blood pressure (hypotension or hypertension)
      (5) Hypoxia
      (6) Hypercapnia
      (7) CPB
      (8) Aortic cross-clamp removal

B. **Humoral mediators** and the systemic effects of the stress response: (see Table 7.2)

C. **Modification of the stress response**

1. Systemic opioids (high dose)
   a. **Fentanyl (50 to 150 μg/kg)** blunts almost all responses except for prolactin increase and an occasional increase in myocardial lactate production before CPB.

TABLE 7.2 Stress response—mediators and systemic response

Humoral mediators	End organ responses
Adrenocorticotropic hormone (ACTH) ↑ Cortisol ↑	Blood glucose ↑
Catecholamines ↑	Hypertension Tachycardia Dysrhythmias Myocardial O_2 demand ↑ Cerebral metabolic rate ↑ Bronchodilation and dead space ↑ Lactate levels ↑
Insulin (inappropriate ↓ for glucose level) Glucagon ↑	Blood glucose ↑ Inotropy ↑ Fatty acids ↑
Growth hormone (GH) ↑	Protein synthesis ↑
Antidiuretic hormone (ADH) ↑ Renin ↑	Blood volume (preload) ↑ SVR (afterload) ↑ Urine output ↓ Plasma K^+ ↓ Plasma Na^+ ↑ Renal blood flow ↓ Aldosterone ↑
Prolactin ↑ Endorphins ↑	MAC ↓

MAC, minimum alveolar concentration; SVR, systemic vascular resistance.

b. **Sufentanil (10 to 30 μg/kg)** is similar to fentanyl, but some studies have shown increased norepinephrine levels with sternotomy. Free fatty acid levels increase with cannulation but may be associated with heparin.

c. **Disadvantages.** High-dose narcotics will lead to prolonged mechanical ventilation and delayed extubation. They also do not ensure amnesia.

2. Inhalation anesthetics
   a. MAC BAR—inhalation anesthetic partial pressure that blocks adrenergic response in 50% of patients
      (1) MAC BAR is approximately equal to 1.5 MAC.
      (2) Cortisol and growth hormone (GH) levels will increase with the depth of anesthesia.
      (3) To reduce catecholamine responses in 95% of patients, 2 MAC is needed.
      (4) MAC BAR is associated with myocardial depression, decreased blood pressure, and increased pulmonary capillary wedge pressure.
3. Systemic medications that decrease catecholamine effects:
   a. β-blockers
      (1) β-blockers attenuate increases in heart rate and myocardial O_2 demand.
      (2) Adverse effects include:
         (a) Decreased myocardial contractility
         (b) Bronchospasm
   b. Centrally acting α_2-adrenergic agonists (clonidine, dexmedetomidine) [14]
      (1) Both agents decrease peripheral efferent sympathetic activity.
      (2) They cause a decrease in all catecholamine levels (reduced norepinephrine levels are most prominent) and enhance cardiovascular stability.
      (3) They can decrease heart rate, blood pressure, and SVR in the perioperative period.
      (4) Some attenuation of adrenergic response during or after CPB is seen with preoperative dosing.

(5) They may cause bradycardia and hypotension, especially when combined with angiotensin-converting enzyme (ACE) inhibitors or vasodilators. Paradoxically, high doses may cause increases in PVR, hypertension, and decreases in cardiac index.

(6) Dexmedetomidine will produce analgesia and sedation. Infusions often are used after CPB for "fast track" anesthesia.

c. Vasodilators

(1) Vasodilators are used as treatment for increases in SVR, often secondary to elevated norepinephrine levels.

(2) Adverse effects include:

(a) Reflex increase in catecholamines

(b) Reflex increase in heart rate

(c) Inhibition of hypoxic pulmonary vasoconstriction

4. Regional (epidural or subarachnoid) anesthetic techniques [15]

a. Local anesthetics

(1) These drugs decrease GH, adrenocorticotropic hormone (ACTH), antidiuretic hormone (ADH), and catecholamine responses to lower abdominal procedures.

(2) Thoracic epidural anesthesia is inconsistent in blocking the stress response to thoracic surgery, possibly due to insufficient somatic or sympathetic blockade or from unblocked pelvic afferents.

(3) Adverse effects include decreased SVR, bradycardia, decreased inotropy from sympathectomy, and risk of epidural hemorrhage after heparinization.

(4) In elective cardiac surgery, thoracic epidural analgesia combined with general anesthesia followed by patient-controlled thoracic epidural analgesia offers no major advantage with respect to hospital length of stay, quality of recovery, or morbidity when compared with general anesthesia alone followed by patient-controlled analgesia with IV morphine. Time to extubation was shorter and consumption of anesthetics was lower in the patient-controlled thoracic epidural analgesia group. Pain relief, degree of sedation, ambulation, and lung volumes were similar in both the study groups. There was a trend toward lower incidences of pneumonia and confusion in the patient-controlled thoracic epidural analgesia group, whereas lung volumes, and cardiac, renal, and neurologic outcomes were similar between the groups [16].

b. Narcotics

(1) Peridural narcotics poorly block the stress response to surgery.

(2) They provide postoperative analgesia.

III. Treatment of hemodynamic changes.

Treatment of hemodynamic changes. Pressor and vasodilator treatment of any hemodynamic change ideally should involve the use of agents with a very short half-life, for the following reasons: (i) The surgical stimuli and the patient response are usually short lived (after sternotomy, the duration of patient response is usually limited to 5 to 15 min). (ii) Many agents (β-blockers, calcium channel blockers, vasodilators, ACE inhibitors, and phosphodiesterase inhibitors) will affect hemodynamic parameters for longer than 15 min and have half-lives of several hours. Their actions could affect weaning from CPB. For these reasons, the use of short-acting agents (esmolol, nitroglycerin, sodium nitroprusside, phenylephrine, and ephedrine) should be encouraged.

A. Hypotension

1. Causes

a. Mechanical causes must first be ruled out before pharmacologic treatment. Among these are the following:

(1) Surgical compression of the heart

(2) Technical problems with invasive blood pressure measurement (kinked catheter, wrist position, and air bubbles)

b. The most common cause of hypotension is hypovolemia (Table 7.3).

c. Myocardial ischemia is another potentially treatable cause of hypotension.

2. Treatment is outlined in Figure 7.1.

TABLE 7.3 Differential diagnosis of hypotension[a]

I.	Hypovolemia
II.	Deep anesthetic plane for level of stimulation
III.	Decreased venous return
	A. Mechanical compression of the heart or great vessels
	B. Increased airway pressure
	C. Tension pneumothorax
IV.	Impaired myocardial contractility
V.	Ischemia
VI.	Dysrhythmia
	A. Bradycardia
	B. Tachycardia (decrease in diastolic filling time)
	C. Dysrhythmia leading to loss of atrial contraction and its contribution to ventricular filling
VII.	Decrease in SVR
VIII.	Constrictive pericarditis in reoperation cases
IX.	Steroid depletion with chronic steroid administration

[a]Causes of hypotension are listed in order of frequency of occurrence.
SVR, systemic vascular resistance.

B. Hypertension

1. Hypertension is less common in patients with LV dysfunction than in patients with normal contractility, but it still occurs.
2. The most likely cause of hypertension is sympathetic discharge. This is seen most often in younger patients and in those with preoperative hypertension (Table 7.4).
3. Treatment is outlined in Figure 7.2.

C. Sinus bradycardia

1. The most common cause of sinus bradycardia is vagal stimulation, which often results from the vagotonic effects of narcotics (Table 7.5).
2. Treatment
   - **a.** Treatment is indicated for the following:
     - **(1)** Any heart rate decrease associated with a significant decrease in blood pressure.
     - **(2)** Heart rate less than 40 beats/min, even without decrease in blood pressure, if it is associated with a nodal or ventricular escape rhythm.
   - **b.** The underlying cause should be treated.
   - **c.** Atropine, 0.2 to 0.4 mg IV, can cause an unpredictable response.
     - **(1)** It may cause uncontrolled tachycardia and ischemia.
     - **(2)** It is often ineffective.
     - **(3)** Glycopyrrolate (0.1 to 0.2 mg IV), another vagolytic agent, may induce less increase in heart rate, but it is unpredictable and has a longer half-life than atropine.
   - **d.** Pancuronium, 2 to 4 mg IV, is often effective owing to its sympathomimetic activity, but it can be unpredictable.
   - **e.** Ephedrine, 2.5 to 25 mg IV, is indicated if bradycardia is associated with hypotension. The response may be unpredictable.
   - **f.** PA catheters with pacing capabilities and esophageal atrial pacing may provide safe and predictable, although expensive, means of increasing the heart rate.
   - **g.** Atropine and pacing can be used for life-threatening bradycardia. For minimally invasive procedures, placement of external patches may be needed to provide pacing.

D. Sinus tachycardia

5 1. Sinus tachycardia appears to be the most significant risk factor for intraoperative ischemia. Sinus tachycardia greater than 100 beats/min has been associated with a 40%

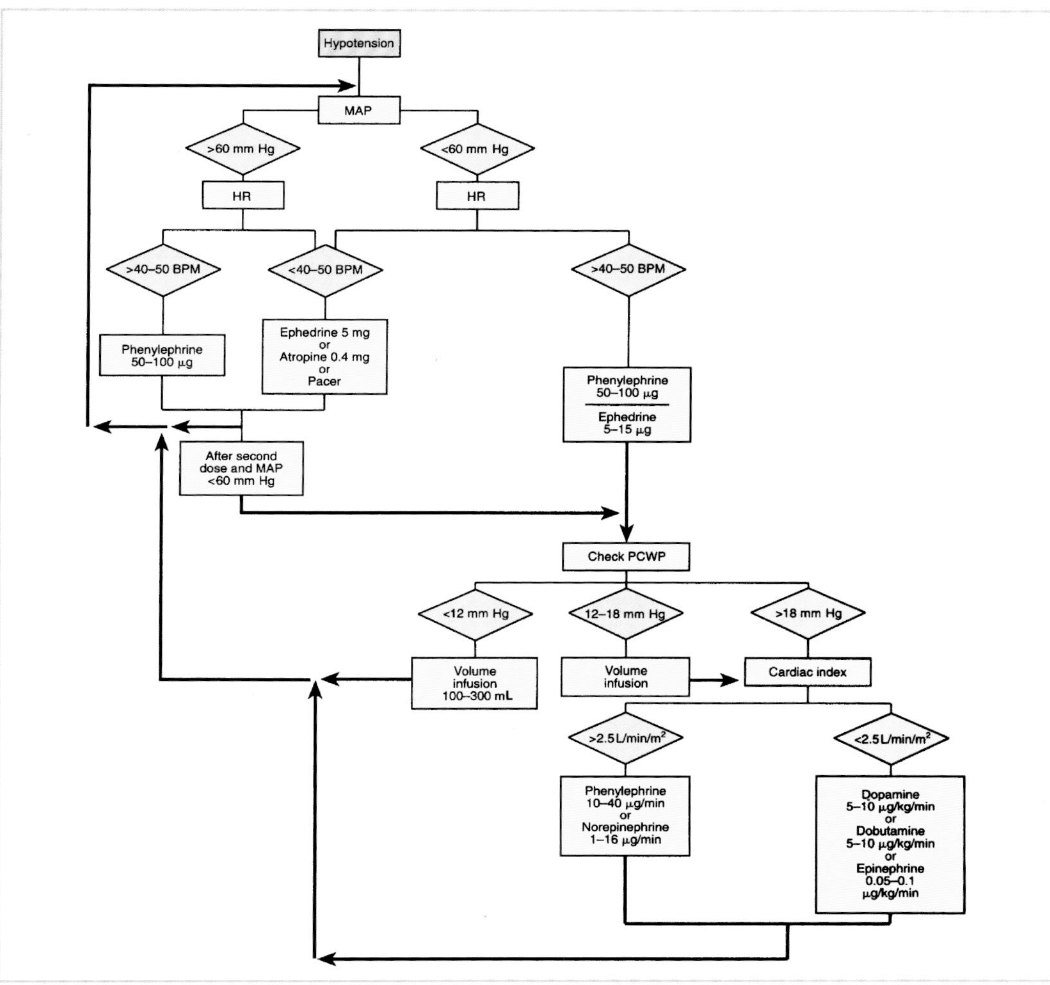

FIGURE 7.1 Treatment of hypotension in the prebypass period. Once hypotension is identified: (i) supply 100% O_2; (ii) check end-tidal carbon dioxide level ($ETCO_2$) and blood gas; (iii) decrease inhalation agent concentration; (iv) rule out dysrhythmias and technical or mechanical factors. Treat per algorithm. *HR,* heart rate; *MAP,* mean arterial pressure; *PCWP,* pulmonary capillary wedge pressure.

incidence of ischemia. Heart rate greater than 110 beats/min was associated with a 32% to 63% incidence of ischemia [17]. The most likely cause is light anesthesia (sympathetic stimulation) (Table 7.6).

2. Treatment

a. Rule out ventilation abnormalities and correct them if present.

b. Increase anesthetic level if other signs of light anesthesia or BIS monitor changes are seen. An empiric small dose of narcotic is often used.

c. Treat the underlying cause.

(1) Give volume infusion if low preload is evident.

(2) Address the other causes of tachycardia listed in Table 7.5.

(3) β-blockade with esmolol can be used, particularly if ischemia is noted.

TABLE 7.4 Differential diagnosis of hypertension[a]

I. Light anesthesia (increased narcotic requirements are noted in patients with chronic tobacco, alcohol, or caffeine use)	
II. Dissection of sympathetic nerves from the aorta in preparation for aortic cannulation	
III. Hypoxia	
IV. Hypercapnia	
V. Hypervolemia	Rare
VI. Withdrawal syndromes	Rare
A. β-blockers	Rare
B. Clonidine	Rare
C. Alcohol	Rare
VII. Thyroid storm	Rare
VIII. Malignant hyperpyrexia	Rare
IX. Pheochromocytoma	Rare

[a]Causes of hypertension are listed in order of frequency of occurrence.

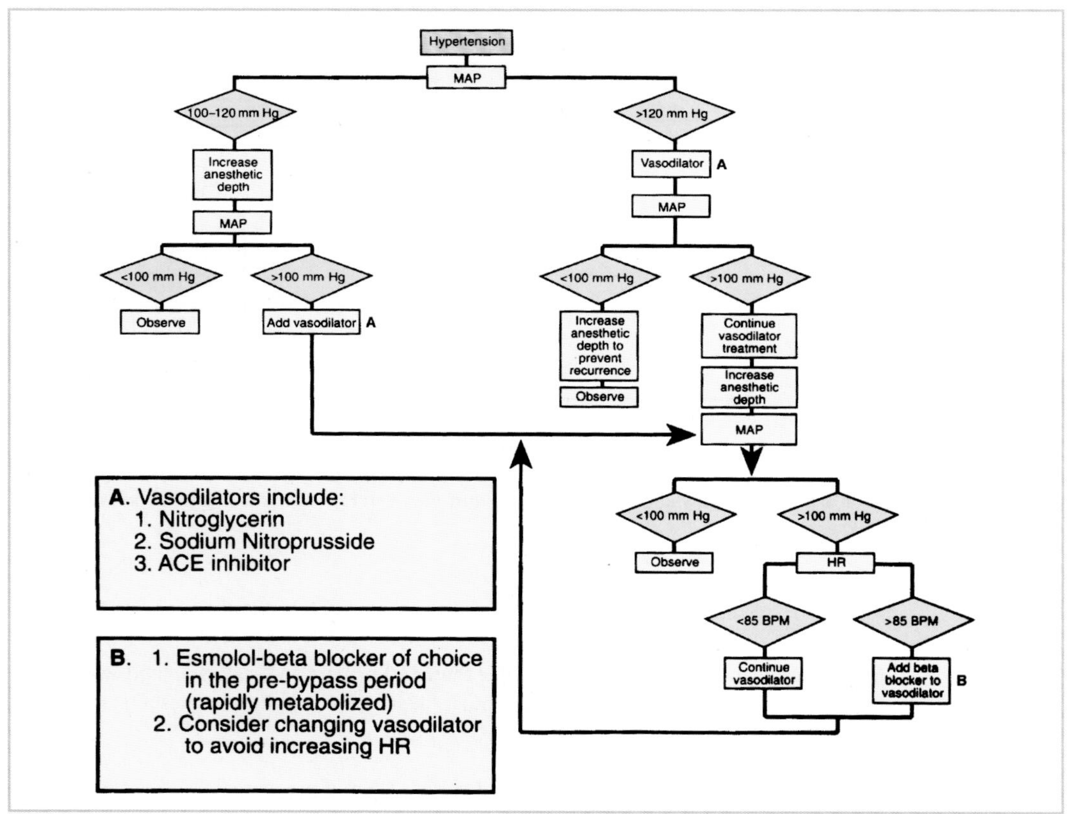

FIGURE 7.2 Treatment of hypertension in the prebypass period. First, rule out technical problems and airway difficulties. HR, heart rate; MAP, mean arterial pressure; ACE, angiotensin converting enzyme.

TABLE 7.5 Differential diagnosis of sinus bradycardia[a]

- **I.** Vagal stimulation
  - **A.** Vagotonic effects of narcotics
  - **B.** Intense surgical stimulation with light plane of anesthesia (e.g., during sternotomy)
    - **1.** Sufentanil more effective than fentanyl, which is more effective than morphine
    - **2.** Associated with rapid administration
    - **3.** Associated with initial dose (less bradycardia occurs with subsequent narcotic doses)
    - **4.** More pronounced when nitrous oxide is not present (nitrous oxide may increase sympathetic tone)
    - **5.** More pronounced with vecuronium, atracurium, or metocurine compared with pancuronium
- **II.** Deep anesthetic levels
- **III.** Hypoxia
- **IV.** β-blockade
- **V.** Calcium channel blockers (verapamil and diltiazem produce greater effects than nifedipine)
- **VI.** Ischemia
- **VII.** Sick sinus syndrome
- **VIII.** Reflex bradycardia secondary to:
  - **A.** Hypervolemia
  - **B.** Hypertension
    - **1.** Secondary to vasoconstrictor use
    - **2.** Secondary to other causes of hypertension (see Table 7.3)

[a]Causes of sinus bradycardia are listed in order of frequency of occurrence.

TABLE 7.6 Differential diagnosis of sinus tachycardia[a]

- **I.** Light anesthesia insufficient for level of surgical stimulation
- **II.** Medications
  - **A.** Pancuronium
  - **B.** Scopolamine
  - **C.** Inotropic agents
  - **D.** Isoflurane
  - **E.** Aminophylline preparations
  - **F.** β-agonists
  - **G.** Monoamine oxidase inhibitors or tricyclic antidepressants
- **III.** Hypovolemia
- **IV.** Ischemia
- **V.** Hypoxia
- **VI.** Hypercapnia
- **VII.** Congestive heart failure
- **VIII.** Withdrawal syndromes (Rare)
  - **A.** β-blockers (Rare)
  - **B.** Clonidine (Rare)
  - **C.** Alcohol (Rare)
- **IX.** Thyroid storm (Rare)
- **X.** Malignant hyperpyrexia (Rare)
- **XI.** Pheochromocytoma (Rare)

[a]Causes of sinus tachycardia are listed in order of frequency of occurrence.

TABLE 7.7 Common causes of dysrhythmias[a]

I. Mechanical stimulation of the heart (e.g., placement of pursestring sutures, cannulation, vent placement, and lifting the heart to study coronary anatomy)
II. Pre-existing dysrhythmias
III. Increase in catecholamine levels
- **A.** Light anesthesia
- **B.** Hypercapnia
- **C.** Nitrous oxide

IV. Direct and indirect autonomic stimulants
- **A.** Pancuronium
- **B.** Inotropic agents
- **C.** Aminophylline preparations
- **D.** β-agonists
- **E.** Monoamine oxidase inhibitors and tricyclic antidepressants

V. Electrolyte abnormalities including hypokalemia
VI. Hypertension
VII. Hypotension
VIII. Ischemia[b]
IX. Hypoxemia

[a]Causes of dysrhythmias are listed in order of frequency of occurrence.
[b]More frequent in patients with severe coronary disease.

E. Dysrhythmias

6 1. The most likely cause of dysrhythmia in the prebypass period is surgical manipulation of the heart (Table 7.7).
2. Treatment
   a. **Treatment of the underlying cause.** Potassium replacement in the pre-CPB period should be limited to treatment for symptomatic hypokalemia because the cardioplegic solution used during CPB may increase the serum potassium level significantly. Magnesium replacement has been useful in patients who have dysrhythmias and are hypomagnesemic.
   b. **Dysrhythmias causing minor hemodynamic disturbances**
      1. Supraventricular tachycardia (including acute atrial fibrillation or flutter)
         (a) Stop mechanical irritation.
         (b) Use vagal maneuvers, adenosine, digoxin, calcium channel blockers, β-blockers, Neo-Synephrine, or edrophonium.
      2. Premature ventricular contractions
         (a) Stop mechanical irritation.
         (b) Treat with lidocaine, procainamide, β-blockers, and amiodarone.
   c. **Dysrhythmias causing major hemodynamic compromise.** Continue chemical resuscitation as in Section b above, concurrent with the following:
      1. Cardioversion or defibrillation for atrial dysrhythmias, ventricular tachycardia, or ventricular fibrillation
         (a) Internal cardioversion
            (i) Small paddles are applied directly to the heart when the chest is open.
            (ii) Low energy levels (10 to 25 J) are needed for cardioversion (skin impedance is bypassed).
            (iii) Synchronization capabilities are desirable for atrial dysrhythmias and ventricular tachycardia. This may require additional cables or equipment.
            (iv) Defibrillation requires similar energy levels in a nonsynchronized mode.
         (b) External cardioversion
            (i) Usual paddle size is used with the chest closed.
            (ii) Energy levels of 25 to 300 J are needed.

(iii) Sterile external paddles are desirable.
(iv) Defibrillation should be initiated with 300 J.

IV. Preparation for CPB

A. Heparinization [18]

1. Unfractionated heparin is the preferred agent for anticoagulation. It is a water-soluble mucopolysaccharide with an average molecular weight of 15,000 Da.
   a. Mechanism of action
      (1) Binds to antithrombin III (AT III), a protease inhibitor
      (2) Increases the speed of the reaction between AT III and several activated clotting factors (II, IX, X, XI, XII, XIII)
   b. Onset time: Immediate.
   c. Half-life: Approximately 2.5 h at usual cardiac surgery dose.
   d. Metabolism
      (1) 50% by liver (heparinase) or reticuloendothelial system
      (2) 50% unchanged by renal elimination
   e. Potency of different preparations may differ markedly.
      (1) Potency is measured in units (not milligrams).
      (2) Heparin solutions usually contain at least 120 to 140 units/mg, depending on the lot or manufacturer.
   f. Protamine sulfate rapidly reverses heparin activity by combining with heparin to form an inactive compound.
   g. **Dosage**
      (1) The initial dosage of heparin for anticoagulation before CPB is 300 units/kg. This initial dose has been established by many investigators. However, some patients may remain inadequately anticoagulated using this dose, so adequate anticoagulation must be established on an individual basis according to the ACT (see Section 3 below).
      (2) Some institutions use a heparin dose–response titration to establish an initial dose.
2. **Routes of administration.** Heparin must be administered directly into a central vein or into the right atrium, with documentation that heparin is being administered into the intravascular space (aspiration to confirm blood return).
3. ACT technique
   a. The ACT monitors the effect of heparin on coagulation. Two milliliters of blood are placed in a tube that contains diatomite (clay), which causes contact activation of the coagulation cascade. The tube is heated to 37°C, and the solution is mixed continuously. The time from introduction of blood into the tube until the first clot is formed is the ACT. This measurement is now automated.
   b. Normal automated ACT is 105 to 167 s.
   c. An ACT of at least 300 s is safe for initiating CPB, provided the ACT is rechecked immediately after starting CPB and heparin (3,000 to 5,000 units) is included in the pump prime.
   d. An ACT greater than 400 s is known to prevent fibrin monomer appearance during CPB. Some institutions require an ACT of 480 s before CPB.
4. Inadequate ACT
   a. Causes of inadequate ACT are listed in Table 7.8.
   b. Treatment of inadequate ACT
      (1) Check ACT before and after heparin administration.
      (2) If ACT is less than 300 s, do not begin CPB.
      (3) Give more heparin in 5,000- to 10,000-unit increments (from different vials or different lots).
      (4) Recheck ACT.
      (5) AT III concentrates as well as recombinant AT III can be given empirically for treatment of presumed AT III deficiency if ACT less than 300 seconds persists despite administration of large doses of heparin (800 to 1,000 units/kg) and if other causes of inadequate ACT are ruled out (Table 7.8).
         (a) If available, a heparin dose–response curve can indicate heparin resistance early in this process.

TABLE 7.8 Causes of inadequate activated clotting time before initiation of cardiopulmonary bypass

Technical causes
Mislabeled syringe
Heparin not injected intravascularly (extravasation, not injected into right atrium, line disconnection)
Heparin having low activity (old or nonrefrigerated vials)
Type of heparin (bovine vs. porcine)
Source of heparin (intestinal vs. lung)
Heparin resistance (most causes related to low AT III levels)
Previous heparin use or ongoing infusion
Nitroglycerin infusion
Hemodilution
Pregnancy or oral contraceptives
IABP
Shock
Streptokinase
Hereditary AT III deficiency
Low-grade disseminated intravascular coagulation
Infective endocarditis
Intracardiac thrombus
Elderly patient

AT III, antithrombin III; IABP, intra-aortic balloon pump. Modified from Anderson EF. Heparin resistance prior to cardiopulmonary bypass. *Anesthesiology.* 1986;64:505, with permission.

(b) If AT III is not available, 2 to 3 units of fresh frozen plasma (FFP) should be given to increase the levels of AT III that presumably are depleted.

(c) Recheck ACT after AT III or FFP is given.

(d) Various alternative anticoagulation regimens have been used in cases of intolerance to unfractionated heparin, including extreme hemodilution, low–molecular-weight heparins, danaparoid, ancrod, r-hirudin, abciximab, tirofiban, argatroban, and others.

B. Cannulation (Fig. 7.3)

1. A pericardial sling is created before cannulation to increase working space and to provide a dam for external cooling fluid and ice slush solution. The sling may lift the heart, which can decrease venous return and lead to hypotension.
2. Pursestring sutures are used to keep the aortic and venous cannulae in place during surgery and to close the incisions after decannulation.
3. Nitrous oxide is discontinued to avoid enlargement of air emboli.
4. Heparin is **always** given before cannulation.
5. The aortic cannula is inserted first to allow infusion of volume in case of hemorrhage associated with venous cannulation. Systolic blood pressure should be decreased to 90 to 100 mm Hg to reduce the risk of aortic dissection and to facilitate cannulation. If necessary, emergency CPB can be instituted using cardiotomy suckers to deliver venous return (the so-called "sucker bypass").
6. The surgical and anesthesia teams both should check the aortic cannula for air bubbles as it is filled with saline and connected to CPB tubing. A test transfusion of 100 mL should be performed to ensure proper placement and functioning of the cannula.
7. If you request an infusion of volume before CPB, make sure the surgical team or the perfusionist does not have any clamps on the tubing.
8. PEEP may be applied to increase intracardiac pressures to avoid air entrainment during cannulation of the right atrium and LV (vent insertion).
9. Complications of cannulation

   a. Aortic cannulation

   (1) Embolic phenomena from air or atherosclerotic plaque dislodgment can occur. Epiaortic echocardiography is sometimes used to identify intimal plaque and to find a "safe" location for the cannula.

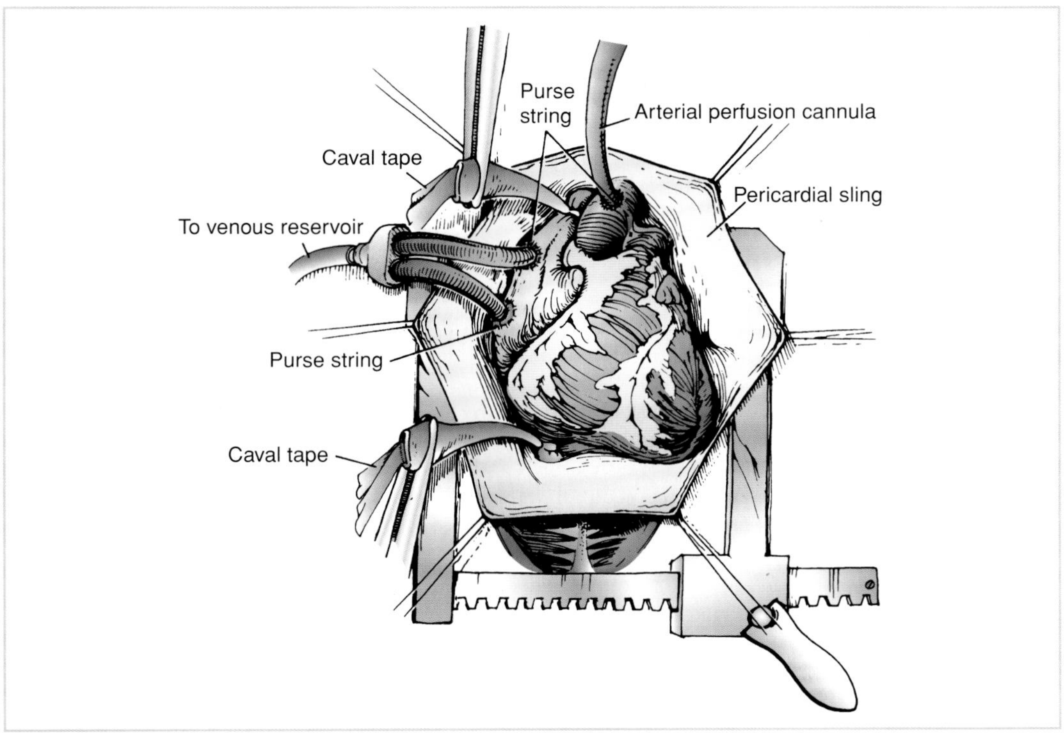

FIGURE 7.3 View of an open chest with formation of a pericardial sling (see text). Note arterial and venous cannulation sites. Caval tapes, placed around the superior and inferior vena cava, are tightened to institute complete CPB (see Chapter 7 for a discussion of complete and partial CPB).

(2) Hypotension

(a) Hypotension is usually secondary to hypovolemia (blood loss).

(b) It may result from mechanical compression of the heart.

(c) A partial occlusion clamp used for cannulation may narrow the aortic lumen (more common in children). Check the aortic pressure immediately when the clamp is applied.

(3) Dysrhythmias are most likely due to surgical manipulation.

(4) Aortic dissection can occur due to cannula misplacement. A pulsatile pressure from the aortic cannula that correlates with the radial mean arterial blood pressure effectively rules out dissection (see Chapter 8 Anesthetic Management during Cardiopulmonary Bypass).

(5) Bleeding

(a) Minor bleeding is not uncommon with cannulation.

(b) Major bleeding may occur if the aorta is torn.

(c) Treatment consists of infusion of volume as needed or initiation of CPB.

(6) Rarely, air entrainment around the cannula occurs, with resultant systemic embolization.

b. Venous cannulation

(1) Hypotension

(a) If hypotension is due to hypovolemia, give volume in 100-mL increments for adults and 10 to 25 mL for pediatric patients through the aortic line as needed.

(b) Mechanical compression of the heart may cause hypotension, especially during inferior vena caval cannulation.

(2) Bleeding
  (a) Bleeding can occur from a tear of the right atrium or the superior or inferior vena cava.
  (b) Treatment is accomplished by infusing volume or initiating emergency CPB.
(3) Dysrhythmias
  (a) Dysrhythmias usually result from surgical manipulation.
  (b) No treatment is required if they do not cause hemodynamic deterioration.
  (c) Cessation or limitation of mechanical stimulation may be all that is necessary.
  (d) Treatment consists of medications, cardioversion, or initiating CPB (see Section III.E).
(4) Air entrainment
  (a) Air entrainment from around the cannula with subsequent signs of pulmonary embolization is possible.

C. Autologous blood removal

1. **Sequestration of platelets and clotting factors.** Autologous blood may be removed to sequester platelets and clotting factors from damage during CPB, with return at the conclusion of CPB. Some practitioners believe this practice enhances coagulation after CPB and decreases the need for transfusion of homologous blood and blood products during this period. However, there is controversy in the literature regarding the benefits of this procedure. Sequestration of platelets and clotting factors can be accomplished in a variety of ways.
2. Techniques
   - **a.** Blood, 500 to 1,000 mL, can be withdrawn in the pre-CPB period and stored in a citrate phosphate dextrose (CPD) solution, similar to banked blood.
   - **b.** Before initiation of bypass, 500 to 1,000 mL of heparinized blood can be removed from the venous bypass drainage line and saved for later infusion.
   - **c.** Plateletpheresis cell salvage equipment can be used in the prebypass period to remove blood, if necessary, from a central venous catheter. After centrifugation, the red cells are returned to maintain hemoglobin levels and O_2 transport. The platelet-poor fraction may be returned to maintain intravascular volume or reserved along with the platelet-rich fraction for later infusion after bypass.
3. **Risks**
   - **a.** Hypotension secondary to hypovolemia. Treat with vasopressors and decrease the withdrawal rate while increasing the infusion rate.
   - **b.** Decreased O_2-carrying capacity, as evidenced by decreased mixed venous oxygenation saturation. Treat with 100% FiO_2, halt blood removal, return red cells as needed, and begin CPB as soon as possible.
   - **c.** **Infection.** Maintain sterile technique for removal and return of blood.
   - **d.** Relative contraindications
     (1) Left main coronary disease or equivalent
     (2) LV dysfunction
     (3) Anemia with hemoglobin less than 12 g/dL
     (4) Emergent surgery

REFERENCES

1. O'Connor JP, Ramsey JG, Wynands JE, et al. The incidence of myocardial ischemia during anesthesia for coronary artery bypass surgery in patients receiving pancuronium or vecuronium. *Anesthesiology.* 1989;70:230–236.
2. Sharma AD, Parmley CL, Sreeram G, et al. Peripheral nerve injuries during cardiac surgery: Risk factors, diagnosis, prognosis, and prevention. *Anesth Analg.* 2000;91:1358–1369.
3. Gandhi GY, Nuttall GA, Abel MD, et al. Intraoperative hyperglycemia and perioperative outcomes in cardiac surgery patients. *Mayo Clin Proc.* 2005;80:862–866.
4. Edwards FH, Engelman RM, Houck P, et al. The Society of Thoracic Surgeons Practice Guidelines Series: Antibiotic prophylaxis in cardiac surgery, part I: Duration. *Ann Thorac Surg.* 2006;81:397–404.
5. Engelman R, Shahian D, Shemin R, et al. The Society of Thoracic surgeons Practice Guideline Series: Antibiotic prophylaxis in cardiac surgery, part II: Antibiotic choice. *Ann Thorac Surg.* 2007;83:1596–1576.

6. Fergusson DA, Hebert PC, Mazer CD, et al. A comparison of aprotinin and lysine analogues in high-risk cardiac surgery. *N Engl J Med.* 2008;358:2319–2331.
7. Martin K, Knorr J, Gertler R, et al. Seizures after open heart surgery: Comparison of Σ-aminocaproic acid and tranexamic acid. *J Cardiothorac Vasc Anesth.* 2011;25:20–25.
8. Perrault LP, Kollpainter R, Page R, et al. Techniques, complications, and pitfalls of endoscopic saphenectomy for coronary artery bypass grafting. *J Card Surg.* 2005;20:393–402.
9. Aronson S, Blumenthal R. Perioperative renal dysfunction and cardiovascular anesthesia: Concerns and controversies. *J Cardiothorac Vasc Anesth.* 1998;12:567–586.
10. Bovill JG, Sebel PS, Stanley TH. Opioid analgesics in anesthesia: With special reference to their use in cardiovascular anesthesia. *Anesthesiology. 1984;61:731–755.*
11. Leslie K, Myles PS, et al. Nitrous oxide and long-term morbidity and mortality in the ENIGMA trial. *Anesth Analg.* 2011; 112:387–393.
12. Sabik JF 3rd, Blackstone EH, Houghtaling PL, et al. Is reoperation still a risk factor in coronary artery bypass surgery? *Ann Thorac Surg.* 2005;80:1719–1727.
13. Bates ER. Ischemic complications after percutaneous transluminal coronary angioplasty. *Am J Med.* 2000;108:309–316.
14. Kamibayashi T, Maze M. Clinical uses of [alpha]2-adrenergic agonists. *Anesthesiology.* 2000;93:1345–1349.
15. Liu S, Carpenter RL, Neal JM. Epidural anesthesia and analgesia: Their role in postoperative outcome. *Anesthesiology.* 1995;82:1474–1506.
16. Hansdottir V, Philip J, Olsen MF, et al. Thoracic epidural versus intravenous patient-controlled analgesia after cardiac surgery: A randomized controlled trial on length of hospital stay and patient-perceived quality of recovery. *Anesthesiology.* 2006;104:142–151.
17. Slogoff S, Keats AS. Randomized trial of primary anesthetic agents on outcome of coronary artery bypass operations. *Anesthesiology.* 1989;70:179–188.
18. Despotis GJ, Gravlee G, Kriton F, et al. Anticoagulation monitoring during cardiac surgery: A review of current and emerging techniques. *Anesthesiology.* 1999;91:1122–1129.

8 Anesthetic Management during Cardiopulmonary Bypass

Neville M. Gibbs and David R. Larach

KEY POINTS

1. Prior to cannulation for cardiopulmonary bypass (CPB), the anesthesiologist must assure that adequate heparin-induced anticoagulation has been achieved, which is typically diagnosed as an activated clotting time (ACT) >400 s.
2. At commencement of CPB, the anesthesiologist should confirm full bypass (typically by loss of pulsatile arterial waveform), discontinue mechanical ventilation, and assess adequacy of perfusion pressure and flow. Other tasks include assessment of adequacy of anesthesia and

neuromuscular blockade, emptying of urine, withdrawing the pulmonary artery (PA) catheter to the proximal PA, and assessment of adequacy of other monitors such as central venous pressure (CVP), electrocardiogram (ECG), and temperature measurement devices.

3. During cardioplegic arrest, the anesthesiologist monitors the adequacy of left ventricular emptying via direct observation of the heart, by ensuring of low cardiac filling pressures, and by the presence of electrical silence on the ECG.
4. Anesthesia during CPB can be maintained with various combinations of volatile agents, opioids, and hypnotic agents (e.g., propofol, midazolam). Especially during hypothermia, maintaining neuromuscular blockade is important in order to avoid spontaneous breathing and visible or subclinical shivering. Anesthetic requirements are reduced during hypothermia.
5. Appropriate perfusion flows and pressures during CPB are controversial, but for most patients a normothermic perfusion index of 2.4 L/min/M^2 and mean arterial pressures (MAPs) of 50 to 70 mm Hg suffice. Continuous monitoring of mixed venous oxygen saturation is useful to assess global perfusion adequacy, as are intermittent arterial blood gas measurements.
6. Moderate hemodilution is useful during CPB, as aided by clear CPB circuit priming solutions. Minimum safe hemoglobin (Hb) concentrations during CPB are controversial, but for most patients Hb ≥ 6.5 g/dL (hematocrit [Hct] ≥ 20%) is safe in the absence of evidence for inadequate oxygen delivery (e.g., metabolic acidosis, low SVO_2).
7. Hypothermia is commonly used during CPB to reduce oxygen consumption and metabolism and to confer organ protection. Often temperatures of 32 to 34°C are used in combination with alpha-stat arterial blood gas management. Rewarming should be accomplished slowly and should not proceed beyond a core temperature of 37°C.
8. Cardioplegic solutions have a variety of "recipes," but most contain a hyperkalemic solution at a low temperature as well as a combination of crystalloid and blood. Cardioplegia can be administered in an antegrade (via coronary arteries) or retrograde (via coronary sinus) direction.
9. CPB can produce catastrophic events such as aortic dissection, cerebral ischemia from aortic cannula malposition, regional venous congestion from venous cannula malposition, venous obstruction from air lock, massive air embolism, pump or oxygenator failure, and blood clots in the extracorporeal circuit.
10. A variety of unusual conditions such as sickle cell disease, cold agglutinin disease, malignant hyperthermia (MH), and angioedema may present during or influence the management of CPB.

I. Preparations for CPB

This requires close communication and coordination between surgeon, perfusionist, and anesthesiologist.

A. Assembling and checking the CPB circuit

The perfusionist assembles the CPB circuit (Fig. 8.1) before commencement of surgery, so that CPB can be instituted rapidly if necessary. The circuit components [e.g., pump (roller or centrifugal), tubing (e.g., standard or heparin-bonded), reservoir (venous and possibly arterial), oxygenator, filters, and safety monitors] are usually decided by institutional preference, but should comply with guidelines of professional organizations. Similarly, the type and volume of CPB prime are decided by the perfusionist in consultation with surgeon and anesthesiologist. The perfusionist checks all components using an approved checklist. See Chapter 21 for details on CPB circuit design and use.

B. Anesthesiologist pre-CPB checklist (Table 8.1)

1 A separate pre-CPB checklist is undertaken by the anesthesiologist (Table 8.1). This includes ensuring that anticoagulation is sufficient for cannulation and CPB (e.g., **ACT > 400 s),** adequate anesthesia will be provided during CPB, fluid infusions are ceased, and monitors are withdrawn to safe positions for CPB (e.g., Swan Ganz catheter, if present, is withdrawn into the proximal PA and a transesophageal echocardiography [TEE] probe, if present, is returned to a neutral position within the esophagus). This is also an appropriate time to empty the urinary catheter drainage bag, and to check the patient's face and pupils so that any changes occurring as a result of CPB can be recognized.

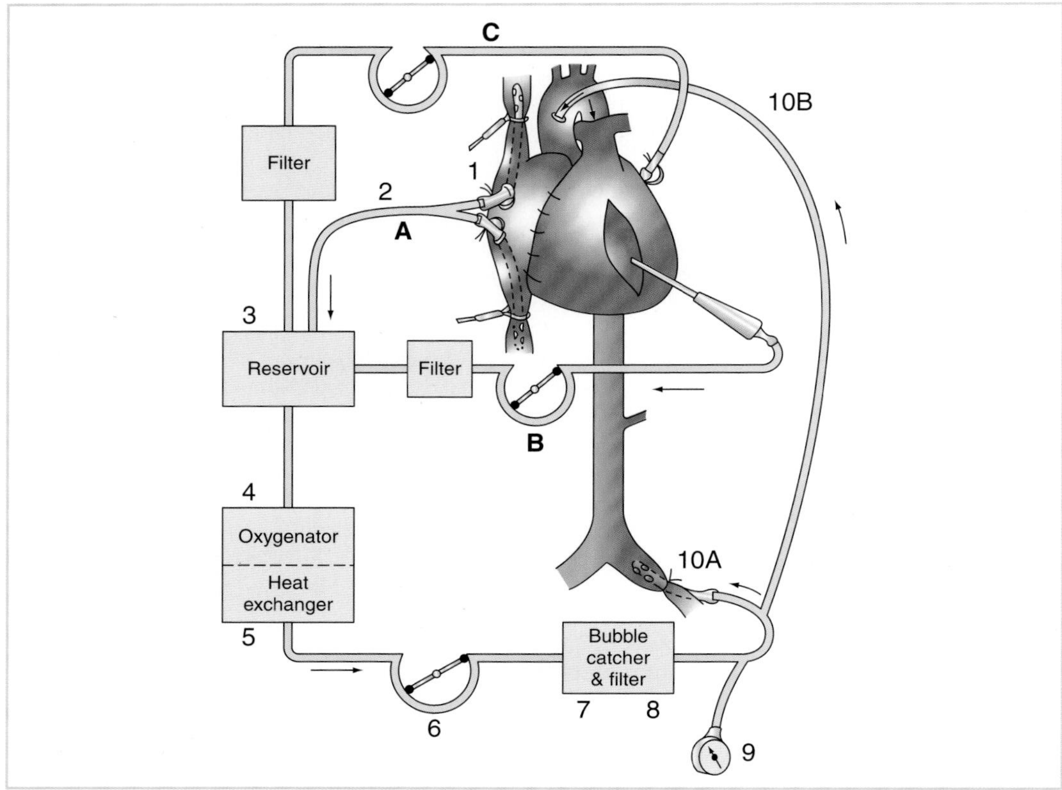

FIGURE 8.1 CPB circuit (example). Blood drains by gravity (or with vacuum assistance) **(A)** from venae cavae (1) through venous cannula (2) into venous reservoir (3). Blood from surgical field suction and from vent is pumped **(B, C)** into cardiotomy reservoir (not shown) and then drains into venous reservoir (3). Venous blood is oxygenated (4), temperature adjusted (5), raised to arterial pressure (6), filtered (7, 8), and injected into either aorta (10B) or femoral artery (10A). Arterial line pressure is monitored (9). Note that items 3, 4, and 5 often are single integral units. (Modified from Nose Y. *The Oxygenator.* St. Louis, MO: Mosby; 1973: 53.)

C. Management of arterial and venous cannulation

In most cases, the arterial cannulation site will be the distal ascending aorta. Prior to cannulation, adequate anticoagulation must be confirmed, and nitrous oxide, if used, must be ceased (to avoid the expansion of any air bubbles inadvertently introduced during cannulation). The anesthesiologist typically reduces the systemic systolic blood pressure to about 80 to 100 mm Hg to reduce the risk of arterial dissection while the cannula is placed. The perfusionist then

TABLE 8.1 Prebypass checklist
Anticoagulation—adequate?
Anesthesia—adequate?
Cannulation—proper and patent?
Infusions turned off
Monitoring in place and checked Pressure transducers Temperatures Urine catheter
Pupils inspected

can check that the pressure trace through the arterial cannula matches the systemic blood pressure trace, which ensures that the **arterial cannula has been placed within the aortic lumen.** If a two-stage venous cannula is selected, the surgeon then inserts the venous cannula into the right atrium and guides the distal stage of the cannula into the inferior vena cava. A separate smaller cannula is guided via the right atrium into the coronary sinus if retrograde cardioplegia is planned. Femoral arterial cannulation may be used if access to the distal ascending aorta is limited, but axillary artery cannulation has become popular in this situation, because this avoids retrograde flow in the often-atherosclerotic thoracic and abdominal aorta. The venous cannula can also be inserted through a femoral vein if necessary, but must be advanced to the right atrium for adequate drainage. In these cases, TEE is required to confirm satisfactory venous cannula position.

II. Commencement of CPB

A. Establishing "full" flow

Once the cannulas are in place and all other checks and observations are satisfactory, the surgeon indicates that CPB should commence. The perfusionist gradually increases the flow of oxygenated blood through the arterial cannula into the systemic circulation. If an arterial cannula clamp is present, this must first be released. At the same time, the venous clamp is gradually released, allowing an increasing proportion of systemic venous blood to drain into the CPB reservoir. Care is taken to match the arterial flow to the venous drainage. Typically, the arterial inflow is increased to equate to a normal cardiac output (CO) for the patient over about 30 to 60 s. The "normal" CO is usually based on a cardiac index of about 2.4 L/min/M^2. This is known as "full flow." At this stage the left ventricle (LV) will have ceased to eject, and the CVP will be close to zero.

B. Initial bypass checklist (Table 8.2)

2 As CPB commences, the anesthesiologist should check the patient's face for asymmetry of color and the patient's pupils for asymmetry of size. Satisfactory oxygenator function should be confirmed by checking the color of the arterial blood and, if available, the in-line PaO_2 or oxygen saturation monitor. Adequate venous drainage is confirmed by the absence of pulsatility in the arterial waveform and low CVP (typically <5 mm Hg).

C. Cessation of ventilation

If the observations of the initial CPB checklist are satisfactory and full flow is established, ventilation of the lungs is ceased, and the airway pressure release valve is opened fully to avoid inflation of the lungs. It is not necessary to disconnect the anesthesia circuit from the anesthesia machine.

D. Monitoring. Patient monitoring during CPB includes continuous **ECG, MAP, CVP, core**
3 **temperature (e.g., nasopharyngeal, tympanic membrane, bladder), blood temperature, and urine output.** Continuous monitoring of arterial and **venous oxygen saturations** and in-line monitoring of arterial blood gases, pH, electrolytes, and Hct are also recommended. Measurement errors may lead to inappropriate management with potentially disastrous consequences, so frequent checks confirming accuracy are advised. Intermittent monitoring of **coagulation (e.g., ACT), laboratory arterial blood gases, electrolytes (including calcium,**

TABLE 8.2 Initial Cardiopulmonary bypass checklist

Face: Examine for color, temperature, plethora, edema, and symmetry
Eyes: Examine pupils for size and symmetry and conjunctiva for chemosis (edema) and injection
Pump lines: Arteriovenous color difference should be visible
Arterial blood pressure: Normally 30–60 mm Hg initially
PA pressure: If monitored, should be <15 mm Hg mean
Central venous pressure: Should be <5 mm Hg
Examine the heart: Distention, contractility
Stop ventilation when aortic ejection by the heart ceases

potassium, blood glucose, and possibly lactate), and Hb are also appropriate. Estimates of Hb and blood glucose can be obtained rapidly using **point-of-care devices.**

III. Typical CPB sequence

A. Typical coronary artery bypass graft (CABG) operation. A typical CABG operation proceeds as follows. Total CPB is initiated and mild-to-moderate hypothermia is either actively induced (30 to 34°C) or permitted to occur passively (sometimes called "drifting"). The aorta is cross-clamped and cardioplegic solution is infused antegrade through the aortic root and/or retrograde via the coronary sinus to arrest the heart. The distal saphenous vein grafts are placed on the most severely diseased coronary arteries first, to facilitate administration of additional cardioplegic solution (via the vein graft) distal to the stenoses. The internal mammary artery anastomosis (if used) is often constructed last because of its fragility and shorter length. Rewarming typically begins when the final distal anastomosis is started. The aorta is unclamped and either an aortic side clamp is applied or an internal occlusive device is used to permit construction of proximal vein graft anastomoses while cardioplegic solution is being washed out of the heart. When it is sufficiently warm, the heart is defibrillated if necessary. Alternatively, the proximal anastomoses are completed with the aortic clamp in place, in order to reduce instrumentation of the aorta (with the risk of dislodging of atheroma). Total CPB continues until the heart is reperfused from its new blood supply. Finally, when the patient is adequately rewarmed and the coronary artery grafts are completed, epicardial pacing wires are placed, and CPB is then terminated.

B. Typical aortic valve replacement or repair operation. After initiation of CPB and application of the aortic cross-clamp, the aortic root is opened, and cardioplegic solution is infused into each coronary ostium under direct vision (to prevent retrograde filling of the LV with cardioplegic solution through an incompetent aortic valve). Commonly, cardioplegia is administered retrograde via the coronary sinus either instead of or in addition to antegrade cardioplegia. The valve is repaired or replaced. Rewarming commences toward the end of valve replacement. The heart is irrigated to remove air or tissue debris, and the aortotomy is closed except for a vent. The aortic cross-clamp is removed (often with the patient in a head-down position) and the heart is defibrillated if necessary. Final de-airing occurs as venous drainage to the pump is retarded, the heart fills and begins to eject (partial CPB), and air is aspirated through the aortic vent, an LV vent, or a needle placed in the apex of the heart. During de-airing, the lungs are inflated to help flush bubbles out of pulmonary veins and the heart chambers, and TEE is viewed to monitor air evacuation.

C. Typical mitral valve replacement or repair operation. This operation is similar to aortic valve surgery (see Section **2** above), except that the left atrium (or right atrium for a trans-atrial septal approach) is opened instead of the aorta and the cardioplegia infusion can take place through the aortic root and the coronary sinus. The valve is replaced or repaired, and a large vent tube is passed through the mitral valve into the LV to prevent ejection of blood into the aorta until de-airing is completed. After thorough irrigation of the field and closure of the atriotomy except for the LV vent, the aortic cross-clamp is removed, often with the patient in a head-down position. The heart is defibrillated if necessary, and de-airing occurs as described above. Finally, the LV vent is removed, and de-airing is completed.

D. Typical combined valve–CABG operation. Usually the distal vein–graft anastomoses are created first, to permit cardioplegia of the myocardium distal to severe coronary stenoses. Also, lifting the heart to access the posterior wall vessels can disrupt myocardium if an artificial valve has been inserted, especially in the case of mitral valve replacement. Next, the valve is operated on, and the operation proceeds as described above.

IV. Maintenance of CPB

A. Anesthesia

1. **Choice of agent and technique.** Just as in the pre-CPB period, anesthesia is typically provided by a **potent volatile agent** or an infusion of **intravenous anesthetic** (e.g., propofol) on a background of **opiates** (e.g., fentanyl, sufentanil) and other **sedative drugs** (e.g., benzodiazepines). Volatile agents have a more defined role in myocardial protection than other anesthetics through ischemic preconditioning and reduction of reperfusion injury [1].

2. **Potent volatile agent via pump oxygenator.** This requires a vaporizer mount in the gas inlet line to the oxygenator. A flow- and temperature-compensated vaporizer, often containing isoflurane, is then attached to the mount. The concentration of agent is typically 0.5 to 1.0 MAC at normothermia, depending on the amount of supplementary opiates and sedatives, and is reduced with hypothermia. With most oxygenators, uptake and elimination of the volatile agent are more rapid than that observed via an anesthesia machine, breathing circuit, and normal lungs and heart. Volatile agent administration can be confirmed by disconnecting the gas analysis line from the airway circuit and reconnecting it to the oxygenator outlet [2]. If volatile agents are used, appropriate scavenging of the oxygenator outlet should be ensured. Nitrous oxide is never used, because of its propensity to enlarge gas-filled spaces, including micro- and macro-gas emboli.
3. **Total intravenous anesthesia.** Total intravenous anesthesia (TIVA) can be provided during CPB using a combination of opiates and sedatives, either by intermittent bolus or by infusion. For propofol, the typical infusion rates are 3 to 6 mg/kg/h or a target plasma concentration of 2 to 4 μg/mL, depending on the use of other IV agents and the patient's temperature. The advantages of TIVA are simplicity, less myocardial depression, and the absence of a need for oxygenator scavenging. However, as with all forms of TIVA, ensuring adequate depth is more difficult, providing greater justification for anesthesia depth monitoring (e.g., bispectral index, entropy) [3,4].
4. **Muscle relaxation.** Movement of the patient during CPB risks cannula dislodgement and should be avoided. If additional muscle relaxants are not used, adequate anesthesia to prevent movement must be ensured. As in the pre-CPB period, train-of-four monitoring can be titrated to a level of approximately one twitch. Similarly, spontaneous breathing must be avoided, as this risks the development of negative vascular pressures and potential air entrainment.
5. **Effect of temperature.** Anesthetic requirements fall as temperature drops. However, due to its relatively high blood supply, brain temperature changes faster than core temperature. For this reason, particular care should be taken to ensure **adequate anesthesia** as soon as **rewarming commences,** and additional opiates or sedatives may be required. When the patient is normothermic, anesthetic requirements are the same as the pre-CPB phase, although the context-sensitive half-time for most anesthetic drugs increases substantially during and after CPB.
6. **Monitoring anesthetic depth. Awareness** may be difficult to exclude clinically due to the use of high-dose opiates, cardiovascular drugs (e.g., β-adrenergic blockers), and muscle relaxants. Moreover, hemodynamic cues cannot be used during CPB. The patient should be checked for pupillary dilation and sweating, but these signs may be affected by opiate medication and rewarming. Therefore, emphasis should be placed on ensuring delivery of adequate anesthesia, or the use of depth-of-anesthesia monitors [3,4].
7. **Altered pharmacokinetics and pharmacodynamics.** The onset of CPB increases the circulating blood volume by the amount of the priming solution for the extracorporeal circuit, but the percentage change in the total volume of distribution of most anesthetic agents is minimal. Neuromuscular blockers constitute an exception to this; hence, they may require supplementation at the onset of CPB. Hemodilution reduces the concentration of plasma proteins, increasing the unbound active proportion of many drugs (e.g., propofol) to offset the reduced total plasma concentration induced by the increased circulating blood volume [5]. A small proportion of some agents (e.g., fentanyl, nitroglycerin) may be absorbed onto the foreign surfaces of the CPB circuit. Hypothermia reduces the rate of drug metabolism and elimination, as does reduction in blood flow to the liver and kidneys. Bypassing the lungs reduces pulmonary metabolism and sequestration of certain drugs and hormones. Reduced blood supply to vessel-poor tissues such as muscle and fat may result in sequestration of drugs given pre-CPB. The response to drugs may also be altered by hypothermia and hemodynamic alterations associated with CPB. The combined effect of these pharmacological changes may be difficult to predict, so the **principle of titrating drugs** to achieve a certain endpoint is particularly important during CPB.

B. Hemodynamic management. See also Chapter 19.

1. **Systemic perfusion flow rate.** The most fundamental hemodynamic change during CPB is the generation of the CO by the CPB pump rather than the patient's heart. The perfusionist regulates the CPB pump to deliver the desired perfusion flow rate for the patient. This is usually based on a nomogram taking into consideration the patient's height
5 and weight and the core temperature. Typically the perfusion flow rate is set to deliver an effective perfusion flow rate of **2.4 L/min/M^2 at 37°C and about 1.5 L/min/M^2 at 28°C.** The amount delivered by the CPB pump is usually set slightly higher than the target flow rate to account for any recirculation within the CPB circuit. For example, a continuous flow of about 200 mL/min from the arterial line filter may be returned to the reservoir through a purge line to provide a mechanism for purging trapped microbubbles. An **inadequate perfusion flow rate** will result in a **low venous Hb oxygen saturation** (continuously monitored in the CPB venous return), and the development of a **metabolic acidosis** due to anaerobic metabolism and the accumulation of **lactic acid.** If other causes for a low venous Hb oxygen saturation can be excluded (e.g., excessive hemodilution, inadequate anesthesia, over-rewarming to increase metabolism), the perfusion flow rate should be increased accordingly. Unfortunately, a normal venous oxygen saturation does not confirm adequate perfusion of all tissues. **Shunting** may occur leaving some tissue beds underperfused. An increased metabolic rate due to shivering, which may be subclinical during hypothermia, or to much more unlikely causes such as thyrotoxicosis or MH, may also reduce venous HbO_2 saturations despite normal flow rates.
2. **MAP.** The optimum MAP during CPB is not known. Systolic and diastolic pressures are generally of no concern, because the vast majority of CPB is conducted using nonpulsatile flow. If an adequate perfusion flow rate is delivered, the MAP *may* be irrelevant, so long as the **limits of autoregulation** have not been exceeded, and also there is **no critical stenosis** in the arterial supply to individual organs. A higher MAP than necessary should be avoided to reduce noncoronary collateral blood flow (which may wash out cardioplegia). In adults, a conservative approach is usually taken, maintaining the MAP between **50 and 70 mm Hg.** Higher levels may be required in patients with **pre-existing hypertension** or known **cerebrovascular disease.** Lower levels may be tolerated in children. This range of MAP assumes a CVP < 5 mm Hg. The possibility of **measurement error due to inappropriate position of the pressure transducers or zero drift should be checked frequently.**
3. **Hypotension.** The most important consideration in the management of hypotension is to ensure that an adequate perfusion flow rate is being delivered. While a transient reduction of perfusion flow rate (such as may be requested by the surgeon at particular stages of the procedure) is of little consequence, sustained reductions must be avoided. Once adequate perfusion flow rate is confirmed, the MAP may be corrected by increasing the systemic vascular resistance (SVR) with the use of vasoconstrictors such as phenylephrine (0.5 to 10 μg/kg/min, or noradrenaline 0.03 to 0.3 μg/kg/min), on the basis of the following relationship:

$$\mathbf{SVR = (MAP - CVP)/effective\ perfusion\ flow\ rate\ (L/min)}$$

where MAP is expressed in mm Hg, CVP in mm Hg, and SVR in mm Hg/L/min (to convert to dyne.s.cm^{-5}, multiply by 80).

As there is substantial individual variability in response to vasoconstrictors, especially during CPB, the dose should be titrated, commencing with less potent agents (e.g., phenylephrine) or smaller doses, and progressing to higher doses of more potent agents (e.g., noradrenaline) if required. Occasionally vasopressin (e.g., 0.01 to 0.05 units/min) is required. The perfusion flow rate can be increased above normal to correct hypotension temporarily (e.g., while vasoconstrictors take effect), but this is not an appropriate strategy to correct persistent hypotension. The onset of CPB is typically associated with sudden **hemodilution,** which decreases SVR. **Cardioplegia solution** entering the circulation also reduces SVR and is a common cause of hypotension. Reperfusion of the myocardium after release of the aortic cross-clamp is another common cause of transient hypotension. For these reasons, the use of vasoconstrictors during CPB is common. (Reduced SVR constitutes an oft-underutilized opportunity for communication between the perfusionist and the anesthesia team. Perfusionists can at times create a "roller coaster" with frequent intermittent boluses of phenylephrine at times when MAP management would be smoother if the anesthesiologist would initiate a continuous phenylephrine infusion.)

4. **Hypertension.** Hypertension is usually the result of an increase in SVR, which may be due to endogenous sympathetic stimulation or hypothermia. Before treating hypertension with direct vasodilators (e.g., nitroglycerin 0.1 to 10 μg/kg/min, sodium nitroprusside 0.1 to 2 μg/kg/min, nicardipine 2 to 5 mg/h), **adequate anesthesia** should be ensured. Artifactual hypertension due to aortic cannula malposition should also be excluded (see I.C and VII.A). The perfusion flow rate can be decreased below normal to correct hypertension temporarily (e.g., while vasodilators take effect), but not to correct persistent hypertension. Hypertension should be avoided during all **aortic cross-clamp manipulations,** including the application and release of side-biting clamps.
5. **Central venous pressure.** With appropriate venous drainage, the CVP should be low (0 to 5 mm Hg). A persistently high CVP indicates poor venous drainage, which may require adjustment of the venous cannula or cannulas by the surgeon. Venous drainage can also be improved slightly by raising the operating table height, thereby increasing the hydrostatic gradient between the heart and the venous reservoir. Increasingly in recent years, suction (vacuum-assisted venous drainage) is applied to the venous reservoir, especially for miniaturized circuits (see Chapter 21), during which one should suspect excessive suction if the CVP reading should fall to levels below −5 mm Hg. As the CVP is a low-range pressure, it is very sensitive to measurement errors (e.g., hydrostatic gradient between transducer and right atrium). Care should also be taken to ensure that the catheter measuring the CVP is in a large central vein and is not snared by surgical tapes.

C. **Fluid management and hemodilution**

1. **CPB Prime.** The CPB circuit is "primed" with a balanced isotonic crystalloid solution, to which colloids, mannitol, or buffers may be added, depending on perfusionist, anesthesiologist, and surgical preference (see Chapter 21). CPB prime also contains a small dose of heparin (e.g., 5,000 to 10,000 units) and a dose of the antifibrinolytic agent being used (e.g., aminocaproic acid 5 g). The volume of the prime depends on the circuit components, but is typically about 800 to 1,200 mL for adults, and can be even lower when a miniaturized system is used (see Chapter 21).
2. **Hemodilution.** The use of a non-sanguineous prime inevitably results in hemodilution. The degree of hemodilution on commencement of CPB can be estimated prior to CPB by multiplying the Hb concentration (or Hct) prior to CPB by the ratio of the patient's estimated blood volume to the patient's estimated blood volume *plus* the CPB prime volume. Moderate hemodilution is usually well tolerated, because oxygen delivery remains adequate and oxygen requirements are often reduced during CPB, especially if hypothermia is used. Moderate hemodilution may also be beneficial, because it reduces blood viscosity, which counters the increase in blood viscosity induced by hypothermia.
3. **Limits of hemodilution.** While the safe limit of hemodilution during CPB in individual patients is not known, a conservative approach is to **avoid Hb levels <6.5 g/dL (approximately an Hct of 20%).** If the estimated degree of hemodilution on commencement of CPB is too low, allogeneic red blood cells (RBCs) can be added to the CPB prime. This is particularly important for smaller patients (due to their lower estimated blood volumes) (e.g., pediatric patients), and anemic patients. If venous oxygen saturations are low during CPB despite normal effective perfusion flow rates, excessive hemodilution as a cause should be considered, and additional RBCs added if necessary. Similarly, inadequate oxygen delivery will result in anaerobic metabolism and the development of **acidosis.** Patients with **known stenoses** of cerebral or renal arteries may be **less tolerant** of hemodilution.
4. **Time course of hemodilution.** During the course of CPB, crystalloid fluid will diffuse from the vascular to the extracellular space and also will be filtered by the kidney, gradually reducing the extent of hemodilution. However, **crystalloid cardioplegia** returning to the

circulation will increase hemodilution, as will the addition of other crystalloids or colloids used to replace blood loss or redistribution of fluid into nonvascular compartments.

5. **Monitoring hemodilution.** The Hb (or Hct) should be measured frequently (e.g., every 30 to 60 min) (if possible, it should be monitored continuously), especially if there is ongoing blood loss, or low mixed venous oxygen saturations.
6. **Acute normovolemic hemodilution.** In adult patients with average (or greater) body size and normal preoperative Hb, acute normovolemic hemodilution prior to, or at the time of commencement of, CPB should be considered. Typically, 1 to 2 units of anticoagulated blood are collected, and replaced with colloids or a combination of crystalloids and colloids. This blood, containing pre-CPB Hb, platelet, and clotting factor levels can be re-infused post-CPB.
7. **Allogeneic blood transfusion.** The trigger for allogeneic RBC transfusion varies between institutions, and will depend also on patient and surgical factors. Conservative triggers are an Hb <6.5 g/dL during the maintenance phase of CPB, and <8.0 g/dL at the time of separation, although **lower levels** may be tolerated in selected patients.
8. **Cardiotomy suction.** Shed blood may be returned to the CPB circuit using cardiotomy suction. However, shed blood often contains activated coagulation and fibrinolytic factors, especially if exposed to the pericardium. Excessive cardiotomy suction may also be associated with hemolysis, especially if there is co-aspiration of air. For this reason, some choose to return only brisk blood loss to the CPB circuit. An alternative is separate cell salvage with washing of RBCs before returning them to the CPB circuit.
9. **Fluid replacement.** Fluid may be lost from the circuit through blood loss, redistribution to other compartments, and filtration by the kidney. A reduction in the circulating blood volume will manifest as a fall in the CPB reservoir fluid level. A falling CPB reservoir fluid level is dangerous, as it reduces the margin of safety for air embolism. In many circuits an alarm will be activated if the reservoir volume falls to unsafe levels. The replacement fluid is typically crystalloid with colloid added depending on perfusionist, surgeon, and anesthesiologist preference.
10. **Diuresis and ultrafiltration.** Occasionally the return of cardioplegia solution to the CPB circuit, or contraction of the vascular space by vasoconstrictors or hypothermia, will cause reservoir level to increase. If high levels persist, diuresis can be encouraged by the use of diuretic agents such as furosemide or mannitol. Alternatively, an ultrafiltration device can be added to the circuit to remove water and electrolytes (see Chapter 21).
11. **Urine production** should be identified and quantified as a sign of adequate renal perfusion and to assist in appropriate fluid management. Very high urine flow rates (e.g., >300 mL/h) may be seen during hemodilution (due to low plasma oncotic pressure), especially if mannitol is also present in the priming solution. Oliguria (less than 1 mL/kg/h) should prompt an investigation, because it may indicate inadequate renal perfusion. However, some hypothermic patients demonstrate oliguria without an apparent cause. Kinking of urinary drainage catheters should be excluded.

D. **Management of anticoagulation** (see also Chapter 19)

1. **Monitoring anticoagulation.** The ACT or a similar rapid test of anticoagulation must periodically confirm adequate anticoagulation (e.g., ACT > 400 s; see also Chapter 19). The ACT should optimally be checked after initiating CPB and every 30 min thereafter. The ACT can be checked within 2 min of administering heparin [6]. As the ACT falls over time, often a higher target is chosen (e.g., >500 s), so that the lowest ACT remains >400 s. During periods of **normothermia,** heparin elimination is faster, so a requirement for heparin supplementation is more likely.
2. **Additional heparin** is usually given in 5,000 to 10,000 unit increments, and the ACT is repeated to confirm an adequate response. Use of fully heparin-coated circuits does not eliminate the need for heparin; an ACT of 400 s or greater is often recommended [7].
3. **Heparin resistance** is a term used to describe the inability to achieve adequate heparinization despite conventional doses of heparin. It may be due to a variety of causes, but it is most common in patients who have received heparin therapy for several days

preoperatively. Most cases will respond to **increased doses of heparin.** However, if an ACT > 400 s cannot be achieved despite heparin > 600 units/kg, consideration should be given to administering **supplemental antithrombin III** (AT-III). A dose of 1,000 units of AT-III concentrate will increase the AT-III level in an adult by about 30%. Fresh frozen plasma, 2 to 4 units, is a less expensive alternative, but it is less specific and carries the risk of infective and other complications. For a detailed discussion of heparin resistance and AT-III deficiency, see Chapter 19.

E. **Temperature management**

1. **Benefits of hypothermia.** Hypothermia during CPB reduces metabolic rate and oxygen requirements and provides organ protection against ischemia.
2. **Disadvantages of hypothermia.** Hypothermia may promote coagulation abnormalities, and may increase the risk of microbubble formation during rewarming. Hypothermia shifts the Hb oxygen saturation curve to the left, reducing peripheral oxygen delivery, but this is countered by the reduced oxygen requirements.
3. **Choice of maintenance temperature.** The optimal temperature during the maintenance phase of CPB is not known. Typically the patient's core temperature at the onset of CPB is 35 to 36°C. Core temperature is usually measured in the **nasopharynx or tympanic**
7 **membrane,** but the bladder or esophagus may also be used. The target temperature is chosen on the basis of the type and length of surgical procedure, patient factors, and surgical preference. Often the temperature is allowed to drift lower without active cooling. Alternatively, the heat exchanger is used to provide moderate hypothermia, which may be as low as 28°C, but is more often 32°C or above. If there is a concern about the adequacy of myocardial protection, lower temperatures may be used (see also Chapter 23).
4. **Slow cooling.** Lack of response of the **nasopharyngeal or tympanic temperature** during the cooling phase may indicate **inadequate brain cooling,** and should prompt investigation of the cause (e.g., ineffective heat, exchanger, inadequate cerebral perfusion). The position and function of the temperature monitor should also be checked to exclude artifactual causes.
5. **Deep hypothermic circulatory arrest** (DHCA). For certain surgical procedures in which circulatory arrest is required (e.g., repairs of the aortic arch), deep hypothermia is used as part of a **strategy to prevent cerebral injury.** The typical target temperature prior to circulatory arrest is about 15 to 17°C. Other strategies to minimize injury include limiting the period of circulatory arrest to as short a time as possible, **anterograde or retrograde cerebral perfusion** during the period of DHCA, and **pharmacological protection** using **barbiturates** (e.g., thiopental 10 mg/kg), **corticosteroids** (e.g., methylprednisolone 30 mg/kg), and **mannitol** (0.25 to 0.5 g/kg). These must be given before DHCA is commenced (see also Chapter 25). Achieving deep neuromuscular blockade (0–1 twitches on train-of-four) prior to DHCA is advisable.
6. **Rewarming.** Rewarming commences early enough to ensure that the patient's core temperature has returned to 37°C by the time the surgical procedure is completed, so that separation from CPB is not delayed. The surgeon will usually advise the perfusionist when rewarming should commence, taking into account the patient's core temperature at the time, how long the patient has been at this temperature, and the patient's body size. The rate of rewarming is limited by the **maximum safe temperature gradient** between the water temperature in the heat exchanger and the blood (<10°C, some centers use a maximum of 6 to 8°C). Higher gradients risk the formation of microbubbles. Typically, patients' core temperature rises no faster than 0.3°C/min. Vasodilators may facilitate rewarming by improving distribution of blood and permitting higher pump flow rates.
7. **Hypothermia and arterial blood gas analysis.** Hypothermia increases the solubility of oxygen and carbon dioxide, thereby reducing their partial pressures. However, arterial blood gas measurement is performed at 37°C, so the values have to be "temperature corrected" to the patient's blood temperature if the values at the patient's blood temperature are required. The reduced PaO_2 is of limited clinical significance, so long as increased fractions of oxygen are administered ($FiO_2 > 0.5$). However, the reduced $PaCO_2$ produces an apparent

respiratory alkalosis when temperature-corrected values are used. To keep the pH normal **(pH stat)** it would be necessary to add CO_2 to the oxygenator. The alternative is to avoid temperature correction of arterial blood gases and accept that the **degree of dissociation of H^+** also varies with temperature **(alpha stat).** With this strategy there is no requirement to add CO_2 to maintain neutrality. These complex biochemical considerations are avoided by using **non–temperature-corrected values,** and making decisions based on the values measured at 37°C, irrespective of the patient's blood temperature. See Chapter 24 for detailed discussion of arterial blood gas management.

8. **Shivering.** Shivering should not occur if adequate anesthesia is provided, especially if a muscle relaxant is administered.

F. **ECG management.** Isolated atrial and ventricular ectopic beats are common during cardiac manipulation and require no specific intervention. If ventricular fibrillation occurs before aortic cross-clamp placement, defibrillation may be required. Ventricular fibrillation once the aortic cross-clamp has been placed is likely to be short-lived because the delivery of cardioplegia will achieve cardiac standstill. Persistent ventricular fibrillation indicates ineffective cardioplegia. Return of electrical activity after cardioplegic arrest suggests washout of cardioplegia solution. The surgeon should be notified as additional cardioplegia may be required. Ventricular fibrillation may occur during the rewarming phase after the release of the aortic cross-clamp. This often resolves spontaneously, but may require defibrillation, especially if the patient remains hypothermic.

G. **Myocardial protection** (see also Chapter 23)

1. **Cardioplegia.** When the myocardial blood supply is interrupted by the placement of an aortic cross-clamp, cardioplegic arrest of the myocardium is required. The **antegrade technique** is achieved by administering cardioplegia solution into the aortic root between the aortic valve and aortic clamp. The interval between the placement of the cross-clamp and the administration of the cardioplegia is kept to a minimum (no more than a few seconds) to prevent any warm ischemia. The cardioplegia solution is typically high in potassium, arresting the heart in diastole. The solution is typically cold (8 to 12°C) to provide further protection, although warm continuous cardioplegic techniques are used in some institutions. Cardioplegic solutions may be entirely crystalloid or may be mixed with blood **(blood cardioplegia)**. Cardioplegia may also be administered **retrograde** through a catheter in the **coronary sinus.** In patients with aortic regurgitation, administration of cardioplegia directly into the left and right coronary ostia may be required. Cardioplegia is typically given intermittently every 20 to 30 min, but may be given continuously.

8

2. **Cold.** Most myocardial protection techniques involve cold cardioplegia, and ice may be placed around the heart to provide further protection. Systemic hypothermia, if used, contributes to keeping the myocardium cold.
3. **Venting.** During cross-clamping, vents are typically placed in the aortic root to ensure that the heart does not distend. For open-chamber procedures vents are placed also in the left atrium or LV to remove both blood and air. Inadequate venting may result in the **development of tension** in the LV, causing potential ischemia and **subendocardial necrosis.** The coronary perfusion pressure for cardioplegia is also reduced.
4. **Avoiding electrical activity.** See Section IV.F above.

H. **Arterial blood gas and acid–base management**

1. **Alpha stat or pH stat strategy?** (see Section IV.E.7 and Chapter 24)
2. The **arterial PO_2** is maintained between **150 and 300 mm Hg** by adjusting the percentage oxygen in the sweep (analogous to inspired) gas delivered to the oxygenator. **Arterial hypoxemia** may indicate **inadequate oxygenator sweep gas flow** (or leak) or **inadequate oxygen percentage** in the oxygenator sweep gas. Alternatively, it may indicate **oxygenator dysfunction.**
3. The **arterial PCO_2** is maintained at approximately **40 mm Hg** by adjusting the sweep gas flow rate through the oxygenator. There is an inverse relationship between the sweep gas flow rate and the arterial PCO_2. **Hypercapnea** (PCO_2 > 45 mm Hg) should be avoided as it is associated with sympathetic stimulation and **respiratory acidosis.** Hypercapnea may be caused by an inadequate sweep gas flow rate, absorption of CO_2 used to flood

the wound during open chamber procedures [8], or increased CO_2 production. The administration of bicarbonate also increases the P_{CO_2}. **Hypocapnea** (P_{CO_2} < 35 mm Hg) should also be avoided as it is associated with **respiratory alkalosis and left shift of the HbO_2 dissociation curve** (further reducing oxygen delivery), and **cerebral vasoconstriction.**

4. **Metabolic acidosis** (e.g., lactic acidosis) is prevented where possible by ensuring adequate oxygen delivery and tissue perfusion. Severe metabolic acidosis should be corrected cautiously with the use of sodium bicarbonate. If unexplained acidosis occurs with signs of an increased metabolic rate (e.g., low mixed venous oxygen saturations, elevated P_{CO_2}), malignant hyperthermia (MH) should be considered.

I. **Management of serum potassium and sodium**

1. **Hyperkalemia** may occur when cardioplegia solution (which contains high potassium concentrations) enters the circulation. This is usually mild or transient unless **large amounts of cardioplegia** are used, or the patient has **renal dysfunction.** Hyperkalemia more often follows the first dose of hyperkalemia than later ones, because both the volume and potassium concentration are typically higher for the initial cardioplegia solution. Hyperkalemia can cause **heart block, negative inotropy,** and **arrhythmias.** Hyperkalemia can be treated by promoting potassium elimination by loop diuretics (e.g., **furosemide**) or by **ultrafiltration.** Potassium can also be shifted into cells by the administration of **insulin and glucose,** or by creating an **alkalosis.** In rare cases, **hemodialysis** is required. If the patient has severe renal dysfunction or the serum potassium remains above the normal range, the cardioplegia delivery technique should be modified to ensure that cardioplegia is vented separately and not returned to the circulation.
2. **Hypokalemia.** If a patient is hypokalemic, initiating K^+ replacement during CPB is much safer than waiting until after bypass, thus avoiding hypokalemic dysrhythmias during CPB weaning or potential cardiac arrest during rapid K^+ replacement post-CPB.
3. **Sodium.** Serum sodium should be maintained within the normal range where possible. Rapid corrections should be avoided due to the risk of acute changes in **intracranial pressure** as a result of the changes in **plasma osmolality.**

J. **Management of blood glucose**

1. **Hyperglycemia.** Glucose tolerance is often impaired during CPB due to the stress response associated with CPB, as well as from insulin resistance induced by hypothermia. Hyperglycemia may exacerbate neuronal injury and increase the risk of wound infection. Blood glucose should be measured frequently, especially in patients with diabetes mellitus. Glucose containing fluids should be avoided. Blood glucose should optimally be maintained below 180 mg/dL, which may require the infusion of insulin.
2. **Hypoglycemia.** Hypoglycemia should be avoided at all costs during CPB, because severe hypoglycemia is associated with neurological injury within a short period, and the signs of hypoglycemia are masked by both the anesthesia and the hemodynamic changes during CPB. Blood glucose should be measured more frequently if patients are receiving insulin or have received hypoglycemic agents preoperatively on the day of surgery.

V. Rewarming, aortic cross-clamp release, and preparation for weaning

A. **Rewarming.** On commencement of rewarming, **additional anesthetics** may be required, because the brain rewarms faster then the body core. **Additional heparin** may be required, because the rate of metabolism of heparin returns to normal at normothermia. The extent of **hemodilution** should be re-assessed because oxygen requirements increase during rewarming (see also Section IV.E.6 above).

B. **Release of aortic cross-clamp**

1. **De-airing.** Air may collect in the pulmonary veins, left atrium, or LV, particularly during open chamber procedures. This is aspirated through the aortic root vent prior to cross-clamp release or other vents. Temporarily raising the CVP and inflating the lungs will fill the LV and permit easier surgical aspiration of intracavity air. Residual air can be detected using TEE [9]. Flushing the surgical field with CO_2 prior to cardiac chamber closure [8] may reduce residual air, as CO_2 is reabsorbed much faster than air.

2. **Blood pressure.** Hypertension should be avoided at the time of aortic cross-clamp release. Transient hypotension may occur after the release of the cross-clamp due to residual cardioplegia or metabolites returning to the circulation as the myocardium is reperfused.

C. **Preparation for weaning from CPB.** In preparation for weaning from CPB, cardiac **pacing equipment** is attached and checked, **electrolytes and acid–base** disturbances are corrected if necessary, an adequate **Hb** is ensured, and additional **inotropic drug infusions** (e.g., epinephrine, dobutamine) required for the weaning process are prepared and attached to the patient. If **loading doses** of inodilators (e.g., milrinone) or calcium sensitizers (e.g., levosimendan) are required, these should be given before completion of CPB. If the negative inotropic effects of volatile agents are a concern, they should be ceased before weaning commences, and other agents used to maintain adequate anesthesia. Anesthetic management of weaning from CPB is covered in Chapter 9.

VI. Organ protection during CPB

A. **Renal protection.** The most important renal protective strategy is to ensure adequate renal perfusion during CPB by **optimal fluid loading, appropriate pump flow rates,** close attention to the **renal perfusion pressure,** and avoidance of intravascular **hemolysis and hemoglobinuria.** It may be possible to reduce the risk of development of acute renal failure through the use of drugs to increase renal blood flow and urine production, although there is no definitive evidence to support their routine use. **Mannitol,** low-dose dopamine, furosemide, prostaglandin E, and fenoldopam (a selective dopamine-1 receptor agonist) have been advocated for use in high-risk patients during CPB, particularly if oliguria is present. Of these, fenoldopam 0.05 to 0.10 μg/kg/min shows the most promise [10]. *N*-acetylcysteine (a free-radical scavenger) and urinary alkalinization have also been used. **Hemolysis and hemoglobinuria** are managed by correcting the cause where possible, and by promoting a diuresis.

B. **Brain protection** during CPB involves ensuring adequate **cerebral perfusion** pressure (MAP-CVP) and oxygen delivery, and measures to prevent increases in intracranial pressure (which will reduce cerebral perfusion pressure). Mild or moderate **hypothermia** is often used to provide additional protection, and **deep hypothermia** if circulatory arrest is required (see also Section IV.E.5 above). Care is taken to **avoid emboli,** both particulate (e.g., atheroma) and gaseous, by meticulous surgical and perfusion technique. Brain protection is covered in detail in Chapter 24.

C. **Myocardial protection.** See Section IV.G above.

D. **Inflammatory response to CPB.** CPB is one of the main factors contributing to the inflammatory response associated with cardiac surgery. Reactions are usually mild or subclinical, but may be severe in some cases and contribute to brain, lung, renal, or myocardial injury. For a detailed discussion of this inflammatory response to CPB and cardiac surgery, see Chapter 21.

1. **Etiology**

   a. **Exposure of blood to circuit components.** The extensive contact between circulating blood and the extracorporeal circuit results in variable amounts of thrombin generation, activation of complement, release of cytokines, and expression of immune mediators, all of which may contribute to the inflammatory response.

   b. **Return of shed blood to the CPB circuit.** Shed blood is in contact with mediastinal tissues (e.g., pericardium) and air, and is exposed to shear stress when suction is used. It is a potent source of activated coagulation factors and inflammatory mediators and may cause hypotension when returned to the bypass circuit. Unless bleeding is brisk or stasis is minimal, shed blood should not be returned directly to the CPB circuit. A cell saver can be used to conserve red blood cells.

   c. **Ischemia** due to inadequate tissue perfusion or organ protection

   d. **Endotoxemia** due to **splanchnic hypoperfusion**

2. **Prevention**

   Severe reactions are difficult to predict or prevent. Adequate anticoagulation, organ perfusion, and myocardial protection are fundamental. **Biocompatible surface coated circuits** may be beneficial. The use of miniature bypass circuits, steroids, and leuco-depletion filters are controversial. Fibrinolysis can be reduced by the use of **aminocaproic or tranexamic acid.** Novel anti-inflammatory agents (e.g., pexelizumab) [11] remain investigational, but as yet have no proven benefit.

3. **Management**

Low SVR and evidence of capillary leak may be observed during CPB, but most reactions manifest post-CPB. No specific therapy is available and management is supportive.

VII. Prevention and management of CPB catastrophes (see also Chapter 21)

The safe conduct of perfusion requires vigilance on the parts of the perfusionist, anesthesiologist, and cardiac surgeon to ensure that perfusion-related problems are prevented where possible, and diagnosed early and managed quickly if they occur. Appropriate training, expertise, and accreditation of all personnel are required, and adherence to protocols and checklists is encouraged. The following complications must be actively sought during initiation of CPB. They may, however, occur at any time during CPB [12]. **Prevention is paramount.**

A. Malposition of arterial cannula

9 1. **Aortic dissection.** If the cannula orifice is situated within the arterial wall, not in the true lumen, there is a risk of aortic dissection upon commencement of CPB. Therefore, either arterial cannula pressure or pressure in the arterial tubing proximal to it should always be monitored, and **pressure and pulsatility** checked **before starting CPB.** If the pressure in the aortic cannula does not match the systemic pressure, CPB must not commence until the cannula position has been corrected. If the pressure is instead monitored in the arterial tubing, a pressure gradient should be expected across the aortic cannula. If this gradient exceeds the recommended range for the flow/cannula combination, either cannula malposition or aortic dissection should be strongly considered. If CPB has commenced and a dissection has occurred or is suspected, CPB must cease, the aortic cannula be repositioned, and the dissection repaired if necessary.

2. **Carotid or innominate artery hyperperfusion** (Fig. 8.2) can occur if the aortic cannula outflow is too close to the innominate artery or the left carotid artery. Deleterious effects include cerebral edema or possibly even arterial rupture from the high flows and pressures. Prevention is surgical; use of a short aortic cannula with a flange may help prevent this complication. Diagnosis is suggested by facial flushing, pupillary dilation, and conjunctival chemosis (edema). There is likely to be low blood pressure measured by a left radial or femoral arterial catheter. A right radial arterial catheter may show **hypertension** due to innominate artery hyperperfusion. The surgeon must reposition the arterial cannula, and measures to reduce cerebral edema (e.g., mannitol, head-up position) may be required.

B. Reversed cannulation.

Venous drainage connected to the arterial cannula with arterial inflow into the right atrium or vena cava is very unlikely in adults, due to **different size tubing** for arterial and venous drainage. This complication is avoided also by ensuring that arterial pressures are observed in the arterial outflow line before commencing CPB. Reversed cannulation will result in very **low systemic pressures** and **high venous pressures.** More importantly, negative pressure in the aortic cannula risks the **entrainment of air,** which **must be avoided at all costs.** Reverse rotation of roller pumps must also be avoided. Management requires cessation of CPB, placing the patient in a steep head-down position, de-airing the cannulas and executing a massive gas embolism protocol if necessary (Table 8.3).

C. Obstruction to venous return.

Sudden reduced venous drainage from the patient during CPB will **lower the reservoir level,** increasing the risk of **air embolism.** At the same time the venous pressures in the patient will rise, reducing perfusion pressure to organs. To avoid emptying the venous reservoir further, the perfusionist must reduce the perfusion flow rate, further **reducing organ perfusion.** Alternatively, large fluid volumes must be added to the reservoir. For this reason, the cause must be determined immediately and the **venous drainage restored as quickly as possible.** Most centers use electronic monitors for low reservoir volume (see VII.E.1.a).

1. **Air lock.** A sudden reduction in venous blood draining into the venous reservoir may be caused by the presence of large air bubbles within the venous drainage cannula. This creates an "air lock" due to the lower pressure gradient and the surface tension in the air–blood interface. The air lock is overcome by sequentially elevating the venous tubing

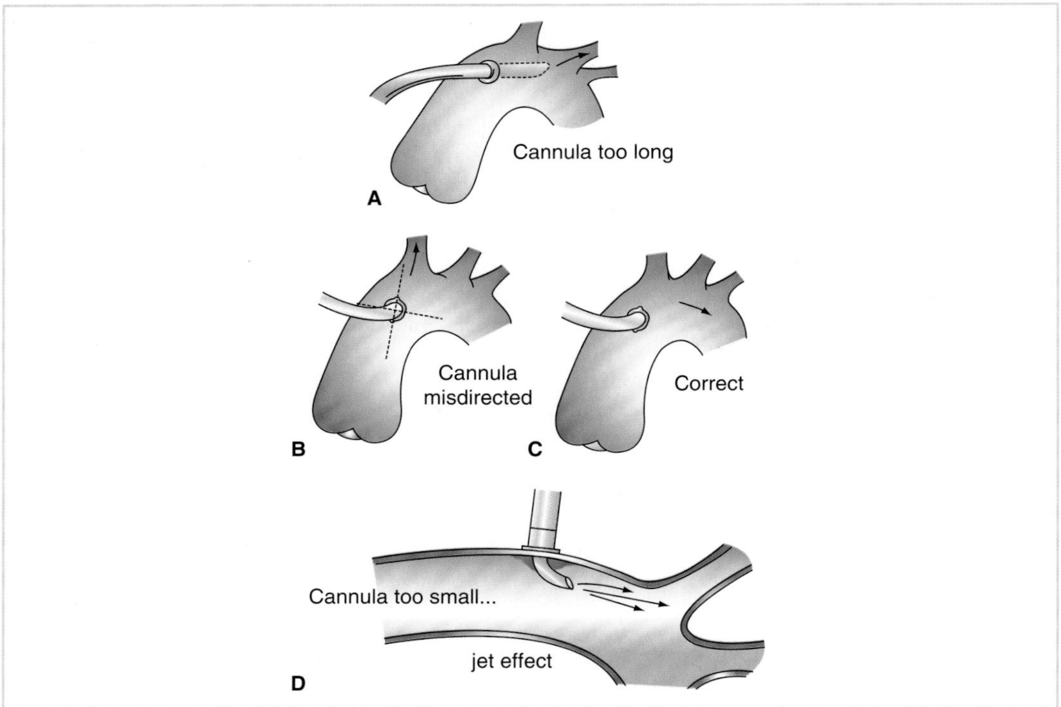

FIGURE 8.2 Potential aortic cannulation problems. **A:** Cannula extends into carotid owing to excessive length, causing excessive carotid flow. **B:** Angle of cannula insertion is improper, which also causes carotid hypoperfusion. **C:** Correct placement. **D:** Cannula diameter is too small; high-velocity jet of blood may damage intima and occlude a vessel. (Redrawn from Moores WY. Cardiopulmonary bypass strategies in patients with severe aortic disease. In: Utley JR, ed. *Pathophysiology and Techniques of Cardiopulmonary Bypass*. Vol. 2. Baltimore, MD: Williams & Wilkins; 1983:190, with permission.)

allowing the air bubble to rise (float to the surface), followed by dropping the tubing to allow the column of blood to force the bubble distally toward the reservoir.

2. **Mechanical.** Lifting of the heart within the chest by the surgeon often impedes venous drainage. The venous cannula may be malpositioned or kinked inadvertently during surgical manipulations. If reduced venous drainage is observed, the surgeon must be notified immediately, and appropriate venous drainage restored urgently.

D. **High pressure in arterial pump line.** Normally, arterial inflow line pressure proximal to the aortic cannula is up to three times the patient's arterial pressure, due to high resistance in the tubing and arterial cannula. However, kinking of the inflow line during pump operation will further increase the pressure, risking disruption of the tubing or connections, especially if the line is inadvertently clamped. For this reason, a high-pressure alarm is used, often with automatic feedback to stop roller pump operation.

E. **Massive gas embolism.** Most massive (macroscopic) gas emboli [12] consist of air, although oxygen emboli can be generated by a defective or clotted oxygenator. (For further discussion of this and CPB safety devices, see Chapter 21.) Use of a vented arterial line filter is an important safety device that can help prevent gas emboli reaching the patient; its routine use is strongly recommended. Because of the high risk of stroke, myocardial infarction, or death after massive gas embolism, **prevention is of utmost importance.**

1. **Etiology**

   a. **Empty or low oxygenator reservoir level.** Air may be pumped from an empty reservoir. Avoiding this scenario is one of the key tasks of the perfusionist. There are also alarms to alert staff when the oxygenator reservoir level is reaching an unsafe level.

TABLE 8.3 Massive gas embolism emergency protocol[a]

I. **Stop CPB** immediately (perfusionist), clamp arterial and venous lines, notify entire operating room team of emergency situation
II. Place patient in steep **head-down** position (anesthesiologist)
III. **Locate and isolate source of air**—if from pressurized CPB component, confirm isolation from patient before purging air (surgeon and perfusionist)
IV. Remove aortic cannula; **vent air** from aortic cannulation site (surgeon)
V. **Deair** arterial cannula and pump line and refill with fluid (perfusionist)

If massive cerebral air embolism seems unlikely:

VI. Confirm sufficient volume in CPB reservoir and consider resuming CPB with aortic root venting, administer vasopressors to raise perfusion pressure (hydrostatic pressure shrinks bubbles; also, bubbles occluding arterial bifurcations are pushed into one vessel, opening the other branch), set blender to 100% O_2
VII. Express coronary air by massage and needle venting
VIII. Consider cooling to 20°C for 45 min (increases gas solubility, decreases metabolic demands)
IX. Complete surgical procedure as appropriate to overall clinical situation, rewarm patient, separate slowly from CPB
X. **Continue ventilating the patient with 100% O_2** for at least 6 h (to maximize the blood–alveolar gradient for elimination of N_2)

If massive air embolism seems likely, initiate retrograde perfusion protocol:

I. Institute hypothermic **retrograde SVC perfusion** by connecting arterial pump line to the SVC cannula with caval tape tightened. Blood at 20–24°C is injected into the SVC at 1–2 L/min or more, and air plus blood is drained from the aortic root cannulation site to the pump (Fig. 8.3). Ensure that retrograde perfusion pressure does not exceed 30 mm Hg
II. **Carotid compression** is performed intermittently during retrograde SVC perfusion to allow retrograde purging of air from the **vertebral** arteries (Fig. 8.4)
III. Maintain retrograde SVC perfusion for at least 1–2 min. Continue for an additional 1–2 min if air continues to exit from aorta
IV. In **extensive** systemic air injection accidents in which emboli to splanchnic, renal, or femoral circulation are suspected, **retrograde IVC perfusion** may be performed **after** head de-airing procedures are completed. This is performed while the **carotid arteries are clamped** and the patient is in **head-up position** to facilitate removal of air through the aortic root vent but prevent re-embolization of the brain
V. When no additional air can be expelled, **resume anterograde CPB** as in steps VI–X above

Medication considerations

I. **Corticosteroids** may be administered, although this is controversial. The usual dose of methylprednisolone is 30 mg/kg
II. **Barbiturate coma** should be considered if the embolism occurred during warm CPB and if the myocardium will be able to tolerate the significant negative inotropy. Thiopental or pentobarbital, 10 mg/kg loading dose plus infusion at 1–3 mg/kg/h, may be used empirically. If EEG monitoring is available, titration of barbiturate to an EEG burst-suppression (1 burst/min) pattern is preferable
III. Consider additional mannitol 12.5–25 g

Postoperative considerations

I. Consider hyperbaric oxygen treatment (6 atm recommended by US Navy diving tables) and make any necessary transportation arrangements
II. Consult a neurologist
III. Consider early awakening for neurologic examination versus sustained barbiturate coma and/or sustained ventilation with 100% O_2
IV. Perform brain CT scan or MRI as advised by neurologist if patient is sufficiently stable.
V. Continue resuscitative efforts unless patient is diagnosed as brain dead or unless sustained support becomes futile for other reasons (e.g., multiorgan failure)

[a]This protocol should be reviewed together by all members of the cardiac team periodically.

CPB, cardiopulmonary bypass; CT, computerized tomography; EEG, electroencephalogram; IVC, inferior vena cava; MRI, magnetic resonance imaging; SVC, superior vena cava.

Modified from Mills NL, Ochsner JL. Massive air embolism during cardiopulmonary bypass: Causes, prevention, and management. *J Thorac Cardiovasc Surg.* 1980;80:712, and from Kurusz M, Mills NL. Management of unusual problems encountered in initiating and maintaining cardiopulmonary bypass. In: Gravlee GP, Davis RF, Kurusz M, et al., eds. *Cardiopulmonary Bypass: Principles and Practice.* 2nd ed. Philadelphia, PA: Lippincott Williams & Wilkins; 2000:596, with permission.

Many such alarms are linked to an automatic cessation of the arterial roller pump. Vortexing can permit air entrainment and embolism when the reservoir blood level is very low but not empty. This is **the most important cause of bypass catastrophes** when utilizing a closed reservoir system. A high-risk period for air embolism or entrainment is at the time of separation from CPB, when the oxygenator reservoir level is often low.

b. **Leaks in the negative pressure part of the CPB circuit** (between the oxygenator reservoir and the arterial pump) may result in air entrainment, e.g., clotted or defective oxygenator, disruption of tubing connections.
c. **Entrainment of air around the aortic cannula.** This may occur during cannula insertion. Entrainment can also occur via this route if negative pressure in the arterial cannula is allowed to develop during periods of no flow (e.g., before or after the onset of CPB). To prevent negative pressure and draining blood from the patient, the aortic cannula must be clamped during all periods when the arterial pump is inactive.
d. **Inadequate de-airing** prior to aortic cross-clamp release. This is particularly important for open-chamber procedures.
e. **Reversed roller pump** flow in vent line or arterial cannula.
f. **Pressurized cardiotomy reservoir** (causing retrograde flow of air through a nonocclusive vent line roller head into heart or aorta)
g. **Runaway pump head** (switch inoperative; must unplug pump and crank by hand)
h. **Other causes** not related specifically to CPB include an improper flushing technique for arterial or left atrial pressure monitoring lines, **paradoxical embolism** of venous air across atrial or ventricular septal defects. Occasionally, a **persistent left** superior vena cava **(SVC)** communicates with the left atrium (IV air from a left-sided IV may enter the systemic circulation through this SVC).

2. **Prevention.** Vigilance is required. Safety devices and alarms must be activated.
3. **Diagnosis.** Gas embolism is diagnosed mostly by visual inspection. The extent of gas embolism can be gauged by signs of myocardial or other organ ischemia.
4. **Management.** A massive gas embolus emergency protocol should be available and followed by all staff [13]. See Table 8.3, Figures 8.3 and 8.4.

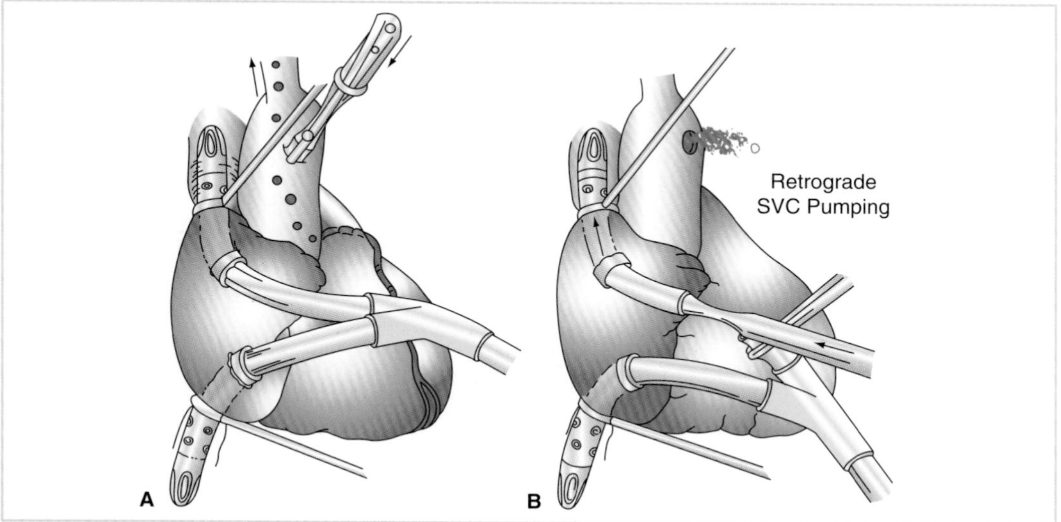

FIGURE 8.3 Retrograde perfusion in the treatment of massive air embolism. **A:** Massive arterial gas embolism has occurred. **B:** Bubbles in the arterial tree are flushed out by performing retrograde body perfusion into the SVC by connecting the deaired arterial pump line to the SVC cannula (and tightening caval tapes). Blood and bubbles exit the aorta from the cannulation wound. (Redrawn from Mills NL, Ochsner JL. Massive air embolism during cardiopulmonary bypass: Causes, prevention, and management. *J Thorac Cardiovasc Surg.* 1980;80:713, with permission.)

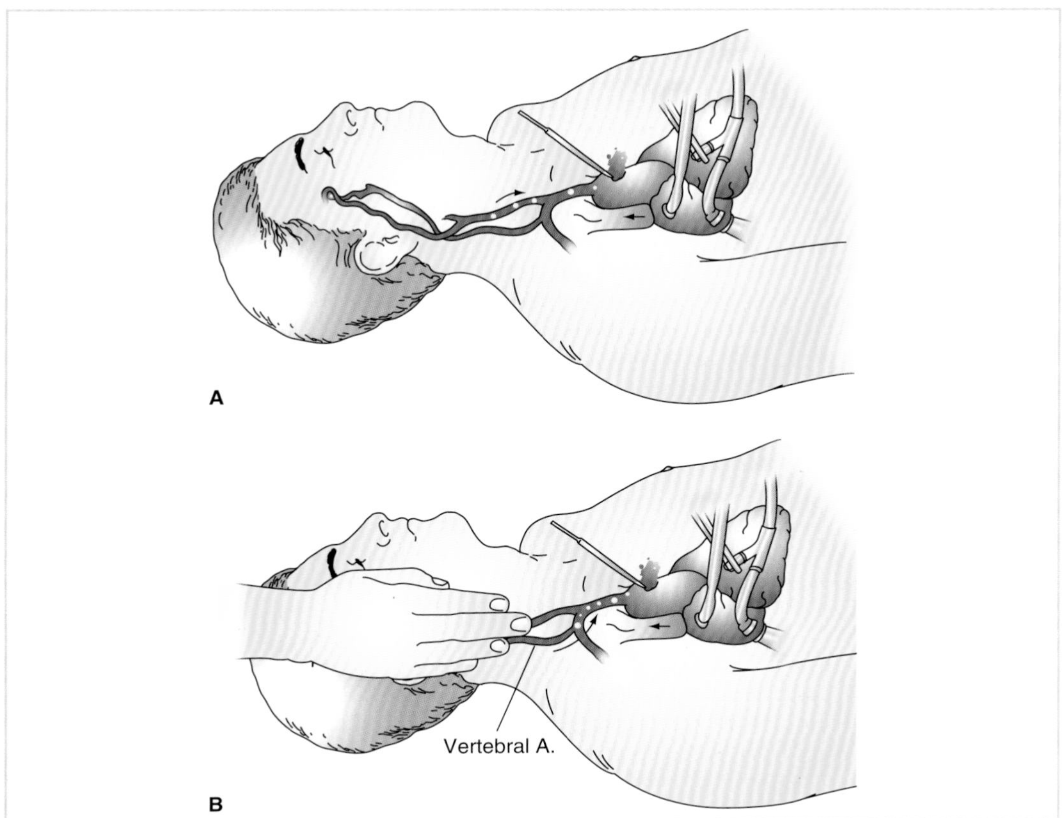

FIGURE 8.4 Carotid **(A)** and vertebral **(B)** artery de-airing during retrograde perfusion. In the management of massive arterial gas embolism, steep head-down position helps to flush bubbles out of the *carotid arteries.* Application of intermittent pressure to the carotid arteries increases retrograde *vertebral artery* flow, which helps to evacuate bubbles. (Redrawn from Mills NL, Ochsner JL. Massive air embolism during cardiopulmonary bypass: Causes, prevention, and management. *J Thorac Cardiovasc Surg.* 1980;80:713, with permission.)

F. **Failure of oxygen supply.** Inadequate oxygenator gas flow or a hypoxic mixture will result in arterial hypoxemia. The blood in the arterial line will appear dark, and the lower PO_2 will register on in-line PO_2 or Hb oxygen saturation monitors. An oxygen analyzer can be incorporated in the oxygenator gas inflow line as an early alert for hypoxic mixtures. The O_2 supply should be restored immediately, connecting a portable O_2 cylinder to the oxygenator if necessary. If a delay is anticipated, either separate from CPB (if still plausible) or cool the patient maximally until O_2 supply is restored. Ventilation with **room air** is preferable to no ventilation at all, if immediate restoration of O_2 supply is not possible.

G. **Pump or oxygenator failure**

1. **Pump failure** may be due to electrical or mechanical failure, tubing rupture or disconnection, or automatic shutoff by a bubble or low reservoir detector. A runaway pump head may raise the pump flow to its maximum inappropriately, and the pump control switch will be inoperative. For systems designed to be used with an electromagnetic or ultrasonic transducer, failure of the sensor can prevent one from knowing the actual pump flow rate. If the occlusion of a roller pump is improperly set, excessive regurgitation occurs (causing hemolysis) and the forward flow is reduced. In the event of electrical failure, CPB pumps can be hand cranked until current is restored. Mechanical failure requires

replacement of the pump. In case of a runaway pump head, the CPB machine must be unplugged and the tubing switched to a different roller head.

2. **Oxygenator failure** may be due to a manufacturing defect, mechanical obstruction from clot, disruption of the oxygenator shell (trauma, spill of volatile liquid anesthetic), or leakage of water from heat exchanger into blood. The diagnosis is based on arterial blood gas abnormalities, acidosis, blood leak, excessive hemolysis, or high premembrane pressures. For severe failure, the oxygenator must be replaced. A protocol should be in place for **rapid oxygenator replacement.** If body perfusion will be low or absent for more than 1 or 2 min and if the patient cannot be immediately weaned from CPB, then hypothermia to 18 to 20°C should be induced if possible and consideration given to brain, myocardial, and renal protection during the oxygenator replacement. Open cardiac massage may be necessary, depending on the stage of the operation.

H. **Clotted oxygenator or circuit.** This serious event can interfere with gas exchange, prevent CPB flow, or cause massive gas embolus. The main cause is **inadequate anticoagulation,** which may result from **inadequate dose, heparin resistance,** or the inadvertent administration of **protamine during CPB.** This potentially lethal catastrophe should not occur if adequate anticoagulation is confirmed before initiating CPB and at frequent intervals thereafter. It can be diagnosed by visual observation of clot in the oxygenator, or high arterial line pressure (evidence of partially clotted arterial line filter). There may also be clues to inadequate heparinization by **the presence of clot in the surgical field.** Management involves cessation of CPB, and replacement of the oxygenator and tubing if necessary. If the patient is not cold, open cardiopulmonary resuscitation and topical hypothermia may be required. The patient should then be reheparinized using a different lot of heparin if possible, and satisfactory anticoagulation confirmed before re-instituting CPB.

VIII. Less-invasive surgical techniques

A. **Port access CPB** is similar to conventional CPB but requires additional instrumentation and monitoring [14,15]. Arterial and venous CPB cannulas are inserted peripherally (e.g., femoral artery and vein). An aortic occlusion catheter is placed in the ascending aorta under fluoroscopic or TEE guidance. An endocoronary sinus catheter is inserted for delivery of retrograde cardioplegia, and a PA vent catheter is inserted to decompress the heart through the left atrium. Correct position of the inflated aortic occlusion catheter balloon should be checked regularly using TEE. Loss of the right radial arterial pressure trace may indicate cephalad migration of the balloon. Frequent interaction among surgeon, perfusionist, and anesthesiologist is required for a successful outcome (see Chapter 13).

B. **Mitral valve surgery through a right minithoracotomy.** In this procedure arterial and venous cannulas are inserted peripherally and CPB is instituted prior to a right minithoracotomy [15]. TEE guidance is used to ensure that the venous cannula enters or crosses the right atrium to drain the SVC as well as the IVC. Due to the increased length and decreased diameter of the venous cannula, suction is typically required to maintain adequate venous drainage. If the right atrium is opened (e.g., for tricuspid valve surgery), a separate SVC cannula (often inserted percutaneously) may be required. With the onset of CPB, ventilation of the lungs is no longer required. Collapse of the right lung on opening of the chest provides surgical access to the heart and great vessels. An aortic root cannula for the administration of cardioplegia can then be placed, followed by an aortic cross-clamp. Access to the mitral valve is obtained through the left atrium. CPB management is otherwise unchanged, although before final separation from CPB, a trial separation is undertaken to ensure satisfactory mitral valve function (as assessed by TEE). For further details see Chapter 13.

IX. Management of unusual or rare conditions affecting bypass

A. **Sickle cell trait and disease** [16–19]. The congenital presence of abnormal Hb S as the trait (heterozygote, Hb-AS) but especially as the disease (homozygote, Hb-SS) allows RBCs to undergo
10 sickle transformation and occlude the microvasculature or lyse. RBC sickling may be induced by exposure to hypoxemia, vascular stasis, hyperosmolarity, or acidosis. Hypothermia produces sickling only by causing vasoconstriction and stasis. Although anesthesia for noncardiac surgery is well tolerated in sickle trait patients, the risks are higher for operations requiring CPB. CPB

may induce sickling by redistributing blood flow, causing stasis, and reducing venous O_2 tensions. **Sickle cell trait** (heterozygous Hb-AS) patients are at low risk for RBC sickling unless the O_2 saturation is below 40%. Djaiani et al. reported a series of 10 sickle cell trait patients who successfully underwent fast-track coronary revascularization using normothermic CPB, although one very high-risk patient died of multiorgan failure after a protracted postoperative course [19]. In contrast, **sickle cell disease** (homozygous Hb-SS or Hb-SC) patients develop RBC sickling at O_2 saturations less than 85% and are at risk for developing potentially fatal thromboses during CPB unless appropriate measures are taken. CPB should be avoided if alternative treatment options are available (e.g., off-pump surgery). If CPB is required, hypothermia should ideally be avoided.

1. **Diagnosis. In the United States, high-risk newborns have been routinely screened for sickle cell disease and trait for over 20 yrs,** so most African-American patients will know if they have sickle cell trait or disease. If not, the rapid "sickle-dex" test or "sickle-prep" is appropriate for screening, whereas Hb electrophoresis yields important quantitative information if the result of a screening test is positive. Expert preoperative hematologic consultation is advised for sickle cell disease patients before CPB.
2. **Management.** Hypoxia, acidosis, and conditions leading to vascular stasis (e.g., hypovolemia, dehydration) should be avoided or minimized in all patients with **sickle cell trait or disease.**
3. **Preoperative transfusion to achieve a total Hb concentration of 10 g/dL or higher is appropriate for sickle cell disease patients,** and possibly higher if the patient will tolerate the intravascular volume. Increasing the Hct improves O_2 carriage, dilutes Hb-SS, and suppresses erythropoiesis, but also increases the risk of alloimmunization [18]. Preoperative Hb concentration for sickle cell patients should optimally exceed 10 g/dL, which may require transfusion.
4. **Preoperative transfusion** with Hb-A donor RBCs is the conservative approach to the management of **sickle cell disease** patients requiring hypothermic CPB. Heiner and colleagues [16] recommended that, prior to CPB with deep hypothermia, patients with sickle trait or sickle disease be transfused with donor cells (containing no Hb-S) until the proportion of native RBCs containing any Hb-S (RBCs) be reduced from 100% to less than 33%.

   If used**, intraoperative exchange transfusion** has an advantage because invasive monitoring may be used to guide transfusion and volume replacement. CPB per se provides an opportunity for limited exchange transfusion because of the necessary priming volume, which most often should contain allogeneic blood in patients with sickle cell disease. For patients with sickle cell disease, it seems sensible to maintain total Hb concentration at 8 g/dL or higher during CPB, and to achieve a total Hb concentration of 10 g/dL or higher at separation from CPB or soon thereafter. Donor Hb-A RBCs can be used to prime the CPB circuit. If additional exchange is desired, upon initiation of CPB, the patient's venous blood can be diverted into a separate reservoir. The diverted blood can then be replaced by further donor HbA transfusion and volume replacement.
5. **CPB management.** Avoid arterial or venous hypoxemia, acidosis, dehydration, hyperosmolarity, and hypothermia if possible. Higher-than-usual pump flow rates theoretically may raise venous oxygen saturations and reduce sickling. Shivering or other factors that increase O_2 consumption and reduce venous oxygen saturation should be avoided. If **cold cardioplegia** is required, crystalloid cardioplegia can be used to flush out Hb-S from the coronary circulation. If blood cardioplegia is used, it should be normothermic and have less than 5% Hb-S.

B. Cold agglutinin disease [20–22]

1. **Pathophysiology**
   a. Autoantibodies against RBCs in patients with cold agglutinin disease are activated by even transient cold exposure. At temperatures below the **critical temperature** for an individual patient, hemagglutination will occur, resulting in **vascular occlusion** with organ ischemia or infarction. Hemagglutination also can fix complement,

leading to **hemolysis** on RBC rewarming. The antibodies are typically immunoglobulin M (IgM).

b. Symptoms usually are of vascular occlusion, manifesting as acrocyanosis on exposure to cold. Signs of hemolytic anemia may be present.

c. Low titers of antibodies with a low critical temperature (e.g., <28°C) are common, but of little clinical relevance. In contrast, patients who have **high titers** of antibodies with a **high critical temperature** are at risk of hemagglutination perioperatively, especially during **hypothermic CPB.**

d. The organ at greatest risk of damage is the myocardium, because RBCs are exposed to extreme hypothermia (4 to 8°C) during the preparation of **blood cardioplegia** solution. Aggregates thus formed may be infused into the coronary vasculature, causing severe microcirculatory occlusion and preventing distribution of cardioplegia.

e. The idiopathic form of cold agglutinin disease is seen most frequently in older patients and probably represents a subclinical form of a lymphoproliferative or immunoproliferative disorder, either of which can induce cold agglutinins. The disease also occurs after mycoplasmal pneumonia, mononucleosis, and other infections.

2. **Diagnosis**

a. Routine **blood cross-matching** using the direct Coombs' test may identify patients with critical temperatures (thermal amplitude) at or above room temperature. However, autoantibodies responding to such warm temperatures are seen rarely (less than 1% of cardiac surgical patients). Direct Coombs' tests run at varying temperatures will characterize the critical temperature of a cold agglutinin.

b. An RBC precipitate (hemagglutination) may form when blood is mixed with a cold high-K^+ solution (e.g., cold blood cardioplegia). A **rapid diagnostic test** has been proposed in which approximately 5 mL of the patient's blood is added to the chilled cardioplegia solution during setup. Routine use of this test has been advocated.

c. Unexplained high aortic root pressure during cold blood cardioplegia infusion may indicate cold agglutinin disease.

d. The sudden appearance of hemolysis with hemoglobinuria during hypothermic CPB or use of blood cardioplegia may be diagnostic.

3. **Management**

a. If cold agglutinins are suspected preoperatively, careful assessment by a hematologist is warranted, including characterizing the type of antibody, its titer, and its critical temperature.

b. The thermal design of the operation should be reviewed and revised if possible. CPB should be avoided if alternative strategies (e.g., off-pump surgery) are feasible. If CPB is required, **systemic temperatures** (including arterial and venous blood values) should be maintained *above* the critical temperature. Systemic temperatures of 28°C or higher are generally safe in asymptomatic patients. **DHCA** is feasible, provided the coldest blood temperature is several degrees warmer than the critical temperature.

c. **Cardioplegia** management includes avoidance of cold blood cardioplegia. Induction of cardiac arrest is achieved with **warm** crystalloid cardioplegia to wash all RBCs out of the myocardium. Subsequently, cold crystalloid cardioplegia can be used to maintain arrest. Alternatives include warm blood cardioplegia or warm ischemic arrest with intermittent reperfusion.

d. **Plasmapheresis.** If a reduction of the patient's core temperature below their critical temperature for hemagglutinin formation is unavoidable, preoperative plasmapheresis may be required, particularly if the patient has high antibody titers. Plasmapheresis removes the majority of IgM antibodies, which are large and mainly intravascular. However, not all IgM antibodies are removed, so limiting cold exposure as much as possible is still required.

C. **Cold urticaria** [23,24]. Patients with this disorder develop systemic histamine release and generalized urticaria in response to cold exposure. Cold CPB should be avoided if possible, because marked histamine release occurs during CPB rewarming and can cause hemodynamic instability. If cold CPB is unavoidable, the cardiovascular responses to histamine can be prevented by pretreatment with H_1- and H_2-receptor blockade; concomitant steroid administration may be useful.

D. Malignant Hyperthermia (MH) [25–27]

An acute MH crisis may occur in susceptible patients exposed to triggering agents, and in rare cases, may manifest for the first time during CPB.

1. **Prevention.** Management of known susceptibility requires the avoidance of triggering agents. During CPB it may be prudent to rewarm the patient gradually, avoid calcium administration unless Ca^{2+} concentration is low, and possibly avoid α-adrenergic agonists.
2. **Diagnosis** of an MH crisis. During CPB the usual early signs of signs of an MH crisis of hyperthermia, rigidity, and tachycardia may be absent due to the use of hypothermia and cardioplegia. However, the increased skeletal muscle metabolism associated with the disorder may cause a mixed metabolic and respiratory acidosis, hyperkalemia, rhabdomyolysis with myoglobinuria (and late renal failure) even during CPB. Recognition of MH crisis can be difficult, particularly during the rewarming phase when temperature is expected to increase. **A high index of suspicion** is required for patients with known MH susceptibility. Monitoring the **rate of CO_2 elimination** (by monitoring oxygenator exhaust gas) or O_2 uptake (by arteriovenous O_2 measurements and pump flow rate) may permit early diagnosis of MH.
3. **Management** involves ceasing triggering agents, cooling to reduce hyperthermia, correction of acid–base and electrolyte changes, and the early administration of dantrolene (1 to 2 mg/kg IV initially, with further doses as required titrated to effect). Active cooling and treatment of other MH complications may be necessary in the post-CPB period.

E. Hereditary angioedema [28,29]. A deficiency or abnormality in function of an endogenous inhibitor of the C1 esterase complement protein leads to exaggerated complement pathway activation. Edema involving the airway, face, gastrointestinal tract, and extremities may follow even minor stresses. CPB can cause fatal complement activation in patients with hereditary angioedema; peak activation follows protamine administration. In the past, management of acute episodes has been mainly supportive, because epinephrine, steroids, and histamine antagonists are of little benefit, and fresh frozen plasma may exacerbate the reaction by providing additional complement substrates. Subacute and chronic therapies include androgens (stanozolol) and antifibrinolytics. A purified human C1 esterase inhibitor replacement protein (C1-INHRP) concentrate (Cinryze, ViroPharma, Exton, PA) is now available for prophylaxis against and treatment of acute episodes, and another purified C1-INH concentrate (Berinert, CSL Behring, King of Prussia, PA) is available for treatment [29]. Other drugs have been introduced recently to block bradykinin B_2 receptors or inhibitor plasma kallikrein and reduce the severity of reactions [29].

F. Pregnancy [30,31]. Cardiac surgery with CPB during pregnancy involves a high risk of fetal demise or morbidity (10% to 50%), although maternal mortality appears to be no greater than in the nonpregnant patient. Longer duration of CPB appears to increase the risk to the fetus.

1. **Physiology.** Placental ischemia may be caused by microembolization, elevated inferior vena cava pressure due to obstructed drainage, or low pump flow rates (pregnant patients have a larger resting CO and require higher than usual flows during CPB). In addition, uterine blood flow is not autoregulated, so hypotension of any origin is likely to cause placental hypoperfusion. Uterine contractions may be induced by CPB, possibly related to rewarming or to dilution of progesterone.
2. **Management**
   a. **Additional monitoring.** Fetal heart rate monitoring is mandatory, although in the first trimester this may not be possible. Uterine contractile activity should be monitored using a tocodynamometer applied to the maternal abdomen.
   b. **Blood pressure and flow.** Maintaining an increased perfusion pressure (e.g., >70 mm Hg) is advocated. Using increases in pump flow to elevate the blood pressure may be preferable to using pressor drugs, due to the risk of uterine artery vasoconstriction with α-adrenergic stimulation. Toward term, left uterine displacement is appropriate.

Fetal bradycardia not related to hypothermia may indicate placental hypoperfusion and should be treated promptly by increasing the pump flow and perfusion pressure.

c. **Metabolic state.** Maintain normal blood gases (including avoiding very high PaO_2 values, ideally keep in 100 to 200 range) and ensure adequate oxygen delivery (Hct > 28%), and maintain normothermia if possible. The duration of CPB should be minimized and pulsatile perfusion should be considered. An adequate blood glucose level must be maintained.

d. **Tocolytic drugs** such as magnesium sulfate, ritodrine, or terbutaline may be necessary.

e. **Inotropic drugs** ideally should not have unbalanced α-vasoconstrictor and uterine-contracting activity. Milrinone, or low-to-moderate doses of epinephrine or dopamine, have theoretical advantages.

G. **Jehovah's Witnesses** rarely accept retransfusion of their own blood if it has left their circulation. Therefore, it is important to ensure continuous circulation of blood from commencement of CPB until full separation.

REFERENCES

1. Frahdorf J, De hert S, Schlack W. Anaesthesia and myocardial ischaemia/reperfusion injury. *Br J Anaesth.* 2009;103:89–98.
2. Graham J, Gibbs NM, Weightman WM. Relationship between temperature corrected oxygenator exhaust PCO_2 and arterial PCO_2 during hypothermic cardiopulmonary bypass. *Anaesth Intensive Care.* 2005;33:457–461.
3. Sebel PS. Central nervous system monitoring during open heart surgery: An update. *J Cardiothorac Vasc Anesth.* 1998; 12:3–8.
4. Baulig W, Seifert B, Schmid ER, et al. Comparison of spectral entropy and bispectral index electroencephalography in coronary artery bypass surgery. *J Cardiothor Vasc Anesth.* 2010;24:544–549.
5. Dawson PJ, Bjorksten AR, Blake DW, et al. The effects of cardiopulmonary bypass on total and unbound plasma concentrations of propofol and midazolam. *J Cardiothorac Vasc Anesth.* 1997;11:556–561.
6. Gravlee GR, Angert KC, Tucker WY, et al. Early anticoagulation peak and rapid distribution after intravenous heparin. *Anesthesiology.* 1988;68:126–129.
7. Aldea GS, O'Gara P, Shapira OM, et al. Effect of anticoagulation protocol on outcome in patients undergoing CABG with heparin-bonded cardiopulmonary bypass circuits. *Ann Thorac Surg.* 1998;65:425–433.
8. Nadolney EM, Svennson LG. Carbon dioxide field flooding techniques for open heart surgery: Monitoring and minimizing potential adverse effects. *Perfusion.* 2000;15:151–153.
9. Oka Y, Inoue T, Hong Y, et al. Retained intracardiac air. Transesophageal echocardiography for definition of incidence and monitoring removal by improved techniques. *J Thorac Cardiovasc Surg.* 1986;63:329–338.
10. Rannucci M, De Benedetti D, Biachini C, et al. Effects of fenoldapam infusion on in complex cardiac operations: A prospective, double-blind, placebo-controlled study. *Minerva Anesthesiol.* 2010;76:249–259.
11. Levy JH, Tanaka KA. Inflammatory response to cardiopulmonary bypass. *Ann Thorac Surg.* 2003;75:S715–S720.
12. von Segesser LK. Unusual problems in cardiopulmonary bypass. In: Gravlee GR, Davis RF, Stammers AH, Ungerleider RM, eds. *Cardiopulmonary Bypass: Principles and Practice.* 3rd ed. Philadelphia, PA: Wolters Kluwer/Lippincott Williams & Wilkins; 2008:608–613.
13. Mills NL, Ochsner JL. Massive air embolism during cardiopulmonary bypass: Causes, prevention, and management. *J Thorac Cardiovasc Surg.* 1980;80:713.
14. Schwartz DS, Ribakove GH, Grossi EA, et al. Single and multivessel port access coronary artery bypass grafting with cardioplegic arrest: Technique and reproducibility. *J Thorac Cardiovasc Surg.* 1997;114:46–52.
15. Walther T, Falk V, Mohr FW. Minimally invasive mitral valve surgery. *J Cardiovasc Surg.* 2004;45:487–495.
16. Heiner M, Teasdale SJ, David T, et al. Aorto-coronary bypass in a patient with sickle cell trait. *Can Anaesth Soc J.* 1979;26:428–434.
17. Koshy M, Weiner SJ, Miller ST, et al. Surgery and anesthesia in sickle cell disease. Cooperative study of sickle cell diseases. *Blood.* 1995;86:3676–3684.
18. Firth PG, Head CA. Sickle cell disease and anesthesia. *Anesthesiology.* 2004;101:766–785.
19. Djaiani GN, Cheng DCH, Carroll JA, et al. Fast-track cardiac anesthesia in patients with sickle cell abnormalities. *Anesth Analg.* 1999;89:598–603.
20. Agarwal SK, Ghosh PK, Gupta D. Cardiac surgery and cold-reactive proteins. *Ann Thorac Surg.* 1995;60:1143–1150.
21. Bratkovic K, Fahy C. Anesthesia for off-pump coronary artery surgery in a patient with cold agglutinin disease. *J Cardiothorac Vasc Anesth.* 2008;22:449–452.
22. Atkinson VP, Soeding P, Horne G, et al. Cold agglutinins in cardiac surgery: Management of myocardial protection and cardiopulmonary bypass. *Ann Thorac Surg.* 2008;85:310–311.
23. Johnston WE, Moss J, Philbin DM, et al. Management of cold urticaria during hypothermic cardiopulmonary bypass. *N Engl J Med.* 1982;306:219–221.
24. Lancey RA, Schaefer OP, McCormick MJ. Coronary artery bypass grafting and aortic valve replacement with cold cardioplegia in a patient with cold-induced urticaria. *Ann Allergy Asthma Immunol.* 2004;92:273–275.

25. Byrick RJ, Rose DK, Ranganathan N. Management of a malignant hyperthermia patient during cardiopulmonary bypass. *Can Anaesth Soc J.* 1982;29:50–54.
26. Larach DR, High KM, Larach MG, et al. Cardiopulmonary bypass interference with dantrolene prophylaxis of malignant hyperthermia. *J Cardiothorac Anesth.* 1987;1:448–453.
27. Metterlein T, Zink W, Haneya A, et al. Cardiopulmonary bypass in malignant hyperthermia susceptible patients: A systematic review of published cases. *J Thorac Cardiovasc Surg.* 2010;141:1488–1495.
28. Jaering JM, Comunale ME. Cardiopulmonary bypass in hereditary angioedema. *Anesthesiology.* 1993;79:1429–1433.
29. Levy JH, Freiberger DJ, Roback J. Hereditary angioedema: Current and emerging option. *Anesth Analg.* 2010;110:1271–1280.
30. Strickland RA, Oliver WC, Chamtigian RC. Anesthesia, cardiopulmonary bypass, and the pregnant patient. *Mayo Clin Proc.* 1991;66:411–429.
31. Chandrasekhar S, Cook CR, Collard CD. Cardiac surgery in the parturient. *Anesth Analg.* 2009;108:777–785.

9 The Postcardiopulmonary Bypass Period: Weaning to ICU Transport

Benjamin N. Morris, Mark E. Romanoff, and Roger L. Royster

KEY POINTS

1. Core temperature (nasopharyngeal or tympanic membrane) should be greater than 36°C before terminating cardiopulmonary bypass (CPB). However, the nasopharyngeal temperature should not exceed 37°C, as this will increase the risk of postoperative central nervous system dysfunction. Using nasopharyngeal temperature to avoid hyperthermia and the rectal/bladder temperature to avoid underwarming may be the safest technique.
2. Visualization of the heart, directly as well as with transesophageal echocardiography (TEE), is important before terminating CPB.
3. "The first attempt to terminate CPB is the best one." Optimize all parameters before CPB termination.
4. When terminating CPB, left ventricular failure is suggested by a decreased pulse pressure.

5. Vasoplegic syndrome is a severe form of post-CPB vasodilation characterized by low arterial pressure, normal to high cardiac output (CO), normal right-side filling pressures, low systemic vascular resistance (SVR) which is refractory to pressor therapy.
6. When evaluating hypoxemia after CPB, the possibility of a right-to-left shunt through a patent foramen ovale must be considered and evaluated with TEE.
7. New onset renal dysfunction requiring dialysis after CPB will increase mortality almost eightfold.

TERMINATING CPB REQUIRES THE ANESTHESIOLOGIST to apply the basic tenets of cardiovascular physiology and pharmacology. The goal is a smooth transition from the mechanical pump back to the heart as the source of blood flow. Weaning from the pump involves optimizing cardiovascular variables including preload, afterload, heart rate (HR), conduction, contractility, and the O_2 supply–demand ratio, as in the pre-CPB period. However, the time period for optimization is compressed to minutes or seconds, and decisions must be made quickly to avoid myocardial injury or damage to the other major organ systems.

I. Preparation for termination of bypass: CVP mnemonic.

The major objectives in preparing for termination of CPB can be remembered with the aid of the mnemonic ***CVP:***

C	V	P
Cold	Ventilation	Predictors
Conduction	Vaporizer	Protamine
Calcium	Volume expanders	Pressure
Cardiac output	Visualization	Pressors
Cells		Pacer
Coagulation		Potassium

1 **A. Cold.** Core temperature (nasopharyngeal or tympanic membrane) should be greater than 36°C before terminating CPB. Rectal or bladder temperature should be at least 35 to 36°C [1]. Ending CPB when cold causes prolonged hypothermia from equilibration of the cooler, vessel-poor group with the warmer and better perfused vessel-rich group. Nasopharyngeal temperature correlates with brain temperature but may be artificially elevated during rapid rewarming and should not be used for determining the temperature at which CPB is discontinued unless it has been stable for 20 to 30 min. Venous return temperature can be used in a similar manner to help confirm core temperature. The nasopharyngeal temperature should not exceed 37°C, as this will increase the risk of postoperative central nervous system dysfunction. Using nasopharyngeal temperature to avoid hyperthermia and the rectal/bladder temperature to avoid under-warming may be the safest technique.

B. Conduction. Cardiac rate and rhythm must be controlled as follows:

1. **Rate**
   - **a.** HR of 80 to 100 beats/min often is needed for adequate CO post-CPB because of reduced ventricular compliance and inability to increase stroke volume. In coronary artery bypass graft (CABG) procedures, complete revascularization allows a higher rate (80 to 100 beats/min) after CPB, with less risk of ischemia than before CPB. Patients with severely limited stroke volume (aneurysmectomy or after ventricular remodeling) may require even higher rates.
   - **b.** Sinus bradycardia may be treated with atropine or an inotropic drug, but epicardial pacing is more reliable.
   - **c.** Sinus tachycardia of more than 120 beats/min should be treated before termination of CPB. Often the act of "filling the heart" and increasing preload will reflexively decrease the HR to an acceptable level. Other etiologies of increased HR must be addressed. Common etiologies include:
     - **(1)** Hypoxia
     - **(2)** Hypercapnia

(3) Medications (inotropes, pancuronium, scopolamine)

(4) Light anesthesia, awareness

(a) "Fast track" anesthesia with its lower medication dosing schedule requires special attention to this complication. An additional dose of narcotic and benzodiazepine, or hypnotic (propofol infusion) should be considered during the rewarming period if tachycardia is present. BIS or depth of anesthesia monitors may be helpful in guiding therapy.

(5) Anemia

(6) **Ischemia:** ST and T-wave changes indicative of ischemia should be treated and the surgeon should be notified. A nitroglycerin (NTG) infusion and/or an increase in the perfusion pressure often improves the situation. Refractory causes include residual air or graft occlusions. If coronary air is suspected, briefly increasing the perfusion pressure to a mean of 90 mm Hg may improve the situation.

2. **Rhythm**

a. Normal sinus rhythm is preferable. In patients with poorly compliant, thick-walled ventricles (associated with aortic stenosis, hypertension, or ischemia), the atrial "kick" may contribute up to 40% of CO, so attaining synchronized atrial contraction (sinus rhythm, atrial or atrioventricular [AV] sequential pacing) is very important before attempting CPB termination. This may require a discussion with the surgeon if they feel ventricular pacing alone is adequate. Atrial pacing is acceptable if there is no AV block, but often atrial and ventricular leads are needed.

b. Supraventricular tachycardias (HR greater than 120 beats/min) such as regular narrow-QRS atrial flutter and atrial fibrillation, should be cardioverted with synchronized internal cardioversion before terminating CPB.

c. Esmolol, verapamil, amiodarone, or adenosine may be used to chemically cardiovert or to control the ventricular response rate. A decrease in contractility is seen with some agents.

d. Third-degree AV block requires pacing, although atropine occasionally may be effective.

e. Ventricular dysrhythmias are treated as indicated (see Chapter 2).

C. **Calcium.** Calcium should be immediately available to treat hypocalcemia and hyperkalemia, which commonly occur after CPB. However, the routine administration of calcium post-CPB is not recommended.

1. **Mechanism of action.** Most studies suggest that calcium produces an elevation in SVR when the ionized Ca^{2+} level is in the low–normal range or higher [2]. Despite this increase in afterload, contractility is maintained. At very low ionized calcium levels (<0.8 mM), contractility is increased by calcium administration. Elevating calcium levels will also help counteract the dysrhythmogenic and negative inotropic actions of hyperkalemia. The usual dose is 5 to 15 mg/kg of CaCl.

2. **Measurement.** Ionized Ca^{2+} levels should be evaluated after rewarming to help direct therapy. Citrated blood cardioplegia reperfusion solutions can lower blood Ca^{2+} levels substantially. The usual range is 1 to 1.3 mmol/dL. Calcium levels are affected by pH: Low pH will increase Ca^{2+} levels, whereas elevated pH will decrease Ca^{2+} levels. **Correction of pH should be attempted before treating abnormal values.**

3. **Risks of calcium administration**

a. Patients taking digoxin may experience life-threatening dysrhythmias.

b. Inhibition of the hemodynamic action of inotropes (e.g., epinephrine, dobutamine) has been reported.

c. Coronary spasm might occur in rare susceptible patients.

d. Augmentation of reperfusion injury is possible. Calcium administration should wait until 15 min after aortic cross-clamp release.

D. **Cardiac output.** Evaluating cardiac function is vital after CPB. CO may be obtained from a pulmonary artery (PA) catheter or contractility may be estimated by using TEE. If a continuous CO PA catheter is used, it may take more than 3 min to obtain the first CO after CPB. If the patient is stable, this is acceptable; if not, the equipment for a manual determination should be used initially.

E. Cells

1. The hemoglobin concentration should be measured after rewarming. If it is less than 6.5 to 7 g/dL before terminating CPB, blood administration should be considered to maintain O_2-carrying capacity after CPB. If the venous reservoir contains a large amount of blood, this blood may be concentrated by a cell saver and given back to the patient after CPB, which could preclude the need for a blood transfusion. Patients with residual coronary stenoses, anticipated low CO, or end-organ damage may benefit from even higher hemoglobin concentrations.
2. Two units of packed red blood cells (PRBCs) should be immediately available for use once the CPB pump volume is exhausted. If excessive bleeding is anticipated (see Section F below), then additional units should be on hand.

F. Coagulation. Anticipation of possible coagulation abnormalities is necessary prior to discontinuation of CPB. Blood components should be administered only after CPB when the heparin has been reversed and all surgical repairs are complete. Blood component therapy should be guided by the clinical situation and laboratory findings (e.g., thromboelastogram, prothrombin time, partial thromboplastin time, platelet count).

1. Patients at risk include:
   a. Patients taking platelet inhibitors (clopidogrel, prasugrel, ticlopidine, aspirin) [3]
   b. Patients having emergency surgery and who have been exposed to:
      (1) Thrombolytic agents (alteplase, tenecteplase)
      (2) Antiplatelet glycoprotein IIb/IIIa agents (abciximab, eptifibatide, tirofiban)
      (3) Direct thrombin inhibitors (bivalirudin, dabigatran, argatroban)
      (4) Coumadin
   c. Patients with chronic renal failure
   d. Long "pump run," e.g., redo or complex operation
   e. Low body mass index (BMI)
   f. Extreme hypothermia on CPB
   g. Excessive bleeding with previous CABG [4]
2. Platelets should be available if indicated (as above).
3. Desmopressin acetate (DDAVP) can be used to increase platelet aggregation in patients with chronic renal failure, acquired von Willebrand disease which occurs with aortic stenosis, or other platelet abnormalities. In patients without pre-existing platelet abnormalities, DDAVP has little effect on blood loss or replacement in CABG patients but may be effective in open-chamber surgery (see Section VI.B.3.b).
4. Fresh frozen plasma or cryoprecipitate should be available if indicated for the treatment of appropriate factor deficiencies.
5. Factor concentrates (specifically rVIIA and prothrombin complex concentrates [PCCs]) have been used in cases of severe refractory bleeding. Possible complications are related to increased risk of thrombosis (coronary occlusion, graft occlusion, stroke).

G. Ventilation

1. Adequate oxygenation and ventilation while the patient is on CPB must be ensured by checking arterial and venous blood gas measurements at routine intervals. Arterial pH should be between 7.3 and 7.5 at normothermia before CPB separation.
2. The lungs should be re-expanded with two to three sustained breaths (15 to 20 s each) to a peak pressure of 30 cm H_2O with visual confirmation of bilateral lung expansion and resolution of atelectasis. In patients with internal mammary artery grafts, care must be taken to prevent lung overdistention, which may cause graft avulsion. Coordinate this maneuver with the surgical team. An estimate of lung compliance should be made (see Section 7). The surgeon may need to evacuate any hemothorax or pneumothorax.
3. Inspired oxygen fraction (FiO_2) should be 100%. If air was used during CPB to prevent atelectasis, it should be discontinued. Nitrous oxide should never be used during or after cannulation to avoid increasing the size of air emboli.

4. Confirm pulse oximeter is working once pulsatile flow returns. The pulse oximeter may not work, however, despite pulsatile flow in a patient who is still cold and peripherally vasoconstricted.
5. All airway monitors should be on line (apnea, PIP, FiO_2, end-tidal CO_2).
6. Mechanical ventilation *must* be started before an attempt to terminate CPB. The timing for commencement of mechanical ventilation while the patient is still on CPB is controversial. Some practitioners believe that ventilation should begin when arterial or pulmonary pulsatile blood flow resumes in order to avoid hypoxemia. However, this may not be necessary in normothermic, nearly full-flow bypass and may cause severe respiratory alkalosis of pulmonary venous blood. The pulse oximeter or the CPB circuit venous oxygen tension also can be used to assess the need for ventilation during partial CPB.
7. Auscultation of breath sounds will confirm air movement and may reveal wheezing, rales, or rhonchi. Visual confirmation of bilateral lung expansion is important. Appropriate treatment (suctioning, bronchodilators) should be instituted before terminating CPB. Bronchoscopy may occasionally be needed.

H. **Vaporizer.** Inhalation agents used during CPB for blood pressure (BP) control ordinarily should be turned down or off at least 10 min before terminating CPB. These agents will decrease contractility and confuse the etiology of myocardial dysfunction postbypass.

I. **Volume expanders.** Colloid or crystalloid solution should be available to increase preload if blood products are not indicated. Hetastarch may be contraindicated if excessive bleeding is anticipated or with impaired renal function.

2 J. **Visualization of the heart is important before terminating CPB.** Primarily. Primarily the right atrium and ventricle are visible in the chest. TEE is helpful in permitting a detailed examination. It is possible to evaluate the following parameters:

1. **Contractility.** An experienced observer can often estimate contractility by just looking at the heart in the chest. Wall-motion abnormalities from ischemia or infarct should be compared to pre-CPB observations.
2. **Distention** of the chambers can be seen with both methods.
3. **Residual air** in left-sided structures (e.g., left atrium [LA], left ventricle [LV], pulmonary veins). Inspection during and after ventilation will confirm the location of residual air.
4. **Conduction.** Direct observation of the atria and ventricles can often help differentiate dysrhythmias easier than using the electrocardiogram (ECG). Visualization of the RA appendage may prove especially helpful in this regard. A four-chamber view is most helpful.
5. **Valvular function** or perivalvular leaks should be identified before attempting CPB termination so that repair can be accomplished if needed.

K. **Predictors and factors contributing to adverse cardiovascular outcome**

1. Assess the patient's risk for difficult weaning from CPB. Risk factors that can be identified before terminating CPB include [5]:
   - **a.** Preoperative ejection fraction (EF) less than 45% or diastolic dysfunction
   - **b.** Renal disease—increased morbidity and mortality with increasing creatinine
   - **c.** Female patient undergoing CABG (tendency for incomplete revascularization due to smaller more diseased coronary arteries)
   - **d.** Elderly patient
   - **e.** Congestive heart failure (usually related to valvular or myocardial dysfunction)
   - **f.** Emergent surgery
     - **(1)** Ongoing ischemia or evolving infarct
     - **(2)** Failed closed intervention (angioplasty/stent/valvuloplasty)
   - **g.** Prolonged CPB duration (more than 2 to 3 hrs)
   - **h.** Inadequate surgical repair
     - **(1)** Incomplete coronary revascularization
       - **(a)** Small vessels (not graftable or poor "runoff")
       - **(b)** Distal disease (especially in diabetic patients)

(2) Valvular disease

(a) Valve replacement with very small valve (high transvalvular pressure gradient post-CPB)

(b) Suboptimal valve repair (residual regurgitation or stenosis)

i. Incomplete myocardial preservation during cross-clamping

(1) ECG not asystolic (incomplete diastolic arrest)

(2) Prolonged ventricular fibrillation before cross-clamping

(3) Warm myocardium

(a) LV hypertrophy (incomplete cardioplegia)

(b) High-grade coronary stenoses (no cardioplegia to that area of heart)

(c) Choice of grafting order (grafts should be performed first in an area of the heart served by a high-grade lesion in the absence of retrograde cardioplegia, so cardioplegia may be infused early)

(d) Noncoronary collateral flow washing out cardioplegia

(e) Poor LV venting causing cardiac distention (aortic insufficiency if using antero-grade cardioplegia)

(f) Inadequate topical cooling

j. Prolonged ventricular failure

k. Impaired myocardial perfusion before and after cross-clamping

(1) Low perfusion pressure on CPB (less than 50 mm Hg)

(2) Ventricular distention

(3) Emboli (air, clot, particulate)

(a) From ventriculotomy or improper de-airing of coronary grafts

2. Additional preparations for high-risk patients

a. One common practice is to have a syringe of ephedrine (5 mg/mL) or dilute epinephrine prepared (4 to 10 μg/mL). Boluses can be used until a decision is made regarding the need for further inotropes.

b. Discuss the need for additional invasive monitoring with the surgeon (i.e., LA or central aortic catheter).

c. Check for immediate availability of other inotropic or vasoactive medications: epinephrine, dopamine, milrinone, norepinephrine, nitric oxide, or inhaled epoprostenol (Flolan).

d. As appropriate to the anticipated level of difficulty separating from CPB, check for immediate availability of an intra-aortic balloon pump (IABP). Consider placement of a femoral arterial catheter prebypass to facilitate its rapid insertion and possibly for improved BP monitoring.

e. Consider starting an inotropic infusion or the IABP before terminating CPB in patients with poor contractility. Note that the Frank–Starling law implies that an empty heart will not beat very forcefully. Often a sluggishly contracting heart will start to "snap" once it is filled.

f. "The first attempt at terminating CPB is the best one." Optimizing all parameters before CPB termination is strongly advised. If in doubt, start an inotrope. Pre-emptive use of milrinone has been shown to improve cardiac function during and after cardiac surgery. A milrinone bolus without an infusion can be sufficient in marginal candidates [6].

g. Ischemic preconditioning/postconditioning. The heart will react to a low level ischemic stress and subsequent exposure to free radicals by becoming more "resistant" to further ischemic injury. This can be attempted in the OR [7,8].

(1) Inhalational agents (isoflurane/sevoflurane have been most studied) can mimic this effect.

(a) This can be accomplished by using the agent at 1 to 2.5 MAC for 5 to 10 min after initiating CPB but before the aortic cross-clamp has been placed. Then a 10-min washout occurs prior to starting cardioplegia.

(b) Others suggest using sevoflurane pre-CPB, during CPB, and post-CPB instead of using a propofol infusion [9].

(2) Ketamine, nicorandil, and the "statins" have also been studied with beneficial results [10].
(3) Postischemic conditioning by brief sequential ischemia and reperfusion episodes has also been suggested in this setting.

L. **Protamine.** The protamine dose should be calculated and drawn up in a syringe or should be ready as an infusion. Premature use of protamine is catastrophic. Protamine should be prominently labeled and should not be placed where routine medications are stored to avoid accidental use. The surgeon, anesthesiologist, and perfusionist must all coordinate the use of this medication.

M. **Pressure.** Check the calibration and zero level of all transducers before terminating CPB.

1. **Arterial pressure.** Recognize that radial artery catheters may underestimate central aortic pressure following rewarming [11]. Femoral artery catheters do not share this limitation. An aortic root vent, if present, may be connected to a transducer also. If the radial arterial catheter is not functioning, a needle placed in the aorta or aortic cannula can be transduced during and after termination of CPB until the cannula is removed.
2. **PA pressure.** Ensure that the catheter has not migrated distally to a wedge position. Often the PA catheter must be withdrawn 3 to 5 cm even if this was done at CPB initiation.

N. **Pressors and inotropes**

1. Medications that are likely to be used should be readily available, including a vasodilator (e.g., NTG, nitroprusside) and a potent inotropic agent (e.g., dopamine, dobutamine, epinephrine, milrinone).
2. NTG and phenylephrine should always be available to infuse after CPB as they are almost always used. Some practitioners use prophylactic NTG infusion (approximately 25 to 50 μg/min) for all coronary revascularization procedures to prevent coronary spasm and to enhance non-coronary collateral flow in cases of incomplete revascularization. It also can be used as a venodilator to allow additional CPB pump volume to be infused in patients after CPB.
3. Volumetric infusion pumps deliver vasoactive substances with the highest accuracy and reproducibility.

O. **Pacer.** An external pacemaker should be in the room, checked, and set to the initial settings by the anesthesiologist. A pacemaker often is needed for treatment of relative bradycardia or asystole. In patients with heart block, an AV sequential pacemaker is strongly advised to retain a synchronized atrial contraction. Use of a DDD pacer, when available, is recommended. Temporary biventricular pacing in patients with reduced EF is used in some centers.

P. **Potassium.** Blood chemistries should be checked before terminating CPB.

1. **Hyperkalemia** may induce conduction abnormalities and decreases in contractility. It is more common after long pump runs when large amounts of cardioplegia solution are used and absorbed, especially in patients with renal dysfunction.
2. **Hypokalemia** can cause dysrhythmias and should be treated if less than 3.5 mEq/L and there is adequate urine output after CPB.
3. **Glucose** levels should be checked and treatment undertaken for hyperglycemia in all patients, not just diabetic patients. Hyperglycemia may contribute to central nervous system dysfunction, poor wound healing, and cardiac morbidity. The optimal glucose level is controversial. Some advocate "aggressive treatment" and suggest a glucose level of 110 mg/dL. Most authors try to maintain a level less than 180 mg/mL due to concerns that more aggressive control may lead to complications related to hypoglycemia and possibly higher mortality [12].
4. Ionized Ca^{2+} levels are discussed in Section I.C above.
5. Other electrolytes should be evaluated as needed. In particular, low levels of magnesium are common after CPB and have been associated with dysrhythmias, coronary vasospasm, and postoperative hypertension. Magnesium (2 to 4 g) can be administered into the pump prior to emergence from CPB [13].

II. **Sequence of events immediately before terminating CPB.** Weaning from bypass describes the transition from total CPB to a final condition in which the heart provides 100% of the work. The transition should be gradual, recognizing that cardiac function post-CPB is not usually normal. At times, though, cardiac function may be improved after bypass if ischemia is relieved or valvular dysfunction repaired.

A. Final checklist before terminating CPB

1. **Confirm**
   a. **Ventilation**
      (1) Lungs are ventilated with 100% O_2, visual confirmation, and $ETCO_2$ present.
      (2) Ventilatory alarms are enabled.
      (3) Breath sounds and heart tones are heard via the esophageal stethoscope.
   b. The patient is sufficiently rewarmed.
   c. The heart, great vessels, and grafts have been properly de-aired.
   d. The patient is in optimal metabolic condition.
   e. All equipment and medications are ready.
2. Do not proceed until these criteria have been met.
3. Weaning from CPB requires the utmost concentration and vigilance by the anesthesiologist, and all distractions should be eliminated. Turn the music down and limit extraneous conversations.

B. What to look at during weaning. Key information can be obtained from four sources: the invasive pressure display, the heart itself, the TEE, and the ECG.

1. **Invasive pressure display**
   a. Pressure waveforms (arterial, central venous pressure [CVP], and PA or LA, if used) are best displayed using overlapping traces, and there are some benefits to the use of an identical scale as well. Advantages of this display format include the following:
      (1) Coronary perfusion pressure is graphically depicted as the vertical height between the arterial diastolic pressure and the filling pressure (PA diastolic or LA mean) during diastole.
      (2) The vertical separation between the PA mean and CVP waveforms estimates right ventricular (RV) work.
      (3) The slope of the rise in central aortic pressure during systole may give some indication of LV contractility and is most easily appreciated if the waveform is not compressed.
      (4) Valvular regurgitation can be diagnosed by examining CVP, pulmonary capillary wedge pressure (PCWP), or LA waveforms (e.g., mitral regurgitation may produce V waves in LA and PCWP tracings) as well as by TEE.
   b. **Arterial pressure.** The systolic and mean systemic arterial pressures should be checked continuously.
      (1) The systolic pressure describes the pressure generated by the heart's own contraction.
      (2) Before CPB separation, the mean pressure describes the work performed by the bypass pump and the vascular tone. After separation, it reflects the cardiac work and vascular tone.
      (3) The diastolic pressure reflects vascular tone and gives an indication of coronary perfusion pressure.
      (4) The pulse pressure reflects the mechanical work done by the heart. As the heart assumes more of the circulatory work, this pressure difference increases. LV failure is suggested by a decreased pulse pressure.
      (5) Difficulty in weaning (poor LV function) may be reflected by a low pulse pressure or systolic minus mean pressure difference in the presence of high atrial filling pressures when the venous return line is partially occluded.
      (6) It is important to remember that a radial artery catheter may not be accurate following CPB. During the first 30 min after CPB, the radial artery tends to underestimate both the systolic and mean central aortic pressures. The surgeon can often confirm that there is a pressure difference by palpating the aorta. Clinically significant radial artery hypotension should be confirmed by a noninvasive BP

reading or with a central aortic or femoral artery pressure measurement before treatment or resumption of CPB.

c. **CVP.** This provides an index of right heart filling before and during weaning.
   (1) **Inspection of the heart visually or by TEE** provides valuable information about contractility, wall-motion abnormalities, conduction, preload, valvular function, and quality of surgical repair.
   (2) **ECG** changes, such as heart block, dysrhythmias, or ischemia, occur frequently, mandating frequent examination.
   (3) **TEE.** The mid-papillary transverse view is best for obtaining EF, filling parameters, and regional wall motion abnormalities. The four-chamber view can reveal valvular function and conduction abnormalities.
   (4) **Ventilation and oxygenation.** Routine airway management issues as well as problems in the other major organ systems must not be overlooked. The partial pressure of carbon dioxide ($PaCO_2$) should be kept at or below 40 mm Hg in the post-CPB period. Minor elevations in $PaCO_2$ can increase pulmonary vascular resistance (PVR) significantly. This is most important when RV failure is noted.

III. Sequence of events during weaning from CPB

A. Step 1: Impeding venous return to the pump

1. **Consequences of partial venous occlusion.** Slowly the venous line is partially occluded (by the surgeon or perfusionist). This increase in venous line resistance causes right atrial pressure to rise and diverts blood flow through the tricuspid valve into the RV instead of drainage into the pump. According to the Frank–Starling law, CO increases as preload rises; therefore, the heart begins to eject blood more forcefully as the heart fills and enlarges.
2. **Preload.** The amount of venous line occlusion is adjusted carefully to attain and maintain a certain optimal preload or **LV** end-diastolic volume (LVEDV).
   a. **Estimating preload.** Unless TEE is in use, LV filling volumes cannot be measured directly. Instead, LVEDV is estimated from a filling pressure (PA diastolic, PCWP, or LA pressure [LAP]). The relationship of LVEDV to LAP and PCWP can be quite variable after bypass secondary to changes in diastolic compliance. Decreased compliance is caused by myocardial edema and ischemia. Therefore, the PCWP is a relatively poor indicator of LVEDV in the post-CPB period.
   b. **Optimal preload** is the lowest value that provides an adequate CO. Preload greater than the optimal value may cause:
      (1) Ventricular distention and increased wall tension (increased myocardial oxygen consumption [Mvo_2])
      (2) Decreased coronary perfusion pressure
      (3) Excessive or decreased CO
      (4) Pulmonary edema
   c. **Typical weaning filling pressures.** For patients with good LV function preoperatively, PCWP of 8 to 12 mm Hg or CVP of 6 to 12 mm Hg often suffices. Abnormal contractility or diastolic stiffness may necessitate much higher filling pressures to achieve adequate filling volumes (20 mm Hg or higher), but in such cases it is imperative to monitor left heart filling by a PA or LA line, or by TEE.
   d. **CVP/LAP ratio.** Normally, the CVP is equal or lower than the LAP, which is usually estimated by the PA diastolic pressure (CVP/LAP ratio less than or equal to 1). If the ratio is elevated (greater than 1), the intraventricular septum may be forced toward the left, limiting LV filling and CO. This "septal shift" often can be diagnosed by TEE as well. In this situation, termination of CPB may be impossible until the ratio is normalized by improving RV function [14].

B. Step 2: Lowering pump flow into the aorta

1. **Attaining partial bypass.** The rise in preload causes the heart to begin to contribute to the CO. This condition is termed *partial bypass* because the venous blood draining into the right atrium divides into two paths: Some goes to the pump, and some passes through the RV and lungs and is ejected into the aorta by the LV.

a. Some institutions advocate keeping the patient on partial CPB for several minutes to wash vasoactive substances from the lungs before terminating CPB.

2. **Reduced pump outflow requirement.** Because two sources of blood are now supplying the aorta, the amount of arterial blood returned from the pump to the patient can be reduced as native CO increases to maintain total aortic blood flow. Therefore, the perfusionist lowers the pump flow rate in increments of 0.5 to 1 L/min. This step is repeated, allowing gradual reductions in pump flow rate while cardiac function and hemodynamics are carefully monitored.

3. **Readjusting venous line resistance.** Some adjustment in the venous line resistance may be needed to maintain a constant filling pressure as the heart is given more work to perform. Also, as arterial pump outflow is reduced, less venous inflow is needed to keep the venous reservoir from being pumped dry. Therefore, the venous line clamp can be progressively tightened to achieve the desired increase in preload.

C. **Step 3: Terminating bypass.** If the heart is generating an adequate systolic pressure (typically 90 to 100 mm Hg for an adult) at an acceptable preload with pump flows of 1 L/min or less, the patient is ready for a trial without CPB, and bypass is terminated. The pump is stopped and the venous cannula is clamped. If hemodynamics are not satisfactory, CPB is reinstituted, and management of cardiovascular decompensation is begun (see Section IV.D. below).

IV. Sequence of events immediately after terminating CPB

A. **Preload: Infusing blood from the pump.** If cardiac performance is inadequate, small increases in preload may be beneficial. For adult patients, volume is transferred in 50- to 100-mL increments from the venous pump reservoir to the patient through the aortic cannula. Before volume infusion, the aortic cannula should be inspected for air bubbles within its lumen. Increments of 10 to 50 mL are used in pediatric patients. During volume infusions from the pump, the BP, filling pressure, and heart should be watched closely. Continuous infusion is contraindicated because overdistention of the heart may occur and the oxygenator reservoir may be emptied, infusing air into the patient.

1. The almost instantaneous infusion of volume by the pump allows for evaluation of LV function. You can assume that during the infusion there is no change in SVR. According to the formula:

$$BP = CO \times SVR$$

If you make SVR a constant, then:

$$BP = CO$$

An increase in BP with a small volume infusion must indicate an increase in CO.

2. **If BP and CO do not change** with increased preload, the patient probably is at the top (flat part) of the Frank–Starling curve, and further volume infusion is unlikely to be of benefit.

3. **If BP does rise**, the rise is probably due to a rise in CO, and further volume administration may be beneficial. In this manner, the optimal preload can be titrated after CPB. The TEE can be helpful here.

4. Three factors often contribute to a need to give volume after CPB:
   a. Continued rewarming of peripheral vascular beds results in vasodilation.
   b. Changes in LV diastolic compliance alter optimal filling pressure.
   c. Continued bleeding.

B. **Measuring cardiac function**

1. Before taking the relatively irrevocable steps of removing the aortic cannula or administering protamine, cardiac function should be assessed because an adequate BP may be the result of a low CO and a high SVR. Cardiac function may be assessed by measuring CO or by TEE. The derived cardiac index (CO/body surface area) should be calculated. Generally, a cardiac index of more than 2 L/min/m^2 should be present to consider permanent termination of CPB, although an index of greater than 2.2 usually is considered "normal." If

HR is high, a normal CO can exist despite a low stroke volume. Therefore, a calculation of the stroke volume index (cardiac index/HR) can be useful (normal is greater than 40 mL/beat/m^2).

2. **Measuring patient perfusion.** Signs of adequate tissue perfusion after CPB should be sought. Within the first 5 to 10 min after terminating CPB, arterial blood gases and pH should be measured, looking for lactic acidosis or gas exchange abnormalities. Mixed venous oxygen saturation (SVO_2) indicates global body O_2 supply–demand balance. Urine output indicates adequacy of renal perfusion and normally rises after CPB, and lack of such a rise should be evaluated and treated immediately. The ideal perfusion pressure for adequate tissue perfusion should be individualized. Patients with renal insufficiency, cerebrovascular disease, or hypertension may require higher perfusion pressures, although the increased BP may worsen bleeding.
3. **Afterload and aortic impedance.** In the presence of good LV function (and the absence of myocardial ischemia), the anesthesiologist should avoid elevated afterload (as reflected by systolic BP) to prevent excessive stress on the aortic suture lines and to reduce surgical bleeding. In adults, the usual desired range for systolic BP is 100 to 130 mm Hg.

   With impaired LV function or valvular regurgitation, SVR should be reduced to the lowest level possible while maintaining adequate BP for organ perfusion. Reducing the aortic impedance improves LV ejection and lowers systolic LV wall stress and myocardial O_2 demand. Impedance is related to BP and SVR, and lowering SVR can result in increased CO with no change in BP.

C. **Removing the cannulas**

1. **Venous cannula(s).** The presence of a large cannula(s) in the right atrium or in the vena cava will impair venous return to the heart, and if cardiac function is reasonable, the venous cannula should be removed as soon as practical. Removing the cannula will allow the perfusionist to "reprime" the pump and allow for further volume infusion through the aortic cannula.
2. **Aortic cannula.** Removal of the aortic cannula should usually wait until at least half of the protamine dose has been infused and cardiovascular stability confirmed.

D. **Cardiovascular decompensation**

1. Refer to Chapter 2 for specific drug pharmacology and doses.
2. Failure of the LV or RV, both of which are recovering from the insult of CPB, together with low SVR are the most common causes of cardiovascular insufficiency during the weaning process.

   a. **LV failure**

   (1) The differential diagnosis of LV failure after CPB is listed in Table 9.1.

   (2) Treatment of LV failure during weaning from CPB includes:

   (a) Inotropic drug administration. Most commonly epinephrine or milrinone is chosen as a first-line agent, although some institutions advocate the use of dopamine or dobutamine initially. Regardless of choice, ephedrine 5 to 20 mg or a 4 to 10 μg bolus of epinephrine is given to increase contractility and BP while commencing infusion of an inotrope.

   (i) Epinephrine or dopamine may be appropriate if HR is normal and SVR is low or normal.

   (ii) Dobutamine or milrinone may be more appropriate if SVR is increased.

   (iii) Low-dose epinephrine or milrinone may be appropriate if HR is elevated.

   (iv) Dobutamine or dopamine may be more appropriate if HR is low and pacing is not being used.

   (v) Norepinephrine or phenylephrine may be appropriate if SVR is low and CO is normal or elevated.

   (vi) Milrinone will significantly reduce SVR, so the use of an arterial vasoconstrictor (phenylephrine, norepinephrine) often is necessary.

   (b) Start NTG if ischemia is present (consider use of short-acting beta-blockers).

TABLE 9.1 Differential diagnosis of LV failure after CPB

I. Ischemia
- **A.** Graft failure
  - **1.** Clot, particulate in graft
  - **2.** Distal suture causing constriction
  - **3.** Kinking of graft
  - **4.** Air in graft
  - **5.** Graft sewn in backward (no flow through valves)
  - **6.** Inadequate flow through internal mammary artery
- **B.** Inadequate coronary blood flow
  - **1.** Incomplete revascularization (secondary to distal disease or inoperable vessels)
  - **2.** Inadequate coronary perfusion pressure
  - **3.** Emboli in native coronary arteries—air or particulate matter (clot, atherosclerotic plaque)
  - **4.** Coronary spasm
  - **5.** Tachycardia (decreased diastolic filling time)
  - **6.** Increased myocardial O_2 demand
  - **7.** Surgical injury to native coronary artery
- **C.** Myocardial ischemia leading to myocardial damage
  - **1.** Incomplete myocardial preservation during CPB
  - **2.** Evolving myocardial infarction

II. Valve failure
- **A.** Prosthetic valve
  - **1.** Sewn in backward
  - **2.** Perivalvular leak
  - **3.** Mechanical obstruction (immobile disk)
- **B.** Native valve—acute mitral regurgitation (papillary muscle ischemia or rupture)

III. Inadequate Gas exchange
- **A.** Hypoxemia
  - **1.** Inadequate Fio_2
  - **2.** Residual atelectasis
  - **3.** Mechanical ventilator failure
  - **4.** Airway disconnection
  - **5.** Severe bronchospasm
  - **6.** Pulmonary edema ("pump lung" or adult respiratory distress syndrome)
- **B.** Hypoventilation

IV. Preload
- **A.** Inadequate preload
  - **1.** Hypovolemia
  - **2.** Loss of atrial contraction
- **B.** Excessive preload (can lead to distention of cardiac structures)

V. Reperfusion injury

VI. Ventricular septal defect

VII. Miscellaneous causes of decreased contractility
- **A.** Medications
  - **1.** β-blockade
  - **2.** Calcium channel blockers
  - **3.** Inhalational agents
- **B.** Acidemia
- **C.** Electrolyte abnormalities
  - **1.** Hyperkalemia
  - **2.** Hypocalcemia
- **D.** Pre-existing LV failure

CPB, cardiopulmonary bypass.

b. RV failure

(1) Diagnosis

(a) Active pumping by the RV is mandatory for optimal cardiovascular function, particularly in the presence of elevated PA pressures.

(b) Patients most at risk include those with

(i) Pulmonary hypertension

(a) Chronic mitral valve disease

(b) Left-to-right shunts (atrial septal defect, ventricular septal defect)

(c) Massive pulmonary embolism

(d) Air embolism

(e) Primary pulmonary hypertension

(f) Acute or chronic mitral regurgitation

(i) Valvular dysfunction

(ii) Papillary muscle rupture

(g) Diastolic LV dysfunction

(i) RV ischemia or infarct

(ii) RV outflow obstruction

(iii) Tricuspid regurgitation

(c) Physiologic findings

(i) Depressed cardiac index (CI)

(ii) Inappropriate elevation in CVP compared to PCWP (unless biventricular failure exists)

(iii) Increased PVR (more than 2.5 Wood units or greater than 200 dynes · sec/cm^5)

(iv) Pulmonary hypertension

(v) Reduced PA minus CVP mean pressure difference to less than 5 mm Hg.

(2) Treatment

(a) Treat signs of ischemia.

(i) Start NTG infusion if systemic BP permits.

(ii) Increase coronary perfusion pressure.

(b) Increased preload usually is required.

(c) Increase inotropic support. Milrinone, dobutamine, and isoproterenol are often effective because any of these will increase RV contractility and decrease PVR.

(d) Use adjuncts to decrease PVR [15].

(i) Hyperventilation will induce hypocapnia and decrease PVR. This should be accomplished by means of a high respiratory rate rather than an increase in inflation pressure, which may increase PVR.

(ii) Avoid hypoxemia, which will induce pulmonary vasoconstriction.

(iii) Avoid acidemia.

(iv) Maintain normal core temperature.

(v) Use pulmonary vasodilators (nitroglycerin, nitroprusside, epoprostenol [Flolan]) [16].

(e) Administer nitric oxide (NO) by inhalation (10 to 40 ppm).

(f) Prostaglandin E_1 Prostacyclin (PGE_1 Flolan—epoprostenol) infusion through a right atrial line will induce pulmonary vasodilation. This often requires concomitant norepinephrine infusion into the systemic circulation through an LA catheter to avoid marked SVR reduction. Inhaled iloprost is another alternative [16].

(g) Sildenafil has been suggested.

(h) Use an RV assist device.

E. **Inappropriate vasodilation** may prevent achievement of an adequate BP despite an acceptable or elevated CI.

1. Causes include:

a. Pre-existing medications (calcium channel blockers, ACE inhibitors)

   b. Electrolyte abnormalities
   c. Acid–base disturbances
   d. Sepsis
   e. Pre-existing diseases (cirrhosis, dialysis fistula)
   f. Hyperthermia
   g. Idiopathic condition (poorly characterized factors related to CPB)
2. Excessive hemodilution decreases viscosity and lowers the apparent SVR.
3. Management includes vasoconstrictors (e.g., phenylephrine or norepinephrine) and red blood cell (RBC) transfusion when appropriate.
4. **Vasoplegic syndrome** is a severe form of post-CPB dilation characterized by low mean arterial pressure (MAP), normal to high CO, normal right-sided filling pressures, low SVR which is refractory to pressor therapy. Pre-CPB risk factors including patient Euroscore, preoperative use of beta-blockers and ACE inhibitors, pre-CPB hypotension and pressor use, as well as unexpected hypotension after starting CPB may predict this syndrome [17]. The syndrome is associated with an increased overall mortality. Nitric oxide inhibition with methylene blue has been used as salvage therapy in these cases. A dose of 2 mg/kg can be given over 20 min. There is some data suggesting that administration pre-CPB may be more beneficial [18].

5

F. **Resumption of CPB**

1. The decision to resume CPB after a trial of native circulation must not be made prematurely because there are dangers to resuming CPB (inadequate heparinization, hemolysis), but CPB must be restarted before permanent ischemic organ damage occurs (heart, brain, kidneys). Inserting a **TEE** probe, if not present, can rapidly facilitate diagnosis and treatment, preventing the resumption of CPB. There is a risk of bleeding as the patient is still fully heparinized. If severe cardiovascular derangements continue for 3 to 5 min, reinstitution of CPB is indicated. While the patient is on CPB, diagnosis and treatment should continue but may proceed without markedly increasing the risk of organ failure.
2. Heparin should be given as needed based on the last activated clotting time measurement made while the patient was on CPB. (If any protamine was given, a full dose of heparin, 300 units/kg, is needed before resuming CPB.)
3. During the period that it takes to reestablish CPB, it is important to maintain coronary and cerebral perfusion with inotropes and vasopressors. In extreme circumstances, it may be necessary for the surgical assistant to initiate open-chest massage if the cannulas were already removed.
4. When CPB is initiated, all inotropes and vasopressors should initially be stopped, because patients in this situation frequently become hypertensive. If BP elevation is marked, the perfusionist can lower pump flow briefly while appropriate vasodilator therapy is given. Resumption of extracorporeal circulation will significantly lower myocardial oxygen requirements. Maintenance of a reasonable perfusion pressure is critical to allow adequate O_2 delivery to potentially ischemic cells. This should be achieved with a pure alpha-agent such as phenylephrine. Despite lower O_2 requirements and adequate supply, the ischemic cell may not be able to utilize O_2 efficiently. This has resulted in the use of secondary cardioplegia.
5. Additional recovery and reversal of damage can occur if the heart is rearrested with warm-blood–enriched cardioplegia for a brief period.
6. Any mechanical factors that could compromise cardiac performance must be sought and surgically corrected.
   a. Ongoing ischemia based on ECG changes or TEE wall-motion abnormalities may indicate graft occlusion and may require surgical reevaluation for graft patency. A Doppler probe can be used to assess flow.
   b. Valvular abnormalities may be inferred from the PA trace or more specifically by TEE. Evaluation for perivalvular leaks, prosthetic valve function, or residual stenosis/regurgitation should be undertaken at this time, if indicated.
7. Unsuccessful weaning will necessitate the addition of more aggressive inotropic support.

8. **Increase monitoring.** LA pressure is a better estimate of LV end-diastolic pressure than PA pressures. Aortic or femoral arterial pressures may be more accurate than radial pressures. TEE or epicardial echocardiography can provide valuable data on function and filling.
9. Consideration of separation from bypass should be made only after the surgeon is assured that technical difficulties did not account for impaired myocardial performance and that the heart is "adequately rested." If the second attempt to wean is unsuccessful, continue to optimize preload and afterload with vasodilators or volume infusion as needed.
   a. **IABP** will augment diastolic BP, increase coronary perfusion, and decrease afterload, and should be considered. It is contraindicated in aortic surgery.
   b. Chest closure may adversely affect hemodynamics (see Section V.E)
   c. If available, ventricular assist devices can be life saving after multiple failed attempts to separate the patient from CPB. These are generally used either to rest the "stunned myocardium" or as a bridge to heart transplantation (see Chapter 20).

V. Cardiovascular considerations after successful weaning from CPB

The post-CPB period represents a time in which the myocardium is recovering from the insult of surgery, CPB, and its attendant inflammatory effects. During this period, major physiologic and surgical changes occur and they need to be understood in order to develop proper therapeutic approaches in patient management. The extent of these physiologic alterations and the time to recovery depend on numerous patient and surgical factors that have been described in Section I.K.

A. Reperfusion injury

Reperfusion injury describes a series of functional, structural, and metabolic alterations that result from reperfusion of myocardium after a period of temporary ischemia. The potential for this type of injury exists for all cardiac procedures where the aorta is clamped. The damage is characterized by:

1. Cytosolic accumulation of calcium
2. Marked cell swelling (myocardial edema), which decreases postischemic blood flow and ventricular compliance
3. Generation of free radicals resulting from reintroduction of O_2 during reperfusion. These oxygen free radicals can cause membrane damage by lipid peroxidation. Various strategies are used to minimize injury, including re-oxygenation with warm blood to start aerobic metabolism as well as other evolving strategies [19].

B. Decannulation. When the patient is hemodynamically stable after separation from CPB, the venous cannula(s) is (are) removed. Blood loss and atrial dysrhythmias are the most common complications during repair of the atrial cannula site. After infusion of the appropriate volume of blood from the pump, the aortic cannula is clamped and removed. To minimize blood loss and prevent possible aortic disruption, the BP is frequently lowered (usually less than 100 mm Hg) to reduce tension on the aortic wall. If, during aortic cannula removal, there is significant blood loss resulting in hemodynamic deterioration, a cannula may quickly be reinserted into the right atrium and the appropriate volume infused to achieve stability. Protamine administration is usually started prior to aortic cannula removal in case it adversely affects hemodynamics (see Section VI.B1).

C. Manipulation of the heart. The heart often is lifted after bypass, to allow examination or repair of the distal anastomotic sites. The sequelae of this action include impaired venous return, atrial and ventricular dysrhythmias, and decreased ventricular ejection, all of which result in systemic hypotension. Manipulation such as this should be limited to brief periods in order to avoid hemodynamic deterioration. Discuss with the surgeon when to put the heart back down. If the heart is slow to recover, you may need to limit cardiac manipulation. Overtreatment of these hypotensive episodes with the administration of catecholamine or calcium boluses should be avoided, as it usually results in major hypertension when manipulation is stopped. Very high BP at this stage can lead to graft disruption and increased bleeding.

D. Myocardial ischemia

1. **Coronary artery spasm.** Ischemia in the postbypass period may be secondary to spasm of the native coronary vessels or internal mammary artery. This typically manifests as

ST-segment elevation, although dysrhythmias, severe hypotension, and cardiac arrest may also occur as sequelae. Mechanisms that have been proposed include intense coronary vasoconstriction from hypothermia, local trauma, respiratory alkalosis, excess sympathetic stimulation of the α-receptors on the coronary vessels, release of vasoconstricting agents from platelets (thromboxane), and injury to native vascular endothelium with the loss of endogenous vascular relaxing factors (i.e., endothelium-derived relaxing factor and prostacyclin). Therapeutic modalities that have been used successfully to treat coronary spasm include intracoronary administration of drugs including nitroglycerin and papaverine, or systemic administration of nitroglycerin; calcium channel blockers (e.g., nicardipine); and other phosphodiesterase inhibitors (milrinone).

2. **Mechanical obstruction.** Compression of vein or internal mammary artery grafts can produce myocardial ischemia and should be considered. Ventilation with large tidal volumes can intermittently impair internal mammary artery graft flow and the distended lung can lead to disruption of the graft at the anastomotic site.
3. **Inadequate revascularization**

E. Chest closure. During chest closure, hemodynamic deterioration may ensue. In general, patients with normal LV function and adequate intravascular volume tolerate closure without problems. Some patients experience mild hypotension and will respond promptly to volume administration. In individuals with poor ventricular function or patients currently receiving inotropic agents, additional volume or inotropic support may be required to maintain similar hemodynamics. If these interventions fail, the surgeon may be required to reopen the chest. The TEE can be especially useful to determine the causes of hemodynamic instability, including myocardial ischemia with new wall-motion abnormalities or hypovolemia.

Chest closure may cause cardiovascular deterioration for the following reasons.

1. In patients who have significant myocardial edema, closure will impair RV contractility and venous return.
2. Edematous, overdistended lungs can lead to a tamponade-like effect after closure in patients with severe chronic obstructive lung disease (COPD).
3. A source of bleeding not identified before adaptation of the sternal borders can lead to cardiac tamponade.
4. Finally, closure may result in a vein or internal mammary artery graft becoming kinked with the development of ischemia in the area of the jeopardized myocardium. If these mechanical problems are eliminated and hemodynamics remain compromised, the chest may need to be left opened temporarily. A sterile dressing can be placed over the open chest and the patient brought to the ICU in this condition. The chest can be closed in the future.

F. Management of hemodynamics in the postbypass period. Proper management of patients in the postbypass period involves continuous assessment of five hemodynamic variables as summarized in Figure 9.1. These are preload, rate, rhythm, contractility, and afterload. Although profound cardiovascular collapse after bypass is uncommon, it is likely that a technical problem (ischemia, valvular dysfunction) or severe metabolic derangement exists, and TEE can help make the correct diagnosis. If cardiovascular deterioration is unresponsive to maximal inotropic therapy [20] and no immediate reversible cause can be identified, then reinstitution of CPB will be necessary.

VI. Noncardiovascular considerations

A. Respiratory system

1. Pulmonary edema

a. **Post-CPB pulmonary dysfunction.** Pulmonary dysfunction after CPB is a common event; however, the extent and severity often vary. The alveolar-arterial (A-a) O_2 gradient increases after bypass and becomes maximal at approximately 18 to 48 hrs postoperatively. The etiology of this ventilation–perfusion mismatch is presumed to be an increase in pulmonary interstitial fluid and results in hypoxemia and hypercapnia. In its most severe state, a form of adult respiratory distress syndrome develops and is referred to as *postperfusion lung syndrome*.

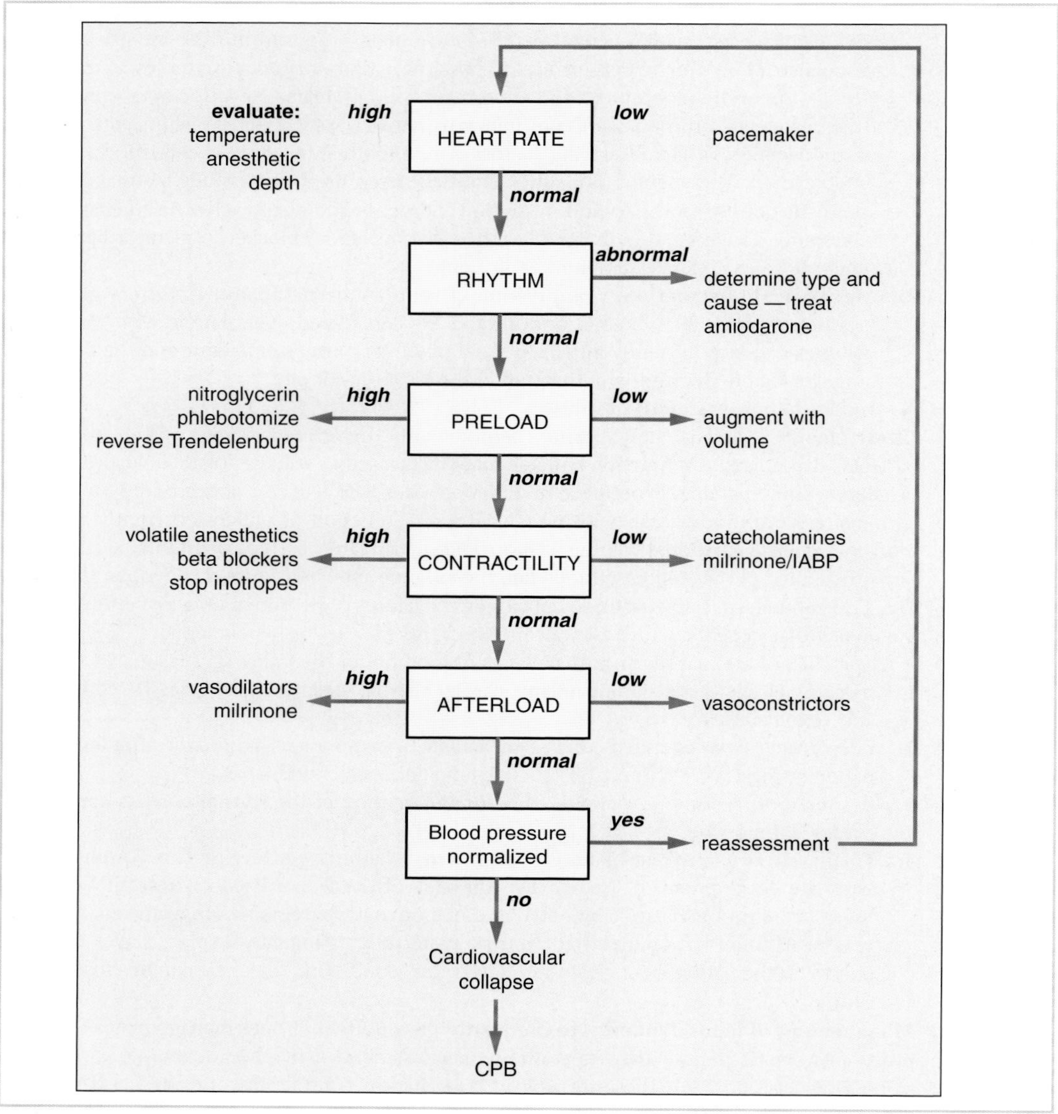

FIGURE 9.1 Management scheme for cardiovascular dysfunction in the postbypass period. CPB, cardiopulmonary bypass; IABP, intra-aortic balloon pump.

(1) Etiologic factors include:
- **(a)** Loss of surfactant
- **(b)** Hypoxic damage to lung tissue, and pulmonary vasculitis caused by:
  - **(i)** Hemolyzed blood
  - **(ii)** Protein denaturation
  - **(iii)** Multiple pulmonary emboli
- **(c)** Accumulation of activated neutrophils in the lungs. Lysosomal enzymes produce pulmonary capillary damage and subsequent leakage of plasma.
- **(d)** Transfusion reactions and transfusion-related acute lung injury.

(e) Postperfusion lung syndrome has virtually been eliminated today with the use of membrane oxygenators, which has greatly diminished blood trauma.

b. **LV dysfunction.** Poor ventricular function in the postbypass period will result in elevated pulmonary venous pressures. This, combined with reduced colloid osmotic pressure secondary to hemodilution, will result in increased pulmonary interstitial fluid.

c. **Pre-existing pulmonary edema.** The individuals presenting for surgery with pulmonary edema represent a significant risk. These patients may be extremely difficult to oxygenate or ventilate after CPB. Techniques that may improve oxygenation include ultrafiltration and aggressive diuresis while on bypass.

d. **Treatment options**
   (1) Decrease preload (nitroglycerin infusion)
   (2) Decrease afterload (sodium nitroprusside, reduce vasoconstrictors if in use)
   (3) Diuresis
   (4) Increase contractility
   (5) Increase positive end-expiratory pressure (PEEP)
   (6) Increase tidal volume or FiO_2

e. **Anaphylactic reactions.** Certain drugs, such as protamine, and administration of blood products or colloid volume expanders may, on rare occasions, cause an increase in pulmonary capillary permeability.

2. **Mechanical factors**

a. **Pneumothorax** occurs most commonly when the pleural cavity is entered during dissection of the internal mammary artery. Other etiologic factors include barotrauma from excess positive-pressure ventilation, particularly in patients with low lung or chest wall compliance, and entry into the pleural space as a complication of central venous access. A pneumothorax may manifest itself only after chest closure.

b. **Hemothorax.** Accumulation of blood in the pleural cavity can occur during bypass as blood from the mediastinum frequently overfills the pericardial sling. It also may occur with dissection of the internal mammary artery before administration of heparin, which results in the collection of clot in the pleural space. The pleural space should be examined, and adequate removal of blood and clot is imperative before termination of CPB and before chest closure.

c. **Movement of the endotracheal tube.** Draping the patient for cardiac procedures will often result in part of the head and endotracheal tube being obscured from direct vision. Even when the endotracheal tube is visualized, the surgeon will frequently push on this tube in an attempt to gain better surgical exposure, which may result in its displacement. Therefore, it is important, intermittently, to reconfirm proper positioning by checking all connections, observing bilateral chest movement, and visualizing one or both lung fields if the pleural cavities are exposed.

d. **Obstruction of the tracheobronchial tree**
   (1) **Mucous plug.** Dry inspissated secretions may accumulate in the tracheobronchial tree or endotracheal tube, and partially or completely obstruct the airway. In most cases, this can be diagnosed and managed by suctioning the airway with a small catheter.
   (2) **Blood.** Injury to the upper airway or trachea due to laryngoscopy, placement of an endotracheal tube, or an unrecognized pre-existent airway lesion followed by heparinization may result in aspiration of blood. If significant, this can result in varying degrees of airway obstruction. More likely, however, the blood will be aspirated into the distal airways and alveoli, causing marked ventilation–perfusion mismatch. Blood also may appear in the airway due to perforation of the PA secondary to inappropriate management of the PA catheter. Risk factors for inadvertent PA displacement include surgical manipulation of the heart, advanced patient age, anticoagulation, hypothermia, and pulmonary hypertension.

3. **Increase in dead space**

a. The most common cause is air trapping from bronchospasm but may be related to other factors. The end tidal CO_2 tracing can help confirm an obstructive pattern. A change will be noted in the $ETCO_2$–$PaCO_2$ difference. In severe cases the gradient may be 15 to 25 torr.

b. **Etiology**
   (1) Bronchospasm
      (a) Pre-existing asthma or COPD
      (b) New onset
         (i) Mechanical
            (a) Endotracheal tube (carinal irritation)
            (b) Secretions or blood
         (ii) Chemical
            (a) Medications
            (b) Histamine release
            (c) Inflammation
            (d) Anaphylaxis
   (2) ARDS
   (3) Transfusion-related
   (4) Decreased CO
   (5) Pulmonary embolus
      (a) Thrombus unlikely, but possible after protamine administration
      (b) Air entrainment

c. **Treatment for bronchospasm**
   (1) Remove the offending agent
   (2) Inhaled $beta_2$ agonists (albuterol, salmeterol)
   (3) Inhaled anticholinergic agents—ipratropium bromide
   (4) Epinephrine
   (5) Corticosteroids (IV or inhaled)
   (6) Theophylline in chronic patients
   (7) Ventilatory changes (longer expiratory time, lower respiratory rate)
   (8) Inhalational agents if CI is adequate

4. **Intrapulmonary shunt**
   a. **Atelectasis.** Perhaps the most common cause of decreased arterial oxygenation postbypass is atelectasis. Although diffuse, chest radiographs postoperatively frequently reveal a pattern of left lower lobe infiltration and atelectasis. The likely explanation is that application of ice causes temporary phrenic nerve injury with subsequent paralysis of the left leaf of the diaphragm. For this reason many have ceased using topical ice slush. During CPB or post-CPB you may be asked to limit tidal volume to improve surgical exposure and visualization. Increasing tidal volume back to normal or the addition of PEEP can improve oxygenation.
   b. **Inhibition of hypoxic pulmonary vasoconstriction.** Hypoxic pulmonary vasoconstriction is the mechanism believed to be responsible for the increase in PVR in regions of atelectasis. This protective mechanism can be attenuated or inhibited by the use of vasodilators (nitroprusside, nitroglycerin) and inotropes used to improve hemodynamic status.

5. **Intracardiac shunt.** When evaluating hypoxemia after CPB, the possibility of a right-to-left shunt must always be considered. Decreased RV contractility and compliance after CPB, in the presence of increased PVR associated with PEEP, will frequently elevate right atrial pressures above those on the left side. This equalization or reversal of pressure is the mechanism by which a patent foramen is opened. A helpful diagnostic tool in detecting a

6 right-to-left shunt at the atrial level is TEE.

B. **Hematologic system**

Management of the coagulation system and blood conservation are just below cardiovascular stability in terms of priority and decision making during this time period. Protamine dosing is important and complications can be significant. The optimal hemoglobin level or blood-carrying capacity is also subject to interpretation post-CPB. RBC transfusion, commonly recommended for almost all patients in the past, has now progressed to a joint decision by the surgical, intensive care, and anesthesia teams.

1. **Protamine**
   a. **Pharmacology.** Protamine is a highly alkaline polycationic protein derived from salmon sperm that is predominantly arginine. Protamine binds the polyanionic glycosaminoglycan heparin and neutralizes its effect.
   b. **Dose.** Various methods have been used to determine the appropriate dose of protamine needed to reverse the effects of heparin. Some of these are detailed here.

      In 1975, Bull et al. [21] recommended the quantitative neutralization of heparin. By using the *heparin dose–response curve based on activated clotting time* (ACT) just before separation from CPB, one could determine the amount of circulating heparin remaining. Bull et al. recommended that 1.3 mg of protamine would adequately neutralize 100 units of circulating heparin in most individuals. However, this technique greatly overestimates the amount of protamine required at the end of CPB. Some clinicians still use *fixed dosing of protamine* for neutralizing heparin, which is based on a fixed protamine/heparin ratio determined by the total heparin administered during the initiation of CPB. The ratio used is 0.5 to 1 mg of protamine for every 100 units of heparin given to the patient. Lower doses often are all that is required to reverse heparin, because heparin levels decrease with time.

      The automated heparin protamine titration test represents a more precise method for determining the residual heparin concentration at the termination of bypass. Using this technique, the total dose of protamine administered is less than that using a fixed protamine–heparin regimen [22].
   c. **Route and rate.** Protamine may be administered safely by either a central or a peripheral route. The most important factor in keeping hemodynamic changes at their lowest possible level is the rate of administration. Although this rate varies considerably among institutions, a suggested interval for the initial dose of protamine is as an infusion over 10 to 15 min, but no faster than 25 to 50 mg/min. Infusing protamine over 30 min may reduce the incidence of heparin rebound compared with administration over 5 min, but is rarely done so slowly.
   d. **Classification of protamine reactions.** Multiple reactions to protamine have been described. The most life-threatening types of reactions are related to *anaphylaxis* [23]. Prior exposure to protamine or similar antigen is required to produce sensitization. On re-exposure, cells will release histamine, prostaglandins, and chemotactic factors, thereby initiating an anaphylactic response characterized by vascular collapse. *Anaphylactoid reactions* are nonimmunologic and therefore do not require previous exposure to the antigen. Both immunoglobulin G (IgG) antibodies to protamine and heparin–protamine complexes can activate the complement system with the generation of fragments called *anaphylatoxins.* Complement-mediated reactions can range from mild hypotension to acute cardiovascular collapse, pulmonary vasoconstriction, and RV failure. The hemodynamic consequences of catastrophic pulmonary vasoconstriction include a several-fold increase in PA pressure followed by RV distention and hypokinesis. This obstruction to RV outflow results in severe systemic hypotension requiring inotropic support to restore circulatory stability. The presumed mechanism is the activation of complement, which results in the generation of thromboxane causing acute pulmonary vasoconstriction. Therapy for these protamine reactions is listed in Table 9.2.
2. **Blood conservation**
   a. **Autologous transfusions**
      (1) **Preoperative donation.** Although preoperative autologous blood donations in patients undergoing cardiac surgery have been used, this is not practical for the majority of cardiac surgical patients, and it may not be cost-effective.
      (2) **Prebypass phlebotomy/autologous normovolemic hemodilution.** Intraoperative hemodilution by means of phlebotomy may reduce the requirement for

TABLE 9.2 Therapy for idiosyncratic protamine reactions

Initial therapy

1. Stop administration of protamine
2. Maintain airway with 100% O_2
3. Discontinue all anesthetic agents
4. Start intravascular volume expansion (2–4 L of crystalloid/colloid)
5. Give epinephrine (5–10 μg/IV bolus with hypotension, titrate as needed; 0.1–1 mg IV with cardiovascular collapse)
6. Reinstitute CPB for severe reactions to allow time for drug therapy to take effect

Secondary treatment

1. Antihistamines (diphenhydramine 0.5–1 mg/kg)
2. Catecholamine infusions (starting doses)
   a. Epinephrine (5–10 μg/min)
   b. Norepinephrine (5–10 μg/min)
   c. Arginine vasopressin (0.1 units/min)
3. Bronchospasm treatment
   a. Inhaled beta agonists (albuterol, etc.)
   b. Inhaled acetylcholine esterase inhibitors (ipratropium bromide)
   c. Epinephrine
   d. Aminophylline (5–6 mg/kg bolus over 20 min followed by infusion)
4. Corticosteroids (0.25–1 g hydrocortisone; alternatively, 1–2 g methylprednisolone)[a]
5. Sodium bicarbonate (0.5–1 mEq/kg with persistent hypotension or acidosis)

Specific treatment for catastrophic pulmonary vasoconstriction

1. Initial therapy as above
2. Immediate hyperventilation to reduce $PaCO_2$
3. Milrinone
4. Nitroglycerine infusion
5. Inhaled nitric oxide 10–40 ppm
6. Epoprostenol (Flolan)
7. Sildenafil

[a]Methylprednisolone may be the drug of choice if the reaction is suspected to be mediated by complement. IV, intravenous.
Modified from Levy JH. *Anaphylactic Reactions in Anesthesia and Intensive Care.* 2nd ed. Boston, MA: Butterworth-Heinemann; 1992:162.

homologous RBC transfusion. This occurs by sparing platelets from CPB and therefore improving their function when the unit(s) are given after protamine. Patients should have hemoglobin greater than 12 before blood is removed. The amount of removed blood varies from 1 to 2 units (500 to 1,000 mL) and depends on the baseline hematocrit as well as the age of the patient, the patient's body surface area, and the presence of any coexisting diseases. Prebypass phlebotomy may be accomplished before heparinization and the blood placed in citrate phosphate dextrose (CPD) blood bags, or it may be done just before initiation of bypass when blood is collected from the venous line of the CPB circuit. Whether this practice actually reduces allogenic transfusions (especially fibrinolytic agents are used) is controversial. If enough blood is removed to severely reduce the hematocrit on CPB and the blood is reinfused during CPB, then obviously platelet function will be impaired and no benefit will be seen.

Contraindications include:

(a) Ongoing ischemia, emergency operation, or cardiovascular instability
(b) Hematocrit less than 35%
(c) Severe pulmonary, renal, or cerebrovascular disease

(3) Intraoperative blood salvage. Blood that is lost before systemic heparinization or after protamine administration can be retrieved by a system that adds heparin or other anticoagulants. This salvaged blood is washed and filtered such that the remaining product is packed RBCs without heparin. Blood salvage should be used prior to allogenic RBC transfusion.

(4) **Shed blood.** Blood collected from both the mediastinum and pleural cavities in the postoperative period can be reinfused to the patient; however, the product collected from these sites does not clot due to defibrination, has an increased free hemoglobin content, and contains a spectrum of other hemostatic activation products that may not be ideal for reinfusion unless urgently needed or washed and spun as mentioned above. Refer to Chapter 17 (Arrhythmia, Rhythm Management Devices, and Catheter and Surgical Ablation) for more details regarding the etiology and treatment of postbypass bleeding.

(5) **Acceptance of a lower hematocrit.** What constitutes an acceptable postbypass hematocrit in patients undergoing cardiac surgery still remains controversial and varies among institutions. Increased scrutiny of blood transfusion practices are occurring nationwide. Numerous studies suggest a correlation between increased morbidity and mortality and the use of PRBCs [24]. Patients who are healthy and demonstrate good ventricular function after bypass generally tolerate hematocrits in a range from 20% to 25%.

Those individuals who have a reduced capacity to increase CO, who continue to have limited coronary blood flow, or who have increased metabolic demands will require the increased O_2-carrying capacity afforded by a higher hematocrit. Therefore, in patients with ventricular dysfunction, incomplete revascularization, and perhaps older patients, PRBCs should be considered for the treatment of hypovolemia.

A continuous mixed venous PA catheter can help direct therapy. If the SVO_2 is acceptable, the hematocrit can be kept at the lower level with careful monitoring and quick responses to subsequent changes.

3. **Pharmacologic therapy**

a. **ε-Aminocaproic acid or tranexamic acid.** Both ε-aminocaproic acid (EACA) and tranexamic acid are synthetic fibrinolytic inhibitors that act by occupying the lysine-binding sites on plasminogen and plasmin. This, in turn, displaces these proteins from the lysine residues on fibrinogen and fibrin and interferes with the ability of plasmin to split fibrinogen. The use of antifibrinolytics has been shown to result in modest reductions of bleeding after primary coronary bypass procedures.

b. **DDAVP.** DDAVP is believed to exert its effects by increasing the release of Factor VIII(C) and von Willebrand factor. The von Willebrand factor multimers play a role in enhancing platelet adhesiveness. The prophylactic use of DDAVP (0.3 μg/kg administered after CPB) in patients undergoing elective coronary artery bypass grafting was shown not to decrease blood loss or blood product administration. DDAVP may have a beneficial effect in certain subsets of patients including those with pre-existing uremia and aortic stenosis (Section I.F.3).

4. **Other blood products.** As mentioned in Section I.F, blood products should be given for specific abnormalities causing significant surgical bleeding. Therapy can be guided by a number of tests: thromboelastograph (TEG), PT, PTT, and platelet count. It is important to assess the cause of bleeding and the severity. The most common abnormality post-CPB will be thrombocytopenia.

C. **Renal system**

1. **Effects of CPB on the kidneys.** Many of the variables introduced with initiation of CPB have an effect on the renal system. Hemodilution and/or hemolysis reduce renal vascular resistance, resulting in increased flow to the outer renal cortex and subsequent enhanced urine flow. If systemic hypothermia is used as a form of myocardial protection, renal vascular resistance increases and renal blood flow, glomerular filtration rate, and free water clearance all decrease. Nonpulsatile flow, decreased perfusion pressure, and embolic phenomena from aortic plaque on CPB can also decrease renal blood flow. The decrease is most apparent in patients with renal artery stenosis, although one study has not shown an increase in acute renal failure in these patients. CPB-induced inflammation can also worsen renal outcome. It is important to prevent this complication, because new onset renal dysfunction requiring dialysis will increase mortality almost eightfold [25].

7

2. **Postbypass renal dysfunction.** Certain factors have been identified that place patients at risk for renal dysfunction in the postbypass period. These include elevated preoperative serum creatinine, combined valve and bypass procedures, advanced age, and diabetes. Prolonged bypass times and decreased CI post-CPB place patients at risk.
3. **Management.** Pharmacologic therapy may have some benefit in patients with severe pre-existing renal dysfunction or failure. A frequent observation is that urine flow is diminished during bypass compared with the individuals who have normal renal function. Renal insufficiency may result in significant hyperkalemia and accumulation of extracellular fluid.

   Treatment options include:
   - **a.** Furosemide (initial dose 10 to 20 mg) or mannitol (0.5 to 1 mg/kg)
   - **b.** Fenoldopam (0.05 to 0.1 μg/kg/min) will increase renal blood flow and may provide an important therapeutic option. It may cause unacceptable hypotension.
   - **c.** Ultrafiltration can be performed on CPB to remove excess volume.

   Despite these interventions, some patients may require dialysis in the early postoperative period.

D. Central nervous system

1. **Anesthetic depth.** The modern assessment of anesthetic depth with the bispectral index or other monitors may add important information for the proper management of the patient. In the postbypass period, there are varying levels of surgical stimulation, with the highest being the placement of sternal wires and chest closure. If an increase in the depth of anesthesia is needed, the choice of agent(s) will depend primarily on the hemodynamic status of the patient.

   Small doses of opioids or benzodiazepines can be titrated incrementally in patients with stable hemodynamics. Additionally, the judicious use of a volatile agent may be considered, particularly in patients who are hypertensive with a reasonable cardiac index.

   Use of nitrous oxide should be avoided after bypass for several reasons. Nitrous oxide has the capability of enlarging air emboli that may have been generated during bypass. Many patients require high inspired concentrations of O_2 during this period. Finally, nitrous oxide can elevate PA pressures in those with pre-existing pulmonary hypertension and can depress RV function.

   Many institutions are using a propofol infusion with good results during this time period. The infusion can be started upon rewarming and continue till and through the initial ICU stay. An infusion of 25 to 50 μg/kg/min is usually acceptable but can be titrated as indicated.

   It must be remembered that all patients have some degree of postbypass ventricular dysfunction. Even small doses of narcotics and propofol have the potential to cause adverse hemodynamic consequences.
2. **Neuromuscular blockade.** Patients frequently require additional neuromuscular relaxation in the postbypass period. The main objective is to prevent shivering, which in some circumstances can increase O_2 consumption by 500%. The muscle relaxant can be selected for its specific hemodynamic characteristics and duration of action. Frequent monitoring of the train of four is necessary. Renal and hepatic functions can deteriorate in the face of cardiovascular compromise. Temperature changes, blood loss, cardiac function, and adjuvant medications can also affect the pharmacokinetics and plasma levels of neuromuscular relaxants.

   Fast-track protocols in some hospitals allow for muscle relaxant reversal in the OR or after admission to the ICU. Reversal should be used only in stable patients. The cardiovascular side effects of reversal, such as HR changes, should be anticipated.

E. Metabolic considerations

1. **Electrolyte disturbances**
   - **a. Hypokalemia** is a relatively common electrolyte abnormality in the postbypass period. Although the etiologic factors of hypokalemia are numerous, only those unique to bypass will be mentioned. The kidney represents a major source of potassium loss. Both the preoperative and intraoperative use of diuretics, including mannitol administration

TABLE 9.3 Treatment of hyperkalemia

1. Diuresis-loop diuretic (furosemide 10–40 mg), higher dose if patient on chronic therapy
2. Sodium bicarbonate, 1–2 mEq/kg in children and one ampule (50 mEq) in adults
3. Infusion of dextrose and insulin, 1–2 g glucose per kilogram with 0.3 units regular insulin per gram of glucose in children; 25 g (1 ampule of D50) of glucose and 10 units of regular insulin in adults
4. Calcium, 20 mg/kg of calcium gluconate over a 5-min period for children and 5–10 mg/kg of calcium chloride for adults

on bypass, promotes significant potassium wasting. Glucose may be administered as a myocardial substrate during bypass. If significant hyperglycemia occurs, an osmotic diuresis with potassium loss will ensue. Hypokalemia may also result from the shift of potassium to the intracellular space. Such a shift may occur with alkalemia, from either hyperventilation or excess bicarbonate administration and with concomitant administration of insulin in a diabetic patient.

In addition, the use of inotropes capable of stimulating β_2-receptors will promote the intracellular shift of potassium. Treatment will vary depending on the severity of hypokalemia. Commonly, potassium levels tend to rise modestly without treatment due to redistribution and blood product administration. In most instances, intravenous administration up to 10 mEq/hr (in adults) will be effective. In life-threatening situations, potassium may be administered at a rate of 20 mEq/hr with continuous cardiac monitoring. **Adequate renal function**, initially assessed by urine output, should be present prior to any potassium replacement.

b. **Hyperkalemia** occurs uncommonly after bypass. In most cases, hyperkalemia occurs when large doses of cardioplegic agents are administered, particularly in patients with impaired renal function. Hyperkalemia may persist in the postbypass period but generally resolves spontaneously without intervention. Depending on the cardiac rhythm, moderate hyperkalemia (potassium levels between 6 and 7 mEq/L) may require therapy with one of the treatment modalities listed in Table 9.3. With severe hyperkalemia (potassium levels greater than 7 mEq/L), all therapeutic interventions may be needed.

c. **Hypocalcemia** can occur after bypass. Common etiologic factors include hemodilution from the pump prime, particularly in children; acute alkalemia; and calcium sequestration. Alkalemia that occurs with hyperventilation or rapid administration of parenteral bicarbonate results in enhanced binding of calcium to protein. Sequestration of calcium occurs with administration of a large volume of blood that contains the chelating agent citrate. Severe hypocalcemia results in myocardial depression and vasodilation.

Calcium administration after CPB is indicated in the presence of severe hyperkalemia or in cases of hypotension associated with low serum ionized calcium. Calcium may be administered as 10% calcium chloride (272 mg of elemental calcium) in a dose of 5 to 10 mg/kg. The typical adult dose is 500 to 1,000 mg.

d. **Hypomagnesemia** commonly occurs in patients undergoing cardiac surgery. England and colleagues suggested that large quantities of magnesium-free fluids with subsequent hemodilution most likely contribute to this observation. Other etiologic factors include loss of the cation in the extracorporeal circuit and redistribution of magnesium to other body stores. In a randomized, controlled trial (patients in the treatment group receiving 2 g of magnesium chloride after termination of CPB), magnesium-treated patients had a lower incidence of postoperative ventricular dysrhythmias and an increased cardiac index in the early postoperative period [13]. Therefore, many centers will give magnesium prior to terminating CPB.

2. **Hyperglycemia.** All patients are at risk for developing hyperglycemia during cardiac surgery due to the stress of surgery. Diabetics, particularly those who are insulin dependent, usually require an intraoperative insulin infusion to maintain glucose hemostasis (see Chapter 3). Inotropes, particularly epinephrine, may contribute to hyperglycemia after

bypass by stimulating hepatic glycogenolysis and gluconeogenesis. The deleterious effects associated with hyperglycemia include an osmotic diuresis and the resulting electrolyte abnormalities, enhancement of both focal and global ischemic neurologic and cardiac injury, and, if severe, can produce coma. The use of glucose-containing solutions is no longer recommended (see Section I.P above).

F. Postbypass temperature regulation

1. **Hypothermia.** All patients who undergo hypothermic CPB experience variable degrees of hypothermia in the postbypass period, with profound effects on the cardiovascular system, particularly in individuals with borderline cardiac reserve. As the temperature decreases, arteriolar tone will increase, resulting in elevated SVR. The hemodynamic consequences include hypertension, a decrease in CO, and increased myocardial O_2 consumption. Total body O_2 consumption may be increased because of the presence of shivering. Excessive bleeding is also associated with hypothermia.
2. **Etiology of postbypass hypothermia.** Hypothermic CPB results in a vasoconstricted state. During rewarming, many of the peripheral vascular beds (i.e., muscle and subcutaneous fat) do not adequately dilate and therefore act as a reservoir of cold blood, which will eventually equilibrate with the central circulation. Opening and warming these vascular beds with pharmacologic vasodilation will diminish the "after-drop" in core temperature. The drop in temperature usually reaches its nadir 80 to 90 min after bypass.
3. **Prevention and treatment of hypothermia.** The most effective way to attenuate postbypass hypothermia is to be assured that effective rewarming occurs during CPB. If circulatory arrest was used, rewarming will be significantly delayed. Always take the time necessary to properly rewarm.

   The most effective way to maintain temperature postbypass is the forced-air heater. An upper body cover can only be used to cover the arms and neck due to the surgical drapes. Covering the head improves warming. A lower body cover can be used after the vein sites are dressed if necessary. Other techniques that have been suggested to attenuate hypothermia include heating inspired gases, use of an IV fluid warmer, increasing ambient temperature, and using warm irrigation fluids in the chest cavity and warming blankets. The contribution of these techniques to preventing postbypass hypothermia is likely to be minor for the rewarming process but may be of importance in maintaining the patient's temperature until he or she leaves the operating room.
4. **Hyperthermia should be avoided, since it** will exacerbate cerebral ischemic injury, during either aggressive warming on CPB, after CPB, or in the ICU. The core or nasopharyngeal temperature should not exceed 37°C.

VII. Preparing for transport

A. Moving the patient to the transport or ICU bed in the OR

After the chest is closed and all dressings are applied, the patient must be moved to the transport bed. This requires a coordinated effort to minimize the risk of complications. Monitor lines can be lost, inotropic support disconnected, and ventilation can be interrupted with devastating consequences during this seemingly easy, routine process. There is a lapse in cardiovascular monitoring during transfer to a mobile or transport monitor. Disconnect monitoring devices sequentially, so there is always an "active" monitor to assess the patient at all times.

1. Complications of transfer
   - **a.** Extubation
   - **b.** Coronary air embolism from clot dislodgement (after open procedure) leading to ischemia or ventricular fibrillation
   - **c.** Arterial line or PA catheter removal
   - **d.** IABP line disruption
   - **e.** Pacemaker wire dislocation or disconnect
   - **f.** Loss of intravenous lines
   - **g.** Monitors (pulse oximeter probe, ECG lead) pulled off
   - **h.** Patient fall
   - **i.** Corneal injury (e.g., from wires, tubing)

TABLE 9.4 Suggested emergency equipment for transport

Airway equipment
Endotracheal tube
Laryngoscope and blades
Tube changer (optional)
Bag/valve/mask device
Oxygen tank
PEEP valve (not optional if PEEP >10 cm H_2O)
Medications
Neosynephrine for bolus
Ephedrine or epinephrine (4 μg/mL)
Epinephrine (1 mg) vial if unstable
Atropine
Muscle relaxant of choice
Succinylcholine
Narcotic of choice
Personnel
Trained personnel to monitor/troubleshoot IABP or LVAD/RVAD
Adequate personnel to attend to intravenous poles and bed movement

PEEP, positive end-expiratory pressure; IABP, intra-aortic balloon pump; LVAD, left ventricular assist device; RVAD, left ventricular assist device.

j. Loss of vasoactive or inotrope infusions
k. Chest tube, Foley catheter dislodgement
l. Venodilation with resultant hypotension

B. Transport to the ICU

Emergency equipment and medications must be collected prior to transport. The type of equipment necessary is related to the distance traveled. A move 10 floors away from the OR is much different than the one 50 feet away. See Table 9.4 for a suggested list of equipment/medications. Murphy's Law is in play here. There are case reports of cardiac arrest and extubation in compromising situations. We have experienced an IABP failure in an elevator with significant consequences. The patient must be monitored and adequate ventilation ensured during transport no matter the distance transported. Minimum monitoring requirements include: ECG, arterial line, and pulse oximetry.

C. Admission to the ICU

Most institutions will call or fax a report sheet to the ICU prior to transport. This report will document ventilatory settings, inotrope and vasoactive infusions, and vital signs. This information allows time for preparation. Most ICUs will continue to use the infusion bags from the operating room. If your infusion volumes are getting low, ask the unit personnel to have replacement medication infusions available. The loss of a critical inotrope at this juncture can be devastating.

After the patient is safely transferred to the ICU, permanent monitoring is re-instituted (sequentially). Document the pertinent vital signs in the anesthesia record and to whom you gave the report. At this point in time, you know the most about the physiology of this patient. If hemodynamic instability is noted, *you* are in the best position to provide the treatment of choice. **Take control of the situation.**

When giving the report, give those accepting care of the patient any additional information you feel would help them. For example, you may have seen the CI fall when the PA diastolic pressure is less than 15 mm Hg due to diastolic dysfunction. Let the ICU team know, so they won't have to "reinvent the wheel" and find out for themselves, putting the patient in harm's way.

Continued bleeding during transport can induce hypovolemia and increase fluid requirements. Or, LV dysfunction may improve over time and inotropic support, which is necessary in the OR, may need to be weaned to avoid hypertensive complications. Continue your care until you are satisfied that the patient's condition is stable.

ACKNOWLEDGMENT

Acknowledgments to Jerrold H. Levy. Sections V and VI in this chapter are based on his excellent summary in Chapter 9 in the Third Edition of this book.

REFERENCES

1. Nussmeier NA. Management of temperature during and after cardiac surgery. *Tex Heart Inst J.* 2005;32:472–476.
2. Royster RL, Butterworth JF IV, Prielipp RC, et al. A randomized, blinded, placebo-controlled evaluation of calcium chloride and epinephrine for inotropic support after emergence from cardiopulmonary bypass. *Anesth Analg.* 1992;74:3–13.
3. Carroll RC, Chavez JJ, Snider CC, et al. Correlation of perioperative platelet function and coagulation tests with bleeding after cardiopulmonary bypass surgery. *J Lab Clin Med.* 2006;147:197–204.
4. Nuttall GA, Henderson NS, Quinn M, et al. Excessive bleeding and transfusion in a prior cardiac surgery is associated with excessive bleeding and transfusion in the next surgery. *Anesth Analg.* 2006;102:1012–1017.
5. Bernard F, Denault A, Babin D, et al. Diastolic dysfunction is predictive of difficult weaning from cardiopulmonary bypass. *Anesth Analg.* 2001;92:291–298.
6. Kikura M, Sato S. The efficacy of preemptive milrinone or amrinone therapy in patients undergoing coronary artery bypass grafting. *Anesth Analg.* 2002;94:22–30.
7. Riess ML, Stowe DF, Warltier DC. Cardiac pharmacological preconditioning with volatile anesthetics: from bench to bedside? *Am J Physiol Heart Circ Physiol.* 2004;286:H1603–H1607.
8. Cromheecke S, Pepermans V, Hendrickx E, et al. Cardioprotective properties of sevoflurane in patients undergoing aortic valve replacement with cardiopulmonary bypass. *Anesth Analg.* 2006;103:289–296.
9. Tsang A, Hausenloy DJ, Yellon DM. Myocardial postconditioning: reperfusion injury revisited. *Am J Physiol Heart Circ Physiol.* 2005;289:2–7.
10. Zaugg M, Schaub MC, Foëx P. Myocardial injury and its prevention in the perioperative setting. *Br J Anaesthesia.* 2004;93: 21–33.
11. Mohr R, Lavee J, Goor DA. Inaccuracy of radial artery pressure measurement after cardiac operations. *J Thorac Cardiovasc Surg.* 1987;94:286–290.
12. NICE-SUGAR Study Investigators, et al. Intensive versus conventional glucose control in critically ill patients. *N Engl J Med.* 2009;360(13):1283–1297.
13. England MR, Gordon G, Salem M, et al. Magnesium administration and dysrhythmias after cardiac surgery. *JAMA.* 1992;268:2395–2402.
14. Kopman EA, Ferguson TB. Interaction of right and left ventricular filling pressures at the termination of cardiopulmonary bypass. *J Thorac Cardiovasc Surg.* 1985;89:706–708.
15. Haj RM, Cinco JE, Mazer CD. Treatment of pulmonary hypertension with selective pulmonary vasodilators. *Curr Opinion Anaesthesiology.* 2006;19:88–95.
16. De Wet CJ, Affleck DG, Jacobsohn E, et al. Inhaled prostacyclin is safe, effective, and affordable in patients with pulmonary hypertension, right heart dysfunction, and refractory hypoxemia after cardiothoracic surgery. *J Thorac Cardiovasc Surg.* 2004;127(4):1058–1067.
17. Levin MA, Lin HM, Castillo JG. Early-on cardiopulmonary bypass hypotension and other factors associated with vasoplegic syndrome. *Circulation.* 2009;120:1664–1671.
18. Ozal E, Kuralay E, Yildirim V, et al. Preoperative methylene blue administration in patients at high risk for vasoplegic syndrome during cardiac surgery. *Ann Thorac Surg.* 2005;79:1615–1619.
19. Chello M, Patti G, Candura D, et al. Effects of atorvastatin on systemic inflammatory response after coronary bypass surgery. *Crit Care Med.* 2006;34:660–667.
20. Bailey JM, Levy JH, Hug CC. Cardiac surgical pharmacology. In: Edmunds H, ed. *Adult Cardiac Surgery.* New York, NY: McGraw-Hill; 1997:225–254.
21. Bull BS, Huse WM, Brauer FS, et al. Heparin therapy during extracorporeal circulation. *J Thorac Cardiovasc Surg.* 1975;69: 685–689.
22. Despotis GJ, Filos K, Gravlee G, et al. Anticoagulation monitoring during cardiac surgery: a survey of current practice and review of current and emerging techniques. *Anesthesiology.* 1999;91:1122–1151.
23. Levy JH. *Anaphylactic Reactions in Anesthesia and Intensive Care.* 2nd ed. Boston, MA: Butterworth-Heinemann; 1992.
24. Koch CG, Li L, Duncan AI, et al. Morbidity and mortality risk associated with red blood cell and blood-component transfusion in isolated coronary artery bypass grafting. *Crit Care Med.* 2006;34:1608–1616.
25. Cooper WA, O'Brien SM, Thourani VH, et al. Impact of renal dysfunction on outcomes of coronary artery bypass surgery: results from the Society of Thoracic Surgeons National Adult Cardiac Database. *Circulation.* 2006;113:1063–1070.

10 Postoperative Care of the Cardiac Surgical Patient

Breandan Sullivan and Michael H. Wall

KEY POINTS

1. Transport from the operating room (OR) to the intensive care unit (ICU) is a critical period for patient monitoring or vigilance. Emergency drugs and airway equipment should be present, and adequate transportation personnel (typically three people) should accompany the patient during transport.
2. Patient "hand-off" to the ICU should be consistent, careful, and structured, and should not distract caregivers from continuous assessment of hemodynamics, oxygenation, and ventilation.
3. Early postoperative respiratory support ranges from full mechanical ventilation to immediate extubation in the OR, depending upon institutional practice patterns, anesthetic techniques, and patient stability. There is no "best" ventilation mode for cardiac surgery patients.
4. Weaning from mechanical ventilation involves assessment of oxygenation adequacy (typically PaO_2/F_IO_2 >100 on positive end-expiratory pressure [PEEP] 5 cm H_2O or less), hemodynamic stability, patient responsiveness to commands, and measured ventilatory parameters such as vital capacity and the rapid shallow breathing index (RSBI).
5. Fast-tracking protocols designed to extubate cardiac surgery patients within several hours of completion of surgery are common. With such protocols, early postoperative continuous infusions of propofol or dexmedetomidine may be helpful.
6. Early postoperative differential diagnosis of hypotension is often challenging, and includes hypovolemia, heart valve dysfunction, left ventricular (LV) and/or right ventricular (RV) dysfunction, cardiac tamponade, cardiac dysrhythmia, and vasodilation. Once a diagnosis has been made, optimal therapy usually becomes clear.
7. Hypertension is not uncommon and must be acutely and effectively managed to minimize bleeding and other complications such as LV failure and aortic dissection. The differential diagnosis includes pain, hypothermia, hypercarbia, hypoxemia, intravascular volume excess, anxiety, and pre-existing essential hypertension, among others.
8. Acute poststernotomy pain most often is managed by administering intravenous opioids, but other potentially helpful modalities include nonsteroidal anti-inflammatory drugs, intrathecal opioids, and central neuraxial or peripheral nerve blocks.
9. Early postoperative acid–base, electrolyte, and glucose disturbances are common. They should be diagnosed and treated promptly.
10. Postoperative bleeding may be surgical, coagulopathic, or both. Aggressive diagnosis and treatment of coagulation disturbances facilitates early diagnosis and treatment of surgical bleeding (i.e., return to OR for re-exploration) and avoidance of cardiac tamponade.
11. Discharge from the ICU typically occurs in 1 to 2 days. Criteria vary with cardiac surgical procedures and with institutional capabilities for post-ICU patient care (e.g., stepdown ICU beds vs. traditional floor nursing care).
12. Adequate communication with patients' family members and adequate family visitation and support greatly facilitate postoperative recovery.

THE PURPOSE OF THIS CHAPTER is to briefly discuss the transport of the cardiac surgery patient from the OR to the ICU, the hand-off of care from the OR team to the ICU team, and an approach to common problems that occur in the first 24 hrs in the ICU. The reader is referred to standard critical care text books for discussion of more chronic ICU problems such as nutrition, infectious disease, sepsis, and multiple organ failure.

I. Transition from operating room to intensive care unit

A. General principles

1. Movement of a critically ill patient in the immediate postoperative period to the ICU or to an intermediate level post-cardiac surgical recovery area is a risky business. **Inter- or intrahospital transport of critically ill patients is associated with increased**
1 **morbidity and mortality** [1].
2. The American College of Critical Care Medicine (ACCM) guidelines state that "during transport, there is no hiatus in the monitoring or maintenance of a patient's vital signs" [2].

3. The guidelines state there are four major areas to optimize efficiency and safety of patient transport: Communication (or hand-offs), personnel, equipment, and monitoring. Each of these areas will be discussed.

B. **The transport process**

1. **Prior to movement of the patient from OR table to ICU bed**
   a. **Airway/Breathing.** If patients are suitable candidates for fast-tracking (see subsequent section) and meet standard extubation criteria, they can be extubated in the OR, or within 6 to 8 hrs of arrival in the ICU. If the patient is to remain intubated, the endotracheal tube should be checked for position and patency, and should be securely attached to the patient. In addition, all chest tubes and drains should be checked for ongoing bleeding to ensure that immediate transport from the OR is appropriate, and for proper functioning to avoid hemothorax or pneumothorax during transport.
   b. **Circulation.** The patient should be hemodynamically "stable" prior to transport. In general, if the patient requires frequent bolus doses, or increasing doses of vasoactive drugs, it is better to stabilize prior to transport.
      (1) **Pacemaker.** Proper settings and functioning of the pacemaker should be checked at this point (see Chapter 17).
   c. **Coagulation.** Bleeding should be controlled, and a plan for correction of ongoing coagulopathy should be made prior to transport.
   d. **Metabolic.** Metabolic abnormalities (glucose, electrolyte, and acid–base) should be identified and corrected as much as possible prior to the transport.
   e. **Brief Telephone Report.** A brief verbal report to the ICU team should be provided prior to transport (see hand-off section).
   f. **Special Bed.** Patients at high risk for development of pressure ulcers (pre-existing pressure ulcers, poor nutritional status, elderly, poor ventricular function, etc.) should be placed on special beds/mattresses in the OR.
2. **Patient movement from the OR table to the transport bed.** Movement can cause hemodynamic instability, fluid shifts, and arrhythmias. Movement can also cause inadvertent loss of airway, vascular access, and interruption of intravenous infusions. Residual intracardiac air is a complication of many procedures (e.g., valve replacement) and this air may be easily dislodged when moving the patient. In addition, the position of a pulmonary artery catheter (PAC) can be altered during patient movement. Confirmation of the PAC position (i.e., pulmonary artery waveform rather than pulmonary artery occluded or RV waveform) before and after patient movement should be done. Sudden onset of dysrhythmia should trigger examination of the PAC. Ready access to a large-bore intravenous infusion port and to any ongoing or continuous infusions of medications is critical to managing this period safely and being able to respond promptly.
3. **Transport from the OR to the ICU**
   a. **Personnel.** Generally, at least three members of the operative team should transport the patient from the OR to the ICU. This should include a member of the anesthesia care team, surgical team, and a nurse or technician. Additional team members (perfusionists, respiratory therapists, etc.) may be needed for patients on mechanical assist devices, inhaled pulmonary vasodilators, or those with acute lung injury (ALI) who require a transport ventilator.
   b. **Equipment.** ACCM guidelines recommend a minimum of a blood pressure monitor, pulse oximeter, and cardiac monitor/defibrillator for all transports of critically ill patients [1]. An additional monitor to consider is continuous end-tidal CO_2 for intubated patients. Equipment and drugs for emergency airway management should be immediately available. An oxygen (O_2) source with enough O_2 for the duration of transport plus 30 min must be available. Basic emergency advanced cardiac life support (ACLS) drugs should be immediately available. All infusions should be checked and all pumps should be fully charged prior to transport. Supplemental O_2 should be provided to all extubated patients. Bag mask ventilation (with or without PEEP valves) can be used for most patients. Transport ventilators may be needed for patients with ALI or acute respiratory distress syndrome (ARDS). Mechanical support device batteries should be immediately available.

c. **Monitoring.** ACCM guidelines state that critically ill patients should "... receive the same level of basic physiologic monitoring and transport as they had in the ICU ...." The same concept applies to patients leaving the OR [1].

d. **IV Access.** Every effort must be made to avoid a "tangle" of IV tubing. In general, it is best to have one large bore IV identified for rapid administration of fluids or emergency medications. This line should be easily identified and immediately accessible. Bolus medications should ideally be given via a central venous site for faster onset. Finally, all IV fluid bags should be full enough to give fluid boluses as needed.

e. **Sedation/Analgesia.** In extubated patients, it is best *not* to give boluses of narcotics during transport. It is probably better and safer to give analgesics prior to transport, then give additional medications after arrival in the ICU. In intubated patients, it is best to start the postoperative sedation and analgesia plan prior to transport to minimize the need to give bolus medications during transport.

II. Transfer of care to the ICU team

A. **Importance of hand-offs. The hand-off** of care from the OR team to the ICU team is a surprisingly hazardous and dangerous event. **The Joint Commission identified that com-**
2 **munication failure was the root cause of 65% of sentinel events in 2006** [2]. Numerous studies have shown that the best hand-offs occur when they are structured, standardized, and use checklists [3–6]. Recently, many centers are developing hand-off tools from the electronic medical record [7].

B. **Logistics.** Ideally, each member of the OR and ICU teams should have specific tasks and the hand-off should occur in a standardized sequence [3,4]. One simple sequence would be transition from transport to ICU monitor, then initial ventilator settings, then formal structured hand-off.

C. **Transition to ICU monitors.** The patient must be continuously monitored during this process. Ideally, each parameter (ECG, O_2 saturation, etc.) should be transferred from the transport monitor to the ICU monitor in series, as opposed to unhooking all of them at once then hooking them up one at a time. Some systems allow for all the monitors to be almost instantly switched over by removing the entire "brick" at once. In any event, based on local monitors, there should be an orderly transition between both sets of monitors.

D. **Initial ventilator settings.** Intubated patients must have their endotracheal tube evaluated for patency, security, and position. This can be accomplished with a chest x-ray or with a bedside bronchoscopy. Ventilator parameters including ventilator mode, rate, fraction of
3 inspired oxygen (F_iO_2), PEEP, and pressure support must be selected. The patients who have no respiratory effort can be placed on assist-control (AC) or synchronized intermittent mandatory ventilation (SIMV) with an adequate rate, tidal volume, and PEEP. The patients who have regained spontaneous respiratory effort can be placed on SIMV or **pressure support ventilation (PSV).** PSV and SIMV modes can be combined. Excessive use of PEEP impedes venous return and may impair RV performance. The application of PEEP may decrease mediastinal bleeding, although the literature on this topic is inconsistent and this technique must be used with caution, as PEEP's adverse effects on hemodynamics are well established.

E. **The actual hand-off.** Once the monitors have been transferred to the ICU bedside monitor and oxygenation and ventilation have been confirmed, a structured hand-off should occur. This should include the patient's name, age, allergies, medical history, all significant intraoperative events, and the immediate postoperation plan. One structured hand-off form generated from the electronic medical record (EMR) is shown (see Fig. 10.1). Time should be allowed for questions and answers from all members of OR and ICU teams.

1. The **initial review** of the patient upon his or her arrival to the recovery area includes the patient's history, age, height, weight, pre-existing medical conditions, any allergies, a list of preoperative medications, and review of the most current laboratory findings (with special emphasis on potassium and hematocrit). The report should include a detailed review of the patient's cardiac status, including ventricular dysfunction, valvular disease, coronary anatomy, and details of the surgical procedure.

HI-LIGHTED AREAS ARE TO BE COMMUNICATED DURING THE FIRST PHONE CALL

OR/ICU/PACUICU TRANSFER REPORT

☐ OR→ICU ☐ ICU→OR ☐ OR→PACU→ICU

Patient Name______________________________

Pertinent preop info:

Procedure: Date:

Anesthesiologist: Surgeon:

Allergies (confirm per BJ protocol):

Patient Identification Band On? Y / N

Lines

☐ Arterial line ☐ PA ☐ CORDIS + DLIC ☐ CVP ☐ Femoral Art line ☐ IABP ☐ Lumbar drain ☐ Chest Tube

☐ Epidural → Level Placed T__ L __ Drug: __________ Dose: __________ Time Given:__________

Cardiovascular

☐ Hemodynamically Unstable → ____________________ ☐ Rhythm Disturbance → ____________________

Vasoactive drips:_______________/_______________/_______________/_______________

Notable Intra operative: ☐ Hypotension ☐ Hypertension Notable Events on Transport: ____________________

Cross Clamp Time: ________ CPB Time: ________

Respiratory

☐ Anticipated Difficult Airway ☐ Unanticipated Difficult Airway Describe

☐ Extubated ☐ Face Mask/NC O_2% ☐ Transferred Intubated → Why

Notable Airway Events: ______________________________ ☐ Inhaled NO or PGI_2

VENTILATOR: ___TV Rate FiO_2 PEEP PSV

Notable events during transfer______________________________

Neurologic

☐ Ventriculostomy ☐ ICP Monitor ☐ Post OP CT ☐ Burst Suppression ☐ C-Collar

☐ IntraOperative Vessel Occlusion

Spinal Cord: Notable events on IntraOperative Electrophysiologic monitoring ?

Mental Status: awake/follows commands / comatose/other ____________________

Pupils: _______________ GAG: _______________ Cough: _______________

Motor Response: (circle) Follows Commands – Purposeful – Localizes to Pain – Postures to Pain – Unresponsive to Pain

Focal Deficits: **N Y** RUE/RLE LUE/LLE

Fluids

PRBC's _____ PLT's _____ FFP _____ Cell Saver_____ Cryo ____ Colloids:_____ Crystalloids _______________

Other ____________________ EBL: ____________ Urine Output: _______________

Any Reactions? Y N

IntraOp MEDS

Antibiotics: ____________________ Time: ______________ ☐ Lasix/Mannitol → Time: __________ DDAVP________

Last Narcotic: Drug_______________ Dose __________ Time __________ Narcotic TOTAL: ________

Last Neuromuscular: Drug_______________ Dose__________ Time __________ Neuromuscular TOTAL: ______

Last Benzodiazepine Dose:_____________________________ Time:__________

Steroids Drug_______________ Dose __________ Time __________ Steroid TOTAL: ________

Reversal given N Y → Time:____________ **for:** ☐ Paralytics ☐ Narcotics ☐ Benzodiazepines

Other:

Laboratory

LAST

ABG: pH pCO2 PO2 HCO3 K^+ Glucose HCT Plts PT/PTT/INR

Pertinent abnormal laboratory values:

OTHER Pertinent/IntraOperative Events/Information:

Special Request/Needs:

☐ Blood Warmer ☐ Bair Hugger ☐ Rapid Transfusers ☐ Propofol IMED Pump ☐ SCD ☐ Isolation & Reason__________

PACU UPDATES: Given By:_____ Taken By:_____

Recorded by:____________________ Recorders contact Number/Beeper: ____________________

Information Provided by: ____________________ Information Providers contact Number/Beeper ____________________

CALLS: 56ICU Ext: 2-5812 84ICU Ext: 2-8493 104ICU 450-0741

FIGURE 10.1 Structured hand-off form generated from electronic medical records.

2. An **anesthetic review** should be presented, which includes types and location of intravenous catheters and invasive monitors, along with any complications that occurred during their placement. A brief description of the anesthetic technique should be discussed to help plan for a smooth emergence. Any difficulties with airway management should be emphasized, particularly when weaning and extubation protocols are utilized. The presence or absence of obstructive sleep apnea should be discussed and the need for continuing patients' home continuous positive airway pressure (CPAP) or bi-level positive airway pressure (BiPAP) should be addressed. A post-cardiopulmonary bypass synopsis should be reported, including the use of vasoactive, inotropic, and antiarrhythmic drugs, as well as any untoward events such as arrhythmias and presumed drug reactions. This should also include an update on the presence or absence of bleeding prior to chest closure.
3. Early upon arrival to the ICU, the patient's **heart rate, rhythm, and blood pressure** should be determined. If the heart is being paced, the settings should be reviewed and all electrodes identified and secured, as the patient may be dependent on the device.
   a. If the patient has a permanent pacemaker or defibrillator, the settings should also be reviewed. The devices should be interrogated in the ICU and antitachycardia treatment should be activated. While waiting for the device to be activated, external defibrillator pads should be placed on the patient and a defibrillator should be immediately available [8].
   b. If the patient has a ventricular assist device (VAD), the monitor should be attached to a wall-based energy supply and the output of the device should be attached to the display module. The settings of the device and the position and location of the cannula should be reviewed.
   c. For patients on extracorporeal membrane oxygenation (ECMO), the O_2 and air supplies should be attached to the wall outlet supplies, and back-up tanks should be available.

F. **Laboratory Tests/electrocardiogram (ECG)/chest radiograph (CXR).** After the hand-off is complete and questions are answered, baseline ECG, CXR, and labs should be obtained. An initial arterial blood gas (ABG) should be drawn to ensure the adequacy of oxygenation and ventilation, whether the patient is on a mechanical ventilator or breathing spontaneously. Potassium, blood glucose, and hematocrit levels should be obtained. Acid–base status should be reviewed from ABGs. Baseline coagulation parameters, including prothrombin time (PT), activated partial thromboplastin time (aPTT), and platelet count should be acquired if the patient is bleeding excessively.

III. Mechanical ventilation after cardiac surgery

A. **Hemodynamic response to positive-pressure ventilation (PPV).** Heart–lung interactions of PPV are complex [9,10]. In patients with normal LV function, PPV increases intrathoracic pressure (ITP), which reduces venous return, afterload, and stroke volume (SV) and cardiac output (CO) (see Figure 10.2). On the other hand, in patients with LV dysfunction, decreased preload and afterload actually can *improve* LV performance and CO (see Fig. 10.3). PEEP further increases ITP and decreases venous return.

B. **Pulmonary changes after sternotomy and thoracotomy.** Cardiac surgery requires either a midline sternotomy or a thoracotomy. Both of these approaches temporarily compromise the function of the thoracic cage, which acts as a respiratory pump. One week after cardiac surgery, there is a significant reduction in total lung capacity, inspiratory vital capacity, forced expiratory volumes, and functional residual capacity compared to preoperative values [11]. Even at 6 wks postoperatively, total lung capacity, inspiratory vital capacity, and forced expiratory volume remained significantly below preoperative values. These findings suggest a marked tendency toward postoperative atelectasis and the possibility of hypoxemia from increased physiologic shunting. These changes in chest wall function can increase physiologic shunt to as much as 13% (compared to a baseline normal value of 5%).

In addition to these changes in mechanics and volumes, there are also abnormalities in gas exchange, compliance, and work of breathing [12]. The cause of these abnormalities is multifactorial and may include inflammation, reperfusion, and other mechanisms.

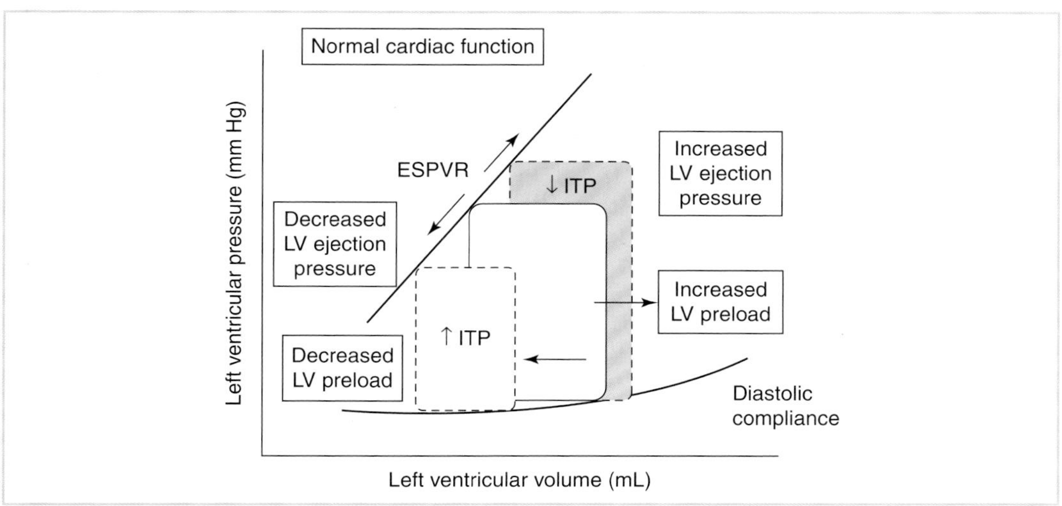

FIGURE 10.2 The effect of increasing and decreasing intrathoracic pressure (ITP) on the pressure-volume loop of the cardiac cycle. The slope of the LV end-systolic pressure–volume relationship (ESPVR) is proportional to contractility. The slope of the diastolic LV pressure–volume relationship defines diastolic compliance [10].

C. **Choosing modes of ventilation**

1. **Extubated patient.** If the patient was **extubated in the OR,** supplemental oxygen may be all that is necessary postoperatively. Following a general anesthetic, patients will exhibit a mild increase in the $PaCO_2$. Aggressive pulmonary toilet and frequent incentive spirometry must be performed to prevent the atelectasis and hypoxemia that may develop from changes in chest wall function.
2. **Noninvasive ventilation (NIV).** NIV can be used to treat or prevent postoperative respiratory failure, and has been shown to prevent reintubation, decrease ventilator-

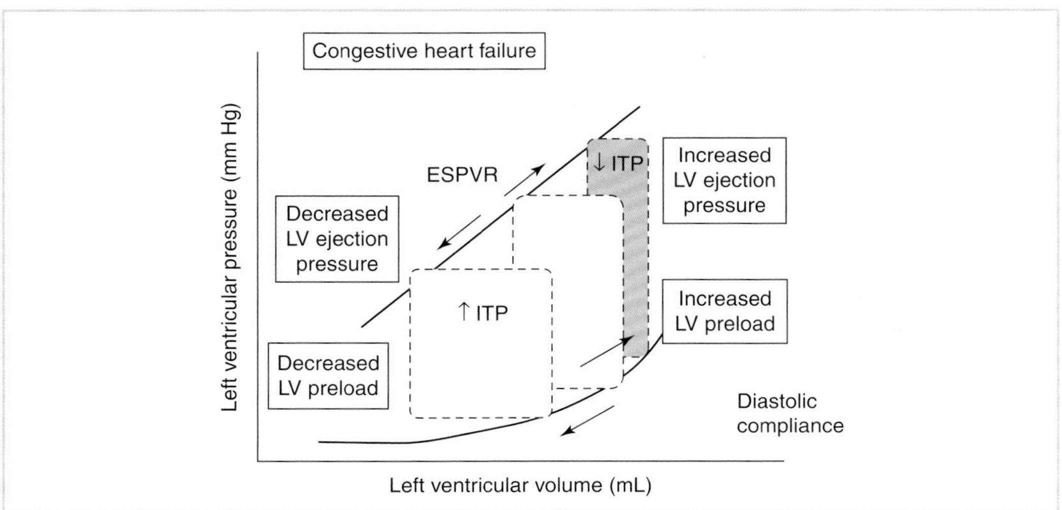

FIGURE 10.3 The effect of increasing and decreasing intrathoracic pressure (ITP) on the LV pressure–volume loop of the cardiac cycle in congestive heart failure when LV contractility is reduced and intravascular volume is expanded. The slope of the LV ESPVR is proportional to contractility. The slope of the diastolic LV pressure–volume relationship defines diastolic compliance [10].

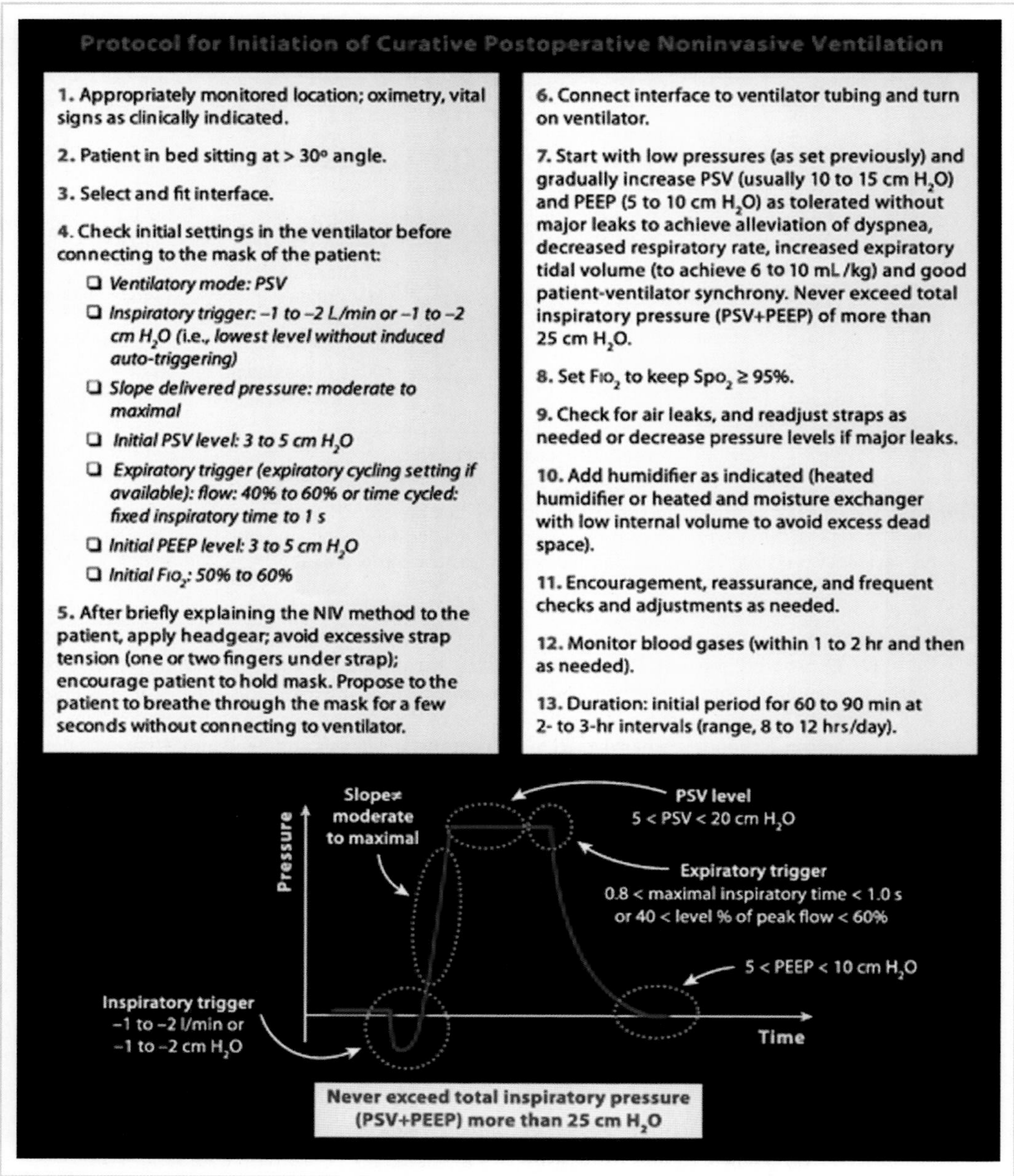

FIGURE 10.4 Protocol for initiation of curative postoperative NIV. *PSV,* pressure support ventilation; *PEEP,* positive end expiratory pressure. F_iO_2, fraction of inspired oxygen; S_{PO_2}, pulse oximetry saturation [13].

associated pneumonia, and improve outcomes [13,14]. A sample protocol for the use of NIV is shown in Figure 10.4. Contraindications are shown in Table 10.1. Two types of NIV are commonly used:

a. CPAP, where constant airway pressure is applied during both inspiration and expiration.

b. BiPAP, where PSV is applied during inspiration and PEEP is applied during expiration.

TABLE 10.1 Contraindications to noninvasive positive-pressure ventilation

Absolute
Cardiac or respiratory arrest
Nonrespiratory organ failure Severe encephalopathy (e.g., Glasgow Coma Score <10) Severe upper gastrointestinal bleeding Hemodynamic instability or unstable cardiac dysrhythmia
Facial surgery, trauma, or deformity
Upper airway obstruction
Inability to cooperate
Inability to clear respiratory secretions
High risk for aspiration
Postoperative esophageal or gastric surgery
Relative
Mildly decreased level of consciousness
Progressive severe respiratory failure
Patient who cannot be calmed or comforted

Modified from: Jaber SD, Chanques G, Jung B. Postoperative noninvasive ventilation. *Anesthesiology.* 2010;112:453–461.

3. **Intubated patient**
   a. If a patient returns from the OR with an **endotracheal tube in place,** an individualized plan of care should be developed for that patient. The choice of mechanical ventilation mode is based on the patient's inherent respiratory effort. If a patient demonstrates an inspiratory effort, PSV or SIMV can be used.

      If a patient is not demonstrating spontaneous respiratory effort, AC or SIMV should be selected. In AC, a set respiratory rate is delivered regardless of the patient's respiratory effort. If a spontaneous breath is initiated, the ventilator detects the trigger and delivers a set tidal volume (or pressure if on pressure control ventilation). In SIMV, a set respiratory rate is also delivered, but spontaneous breaths over the set rate are not fully supported (like they are in AC), but are dependent on the patient's effort.
   b. Patients with severe hypoxemia, respiratory failure, ALI, or ARDS will need to be ventilated in a way that minimizes or avoids further "ventilator-induced lung injury" [15]. There have been several recent reviews on the ICU management of ARDS and ALI [16–20].

      Initial ventilator settings in patients with ALI or ARDS would include (ardsnet.org):
      (1) Any ventilator mode.
      (2) Tidal volume (V_T) 8 mL/kg predicted body weight.
      (3) Set respiratory rate (RR) so minute ventilation is adequate.
      (4) Adjust V_T and RR to achieve a goal pH 7.30 to 7.40 and plateau pressure <30 cm H_2O.
4. **Weaning from mechanical ventilation is multifactorial.** In many postoperative environments, this can best be accomplished by using an algorithm so that weaning can proceed methodically and without interruption. Figure 10.5 shows an algorithm that could facilitate efficient weaning. Prior to attempts at weaning, the following parameters must be met:
   a. Normothermia.
   b. Hemodynamically stable.
      (1) Stable vasoactive drug requirements.
      (2) Not requiring increasing doses or boluses of inotropes or vasopressors.
   c. Stable heart rate and rhythm.

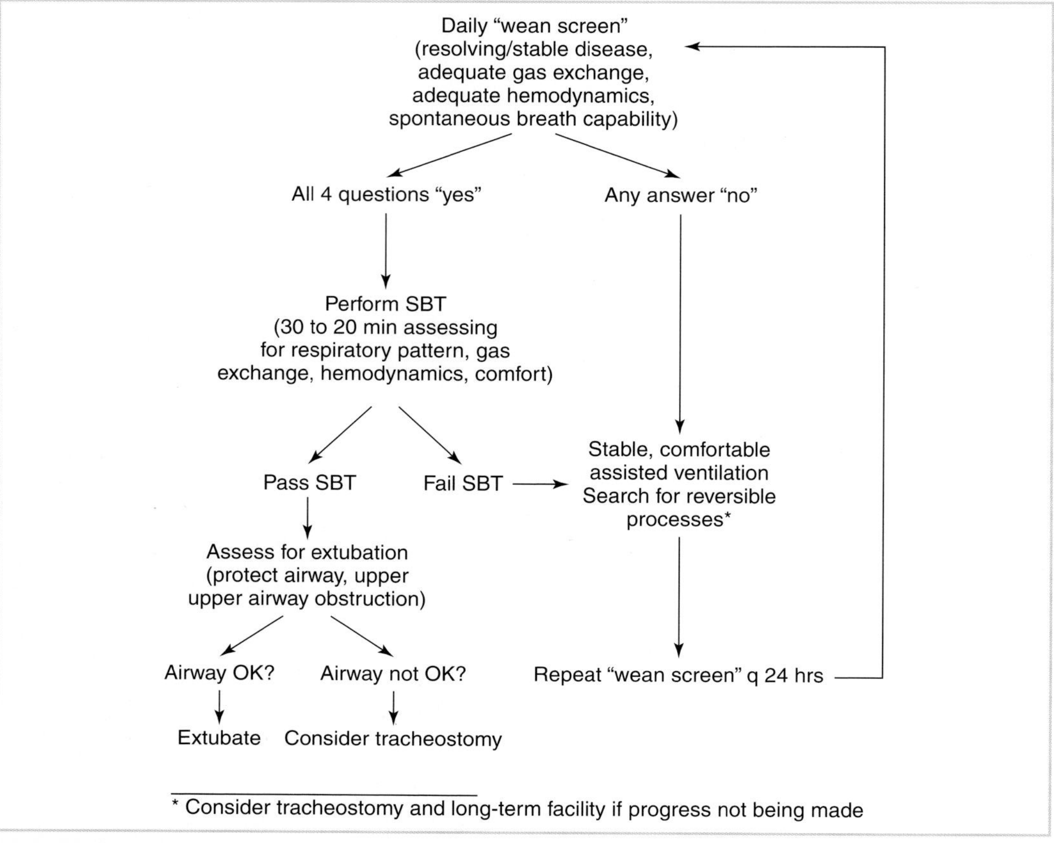

FIGURE 10.5 Protocolized flow chart for ventilator discontinuation [22]. *SBT,* spontaneous breathing trial.

d. Normal acid–base and metabolic state.

e. Not bleeding excessively (criteria vary, but generally <150 mL/hr chest tube drainage).

If these criteria are met, the patient is ready to be liberated from mechanical ventilation.

D. Liberation from mechanical ventilation

1. Current recommendations are that patients should be liberated from mechanical ventilation as quickly as possible, and an attempt should be made at least daily [21,22].
2. The first step is to assess the following to determine "readiness to wean":
   a. $PaO_2/F_iO_2 > 200$ mm Hg with PEEP ≤ 5 cm H_2O.

4

   b. Hemodynamically "stable."
   c. Awake, alert, and following commands.
   d. Able to cough effectively.
   e. Adequate reversal of neuromuscular blockade (negative inspiratory force [NIF] of 30 cm H_2O or more, able to lift head off bed >5 s, no fade on train of 4, vital capacity >15 mL/kg, etc.).
   f. An RSBI (RR/V_T in L) < 80 to 100 breaths/min/L after a 2- to 3-min spontaneous breathing trial.
3. If the patient passes the readiness to wean screen, a trial of spontaneous ventilation via T-piece or with low levels of PSV (5 to 7 cm H_2O) and PEEP (≤7 cm H_2O) for 30 to 120 min is done. At the end of the of the trial, if the RSBI is <80 to 100, the patient should be considered for extubation, if they meet the following final criteria:
   a. Awake and alert.

b. Able to cough and clear secretions.
  (1) The patients who require suctioning more often than every 2 hrs are at a higher risk for reintubation.

c. No airway edema (as judged crudely by edema of tongue and presence of leak when endotracheal tube cuff is deflated).

d. Hemodynamically stable.
  (1) Less than 10% to 20% change in HR, BP, pulmonary artery pressures, cardiac index, etc. during the trial.

e. Normal oxygenation and ventilation.

4. If the patient meets the criteria, extubation can be performed.

5. If the patient does not meet the criteria, correctable causes need to be identified and optimized prior to another attempt.

6. Patients who repeatedly fail spontaneous breathing trials may require more long-term weaning from mechanical ventilation [21].

E. **Incentive spirometry, deep breathing, and coughing maneuvers.** Patients must be encouraged to use **incentive spirometry** and to do **deep breathing** and coughing maneuvers after extubation to reduce atelectasis. There are numerous physiologic causes of hypoxemia. Diffusion abnormality, low F_iO_2, hypoventilation, and V/Q mismatch along with shunt comprise the list of possibilities, with atelectasis (causing shunt) being the most common. If hypoxemia persists and atelectasis is the presumed cause, NIV can be used to improve oxygenation and decrease shunt.

IV. Principles of fast-tracking

A. **Goals of fast-tracking.** Fast-track (FT) cardiac surgery was introduced to speed recovery and increase efficiency of limited resources (ICUs). Early extubation, ambulation, cardiac rehabilitation, and discharge are key goals of an FT program. Numerous randomized controlled trials have shown FT cardiac surgery is safe and less expensive than conventional cardiac anesthesia [23]. Initially, FT protocols were limited to young, low-risk patients; however, it can be used safely in older and higher risk patients as well [24].

5

B. **Methods of fast-tracking.** A variety of anesthetic techniques can be used to facilitate fast-tracking. Shorter-acting intravenous narcotics can be combined with intrathecal opioids to enhance postoperative analgesia [25,26]. Propofol infusions are often used because of a predictable and rapid recovery profile that is almost independent of the duration of infusion. This property makes propofol a very good sedative agent in the early postoperative management of FT cardiac surgery patients, assuming that hemodynamic stability is not compromised by its use. Caution is needed when short-acting agents are used to set the stage for early extubation, as the incidence of intraoperative awareness may be as high as 0.3% [27]. Dexmedetomidine is an intravenous α-2 adrenergic agonist that may facilitate fast-tracking in cardiac surgical patients. Dexmedetomidine possesses both sedative and analgesic properties, and allows patients to follow commands despite adequate sedation, and it most often does not require weaning prior to extubation. Dexmedetomidine does not possess reliable amnestic properties.

Dexmedetomidine has been evaluated in a number of trials in the ICU in both cardiac surgery and non-cardiac surgery patients. When compared to propofol, midazolam, and morphine in separate trials, dexmedetomidine has been shown to provide adjunctive analgesia, induce less delirium, and decrease the duration of mechanical ventilation [28–31].

C. **Fast-tracking in the postanesthesia care unit.** Many institutions prepare for the postoperative management of cardiac surgery patients by developing enhanced step-down or postanesthesia care units (PACUs), where postoperative management can occur safely and efficiently. These units require nurses who understand fast-tracking techniques, so that patients who have undergone cardiac surgery can move smoothly through early extubation in preparation for early transfer to a regular nursing unit. These specialized PACUs can be very effective in providing FT techniques because of their focused effort in caring for FT cardiac surgery patients [32]. Some investigators have even implemented *ambulatory* cardiac surgery programs [33]!

D. **Utilizing protocols.** Developing and utilizing institution-specific FT protocols revolves around systematic plans for weaning patients from ventilators and managing routine postoperative issues to facilitate the progression toward early ICU and hospital discharge. Protocols ideally address most issues before they occur. Fast-tracking protocol development should involve all members of the perioperative care team before implementation.

V. Hemodynamic management in the postoperative period

A. Monitoring for ischemia. Ischemia can be detected by utilizing a continuous ECG with ST segment analysis, although there is a slight delay in diagnosis of ischemia using this method. Many bedside ECG monitoring systems have ST-segment analysis built into their software algorithms, which is a cost-effective method of monitoring for ischemic events. It is important to ensure that the ECG is in diagnostic mode when evaluating potentially ischemic ECG changes. In monitor mode, the ECG filters out some electrical input (to decrease artifact) and may not accurately reflect ischemic changes. If continuous ST segment analysis is chosen, Leads II and V4 or V5 should be monitored, and sensitivity improves if three leads are used (Leads I, II, and V4 or V5, or Leads II, V4, and V5). Other indicators of myocardial ischemia include pulmonary artery pressures and CO, which tend to be less reliable and oftentimes late markers of myocardial ischemia. Transesophageal echocardiogram (TEE) segmental wall-motion abnormalities represent the most sensitive early detector of myocardial ischemia, but continuous monitoring usually is not done because the TEE probe (if used) typically is removed at the end of surgery. It is extremely important for the intensivist to recognize the changes in ECG and hemodynamics that can result from temporary epicardial ventricular pacing. Epicardial ventricular pacing can mimic septal wall dyskinesis that actually represents a pacemaker-induced change in the ventricular depolarization sequence.

Intraoperative and ongoing postoperative ischemia can be detected as soon as 6 hrs after the event begins by examining some specific cardiac markers. The earliest and most useful marker is cardiac troponin I (cTnI). The ability to measure cTnI is particularly useful in cases where ECG monitoring is difficult to interpret, such as with left bundle branch block or LV hypertrophy. Elevated plasma levels of this biologic marker provide clear evidence of ischemia and may suggest a diagnosis of myocardial infarction.

In postoperative cardiac surgical patients, all of the above methods have significant problems. Most often, myocardial ischemia is suspected by ECG changes or unexpected increases in vasoactive drug requirements. The diagnosis is best confirmed by TTE or TEE. Diagnosis may require cardiac catheterization. Treatment options include returning to the OR or medical management.

B. Ventricular dysfunction after cardiac surgery. In addition to pre-existing ventricular dysfunction, postoperative causes of ventricular dysfunction include inadequate **myocardial protection, myocardial stunning, incomplete revascularization, and reperfusion injury.** Preoperative predictors of postoperative ventricular dysfunction include cardiac enlargement, advanced age, diabetes mellitus, female gender, high LV end-diastolic pressures at cardiac catheterization, small coronary arteries (for coronary revascularization procedures), and ejection fraction less than 0.40. Intraoperative predictors include longer cardiopulmonary bypass (CPB) and aortic cross-clamp times. These factors increase the likelihood of needing inotropic support in the postoperative period. The patients who have normal preoperative cardiac performance and short periods of CPB have a much lower likelihood of requiring postoperative inotropic support. The patients who fail to achieve adequate hemodynamics even with pharmacologic support will require mechanical cardiac assistance such as an intra-aortic balloon pump (IABP) or VAD. Recently, Hollenberg has written an excellent review article on **vasoactive drugs** in circulatory shock [34].

The myocardium has both β_1-adrenergic receptors and β_2-adrenergic receptors, which contribute to inotropy and lusitropy (enhanced diastolic relaxation). The β-adrenergic agonists (β-agonists) are often the first-line agents used when there is a need to improve ventricular function after CPB. Depletion of endogenous catecholamines and the resulting β-receptor downregulation can blunt the response to β-agonists. Increased G-inhibitory proteins, reperfusion injury, tachycardia, incomplete revascularization, nonviable myocardium, preoperative use of β-agonists, and acute or chronic heart failure also may attenuate the response to β-agonists.

The inotropic response to β_1/β_2-adrenergic receptor stimulation occurs via activation of the G_s protein and adenylyl cyclase leading to increased intracellular cyclic adenosine monophosphate (cAMP). It is important to recognize that lusitropy is an active, energy-consuming process; impaired ventricular relaxation (diastolic dysfunction) can cause heart failure alone or in combination with systolic dysfunction. Until recently, there have been no head-to-head clinical trials comparing the clinical outcomes of inotropes and vasopressors. In a trial of 30 patients with dopamine-resistant cardiogenic shock, the patients were randomized to receive either epinephrine alone or dobutamine in combination with norepinephrine. Both groups experienced an increase in cardiac index and a decrease in their creatinine. The group receiving epinephrine experienced more arrhythmias, transient lactic acidosis, and a decrease in splanchnic perfusion [35].

Phosphodiesterase Type III inhibitors (amrinone and milrinone) augment β-adrenergic–mediated stimulation by inhibiting the breakdown of cAMP. Phosphodiesterase inhibitors (PDEIs) act either additively or synergistically with β-adrenergic agonists. PDEIs appear to have anti-ischemic effects and may favorably alter myocardial oxygen consumption [36]. PDEIs can be added to β-agonist therapy or employed as a first-line inotrope. Because PDEIs also induce systemic and pulmonary vasodilation (sometimes termed inodilators), clinical paradigms that favor their use include pulmonary hypertension, RV failure, aortic or mitral valvular regurgitation, and acute/chronic β_1/β_2-adrenergric receptor desensitization (long-standing CHF, use of β-agonist therapy preoperatively).

Levosimendan is a novel inotrope that, at this time, is neither FDA-approved nor available in North America. Levosimendan is a myofilament "calcium-sensitizer," which results in increased inotropy by improving the efficiency of the coupling of force-generating myocyte proteins in response to a given level of calcium [37]. Like PDEIs, levosimendan may augment inotropy without significantly increasing myocardial oxygen consumption, thus improving the myocardial oxygen supply/demand balance. In a recent meta-analysis analyzing the use of levosimendan in postoperative coronary artery bypass grafting (CABG), levosimendan was associated with improved mortality and morbidity [38].

B-type natriuretic peptide (nesiritide) has been favored by some for the medical management of CHF [39–42], although some work also associates the use of this agent with increased mortality in that setting. The role of nesiritide in the cardiac surgical population remains ill-defined.

In patients with severely impaired cardiac performance, additional monitoring may be required to ascertain if the patient has optimal myocardial function. Oximetric PACs can provide real-time determinations of mixed venous oxygen saturation (S_VO_2). A normal S_VO_2 value of 75% corresponds to a PaO_2 of approximately 40 mm Hg. Reductions in S_VO_2 result from either decreased oxygen delivery (decreased CO, decreased hemoglobin concentration, or decreased arterial oxygen saturation) or increased oxygen consumption. A sustained S_VO_2 below 40% is associated with increased morbidity and mortality. Similarly, some practitioners choose to use PACs with continuous cardiac output (CCO) determination in such patients, or with both S_VO_2 and CCO.

C. **Fluid management.** Managing postoperative fluids after cardiac surgery can be challenging [43]. The effects of hypothermia (vasoconstriction) and hyperthermia (vasodilation) commonly complicate fluid management especially in the first few hours after cardiac surgery. Central venous pressure (CVP) and PAC are frequently utilized in the cardiac surgical population; however, it is imperative to recognize that these monitors measure pressure as a surrogate estimate of volume and/or cardiac performance. The use of filling pressures (CVP, PAOP, PADP) are poor predictors of assessing total blood volume and volume responsiveness [44]. Volume responsiveness is defined by an increase in cardiac index of >15% in response to a fluid challenge. For mechanically ventilated patients who have a regular respiratory pattern, the pulse pressure variation on an arterial pressure waveform can be a highly useful tool in predicting a hypotensive patient's response to a fluid challenge [45,46].

Cardiac surgical procedures, especially those involving CPB, typically result in fluid sequestration into the interstitial compartment. In addition to the changes in circulating blood volume from blood loss and other factors, fluid shifts into or out of the interstitial or the intracellular compartments can be anticipated in the hours following cardiac surgery. Most cardiac surgery patients reach the recovery area with excess total body fluids present that must eventually be mobilized. Healthy patients who have adequate cardiac and renal function typically diurese these fluids over the first two postoperative days without assistance. Other cardiac surgery patients, such as the elderly or those with renal or cardiac dysfunction, may require diuretic drugs (or possibly dialysis or hemofiltration) to remove excess body water.

Management of blood components, particularly packed red blood cells (PRBC), in the cardiac surgical population is controversial [47,48]. Both transfusion of blood products and anemia are associated with increased perioperative morbidity and mortality. Even though cardiac surgical patients frequently require allogeneic blood products, establishing a transfusion trigger is difficult. Most patients probably require transfusion of PRBC at a hematocrit less than or equal to 21% (hemoglobin less than or equal to 7 g/dL) and few or none require transfusion when the hematocrit is greater than or equal to 30% (hemoglobin greater than or equal to 10 g/dL).

D. **Managing hypotension.** Systematic evaluation of preload, afterload, contractility, and heart rate and rhythm should be performed in the hypotensive patient. If preload is adequate and an acceptable heart rate and a normal cardiac rhythm are present, hypotension represents either inadequate myocardial function or vasodilation. Inadequate cardiac function is managed with inotropes. Vasodilation is managed with vasoconstrictors.

1. **Vasodilatory Shock.** Eight percent of cardiac surgery patients experience refractory vasodilatory shock after CPB. This refractory shock is associated with increased mortality (25% mortality in one case series). These patients do not respond to traditional treatments, vasopressors, or volume expansion. The causes of the problem are usually multifactorial: Long bypass run, preoperative use of angiotensin-converting enzyme inhibitors or angiotensin-receptor blockers, calcium channel blocker agents, heart transplantation, VAD placement, and myocardial dysfunction. Small clinical trials have shown improved morbidity and mortality in this patient population with the use of an intravenous bolus of methylene blue followed by a continuous infusion [49]. Arginine vasopressin may also be useful in this patient population.

   Two other unique causes of hypotension that are difficult to diagnose without the aid of transesophageal echocardiography are systolic anterior motion (SAM) of the mitral valve and cardiac tamponade.
2. **SAM** of the mitral valve should be assessed in the OR in patients undergoing mitral valve repair or septal myectomy. The c-sept distance (see Fig. 10.6) of 2.5 cm or less is associated with a high risk of SAM [50].
3. **Tamponade.** Although this topic is covered elsewhere, post-cardiac surgery tamponade should be addressed and discussed especially if the patient is demonstrating signs of a low CO shock. A large series of patients diagnosed with post-cardiac surgery tamponade demonstrated that the classical diagnostic signs such as equalizing filling pressures, increased jugular venous pressure, and pulsus paradoxus are frequently not present. Echocardiography can aid in the diagnosis; however, tamponade is a constellation of symptoms rather than a single echocardiographic finding [51].

E. **Dysrhythmia management.** Managing postoperative dysrhythmias constitutes an important part of ICU care in cardiac surgery patients. A variety of atrial or ventricular dysrhythmias can occur. The patients with ongoing myocardial ischemia, possibly from incomplete revascularization or myocardial stunning, are predisposed to dysrhythmias. Atrial fibrillation is the most common dysrhythmia to occur after cardiac surgery, and it may occur in as many as half of the patients who undergo myocardial revascularization using CPB. Useful drugs for treating atrial fibrillation include magnesium, digoxin, diltiazem, esmolol, and amiodarone [52].

It has been shown that various preoperative or postoperative pharmacologic prophylactic strategies may reduce the incidence of postoperative atrial fibrillation or other atrial dysrhythmias [53–55]. It is important to identify the patients who are at increased risk for developing perioperative atrial fibrillation. These include the patients who have a previous history of atrial fibrillation, have undergone a combination valve and CABG procedure, are

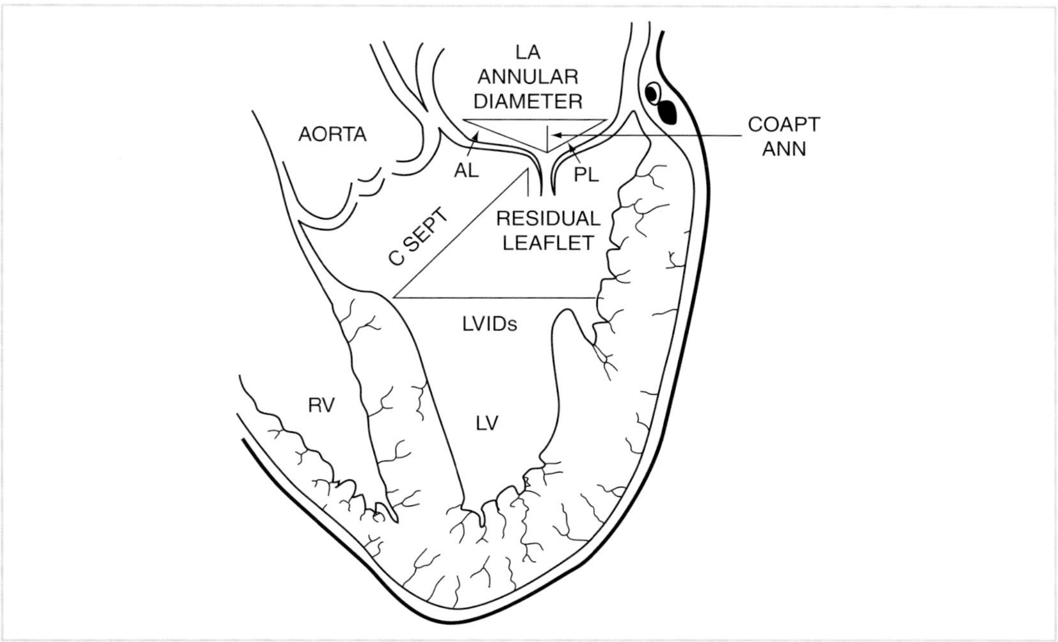

FIGURE 10.6 Schematic demonstrating the transesophageal echocardiographic measurements performed prior to and after mitral valve repair. The biplane image, obtained from the esophageal location at zero degrees, includes the left atrium (LA), left ventricle (LV), mitral valve, and the LV outflow tract. Lengths of the anterior and posterior leaflets were obtained using the middle scallops. *AL,* anterior leaflet length; *CoaptAnn,* distance from the mitral coaptation point to the annular plane; *CSept,* distance from the mitral coaptation point to the septum; *LVIDs,* LV internal diameter in systole; *PL,* posterior leaflet length [50].

receiving inotropic support, or have pre-existing mitral valve disease, lung disease, or congenital heart disease. Prophylaxis against atrial fibrillation may decrease both the number of days spent in the ICU and the total length of stay in the hospital. Administration of a long-acting β-adrenergic receptor antagonist (i.e., atenolol or metoprolol) is frequently initiated on the first postoperative day following cardiac surgery.

The prophylactic use of corticosteroids, in particular, hydrocortisone, has been shown in a recent meta-analysis of randomized controlled trials to be effective in decreasing the incidence of atrial fibrillation in a high-risk patient population [56,57]. It appears that a single dose of steroids during induction of anesthesia is sufficient to provide benefit to the patients.In the context of arrhythmia prevention, it is particularly important to maintain normal **magnesium** and **potassium** concentrations perioperatively [58,59].

F. **Perioperative hypertension.** Perioperative hypertension can result from a number of causes:

1. Etiologies of acute postoperative hypertension include **emergence from anesthesia, hypothermia, hypercarbia, hypoxemia, hypoglycemia, intravascular volume excess, pain, and anxiety.** One must consider iatrogenic causes, such as administration of the wrong medication or use of a vasoconstrictor when it is not necessary.
2. Another cause of postoperative hypertension is withdrawal from preoperative antihypertensive medications. The β-blockers and centrally acting α_2-agonists (clonidine) are known to elicit rebound hypertension upon withdrawal.
3. Unusual causes include intracranial hypertension (from cerebral edema or massive stroke), bladder distention, hypoglycemia, and withdrawal syndromes (e.g., alcohol withdrawal syndrome, withdrawing from chronic opioid use).
4. Rare causes to consider include endocrine or metabolic disorders such as hyperthyroidism, pheochromocytoma, renin–angiotensin disorders, and malignant hyperthermia.

7

G. Pulmonary hypertension. Pulmonary hypertension may occur after cardiac surgery, the causes of which can be divided into new-onset acute pulmonary hypertension and continuation of a more chronic pulmonary hypertensive state. A primary consideration in the evaluation of pulmonary hypertension is the effect on RV performance. Echocardiography is critically important in diagnosing right heart failure. Pulmonary artery pressures may decrease and CVP may increase in the presence of worsening right heart failure. Because of the unique geometry of the right ventricle (RV), traditional echocardiography measurements of LV function cannot be applied to RV performance. Specific validated measurements such as tricuspid annular plane systolic excursion index [60] or Tei index [61,62] should be used to assess the RV function. Pulmonary hypertension and RV failure are particularly problematic following heart or lung transplantation and VAD placement [63].

1. **Chronic pulmonary hypertension** is less responsive than systemic hypertension to traditional therapeutic interventions. Chronic elevation in the pulmonary vascular resistance (PVR) stresses the RV and can lead to RV dysfunction. In addition, the RV hypertrophy associated with chronic pulmonary hypertension enhances susceptibility to inadequate RV oxygen delivery. Chronic pulmonary hypertension is managed by continuing any ongoing medications that the patient has been taking, such as calcium channel blockers, along with utilizing therapeutic agents mentioned below for management of acute pulmonary hypertension.
2. **Acute postoperative pulmonary hypertension** must be managed aggressively to avoid RV failure [64–66]. Parameters that influence pulmonary hypertension (see Table 10.2) should be optimized. There are four major categories of focus in addressing right heart failure associated with acute pulmonary hypertension [67]. See Figure 10.7.
   a. **Volume status of the RV (echocardiography).** Echocardiography will provide a good understanding of the primary problem: Volume versus pressure overload. Chronic pressure overload causes RV hypertrophy, often with normal RV contractility and volume.
   b. **RV function.** Address the need for inotropic support (dobutamine, PDEIs, epinephrine). In addition, optimize the heart rate and rhythm.
   c. **Offload the RV** by correcting any existing acidosis, hypercarbia, or hypoxemia. Consider adding a pulmonary artery vasodilator (inhaled nitric oxide, inhaled prostacyclin, intravenous PDEIs, intravenous nitroglycerin), and minimize any harmful effects of PPV (high peak airway pressures, excessive tidal volumes, ventilator-induced lung injury).
   d. **Maintain an adequate right coronary artery perfusion pressure** by adding a vasopressor (norepinephrine, vasopressin, phenylephrine) or mechanical diastolic pressure support via an IABP.

TABLE 10.2 Factors that contribute to pulmonary hypertension
Mitral Stenosis
Mitral Regurgitation
Clot/Thrombus on prosthetic mitral valve
Peri-vavular leak around prosthetic mitral valve
Acidosis
Atelectasis
Elevated hematocrit
Hypercarbia
Hypoxemia
Increased mean airway pressure (PEEP, hyperinflation)
Increased pulmonary vascular resistance
Mechanical obstruction (e.g., surgical restriction of a main pulmonary artery, pulmonary embolus)
Sympathetic stimulation (pain, inadequate sedation)

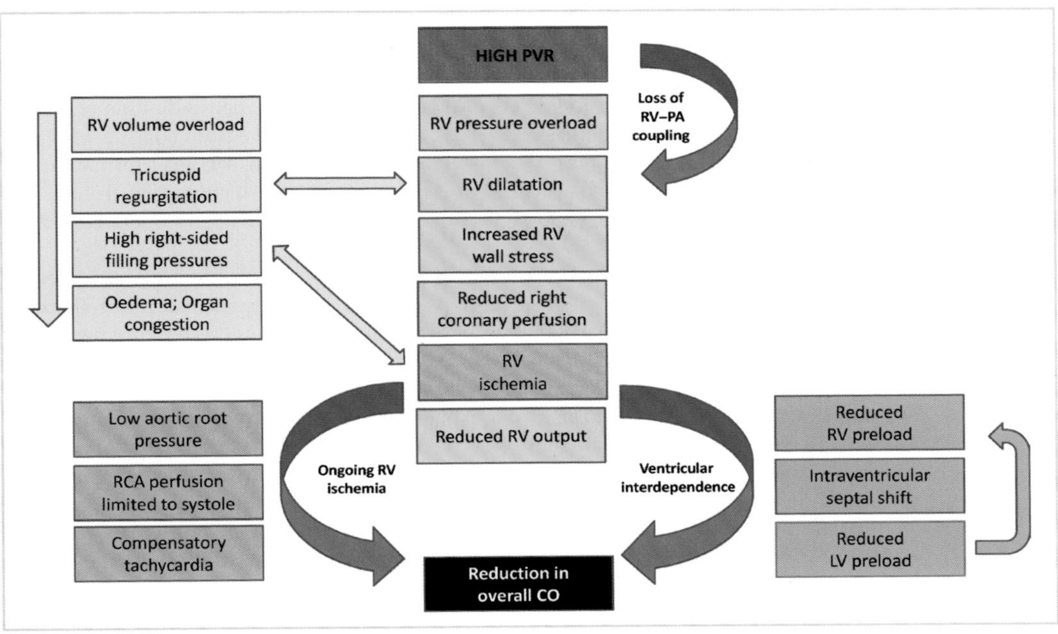

FIGURE 10.7 Pathophysiology of RV failure in the setting of high PVR. *CO,* cardiac output; *LV,* left ventricle; *MAP,* mean arterial pressure; *PVR,* pulmonary vascular resistance; *RV,* right ventricle [67].

VI. Postoperative pain and sedation management techniques

Managing postoperative pain and agitation are paramount in caring for the postoperative cardiac surgery patient. Pain represents a response to nociceptor stimulation from the surgical intervention. Patients may be agitated after cardiac surgery for a variety of reasons. Table 10.3 lists some possible causes of agitation that must be considered because they might be inappropriately "masked" by the administration of a sedative drug, or by residual neuromuscular blockade.

8

A. Systemic opioids. A variety of techniques can be used to manage postoperative pain. It is very useful to initially discern the type, quality, and location of pain before administering an analgesic agent. Commonly used opioids include fentanyl, morphine, and hydromorphone.

TABLE 10.3 Causes of postoperative agitation
Delirium
Alcohol withdrawal syndrome
Electrolyte abnormalities (hyponatremia)
Gastric or urinary retention
Hypercarbia
Hypoxemia
Ischemia or hemorrhage of the central nervous system
Medications (e.g., atropine, cimetidine, propranolol)
Psychological conditions (i.e., anxiety disorder)
Residual anesthetics/emergence from anesthesia
Residual premedication (scopolamine, phenothiazines)
Wernicke encephalopathy
Withdrawal syndrome (i.e., narcotic addiction, chronic benzodiazepine use)

B. **Nonsteroidal anti-inflammatory drugs.** Nonsteroidal anti-inflammatory drugs (NSAIDs) can be helpful when managing postoperative pain in cardiac surgery. A small amount of drug can provide analgesia without excessive sedation and other complications (e.g., respiratory depression) associated with opioid use. A concern with NSAIDs is their inhibition of platelet function and the potential for increased bleeding. NSAIDs also have been considered a poor choice after cardiac surgery because of their tendency to induce gastric ulcer formation and impair renal function. Renal insufficiency, active peptic ulcer disease, history of gastrointestinal bleeding, and bleeding diathesis should exclude the use of NSAIDs in the postoperative cardiac surgery patient [68].

C. **Intrathecal opioids.** In the era of fast-tracking patients through the postoperative period, several regional analgesic techniques have been pursued to improve patient comfort. Systemic (intravenous, intramuscular, transcutaneous, or oral) opioids can cause respiratory depression and somnolence, making them potentially undesirable for fast-tracking. Intrathecal opioids (e.g., morphine 5 to 8 μg/kg up to 1 mg) constitute an alternative to systemic opioids for cardiac surgery [69]. This route has been explored in an attempt to improve patient comfort while minimizing respiratory depression and other side effects. Intrathecal or epidural opioids can facilitate early extubation and discharge from an ICU without compromising pain control or increasing the likelihood of myocardial ischemia [70]. Intrathecal morphine may be useful in attenuating the postsurgical stress response in coronary artery bypass graft (CABG) patients as measured by plasma cortisol and epinephrine concentrations [71]. This evidence suggests that intrathecal opioids may be an excellent pain management choice in preparing the cardiac surgical patient for early extubation and fast-tracking in the ICU. However, this approach has not gained widespread support perhaps because the principal proved advantage is decreased systemic opioid use.

D. **Nerve blocks.** A variety of systemic and intrathecal analgesic techniques have been reviewed. Although these techniques are useful, each has inherent risks and complications. Nerve blocks constitute a potential alternative to these methods. Intercostal nerve blocks can be performed with ease during thoracic surgery procedures, as the intercostal nerves are easily accessible through the surgical field. These blocks can also be performed percutaneously by the anesthesia provider preoperatively or postoperatively. Intercostal nerve blocks do not provide satisfactory analgesia for a median sternotomy. Thoracic epidural analgesia (TEA) for cardiac surgical procedures [69] requiring CPB is considered acceptable by some practitioners and appears to be more accepted in Europe and Asia than in North America. Off-pump coronary artery bypass (OPCAB) procedures may be especially well suited to TEA. TEA decreases the risk of ischemia during cardiac surgery. However, many cardiac anesthesiologists consider the risk of epidural hematoma, however small, to be a deterrent in the face of the hypocoagulable state present during and after CPB. Paravertebral nerve blocks (PVBs) may be an alternative to TEA, which may be associated with less risk of epidural hematoma. PVB and bilateral PVB catheters have been utilized with success in cardiac surgical procedures [72–74]. Recently parasternal nerve blockade has been described and may prove to be useful [75].

E. **Sedation.** It is essential to understand the goals of sedation in a critically ill patient. In the ICU, one should titrate sedatives to the desired effect as precisely as one would titrate vasopressors, inotropes, and oxygen. Light sedation with aggressive analgesic techniques shortens ICU stay, decreases delirium, decreases post-traumatic stress disorder, and probably improves mortality. Sedation should be goal directed. The majority of patients in the ICU should be awake and interactive even if they require mechanical ventilation [76]. Not all postoperative cardiac surgery patients require sedation (see Table 10.4).

1. **Benzodiazepines,** when used as sedatives, have been associated with prolonged mechanical ventilation, delirium, and possibly increased mortality when used as continuous infusions [77,78].
2. **Propofol** is commonly administered as a continuous infusion in the ICU for sedation. It is easily titrated to effect but can produce significant vasodilation or myocardial depression with resultant hypotension. Propofol causes a burning pain during peripheral administration, so central venous administration is advisable if possible. In addition,

TABLE 10.4 ICU sedation

Sedative	Loading dose	Continuous infusion	Special considerations
Dexmedetomidine	1 μg/kg over 10–15 min	0.2–0.7 μg/kg/hr	Hemodynamic stability; treats withdrawal syndromes; no weaning required for extubation, bradycardia
Propofol	None	15–100 μg/kg/min	Sepsis risk; hypotension
Fentanyl (used with midazolam)	1–3 μg/kg	25–250 μg/hr	Potent analgesic; tolerance
Midazolam (used with fentanyl)	0.02–0.05 mg/kg	0.5–3 mg/hr	Amnestic; treats delirium tremens

propofol can be a source for sepsis since the lipid mixture can act as a medium for bacterial growth; strict aseptic technique must be used.

3. **Dexmedetomidine** is a potent α_2-adrenergic agonist that provides sedation, hemodynamic stability, decreased cardiac ischemia, improved pulmonary function, and analgesia, and can therefore be a good choice in cardiac surgical patients [79–82]. Hypotension and bradycardia are occasionally attributed to its use. Dexmedetomidine is unique among sedatives in that patients remain cooperative yet calm and it does not require weaning to permit extubation. Dexmedetomidine activates endogenous sleep pathways, which may decrease agitation and confusion. Dexmedetomidine is administered as a continuous intravenous infusion (0.2 to 0.7 μg/kg/hr) and is approved for use up to 24 hrs. Clinical trials for extended infusion of dexmedetomidine at higher doses (up to1.5 μg/kg/hr) in a diverse ICU population have resulted in more ventilator-free days and more delirium-free days when compared to similar sedation end points with lorazepam or midazolam. Withdrawal syndromes (ethanol, chronic pain narcotic use, illicit drugs) can also be managed with the administration of α_2-adrenergic agonists.

VII. Metabolic abnormalities

Many metabolic abnormalities can occur in the perioperative period. These irregularities result from the physiologic stress response or from the large fluid and electrolyte shifts that can derive from intravenous infusions or from CPB priming or myocardial protectant solutions.

A. Electrolyte abnormalities

1. **Hyperkalemia** can present from cardioplegia, overaggressive replacement, or secondary extracellular shifts associated with respiratory or metabolic acidosis. **Hypokalemia** increases the risk for dysrhythmia following cardiac surgery. Administration of mannitol in the CPB prime, improved renal perfusion, and aggressive treatment of blood glucose with insulin infusion all contribute to hypokalemia. Hypokalemia is more common than hyperkalemia. Potassium supplementation can be infused at a maximum rate of 20 mEq/hr via a central venous catheter. Rapid potassium infusion can induce lethal arrhythmias. The target serum potassium concentration should be 3.5 to 5 mEq/L.
2. **Hypomagnesemia** is a common perioperative electrolyte abnormality and is associated with postoperative dysrhythmia, myocardial ischemia, and ventricular dysfunction [58,83]. Hypomagnesemia may result from dilution by large CPB priming volumes and from urinary excretion. Renal potassium retention requires adequate magnesium concentration and thus magnesium administration should always be considered in hypokalemic patients. If magnesium supplementation is required, it can be given in amounts of 2 to 4 g intravenously over 30 to 45 min. An infusion of 1 g/hr of magnesium sulfate can be used as well to assure a slow, steady infusion of this substance. If given too fast, it may cause hypotension or muscle weakness. In refractory dysrhythmias, particularly of the ventricular type, a normal serum magnesium concentration may not exclude the possibility of decreased total body stores of magnesium. The target serum magnesium concentration should be 2 to 2.5 mEq/L.

3. **Hypocalcemia** may be present and may be related to rapid transfusion of large amounts of citrate-preserved bank blood. Hypocalcemia can be treated with 250 to 1,000 mg intravenous doses of calcium chloride or calcium gluconate, while paying careful attention to the potential for development of dysrhythmias. When following the calcium status, it is important to measure ionized calcium and not total calcium, because low albumin levels may decrease total calcium levels, whereas ionized calcium remains normal.
4. **Hypophosphatemia** is a common problem encountered in the ICU. Hypophosphatemia can contribute to weakness and poor myocardial function, can change the ability of red blood cells to change shape, and can affect oxyhemoglobin dissociation [84,85].

B. Shivering. The exact mechanism of shivering is difficult to discern, but it is thought to be associated with inadequate rewarming and the resulting hypothermic temperature "after-drop." Many patients are hypothermic when they arrive in the ICU and develop shivering as they emerge from anesthesia. Shivering can result in a 300% to 600% increase in oxygen demand, which potentially places unachievable oxygen delivery demand upon a compromised myocardium. The associated increase in CO_2 production may cause respiratory acidosis. In patients with inadequate end-organ oxygen delivery, sustained shivering frequently will require mechanical ventilation and consideration should be given to administration of neuromuscular blockers to abolish the increased metabolic demand of shivering. Effective first-line treatments include active rewarming with forced air blankets and prevention of further temperature loss. Pharmacologic interventions that reduce shivering include intravenous meperidine (12.5 to 25 mg) or dexmedetomidine.

C. Acidosis can be described as respiratory, metabolic, or mixed. Metabolic acidosis is divided into anion gap and non-anion gap acidosis. A complete discussion of acid–base
9 disorders is beyond the scope of this chapter and can be found in standard critical care textbooks. We will briefly discuss the most common causes of acidosis in the early postoperative period.

1. **Respiratory acidosis** results from hypoventilation or increased CO_2 production. Residual anesthetics or an awakening patient with inadequate analgesia combined with impaired respiratory mechanics may lead to hypoventilation. Treatment consists of support of ventilation while treating the underlying cause.
2. **Metabolic acidosis,** when present, is associated frequently with inadequate systemic perfusion because of compromised cardiac function. Treatment is directed at correcting the underlying cause of the acidosis. Metabolic acidosis in a cardiac surgery patient may require administration of sodium bicarbonate as a temporizing measure, especially in patients who are hemodynamically unstable.
3. **Lactic acidosis,** a frequent finding in cardiac surgery patients, needs to be managed by assuring adequate CO and intravascular volume, and avoidance of shivering. There is some evidence that the use of sodium bicarbonate to treat lactic acidosis should be avoided; however, most of the critical care data assessing the effects of buffers in treating acidosis do not include patients with acute pulmonary hypertension or right heart failure. Epinephrine can produce a transient lactic acidosis that does not appear to reflect inadequate perfusion in the patient receiving the drug [35].

D. Glucose management. Glycemic control in the critically ill is a highly controversial topic. Data from 2001 indicated that tight glycemic control in cardiac surgery patients (80 to 110 mg/dL) induced a remarkable improvement in mortality [86]; however, subsequent trials have failed to reproduce this dramatic effect. The most recent multicenter multinational interventional trial of tight glycemic control demonstrated an increase in mortality when hyperglycemia was aggressively managed to maintain a glucose range of 81 to 108 mg/dL [87]. Control of blood glucose levels at less than 150 mg/dL (or some would say less than 180 to 200 mg/dL, as there is no consensus standard) and **avoiding hypoglycemia** with frequent monitoring is a reasonable goal in cardiac surgical patients. Unrecognized hyperglycemia can result in excessive diuresis and the potential for a hyperosmolar or ketoacidotic state. Elevated serum glucose can be managed by using a continuous infusion of regular insulin, often starting at a dose of 0.1 units/kg/hr or less with titration to the desired serum blood glucose level.

VIII. Complications in the first 24 hrs postoperatively

A number of life-threatening complications can occur in the first 24 hrs after cardiac or thoracic surgery.

A. **Respiratory failure.** Respiratory failure may be the most common postoperative complication of cardiac or thoracic surgery. Pulmonary dysfunction develops from the surgical incision and its attendant disruption of the thoracic cage. Postoperative pain exacerbates this effect. Respiratory failure can present as hypoxemia, hypercarbia, or both. Prompt identification and appropriate treatment is essential. Atelectasis is the most common pulmonary complication following cardiac surgery and can usually be managed with the application of PEEP, BiPAP, or CPAP.

B. **Bleeding.** Postoperative hemorrhage from ongoing surgical bleeding or coagulopathy increases a patient's length of stay and mortality [88]. Bleeding typically is monitored by the amount of blood that drains into the chest tubes after surgery. It is critical to differentiate a bleeding diathesis from a surgical bleeding situation requiring reoperation. Consequently, in bleeding patients it becomes essential to determine the status of the coagulation system, which is traditionally done by acquiring (at a minimum) PT, aPTT, fibrinogen concentration, and platelet count in addition to a chest x-ray. This panel of tests does not provide any indication of the functional status of the platelets. Thromboelastogram (TEG) or other platelet functional assays provide useful information about platelet functional status, and the TEG also provides information about plasma clotting function and fibrinolysis. Assessment of platelet function is particularly important in managing the cardiac patients who have received aspirin or other platelet inhibitors (e.g., clopidogrel, glycoprotein IIb/IIIa inhibitors) preoperatively. Transfusion of **platelet concentrates** may be appropriate when one suspects that the bleeding results from platelet dysfunction.

Fresh frozen plasma (FFP) should most often be used to correct abnormalities in PT, INR, or aPTT, although modest elevations in these tests are often clinically insignificant. When associated with clinical bleeding, elevations of PT or aPTT in excess of 1.3 times the upper limit of normal or of INR in excess of 1.5 should probably be treated. Elevated aPTT may occur from deficiencies of plasma coagulation factors or from residual heparin. **Fibrinogen** deficiency (typically less than 75 mg/dL) is treated with cryoprecipitate, and fibrinogen concentrates may be available in some countries.

The role of **activated factor VII** in the cardiac surgical population is controversial. A meta-analysis of 35 randomized clinical trials that included both cardiac surgery and non-cardiac surgery trials showed no statistically significant difference in venous thrombosis after administration of activated factor VII including doses up to 80 mcg/kg. However, there was a statistically significant increase in coronary arterial thromboembolic events when compared to placebo [89].

Surgical bleeding is often considered once coagulopathy has been ruled out, and it may require a return to the OR for mediastinal or thoracic re-exploration to identify and control a bleeding site. Surgical re-exploration commonly fails to identify a specific source for the bleeding. However, irrigation of the pericardium and mediastinum will remove activated plasminogen (from dissolved blood clots), which may markedly decrease bleeding. In general, chest tube drainage greater than 500 mL/hr, sustained drainage exceeding 200 mL/hr, or increasing chest tube drainage justifies surgical re-exploration.

Sudden hemorrhage from a suture line or cannulation site can cause profound hypotension from hypovolemia or tamponade. Rapid infusion of blood products, colloids, or crystalloids is necessary to maintain intravascular volume. Patients who can be quickly stabilized are transferred to the OR. In some instances, emergency sternotomy must be performed in the ICU to control life-threatening hemorrhage or tamponade.

C. **Cardiac tamponade.** Excessive mediastinal bleeding with inadequate drainage or sudden massive bleeding can result in cardiac tamponade. Cardiac tamponade after cardiac surgery may seem impossible if the pericardium has been left open, suggesting to the inexperienced observer that tamponade cannot occur. However, this is not true because *tamponade may occur in localized areas,* affecting an area as circumscribed as the right atrium. As discussed above, it is important to recognize that traditionally described equalization of filling pressures is an unreliable sign of post-cardiac surgery tamponade. The differential diagnosis includes biventricular failure, and TEE or transthoracic echocardiography may be important to making the correct diagnosis. At times, cardiac tamponade is a clinical diagnosis that requires emergent surgical intervention.

D. **Pneumothorax.** Pneumothorax can occur in patients who have undergone sternotomy, thoracotomy, or are undergoing PPV. Most cardiac surgical patients arrive in the recovery or ICU area with one or more chest (intrapleural) tubes in place, in addition to mediastinal tubes. These patients should have a baseline postoperative chest x-ray upon ICU arrival to confirm the adequacy of chest tube placement and the absence of a pneumothorax. Patients who have had a redo sternotomy or who have had an internal mammary artery used for CABG are at particular high risk for a pneumothorax and hemothorax. There is increasing evidence that bedside ultrasound is valuable in diagnosing pneumothorax, hemothorax, and lung consolidation. In some studies, it has higher accuracy than portable chest x-ray when compared to CT scan [90]. An intensivist who is skilled in performing the exam can obtain immediate data and perform repeat exams if needed. Pneumothorax can convert to tension pneumothorax when chest tubes function improperly. The resulting shift of mediastinal structures can obstruct the vena cava or distort the heart to cause a low CO state and hypotension.

E. **Hemothorax.** Hemothorax can occur after coronary artery bypass surgery and must be considered in all patients who have undergone internal mammary artery dissection, which most often involves opening the left intrapleural space. These patients may need to be returned to the OR for surgical management.

F. **Acute graft closure.** Acute coronary graft closure, while uncommon, can result in myocardial ischemia or infarction. If cardiac decompensation occurs and graft closure is the suspected cause, re-exploration should be performed to evaluate graft patency. However, this may be a diagnosis of exclusion, and re-exploration for this reason is uncommon. These patients may need to be taken to the cardiac catheterization laboratory where emergent cardiac catheterization can be performed to discern the presence of an occluded graft. Controversy continues about whether graft patency is similar or different in OPCAB and CPB CABG procedures either acutely or long-term [91,92].

G. **Prosthetic valve failure.** Acute prosthetic valve failure should be suspected when sudden hemodynamic changes occur following open heart surgery, particularly if the rhythm is unchanged and intermittent loss of the arterial waveform is noted on the monitor screen. Immediate surgical correction is necessary. Valve dehiscence with a perivalvular leak usually does not present in the early postoperative period. TEE is the diagnostic modality of choice to evaluate prosthetic valve function in this setting. There is increasing experience and success with closing or reducing perivalvular leaks in the interventional cardiology laboratory using percutaneous atrial septal defect (ASD) and ventricular septal defect (VSD) closure devices.

H. **Postoperative neurologic dysfunction.** Neurologic complications are frequently recognized in the postoperative period and remain one of the most important complications following cardiac surgery [93,94], so an early postoperative neurologic examination is very important. Neurologic complications can be divided into three groups: (1) Focal ischemic injury (stroke), (2) neurocognitive dysfunction (including diffuse encephalopathy), and (3) peripheral nervous system injury. Central nervous system dysfunction after cardiac surgery is discussed in detail in Chapter 22. Brachial plexus injury resulting from sternal retraction can occur, particularly on the left side during internal mammary arterial dissection. A thorough motor exam of the legs is crucial after descending thoracic aortic or thoracoabdominal aneurysm repairs. A delirium assessment, like the Confusion Assessment Method for ICU Patients (CAM-ICU), can identify patients with hypoactive delirium [95]. Hypoactive delirium in the ICU carries an increased morbidity and mortality. Vanderbilt University ICU physicians have developed an excellent resource about delirium for families and clinicians, which can be found at www.icudelirium.org.

IX. Discharge from the intensive care unit

Discharge from the ICU historically has occurred 1 to 3 days after cardiothoracic surgery. Reducing the amount of time spent in the ICU after cardiac surgery recently has become a priority. Many patients are now discharged from the ICU on the morning after routine CABG operations without compromise in patient care or safety. Complications such as those noted earlier often delay ICU discharge. Some centers place routine CABG patients in an ICU-level recovery area for several hours before discharging them to a "step-down" or intermediate care area, or even to a "monitored bed" postoperative nursing unit.

The criteria for ICU discharge vary depending upon the type of surgery. Predicting which patients can leave the ICU in an early FT style can be accomplished by reviewing a variety of preoperative risk factors. Reduced LV ejection fraction is a valid predictor of higher mortality, morbidity, and resource utilization [96]. Other preoperative predictors of prolonged ICU stays include cardiogenic shock, age greater than 80 years, dialysis-dependent renal failure, and surgery performed emergently [97]. These factors and others can be used to predict a patient's length of stay and to plan for resource utilization.

X. The transplant patient. The care of cardiac transplant patients is similar to other cardiac patients with several notable exceptions [98]. Pulmonary hypertension and RV failure are the primary challenges in the early postoperative period following heart or lung transplantation [63]. Heart transplant recipients may have varying degrees of end-organ dysfunction secondary to chronic low CO. Finally, these patients require meticulous attention to medications used to attenuate graft rejection.

XI. Patients with mechanical assist devices (see also Chapter 16)

Recent technologic advances have facilitated the development of mechanical assist devices for cardiac surgery patients with severely impaired RV or LV function. The number of assist devices available continues to grow, resulting in options for LV, RV, or biventricular mechanical assistance [99,100]. Postoperative management of patients with mechanical assist devices requires a thorough understanding of the technology underlying any device that may be chosen. The primary risks with mechanical assistance include thrombosis, bleeding from anticoagulation, infection from percutaneous catheters, and failure to wean from assist devices intended for temporary cardiac support.

A. Intra-aortic balloon pump (IABP). An IABP is typically the first mechanical assist device utilized for cardiogenic shock in cardiac surgical patients [101] (see Chapter 22). The goals of IABP therapy are to acutely decrease the LV afterload, thereby improving forward blood flow, and to augment the LV coronary artery perfusion during diastole. Coronary blood flow is only augmented in patients with hypotension associated with their cardiogenic shock [102]. The IABP is most often placed percutaneously via the femoral artery into the descending thoracic aorta. There are two management strategies for weaning IABP support. Some clinicians wean pharmacologic support prior to IABP; this allows them to resume inotropic support should the patient decompensate after IABP removal. Other clinicians wean IABP support first due to concerns about lower extremity ischemia from arterial occlusion of the femoral and/or iliac arteries. Despite the clear risk of lower extremity ischemia from arterial occlusion, there is no decrease in embolic or thrombotic complications when the patient undergoes systemic anticoagulation [103]. In either strategy, the IABP is weaned from a 1:1 setting (each cardiac contraction triggers an IABP deflation/inflation cycle) to 1:2, then a brief trial at 1:3 precedes IABP removal.

B. Ventricular assist device (VAD) (see Chapter 22). VAD can be utilized for support of the left (LVAD), right (RVAD), or both (BiVAD) ventricles [99,100]. There are three indications for VAD therapy:

1. Temporary support (less than 14 days) in patients who fail to wean from CPB but are expected to recover sufficient cardiac function for removal of the VAD.
2. Bridge to cardiac transplantation.
3. Destination VAD therapy; patients who require long-term or permanent VAD support with the expectation that they will be discharged from the hospital with the VAD.

In patients with LVADs, the possibility that LV decompression will result in geometric alterations and precipitation of right heart failure must be considered. Other considerations that must be addressed during the ICU period include adequate oxygenation and ventilation using a mechanical ventilator, along with maintenance of temperature, nutrition, acid–base balance, and electrolyte balance. The patients with mechanical assist devices can be weaned from the ventilator using standard weaning protocols depending upon their hemodynamic status, blood gas exchange, and neurologic stability. If a VAD has been implanted as short-term support with an anticipated return to the OR within a few days to remove the device, this tends to discourage endotracheal extubation.

XII. Family issues in the postoperative period

Interaction with families is important in communicating any patient's status and in giving appropriate expectations about recovery.

A. **The preoperative discussion.** In the preoperative discussion, it is important for the surgeon and anesthesiologist to give a detailed description of what to anticipate in the postoperative period. This information can be relayed either through preoperative visits or through video or website access describing typical postoperative events. Detailed discussions about planned extubation in the OR or in the ICU may prevent patients from misinterpreting early postoperative intubation as being awake during surgery. It is also important to discuss the goals of general anesthesia versus sedation in the ICU. Caution should be used when assuring the patient that they will have complete amnesia of the OR or being intubated. Family members should be told to expect that the cardiac surgical patient will have invasive monitors and may have significant edema, which alters their appearance. Reassurance that these are temporary cosmetic changes will provide comfort. Preoperative visits allow patients and their families the opportunity to ask questions and to understand the plan of movement through the postoperative course in a more relaxed setting than the preanesthesia holding area. Many times, anesthesiology preoperative visits may be compromised or precluded by admission day surgery patterns whereby cardiac surgery patients arrive at the hospital on the day of surgery. In these circumstances, opportunities for discussions with anesthesia care providers can be limited and should be anticipated at the preoperative visit with the surgeon, when information can be disseminated and questions can be answered. Some centers compensate for this practice pattern with anesthesia-specific pamphlets or web-based videos, often with a Frequently Asked Questions section.

B. **Family visitation.** Family visitation occurs in the ICU or recovery room for many postoperative cardiac and thoracic surgery patients. This provides reassurance about the patient's clinical course progression as well as encouragement toward subsequent postoperative care. Family members can be very important in encouraging adequate pulmonary toilet, coughing, deep breathing, and early ambulation to improve postoperative outcomes. Most cardiac surgery programs have designated personnel for the liaison between the professional staff caring for postoperative cardiac surgery patients and the family members who need education, encouragement, and the opportunity to assist in postoperative care.

C. **The role of family support.** Family support is a vital link toward the early success of a fast-tracking program. Family members need adequate education by surgical and anesthesia staff, who can outline the expected early postoperative events. The role of family support is heightened when patients spend very short periods in postoperative areas such as the recovery room or ICU. Family members who are educated about the expected postoperative course can facilitate postoperative care and smooth the transition from the ICU to a regular nursing floor and finally to the patient's home.

ACKNOWLEDGMENTS

The authors would like to thank Mark Gerhardt, MD, the author of the previous edition of this chapter, and Jennifer Olin for her editorial assistance.

REFERENCES

1. Warren J, Fromm REJ, Orr RA, et al. Guidelines for the inter- and intrahospital transport of critically ill patients. *Crit Care Med.* 2004;32:256–262.
2. Commission J. Improving America's hospitals: The Joint Commission's annual report on quality and safety. http//wwwjointcommissionreportorg/pdf/JC_2006_Annual_Reportpdf 2006.
3. Dunn W, Murphy JG. The patient handoff. *Chest.* 2008;134:9–12.

4. Saver C. Handoffs: what ORs can learn from Formula One race crews. *OR Manager.* 2011;27:1–13.
5. Logio LS, Djuricich AM. Handoffs in teaching hospitals: situation, background, assessment, and recommendation. *Am J Med.* 2010;123:563–567.
6. Cohen MD, Hilligoss PB. The published literature on handoffs in hospitals: deficiencies identified in an extensive review. *Qual Safety Health Care.* 2010;19:493–497.
7. Raptis DA, Fernandes C, Weiliang Chua, et al. Electronic software significantly improves quality of handover in a London teaching hospital. *Health Inform J.* 2009;15:191–198.
8. Apfelbaum JL, Belott R, Connis RT. Practice advisory for the perioperative management of patients with cardiac implantable electronic devices: pacemakers and implantable cardioverter-defibrillators: an updated report by the American Society of Anesthesiologists Task Force on Perioperative Management of Patients with Cardiac Implantable Electronic Devices. *Anesthesiology.* 2011;114:247–261.
9. Frazier SK. Cardiovascular effects of mechanical ventilation and weaning. *Nurs Clin North Am.* 2008;43:1–15.
10. Singh I, Pinsky MR. *Mechanical Ventilation.* Philadelphia, PA: Saunders Elsevier; 2008.
11. van Belle AF, Wesseling GJ, Penn OCKM, et al. Postoperative pulmonary function abnormalities after coronary artery bypass surgery. *Resp Med.* 1992;86:195–199.
12. Cox CM, Ascione R, Cohen AM, et al. Effect of cardiopulmonary bypass on pulmonary gas exchange: a prospective randomized study. *Ann Thor Surg.* 2000;69:140–145.
13. Jaber SD, Chanques G, Jung B. Postoperative noninvasive ventilation. *Anesthesiology.* 2010;112:453–461.
14. Burns KEA, Adhikari NKJ, Keenan SP, et al. Use of non-invasive ventilation to wean critically ill adults off invasive ventilation: meta-analysis and systematic review. *BMJ.* 2009;338.
15. Gattinoni L, Protti A, Caironi P, et al. Ventilator-induced lung injury: the anatomical and physiological framework. *Crit Care Med.* 2010;38(10) Proceedings of a Round Table Conference in Brussels, Belgium, March 2010:S539–S548.
16. Diaz JV, Brower R, Calfee CS, et al. Therapeutic strategies for severe acute lung injury. *Crit Care Med.* 2010;38:1644–1650.
17. Esan A, Hess DR, Raoof S, et al. Severe hypoxemic respiratory failure. *Chest.* 2010;137:1203–1216.
18. Raoof S, Goulet K, Esan A, et al. Severe hypoxemic respiratory failure. *Chest.* 2010;137:1437–1448.
19. Liu LL, Aldrich JM, Shimabukuro DW, et al. Rescue therapies for acute hypoxemic respiratory failure. *Anesth Analg.* 2010;111:693–702.
20. Sud S, Sud M, Friedrich JO, et al. High frequency oscillation in patients with acute lung injury and acute respiratory distress syndrome (ARDS): systematic review and meta-analysis. *BMJ.* 2010;340.
21. Brochard L, Thille AW. What is the proper approach to liberating the weak from mechanical ventilation? *Crit Care Med.* 2009;37:S410–S415.
22. MacIntyre N. Discontinuing mechanical ventilatory support. *Chest.* 2007;132:1049–1056.
23. Constantinides VA, Tekkis PP, Fazil A, et al. Fast-track failure after cardiac surgery: development of a prediction model. *Crit Care Med.* 2006;34:2875–2882.
24. Kogan A, Ghosh P, Preisman S, et al. Risk factors for failed "fast-tracking" after cardiac surgery in patients older than 70 years. *J Cardiothor Vasc Anesth.* 2008;22:530–535.
25. Zarate E, Latham P, White PF, et al. Fast-track cardiac anesthesia: use of remifentanil combined with intrathecal morphine as an alternative to sufentanil during desflurane anesthesia. *Anesth Analg.* 2000;91:283–287.
26. Latham P, Zarate E, White PF, et al. Fast-track cardiac anesthesia: a comparison of remifentanil plus intrathecal morphine with sufentanil in a desflurane-based anesthetic. *J Cardiothor Vasc Anesth.* 2000;14:645–651.
27. Dowd NP, Cheng DCH, Karski JM, et al. Intraoperative awareness in fast-track cardiac anesthesia. *Anesthesiology.* 1998;89:1068–1073.
28. Maldonado JR, Wysong A, van der Starre PJA, et al. Dexmedetomidine and the reduction of postoperative delirium after cardiac surgery. *Psychosomatics.* 2009;50:206–217.
29. Shehabi Y, Grant P, Wolfenden H, et al. Prevalence of delirium with dexmedetomidine compared with morphine based therapy after cardiac surgery: a randomized controlled trial (dexmedetomidine compared to morphine-DEXCOM study). *Anesthesiology.* 2009;111:1075–1084.
30. Herr DL, Sum-Ping STJ, England M. ICU sedation after coronary artery bypass graft surgery: dexmedetomidine-based versus propofol-based sedation regimens. *J Cardiothor Vasc Anesth.* 2003;17:576–584.
31. Riker RR, Shehabi Y, Bokesch PM, et al. dexmedetomidine vs midazolam for sedation of critically ill patients. *JAMA: J Am Med Assoc.* 2009;301:489–499.
32. Novick R, Fox S, Stitt L, et al. Impact of the opening of a specialized cardiac surgery recovery unit on postoperative outcomes in an academic health sciences centre. *Can J Anesth.* 2007;54:737–743.
33. Srivastava AR, Banerjee A, Tempe DK, et al. A comprehensive approach to fast tracking in cardiac surgery: ambulatory low-risk open-heart surgery. *Eur J Cardio-Thor Surg.* 2008;33:955–960.
34. Hollenberg SM. Vasoactive drugs in circulatory shock. *Am J Respir Crit Care Med.* 2011;183:847–855.
35. Levy B, Perez P, Perny J, et al. Comparison of norepinephrine-dobutamine to epinephrine for hemodynamics, lactate metabolism, and organ function variables in cardiogenic shock. A prospective, randomized pilot study. *Crit Care Med.* 2011;39:450–455.
36. Prielipp RC, MacGregor DA, Butterworth JF, et al. Pharmacodynamics and pharmacokinetics of milrinone administration to increase oxygen delivery in critically ill patients. *Chest* 1996;109:1291–1301.
37. Toller WG, Stranz C. Levosimendan, a new inotropic and vasodilator agent. *Anesthesiology.* 2006;104:556–569.
38. Maharaj R, Metaxa V. Levosimendan and mortality after coronary revascularisation: a meta-analysis of randomised controlled trials. *Crit Care.* 2011;15:R140–R150.
39. Arroll B, Doughty R, Andersen V. Investigation and management of congestive heart failure. *Br J Anaesth.* 2010;341:C3657.

40. Ezekowitz JA, Hernandez AF, Starling RC, et al. Standardizing care for acute decompensated heart failure in a large megatrial: The approach for the Acute Studies of Clinical Effectiveness of Nesiritide in Subjects with Decompensated Heart Failure (ASCEND-HF). *Am Heart J.* 2009;157:219–228.
41. Krum H, Teerlink J. Medical therapy for chronic heart failure. *Lancet.* 2011;378:713–721.
42. Shah AM, Mann DL. In search of new therapeutic targets and strategies for heart failure: recent advances in basic science. *Lancet.* 2011;378:704–712.
43. Chappell D, Jacob M, Hofmann-Kiefer K, et al. A rational approach to perioperative fluid management. *Anesthesiology.* 2008;109:723–740.
44. Marik PE, Baram M, Vahid B. Does central venous pressure predict fluid responsiveness?. *Chest.* 2008;134:172–178.
45. Michard F, Teboul J. Using heart-lung interactions to assess fluid responsiveness during mechanical ventilation. *Crit Care.* 2000;4:282–289.
46. Marik PE, Cavallazzi R, Vasu T, et al. Dynamic changes in arterial waveform derived variables and fluid responsiveness in mechanically ventilated patients: a systematic review of the literature. *Crit Care Med.* 2009;37:2642–2647.
47. Ferraris VA, Brown JR, Despotis GJ, et al. 2011 update to The Society of Thoracic Surgeons and The Society of Cardiovascular Anesthesiologists blood conservation clinical practice guidelines. *Ann Thoracic Surg.* 2011;91:944–982.
48. Varghese R, Myers ML. Blood conservation in cardiac surgery: let's get restrictive. *Semin Thor Cardiovasc Surg.* 2010;22: 121–126.
49. Levin RL, Degrange MA, Bruno GF, et al. Methylene blue reduces mortality and morbidity in vasoplegic patients after cardiac surgery. *Ann Thoracic Surg.* 2004;77:496–499.
50. Maslow AD, Regan MM, Haering JM, et al. Echocardiographic predictors of left ventricular outflow tract obstruction and systolic anterior motion of the mitral valve after mitral valve reconstruction for myxomatous valve disease. *J Am Coll Cardiol.* 1999;34:2096–2104.
51. Russo AM, O'Connor WH, Waxman HL. Atypical presentations and echocardiographic findings in patients with cardiac tamponade occurring early and late after cardiac surgery. *Chest.* 1993;104:71–78.
52. Rho RW. The management of atrial fibrillation after cardiac surgery. *Heart.* 2009;95:422–429.
53. Bradley D, Creswell LL, Hogue CW, et al. Pharmacologic prophylaxis: American College of Chest Physicians guidelines for the prevention and management of postoperative atrial fibrillation after cardiac surgery. *Chest.* 2005;128:39S–47S.
54. Halonen J, Loponen P, Järvinen O, et al. Metoprolol versus amiodarone in the prevention of atrial fibrillation after cardiac surgery. *Ann Intern Med.* 2010;153:703–709.
55. Chen WT, Krishnan GM, Sood N, et al. Effect of statins on atrial fibrillation after cardiac surgery: A duration- and dose-response meta-analysis. *J Thor Cardiovasc Surg.* 2010;140:364–372.
56. Marik PE, Fromm R. The efficacy and dosage effect of corticosteroids for the prevention of atrial fibrillation after cardiac surgery: a systematic review. *J Crit Care.* 2009;24:458–463.
57. Ho KM, Tan JA. Benefits and risks of corticosteroid prophylaxis in adult cardiac surgery. *Circulation.* 2009;119:1853–1866.
58. Booth JV, Phillips-Bute B, McCants CB, et al. Low serum magnesium level predicts major adverse cardiac events after coronary artery bypass graft surgery. *Am Heart J.* 2003;145:1108–1113.
59. Cook RC, Humphries KH, Gin K, et al. Prophylactic intravenous magnesium sulphate in addition to oral β-blockade does not prevent atrial arrhythmias after coronary artery or valvular heart surgery. *Circulation.* 2009;120:S163–S169.
60. Forfia PR, Fisher MR, Mathai SC, et al. Tricuspid annular displacement predicts survival in pulmonary hypertension. *Am J Respir Crit Care Med.* 2006;174:1034–1041.
61. Tei C, Dujardin KS, Hodge DO, et al. Doppler echocardiographic index for assessment of global right ventricular function. *J Am Society Echocardiogr.* 1996;9:838–847.
62. Meluzín J, Špinarová L, Bakala J, et al. Pulsed Doppler tissue imaging of the velocity of tricuspid annular systolic motion;. a new, rapid, and non-invasive method of evaluating right ventricular systolic function. *Eur Heart J.* 2001;22:340–348.
63. Rosenberg AL, Rao M, Benedict PE. Anesthetic implications for lung transplantation. *Anesthesiol Clin North Am.* 2004;22:767–788.
64. Taylor MB, Laussen PC. Fundamentals of management of acute postoperative pulmonary hypertension. *Pediatr Crit Care Med.* 2010;11:S27–S29.
65. Gordon C, Collard CD, Pan W. Intraoperative management of pulmonary hypertension and associated right heart failure. *Curr Opin Anesthesiol.* 2010;23:49–56.
66. Lahm T, McCaslin CA, Wozniak TC, et al. Medical and surgical treatment of acute right ventricular failure. *J Am Coll Cardiol.* 2010;56:1435–1446.
67. Price LC, Wort SJ, Finney SJ, et al. Pulmonary vascular and right ventricular dysfunction in adult critical care: current and emerging options for management: a systematic literature review. *Crit Care.* 2010;14:R169–R191.
68. Hynninen M, Cheng D, Hossain I, et al. Non-steroidal anti-inflammatory drugs in treatment of postoperative pain after cardiac surgery. *Can J Anesth.* 2000;47:1182–1187.
69. Chaney MA. Intrathecal and epidural anesthesia and analgesia for cardiac surgery. *Anesth Analg.* 2006;102:45–64.
70. Shroff A, Rooke GA, Bishop MJ. Effects of intrathecal opioid on extubation time, analgesia, and intensive care unit stay following coronary artery bypass grafting. *J Clin Anesth.* 1997;9:415–419.
71. Hall R, Adderley N, MacLaren C, et al. Does intrathecal morphine alter the stress response following coronary artery bypass grafting surgery? *Can J Anesth.* 2000;47:463–466.
72. Ganapathy S, Murkin JM, Boyd DW, et al. Continuous percutaneous paravertebral block for minimally invasive cardiac surgery. *J Cardiothor Vasc Anesth.* 1999;13:594–596.
73. Cantó M, Sánchez MJ, Casas MA, et al. Bilateral paravertebral blockade for conventional cardiac surgery. *Anaesthesia.* 2003;58:365–370.

74. Dhole S, Mehta Y, Saxena H, et al. Comparison of continuous thoracic epidural and paravertebral blocks for postoperative analgesia after minimally invasive direct coronary artery bypass surgery. *J Cardiothor Vasc Anesth.* 2001;15:288–292.
75. McDonald SB, Jacobsohn E, Kopacz DJ, et al. Parasternal block and local anesthetic infiltration with levobupivacaine after cardiac surgery with desflurane: the effect on postoperative pain, pulmonary function, and tracheal extubation times. *Anesth Analg.* 2005;100:25–32.
76. Jackson DL PC, Cann KF, Walsh T. A systematic review of the impact of sedation practice in the ICU on resource use, costs and patient safety. *Crit Care.* 2010;14:R59.
77. Pandharipande P, Shintani A, Peterson J, et al. Lorazepam is an independent risk factor for transitioning to delirium in intensive care unit patients. *Anesthesiology.* 2006;104:21–26.
78. Pandharipande P, Cotton BA, Shintani A, et al. Prevalence and risk factors for development of delirium in surgical and trauma intensive care unit patients. *J Trauma.* 2008;65:34–41.
79. Wijeysundera DN, Naik JS, Scott BW. Alpha-2 adrenergic agonists to prevent perioperative cardiovascular complications: a meta-analysis. *Am J Med.* 2003;114:742–752.
80. Dasta JF, Jacobi J, Sesti A-M, et al. Addition of dexmedetomidine to standard sedation regimens after cardiac surgery: an outcomes analysis. *Pharmacotherapy.* 2006;26:798–805.
81. Finfer S, Bellomo R, Boyce N. A comparison of albumin and saline for fluid resuscitation in the intensive care unit. *N Engl J Med.* 2004;350:2247–2256.
82. Aantaa R, Jalonen J. Periopertive use of alpha2-adrenoceptor agonists and the cardiac patient. *Eur J Anaesthesiol.* 2006;23: 361–372.
83. Chakraborti S, Chakraborti T, Mandal M, et al. Protective role of magnesium in cardiovascular diseases: a review. *Mol Cell Biochem.* 2002;238:163–179.
84. Brown G, Greenwood J. Drug- and nutrition-induced hypophosphatemia: mechanisms and relevance in the critically ill. *Ann Pharmacother.* 1994;28:626–632.
85. Davis SV, Olichwier KK, Chakko SC. Reversible depression of myocardial performance in hypophosphatemia. *Am J Med Sci.* 1988;295:183–187.
86. Van den Berghe G, Wouters P, Weekers F, et al. Intensive insulin therapy in critically ill patients. *N Engl J Med.* 2001;345: 1359–1367.
87. Finfer S, Chittock DR, Su YS. Intensive versus conventional glucose control in critically ill patients. *N Engl J Med.* 2009;360:1283–1297.
88. Hein OV, Birnbaum J, Wernecke KD, et al. Three-year survival after four major post-cardiac operative complications. *Crit Care Med.* 2006;34:2729–2737.
89. Levi M, Levy JH, Andersen HF, et al. Safety of recombinant activated factor VII in randomized clinical trials. *N Engl J Med.* 2010;363:1791–1800.
90. Xirouchaki N, Magkanas E, Vaporidi K, et al. Lung ultrasound in critically ill patients: comparison with bedside chest radiography. *Intens Care Med.* 2011;37:1488–1493.
91. Puskas JD, Williams WH, Mahoney EM, et al. Off-Pump vs conventional coronary artery bypass grafting: early and 1-year graft patency, cost, and quality-of-life outcomes. *JAMA: J Am Med Assoc.* 2004;291:1841–1849.
92. Parolari A, Alamanni F, Polvani G, et al. Meta-analysis of randomized trials comparing off-pump with on-pump coronary artery bypass graft patency. *Ann Thoracic Surg.* 2005;80:2121–2125.
93. Stroobant N, Van Nooten G, Van Belleghem Y, et al. The effect of CABAG on neurocognitive functioning. *Acta Cardiologica.* 2010;65:557–564.
94. Deiner S, Silverstein JH. Postoperative delirium and cognitive dysfunction. *Br J Anaesth.* 2009;103:i41–i46.
95. Ely EW, Inouye SK, Bernard GR, et al. Delirium in mechanically ventilated patients. *JAMA: J Am Med Assoc.* 2001;286: 2703–2710.
96. Kay GL, Sun G-W, Aoki A, et al. Influence of ejection fraction on hospital mortality, morbidity, and costs for CABG patients. *Ann Thoracic Surg.* 1995;60:1640–1651.
97. Doering LV, Esmailian F, Laks H. Perioperative predictors of ICU and hospital costs in coronary artery bypass graft surgery. *Chest.* 2000;118:736–743.
98. Sista RR, Wall M. Postoperative care of the patient after heart or lung transplantation. *Postoperative Cardiac Care.* Richmond, VA: Society of Cardiovascular Anesthesiologists; 2011.
99. Thunberg CA, Gaitan BD, Arabia FA, et al. Ventricular assist devices today and tomorrow. *J Cardiothor Vasc Anesth.* 2010;24:656–680.
100. Naidu SS. Novel percutaneous cardiac assist devices. *Circulation.* 2011;123:533–543.
101. Trost JC, Hillis LD. Intra-aortic balloon counterpulsation. *Am J Cardiol.* 2006;97:1391–1398.
102. Williams D, Korr K, Gewirtz H, et al. The effect of intraaortic balloon counterpulsation on regional myocardial blood flow and oxygen consumption in the presence of coronary artery stenosis in patients with unstable angina. *Circulation.* 1982;66: 593–597.
103. Jiang CY, Zhao LL, Wang JA, et al. Anticoagulation therapy in intra-aortic balloon counterpulsation: does IABP really need anti. *J Zhejiang Univ Sci.* 2003;4:607–611.

III ANESTHETIC MANAGEMENT OF SPECIFIC CARDIAC DISORDERS

11 Anesthetic Management of Myocardial Revascularization

Michael S. Green, Gary S. Okum, and Jay C. Horrow

KEY POINTS

1. The total annual cost of cardiovascular disease in the U.S. is close to 400 billion representing 17% of the total health care costs due to major illness.
2. Risk factors for myocardial revascularization surgery include history of CHF, EF <30%, advanced age, obesity, emergency surgery, concomitant valve surgery, prior cardiac surgery, DM, and renal failure.
3. Supply of oxygen to the myocardium is determined by arterial oxygen content of blood and coronary blood flow.
4. A doubling of heart rate more than doubles the myocardial O_2 demand. The reason is heart rate causes a concomitant small increase in contractility.
5. Elevated wall stress also increases myocardial O_2 demand. This is related by the formula: Wall stress = pressure × Radius/(2 × wall thickness).
6. Regional wall motion abnormalities develop in less than 1 minute after the onset of ischemia: sooner than ECG evidence of ischemia.

(continued)

7. Off-pump coronary bypass compared to conventional CABG shows no difference in mortality and quality of life variables. However, duration of ventilation, hospital stay, and morbidity are decreased with off-pump coronary bypass.
8. Multiple causes of myocardial ischemia can occur during the prebypass, bypass, and postbypass periods.
9. A brief period of myocardial ischemia may protect against the damage caused by subsequent prolonged ischemia and tissue reperfusion. This ischemic preconditioning has been demonstrated in both animal and human studies.

I. Introduction

A. Prevalence and economic impact of coronary artery disease. Although the death rate for coronary heart disease has declined over the last several decades, it is still the leading cause of death in the United States. In the United States, more than 16 million people have a history of angina pectoris, myocardial infarction, or both [1]. More than 400,000 coronary artery bypass graft (CABG) revascularization procedures are performed annually [1].

The economic consequence of coronary heart disease is enormous. It is estimated that the
1 total annual cost of cardiovascular disease in the United States is close to $400 billion, which represents almost 17% of the total health-care costs due to major illnesses [2]. Additionally, coronary heart disease accounts for almost a fifth of all disability disbursements by the Social Security Administration [1].

B. Symptoms and progression of coronary artery disease. A complete description of angina pectoris and other symptoms related to coronary artery disease is given in Chapter 3. Unlike the usually predictable time course and progression of symptoms in patients with valvular heart disease, patients with coronary artery disease may have variable onset of symptoms as well as progression of disease characterized by discrete events such as angina or myocardial infarction. Many patients suffer ischemia without symptoms; these "silent" ischemic events require diligence for detection and prompt treatment before and after operation. Only 18% of myocardial infarctions are preceded by longstanding angina [1]. All aspects of preoperative evaluation of these patients (i.e., exercise stress testing and cardiac catheterization) are discussed in Chapter 3.

C. Historical perspective of CABG. Early unsuccessful or suboptimal attempts at myocardial revascularization took place before the 1960s. In 1967, Favalaro and Effler at the Cleveland Clinic began performing reversed saphenous vein bypass grafting procedures. In 1968, Green performed an anastomosis of the internal mammary artery (IMA) directly to a coronary artery. There was a resurgence of interest in the IMA grafting procedure in the late 1970s and early 1980s after a number of studies showed far greater graft patency rates for IMA grafts compared with saphenous vein grafts. In addition, better long-term survival was evident in patients receiving IMA grafts, regardless of ventricular function.

An interest in enhanced recovery ("fast track") cardiac surgery, fueled perhaps by concern over resource utilization, led to recognized improvements in clinical outcome [3]. In select cases, the advent of new myocardial stabilization devices obviated the need for exposure to cardiopulmonary bypass for myocardial revascularization. In the 1990s, many centers experimented with minimally invasive revascularization techniques and transmyocardial revascularization. During this time, transesophageal echocardiography (TEE) established an increasing role during coronary revascularization.

The extent of physiological derangement of patients presenting for cardiac surgery continues to increase, due to an aging patient population, increasing frequency of reoperations, and application of multivessel angioplasty and intracoronary stents to those with lesser degrees of disease.

D. Evaluating risk of morbidity and mortality for CABG surgery

1. **Introduction.** A comprehensive review of the myriad risk stratification schema for CABG surgery is beyond the scope of this text; however, a brief discussion of some of the more popular risk stratification tools follows.

2 2. **Risk factor models.** Although risk stratification tools may differ in the specific weights assigned to certain risk factors and not all of the risk factors appear in every study, certain

TABLE 11.1 Risk factor inclusion in various risk stratification models for coronary artery bypass grafting

	Montreal	Cleveland	Newark	New York	Northern new England	Society of thoracic surgery
Emergency	+	+	+	+	+	+
Poor LV function/ congestive heart failure	+	+	+	+	+	+
Redo operation	+	+	+	+	+	+
Gender/small size	–	+	+	+	+	+
Valve disease	–	+	+	+	–	–
Advanced age	+	+	+	+	+	+
Renal disease	–	+	+	+	+	–
Obesity	+	–	+	–	–	–

factors appear associated with increased risk of morbidity and mortality. These factors include poor left ventricular (LV) function (history of congestive heart failure or LV ejection fraction less than 30%), advanced age, obesity, emergency surgery, concomitant valve surgery, prior cardiac surgery, history of diabetes, and history of renal failure [4,5].

The composite score of the individually weighted risk factors is associated with a certain predicted risk of short- and long-term morbidity and mortality, length of stay, and hospital costs. Table 11.1 presents several risk stratification tools.

3. **Model evaluation.** No model can completely capture the risk of caring for sicker patients. The ACC/AHA assigns a level IIa recommendation (level of evidence C) to the use of models for prediction of morbidity and mortality [6]. Some models do not allow for adequate flexibility with regard to the dynamic nature of the patient's physiology during the preoperative period. For example, a patient's LV ejection fraction at the time of cardiac catheterization will be used in the evaluation process instead of that derived from TEE at the time of surgery.

II. Myocardial oxygen supply

A. Introduction. The viability and function of the heart depend upon the relatively delicate balance of oxygen supply and demand. The cardiac anesthesiologist must understand the intricacies of this relationship so as to manipulate their determinants perioperatively. The myocardium maximally extracts O_2 from arterial blood at rest: Coronary sinus blood PO_2 is 27 mm Hg and its saturation is less than 50%. With exertion or hemodynamic stress, the only way the O_2 supply can increase acutely to meet the myocardial energy demand is by increasing coronary blood flow (CBF). Ischemia occurs when CBF does not increase to a level sufficient to meet myocardial demand, leading to anaerobic metabolism. The following approach achieves the clinical goal of ensuring that O_2 supply at least matches demand:

1. Optimize the determinants of myocardial O_2 supply and demand
2. Select anesthetics and adjuvant agents and techniques according to their effects on O_2 supply and demand
3. Monitor for ischemia to detect its occurrence early and intervene rapidly

B. Coronary anatomy

1. **Left main coronary artery.** A thorough understanding of the coronary artery anatomy and the distribution of myocardial blood flow allows an understanding of the extent and degree of myocardium at risk for ischemia and infarction during surgery. The blood supply to the myocardium derives from the aorta through two main coronary arteries (see Fig. 11.2), the left and right coronary arteries. The left main coronary artery extends for a short distance (0 to 40 mm) before dividing between the aorta and the pulmonary artery into the left anterior descending artery and the circumflex coronary artery.
2. **Left anterior descending coronary artery.** The left anterior descending artery begins as a continuation of the left main coronary artery and courses down the interventricular

groove, giving rise to the diagonal and septal branches. The septal branches vary in number and size, and provide the predominant blood supply to the interventricular septum. The septal branches also supply the bundle branches and the Purkinje system. One to three diagonal branches of variable size distribute blood to the anterolateral aspect of the heart. The left anterior descending artery usually terminates at the apex of the LV.

3. **Circumflex coronary artery.** The circumflex artery courses the left atrioventricular groove giving rise to one to three obtuse marginal branches, which supply the lateral wall of the LV. In 15% of the patients, the circumflex artery gives rise to the posterior descending coronary artery ("left dominant"). In 45% of the patients, the sinus node artery arises from the circumflex distribution.
4. **Right coronary artery.** The right coronary artery traverses the right atrioventricular groove. It gives rise to acute marginal branches that supply the right anterior wall of the right ventricle (RV). In approximately **85% of the individuals** with **a right dominant system,** the right coronary artery gives rise to the **posterior descending artery** to supply the posterior inferior aspect of the LV. Thus, in the majority of the population, the right coronary artery supplies a significant portion of blood flow to the LV, while in the other 15% of the population, the posterior-inferior aspect of the LV is supplied by the circumflex coronary artery (left dominant system) or both right coronary and circumflex arteries (codominant system). The sinus node artery arises from the right coronary artery in 55% of patients. The atrioventricular node artery derives from the dominant coronary artery and is responsible for blood supply to the node, the bundle of His, and the proximal part of the bundle branches.

3 C. **Determinants of myocardial oxygen supply.** In broad terms, the supply of oxygen to the myocardium is determined by the arterial oxygen content of the blood and the blood flow in the coronary arteries.

1. **O_2 content = (hemoglobin) (1.34) (% saturation) + (0.003) (Po_2)**

   Ensuring maximal O_2 content therefore involves having a high hemoglobin level, highly saturated blood, and a high Po_2. Normothermia, normal pH, and high levels of 2,3-diphosphoglyceric acid all favor tissue release of O_2.
2. **Determinants of blood flow in normal coronary arteries.** CBF varies directly with the **pressure differential** across the coronary bed (coronary perfusion pressure [CPP]) and inversely with coronary vascular resistance (CVR): CBF = CPP/CVR. However, CBF is autoregulated (i.e., resistance varying directly with perfusion pressure) so that flow is relatively independent of CPP between 50 and 150 mm Hg but is pressure dependent outside of this range. Metabolic, autonomic, hormonal, and anatomic parameters alter CVR, and hydraulic factors influence CPP. Coronary stenoses also increase CVR.
   a. **Control of CVR.** Factors affecting CVR are outlined in Table 11.2.

TABLE 11.2 Control of coronary vascular resistance

	Increase CVR	Decrease CVR
Metabolic	↑ O_2, ↓ CO_2, ↓ H^+	↓ O_2, ↑ CO_2, ↑ H^+ Lactate Adenosine
Autonomic nervous system	↑ α-Adrenergic tone ↑ Cholinergic tone	↑ β-Adrenergic tone
Hormonal	↑ Vasopressin (antidiuretic hormone) ↑ Angiotensin ↑ Thromboxane	↑ Prostacyclin
Endothelial modulation		↑ Nitric oxide ↑ Endothelium-derived hyperpolarizing factor ↑ Prostaglandin I_2

↑, increased; ↓, decreased; CVR, coronary vascular resistance; PGI_2, Prostaglandin I_2.

(1) **Metabolic factors.** When increased coronary flow is required secondary to increased myocardial workload, metabolic control factors are primarily responsible. Hydrogen ion, CO_2, lactate, and adenosine all may play a role in metabolic regulation of CBF by inducing changes in CVR [7].

(2) **Autonomic nervous system.** The coronary arteries and arterioles possess α- and β-receptors. In general, α_1-receptors are responsible for coronary vasoconstriction, whereas β-receptors mediate a vasodilatory effect. α_2-Receptors on endothelial cells and muscarinic signaling appear to be involved in a nitric oxide-mediated decrease in coronary vascular tone [8]. An increased population of α-receptors may cause episodes of coronary spasm in individuals with nonobstructed coronaries. α_1-Mediated constriction of the coronary circulation may counter some of the metabolic vasodilation, especially in the resting basal state. However, under most circumstances such as increasing demand or ischemia, metabolic control factors will over-ride α-mediated vasoconstriction.

(3) **Hormonal factors.** Two stress hormones, vasopressin (antidiuretic hormone) and angiotensin, are potent coronary vasoconstrictors. However, blood levels of these hormones during major stress may be insufficient to produce significant coronary vasoconstriction. Thromboxane participates in thrombosis and coronary vasospasm during myocardial infarction. Prostaglandin I_2 (PGI_2) decreases coronary vascular tone.

(4) **Endothelial modulation.** Nitric oxide triggers a cyclic guanosine monophosphate (c-GMP)–mediated vasodilatory effect on vascular smooth muscle, and may also contribute to vessel patency and blood flow by inhibiting platelet adhesion. PGI_2 and endothelium-derived hyperpolarizing factor also cause relaxation of vascular smooth muscle.

(5) **Anatomic factors**

(a) **Capillary/myocyte ratio.** Only three- to four-fifths of available myocardial capillaries function during normal conditions. During exercise, episodes of hypoxia, or extreme myocardial O_2 demand, the additional unopened capillaries are recruited and increase blood flow, causing a decrease in CVR and in diffusion distance of O_2 to a given myocyte. This adaptation, along with coronary vasodilation, contributes to coronary vascular reserve.

(b) **Coronary collaterals.** Coronary collateral channels exist in the human myocardium. Under most circumstances, they are nonfunctional. However, in the presence of impeded CBF, these coronary channels may enlarge over time and become functional.

(6) **Other factors affecting CVR.** CVR may be partly regulated by myogenic control of vessel diameter, which dynamically responds to the distending pressure inside the vessel. CVR increases with the increased blood viscosity caused by high hematocrit or hypothermia. Thus, hemodilution should accompany induced hypothermia. There is a transmural gradient of vascular tone, with vascular resistance being lower in the subendocardium than in the subepicardium [7].

b. Hydraulic factors and subendocardial blood flow

(1) **LV subendocardial blood flow.** Unlike CBF in the low-pressure RV system, LV subendocardial blood flow is intermittent and occurs only during diastole. Because of the increased intracavitary pressure and excessive subendocardial myocyte shortening, subendocardial arterioles are essentially closed during systole. **Of the total LV coronary flow, 85% occurs during diastole and 15% occurs in systole (primarily in the epicardial region).** Thus, the majority of blood flow to the epicardial and middle layers of the LV and all the blood flow to the endocardium occur during diastole.

(2) **CPP.** Equals the arterial driving pressure less the back-pressure to flow across the coronary bed. For the LV, the driving pressure is the aortic blood pressure during diastole. The back-pressure to flow depends on the area of myocardium under

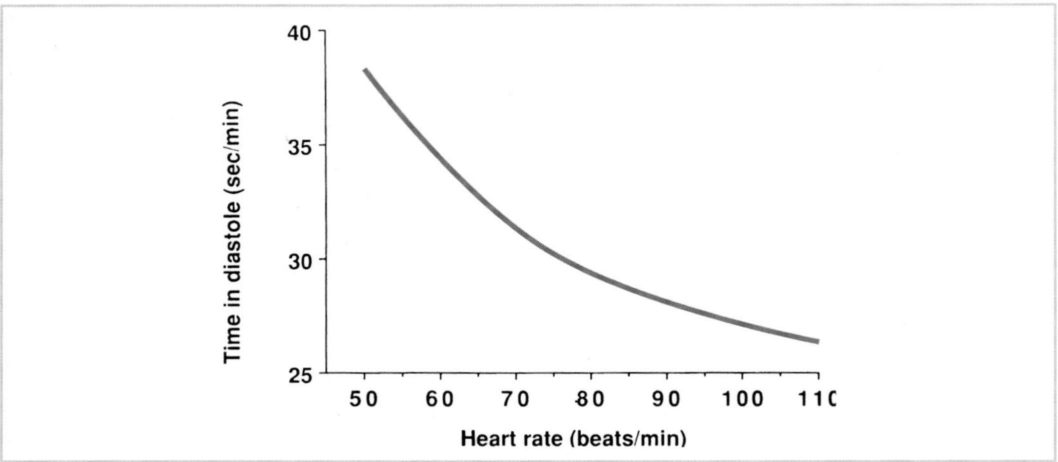

FIGURE 11.1 Total time spent in diastole each minute is plotted as a function of heart rate in beats per minute (beats/min). The reduction in diastolic interval leads to diminished LV blood flow as heart rate increases.

consideration. Because the endocardium is the area most prone to ischemia, attention focuses on its flow, and thus the usual formula for CPP uses left ventricular end-diastolic pressure (LVEDP) as back-pressure instead of right atrial pressure, despite the fact that most blood returns to the heart via the coronary sinus:

$$\text{CPP} = \text{aortic diastolic pressure} - \text{LVEDP}$$

Because diastole shortens relative to systole as heart rate increases, subendocardial blood flow is decreased at extremely rapid heart rates. Figure 11.1 demonstrates the total time per minute spent in diastole as a function of heart rate. Elevations in LVEDP (e.g., heart failure, ischemia) also will impede subendocardial blood flow. **Thus, to optimize CPP, one should aim for normal-to-high diastolic blood pressure, low LVEDP, and low heart rate.**

3. **Determinants of myocardial blood flow in stenotic coronaries.** In addition to the physiologic determinants of myocardial blood flow in normal coronary arteries, stenotic vessels add pathologic determinants of myocardial blood flow. Stenoses increase CVR and decrease CBF. Reduction in CBF in stenotic vessels is a function of the length and degree of stenosis, presence or absence of collaterals, pattern of stenosis, and presence of certain coexisting disease states, such as diabetes mellitus and hypertension, which cause predisposition to microcirculatory pathology and ventricular hypertrophy, respectively.

   In particular, some patients present with a vasospastic component, which may aggravate a fixed lesion or even create anginal symptoms in patients with angiographically clear vessels.

   a. Poiseuille's law determines the hemodynamic significance of a coronary obstruction in long (segmental) lesions. Given the same decrease in cross-sectional area, a longer segmental stenosis of a coronary artery reduces flow more than a short one.
   b. Because CBF is reduced in proportion to the fourth power of the vessel diameter, a 50% diameter decrease in lumen size decreases flow to 1/16th its initial value, which is hemodynamically consistent with symptoms of angina on exertion. A 75% reduction in diameter at angiography corresponds to a greater than 98% reduction in flow, and corresponds clinically to symptoms of angina at rest.
   c. Sequential lesions in the same coronary artery impact coronary flow in an additive fashion.
   d. With longstanding coronary obstruction, collateral circulation often develops. For low-grade obstructive lesions, these channels supply enough blood flow to prevent

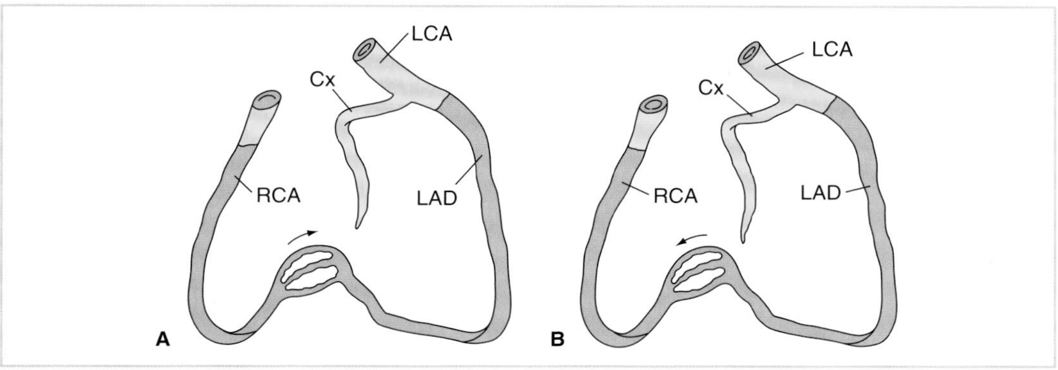

FIGURE 11.2 Two examples of possible left main "equivalency." Two-vessel coronary disease with an occluded left anterior descending coronary artery (LAD) and myocardium jeopardized by a right coronary artery (RCA) stenosis **(A)** or an occluded RCA and myocardium jeopardized by a stenotic LAD **(B)**. Cx, circumflex coronary artery; LCA, left coronary artery. (From Hutter AM Jr. Is there a left main equivalent? *Circulation.* 1980;62:209, with permission.)

ischemia. However, as the degree of coronary stenosis increases, the collateral channels may not be adequate.

e. Certain patterns of stenoses have important clinical implications related to the amount of myocardium supplied and placed in jeopardy by the stenotic lesion(s). A left main coronary stenosis limits blood flow to a large amount of the LV muscle mass. High-grade, very proximal stenotic lesions of both the circumflex and left anterior descending systems have the same physiologic implications as does a left main stenosis. Prognostically, however, a left main stenosis is grimmer because rupture of a single atheroma will compromise a large amount of myocardium. In addition, similar "left main equivalent" situations may exist when a severely stenosed coronary provides collateral blood flow to a region with a totally occluded vessel (Fig. 11.2). In addition to discrete focal and segmental coronary lesions in graftable vessels, diffuse distal disease may lessen the effectiveness of bypassing proximal coronary obstructions.

III. Myocardial oxygen demand. Direct measurement of myocardial oxygen demand is not feasible in the clinical setting. The three major determinants of myocardial O_2 demand are heart rate, contractility, and wall stress.

A. Heart rate. If a relatively fixed amount of O_2 were consumed per heartbeat, one would expect
4 the O_2 demand per minute to increase linearly with heart rate. Thus, a doubling of heart rate would yield a doubling of O_2 demand. In fact, demand more than doubles with a two-fold increase in heart rate. The source of this additional O_2 demand is the staircase phenomenon, in which increased heart rate causes a small increase in contractility and increases in contractility mean more consumption of O_2 (see Section B below).

B. Contractility. More O_2 is used by a highly contractile heart compared to a more relaxed heart.

1. Quantitative assessment. Strictly defined, the contractile state of the heart is a dynamic intrinsic characteristic that is not influenced by preload or afterload. Previous attempts to measure contractility using physiologic variable include the rate of rise of LV pressure, (dP/dt), and its value normalized to chamber pressure, ($[dP/dt]/P$). Neither succeeds. Clinically, it is possible to quantify dP/dt echocardiographically by measuring the rate of rise in the velocity of the mitral regurgitant jet using Doppler technology. Unfortunately, loading conditions and chamber compliance significantly affect the acceleration of the mitral regurgitant jet. Additionally, although mitral regurgitation is frequently observed echocardiographically, it is not universally present. Contractility can be approximated in a load-independent fashion using the slope of the end-systolic pressure–volume relationships of a family of LV pressure–volume loops. This method is usually not available in clinical settings.

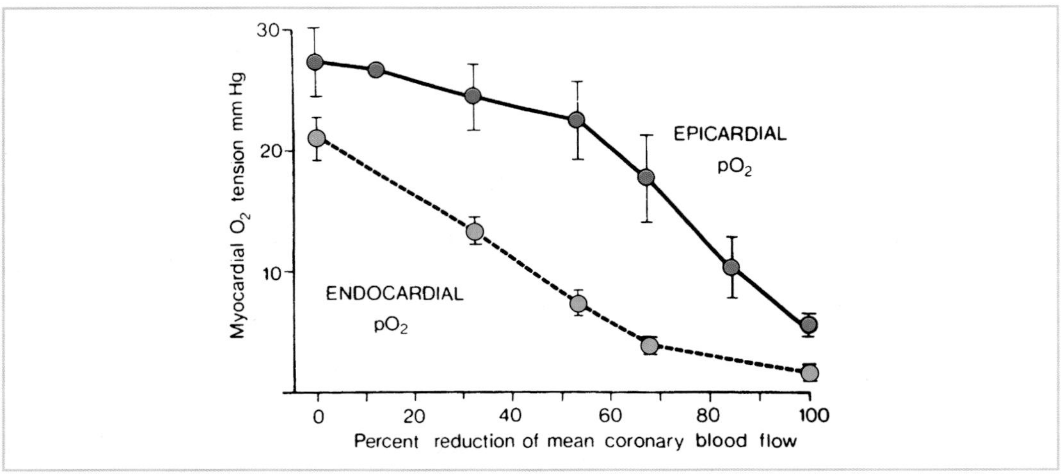

FIGURE 11.3 Relationship of subendocardial O_2 supply (represented by myocardial O_2 tension) to reductions in CBF. Demonstrated is the increased vulnerability of the subendocardial zone compared to the epicardial zone. (Modified from Winbury MM, Howe BB. Stenosis: regional myocardial ischemia and reserve. In: Winbury MM, Abiko Y, eds. *Ischemic Myocardium and Antianginal Drugs*. New York, NY: Raven; 1979:59.)

2. **Qualitative measures.** One can easily observe the contractile state of the heart when the pericardium is open. Remember, though, that the RV is more easily and most often viewed this way, whereas the left is more obscured. TEE provides a means for qualitative estimation of LV contractility. Clinically, we infer good contractility when the arterial pressure tracing rises briskly. However, the shape of the radial arterial tracing is heavily influenced by the system's resonant frequency, damping by air bubbles, compliance of the arterial tree, reflections of pressure waves from arterioles, and other confounders.
3. **Increased subendocardial myocyte shortening.** Myocytes in the subendocardial region undergo more shortening than those in other areas because of geometric factors. Because they operate at a higher contractile state, they have greater oxidative metabolism. Subendocardial vessels, already maximally dilated, cannot respond to increased demand and intermittent limitations of blood flow in the subendocardial region. Thus, myocardial O_2 tension falls first here (Fig. 11.3), and this region is more susceptible to ischemia.

5 C. **Wall stress.** The stress in the ventricular wall depends on the pressure in the ventricle during contraction (afterload), the chamber size (preload), and the wall thickness. The calculation for a sphere (which we shall assume for the shape of the ventricle, for the sake of simplicity) comes from LaPlace's Law:

$$\text{Wall stress} = \text{pressure} \cdot \text{radius}/(2 \cdot \text{wall thickness})$$

1. **Chamber pressure.** Oxygen demand increases with chamber pressure. Doubling the pressure doubles the O_2 demand. Systemic blood pressure usually reflects the chamber pressure; thus, we equate systemic blood pressure with LV afterload. The heart's true afterload is more complex because elastic and inertial components also affect ejection. **Mean systemic pressure, not peak systolic pressure, correlates with O_2 demand.** In aortic stenosis, however, the LV experiences very high chamber pressures despite more modest systemic pressures. The clinical goal is to keep afterload (and thus wall stress) low.
2. **Chamber size.** Doubling the ventricular volume increases the radius by only 26% (volume varies with the radius cubed). Thus, increased chamber size is associated with more modest increases in O_2 demand. Nevertheless, because preload determines ventricular size, we desire a low preload to keep wall stress (and thus O_2 demand) low. Much of the benefit of nitroglycerin stems from venodilation and its attendant decrease in preload.

TABLE 11.3 Regulation of O_2 supply and demand

Parameter	Demand	Supply	O_2 balance
Low heart rate	↓	↑	Positive
Low RAP or PCWP	↓	↑[a]	Positive
High heart rate	↑	↓	Negative
High RAP or PCWP	↑	↓	Negative
High temperature	↑	0	Negative
Low temperature	↑↓	↓	Variable
Low MAP	↓	↓	Variable
High MAP	↑	↑	Variable
Low hemoglobin	↓	↓↑	Variable
High hemoglobin	↑	↑↓	Variable

[a]However, a drastic decrease in filling pressure will decrease cardiac output.
↑, increased; ↓, decreased; ↑ ↓, may increase or decrease; 0, unchanged; MAP, mean arterial pressure; PCWP, pulmonary capillary wedge pressure; RAP, right atrial pressure.

3. **Wall thickness.** A thicker wall means less stress over any part of the wall. Ventricular hypertrophy serves to decrease wall stress, although the additional tissue requires more O_2 overall. Hypertrophy occurs in response to the elevated afterload that occurs in chronic systemic hypertension or aortic stenosis. Although wall thickness is essentially uncontrollable clinically, its effects should be considered. LV aneurysms, seen after transmural infarction, increase wall stress because of their effect on LV volume (radius) and reduced wall thickness.

D. **Summary. The factors that increase O_2 demand are increases in heart rate, chamber size, chamber pressure, and contractility.** Table 11.3 and Figure 11.4 summarize the relationship between myocardial supply and demand. **Note that tachycardia and increases in LVEDP both lead to increased demand and decreased supply of oxygen.**

IV. Monitoring for myocardial ischemia

A. **Introduction.** Monitoring for cardiac surgery is discussed in Chapter 4. Typical monitoring for CABG surgery includes the standard American Society of Anesthesiology (ASA) monitors and invasive arterial blood pressure monitoring. Although TEE is used more frequently in current practice, the most recent ASA/SCA practice guidelines uphold guidelines published in 1996 classifying use in patients with increased risk for myocardial infarction as a category II indication [9]. The use of pulmonary arterial (PA) catheters for routine CABG is also controversial. Detection and treatment of intraoperative ischemia are critically important because intraoperative ischemia is an independent predictor of postoperative myocardial infarction [10]. Only half of the intraoperative ischemic events can be related to a hemodynamic alteration and none can be detected by the presence of angina in anesthetized patients. Lactate extraction of a regional myocardial circulatory bed, while diagnostic of ischemia, cannot be routinely measured. Thus, we seek clues that ischemia leaves in its wake: Changes on the electrocardiogram (ECG), PA pressure (PAP) changes, and myocardial wall-motion abnormalities.

B. **ECG monitoring**

1. **Introduction.** The detection of wall-motion abnormalities by TEE has not led to the replacement of continuous multilead ECG monitoring as a standard monitor of intraoperative ischemia. ECG monitoring is inexpensive, easy to use and read, can be automated, and is available before and during the induction of anesthesia, when the TEE probe is not in place, and may be carried through to the ICU setting, where TEE monitoring is impractical. ECG changes are less sensitive to ischemia: They occur later in the temporal cascade of events that follow myocardial ischemia, especially with less dramatic coronary supply/demand inequality.
2. **ST-segment analysis.** Depression of the ST segment of the ECG denotes endocardial ischemia and elevation denotes transmural ischemia. **ST-segment changes occur at least**

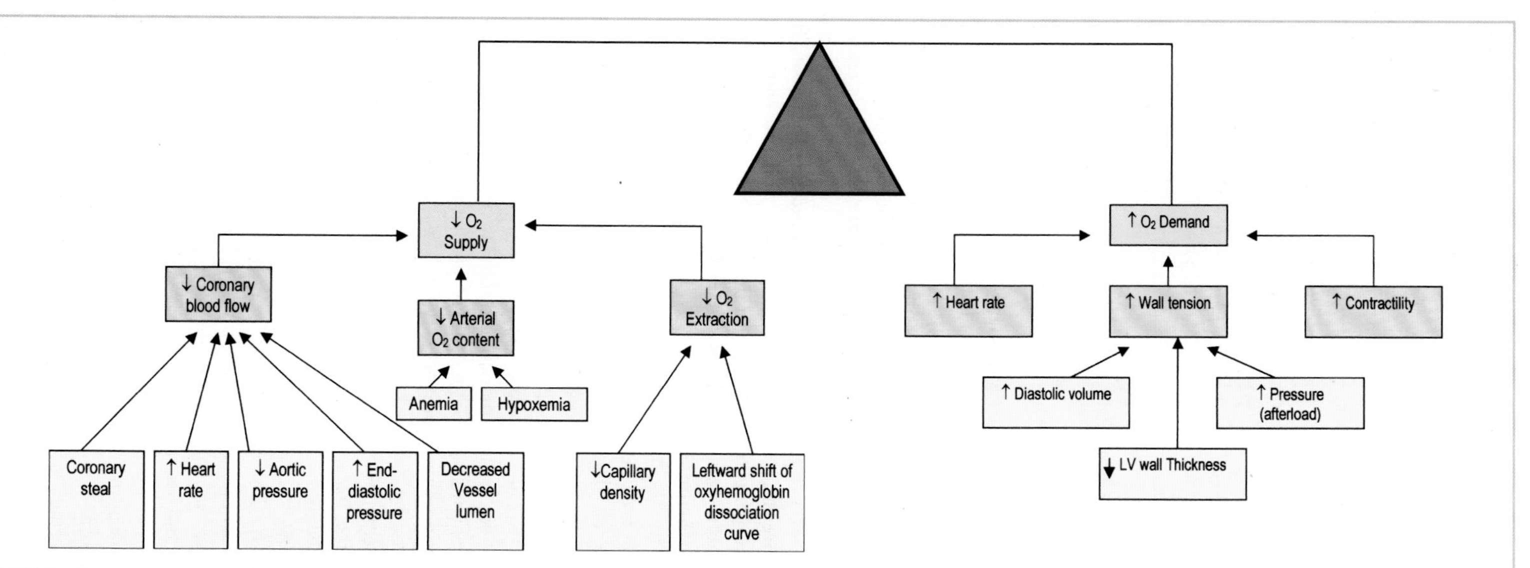

FIGURE 11.4 Summary of factors that affect myocardial oxygen supply and demand. (Adapted from Crystal GJ. Cardiovascular physiology. In: Miller RD, ed. *Atlas of Anesthesia: Vol. VIII. Cardiothoracic Anesthesia.* Philadelphia, PA: Churchill Livingstone; 1999;1:1, with permission.)

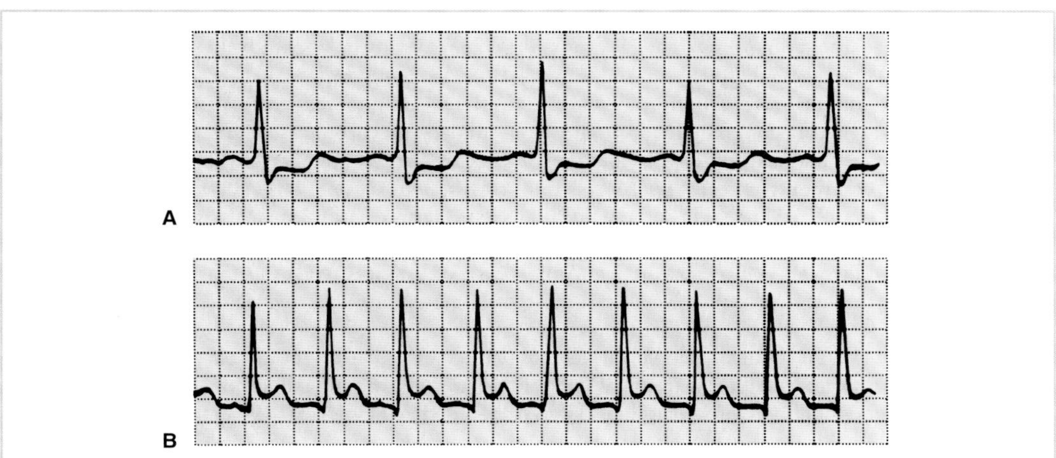

FIGURE 11.5 **A:** ST-segment depression, an indicator of subendocardial ischemia. **B:** Transmural ischemia, one cause of ST-segment elevation, produces the pattern appearing in the lower tracing.

60 to 120 s after the start of ischemia. The reference for the ST segment is usually taken as 80 ms after the J-point, which is the end of the QRS wave (Fig. 11.5). Significant changes are usually defined as 0.1 mV or 1 mm of ST-segment elevation or depression at normal gain. ECG monitoring systems include automated real-time ST-segment analysis. Although this feature constitutes a definite advance in the "human engineering" aspects of ischemia monitoring, the machine is only as smart as the person interpreting its data. Beware of intraventricular conduction delays, bundle branch blocks, and ventricular pacing, all of which can render ST-segment analysis invalid. Check the machine's determination of where the ST segment occurs: 80 ms after the J-point is not always appropriate.

a. **Differential diagnosis of ST-segment changes.** ST-segment elevation may arise from the several causes of transmural ischemia (atherosclerotic disease, coronary vasospasm, intracoronary air), or from pericarditis or ventricular aneurysm (Fig. 11.5). One must also consider improper lead placement, particularly reversal of limb and leg leads, and improper selection of electronic filtering. **The diagnostic mode should always be chosen on machines equipped with a diagnostic–monitor mode selection switch.**

3. **T-wave changes.** New T-wave alterations (flipped or flattened) may indicate ischemia. These may not be detected by viewing the ST segment alone. Likewise, pseudonormalization of the ST segment or T wave (an ischemic-looking tracing in a patient without ischemia changing to a more normal-looking one) may indicate a new onset of ischemia and should be treated appropriately.
4. **Multilead ECG monitoring.** Simultaneous observation of an inferior lead (II, III, or aVF) and an anterior lead (V_5) provides detection superior to single-lead monitoring, detecting approximately 90% of ischemic events. Ischemia limited to the posterior of the heart is difficult to detect with standard ECG monitoring. Modified chest leads may be necessary when the surgical incision precludes usual placement.

C. **PAP monitoring**

1. **General indications for a PA catheter for revascularization procedures.** PA catheters provide a conduit for infusions, measurement of blood temperature and chamber pressures, and calculations of cardiac output, vascular resistance, and RV ejection fraction (with special catheters equipped with particularly fast thermistors). Some catheters also measure mixed venous oxygen saturation. Observational studies concluding that PA catheterization does not affect outcome [11,12] remain unconvincing until randomized studies provide

validation. Although perhaps unnecessary for the intraoperative management of routine coronary bypass surgery, PA catheters achieve utility postoperatively, when TEE cannot be utilized.

2. **Detection of ischemia: PAPs.** The absolute PAP is not diagnostic of ischemia. Pulmonary hypertension, whether primary or secondary to chronic ischemia, hypertension, or to valvular heart disease, is not uncommon. PAPs or pulmonary capillary occlusion pressures commonly exceed upper levels of normal due to chronic obstructive pulmonary disease (COPD), dependent catheter locations in the lung, or mitral stenosis, making measurement less reliable in the absence of ischemia [13]. The shape of the transduced pressure waveform, however, is more predictive. Appearance of a new V wave on the pulmonary capillary occlusion pressure waveform indicates functional mitral regurgitation, which is due to "new" ischemic papillary muscle dysfunction. It may occur before or even in the absence of ECG changes. However, detection of changes on the pulmonary capillary occlusion waveform requires frequent balloon inflation, introducing additional risk because of the possibility of vessel rupture. Often ischemia may be detected by a change in the shape of the PA tracing, obviating the need for frequent wedging.

D. TEE

1. **General indications for TEE during revascularization procedures.** TEE can assess ventricular preload and contractility, detect myocardial ischemia-induced regional wall-motion abnormalities (RWMAs), evaluate the aortic cannulation site, detect concomitant valve pathology, detect the presence and pathophysiologic effect of pericardial effusion, aid the placement of intra-aortic balloon catheters and coronary sinus catheters, and detect the presence of ventricular aneurysms and ventricular septal defects. TEE has become an invaluable clinical tool and has achieved routine use at many institutions. New RWMAs after bypass correlate with adverse outcomes. See Chapter 5 for a detailed discussion of intraoperative TEE.

2. **Detection of myocardial ischemia with TEE**

6 a. **RWMAs**

(1) **Introduction.** The heart **develops abnormal motion in less than 1 min following perfusion defects [14].** RWMAs resulting from myocardial ischemia temporally precede both ECG and PAP changes. TEE simultaneously interrogates regions of the heart representative of all three major coronary arteries, including the posterior wall, which are not easily monitored with ECG. This is, perhaps, most easily accomplished in the short-axis, midpapillary muscle view. Ischemia confined to nonvisualized regions will escape detection. Proper interrogation of the heart requires a comprehensive examination in multiple planes.

(2) **Limitations of monitoring RWMA**

(a) **Tethering.** Nonischemic tissue that is adjacent to ischemic tissue may move abnormally simply because it is attached to tissue exhibiting an RWMA. This tends to exaggerate the RWMA.

(b) **Pacing/bundle branch blocks.** Abnormal ventricular depolarization sequences not only affect ST-segment analysis (see Section IV.B.2), but also alter wall motion and can mimic RWMA.

(c) **Interventricular septum.** Normal septal motion depends on appropriate ventricular loading conditions, the presence of pericardium, and normal electrical conduction.

(d) **Stunned myocardium.** Adequately perfused myocardium may exhibit RWMA if recovering from recent ischemia, thus prompting inappropriate therapeutic intervention.

(e) **Induction/ICU.** TEE use is not practical during induction of anesthesia or for continuous ICU monitoring.

b. **Diastolic LV filling patterns.** Unfortunately, ventricular filling patterns depend on ventricular loading conditions and the site of Doppler interrogation within the ventricular inflow tract, limiting utility to monitor ischemia.

c. **Intraoperative stress TEE.** Low-dose dobutamine (2.5 μg/kg/min), when administered for 3 to 5 min, improves coronary flow without significantly affecting demand. The resultant improved myocardial energetics improves existing wall-motion abnormalities. Demonstration of contractile reserve using intraoperative stress echo then directs revascularization efforts to regions of myocardium able to benefit from the additional blood supply.

d. **Contrast echocardiography.** Intracoronary injection of sonicated albumin allows imaging of perfused myocardium, providing a tool to identify stunned myocardium, thus avoiding needless therapeutic intervention. At present, contrast agents are not approved by the U.S. Food and Drug Administration for this indication. Additionally, there are some technical imaging issues that must be resolved before this technique can become a real clinical tool. A microbubble contrast injection technique has also been described [15].

e. **Detection of infarction complications.** TEE can detect complications of ischemia/infarction such as acute mitral insufficiency, ventricular septal defect, and pericardial effusion.

V. Anesthetic effects on myocardial oxygen supply and demand. Outcome studies in cardiac surgery fail to reveal an effect of particular anesthetic agents [16,17]. Cardiac anesthesiologists, keenly aware of the impact of anesthetic agents on myocardial oxygen supply/demand dynamics, effectively monitor for and treat myocardial ischemia, thus accommodating for any such effects.

A. Intravenous (IV) nonopioid agents

1. **Thiopental and thiamylal.** Induction doses of ultrashort-acting barbiturates **decrease systemic vascular resistance (SVR) and cardiac contractility and increase heart rate.** Oxygen demand decreases from the first two effects and increases from the third. All three decrease oxygen supply. The net effect on myocardial O_2 balance depends on the initial conditions. The hyperdynamic, hypertensive patient benefits from the restoration of more physiologic blood pressure and contractility, whereas a patient with a normal heart rate may respond to the resultant tachycardia with ischemia.
2. **Propofol.** The cardiovascular effects of induction doses of propofol are similar to those of the thiobarbiturates: **Systemic blood pressure, SVR, and cardiac contractility decrease.** Heart rate may increase less with propofol compared to thiopental.
3. **Ketamine.** Ketamine increases sympathetic tone, leading to **increases in SVR, filling pressures, contractility, and heart rate.** Myocardial O_2 demand strongly increases, whereas O_2 supply only slightly augments, thus producing ischemia. However, the patient already maximally sympathetically stimulated responds with decreased contractility and vasodilation. Ketamine is not recommended for routine use in patients with ischemic heart disease. However, it is sometimes used in patients with cardiac tamponade, because of its ability to preserve heart rate, contractility, and SVR; see Chapter 18.
4. **Etomidate.** Induction doses of etomidate (0.2 to 0.3 mg/kg) **do not alter heart rate or cardiac output,** although mild peripheral vasodilation may lower blood pressure slightly. As such, it is an ideal drug for rapid induction of anesthesia in patients with ischemic heart disease. Etomidate offers little protection from the increases in heart rate and blood pressure that accompany intubation. It is usually necessary to supplement etomidate with other agents (e.g., opioids, benzodiazepines, volatile agents, β-blockers, and nitroglycerin) in order to control the hemodynamic profile and prevent myocardial oxygen supply/demand imbalance. An induction dose blocks adrenal steroidogenesis for 6 to 8 h.
5. **Benzodiazepines.** Midazolam (0.2 mg/kg) or diazepam (0.5 mg/kg) may be used to induce anesthesia. Although both agents are compatible with the goal of maintaining hemodynamic stability, blood pressure may decrease more with midazolam because of more potent peripheral vasodilation. Negative inotropic effects are inconsequential. Blood pressure and filling pressures decrease with induction, whereas the heart rate remains essentially unchanged. Addition of induction doses of a benzodiazepine to a moderate-dose opioid technique, however, may result in profound peripheral vasodilation and hypotension.
6. **α_2-Adrenergic agonists.** Centrally acting α_2-adrenergic agonists result in a reduction in stress-mediated neurohumoral responses and therefore are associated with decreases in

heart rate and blood pressure [18]. These agents are typically used during maintenance of anesthesia or postoperatively. Preoperative oral clonidine reduces perioperative myocardial ischemia in patients undergoing CABG surgery, but occasionally results in significant intraoperative hypotension. Dexmedetomidine possesses greater α_2 selectivity than clonidine. Both agents have sedative and antinociceptive properties. Use of α_2-adrenergic agonists is associated with a reduced opioid requirement. Additionally, α_2-adrenergic agonists do not result in respiratory depression.

B. **Volatile agents.** In general, **volatile anesthetics decrease both O_2 supply and demand. The net effect on the myocardial supply/demand balance depends upon the hemodynamic profile that prevails at the time of administration.**

1. **Heart rate.** Sevoflurane has negligible effect on heart rate. Desflurane and isoflurane often increase heart rate, although isoflurane decreases heart rate if its associated decrease in SVR is not profound, if the carotid baroreceptor function is impaired, or if the patient is fully β-blocked. In the steady state, the cardiovascular actions of desflurane are similar to those of isoflurane. However, during induction without opioids, heart rate and systemic and PA blood pressures may increase and require therapeutic intervention.

   Desflurane use for inhalation induction is unwise due to a significant increase in heart rate, particularly with rapid escalation of the inspired concentration. Junctional rhythms may occur with any volatile agent; they deprive the heart of an atrial kick, leading to decreased stroke volume, cardiac output, and CBF, offsetting the salubrious effects of low heart rate.
2. **Contractility.** All volatile anesthetics decrease contractility, lowering O_2 demand. However, isoflurane, desflurane, and sevoflurane cause less depression than halothane or enflurane. In decompensated hearts, all volatile anesthetics impair ventricular function.
3. **Afterload.** Decreases in cardiac output and SVR with volatile anesthesia result in decreased systemic blood pressure. Venodilation and blunted contractility account for the decrease in cardiac output. SVR decreases most with isoflurane and desflurane, moderately with enflurane and sevoflurane, but not at all with halothane administration. Both O_2 supply and O_2 demand decrease.
4. **Preload.** Volatile agents maintain filling pressures. Therefore, CPP (diastolic aortic pressure minus LVEDP) may decrease during volatile anesthesia.
5. **Coronary steal.** A coronary "steal" phenomenon has been described in which dilation of normal vascular beds diverts blood away from other beds that are ischemic and thus maximally dilated (Fig. 11.6). Steal-prone anatomy may exist in 23% of the patients undergoing

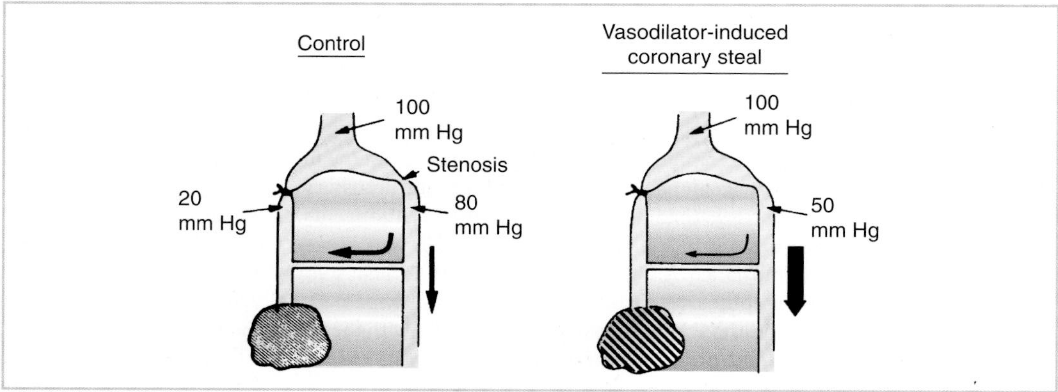

FIGURE 11.6 Theoretical basis of coronary steal. The shaded, marginally ischemic area normally receives barely enough flow **(left)**. A potent vasodilator improves flow to the normal myocardium but does not affect the already maximally dilated area in jeopardy. This process decreases flow through the collateral from the nonischemic bed. This further impoverishment of the marginally ischemic area produces frank ischemia **(right)**. (Modified from Becker LC. Conditions for vasodilator-induced coronary steal in experimental myocardial ischemia. *Circulation.* 1978;57:1108.)

CABG [19]. Coronary steal has been observed in canine models of steal-prone coronary anatomy with isoflurane administration under circumstances that caused collateral flow which is pressure dependent. It is doubtful that isoflurane-induced coronary steal is of significant clinical importance to patients undergoing coronary revascularization surgery as long as hypotension and consequent pressure-dependent coronary artery perfusion are avoided. Coronary steal has not been observed with halothane, enflurane, or desflurane.

6. **Preconditioning.** Volatile anesthetics may confer a degree of preconditioning-like protective effect against ischemia-reperfusion injury in human myocardial tissue [20] and improve late cardiac events following cardiac surgery [21] (see Section VII.D.6).

C. **Nitrous oxide.** The mild negative inotropic effects of nitrous oxide decrease contractility, producing a reduction in both O_2 supply and demand. Nitrous oxide inhibition of norepinephrine uptake in the lung may explain the increased plasma norepinephrine levels and associated increase in pulmonary vascular pressures and resistance seen with nitrous oxide administration [22]. Adding nitrous oxide to an opioid-oxygen anesthetic decreases SVR due, in part, to the removal of the vasoconstrictive effects of 100% O_2. The sympathomimetic effects of nitrous oxide counterbalance any direct depression of contractility except in patients with poor LV function in whom the myocardium already is highly stimulated intrinsically.

If nitrous oxide is used in a technique that provides a "light" anesthetic that is inadequate to cover attendant stimulation, increases in SVR and afterload ensue.

D. **Opioids**

1. **Heart rate.** All opioids except meperidine decrease heart rate by centrally mediated vagotonia; meperidine has an atropine-like effect. The dose of drug and speed of injection affect the degree of bradycardia. The result is decreased O_2 demand. By releasing histamine, morphine or meperidine may elicit a reflex tachycardia that decreases O_2 supply and increases O_2 demand.
2. **Contractility.** Aside from meperidine, which decreases contractility, the opioids have little effect on contractility in clinical doses.
3. **Afterload.** In compromised patients, who often depend on elevated sympathetic tone to maintain cardiac output and systemic resistance, the loss of sympathetic tone associated with opioid induction of anesthesia may result in a sudden drop in blood pressure and consequent decreases in both O_2 supply and demand. Concomitant midazolam use augments the decreased SVR with opioid induction.
4. **Preload.** Despite a lack of histamine-releasing properties, fentanyl and sufentanil reduce preload when administered in either moderate doses (25 μg/kg for fentanyl) or larger doses by decreasing intrinsic sympathetic tone. Oxygen demand is decreased.
5. **Hyperdynamic state.** Elevations of heart rate, blood pressure, and cardiac output with or without decreased filling pressures are common during pure opioid-oxygen anesthetic techniques in patients with good ventricular function. This high-supply/high-demand state may be less preferable than the low-supply/low-demand state achieved with volatile anesthesia. Additional opioid, which often fails to treat the hypertension associated with a hyperdynamic cardiac state, frequently decreases systemic blood pressure excessively when hypertension originates from increased SVR alone.

E. **Muscle relaxants**

1. **Succinylcholine.** This drug may cause a variety of **dysrhythmias** (bradycardia, tachycardia, extrasystoles), which negatively affect myocardial O_2 balance.
2. **Pancuronium.** Heart rate increases 20% when pancuronium accompanies a volatile anesthetic. With high-dose opioid anesthesia, heart rate remains stable. Occasionally, a patient will develop tachycardia and ischemia during induction or intubation. The latest available survey data indicate pancuronium as the neuromuscular blocker most commonly used in cardiac anesthesia [23].
3. **Vecuronium.** Vecuronium has a **flat cardiovascular profile** that is ideal with a low- or moderate-dose opioid anesthetic supplemented by volatile agent. Bradycardia occurs when it accompanies the **rapid** injection of high doses of the highly lipid-soluble opioids.

4. **Rocuronium.** Vagolytic action lies intermediate to that of vecuronium and pancuronium. Consequently, tachycardia is possible but less likely than with pancuronium. Rocuronium administration does not result in significant perturbations in other hemodynamic parameters.
5. **Cisatracurium.** An isomer of atracurium, lacks significant cardiovascular effects with manifestations of histamine release not seen. The majority of metabolism is via Hofmann elimination with ester hydrolysis making a minor contribution. Evidence supports faster neuromuscular recovery with cisatracurium use versus rocuronium or vecuronium in both adults and children [24,25].

F. **Summary.** Volatile anesthesia provides a **low-supply/low-demand** environment. The opioid-oxygen technique provides a **high-supply/high-demand** environment. Success with either technique depends on maintaining proper balance, with O_2 supply exceeding demand.

VI. Anesthetic approach for myocardial revascularization procedures

A. Fast-track cardiac anesthesia

1. **Historical perspective**
   a. **High-dose narcotic technique.** Until the 1990s, anesthesia for cardiac surgery largely utilized a high-dose narcotic technique compatible with minimal impairment of cardiac function and, therefore, conducive to the maintenance of perioperative hemodynamic stability. Additionally, it was believed that the delayed awakening associated with high-dose narcotic technique allowed time for the heart to recover from the obligatory ischemia suffered during cardiopulmonary bypass, decreased the release of stress hormones and attendant myocardial ischemia in the immediate postoperative period, and allowed time requisite for temperature and hemostatic homeostasis [26].
      (1) **Anesthetic management for high-dose narcotic technique.** Typical premedication consists of morphine (0.1 mg/kg administered intramuscularly [IM]) and scopolamine (0.3 to 0.4 mg, IM). Fentanyl (25 to 100 μg/kg) induces anesthesia. Maintenance consists of fentanyl (total cumulative dose of approximately 100 μg/kg) and long-acting muscle relaxant, supplemented as needed with volatile agent, benzodiazepine, or both.
      (2) **Indications for high-dose narcotic technique.** This technique applies when early extubation is not a realistic goal and when precipitous changes in hemodynamic conditions must be scrupulously avoided, such as when there are surgical concerns about anastomotic or aortic cannulation site integrity.
   b. **Impetus for change.** Responding to pressure to reduce hospital stays and costs, clinicians developed a technique based on sharply reduced doses of opioids supplemented by volatile agents or short-acting IV agents [27]. Heavy postoperative sedation, a feature of earlier schema thought necessary to avoid myocardial ischemia, has likewise fallen into disfavor [28]. New surgical techniques, improved myocardial protection, warmer bypass temperatures (32 to 34°C), improvements in anesthetic technique, management of perioperative coagulopathy, and temperature homeostasis (e.g., warmer operating room temperatures and use of active warming devices) have supported development of this "fast-track" cardiac anesthesia.
2. **Inclusion guidelines.** Early fast-track initiatives excluded patients with obesity, moderate-to-severe pulmonary disease, emergency operations, poor ventricular function, combined procedures, redo operations, or advanced age—about 40% to 60% of surgical revascularization patients. Application to sicker and riskier patients has progressed the technique, so that most patients now have an opportunity for early extubation, the exceptions usually being those with hemodynamic compromise or difficult airways.
3. **Anesthetic management** (Table 11.4)
   a. **Premedication.** Long-acting agents such as scopolamine are preferentially avoided. Same-day admission patients may not have adequate time for proper sedation with slow-onset agents. Midazolam (0.03 to 0.07 mg/kg IV) usually suffices to allay anxiety.
   b. **Intraoperative anesthetic agent management**
      (1) **Induction of anesthesia.** Etomidate, propofol, or thiopental accomplishes induction. Etomidate often requires adjuvant agents, such as volatile agent or low-dose opioid, to avoid tachycardia and hypertension with intubation. Esmolol or

TABLE 11.4 Typical fast-track cardiac anesthetic at Robert Wood Johnson Medical School

Induction	Etomidate[a]	0.3 mg/kg
	Fentanyl	0–10 μg/kg
	Midazolam	0–0.05 mg/kg
	Pentothal[a]	5 mg/kg
	Propofol[a]	2–3 mg/kg
	Succinylcholine	1.5–2 mg/kg
Maintenance	Fentanyl	5–10 μg/kg
	Midazolam	0.05 mg/kg
	Rocuronium	As needed by train-of-four monitoring
	Propofol	0–30 μg/kg/min
	Volatile agent	0.5–1 minimum alveolar concentration
Intensive care unit	Propofol	0–30 μg/kg/min

[a]It is typical to use one of these three induction agents, depending on hemodynamic status and ventricular function.

nitroglycerine can help prevent or treat a hyperdynamic state that breaks through low doses of opioids.

Intrathecal or epidural analgesia, placed preoperatively, facilitates recovery by decreasing the perioperative opioid requirements [29]. Concern about neuroaxial hematoma formation in the presence of systemic anticoagulation limits the clinical application of regional anesthesia.

(2) **Maintenance of anesthesia.** Volatile agents are used freely to limit the total opioid dose to 10 to 15 μg/kg fentanyl IV. The ultrashort-acting opioid remifentanil provides good hemodynamic stability, adequate attenuation of the neurohumoral stress response, and early awakening. However, its short half-life necessitates providing analgesia in the postoperative period. Reduce reliance on a volatile agent in advance of patient transport to the ICU, lest the patient becomes acutely hyperdynamic upon arrival, prompting the use of long-duration sedatives by the ICU staff.

α_2-Agonists (e.g., dexmedetomidine and clonidine) are used adjunctively to reduce the neurohumoral stress response and for their sedative and antinociceptive properties. These agents reduce the anesthetic requirement and thus facilitate more rapid emergence.

c. **Intraoperative awareness.** Significant intraoperative awareness occurs in 0.3% of fast-track patients, similar to that observed in general surgery [30]. When using moderate doses of opioids, matching the depth of anesthesia to the operative stimulus at different times will avoid harmful hemodynamic responses; volatile agent provides this flexibility. A vaporizer attached to the cardiopulmonary bypass circuit facilitates appropriate anesthetic depth during bypass with moderate hypothermia. The role of the bispectral index (BIS, Aspect Medical Systems, Natick, MA, USA) remains unclear, although many centers have embraced its use.

d. **Temperature homeostasis.** Early extubation is unwise in the hypothermic patient: Arrhythmia, coagulopathy, shivering, and increased oxygen consumption complicate postoperative care and delay discharge [31]. Fluid-filled warming blankets and heated-humidified breathing circuits fail to preserve heat in the face of the huge caloric deficits of cardiac surgical patients. IV fluid warmers significantly impact body heat during cardiac surgery where infused volumes are substantial [32]. The cardiopulmonary bypass circuit heat exchanger provides the best means of restoring body temperature. Target a PA blood temperature greater than 37°C and a bladder temperature greater than 34°C. Forced hot-air convective warming helps during off-bypass revascularization, despite the minimal body surface available. Maintain operating room temperature as warm as is reasonably tolerated by operative personnel to prevent heat loss.

e. **Hemostatic homeostasis.** To prevent bleeding after operation, supplement a scrupulous surgical attention to hemostasis with pharmacologic hemostatic agents such as aminocaproic acid or aprotinin (see Chapter 17). Use of these agents is generally restricted to revascularization that involves the use of bypass.

f. **Intraoperative extubation.** In the absence of ventricular impairment, hemodynamic instability, hypothermia, or significant coagulopathy, consider extubation in the operating room prior to transport. In one nonrandomized, underpowered study, intraoperative extubation did not reduce the length of stay in the ICU [33]. A more recent study showed that with careful patient selection, immediate extubation offers the opportunity for shorter ICU and hospital stays [34]. Strategic use of opioids at induction and judicious use after sternal wiring produce adequate ventilation and analgesia. One technique combines intrathecal morphine (300 to 500 μg) prior to induction using sufentanil (150 to 250 μg IV) with morphine (0 to 10 mg IV) at sternal reapposition. Rapid awakening depends upon discontinuation of isoflurane or sevoflurane upon placement of sternal wires with substitution by nitrous oxide or desflurane. ICU personnel must tolerate the mild to moderate respiratory acidosis seen in patients with adequate analgesia immediately after extubation. Patients remaining intubated need adequate sedation/anesthesia to last through the transport and for at least 30 min beyond, to avoid hypertension, tachycardia, and bucking in the semicontrolled environment of tangled access lines and rolling beds.

4. **ICU management.** Maintain a degree of sedation with a relatively short-acting agent devoid of significant hemodynamic effect until the patient is ready for extubation. For an uncomplicated patient not extubated in the operating room, tailor the level of sedation for extubation 4 to 6 h after arrival, during which time the patient recovers from inadequate myocardial protection during bypass, achieves normothermia, and demonstrates perioperative hemostasis (Fig. 11.7).

Propofol provides a smooth transition from intraoperative anesthesia to postoperative sedation. It is easy to titrate, with quick onset and offset of action, and minor hemodynamic effects. Supplemental nitroglycerin or nitroprusside infusions titrate blood pressure rapidly.

Dexmedetomidine is an effective medication in the postoperative period. When administered as a continuous infusion, dexmedetomidine produces sedation that mimics natural sleep. It significantly reduces the use of analgesics, β-blockers, antiemetics, epinephrine, and diuretics [35].

The literature provides conflicting evidence regarding the relative safety and efficacy of dexmedetomidine compared to propofol for ICU sedation, including endpoints such as

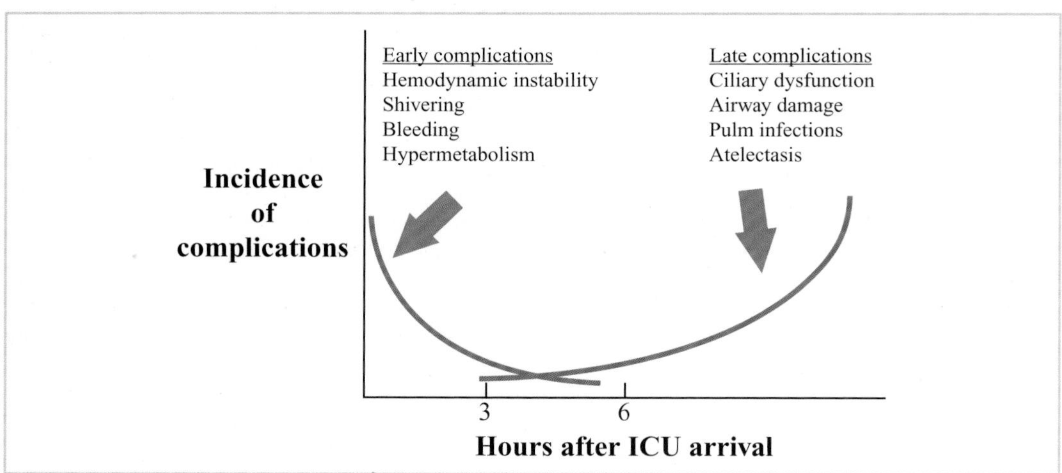

FIGURE 11.7 Early and late complications seen in patients undergoing coronary revascularization in the immediate postoperative period. (Adapted from Higgins T. Pro: Early endotracheal extubation is preferable to late extubation in patients following coronary artery surgery. *J Cardiothorac Vasc Anesth.* 1992;6:488–493.)

analgesic requirement reduction and hemodynamic changes [35,36]. Studies indicate no difference in ventilator weaning time [35].

Special versions of sedation and weaning protocols for fast-track patients facilitate the goal of early ICU discharge. Point-of-care arterial blood gas monitoring permits rapid decisions regarding weaning from mechanical ventilation. Many institutions use the fast-track anesthesia program as a continuing performance improvement project.

5. **Clinical and economic benefits**
   a. **Clinical benefits of enhanced recovery.** Early extubation may be associated with reduced postoperative lung atelectasis and improved pulmonary shunt fraction [37]. Positive-pressure ventilation has deleterious effects on cardiac output and organ perfusion that may be minimized by early extubation. Early chest tube removal facilitates patient mobilization. Early extubation yields greater patient satisfaction as long as appropriate analgesia is maintained.
   b. **Economic benefits.** Early extubation protocols reduce ICU stay, hospital stay, and the cost of hospitalization by as much as 25% [34,38,39].

B. **Off-bypass revascularization**

Off-pump coronary artery bypasses (OPCAB) utilize venous or arterial conduits to the coronary arteries via sternotomy but without CPB. See Section VI.D.2 for a discussion of port-access surgery and Section VI.D.3 for minimally invasive directed coronary artery bypasses (MIDCAB).

1. **Technique.** Following sternotomy and anticoagulation, the surgeon places distal anastomoses using myocardial stabilizers. With the heart continuing to fill, beat, and contract, a section is immobilized sufficiently to permit vascular sutures for distal anastomoses. An aortic side clamp permits placement of proximal anastomoses. Reapproximation of the sternum and layered closure complete the surgical procedure.
2. **Advantages and disadvantages**
   a. **Graft patency.** Randomized studies comparing OPCAB to conventional CABG with CPB yield differing results [40,41] with respect to short- and long-term graft patency. Grafts to the right coronary circulation appear more likely to lose patency with OPCAB.
   7 b. Level-IA evidence-based criteria suggest that mortality and quality-of-life markers do not differ, whereas the duration of ventilation, length of stay in the hospital, and overall morbidity decrease with OPCAB.
   c. Somewhat weaker evidence supports decreased blood loss and transfusion requirements, less myocardial enzyme release up to 24 h, less renal dysfunction, coagulation abnormalities, incidence of atrial fibrillation, and impairment of cognitive function with OPCAB [42]. More large randomized studies will better define outcomes.
   d. **Hemodynamic instability.** Despite frequent manipulation of patient position, volume status, and vasopressors, maintaining a regular rhythm, cardiac output, and blood pressure during performance of circumflex or inferior anastomoses may prove difficult owing to torsion of the heart or geometry incompatible with effective ejection. Ventricular fibrillation may occur suddenly during this time.
3. Patient selection for OPCAB varies widely among institutions:
   a. Patients with anterior lesions only, thus limiting the risks of hemodynamic compromise and potential subsequent graft occlusion associated with inferior anastomoses
   b. Avoidance of CPB to minimize the risk for stroke and renal failure (i.e., for those patients with large amounts of aortic plaque, severe vascular disease in general, or with renal insufficiency)
   c. **None or all.** Selection occurs when the patient or referring physician selects the surgeon, who performs all procedures as OPCAB or conventionally.
4. **Preoperative assessment.** Infinitely more so than with conventional CABG, with OPCAB, knowledge of the intended placement of grafts and functional reserve of myocardium prepares the anesthesia team for the extent of physiologic trespass and expected impact on homeostasis.

a. Interruption of flow when grafting proximal stenoses can impact a large amount of myocardium.
b. Interruption of flow to vessels with high-grade lesions may have little impact owing to formation of collateral circulation.

5. Monitoring of a given patient for OPCAB should be at least as extensive as for conventional CABG due to the added stresses of cumulative myocardial ischemia during vessel occlusion and grafting. Twisting or flipping the heart changes its electrical axis, making difficult the determination of ischemia via ECG criteria, and also thwarts acquisition of standard images using TEE. Thermodilution will still accurately measure cardiac output.
6. **Fast-track criteria apply.** See Section VI.A regarding choice of anesthetic agents and techniques to facilitate early extubation, awakening, and safe transfer from intensive care environments. Occasionally, an OPCAB case converts to one using CPB; for this reason, some caregivers avoid techniques they would not employ in the presence of full heparinization, such as epidural anesthesia.
7. **Temperature.** Without the heat exchanger of the CPB machine to transfer calories to the patient, temperature management focuses on prevention of heat loss and use of forced air on available surface, even if only head and shoulders. See Section VI.A.3.d for additional guidance.
8. Heparin management varies among institutions. Some target an ACT twice that of baseline, as for noncoronary vascular surgery. Others aim for a minimum of 300 s, representing twice the upper limit of normal, whereas some administer doses as they would for the conduct of CPB. Protamine doses should aim to neutralize the heparin administered, because bleeding with OPCAB remains as much a threat to successful surgery as it does with conventional CABG. However, CPB affects platelet function adversely and activates the fibrinolytic system more than does OPCAB.
9. Specific maneuvers to provide adequate hemodynamics
   a. Intravascular volume loading and head-down tilt (modified Trendelenburg's position) augment preload to counter obstructed venous return from torqued or flipped cardiac positioning during performance of distal anastomoses.
   b. Vasoconstrictors (phenylephrine or norepinephrine) likewise maintain CPP, maintaining collateral flow during vessel occlusion.
   c. **Controlled hypotension.** When the surgeon sutures the proximal anastomoses using an aortic side clamp, systolic pressures less than 100 mm Hg will help prevent aortic dissection. Use vasodilators and volatile anesthetics with normovolemia and head-up tilt to accomplish this.

C. Regional anesthesia adjuncts

1. **Intrathecal opioid.** Placement of 200 to 400 μg of preservative-free morphine via lumbar puncture immediately prior to induction of general anesthesia provides lasting, preemptive analgesia. Larger doses increase the risks of postoperative pruritus, nausea, and ventilatory depression, peaking around 6 to 10 h after administration. Minimize the possibility of neuraxial bleeding and compression as follows:
   a. Time the administration of heparin to occur at least 1 h following puncture, especially if blood returns in the spinal needle. Some centers delay the operation by 24 h if a large-bore needle has been used.
   b. Use a small-gauge spinal needle—24 G or smaller.
   c. Do not persist if identification of the intrathecal space proves difficult.
2. **Epidural opioid.** After identifying the epidural space, up to 5 mg of preservative-free morphine can provide preemptive analgesia. The larger epidural needle increases the risk of bleeding and of significant hematoma formation.
3. **Precautions.** Potent antiplatelet therapy (e.g., clopidogrel) not halted at least 7 days before the day of surgery raises concern in performing neuraxial procedures, as does a therapeutic international normalized ratio (greater than 1.5) from vitamin K antagonist therapy.
4. Neuraxial preemptive analgesia may facilitate early extubation by facilitating adequate ventilation. Nevertheless, expect a patient breathing spontaneously immediately after a

very-early-extubation technique to have an arterial Pco_2 of 50 mm Hg, which is similar to that of noncardiac surgical patients with adequate opioid-based analgesia in the PACU.

D. Special circumstances

1. **Radial artery conduits.** Confirm before placing monitoring catheters whether or not the surgeon intends to utilize this conduit, and, if so, mark the operative side clearly to avoid placing either IV or radial arterial catheters there. Some plans call for diltiazem infusions as prophylaxis against arterial spasm in the radial graft; be aware of the accompanying systemic vasodilation.
2. **Port-access surgery.** This approach utilizes a small thoracotomy incision, endoscopic instruments inserted through small ports, and TEE placement of endovascular devices to facilitate CPB. This technique is more frequently employed when valvular surgery is performed rather than coronary revascularization.
3. **MIDCAB.** The anterior thoracotomy incision permits access for harvesting of the left IMA and its anastomosis to the LAD coronary artery without CPB.
4. **Urgent CABG**
   a. **Patient profile.** Patients who present for urgent coronary artery bypass surgery usually have ongoing ischemia, including actively infarcting tissue, frequently with hemodynamic instability.
   b. **Induction and monitoring.** If the patient's condition requires rapid establishment of CPB, utilize existing femoral catheters for monitoring and IV access rather than delayed surgery.
   c. **Anesthetic management.** In the hypotensive patient, consider etomidate for induction and potent amnestics like scopolamine as adjuncts. Make every effort to institute CPB without delay.
5. Patients with poor ventricular function (ejection fraction less than 35%) receive reduced or no premedication. Severe ventricular compromise may require inotrope administration before induction. Popular induction techniques employ etomidate or slow titration of opioids (150 to 250 μg fentanyl every 30 s).
6. **Left main disease or its equivalent.** These patients generally fare better with a high-supply/high-demand anesthetic technique rather than a low-supply/low-demand technique (see Section V.F). Maintain diastolic blood pressure during induction and until revascularization is completed with phenylephrine or other vasopressors to ensure adequate oxygen balance.
7. **CABG for patients previously treated with antiplatelet medications.** Patients treated with potent antiplatelet agents (platelet glycoprotein receptor antagonists or clopidogrel) are at risk for significant coagulopathy and consequent bleeding. Empirical platelet infusions can avoid catastrophic blood loss and high transfusion requirements.
8. **CABG for patients with heparin-induced thrombocytopenia.** See Chapter 17.
9. **Redo CABG procedures.** More bleeding, perioperative ischemia, infarction, and pump failure accompany repeat operations. Adherence of the RV to the sternum may result in sudden, extensive hemorrhage during surgical dissection. Table 11.5 summarizes these special concerns, their causes, and appropriate perioperative anesthetic management.
10. Concomitant acute ischemic mitral regurgitation arises from ischemic papillary muscle dysfunction or ruptured chordae tendineae, with hemodynamic instability. Operation is nearly always urgent (see Section VI.D.4). The accompanying tachycardia, high LVEDP, and increased contractility all worsen myocardial oxygen supply/demand balance. Intra-aortic balloon counterpulsation frequently stabilizes these patients sufficiently to permit survival until the institution of CPB.

VII. Causes and treatment of perioperative myocardial ischemia (Table 11.6)

A. Causes of ischemia in the prebypass period

1. **Specific high-risk anesthetic-surgical events.** Events precipitating ischemia in the prebypass period include endotracheal intubation, surgical stress (skin incision, sternal split), cannulation, and initiation of bypass [10]. Episodes of ischemia may occur during these high-risk events even in the absence of hemodynamic changes [10].

TABLE 11.5 Perioperative management of the myocardial revascularization reoperation patient

Perioperative problem	Cause	Management
Bleeding	Pericardial adhesions Preoperative antiplatelet or anticoagulant medication	Large-bore IV access Blood readily available and checked in the OR Careful dissection on reopening chest Femoral area exposed and ready for emergency cannulation Anticipated need for clotting factors and platelets in the postbypass period Availability of blood salvage equipment (cell saver) Prophylactic antifibrinolytic therapy
Ischemia or infarction	Increased incidence of unstable angina Long period before bypass instituted Thrombus in vein grafts embolize to native vessels Interruption of vein graft flow (associated with 50%–60% mortality) Longer bypass and cross-clamp times Increased amount of noncoronary collateral flow	Close monitoring of ischemia (ECG, PA catheter, two-dimensional TEE) Expeditious treatment of ischemia once detected Careful manipulation of vein grafts; retrograde cardioplegia Careful dissection around vein grafts Minimal cross-clamp time Mean perfusion pressure <60 mm Hg when cross-clamp is applied to limit noncoronary flow
Pump failure after bypass	Perioperative ischemia and infarction	Same as above Treat ischemia aggressively after bypass to improve myocardial function Anticipate need for IV inotropic and mechanical support

ECG, electrocardiogram; IV, intravenous; OR, operating room; PA, pulmonary artery; TEE, transesophageal echocardiography.

2. **Hemodynamic abnormalities.** Some episodes of ischemia during high-risk periods arise from hemodynamic abnormalities, especially tachycardia (greater than 100 beats/min). Minimize hemodynamic alterations to prevent myocardial ischemia. Intraoperative ischemia triples the likelihood of perioperative infarction.
3. **Coronary spasm.** Coronary spasm in a normal vessel or around an atherosclerotic lesion causes ischemia. Intense sympathetic stimulation, light levels of anesthesia, and surgical manipulation may theoretically trigger coronary vasospasm.

8 **TABLE 11.6** Causes of perioperative ischemia in the myocardial revascularization patient

Prebypass	Bypass	Postbypass
Hemodynamic alterations[a]	Hemodynamic alterations[a]	Hemodynamic alterations[a]
Coronary spasm	Coronary spasm Cardioplegic arrest	Coronary spasm
Thrombus formation	Emboli (air, thrombus, particulate matter)	Thrombus (native vessel, graft)
High-risk anesthetic-surgical events[b]	Ventricular fibrillation Ventricular distention Surgical complications[b]	Surgical complications[b] Incomplete revascularization Excessive use of inotropes Distention of the lungs leading to occlusion of IMA graft flow

[a]Includes tachycardia, hypotension, hypertension, and ventricular distention.
[b]See text for details.

4. **Spontaneous thrombus formation.** Atherosclerotic plaque rupture with thrombus formation occludes coronary vessels. Although uncommon, this may occur at any time, including in the operating room prior to revascularization.

B. **Causes of ischemia during bypass**

1. **Periods without aortic cross-clamp.** Hemodynamic alterations rarely lead to ischemia during CPB. However, mechanical factors and ventricular fibrillation can sharply decrease oxygen supply or increase its demand, respectively. Air or particulate microemboli (thrombus, plastic, and other foreign materials) present in the CPB circuit may embolize to the coronary circulation. Whenever the heart or aorta is opened, air embolism to the native coronary circulation can occur.
2. **During aortic cross-clamp.** Ischemia occurs regardless of the myocardial preservation technique. The potential for ischemic injury and subsequent infarction increases with cross-clamp time. Washout of cold cardioplegic solution owing to excessive noncoronary collateral flow may lead to ischemia. Electrical and mechanical quiescence during this period precludes monitoring for ischemia.
3. **After cross-clamp removal**
   a. **Surgical and technical complications**
      (1) Inadvertent incision of the coronary back wall, leading to coronary dissection
      (2) Improper handling of the vein graft with endothelial cell loss, leading to graft thrombus formation
      (3) Twisting of vein grafts
      (4) Anastomosis of the vein graft to the coronary vein
      (5) Suturing the artery closed while grafting or poor-quality anastomoses
      (6) Inadequate vein graft length, leading to stretching of the vein when the heart is filled
      (7) Excess length of vein graft, leading to vein kinking
   b. Etiology of ST-segment elevation after cross-clamp removal. This arises from residual electrophysiologic effects of cardioplegia, coronary air or atheromatous debris embolus, or coronary artery spasm. Appearance in the inferior leads (i.e., right coronary distribution) implicates air embolism, because air seeks the high location of the right coronary ostium. Ventricular aneurysm and pericarditis also cause persistent ST-segment elevations.

C. **Causes of ischemia in the postbypass period**

1. **Incomplete revascularization**
   a. Ungraftable vessels. The region of myocardium supplied by the unrevascularized stenotic vessel may develop ischemia after CPB because of the added insult of ischemic arrest.
   b. Diffuse distal disease and diabetes. Revascularization rarely restores effective flow in this scenario. Early vein graft closure owing to poor runoff in the small distal vessels further complicates care.
   c. Stress. Ischemia occurrence depends on attention to oxygen supply and demand balance, rather than the degree of analgesia or sedation provided to patients [28]. This includes inappropriate inotrope use, including calcium, during separation from CPB or thereafter.
2. **Coronary spasm.** Coronary spasm can occur in the postbypass period, most commonly in the right coronary arteries that are not diseased. Surgical manipulation and exogenous and endogenous catecholamines contribute to this problem.
3. **Mechanical factors.** These include vein graft kinking or stretching, or occlusion of IMA flow secondary to overinflation of the lungs.
4. **Thrombus formation.** See Section VII.A.4. Postsurgical hypercoagulability may contribute to clot formation.

D. **Treatment of myocardial ischemia** (Table 11.7)

1. **Treatment of ischemia secondary to hemodynamic abnormalities**
   a. Increase or decrease anesthetic depth.

TABLE 11.7 Treatment of ischemia

Adequate oxygenation
Hemodynamic stability (e.g., adequate anesthetic depth)
Surgical correction
Specific pharmacologic treatment Nitroglycerin Calcium-channel blockers β-Blockers (esmolol) Heparin
Inotropic support (ischemia secondary to a failing ventricle)
Mechanical support Intra-aortic balloon pump LV assist device RV assist device

b. Administer vasodilators or vasopressors when SVR is either high or low, respectively, assuming euvolemia.
c. Administer a β-blocker, specifically esmolol, to treat tachycardia.
d. Use atrioventricular sequential pacing. (Specifically in the postbypass period, this can be extremely beneficial to improve rate, rhythm, and hemodynamic stability.)
e. Use inotropes for ventricular failure, diagnosed by decreased cardiac output and increased ventricular filling pressures. (Pump failure leads to severe decreases in CPP because diastolic blood pressure is decreased and LVEDP is increased.) ***Note:*** Indiscriminate use of inotropes may aggravate ischemia. Therefore, preload and heart rate and rhythm should be optimized before using inotropes.

2. **Correction of surgical complications and mechanical problems**
   a. Avoid overinflation of the lungs when an IMA graft is present.
   b. Increasing systemic blood pressure with a vasoconstrictor such as phenylephrine can push intracoronary air through the vasculature, and restore blood flow to regions not perfused because of the intravascular air lock.
3. **Treatment of coronary spasm.** IV nifedipine, nitroglycerin, diltiazem, and nicardipine can treat coronary spasm. For specific doses of each drug for this indication, refer to Chapter 2.
4. **Specific pharmacologic treatment of ischemia.** This treatment includes (a) nitroglycerin, (b) β-blockers, and (c) calcium-channel blockers. See Chapter 2. Prophylactic IV nitroglycerin finds use after CPB in incompletely revascularized patients, patients with severe distal coronary disease, and diabetic patients. Because ischemia frequently occurs from thrombus formation on atheroma, many nonsurgical patients receive heparin as acute therapy and antiplatelet agents (most commonly aspirin) for long-term prophylaxis. These agents should be withheld after bypass until the threat of surgical hemorrhage ceases.
5. **Mechanical support.** Refer to Chapter 20 for a complete discussion of circulatory assist devices.
   a. **Intra-aortic balloon pumps.** Intra-aortic balloon counterpulsation increases CPP and decreases afterload for LV ejection. Patients with impaired ventricular function benefit from improved pump performance in addition to relief of ischemia.
   b. **Right and LV assist devices.** These devices may be useful for treating severe ischemia caused by myocardial failure or ischemia that led to myocardial failure. Data on their use in treatment of ischemia are still in question.
6. **Ischemic preconditioning**
   a. **Myocardial injury.** Tissue injury results from ischemia, and subsequent tissue reperfusion may involve a reduction in adenosine triphosphate (ATP) levels, free oxygen

radicals, calcium-mediated injury, nitric oxide, heat shock proteins, a form of protein kinase C, mitogen-activated protein kinases, and mitochondrial ATP-dependent potassium channels.

9 **b.** A brief period of tissue ischemia may protect against the damage caused by subsequent prolonged ischemia and tissue reperfusion. This ischemic preconditioning occurs in both experimental animals and humans. Endogenously produced adenosine may mediate ischemic preconditioning via enhanced preservation of ATP, inhibition of platelet and neutrophil-mediated inflammatory tissue injury, vasodilation, and decreased basal cellular energy requirements related to intracellular hyperpolarization [20].

c. Early versus late preconditioning. The early, classic form lasts 2 to 3 h after the ischemic event. It is followed by a secondary period that begins 24 h hence and lasts up to 2 to 3 days. Typically, the period of ischemia and subsequent period of reperfusion each last about 5 min. Four such cycles reduce the infarct size from a subsequent 40-min ischemic period by 75% [41]. The required 40 min of preconditioning time per anastomosis to mitigate sequelae from 15 min of vessel occlusion create logistic challenges in clinical practice.

d. Role of inhalational anesthetics. Halothane, isoflurane, desflurane, and sevoflurane decrease the deleterious effects of ischemia, in a manner similar to ischemic preconditioning.

REFERENCES

1. Roger VL, Go AS, Lloyd-Jones DM, et al. Heart disease and stroke statistics-2011 update. A report from the American Heart Association. *Circulation.* 2011;123:e18–e209.
2. National Institutes of Health. *Disease Statistics, Fact Book, Fiscal Year 2000.* Bethesda, MD: National Heart, Lung, and Blood Institute.
3. Cheng DC, Wall C, Djaiani G, et al. Randomized assessment of resource use in fast-track cardiac surgery 1-year after hospital discharge. *Anesthesiology.* 2003;98:651–657.
4. Higgins T. Quantifying risk and assessing outcome in cardiac surgery. *J Cardiothorac Vasc Anesth.* 1998;12:330–340.
5. Dupuis J, Feng W, Nathan H, et al. The cardiac anesthesia risk evaluation score. *Anesthesiology.* 2001;94:194–204.
6. Eagle KA, Guyton RA, Davidoff R, et al. ACC/AHA 2004 guideline update for coronary artery bypass graft surgery: Summary article: A report of the American College of Cardiology/American Heart Association Task Force on Practice Guidelines. *Circulation.* 2004;110:1168–1176.
7. Dole W. Autoregulation of the coronary circulation. *Prog Cardiovasc Dis.* 1987;29:293–323.
8. Berkowitz DE. Vascular function: From human physiology to molecular biology. In: Schwinn DA, ed. *New Advances in Vascular Biology and Molecular Cardiovascular Medicine.* Baltimore, MD: Williams & Wilkins; 1998:25–47.
9. Thys DM, Brooker RF, Cahalan MK, et al. Practice guidelines for perioperative transesophageal echocardiography. A report by the American Society of Anesthesiologists and the Society of Cardiovascular Anesthesiologists Task Force on Transesophageal Echocardiography. *Anesthesiology.* 2010;112(5):1084–1096.
10. Slogoff S, Keats A. Does perioperative ischemia lead to postoperative myocardial infarction? *Anesthesiology.* 1985;62:107–114.
11. Tuman KJ, McCarthy RJ, Spiess BD, et al. Effect of pulmonary artery catheterization on outcome in patients undergoing coronary artery surgery. *Anesthesiology.* 1989;70:199–206.
12. Connors A, Speroff T, Dawson NV, et al. The effectiveness of right heart catheterization in the initial care of critically ill patients. *JAMA.* 1996;276:889–896.
13. American Society of Anesthesiologists Task Force on Pulmonary Artery Catheterization. Practice guidelines for pulmonary artery catheterization: An updated report by the American Society of Anesthesiologists Task Force on Pulmonary Artery Catheterization. *Anesthesiology.* 2003;99:988–1014.
14. Shanewise JS. How to reliably detect ischemia in the intensive care unit and operating room. *Semin Cardiothorac Vasc Anesth.* 2006;10:101–109.
15. Ward R, Parker MD. Myocardial contrast echocardiography in acute coronary syndromes. *Curr Opin Cardiol.* 2002;17:455–463.
16. Slogoff S, Keats A. Randomized trial of primary anesthetic agents on outcome of coronary artery bypass operations. *Anesthesiology.* 1989;70:179–188.
17. Tuman KJ, McCarthy RJ, Spiess BD, et al. Does choice of anesthetic agent significantly affect outcome after coronary artery surgery? *Anesthesiology.* 1989;70:189–198.
18. Mukhtar AM, Obayah EM, Hassona AM. The use of dexmedetomidine in pediatric cardiac surgery. *Anesth Analg.* 2006;103: 52–56.
19. Buffington CW, Davis KB, Gillispie S, et al. The prevalence of steal-prone anatomy in patients with coronary artery disease: An analysis of the Coronary Artery Surgery Study Registry. *Anesthesiology.* 1988;69:721–727.
20. Lee T. Mechanisms of ischemic preconditioning and clinical implications for multiorgan-reperfusion injury. *J Cardiothorac Vasc Anesth.* 1999;13:78–91.

21. Garcia C, Julier K, Bestmann L, et al. Preconditioning with sevoflurane decreases PECAM-1 expression and improves one-year cardiovascular outcome in coronary artery bypass graft surgery. *Br J Anaesth.* 2005;94:159–165.
22. Rorie DK, Tyce GM, Sill JC. Increased norepinephrine release from dog pulmonary artery caused by nitrous oxide. *Anesth Analg.* 1986;65:560–564.
23. Murphy GS, Szokol JW, Vender JS, et al. The use of neuromuscular blocking drugs in adult cardiac surgery: Results of a national postal survey. *Anesth Analg.* 2002;95(6):1534–1539.
24. Reich DL, Hollinger I, Harrington DJ, et al. Comparison of cisatracurium and vecuronium by infusion in neonates and small infants after congenital heart surgery. *Anesthesiology.* 2004;101(5):1122–1127.
25. Jellish WS, Brody M, Sawicki K, et al. Recovery from neuromuscular blockade after either bolus and prolonged infusions of cisatracurium or rocuronium using either isoflurane or propofol-based anesthetics. *Anesth Analg.* 2000;91:1250.
26. Mangano DT, Siliciano D, Hollenberg M, et al. Postoperative myocardial ischemia: Therapeutic trials using intensive analgesia following surgery. *Anesthesiology.* 1992;76:342–353.
27. Prakash O, Johson B, Meij S, et al. Criteria for early extubation after intracardiac surgery in adults. *Anesth Analg.* 1977;56:703–708.
28. Hall R, MacLaren C, Smith M, et al. Light versus heavy sedation after cardiac surgery: Myocardial ischemia and the stress response. *Anesth Analg.* 1997;85:971–978.
29. Scott NB, Turfrey DJ, Ray D, et al. A prospective randomized study of the potential benefits of thoracic epidural anesthesia and analgesia in patients undergoing coronary artery bypass grafting. *Anesth Analg.* 2001;93:528–535.
30. Dowd N, Cheng D, Karski J, et al. Intraoperative awareness in fast track cardiac anesthesia. *Anesthesiology.* 1998;89:1068–1073.
31. Leslie K, Sessler D. The implications of hypothermia for early extubation following cardiac surgery. *J Cardiothorac Vasc Anesth.* 1998;12:30–34.
32. Ginsberg S, Solina A, Papp D, et al. A prospective comparison of three heat preservation methods for patients undergoing hypothermic cardiopulmonary bypass. *J Cardiothorac Vasc Anesth.* 2000;14:501–505.
33. Her DL, Sum-Ping ST, England M. ICU sedation after coronary artery bypass graft surgery: Dexmedetomidine-based versus propofol-based sedation regimens. *J Cardiothorac Vasc Anesth.* 2003;17:576.
34. Anger KE, Szumita PM, Baroletti SA, et al. Evaluation of dexmedetomidine versus propofol-based sedation therapy in mechanically ventilated cardiac surgery patients at a tertiary academic medical center. *Crit Path Cardiol.* 2010;9(4):221–226.
35. Montes F, Sanchez S, Giraldo J, et al. The lack of benefit of tracheal extubation in the operating room after coronary artery bypass surgery. *Anesth Analg.* 2000;91:776–780.
36. Chamchad D, Horrow J, Nachamchik L, et al. The impact of immediate extubation in the operating room after cardiac surgery on intensive care and hospital lengths of stay. *J Cardiothorac Vasc Anesth.* 2010;24:780–784.
37. Cheng D, Karski J, Peniston C, et al. Morbidity outcome in early versus conventional tracheal extubation after coronary artery bypass grafting: A prospective randomized trial. *J Thorac Cardiovasc Surg.* 1996;112:755–764.
38. Hawkes CA, Dhileepan S, Foxcroft D. Early extubation for adult cardiac surgical patients. *Cochrane Database Syst Rev.* 2003;4:CD003587.
39. Cheng D, Karski J, Peniston C, et al. Early tracheal extubation after coronary artery bypass graft surgery reduces costs and improves resource use. *Anesthesiology.* 1996;85:1300–1310.
40. Khan NE, DeSouza A, Mister R, et al. A randomized comparison of off-pump and on-pump multivessel coronary-artery bypass surgery. *N Engl J Med.* 2004;350:21–28.
41. Puskas JD, Williams WH, Mahoney EM, et al. Off-pump vs conventional coronary artery bypass grafting. Early and 1-year graft patency, cost, and quality-of-life outcomes. A randomized trial. *JAMA.* 2004;291:1841–1849.
42. Sellke FW, DiMaio JM, Caplan LR, et al. American Heart Association. Comparing on-pump and off-pump coronary artery bypass grafting: Numerous studies but few conclusions: A scientific statement from the American Heart Association Council on cardiovascular surgery and anesthesia in collaboration with the interdisciplinary working group on quality of care and outcomes research. *Circulation.* 2005;111(21):2858–2864.

12 Anesthetic Management for the Surgical Treatment of Valvular Heart Disease

Matthew M. Townsley and Donald E. Martin

KEY POINTS

1. Increasing utilization of intraoperative transesophageal echocardiography (TEE) has greatly expanded the role of the cardiac anesthesiologist in operations for valve repair and replacement.
2. Because atrial contraction contributes up to 40% of left ventricular (LV) filling in patients with aortic stenosis (AS) and with hypertrophinc obstructive cardiomyopathy, it is essential to maintain sinus rhythm and treat arrhythmias aggressively in both of these conditions.
3. In patients with AS, the early use of α-adrenergic agonists such as phenylephrine is indicated to prevent drops in blood pressure that can lead quickly to sudden death.
4. Patients with severe acute aortic regurgitation are not capable of maintaining sufficient forward stroke volume (FSV) and often develop sudden and severe dyspnea, cardiovascular collapse, and deteriorate rapidly. Patients with chronic aortic regurgitation may be asymptomatic for many years.
5. In patients with mitral stenosis, particular attention should be paid to avoiding any increases in pulmonary artery pressure (PAP) due to inadequate anesthesia or inadvertent acidosis, hypercapnia, or hypoxemia.
6. Bradycardia is harmful in patients with mitral regurgitation, leading to an increase in LV volume, reduction in forward cardiac output, and an increase in regurgitant fraction (RF). The heart rate should be kept in the normal to elevated range.
7. In patients with tricuspid regurgitation (TR), high airway pressures during pulmonary ventilation and agents that can increase pulmonary arterial (PA) pressure should be avoided. If inotropic support is necessary, dobutamine, isoproterenol, or milrinone, which dilate the pulmonary vasculature, should be used.
8. Hypertrophy and pressure within the right ventricle with pulmonic stenosis limit right ventricular (RV) subendocardial blood flow to diastole. Coronary perfusion pressure (CPP) must be maintained to provide an adequate RV subendocardial coronary blood supply.
9. The hemodynamic requirements for AS and mitral regurgitation are contradictory. Because AS will most frequently lead these patients into deadly intraoperative situations, it should be given priority when managing the hemodynamic variables.

I. Introduction

Following the "golden age" of cardiac surgery in the 1980s and 1990s, recent years have seen an overall decline in cardiac surgery volume. Surgery is no longer the preferred option for treating many forms of cardiac disease, especially in the case of coronary artery disease (CAD). The number of coronary artery bypass grafting (CABG) operations has undergone a noticeable decline, in large part due to continuing advances in the field of interventional cardiology. However, the same does not hold true for the surgical treatment of valvular heart disease, as the volume of valve surgery remains steady and now represents 10% to 20% of all cardiac surgical procedures in the United States [1]. In the majority of these cases, surgery remains the best, and often only effective, approach to treatment. Valve surgery should continue to thrive with an aging patient population and continued improvements in surgical techniques, available prosthetic valves, and patient outcomes following these procedures. Approximately 66% of valvular surgery is on the aortic valve, most often because of AS [1].

The prevalence of valvular heart disease remains relatively constant at about 2.5% of the population in industrialized countries because an increase in the frequency of degenerative valvular disease has balanced the decrease in rheumatic disease. Further, the widespread use of echocardiography improves the detection and may increase the apparent incidence of disease. In Nkomo's large echo-based series in Minnesota, the two most common valvular lesions were mitral regurgitation and AS, and the prevalence of disease increased markedly with age, ranging from less than 2% before age 65, to 8.5% in patients age 65 to 75, to 13.2% in patients older than 75 yrs [2]. Further, almost one-third of patients presenting for surgical management have had a prior medical or surgical intervention [3]. The mortality of valve surgery ranges from 0% to 3% for isolated mitral valve repair to 6% to 11% in patients undergoing multiple valve replacement, depending on the severity of the patient's cardiac disease as well as their age and general health [4].

The anesthetic management of valvular surgical patients is often quite challenging. These lesions may lead to pathophysiologic changes in the heart with profound hemodynamic consequences, particularly in the setting of general anesthesia and surgical stress. A well-planned anesthetic must compensate for these stresses by manipulating several hemodynamic variables. The most important variables to consider include heart rate and rhythm, preload, afterload, and contractility. In addition, it is critical to consider the time course of the disease, as the clinical presentation and management will vary dramatically in the setting of acute versus chronic valvular disorders.

1 Increasing utilization of intraoperative TEE has greatly expanded the role of the cardiac anesthesiologist in operations for valve repair and replacement. In the setting of valve surgery, the anesthesiologist is frequently consulted by the surgeon to provide diagnostic interpretation of the echo findings to help guide the operative approach. The echo exam is also critical to immediately assess the adequacy of a valve repair or replacement and, if necessary, alert the surgeon to any complications that may require further attention and correction. There are few other settings in which an anesthesiologist's diagnostic skills play such an integral role in surgical decision making as in the cardiac operating room during valve surgery.

This chapter will review the physiologic implications of the most common types of valvular heart disease and the practical approach to the anesthetic management of these patients. All four cardiac valves will be discussed, focusing on the stenotic and regurgitant lesions of each. A section addressing prosthetic valves will conclude the chapter with a review of each of the different types of prostheses most frequently used for valve replacement.

II. Stenotic versus regurgitant lesions

A. Valvular stenosis. Stenotic lesions lead to pathology associated with pressure overload. Narrowing of the orifice of a cardiac valve will ultimately lead to obstruction of blood flow through the valve. This obstruction translates into an increase in blood flow velocity as it approaches the stenotic valve orifice. The pattern of blood flow is distinctly different in the regions proximal and distal to a stenotic valve. The high-velocity flow proximal to the stenosis is laminar and organized, whereas distal to the stenosis, it becomes turbulent and disorganized. In addition, the increased blood flow velocities observed in valvular stenosis translate into an increase in the pressure gradient across the valve. The simplified Bernoulli equation helps explain this relationship. In this equation, the pressure gradient through the stenotic valve can be estimated by multiplying the velocity squared times four:

$$\text{Pressure gradient } (\Delta) = 4 * \text{Blood Flow Velocity } (v) \text{ squared}$$

$$(\Delta P = 4v^2)$$

The simplified Bernoulli equation allows blood flow velocities measured by Doppler echocardiography to be converted into pressure gradients that can be used to quantify the severity of valvular stenosis [5]. It is also important to understand that valvular obstruction can be of two primary types: Fixed versus dynamic. In fixed obstruction (i.e., true valvulvar AS, subaortic membrane), the degree of obstruction to blood flow remains constant throughout the cardiac cycle and is not affected by the loading conditions of the heart. With dynamic obstruction (i.e., HOCM with dynamic subaortic stenosis), obstruction is only present for part of the cardiac cycle, primarily occurring in mid- to late systole. The degree of obstruction is highly dependent on loading conditions, changing in severity as loading conditions change.

B. Valvular regurgitation. Regurgitant lesions lead to pathology associated with volume overload, resulting in chamber dilatation and eccentric hypertrophy. Clinically, although this chamber remodeling will initially allow the left ventricle to compensate for the increased volume load, it will lead to an eventual decline in LV systolic function that can ultimately lead to irreversible LV failure. Effective perioperative management of valvular regurgitation is facilitated by understanding how preload, afterload, and heart rate each affect the contributions of the FSV (flow reaching the peripheral circulation) and regurgitant stroke volume (retrograde flow back across the valve) to the overall total stroke volume (TSV) of the ventricle [5]. Hemodynamic management of these patients should aim to optimize the FSV while minimizing the amount of regurgitant stroke volume.

III. Structural and functional response to valvular heart disease. The anesthetic management of patients undergoing valvular heart surgery requires a thorough understanding of the hemodynamic changes associated with valvular heart disease, as well as the cardiac remodeling imposed by abnormal valves.

A. **Cardiac remodeling** includes changes in the size, shape, and function of the heart in response to an acute or chronic cardiac injury. In valvular heart disease, cardiac injury is usually caused by alterations in ventricular loading conditions. Depending on the nature of the valvular pathology, the ventricle will be subject to either pressure or volume overload, or both. This leads to cardiac remodeling in the form of chamber dilation and ventricular hypertrophy. In addition to mechanical stress, cardiac remodeling results from the activation of neurohumoral factors, enzymes such as angiotensin II, ion channels, and oxidative stress [6]. Intended initially as an adaptive response to maintain cardiac performance, remodeling eventually leads to decompensation and deterioration in ventricular function. Ventricular hypertrophy is defined as increased LV mass. Ventricular hypertrophy can be either concentric or eccentric. Pressure overload usually results in concentric ventricular hypertrophy, which means that ventricular mass is increased by myocardial thickening, whereas ventricular volume is not increased. Its adaptive purpose is to reduce the increased wall stress that results from the chronic pressure overload. Recall the law of LaPlace to understand how this compensatory hypertrophy results in reduced wall stress, where:

$$\text{LV wall stress} = (\text{LV pressure} * \text{LV radius})/2 * \text{LV wall thickness}$$

The increased afterload results in an elevated LV pressure, which translates into an increase in LV wall stress. The resulting increase in wall thickness, seen in the denominator of the above equation, will have the beneficial effect of reducing LV wall stress and avoiding a significant decline in LV systolic function. The cost of LV hypertrophy is a reduction in LV compliance, which leads to diastolic dysfunction with an increase in LV end-diastolic pressure (LVEDP) and subendocardial ischemia.

Volume overload, on the other hand, leads to eccentric hypertrophy, which means that ventricular mass is increased by an increase in ventricular volume, whereas myocardial thickness remains unchanged [3].

B. **Ventricular function.** To anticipate the effect of valvular lesions on ventricular function, it is helpful to separate ventricular function into its two distinct components [3].

1. **Systolic function** represents the ventricle's ability to contract and eject blood. Normal systolic function means that ventricular contractility is normal.
    a. **Contractility** can be defined as the intrinsic ability of the myocardium to contract and generate force. Contractility itself is independent of preload and afterload. Normal contractility means that a ventricle of normal size and normal preload can generate sufficient stroke volume at rest and during exercise.
    b. **Preload** can be defined as the load placed on myocardium before the contraction. This load results from a combination of diastolic volume and filling pressure and can be expressed as end-diastolic stress.
    c. **Afterload** is the load placed on the myocardium during contraction. This load results from the combination of systolic volume and generated pressure and can be expressed as end-systolic stress.
2. **Diastolic function** represents the ventricle's ability to accept inflowing blood. Diastolic function consists of a combination of relaxation and compliance. In general, normal diastolic function means that the ventricle accepts normal diastolic volume at normal filling pressure. When diastolic dysfunction occurs, maintaining normal ventricular diastolic volume requires elevated ventricular filling pressure. Both systolic and diastolic functions require energy and can be compromised by ventricular ischemia.

IV. Pressure–volume loops may be utilized to illustrate LV function and performance. These loops are constructed by plotting ventricular pressure (y-axis) versus ventricular volume (x-axis) over

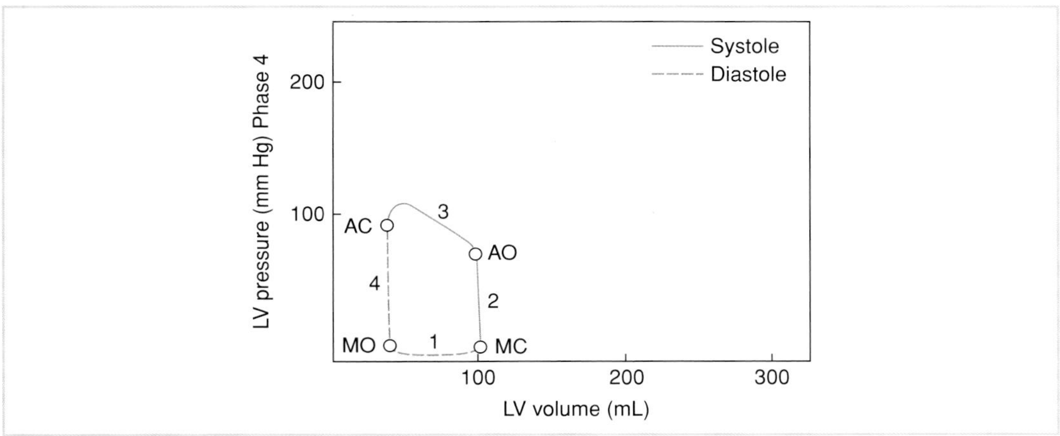

FIGURE 12.1 Normal pressure–volume loop. The first segment of the ventricular pressure–volume loop (Phase 1) represents diastolic filling of the left ventricle. The next two segments represent the two stages of ventricular systole: Isovolemic contraction (Phase 2) and ventricular ejection (Phase 3). The final segment of the loop corresponds to isovolemic relaxation of the left ventricle, which precedes ventricular filling and the start of the next cardiac cycle. The isovolemic relaxation and ventricular filling phases constitute the two phases of diastole. Both end-systolic volume at the time of aortic valve closure (AC), and end-diastolic volume at the time of mitral valve closure (MC), are represented as distinct points on the loop. MO, mitral valve opening; AO, aortic valve opening. [Modified from Jackson JM, Thomas SJ, Lowenstein E. Anesthetic management of patients with valvular heart disease. *Semin Anesth.* 1982;1:240.]

the course of a complete cardiac cycle (Fig. 12.1). The presence of valvular heart disease alters the normal pressure–volume loop tracing, representing changes in ventricular physiology and loading conditions imposed by valvular pathology. The ventricle adapts differently to each valvular lesion and characteristic patterns of the pressure–volume loop help illustrate these changes.

V. Aortic stenosis (AS)

A. Natural history

1. **Etiology.** The normal adult aortic valve has three cusps, with an aortic valve area of 2.6 to 3.5 cm^2, representing a normal aortic valve index of 2 cm^2/m^2. AS may result from congenital or acquired valvular heart disease. Congenital AS is classified as valvular, subvalvular, or supravalvular based on the anatomic location of the stenotic lesion. Subvalvular and supravalvular AS are usually caused by a membrane or muscular band. Congenital valvular AS may occur with a unicuspid, bicuspid, or a tricuspid aortic valve with partial commissural fusion.

   A congenitally bicuspid aortic valve occurs in approximately 1% to 2% of the general population, making it the most common congenital valvular malformation. Calcification of a congentially bicuspid valve results in the early onset of AS, and represents the most common cause of AS among patients younger than 70 yrs of age [7]. Currently, bicuspid aortic valve disease accounts for approximately 50% of all valve replacements for AS in the United States and Europe [8]. Commonly associated findings in patients with bicuspid aortic valves include abnormalities of the aorta, including aortic coarctation, aortic root dilatation, and an increased risk of aortic dissection.

   Of the acquired aortic stenoses, senile degeneration is the most common cause in the developed world, with 30% patients older than 85 yrs demonstrating significant degenerative aortic valve changes on autopsy. The calcification seen with senile degeneration of the aortic valve also appears to have an inflammatory component as well, similar to that observed in CAD [3]. While rheumatic AS is now rarely seen in the developed world, it remains the most common cause of AS worldwide. Additionally, rheumatic AS is usually associated with some degree of aortic regurgitation and frequently affects the mitral valve as well. Less frequent causes of AS include atherosclerosis, end-stage renal disease, and rheumatoid arthritis.

A characteristic finding of senile valvular degeneration is progression of the calcification from the base of the valve toward the edge, as opposed to rheumatic degeneration, in which calcification spreads from the edge toward the base.

2. **Symptoms.** Unicuspid AS often presents in infancy. Patients with rheumatic AS may be asymptomatic for 40 yrs or more. Congenital bicuspid aortic valves in the majority of cases must undergo calcific degeneration to become stenotic. The time of onset and speed of progression of calcific degeneration varies from patient to patient. This is why patients with congenitally bicuspid aortic valves may develop symptomatic AS anytime between the ages of 15 and 65, and even later in life. Degenerative stenosis of a tricuspid aortic valve usually develops in the seventh or eighth decade of life. Asymptomatic patients with AS have an excellent prognosis [3]. Patients with even severe AS may stay asymptomatic for many years and carry a small risk of sudden death, which does not exceed the risk of operation. However, the onset of any one of the following triad of symptoms is an ominous sign and indicates a life expectancy of less than 5 yrs:
   a. **Angina pectoris.** Angina is the initial symptom in approximately two-thirds of patients with severe AS. Angina and dyspnea secondary to AS alone initially occur with exertion [1]. Life expectancy when angina develops is about 5 yrs.
   b. **Syncope.** Syncope is the first symptom in 15% to 30% of patients. Once syncope appears, the average life expectancy is 3 to 4 yrs.
   c. **Congestive heart failure.** Once signs of LV failure occur, the average life expectancy is only 1 to 2 yrs.

B. **Pathophysiology**

1. **Heart remodeling.** As stenosis progresses, the maintenance of normal stroke volume is associated with an increasing systolic pressure gradient between the LV and the aorta. The LV systolic pressure increases to as much as 300 mm Hg, whereas the aortic systolic pressure and stroke volume remain relatively normal. This pressure gradient results in a compensatory concentric LV hypertrophy. As stenosis progresses, eccentric LV hypertrophy may develop. This is usually associated with low LV ejection fraction, indicating a compromise of LV contractility.
2. **Hemodynamic changes**
   a. **Arterial pressure.** In severe AS, the arterial pulse pressure usually is reduced to less than 50 mm Hg. The systolic pressure rise is delayed with a late peak and a prominent anacrotic notch. As stenosis increases in severity, the anacrotic notch occurs lower in the ascending arterial pressure trace. The dicrotic notch is relatively small or absent.
   b. **PA wedge pressure.** Because of the elevated LVEDP, which stretches the mitral valve annulus, a prominent V wave can be observed, but with progression of the disease and the development of left atrial hypertrophy, a prominent A wave becomes the dominant feature.
3. **Pressure–Volume Loop in AS.** (Fig. 12.2)

C. **Assessment of severity (echocardiographic criteria;** see Table 12.1**)**

1. **Transthoracic echocardiography.** Echocardiography is now the standard modality for quantifying the severity of AS. With the exception of rare cases where echocardiography is non-diagnostic or discrepant with clinical data, cardiac catheterization is no longer recommended for this purpose. The most commonly utilized methods for quantifying AS severity with echocardiography include measurement of the peak blood flow velocity of the AS jet, mean gradient across the aortic valve, and determination of aortic valve area. In AS, the valve area can be measured by the direct planimetry and continuity equation methods. The pressure gradient can be measured using a simplified Bernoulli equation. (Fig. 12.3) Cardiac remodeling is assessed by measurement of left atrial size, LV end-systolic and end-diastolic dimensions, and LV myocardial thickness.
2. **Transesophageal echocardiography (TEE).** TEE is useful in patients with a poor transthoracic window or in patients with complex cardiac pathology (e.g., a combination of subaortic and valvular stenosis). It is also useful when precise planimetry of the aortic valve area is necessary or when infective endocarditis is suspected.

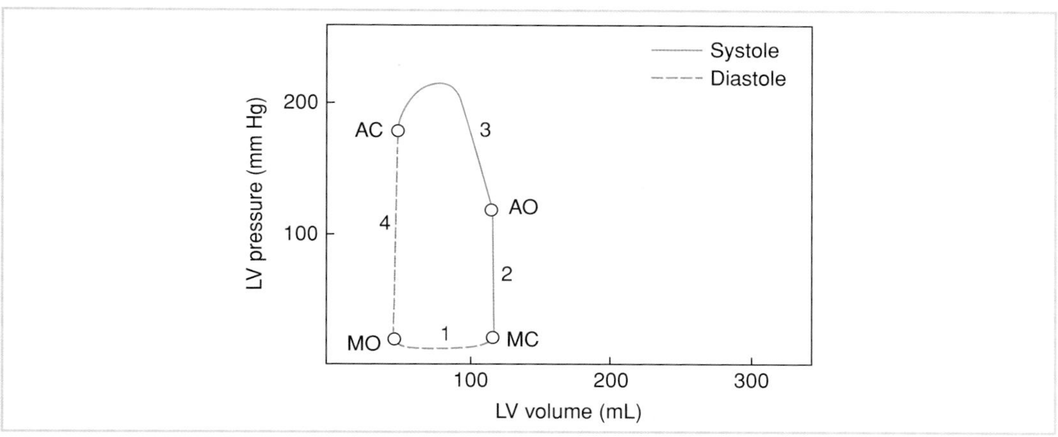

FIGURE 12.2 Pressure–volume loop in AS. In comparison to the normal loop, note the elevated peak systolic pressure necessary to generate a normal stroke volume in the face of the elevated pressure gradient through the aortic valve. Also, end-diastolic pressure is elevated with a steeper diastolic slope, reflecting diastolic dysfunction with altered LV compliance. Phase 1, Diastolic filling; Phase 2, Isovolumetric contraction; Phase 3, Ventricular ejection; Phase 4, Isovolumetric relaxation; MO, Mitral valve opening; MC, Mitral valve closure; AO, Aortic valve opening; AC, Aortic valve closure. [Modified from Jackson JM, Thomas SJ, Lowenstein E. Anesthetic management of patients with valvular heart disease. *Semin Anesth.* 1982;1:241.]

3. **Dobutamine stress echocardiography** is useful in patients with apparently severe AS on the echocardiogram that is combined with severe LV dysfunction and low cardiac output. Low cardiac output will not allow the generation of elevated blood flow velocities and pressure gradients commonly observed in AS. This combination of findings may be explained either by primary severe valvular AS causing LV dysfunction or by severe LV dysfunction independent of some degree of AS. In this case, the aortic valve does not open to its full extent due to low stroke volume and low generated pressure, which imitates severe AS. If with dobutamine infusion the transvalvular pressure gradient increases and the aortic valve area on the echocardiogram does not change, then AS is probably fixed and has caused the LV dysfunction. In this case, the patient will most likely benefit from surgical intervention [9]. If, however, the apparent aortic valve area increases with dobutamine, then ventricular dysfunction is likely the prime factor and valve replacement would have little benefit.
4. If cardiac catheterization data is utilized, the mean pressure gradient may be measured from a direct transaortic measurement and the aortic valve area may be calculated using the Gorlin formula.

D. **Timing and type of intervention**
1. Due to the high risk of sudden death and limited life expectancy, symptomatic patients should undergo surgery. Asymptomatic patients with severe AS may be monitored closely

TABLE 12.1

Measurement	Aortic sclerosis	Mild aortic stenosis	Moderate aortic stenosis	Severe aortic stenosis
Aortic valve area (cm^2)	2.6–3.5	>1.5	1.0–1.5	<1.0
Mean gradient (mm Hg)	<10	<20	20–40	>40
Indexed aortic valve area (cm^2/m^2)	2.0	>0.85	0.60–0.85	<0.6
Peak velocity of blood flow through aortic valve (m/s)	<2.6	2.6–3.0	3–4	>4

Adapted from: Baumgartner H, Hung J, Bermejo J, et al. Echocardiographic assessment of valve stenosis: EAE/ASE recommendations for clinical practice. *J Am Soc Echocardiogr.* 2009;22:1–23.

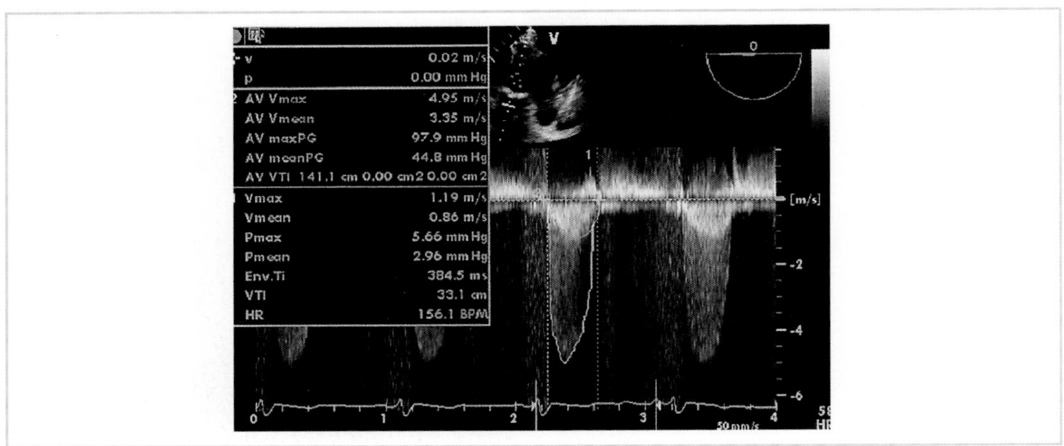

FIGURE 12.3 Severe AS, showing determination of valve gradient using the Bernoulli equation. This image displays a deep transgastric long-axis TEE view with a continuous wave Doppler beam aligned through the left ventricular outflow tract (LVOT) and aortic valve (AV). Tracing 2 on the spectral display (outer envelope) demonstrates blood flow through the severely stenotic aortic valve, with a maximum velocity (AV Vmax) of 4.95 m/s and peak AV pressure gradient (AV max PG) of 97.9 mmHg. Tracing 1 (inner envelope) demonstrates blood flow through the LVOT, with a maximum velocity (Vmax) of 1.19 m/s and peak LVOT pressure gradient (Pmax) of 5.66 mmHg. Additional parameters: AV Vmean, Mean velocity of blood flow across the aortic valve; AV meanPG, Mean pressure gradient across the aortic valve; AV VTI, Aortic valve velocity-time integral; V mean, Mean velocity of blood flow in LVOT; Pmean, Mean pressure gradient in LVOT; VTI, LVOT velocity-time integral in LVOT; HR, Heart Rate. [ECHO Image from Perrino AC, Reeves ST, eds. *A Practical Approach to Transesophageal Echocardiography.* 2nd ed. Philadelphia, PA: Lippincott Williams & Wilkins; 2008:246, Figure 12.2.]

until symptoms develop. However, the risk of waiting should be carefully weighted against the risk of surgery. For example, prior to elective noncardiac surgery under general or neuraxial anesthesia, asymptomatic patients with severe AS should be considered for aortic valve surgery.

2. Patients with moderate AS should have aortic valve surgery if they happen to require another cardiac operation, such as CABG, because the rate of progression of AS is approximately 0.1 cm^2/yr and the risk of having to redo cardiac surgery is substantially higher than the risk of the primary operation. Similarly, if a patient undergoing aortic valve surgery has significant CAD, CABG should be performed simultaneously. In patients over age 80 yrs, the risk of aortic valve replacement (AVR) alone is approximately the same as the risk of combined AVR and CABG [10].
3. A commissural incision or balloon aortic valvuloplasty is often the first procedure performed in young patients with severe noncalcific aortc valve stenosis, even if they are asymptomatic [1]. This operation frequently results in some residual AS and aortic regurgitation. Eventually, most patients require a subsequent prosthetic valve replacement. In older adult patients with calcific AS, valve replacement is the primary operation. In young adults, a viable alternative to AVR is the Ross (switch) procedure. In the Ross procedure, the diseased aortic valve is replaced with a patient's normal pulmonary valve and the pulmonary valve is replaced with a pulmonary homograft. This more complex procedure avoids the need for systemic anticoagulation and extends the time until reoperation is required by several decades.
4. Surgical intervention should not be denied to patients, almost no matter how severe the symptoms, because irreversible LV failure occurs only very late in the disease process.
5. **Balloon aortic valvuloplasty** in adults with advanced disease often results in significant aortic regurgitation and early restenosis, and is reserved for patients with severe comorbidity. Percutaneous AVR is a treatment modality with potential applications for high-risk patients deemed not suitable candidates for surgery. Transapical AVR, involving a small thoracotomy incision and insertion of the valve via the LV apex, has shown similar promise

TABLE 12.2

	LV preload	Heart rate	Contractility	Systemic vascular resistance	Pulmonary vascular resistance
Aortic stenosis	↑	↓ (sinus)	Maintain constant	↑	Maintain constant

in this same high-risk patient population. Both techniques require brief cessation of the patient's cardiac output via rapid pacing during positioning of the device. Hemodynamic instability is common and necessitates prompt recognition and treatment. These techniques have demonstrated improved rates of procedural success and clinical outcomes, with an overall 94% success rate and an 11.3% 30-day mortality [11].

E. Goals of perioperative management

1. **Hemodynamic profile** (Table 12.2)
   a. **LV preload.** Due to the decreased LV compliance as well as the increased LVEDP and LV end-diastolic volume (LVEDV), preload augmentation is necessary to maintain a normal stroke volume.
   b. **Heart rate.** Extremes of heart rate are not tolerated well. A high heart rate can lead to decreased coronary perfusion. A low heart rate can limit cardiac output in these patients with a fixed stroke volume. If a choice must be made, however, low heart rates (50 to 70 beats/min) are preferred to rapid heart rates (greater than 90 beats/min) to
2 allow time for systolic ejection across a stenotic aortic valve. Because atrial contraction contributes up to 40% of LV filling, due to decreased LV compliance and impaired early filling during diastole, it is **essential to maintain a sinus rhythm.** Supraventricular dysrhythmias should be treated aggressively, if necessary, with synchronized DC shock, because both tachycardia and the loss of effective atrial contraction can lead to rapid reduction of cardiac output.
   c. **Contractility.** Stroke volume is maintained through preservation of a heightened contractile state. The β-blockade is not well tolerated and can lead to an increase in LVEDV and a decrease in cardiac output, significant enough to induce clinical deterioration.
   d. **Systemic vascular resistance.** Most of the afterload to LV ejection is caused by the stenotic aortic valve itself and thus is fixed. Systemic blood pressure reduction does little to decrease LV afterload. In addition, patients with hemodynamically significant AS cannot increase cardiac output in response to a drop in systemic vascular resistance. Thus, arterial hypotension may rapidly develop in response to the majority of anesthetics. Finally, when hypotension develops, the hypertrophied myocardium of the patient with AS is at great risk for subendocardial ischemia because coronary perfu-
3 sion depends on maintenance of an adequate systemic diastolic perfusion pressure. Therefore, the early use of α-adrenergic agonists such as phenylephrine is indicated to prevent drops in blood pressure that can lead quickly to sudden death.
   e. **Pulmonary vascular resistance (PVR).** Except for end-stage AS, **PAPs remain relatively normal.** Special intervention for stabilizing PVR is not necessary.
2. **Anesthetic techniques**
   a. **Light premedication** is necessary to provide a calm patient without tachycardia. An experienced cardiac surgeon should be present, and perfusionists should be prepared, before induction of anesthesia should rapid cardiovascular deterioration necessitate emergency use of cardiopulmonary bypass.
   b. **Placement of external defibrillator pads** should be considered to allow for rapid defibrillation if cardiovascular collapse occurs on induction or prior to sternotomy.
   c. **Preinduction arterial line placement** is standard practice at most institutions and is generally well tolerated with light premedication and local anesthetic infiltration. Invasive blood pressure monitoring facilitates early recognition and intervention if any hemodynamic instability occurs during induction.

d. During induction of anesthesia, in order to maintain hemodynamic stability, medications should be carefully titrated to a fine line between a reasonable depth of anesthesia and hemodynamic stability.

e. During the maintenance stage of anesthesia, anesthetic agents causing myocardial depression, blood pressure reduction, tachycardia, or dysrhythmias can lead to rapid deterioration. A narcotic-based anesthetic is usually chosen for this reason. Low concentrations of volatile anesthetics are usually safe.

f. If the patient develops signs or symptoms of ischemia, nitroglycerin should be used with caution because its effect on preload or arterial pressure may actually make things worse.

g. **Thermodilution cardiac output.** Pulmonary artery catheters are helpful in evaluating the cardiac output of patients prior to repair of the aortic valve. The pulmonary capillary wedge pressure (PCWP), however, may overestimate preload of a noncompliant LV. Mixed venous oxygen saturation monitoring via an oximetric PA catheter may be used to provide a continuous index of cardiac output. However, because the postbypass management is not likely to be marked by myocardial failure or low output states, this technique may be best reserved for other patients who may be at higher risk of postbypass hemodynamic complications.

There is also a small risk of life-threatening arrhythmias leading to drug-resistant hypotension during passage of a pulmonary artery catheter through the right atrium and ventricle. In the absence of pre-existing left bundle branch block (LBBB) or tachyarrhythmias, a pulmonary artery catheter may be placed under continuous rhythm monitoring, perhaps after placement of transcutaneous pacing electrodes. In the presence of pre-existing abnormal rhythms or conduction disturbances, however, the most conservative approach dictates leaving the catheter tip in a central venous position until the chest is open, when internal defibrillator pads can be easily applied and cardiopulmonary bypass can be initiated within a few minutes if necessary.

h. **Omniplane TEE** is useful for intraoperative monitoring of LV function, preload, and afterload. TEE can predict prosthetic aortic valve size based on the LV outflow tract width. It is also very helpful in the detection of air and facilitating deairing prior to weaning from cardiopulmonary bypass. TEE is the method of choice for the postbypass assessment of a prosthetic valve for paravalvular regurgitation and prosthetic valve stenosis. It is important to remember that Doppler-derived blood flow velocities and pressure gradient must be interpreted in light of the altered loading conditions seen in the dynamic operating room setting.

i. In the presence of myocardial hypertrophy, adequate myocardial preservation with cardioplegic solution during bypass is a challenging task. A combination of antegrade cardioplegia administered via coronary ostia and retrograde cardioplegia via the coronary sinus has an important role in preserving myocardial integrity.

j. In the absence of preoperative ventricular dysfunction and associated coronary disease, inotropic support often is not required after cardiopulmonary bypass because valve replacement decreases ventricular afterload.

F. **Postoperative care.** After a sharp drop in the aortic valve gradient, PCWP and LVEDP immediately decrease and stroke volume rises. Myocardial function improves rapidly, although the hypertrophied ventricle may still require an elevated preload to function normally. Over a period of several months, LV hypertrophy regresses. It must be remembered that a prosthetic aortic valve may cause a mean pressure gradient of 7 to 19 mm Hg.

VI. Hypertrophic cardiomyopathy

A. Natural history

1. **Etiology and classification.** Hypertrophic cardiomyopathy (HCM) is a relatively uncommon genetic disorder affecting approximately 0.2% of the general population. The inheritance pattern is autosomal dominant with variable penetrance, making it a heterogeneous condition with a highly variable presentation. Historically, several names have been given to this disorder, such as idiopathic hypertrophic subaortic stenosis (IHSS) and asymmetric

septal hypertrophy. Since ventricular hypertrophy may occur in multiple patterns, not just confined to the septum, the term HCM is now used to describe this disorder. Additionally, despite the classic association of HCM with obstruction to systolic outflow through the left ventricular outflow tract (LVOT), only 25% of patients with HCM exhibit this subvalvular obstruction. The term HOCM is used to refer to this subset of HCM patients.

2. **Symptoms.** Patients with HCM may present with a wide range of symptoms, with many having no symptoms at all. The most common presenting symptom is dyspnea on exertion with poor exercise tolerance. Patients may also experience syncope, presyncope, chest pains, fatigue, and palpitations. Though LVOT obstruction may cause symptoms, there is no clear relationship between the degree of LVOT obstruction and the occurrence or severity of the symptoms. Other equally important causes of symptoms include diastolic dysfunction, dysrhythmias, mitral regurgitation, and an imbalance of myocardial oxygen supply and demand. Unfortunately, the initial presenting symptom in many patients is sudden cardiac death, usually due to ventricular fibrillation. Though all patients with HCM are at risk for sudden death, the highest-risk groups include those with a family history of HCM and young patients undergoing significant physical exertion. This has led to increased and improved measures to screen for HCM in young athletes and patients with a family history of the disorder.

B. **Pathophysiology.** By definitition, HCM involves an abnormal thickening of the myocardium without an identifiable cause of hypertrophy. There is an absence of chamber dilation and, in most cases, normal to hyperdynamic LV systolic function. In addition, there are important histological derangements, including abnormal cellular architecture and disarray of the cardiac myocytes, interstitial fibrosis, increased connective tissue, and patchy myocardial scarring. These cellular abnormalities contribute significantly to the common, and potentially catastrophic, dysrhythmias seen in these patients. HCM patients are prone to both atrial and ventricular dysrhythmias, with ventricular fibrillation as the most common cause of sudden death.

In the subset of patients with HOCM, hypertrophy occurs disproportionately in the ventricular septum. As the septum enlarges, it extends into and narrows the LVOT, whose borders are formed by the ventricular septum and the anterior leaflet of the mitral valve. During systole, there is further narrowing of the LVOT due to inward septal movement with ventricular contraction, leading to increased blood flow velocities and pressure gradients through the narrowed outflow tract. Rapid blood flow creates hydraulic forces (Venturi effect) capable of pulling the anterior mitral leaflet into the LVOT, causing further narrowing and obstruction. This abnormal systolic anterior motion (SAM) of the mitral valve leads to dynamic obstruction, in which the degree of obstruction varies based upon cardiac loading conditions and contractility. The obstruction occurs proximal to the aortic valve (subaortic) and occurs only in mid- to late systole. The degree of obstruction is directly proportional to LV contractility and inversely proportional to LV preload and afterload.

While dynamic LVOT obstruction is seen in only a subset of HCM patients, most of them exhibit diastolic dysfunction secondary to ventricular hypertrophy, as well as hypertrophy and disarray of the myocytes. Early diastolic filling is impaired secondary to this poor diastolic compliance, making atrial contraction, and thus maintenance of sinus rhythm, critical for adequate diastolic filling. Mitral regurgitation can be significant, as SAM does not allow for normal coaptation of the mitral valve, creating a regurgitant orifice as the anterior mitral valve leaflet is pulled into the LVOT. Mismatch of oxygen supply and demand is a frequent occurrence in HCM that predisposes to ischemia. The hypertrophied myocardium represents a large muscle mass and there is increased oxygen demand associated with elevated ventricular pressures and wall tension [3].

C. **Preoperative evaluation and assessment of severity.** Echocardiography allows for assessment of the location and severity of hypertrophy and helps determine the necessity and feasibility of potential surgical intervention. It demonstrates the degree of LVOT narrowing, as well as the presence or absence of SAM. Doppler measurements in the LVOT help determine the presence and severity of subaortic obstruction, with outflow gradients of >30 mm Hg representing significant obstruction. In addition to the mitral coaptation defect associated with

TABLE 12.3

	LV preload	Heart rate	Contractility	Systemic vascular resistance	Pulmonary vascular resistance
Dynamic subaortic stenosis	↑	↓	↓	↑	Maintain constant

SAM, the mitral apparatus itself may be abnormal in HCM patients and should be thoroughly examined. LV systolic function is typically normal or hyperdynamic and diastolic function is almost always abnormal.

D. **Timing and type of intervention.** The mainstay of medical therapy for HCM involves treatment with β-blockers, which help reduce LVOT obstruction due to their negative inotropic effects and reduction in heart rate. Calcium channel blockers are also frequently utilized for their favorable effect on diastolic compliance. The most critical intervention in patients identified as high risk for malignant dysrthythmias is placement of an automated implantable cardioverter-defibrillator. Other non-surgical approaches to decrease outflow obstruction include dual-chamber pacing and ethanol ablation of the ventricular septum. Surgical treatment involves removal of septal muscle tissue to widen the LVOT via septal myomectomy and may occasionally involve modification of the mitral valve apparatus or mitral valve repair/replacement.

E. **Goals of perioperative management**

1. **Hemodynamic profile** (Table 12.3)

   a. **LV preload.** Any condition that leads to a decrease in LV cavity size can potentially exacerbate dynamic LVOT obstruction, as this places the septum and anterior mitral leaflet in closer proximity, narrowing the outflow tract and increasing the potential for SAM and obstruction. In this regard, preload augmentation is essential to help maintain ventricular volume. Additionally, like in AS, diastolic dysfunction will lead to decreased LV compliance with increased LVEDP, which will necessitate adequate preload to maintain a normal stroke volume. Treatment with nitroglycerin, or other vasodilators, should be avoided as it may dangerously reduce cardiac output.

   b. **Heart rate.** It is essential to avoid tachycardia in patients with HCM because it leads to a reduction in ventricular volume, exacerbation of dynamic LVOT obstruction, and increased oxygen demand. Decreased heart rates are beneficial as this prolongs diastole and allows more time for ventricular filling. Maintenance of sinus rhythm is essential, as the atrial contraction component of ventricular filling is critical due to reduced early diastolic filling because of reduced LV compliance.

   c. **Contractility.** Decreases in myocardial contractility help reduce outflow obstruction. The β-blockade, volatile anesthetics, and avoidance of sympathetic stimulation are all beneficial. The use of intraoperative inotropic agents can increase contractility, worsen LVOT, lead to severe hemodynamic instability, and must be avoided.

   d. **Systemic vascular resistance.** Decreases in afterload must be promptly and aggressively treated with vasopressors such as phenylephrine or vasopressin. Hypotension can be especially detrimental in this population because diastolic dysfunction leads to increased LVEDP, requiring an increased blood pressure to provide adequate CPP:

   $$\text{CPP} = \text{Diastolic blood pressure (aorta)} - \text{LVEDP}$$

   e. **PVR.** PAPs remain relatively normal in this patient population. Special intervention for stabilizing PVR is not necessary.

2. **Anesthetic technique**

   a. **Premedication.** Many of these patients are on maintenance therapy with β-blockers or calcium channel blockers, which should be given on the day of surgery and continued throughout the perioperative period.

   b. **Induction and maintenance of anesthesia.** During induction and laryngoscopy, careful attention is required to avoid decreases in afterload, as well as sympathetic stimulation leading to increases in heart rate and contractility. Adequate preload must be maintained and all blood or fluid losses must be aggressively replaced. The direct myocardial depression of volatile anesthetics is advantageous.

c. **Patients with HCM** are at risk for atrial and ventricular tachyarrythmias during surgery. Preparation must be in place for immediate cardioversion or defibrillation.

d. **Intraoperative TEE,** like preoperative echocardiography, allows visualization of the location and extent of hypertrophy in the septum, the degree SAM, the degree of obstruction, and quantification of the degree of mitral regurgitation. Since CVP and PCWP measurements will overestimate true volume status, TEE is the most reliable means of accurately assessing volume. The ability to monitor LV systolic function and wall motion is useful, as the oxygen supply–demand relationship is tenuous in these patients, making them prone to ischemia. The adequacy of surgical repair and any post-repair complications can be immediately assessed.

e. **Postoperative care.** Potential complications in the immediate postoperative period following septal myomectomy include residual LVOT obstruction, residual SAM, residual mitral regurgitation, complete heart block, and the creation of a ventricular septal defect.

VII. Aortic regurgitation

A. Natural history

1. **Etiology.** Aortic insufficiency can be caused by aortic valve disease, aortic root dilation, or a combination of both [1]. Examples of causes of chronic aortic valve insufficiency include rheumatic fever, infective endocarditis, congenital bicuspid valve, and rheumatoid arthritis. Aortic root dilation can be caused by degenerative aortic dilation, syphilitic aortitis, Marfan's syndrome, and aortic dissection. Acute aortic insufficiency is usually caused by aortic dissection, trauma, or aortic valve endocarditis.

4 2. **Symptoms.** Patients with severe **acute aortic regurgitation** are not capable of maintaining sufficient FSV and often develop sudden and severe dyspnea, cardiovascular collapse, and deteriorate rapidly. Patients with **chronic aortic regurgitation** may be asymptomatic for many years. Symptoms such as shortness of breath, palpitations, fatigue, and angina usually develop after significant dilatation and dysfunction of the LV myocardium. The 10-yr mortality for asymptomatic aortic regurgitation varies between 5% and 15%. However, once symptoms develop, patients progressively deteriorate and have an expected survival of only 5 to 10 yrs.

B. Pathophysiology

1. **Pathophysiology and natural progression**

a. **Acute aortic regurgitation.** The sudden occurrence of acute aortic regurgitation places a major volume load on the LV. The immediate compensatory mechanism for the maintenance of adequate forward flow is increased sympathetic tone, producing tachycardia and an increased contractile state. Fluid retention increases preload. However, the combination of increased LVEDV and increased stroke volume and heart rate may not be sufficient to maintain a normal cardiac output. Rapid deterioration of LV function can occur, necessitating emergency surgical intervention.

b. **Chronic aortic regurgitation.** The onset of aortic regurgitation leads to LV systolic and diastolic volume overload. The increased volume load causes an increase in the size of the ventricular cavity, or eccentric ventricular hypertrophy. Because the LVEDV increases slowly, the LVEDP remains relatively normal. Forward flow is aided by the presence of chronic peripheral vasodilation, which occurs along with a large stroke volume in patients with mild aortic regurgitation. As the LV dilation and hypertrophy progresses, coronary perfusion finally decreases leading to irreversible LV myocardial tissue damage and dysfunction. The onset of LV dysfunction is followed by an increase in PAP with symptoms of dyspnea and congestive heart failure. As a compensatory mechanism for the poor cardiac output and poor coronary perfusion, sympathetic constriction of the periphery occurs to maintain blood pressure, which in turn leads to further decreases in cardiac output.

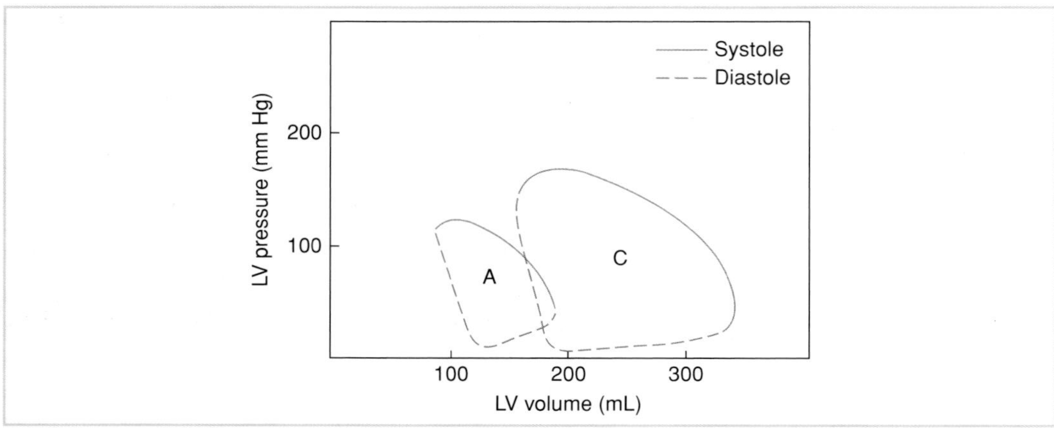

FIGURE 12.4 Pressure–volume loop in acute and chronic aortic regurgitation. Note the rightward shift of the loop in chronic aortic regurgitation (C), reflecting elevated LV volume without a dramatic elevation in filling pressure. In acute aortic regurgitation (A), LV volumes are also increased; however, the ventricle has not adapted to accommodate the increased volumes without elevation of filling pressures. [Modified from Jackson JM, Thomas SJ, Lowenstein E. Anesthetic management of patients with valvular heart disease. *Semin Anesth.* 1982;1:247.]

2. **Pressure wave disturbances**
   a. **Arterial pressure.** Incompetence of the aortic valve leads to regurgitant blood flow from the aorta back into the LV during diastole. This causes a pronounced decline in aortic diastolic blood pressure, translating into a wide pulse pressure. Patients with aortic regurgitation, therefore, show a wide pulse pressure with a rapid rate of rise, a high systolic peak, and a low diastolic pressure. The pulse pressure may be as great as 80 to 100 mm Hg. The rapid upstroke is due to the large stroke volume, and the rapid downstroke is due to the rapid flow of blood from the aorta back into the ventricle and into the dilated peripheral vessels. The occurrence of a double-peaked or bisferiens pulse trace is not unusual due to the occurrence of a "tidal" or backwave.
   b. **Pulmonary capillary wedge trace.** Stretching of the mitral valve annulus may lead to functional mitral regurgitation, a prominent V wave, and a rapid Y descent. In patients with acute aortic regurgitation associated with poor ventricular compliance, LV pressure may increase fast enough to close the mitral valve before end diastole. In this situation, the continued regurgitation of blood raises the LVEDP above left atrial pressure, and the PCWP can significantly underestimate the true LVEDP.
3. **Pressure–volume loop in aortic regurgitation** (Fig. 12.4)

C. **Assessment of severity**
1. Traditionally, the amount of aortic regurgitation is estimated based on angiocardiographic clearance of dye injected into the aortic root. Currently, echocardiography is the method of choice for qualitative, semiquantitative, and quantitative assessment of aortic regurgitation.
   a. **Echocardiographic assessment of aortic regurgitation**
   The severity of aortic regurgitation can be assessed with echocardiography by several qualitative, quantitative, and semiquantitative techniques (Table 12.4). Qualitative assessment includes the two-dimensional analysis of the aortic valve anatomy, with particular attention to any structural abnormalities of the leaflets. The aortic root and LV cavity should be closely examined for evidence of dilation. Color flow Doppler allows visualization of the regurgitant jet, originating at the aortic valve and extending back into the LVOT in diastole. An experienced echocardiographer can often accurately estimate the degree of regurgitation with this initial observation; however, quantitative measurements can be made to assess the severity more accurately. The vena contracta is perhaps the most widely utilized measurement. It represents the

TABLE 12.4

Grade	Mild	Moderate	Severe
Left ventricular size	Normal[a]	Normal or dilated	Usually dilated[b]
Jet deceleration rate/Pressure half-time (milliseconds)[c]	Slow (>500)	Medium (500–200)	Steep (<200)
Diastolic flow reversal in descending thoracic aorta	Brief, early diastolic reversal	Intermediate	Prominent holodiastolic reversal
Vena contracta width (cm)	<0.3	0.3–0.6	>0.6

Grade	Mild (1+)[d]	Mild–moderate (2+)	Moderate–severe (3+)	Severe (4+)
Jet width/LVOT width (%)	<25	25–45	46–64	≥65
Jet CSA/LVOT CSA (%)	<5	5–20	21–59	≥60
Regurgitant volume (mL/beat)	<30	30–44	45–59	≥60
Regurgitant fraction (%)	<30	30–39	40–49	≥50
EROA (cm^2)	<0.10	0.10–0.19	0.20–0.29	≥3.0

CSA, cross-sectional area; EROA, effective regurgitant orifice area.
[a]Unless there are other reasons for LV dilation.
[b]The LV is usually dilated in chronic aortic regurgitation. In acute aortic regurgitation, the LV size is often normal since the ventricle has not had time to dilate.
[c]Pressure half-time is shortened with increasing LV diastolic pressure and vasodilator therapy. It may be prolonged with chronic adaptation to severe aortic regurgitation.
[d]Note that there are several echocardiographic parameters that can subclassify regurgitation severity into mild, mild-moderate, moderate-severe, and severe. These subclassifications correspond to the angiographic grades of 1+, 2+, 3+, and 4+, respectively.
Adapted from: Bonow RO, Carabello BA, Chatterjee K, et al. ACC/AHA 2006 guidelines for the management of patients with valvular heart disease: a report of the American College of Cardiology/American Heart Association Task Force on Practice Guidelines (writing Committee to Revise the 1998 guidelines for the management of patients with valvular heart disease) developed in collaboration with the Society of Cardiovascular Anesthesiologists endorsed by the Society for Cardiovascular Angiography and Interventions and the Society of Thoracic Surgeons. *J Am Coll Cardiol.* 2006;48(3):e1–e148. and Zoghbi WA, Enriquez-Sarano M, Foster E, et al. Recommendations for evaluation of the severity of native valvular regurgitation with two-dimensional and Doppler echocardiography. *J Am Soc Echocardiogr.* 2003;16(7):777–802.

narrowest point of the regurgitant jet and corresponds to the size of the regurgitant orifice. It is a relatively easy measurement to obtain and is also not affected by changes in preload or afterload (Fig. 12.5). Severity of regurgitation can also be estimated by determining the extent to which the regurgitant jet occupies the LVOT. The ratio of jet width to LVOT width, or jet area to LVOT area, has been found to correlate

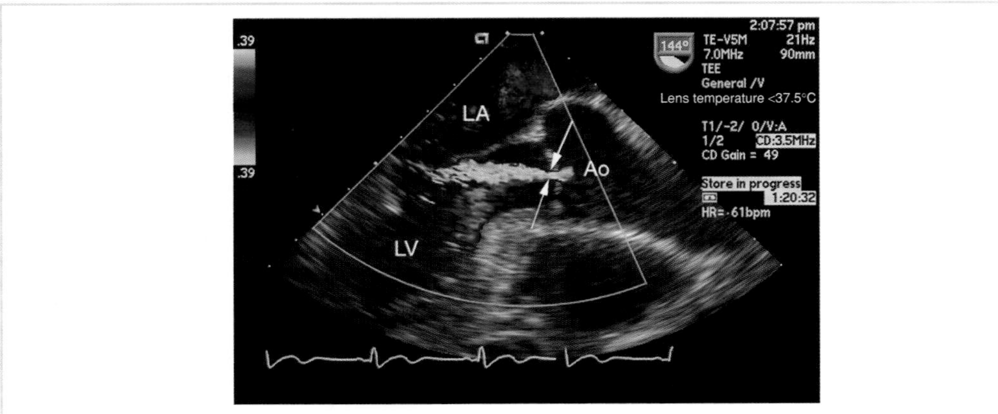

FIGURE 12.5 Vena Contracta. Caliper measurement of the narrowest portion of the aortic regurgitant jet, which corresponds to an approximation of the regurgitant orifice area. LA, Left atrium; LV, Left ventricle; Ao, aorta. [ECHO image from Perrino AC, Reeves ST, eds. *A Practical Approach to Transesophageal Echocardiography.* 2nd ed. Philadelphia, PA: Lippincott Williams & Wilkins, 2008:232, Figure 11.4.]

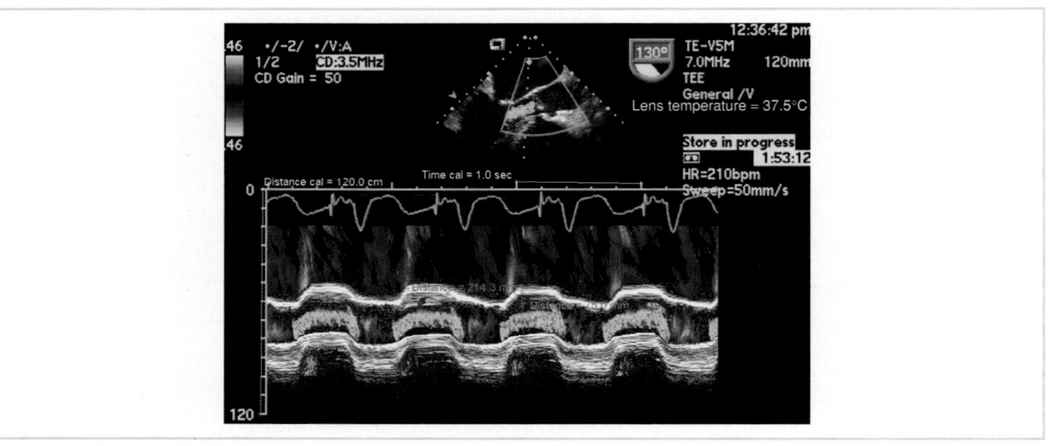

FIGURE 12.6 Color M-mode assessment of aortic regurgitation. Utilizing a midesophageal aortic long-axis view, the width of the regurgitant jet and the LVOT are measured. The ratio of jet width:LVOT width can be used to estimate the severity of the aortic regurgitation. [ECHO image from Perrino AC, Reeves ST, eds. *A Practical Approach to Transesophageal Echocardiography.* 2nd ed. Philadelphia, PA: Lippincott Williams & Wilkins, 2008:229, Figure 11.2.]

well with angiocardiographic assessment. (Fig. 12.6) Continuous-wave Doppler can be used to measure the deceleration rate of the regurgitant jet and the pressure half-time (PHT). These measurements are based on the rate of equilibration between aortic and LV pressures. As regurgitant severity increases (i.e., regurgitant orifice becomes larger), these pressures will equilibrate more quickly. Thus, significant aortic regurgitation corresponds to a steep slope of the jet deceleration rate and a short PHT. Severe aortic regurgitation may also be associated with holodiastolic flow reversal in the descending thoracic aorta seen on a pulsed-wave Doppler exam.

b. **Quantitative assessment of aortic regurgitation—calculation of regurgitant volume and RF.** A quantitative estimate of the severity of aortic regurgitation may be obtained by calculating the regurgitant volume and RF. The TSV in a patient with aortic regurgitation is the regurgitant volume plus the FSV actually ejected into the circulation. The regurgitant volume is the amount of blood that flows back through the incompetent aortic valve during each cardiac cycle. It is quantified as the difference between the TSV flowing through the aortic valve and the total FSV through a different valve. This reference valve is most commonly the mitral valve, with Doppler echocardiography being used to calculate the transmitral stoke volume. Total LV stroke volume can be determined with either Doppler echocardiography measurement of flow through the LV outflow tract or derived from left ventriculogram on cardiac catheterization. The RF, or fraction of each stroke volume flowing back into the LV, equals the ratio of the regurgitant volume to the TSV through the regurgitant aortic valve. These relationships can be summarized using the following equations:

$$\text{TSV} = \text{Regurgitant Volume} + \text{FSV}$$

$$\text{Regurgitant Volume} = \text{TSV} - \text{FSV}$$

$$\text{RF} = \text{Regurgitant Volume}/\text{TSV}$$

D. **Timing and type of intervention**

1. **Acute aortic regurgitation.** Urgent surgical intervention is often indicated in acute aortic regurgitation due to a high incidence of hemodynamic instability. Inotropic support is frequently needed to maintain cardiac output.
2. **Chronic aortic regurgitation.** Symptomatic patients with severe and moderately severe chronic aortic regurgitation should have surgery. Asymptomatic patients with severe and

TABLE 12.5

	LV Preload	Heart rate	Contractile state	Systemic vascular resistance	Pulmonary vascular resistance
Aortic regurgitation	↑	↑	Maintain	↓	Maintain

moderately severe chronic aortic regurgitation and normal LV function should be examined clinically and echocardiographically every 6 months. These patients should have surgical intervention at the earliest sign of LV dysfunction, as overall outcomes are significantly improved when surgery is performed prior to deterioration of ventricular function. Additionally, evidence of ventricular dilatation should prompt consideration for surgery, even in the presence of normal LV function. Patients with mild and moderate aortic regurgitation should be followed on a 12- to 24-month basis.

3. **Surgical intervention.** Surgical treatment of aortic regurgitation is most frequently provided through the use of valvular replacement with a prosthetic valve. However, techniques for surgical repair are becoming more widely accepted, with reports of an in-hospital mortality of 1%, late mortality rate of 4%, and the development of functional classifications of valve lesions to guide selection of surgical technique. Techniques include annuloplasty or commissural plication in the case of annular dilation, and leaflet resuspension or patch. [12]. Aortic valve repair may also be particularly beneficial in patients with aortic regurgitation secondary to bicuspid aortic valve disease, especially considering the younger age at which these patients typically present for surgical intervention. This avoids the need for anticoagulation following mechanical valve placement and may potentially provide more long-term valve integrity than a prosthetic valve. The long-term results of some of the more experimental techniques of aortic valve repair are still not known.

E. **Goals of perioperative management**

1. **Hemodynamic management** (Table 12.5)
   a. **LV preload.** Due to the increased LV volumes, maintenance of forward flow depends on preload augmentation. Pharmacologic intervention that produces venous dilation may significantly impair cardiac output in these patients by reducing preload.
   b. **Heart rate.** Patients with aortic regurgitation show a significant increase in forward cardiac output with an increase in heart rate. The decreased time spent in diastole during tachycardia leads to a decreased RF. Actual improvement in subendocardial blood flow is observed with tachycardia owing to a higher systemic diastolic pressure and a lower LVEDP. This explains why a patient who is symptomatic at rest may show an improvement in symptoms with exercise. A heart rate of 90 beats/min seems to be optimal, improving cardiac output while not inducing ischemia.
   c. **Contractility.** LV contractility must be maintained. In patients with impaired LV function, use of pure β-agonists or phosphodiesterase inhibitors can increase stroke volume through a combination of peripheral dilation and increased contractility.
   d. **Systemic vascular resistance.** The forward flow can be improved with afterload reduction. Increases in afterload result in increased stroke work and can significantly increase the LVEDP.
   e. **PVR.** Pulmonary vascular pressure remains relatively normal except in patients with end-stage aortic regurgitation associated with severe LV dysfunction.
2. **Anesthetic technique**
   a. **Premedication.** Light premedication is recommended.
   b. **Induction and maintenance.** Serious hemodynamic instability during induction of general anesthesia is less likely with severe aortic insufficiency than with severe AS because arterial vasodilation, which is a major effect of most of the induction drugs, is beneficial in aortic insufficiency and transient hypotension is well tolerated. However,

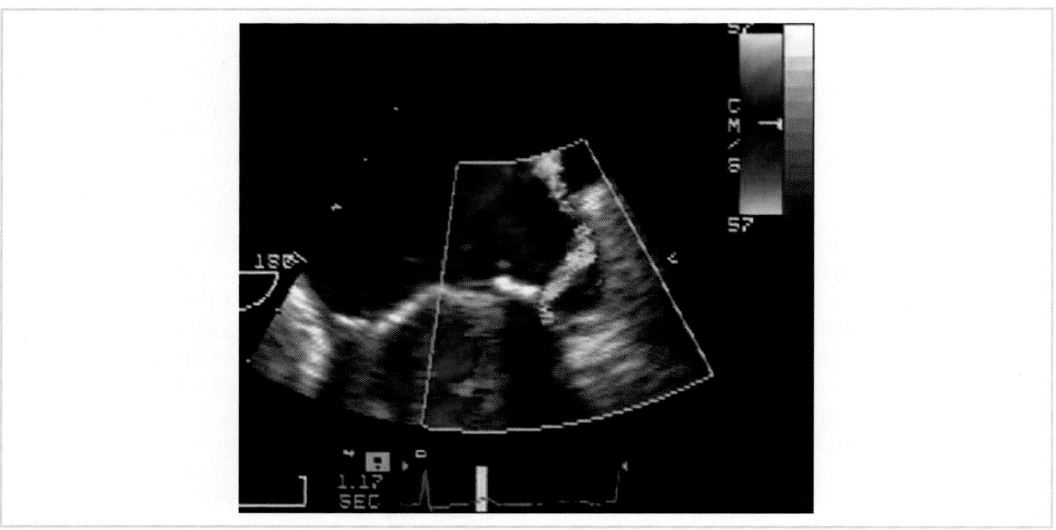

FIGURE 12.7 Color flow Doppler image of a mechanical bileaflet prosthetic valve in the mitral position with a paravalvular leak. [ECHO Image from Perrino AC, Reeves ST, eds. *A Practical Approach to Transesophageal Echocardiography.* 2nd ed. Philadelphia, PA: Lippincott Williams & Wilkins, 2008:271, Figure 13.14.]

the importance of careful titration of induction agents in combination with adequate hydration should not be underestimated. Particular caution is warranted with acute aortic insufficiency where ventricular decompensation is more likely to occur. The hemodynamic goals for induction and maintenance of anesthesia should be directed at preserving the patient's preload and contractility, maintaining the peripheral arterial dilation, and keeping the heart rate near 90 beats/min.

c. A pulmonary artery catheter is helpful in evaluating the cardiac output of patients prior to repair of the aortic valve and especially in the postbypass period for monitoring and optimizing preload and myocardial function.

d. **Omniplane TEE** is beneficial for monitoring LV function and assessment of the severity of regurgitation prior to valve repair. Specific pathology of the aortic valve leaflets and aortic root can be easily assessed. It is also useful in predicting the appropriate size of a prosthetic valve based on the diameters of the aortic annulus and LV outflow tract. If aortic valve repair is performed, TEE is valuable for providing immediate feedback concerning the integrity of valvular function. In AVR, TEE allows assessment of perivalvular regurgitation and the pressure gradient across the prosthetic valve (Fig. 12.7).

e. **Use of an intra-aortic balloon pump is contraindicated** in the presence of aortic regurgitation because augmentation of the diastolic pressure will increase the amount of regurgitant flow.

f. **Weaning from cardiopulmonary bypass** may be complicated by LV dysfunction secondary to suboptimal myocardial protection and coronary air embolism. AVR leads to a mild transvalvular gradient because a majority of prosthetic valves are intrinsically stenotic. Mild AS in combination with a significantly dilated LV may result in increased afterload, low cardiac output, and may contribute to the LV dysfunction. Inotropic support may be indicated in order to maintain cardiac output and avoid further LV dilation and dysfunction. Preload augmentation must be continued to maintain filling of the dilated LV.

3. **Postoperative care.** Immediately following AVR, the LVEDP and LVEDV decrease. However, the LV dilation and eccentric hypertrophy persist. In the early postoperative period, a decline in LV function may necessitate inotropic or intra-aortic balloon pump support. If surgical intervention is delayed until major LV dysfunction has occurred, the prognosis for long-term survival is not good. The 5-yr survival rate for patients whose

hearts do not return to a relatively normal size within 6 months following surgical repair is only 43%. If surgery is performed early enough, the heart will return to relatively normal dimensions, and a long-term survival rate of 85% to 90% after 6 yrs can be expected [3].

VIII. Mitral stenosis

A. Natural history

1. **Etiology.** In adults, mitral stenosis is predominately secondary to rheumatic heart disease, which leads to scarring and fibrosis of the free edges of the mitral valve leaflets. Rheumatic changes are present in 99% of surgically excised stenotic mitral valves [1]. Women are affected twice as frequently as men. Rheumatic heart disease commonly affects multiple cardiac valves and is often associated with both valvular stenosis and regurgitation.
2. **Symptoms.** In rheumatic mitral stenosis, patients are frequently asymptomatic for 20 yrs or more following an acute episode of rheumatic fever. However, as stenosis develops, symptoms appear, associated at first with exercise or high cardiac output states. Without surgical intervention, 20% of the patients, in whom the diagnosis of mitral stenosis is made, die within 1 yr and 50% die within 10 yrs following the diagnosis. The natural history is a slow, progressive downhill course with repeated episodes of fatigue, chest pains, palpitations, shortness of breath, paroxysmal nocturnal dyspnea, pulmonary edema, and hemoptysis, as well as hoarseness due to compression of the left recurrent laryngeal nerve by a distended left atrium and enlarged pulmonary artery. Symptoms often become apparent with the onset of atrial fibrillation, and patients in atrial fibrillation are at an increased risk of forming left atrial thrombi and subsequent cerebral or systemic emboli. Chest pain may occur in 10% to 20% of patients with mitral stenosis. However, it is a poor predictor of the coexistence of CAD, probably because symptoms also may be caused by coronary thromboembolism or pulmonary hypertension.

B. Pathophysiology

1. **Natural progression.** The normal mitral valve is composed of anterior and posterior leaflet, with an area of 4 to 6 cm^2 (mitral valve index: 4 to 4.5 cm^2/m^2). When the valve area decreases to <2.5 cm^2 (or valve index to less than 2 cm^2/m^2), moderate exercise may induce dyspnea. Further progression of mitral stenosis leads to increases in left atrial pressure and volume that are reflected back into the pulmonary circuit. Increased left atrial pressure results in atrial enlargement, which predisposes these patients to atrial fibrillation. Between a valve area of 1 to 1.5 cm^2, increasing symptoms appear with mild to moderate exertion. Severe congestive failure can be induced either by the onset of atrial fibrillation or by a variety of disease processes leading to high cardiac output states such as thyrotoxicosis, pregnancy, anemia, or fever. In all these conditions, the left atrial and PAPs suddenly rise as a result of the increased cardiac demand. Because atrial contraction contributes about 30% of LV filling in mitral stenosis, the onset of atrial fibrillation can lead to significant impairment in cardiac output. With a valve area below 1 cm^2, a patient is considered to have severe mitral stenosis, and symptoms are present even at rest. Not only are left atrial pressures sufficient to produce congestive heart failure, but cardiac output may also be reduced. The increase in PVR in response to a high left atrial pressure can eventually lead to RV dilation and failure. PA constriction, pulmonary intimal hyperplasia, and pulmonary medial hypertrophy eventually result in chronic PA hypertension associated with restrictive lung disease. The dilated RV can cause a leftward shift of the interventricular septum, thereby limiting the already reduced LV size and further impairing stroke volume. With further RV dilation, TR results, leading to signs of peripheral congestion. A mitral valve area of 0.3 to 0.4 cm^2 is the smallest area compatible with life.
2. **Intracardiac hemodynamics and cardiac remodeling.** Due to the restriction of flow from the left atrium to the left ventricle, patients with significant mitral stenosis have a reduced LVEDV and LVEDP. Stroke volume is also reduced. The actual LV contractility is usually normal, but may be reduced due to chronic LV deconditioning. The limitation of stroke volume in these patients is due to inadequate filling of the LV. Patients with severe mitral stenosis typically have a dilated left atrium, normal or diminished LV size, and a dilated RV and right atrium.

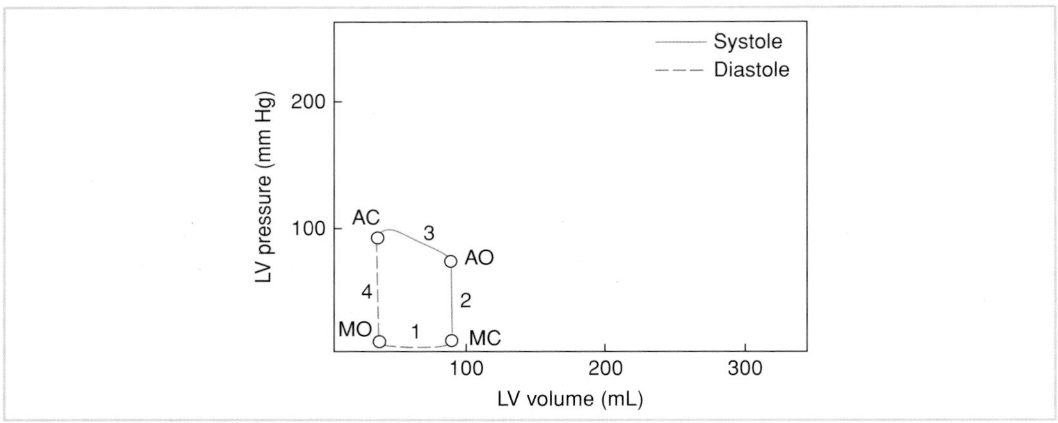

FIGURE 12.8 Pressure–volume loop in mitral stenosis. Both end-diastolic and end-systolic volumes, as well as LV filling pressures, are reduced, resulting in a decreased stroke volume. AO, aortic valve opening; MC, mitral valve closure; MO, mitral valve opening. Phase 1, Ventricular filling; Phase 2, Isovolumetric contraction; Phase 3, Ventricular ejection; Phase 4, Isovolumetric relaxation. [Modified from Jackson JM, Thomas SJ, Lowenstein E. Anesthetic management of patients with valvular heart disease. *Semin Anesth.* 1982;1:244.]

3. **Pressure wave disturbances.** Mitral stenosis produces a large A wave on the PCWP tracing in patients with preserved sinus rhythm. If the mitral stenosis is associated with mitral regurgitation, a prominent V wave is also present. With increased impairment of left atrial contractility secondary to severe mitral obstruction, the A wave may become small. In the presence of atrial fibrillation, the A wave is obviously absent.
4. **Pressure–volume loop in mitral stenosis** (Fig. 12.8).
5. **TEE findings.** Patients with rheumatic mitral stenosis exhibit several characteristic echocardiographic findings. The valve leaflets appear thickened, calcified, and have limited mobility (Fig. 12.9). In particular, the body of the anterior mitral valve leaflet exhibits diastolic doming and is often described as having a "hockey-stick" appearance. Additional findings may include mitral regurgitation and left atrial enlargement. Spontaneous echo

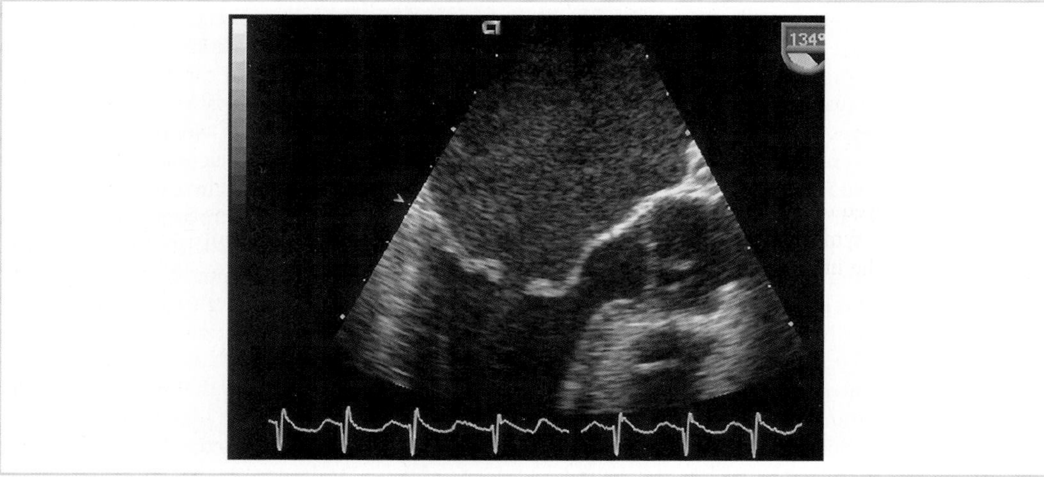

FIGURE 12.9 Classic echocardiographic appearance of rheumatic mitral stenosis, including thickened mitral leaflets with diastolic doming of the anterior leaflet. [ECHO Image from Perrino AC, Reeves ST, eds. *A Practical Approach to Transesophageal Echocardiography.* 2nd ed. Philadelphia, PA: Lippincott Williams & Wilkins, 2008:192, Figure 9.3.]

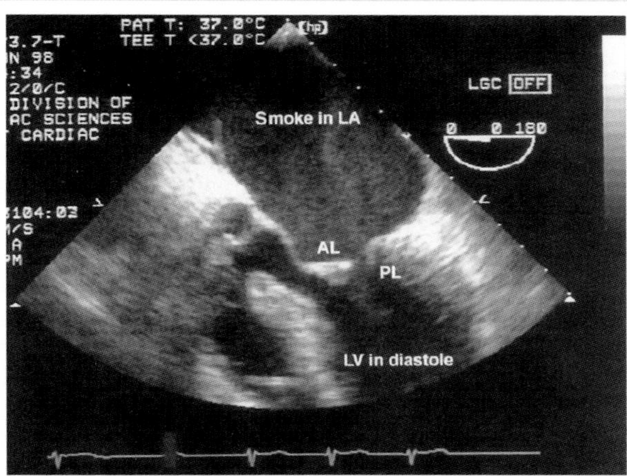

FIGURE 12.10 Mitral stenosis. The left atrium is significantly enlarged, with spontaneous echo contrast ("smoke") demonstrating low flow state. LA, Left atrium; LV, Left ventricle; AL, Anterior leaflet; PL, Posterior leaflet. [ECHO Image from Perrino AC, Reeves ST, eds. *A Practical Approach to Transesophageal Echocardiography.* 2nd ed. Philadelphia, PA: Lippincott Williams & Wilkins, 2008:217, Figure 10.10.]

contrast, indicating a low flow state in the enlarged left atrium, is frequently seen and should prompt examination for thrombus formation (Fig. 12.10). The most likely location for atrial thrombus is the left atrial appendage.

C. **Assessment of severity** of mitral stenosis can be done by the calculation of mitral valve area or a diastolic pressure gradient across the mitral valve using echocardiography or, infrequently, cardiac catheterization. Assessment of mitral stenosis by the pressure gradient is less accurate than the area method because pressure gradient depends on transmitral flow (Table 12.6).

Mitral stenosis severity can also be graded by the PHT method, in which prolongation of the PHT correlates with a reduction in mitral valve orifice area. A normal PHT, measured with continuous wave Doppler, is relatively short, corresponding to rapid early diastolic filling of the LV and the associated rapid decline in the LA to LV pressure gradient during this early filling phase. Since this LA to LV pressure gradient remains elevated for a longer period in mitral stenosis, the PHT will become more prolonged as the degree of stenosis worsens [13]. A PHT greater than 220 ms corresponds to severe mitral stenosis, as the valve area will be less than 1.0 cm^2 as seen by the following equation:

$$\text{Mitral valve area} = 220/\text{PHT}$$

D. **Timing and type of intervention.** Surgical intervention should occur prior to the development of severe symptoms because irreversible ventricular dysfunction may result if surgery is delayed too long. Surgery is not recommended for the asymptomatic patient. In patients with mild symptoms, the decision about surgical intervention should be individualized and based on the lifestyle desired, mitral valve orifice size, evidence of systemic embolization, and risk of the procedure. The presence and severity of pulmonary hypertension should also guide the

TABLE 12.6

Grade	Mild	Moderate	Severe
Mitral valve area (cm^2)	>1.5	1.0–1.5	<1.0
Mean pressure gradient (mm Hg)	<5	5–10	>10
Pressure half-time (milliseconds)	90–150	150–219	>220

Adapted from: Baumgartner H, Hung J, Bermejo J, et al. Echocardiographic assessment of valve stenosis: EAE/ASE recommendations for clinical practice. *J Am Soc Echocardiogr.* 2009;22:1–23.

TABLE 12.7

	LV preload	Heart rate	Contractile state	Systemic vascular resistance	Pulmonary vascular resistance
Mitral stenosis	↑	↓	Maintain	Maintain	↓

decision-making process. Surgical intervention is likely warranted once the pulmonary artery systolic pressure exceeds 50 mm Hg [4]. Four types of interventions are available for rheumatic mitral stenosis: (i) Mitral valve replacement, (ii) open mitral commissurotomy, (iii) closed commisurotomy, and (iv) balloon mitral valvuloplasty. Closed mitral comissurotomy can be performed without cardiopulmonary bypass in a carefully selected group of patients without atrial thrombosis, significant valvular calcification, or chordal fusion. It is rarely done in the United States, being almost completely replaced by the balloon mitral valvuloplasty. Balloon mitral valvuloplasty is performed by interventional cardiologists in the cardiac catheterization laboratory. It consists of the advancement of a balloon catheter through the interatrial septum and its inflation at the mitral orifice. This procedure may be complicated by severe mitral regurgitation, systemic embolism, and residual atrial septal defect. Commissurotomy and balloon mitral valvuloplasty do not totally relieve the stenosis, but rather make it less severe. In addition, they carry significant risk of restenosis. Nevertheless, they can delay the ultimate procedure. During this time, the patient does not require anticoagulation and is at risk for less morbidity than with an indwelling prosthetic valve. If the valve is not amenable to balloon mitral valvuloplasty or commissurotomy, mitral valve replacement should be performed. When chronic atrial fibrillation is present, scar tissue can be created surgically in the left atrium during open heart surgery in order to disrupt re-entry circuits of atrial fibrillation in what is called maze procedure.

E. **Goals of perioperative management**

1. **Hemodynamic management** (Table 12.7)

a. **LV preload.** Forward flow across the stenotic mitral valve is dependent on adequate preload. On the other hand, patients with mitral stenosis already have elevated left atrial pressures and are prone to pulmonary vascular congestion, so that overly aggressive use of fluids can easily send a patient who is in borderline congestive heart failure into florid pulmonary edema. Intraoperative TEE is often the best method to assess volume status. However, other invasive monitoring techniques (i.e., the pulmonary artery catheter) can also be used.

b. **Heart rate.** Blood flow across the mitral valve occurs during ventricular diastole, so slower heart rates are hemodynamically beneficial. At the same time, excessive bradycardia can be dangerous because stroke volume is relatively fixed.

If atrioventricular pacing is initiated in these patients, a long PR interval of 0.15 to 0.20 ms is optimal to allow blood adequate time, after atrial contraction, to cross the stenotic mitral valve. Decreases in the PR interval will drop diastolic flow and result in reduced cardiac output.

c. **Contractility.** Adequate forward flow depends on adequate RV and LV contractility. Chronic underfilling of the LV, however, may lead to a deconditioning with depressed ventricular contractility even in the face of restored filling. In end-stage mitral stenosis, depression of LV contractility may lead to severe congestive heart failure. Depression of RV contractility limits left atrial filling and, eventually, cardiac output. Many patients will require inotropic support before and especially after cardiopulmonary bypass.

d. **Systemic vascular resistance.** To maintain blood pressure in the presence of a limited cardiac output, patients with mitral stenosis usually develop an increased systemic vascular resistance. Afterload reduction is not helpful in improving forward flow because the limiting factor for cardiac output is the stenotic mitral valve. It is recommended that the afterload be kept in the normal range for these patients.

5 e. **PVR.** These patients frequently have elevated PVR and are prone to exaggerated pulmonary vasoconstriction in the presence of hypoxia. Particular attention should be

paid to avoiding any increases in PAP due to inadequate anesthesia or inadvertent acidosis, hypercapnia, or hypoxemia.

2. **Anesthetic technique**
   a. **Premedication** should be light to avoid either an acute decrease in preload or the possibility of oversedation with resultant hypoxemia and hypercapnia, with subsequent exacerbation of any preexisting pulmonary hypertension. Use of cardioversion is recommended if new atrial fibrillation should occur.
   b. **Pulmonary artery catheters** are useful for perioperative management. However, because of dilated pulmonary arteries, special care should be taken in the placement of these catheters due to the increased risk of pulmonary artery rupture. Because of the risk of pulmonary artery rupture and the questionable information obtained from a wedge pressure, placement of the pulmonary artery catheter in a wedge position is usually not necessary.
   c. **TEE evaluation** is particularly helpful in monitoring the adequacy of mitral valve repair. Mitral commissurotomy may result in significant mitral regurgitation, which can be identified in the immediate postbypass period in order to provide further surgical intervention for the patient. In addition, complications associated with mitral valve replacement, such as paravalvular regurgitation and SAM of the anterior mitral valve leaflet, may also be rapidly identified and repaired while still in the operating room. TEE is also helpful for the assessment of the RV and LV loading conditions and contractility.
   d. **Immediately following cardiopulmonary bypass,** even patients with seemingly normal preoperative LV function may have major depression of myocardial contractility due to their underlying myocardial dysfunction exacerbated by ischemic arrest. Subsequently, volume therapy should be used carefully to avoid LV and RV failures. Inotropes and pressors may be required to maintain cardiac output and to avoid volume overload. In patients previously in chronic atrial fibrillation, especially after the maze procedure, prophylactic use of amiodarone is indicated.
3. **Postoperative course.** In spite of the fact that following prosthetic valve placement, a mean pressure gradient of 4 to 7 mm Hg across the mitral valve persists, successful surgical intervention leads to a drop in PVR, PAP, and left atrial pressure while increasing cardiac output in the first postoperative day. PVR in most patients will continue to decrease with time following surgery. Failure of the PAP to decrease is usually indicative of irreversible pulmonary hypertension and/or irreversible LV dysfunction, either of which places the patient in a prognostically poor group.

IX. Mitral regurgitation

A. **Natural history.** The spectrum of mitral regurgitation varies from acute forms, in which rapid deterioration of myocardial function can occur, to chronic forms that have slow indolent courses. Mitral regurgitation may result from mitral valve leaflet abnormalities, mitral annulus dilation, chordate rupture, papillary muscle disorder, global LV dysfunction, or disproportional LV enlargement [1].

1. **Acute mitral regurgitation.** Acute mitral regurgitation may result from papillary muscle dysfunction due to myocardial ischemia, or papillary muscle rupture due to myocardial infarction or blunt chest trauma. Chordae tendineae rupture can be caused by myxomatous disease of the mitral valve or acute rheumatic fever. A mitral valve leaflet can acutely deteriorate as a result of infective endocarditits, balloon valvuloplasty, or a penetrating chest injury.
2. **Chronic mitral regurgitation**
   a. **Mitral annulus dilatation** may result from LV dilatation due to dilated or ischemic cardiomyopathy or aortic insufficiency. It can also develop from left atrial enlargement in patients with diastolic dysfunction, e.g., AS or systemic hypertension. Finally, mitral annulus dilatation will eventually exacerbate mitral regurgitation of any other cause secondary to left atrial and LV enlargement and stretching of the annulus.
   b. **Disorders of mitral leaflets** include mitral valve prolapse that may be idiopathic or caused by rheumatic fever or myxomatous degeneration; mitral leaflet damage by

infective endocarditis; and restrictive changes due to thickening or calcification from any inflammatory or degenerative processes. Restriction can also be caused by disproportional enlargement of the LV in relation to papillary muscles and chordae tendineae causing incomplete mitral valve closure. This occurs in a majority of cases of ischemic mitral regurgitation.

c. **Disorders of subvalvular apparatus.** Rupture or elongation of chordae tendineae may occur in myxomatous degeneration. Rheumatic heart disease may lead to chordae tendineae rupture, thickening, and calcium deposition in subvalvular apparatus. Depending on the type and number of chordae ruptured, subsequent mitral regurgitation may range from acute to chronic and from mild to severe.

d. **Functional mitral regurgitation.** Mitral regurgitation that occurs in the setting of normal leaflets and chordal structures is frequently due to functional mitral regurgitation. This phenomenon is not fully understood, but is most likely the result of global LV dysfunction, which results in disruption of the normal geometric relationship between the mitral valve leaflets, papillary muscles, and LV. The LV dysfunction results in ventricular dilatation and a more spherical appearance of the LV, which ultimately disrupts the normal structure and function of the entire mitral apparatus [13]. Ischemic mitral regurgitation is a type of functional mitral regurgitation that is caused by ischemic heart disease.

3. **Carpentier classification.** This widely recognized classification scheme is used to describe differing mechanisms of mitral regurgitation based upon the leaflet motion of the valve (Table 12.8) [14].

B. **Pathophysiology**

1. **Natural progression**

a. **Acute.** Sudden development of mitral regurgitation leads to marked left atrial volume overload. Because of the normal compliance of the left atrium, the sudden volume overload leads to significant increases in left atrial pressure that are passed on to the pulmonary circuit. As immediate compensation for a decreased cardiac output, sympathetic stimulation increases ventricular contractility and produces tachycardia. In addition, the LV functions on a higher portion of the Frank–Starling curve owing to increased LV volume. Increased LV volume leads to increased LVEDP, which in combination with tachycardia can cause ischemia and LV dysfunction. The acute increases in left atrial and PAPs can lead to pulmonary congestion, pulmonary edema, and RV failure. Thus, acute mitral regurgitation often presents as biventricular failure.

b. **Chronic.** During the slow development of chronic mitral regurgitation, left atrial dilatation and eccentric hypertrophy of the LV develops. At early stages, the dilation of the LV allows the preservation of a relatively normal LVEDP despite a markedly increased LVEDV. The forward cardiac output is preserved by an overall increase in total LV stroke volume (combined FSV and regurgitant stroke volume). Left atrial enlargement, however, may lead to the development of atrial fibrillation. In addition, continued left atrial dilation may lead to further increases in regurgitation due to stretching of the mitral annulus. Continued worsening of regurgitation results in an increase in PAP, pulmonary congestion, and eventually RV failure. When LV dilation and hypertrophy

TABLE 12.8

Carpentier classification	Mitral valve motion	Common causes
I	Normal	• Mitral annulus dilation • Leaflet destruction (endocarditis) • Leaflet perforation or cleft
II	Excessive	• Leaflet prolapse • Flail leaflet
IIIa	Restricted abnormal leaflets	• Rheumatic valve disease
IIIb	Restricted normal leaflets	• Dilated left ventricle

can no longer compensate for increasing regurgitation, the FSV is eventually compromised. At this point, the symptoms of forward heart failure, including increased fatigability and generalized weakness, may appear. LV ejection fraction is elevated in patients with mitral regurgitation because of the ease of ejecting blood backward into the low-pressure pulmonary circuit. An ejection fraction of 50% or less indicates the presence of significant ventricular dysfunction in these patients. The depression of ventricular function may become irreversible even after mitral valve replacement.

2. **Intracardiac hemodynamics and remodeling.** In acute mitral regurgitation, LVEDP increases rapidly to dilate the left atrium and maintain stroke volume. In contrast, in chronic mitral regurgitation, compensatory dilation occurs slowly and the LVEDP may remain relatively normal until the disease is far advanced. The eccentric hypertrophy of the ventricle allows preservation of FSV by increasing TSV.
3. **Pressure wave disturbances.** On pulmonary capillary wedge tracing, the size of the regurgitant wave, or "giant V wave," depends on the compliance of the left atrium, the compliance of the pulmonary vasculature, the amount of pulmonary venous return, and the regurgitant volume. In patients with sudden onset of mitral regurgitation, a relatively noncompliant left atrium leads to large V waves. Patients with chronic mitral regurgitation have a large compliant left atrium that can accept the regurgitant volume without passing the pressure wave on to the pulmonary circuit.
4. **Pressure–volume loop in mitral regurgitation** (Fig. 12.11).
5. **TEE.** The baseline TEE exam in the operating room should focus on identifying the specific underlying pathology. A thorough examination of the structure and function of the leaflets is critical, as is a close examination of the subvalvular apparatus and LV function and shape (Fig. 12.12). This initial intraoperative assessment is often needed by the surgeon to help formulate the ultimate surgical plan (i.e., in determining whether the mitral valve is suitable for an attempt at valve repair). If mitral repair is to be attempted, the baseline TEE exam should focus on identifying any predictors of post-repair SAM, which is a noted complication of this procedure. The ratio of the anterior leaflet to posterior mitral leaflet, expressed as the **AL:PL ratio**, should be assessed. A longer posterior leaflet will push the normal leaflet coaptation point toward the LVOT and increase the risk of post-repair SAM. This distance between the coaptation point and the LVOT, at the border of the anterior ventricular septum, is called C-sept distance and should also be measured.

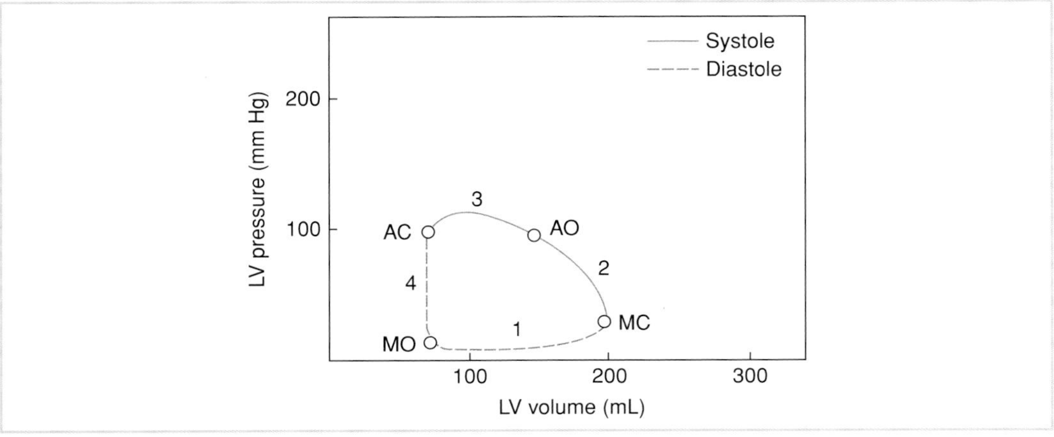

FIGURE 12.11 Pressure–volume loop in acute and chronic mitral regurgitation. With chronic mitral regurgitation, end-diastolic volume is elevated without significant elevation of LV filling pressures. In contrast, with acute mitral regurgitation LVEDV is increased, but is accompanied by an increase in LV filling pressure. AC, aortic valve closure; AO, aortic valve opening; MC, mitral valve closure; MO, mitral valve opening. Phase 1, ventricular filling; Phase 2, isovolumetric contraction; Phase 3, ventricular ejection; Phase 4, isovolumetric relaxation. [Modified from Jackson JM, Thomas SJ, Lowenstein E. Anesthetic management of patients with valvular heart disease. *Semin Anesth.* 1982;1:248.]

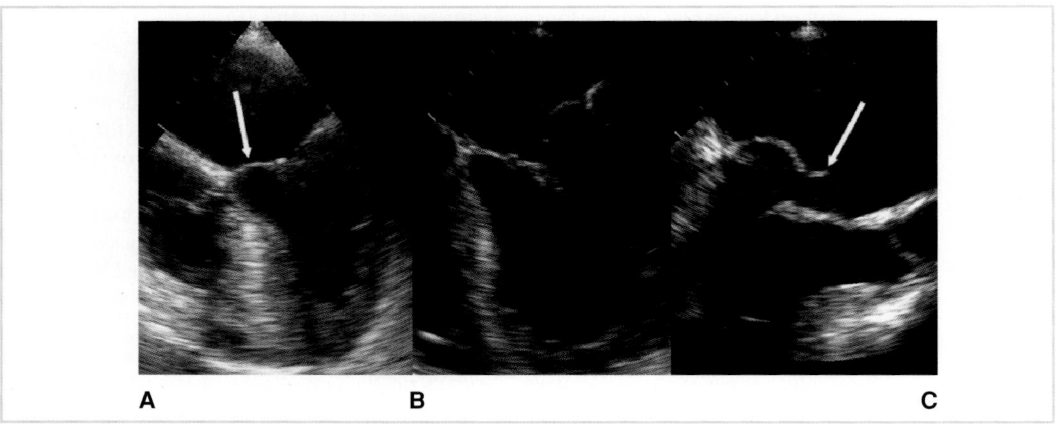

FIGURE 12.12 The 2D images of excessive mitral valve motion. **A:** billowing. **B:** prolapse. **C:** Flail. [Echo Image from Perrino AC, Reeves ST, eds. *A Practical Approach to Transesophageal Echocardiography.* 2nd ed. Philadelphia, PA: Lippincott Williams & Wilkins, 2008:175, Figure 8.4.]

Assessing the severity of mitral regurgitation is not always reliable in the operating room setting, as the severity of mitral regurgitation may be significantly underestimated under the altered loading conditions of general anesthesia. In this regard, it is more appropriate to grade the severity of mitral regurgitation using the preoperative echo exam as opposed to an exam performed under general anesthesia [13].

C. **Assessment of severity.** As with aortic regurgitation, estimation of mitral regurgitation by angiocardiographic dye clearance has been almost completely replaced by echocardiography.

1. **Echocardiographic assessment of mitral regurgitation** (Table 12.9)
2. **Quantitative assessment of mitral regurgitation—calculation of RF** (Fig. 12.13). A quantitative estimate of the severity of mitral regurgitation may be obtained by calculation of the regurgitant volume and RF. As for patients with aortic regurgitation, RF is defined as a fraction of regurgitant volume in relation to TSV. FSV can be obtained by thermodilution from a PA catheter or by measurement of stroke volume in the LV outflow tract by echocardiogram with Doppler (in the absence of aortic regurgitation). Total LV stroke volume can be derived from the LV angiogram or measured by echocardiogram with Doppler as the diastolic volume of blood flowing through the mitral valve, and the regurgitant volume and RF calculated as for aortic regurgitation.

   Mitral regurgitation consisting of less than 30% of the total LV stroke volume is considered mild, 30% to 39% is considered moderate, 40% to 49% is considered moderately severe, and greater than 50% is considered severe.

TABLE 12.9

Grade	Mild	Moderate	Severe	
LA size	Normal	Normal or dilated	Usually dilated	
LV size	Normal	Normal or dilated	Usually dilated	
Vena contracta width (cm)	<0.3	0.3–0.69	≥0.7	
Grade	**Mild**	**Mild-moderate**	**Moderate-severe**	**Severe**
Regurgitant volume (mL/beat)	<30	30–44	45–59	≥60
Regurgitant fraction (%)	<30	30–39	40–49	≥50
Effective regurgitant orifice area (cm^2)	<0.20	0.20–0.29	0.30–0.39	≥0.40

Adapted from: Zoghbi WA, Enriquez-Sarano M, Foster E, et al. Recommendations for evaluation of the severity of native valvular regurgitation with two-dimensional and Doppler echocardiography. *J Am Soc Echocardiogr.* 2003;16(7):777–802.

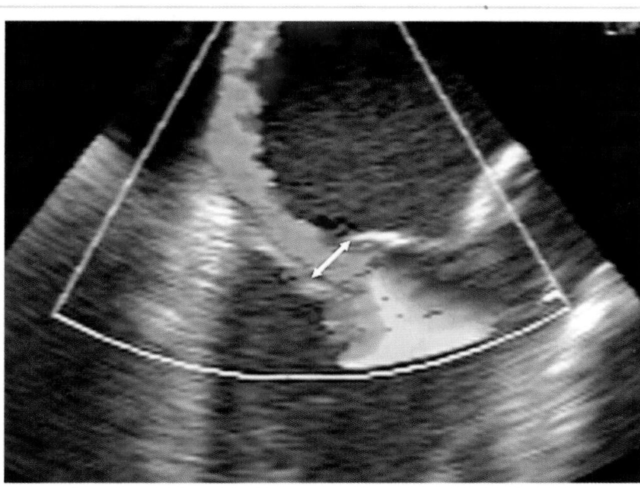

FIGURE 12.13 Vena contracta. Measurement of the narrowest portion of the color flow Doppler jet (*arrow*) corresponds to the severity of mitral regurgitation. [ECHO Image from Perrino AC, Reeves ST, eds. *A Practical Approach to Transesophageal Echocardiography.* 2nd ed. Philadelphia, PA: Lippincott Williams & Wilkins, 2008:176, Figure 8.5.]

D. **Surgical intervention** for mitral regurgitation involves either mitral valve repair or replacement, with many now recommending an attempt at mitral valve repair whenever feasible, assuming the surgeon has appropriate expertise in valve repair surgery and that the mitral valve appears suitable for repair. Benefits of mitral valve repair over replacement include avoidance of chronic anticoagulation (with mechanical valves) and future reoperation for prosthetic valve failure (with bioprosthetic valves). Perhaps more importantly, LV function is better preserved following valve repair. The mitral valve support apparatus is a critical structural and functional component to the left ventricle and any disruption of this apparatus, as can occur during mitral valve replacement, can lead to LV dysfunction. Since mitral repair leaves the mitral apparatus intact, this cause of LV failure can be avoided.

Surgery should be strongly considered in symptomatic patients with New York Heart Association (NYHA) Class II heart failure and/or chronic or recurrent atrial fibrillation resulting from mitral regurgitation. In asymptomatic patients, the benefits of surgery must be weighed carefully against the benefits of waiting. The decision is made based on the presence of LV enlargement, dysfunction, and pulmonary hypertension, with the onset of LV dysfunction being the most important indicator for surgery in asymptomatic patients [15]. When in doubt, stress echo can be done to search for latent LV dysfunction. If chances of repair are good, early surgery is recommended because good long-term results are likely and anticoagulation is not needed. If CABG is indicated and at least moderate ischemic mitral regurgitation is present, mitral valve repair/replacement at the same time as CABG is beneficial. In this scenario, successful mitral valve repair is often straightforward, requiring only placement of an annuloplasty ring [16].

1. **Mitral valve repairability.** In general, mitral valve lesions that are relatively easy to repair include leaflet perforation, mitral valve annulus dilatation, and excessive motion of mitral valve leaflets. Among difficult-to-repair conditions are restricted leaflet motion, severe calcification, and active infection. The greatest likelihood for successful repair involves isolated lesions of the posterior mitral valve leaflet. Pathology of the anterior leaflet only or both mitral leaflets presents a significantly greater challenge to the surgeon and minimizes the chances for successful repair (Table 12.10).

E. **Goals of perioperative management**

1. **Hemodynamic management** (Table 12.11)
   a. **LV preload.** Augmentation and maintenance of preload is frequently helpful to ensure adequate FSV. Unfortunately, a universal recommendation for preload augmentation

TABLE 12.10 Mitral valve repair techniques for specific lesions

Repair technique	Indication
Ring annuloplasty	Mitral valve annulus dilatation, ischemic MR with minimal downward displacement of the coaptation point
Quadrangular resection of the posterior leaflet central portion	Central posterior leaflet prolapsed
Chordae tendinae transfer, artificial chordae, often combined with triangular resection	Central anterior leaflet prolapsed
Paracommissural closure	Paracommissural prolapse of anterior or posterior mitral valve leaflet

cannot be made because, in some patients, dilation of the left atrial and LV compartments dilates the mitral valve annulus and increases the RF. A decision about the best level of preload augmentation for an individual patient should be based on that patient's hemodynamic and clinical response to a fluid load.

6

b. **Heart rate.** Bradycardia is harmful in patients with mitral regurgitation because it leads to an increase in LV volume, reduction in forward cardiac output, and an increase in RF. The heart rate should be kept in the normal to elevated range in these patients. Atrial contribution to preload is important in patients with mitral regurgitation, but not as critical as in those with stenotic lesions. Many of these patients, particularly those with chronic mitral regurgitation, will come to the operating room in atrial fibrillation.

c. **Contractility.** Maintenance of FSV is dependent on systolic function of the eccentrically hypertrophied LV. Depression of myocardial contractility can lead to major LV dysfunction and clinical deterioration. Inotropic agents that increase contractility have a tendency to provide increased forward flow and can actually decrease regurgitation due to constriction of the mitral annulus.

d. **Systemic vascular resistance.** An increase in afterload leads to an increase in RF and reduction in systemic cardiac output. For this reason, careful afterload reduction is normally desired.

e. **PVR.** Patients with severe mitral regurgitation develop elevated pulmonary pressure secondary to increased PVR, as well as elevated left atrial pressure. The importance of each component in elevating PAP can be determined by calculating PVR using the following formula:

$$\text{PVR} = 80 * (\text{mean PAP} - \text{PCWP})/\text{CO}$$

PVR = pulmonary vascular resistance

80 = the conversion factor to dynes.sec/cm^5

PAP = pulmonary artery pressure

PCWP = pulmonary capillary wedge pressure

CO = cardiac output

If elevated PVR is present, caution must be taken to avoid hypercapnia, hypoxia, nitrous oxide, and light anesthesia that might lead to pulmonary constrictive responses.

TABLE 12.11

	LV preload	Heart rate	Contractile state	Systemic vascular resistance	Pulmonary vascular resistance
Mitral regurgitation	↑ or ↓	↑, maintain	Maintain	↓	↓

2. **Anesthetic management**
   a. **Premedication.** Light premedication is indicated.
   b. **Induction and maintenance of general anesthesia.** As with aortic insufficiency, the hemodynamic goals for induction and maintenance of anesthesia should be directed to maintaining peripheral arterial dilation, ventricular contractility, and keeping the heart rate close to 90 beats/min. Careful titration of narcotics, hypnotics, and volatile anesthetics are usually well tolerated. Tracheal intubation in inadequately anesthetized patients may lead to a sudden rise in arterial blood pressure followed by a dramatic increase in RF and, subsequently, pulmonary edema.
   c. **Pulmonary artery catheters** are helpful in guiding fluid management and in the timely detection and treatment of hemodynamic conditions associated with elevated PAP. These conditions include (a) sudden increase in RF (e.g., from LV ischemia or vasoconstriction resulting from inadequate depth of anesthesia) as well as (b) PA vasoconstriction. Nitric oxide, as a specific pulmonary artery dilator, may have an important role in the management of patients with reversible pulmonary hypertension. Hyperventilation, but with minimum increases in intrathoracic pressure, is a second therapeutic modality available for selectively dilating the pulmonary vasculature without affecting the patient's systemic blood pressure. Prostaglandin E1 has also been used but is accompanied by a decrease in systemic pressure as well. Inhaled milrinone may represent a promising alternative, as it avoids the significant systemic hypotension frequently seen with the intravenous form of the drug [17].
   d. **TEE.** Post-bypass, TEE is invaluable for the assessment of the adequacy of valvular repair. When valve replacement is performed, TEE is important in detecting the presence of a paravalvular leak or a hemodynamically significant pressure gradient in the immediate postbypass period. If a large paravalvular leak, significant residual regurgitation, or a hemodynamically significant pressure gradient are seen at this point, it is critical to communicate with the surgical team and discuss the potential need to return to cardiopulmonary bypass to address these issues.
   e. **Weaning from cardiopulmonary bypass.** A primary concern following mitral valve repair or replacement is the need to maintain LV performance. Once the valve is in place, the LV has to eject a full stroke volume into the aorta without the protection of a low-pressure pop-off into the left atrium. The result is an increase in LV wall tension that can compromise ejection fraction. Patients who had mitral valve repair less often require inotropic support than patients after mitral valve replacement. This is because mitral valve replacement introduces more changes in LV structure, particularly when extensive resection of the subvalvular apparatus is performed. Severity of regurgitation, LV ejection fraction, presence of pulmonary hypertension, and aortic cross-clamp time are other factors to consider in determining the postbypass use of inotropes. In some cases, insertion of an intra-aortic balloon pump may be needed to prevent LV dilatation and failure. Immediately following the patient's weaning from cardiopulmonary bypass, an attempt should be made to keep the patient in sinus rhythm, often by treatment with amiodarone. Amiodarone is routinely used if mitral valve surgery was combined with a maze procedure.
3. **Postoperative course.** Following valve replacement, left atrial and PAPs should decrease. Patients with long-standing mitral regurgitation, however, will continue to need an elevated left atrial pressure for maintenance of adequate forward flow.

X. Tricuspid stenosis

A. Natural history

1. **Etiology.** The primary cause of acquired tricuspid stenosis is rheumatic valvulitis [1]. Rheumatic tricuspid stenosis is rare, almost never exists in isolation, and is often associated with concomitant TR. In the majority of cases, the mitral valve is also involved. Other causes for tricuspid stenosis include systemic lupus erythematosus, endomyocardial fibroelastosis, right atrial tumor, and carcinoid syndrome.

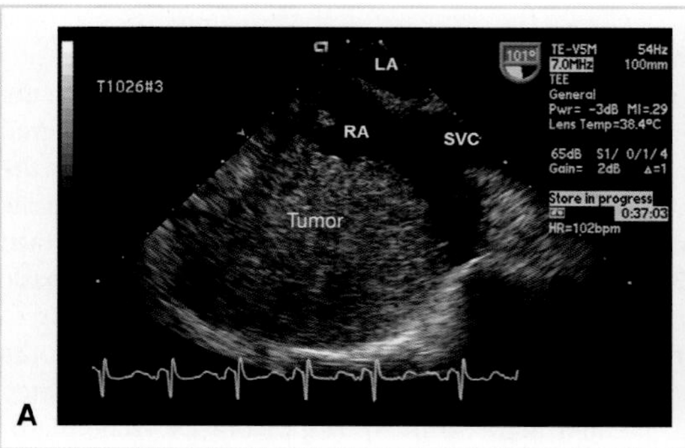

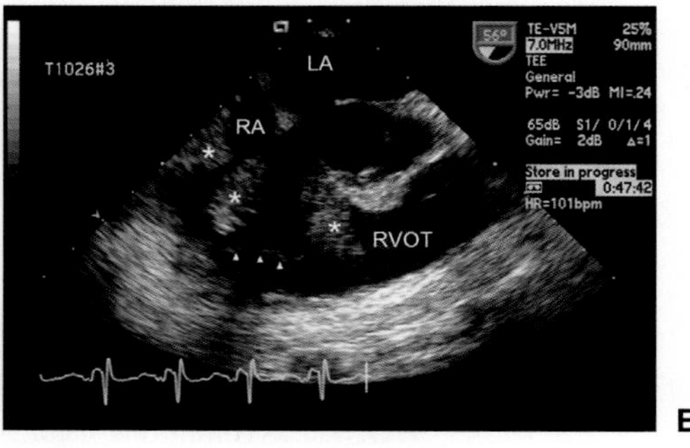

FIGURE 12.14 Right atrial tumor. The tumor occupies the majority of the right atrium **(A)** and obstructs the tricuspid valve **(B)**. *Tumor; LA, Left atrium; RA, Right atrium; RVOT, Right ventricular outflow tract; SVC, Superior vena cava. [ECHO Image from Perrino AC, Reeves ST, eds. *A Practical Approach to Transesophageal Echocardiography.* 2nd ed. Philadelphia, PA: Lippincott Williams & Wilkins, 2008:405, Figure 19.8.]

2. **Symptoms.** Tricuspid stenosis is manifested by the signs and symptoms of right-sided heart failure, including hepatomegaly, hepatic dysfunction, ascites, peripheral edema, and jugular venous distension.

B. **Pathophysiology**

1. **Natural progression.** The tricuspid valve is the largest cardiac valve with a normal area of 7 to 9 cm^2 in the typical adult. It is composed of three leaflets: Anterior, posterior, and septal. The normal gradient across the tricuspid valve is only 1 mm Hg. Significant impairment to forward blood flow does not occur until the valve orifice decreases to less than 1.5 cm^2. Therefore, there is a long asymptomatic period as stenosis develops. A valve area of 1.5 cm^2 usually corresponds to a mean gradient of 3 mm Hg across the tricuspid valve. With progression of the stenosis, the right atrial pressure increases, right atrium dilates, and forward blood flow decreases.
2. **Calculation of severity.** As with left-sided stenotic lesions, the severity of tricuspid stenosis can be determined with cardiac catheterization or echocardiography by the measurement and calculation of orifice area and pressure gradient. A gradient of 5 mm Hg across the tricuspid valve and tricuspid valve area of 1 cm^2 indicate severe stenosis.
3. **TEE.** Patients with rheumatic tricuspid stenosis will demonstrate thickened leaflets with restricted motion and diastolic doming. Fusion of the commissures is also frequently seen. If the cause of tricuspid stenosis is functional stenosis, a right atrial mass responsible for the RV inflow obstruction will be seen (Fig. 12.14). Continuous wave Doppler will allow for the assessment of the previously discussed pressure gradients used to grade stenosis severity.

C. **Surgical intervention.** Salt restriction, digitalization, and diuretics may reduce hepatic congestion, improve hepatic function, delay the surgery, and reduce surgical risks in patients with severe tricuspid stenosis. A majority of patients with tricuspid stenosis have other valvular lesions that require operation. Tricuspid valve intervention is indicated if pressure gradients exceed 5 mm Hg or valvular area is less than 2 cm^2. Commissurotomy of the tricuspid valve is commonly the procedure of choice. However, in cases of extensive calcification, valve replacement with a low-profile prosthetic valve may be necessary.

D. **Goals of perioperative management**

1. **Hemodynamic management** (Table 12.12)

TABLE 12.12

	RV preload	Heart rate	Contractile state	Systemic vascular resistance	Pulmonary vascular resistance
Tricuspid stenosis	↑	↓, maintain	Maintain	↑	Maintain

a. **RV preload.** Adequate forward flow of blood across the stenotic tricuspid valve depends on maintenance of adequate preload.
b. **Heart rate.** Patients with tricuspid stenosis depend on maintenance of sinus rhythm. Supraventricular tachyarrhythmias can cause rapid clinical deterioration and should be controlled with either immediate cardioversion or pharmacologic intervention. At the same time, bradycardia can be harmful because it reduces total forward flow.
c. **Contractility.** RV filling is impeded by tricuspid stenosis. Adequate cardiac output is maintained by an increase in RV contractility. A sudden depression in ventricular contractility can severely limit cardiac output and elevate right atrial pressure.
d. **Systemic vascular resistance.** Systemic vasodilation may lead to hypotension in patients with limited blood flow across the tricuspid valve.
e. **PVR.** Because the limitation to forward flow is at the tricuspid valve, reducing PVR has little positive effect on improving forward flow. Keeping PVR in the normal range is adequate.

2. **Anesthetic technique**
a. Light premedication is indicated.
b. In patients with coexisting mitral valve disease, the anesthetic technique is determined by the mitral valve lesion. In patients with isolated tricuspid stenosis, the primary requirements are to maintain high preload, high afterload, and adequate contractility.
c. Passage of a pulmonary artery catheter through the stenotic tricuspid valve may be difficult and not always justified. In many cases, the catheter can be left in the superior vena cava (SVC) until after bypass and then advanced by a surgeon upon completion of tricuspid valve repair/replacement or floated after weaning from cardiopulmonary bypass. Detailed discussion with the surgeon prior to the beginning of the operation is needed.
d. During **cardiopulmonary bypass,** because no flow into the right atrium is allowed and SVC pressure completely depends on the adequate drainage of the SVC by the SCV cannula, attention must be paid to the SVC drainage in order to avoid elevated SVC pressure, reduced cerebral perfusion pressure, and irreversible brain damage. Central venous pressure monitoring above the SVC tie, as well as intermittent assessment of the patient's head for any signs of edema, is indicated. No drug infusions may be given through any pulmonary artery accessory port since it is isolated from the blood flow during cardiopulmonary bypass.
e. In the postcardiopulmonary bypass period, preload augmentation must be continued. Inotropic support may be necessary if RV failure develops.

XI. Tricuspid Regurgitation

A. **Natural history.** Isolated TR is most frequently seen in association with drug abuse-related endocarditis, carcinoid syndrome, Ebstein's anomaly, connective tissue disorders leading to valve prolapse, or chest trauma. More commonly, however, functional TR develops secondary to RV failure, pulmonary hypertension, or left-sided cardiac abnormalities, such as end-stage aortic or mitral stenosis [1]. With severe aortic or mitral valve disease, elevated PAP leads to RV strain and, eventually, RV failure with TR. The primary mechanism of this functional TR results from dilatation of the tricuspid valve annulus. It may is also often seen with RV dilatation leading to tethering of the tricuspid valve leaflets that restricts their mobility.

B. **Pathophysiology**

1. **Natural progression.** Isolated TR is well tolerated because the RV can compensate for volume overload. Most symptoms associated with TR are directly related to an increased RV afterload. Therefore, when TR is associated with pulmonary hypertension, the impedance to RV ejection produces significant deterioration secondary to decreased cardiac output. Most patients with TR have associated atrial fibrillation due to distension of the right atrium.
2. **TEE evaluation and grading of severity** of TR (Table 12.13).
With functional TR, the TEE exam will often demonstrate RV dysfunction and dilatation, along with dilatation of the tricuspid valve annulus. The valve leaflets may appear

TABLE 12.13

Grade	Mild	Moderate	Severe
Right atrial size	Normal	Normal or dilated	Usually dilated
Jet area (cm^2) for central jets	<5	5–10	>10
Vena contracta width (cm)	Not defined	Not defined, but less than 0.7	>0.7
Hepatic vein flow- pulsed wave Doppler	Systolic dominance	Systolic blunting	Systolic reversal

Adapted from: Zoghbi WA, Enriquez-Sarano M, Foster E, et al. Recommendations for evaluation of the severity of native valvular regurgitation with two-dimensional and Doppler echocardiography. *J Am Soc Echocardiogr.* 2003;*16*(7):777–802.

tethered with restricted motion. In the setting of endocarditis, vegetations and valvular perforation are common. With rheumatic disease, findings will include leaflet thickening and restriction, along with commissural fusion and probable mitral and/or aortic valve involvement. Carcinoid heart disease results in diffuse leaflet thickening and restriction. It may frequently lead to both stenosis and regurgitation, and almost always involves both the tricuspid and pulmonic valves. With Ebstein's anomaly, one or more tricuspid leafltes are positioned abnormally into the RV cavity. The RV is reduced in size and is said to be "atrialized" due to this displacement of the tricuspid leaflets toward the RV apex.

Color flow Doppler, assessing the size of the regurgitant jet, is the primary modality used to grade severity of TR (Fig. 12.15). However, similar to mitral regurgitation, the altered loading conditions induced by general anesthesia may underestimate the true severity of

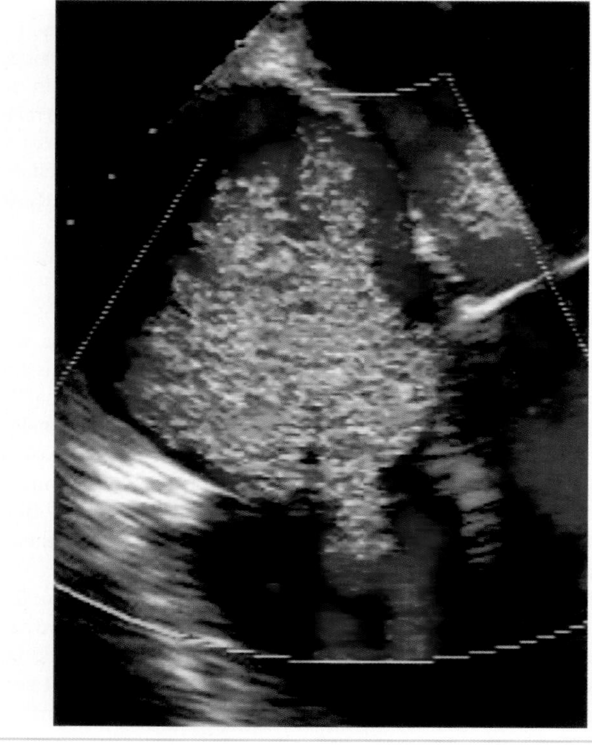

FIGURE 12.15 Color flow Doppler image of severe tricuspid regurgitation. [ECHO Image from Perrino AC, Reeves ST, eds. *A Practical Approach to Transesophageal Echocardiography.* 2nd ed. Philadelphia, PA: Lippincott Williams & Wilkins, 2008:288, Figure 14.8.]

TABLE 12.14

	RV preload	Heart rate	Contractile state	Systemic vascular resistance	Pulmonary vascular resistance
Tricuspid regurgitation	↑	↑, maintain	Maintain	Maintain	↓

the lesion. Alterations in hepatic vein flow, as seen with pulsed wave Doppler, can also be utilized to assist in grading the severity of regurgitation.

3. **Pressure wave abnormalities.** Central venous pressure tracings may show the presence of giant V waves. However, as with mitral regurgitation, the compliance of the right atrium, filling of the right atrium, and regurgitant volume determine the size of the regurgitant wave.

C. **Goals of perioperative management**

1. **Hemodynamic management** (Table 12.14)
   a. **RV preload.** To provide adequate forward flow, preload augmentation is desirable. A drop in central venous pressure can severely limit RV stroke volume.
   b. **Heart rate.** Normal to high heart rates are beneficial in these patients to sustain forward flow and prevent peripheral congestion.
   c. **Contractility.** RV failure is the primary cause of clinical deterioration in patients with TR. Because the RV is designed geometrically to accommodate volume but not pressure loads, positive-pressure ventilation or elevated PVR may lead to RV failure. Suppression of contractility with myocardial depressants may also induce RV failure.
   d. **Systemic vascular resistance.** Variations in systemic afterload have little effect on TR unless there is concurrent aortic or mitral valve dysfunction.
   e. **PVR.** RV function and forward blood flow are improved with decreases in PVR. **Hyperventilation is helpful** in reducing PVR by producing hypocapnia. However,
7 high airway pressures during pulmonary ventilation and agents that can increase PAP should be avoided. If inotropic support is necessary, dobutamine, isoproterenol, or milrinone, which dilate the pulmonary vasculature, should be used. Inhalation of nitric oxide may have an important role in selectively reducing PVR in these patients.

2. **Anesthetic technique**
   a. Light premedication is indicated.
   b. As with tricuspid stenosis, in patients with coexisting mitral valve disease, anesthetic technique is determined by the mitral valve lesion.
   c. Passage of a pulmonary artery catheter through the regurgitant tricuspid valve may be difficult due to the tendency of the regurgitant wave to push the catheter in the opposite direction. Determination of cardiac output in the presence of TR is inaccurate because some of the cold injectate is ejected retrograde into the atrium rather than into the pulmonary artery.
   d. As with tricuspid stenosis, during cardiopulmonary bypass, attention must be paid to the SVC drainage.
   e. If a prosthetic valve is placed, residual tricuspid stenosis may occur because the valve prosthesis is smaller than the native valve, and postbypass preload augmentation may be necessary. In addition, in the immediate postbypass period, the RV will be under increased strain because the entire stroke volume will have to be ejected against the higher PVR with no pop-off pressure lowering back into the right atrium. Therefore, RV failure requiring inotropic support may occur.

XII. Pulmonary stenosis

A. **Natural history**

1. **Etiology.** The majority of pulmonary stenoses are congenital. Rarely, rheumatic heart disease, malignant carcinoid, or extrinsic compression by a tumor or sinus of Valsalva aneurysm may lead to pulmonary stenosis. With both rheumatic heart disease and carcinoid

syndrome, there is almost always involvement of other cardiac valves in addition to the pulmonic valve.

2. **Symptoms.** Patients with pulmonary stenosis may live for extended periods completely without symptoms and frequently survive past the age of 70 yrs without surgical intervention. Symptoms, when they do occur, include tachypnea, syncope, angina, or hepatomegaly and peripheral edema. Intervening bacterial endocarditis or RV failure due to severe stenosis may lead to death.

B. **Pathophysiology**

1. **Natural progression.** The normal pressure gradient across the pulmonary valve orifice is usually under 5 mm Hg. The diagnosis of pulmonary stenosis can be made when the gradient across the pulmonary valve reaches 15 mm Hg. A peak systolic gradient of 36 mm Hg or less is considered mild pulmonary stenosis, between 36 and 64 mm Hg is considered moderate stenosis, and more than 64 mm Hg is considered severe pulmonary stenosis. As the pulmonary stenosis progresses from mild to moderate, concentric hypertrophy of the RV occurs. The increased hypertrophy and pressure within the RV leads to a situation in which RV subendocardial blood flow no longer occurs throughout the cardiac cycle, but only during diastole, similar to the LV. Coronary perfusion pressure must be maintained to provide an adequate RV subendocardial coronary blood supply.
2. **Pressure wave abnormalities**
   a. **PAP trace.** The PAP upstroke is delayed, and there is a late systolic peak owing to impedance to blood flow through the stenotic pulmonary valve.
   b. **Central venous pressure trace.** A prominent A wave is frequently found in the central venous pressure trace.
3. **TEE.** The pulmonic valve is not always visualized with TEE based on its anterior location far from the TEE probe, making 2D imaging and Doppler analysis of the pulmonic valve difficult. When adequate visualization of the valve is obtained, continuous wave Doppler allows for estimation of transvalvular gradients used to grade stenosis severity. The degree of RV dilatation and dysfunction may provide some indirect estimation of the degree of stenosis and obstruction to RV outflow (Fig. 12.16).

C. **Surgical intervention.** Any patient developing significant symptoms, a peak systolic gradient across the pulmonary valve of more than 80 mm Hg, or a peak systolic RV pressure of 100 mm Hg should have surgical intervention. Normally, valvulotomy is all that is necessary. Balloon

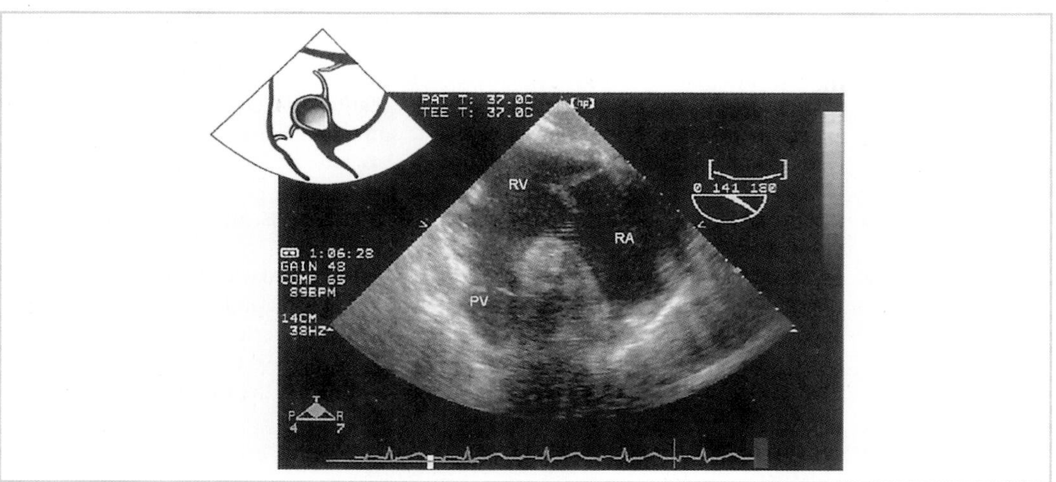

FIGURE 12.16 The 2D image of the pulmonic valve, seen in a transgastric pulmonic valve view. PV, pulmonic valve; RA, right atrium; RV, right ventricle. [ECHO Image from Perrino AC, Reeves ST, eds. *A Practical Approach to Transesophageal Echocardiography.* 2nd ed. Philadelphia, PA: Lippincott Williams & Wilkins, 2008:292, Figure 14.2.]

TABLE 12.15

	RV preload	Heart rate	Contractile state	Systemic vascular resistance	Pulmonary vascular resistance
Pulmonary stenosis	↑	↑	Maintain	Maintain	↓, maintain

valvuloplasty is a viable alternative to valvulotomy. Rarely, the pulmonary valve actually has to be replaced. An attractive alternative to open heart surgery is transluminal balloon angioplasty, which is frequently used for congenital pulmonary valve stenosis.

D. **Goals of perioperative management**

1. **Hemodynamic management** (Table 12.15)
2. **RV preload.** RV performance depends on adequate preload for the RV. Decreases in central venous pressure will lead to inadequate filling of the RV and decreased RV stroke volume.
3. **Heart rate.** As pulmonary stenosis progresses, the patient becomes increasingly dependent on the atrial contraction to provide adequate RV filling. Unfortunately, in severe pulmonary stenosis, TR can develop, leading to right atrial distension and the occurrence of atrial fibrillation. Because blood flow across the stenotic pulmonary valve occurs primarily during ventricular systole, increases in heart rate usually provide increased flow. Rarely, RV hypertrophy in combination with angina symptoms dictates the need for a slower heart rate to allow adequate time in diastole for subendocardial coronary blood flow.
4. **Contractility.** With severe pulmonary stenosis, the RV hypertrophies in response to the pressure load. Depression of the contractile state can lead to RV failure and clinical deterioration. Pharmacologic intervention that depresses RV function should be avoided.
5. **Systemic vascular resistance** should be maintained to provide adequate coronary perfusion to the hypertrophied RV.
6. **PVR.** Because the primary impedance to forward flow is the pulmonary valve, reducing PVR will do little to enhance forward blood flow. However, especially in patients with mild or moderate pulmonary stenosis, major increases in PVR can potentially harm forward blood flow and lead to RV dysfunction. Therefore, PVR should be kept in the low-normal range.

XIII. Pulmonary regurgitation

A. **Natural history**

1. **Etiology.** The majority of patients with acquired pulmonary regurgitation have annular dilatation secondary to pulmonary hypertension of various etiologies [1]. Pulmonary regurgitation also can be associated with congenital valve deformities or primary surgical procedures to correct these deformities. Less commonly, pulmonary regurgitation is caused by connective tissue disorders, trauma, carcinoid syndrome, infective endocarditis, and rheumatic fever.
2. **Symptoms.** Patients without pulmonary hypertension usually are asymptomatic. Patients with pulmonary hypertension and pulmonary regurgitation usually present with RV failure.

B. **Surgical intervention** consists of pulmonary valve replacement and is rarely performed in patients with acquired pulmonary regurgitation.

XIV. Mixed valvular lesions.

For all mixed valvular lesions, management decisions emphasize the most severe or the most hemodynamically significant lesion.

A. **Aortic stenosis and mitral stenosis.** Pathophysiologically, the progression of the disease follows a course similar to that seen in patients with pure mitral stenosis with development of pulmonary hypertension and, eventually, RV failure. Symptoms are primarily referable to the pulmonary circuit, including dyspnea, hemoptysis, and atrial fibrillation. This combination of valvular heart disease may lead to underestimation of the severity of the AS because the aortic valve gradient may be relatively low owing to low aortic valvular flow. Such a combination of lesions can be extremely serious because of the limitation of blood flow at two points.

B. **Aortic stenosis and mitral regurgitation.** This combination is relatively rare, but should be expected in patients with AS who also have left atrial enlargement with atrial fibrillation. Mitral regurgitation can be exacerbated by LV dysfunction due to severe AS. In this situation, the mitral valve does not require replacement, and the mitral regurgitation usually regresses after the aortic valve is replaced.

9 In managing these patients, the hemodynamic requirements for AS and mitral regurgitation are contradictory. Because AS will most frequently lead these patients into deadly intraoperative situations, it should be given priority when managing the hemodynamic variables.

C. **Aortic stenosis and aortic regurgitation.** The combination of aortic regurgitation and AS is not well tolerated because it provides the LV with both severe pressure and volume overloading. These stresses lead to major increases in myocardial oxygen consumption (MVO_2) and, as might be expected, angina pectoris is an early symptom with this combination. Once symptoms develop, the prognosis is similar to that of pure AS.

D. **Aortic regurgitation and mitral regurgitation.** The combination of aortic and mitral regurgitation occurs frequently, and this combination can cause rapid clinical deterioration.

The hemodynamic requirements of aortic regurgitation and mitral regurgitation are similar. The primary problem is providing adequate forward flow and peripheral circulation. The development of acidosis leading to peripheral vasoconstriction and increased impedance to LV outflow can lead to rapid clinical deterioration. Therefore, a low systemic vascular resistance with an adequate perfusion pressure is needed until cardiopulmonary bypass can be initiated.

E. **Mitral stenosis and mitral regurgitation.** Rheumatic mitral stenosis is rarely pure and commonly exists in conjunction with mitral regurgitation. When dealing with patients with combined mitral stenosis and mitral regurgitation, decisions concerning hemodynamic management must consider which lesion is predominant. As a rule of thumb, normalization of afterload, heart rate, and contractility, while avoiding agents or conditions leading to reactive pulmonary constriction and providing adequate preload, leads to optimal hemodynamic stabilization.

F. **Multi-valve surgical procedures.** While the surgical management of multi-valve disease has continued to improve, these patients still represent a significantly higher-risk group than patients presenting for surgery on a single valve.

XV. Prosthetic valves

The decision regarding which prosthetic valve should be used for a particular patient is based upon a variety of factors, including the expected longevity of the patient (mechanical prostheses last longer), the ability of the patient to comply with anticoagulation therapy (mechanical prostheses require ongoing anticoagulation), the anatomy and pathology of the existing valvular disease, and the experience of the operating surgeon [18].

A. **Essential characteristics** of prosthetic heart valves. An ideal prosthetic heart valve is: nonthrombogenic, chemically inert, preserves blood elements, and allows physiologic blood flow. The large number of different prosthetic valves that have been developed means that no ideal valve has yet been found.

B. **Types of prosthetic valves**

1. **Mechanical.** Current mechanical prosthetic valves are durable but thrombogenic. At present, all patients with mechanical prosthetic valves require anticoagulation therapy for the remainder of their lives. Normally, anticoagulation is provided with warfarin sodium, administered at a dose that will elevate the prothrombin time to 1.5 to 2 times control. There are four basic types of mechanical prosthetic valves, the caged ball, caged disc, monocuspid tilting disc, and bicuspid tilting disc valves. Of these, the bicuspid tilting disc valves are in common use to today. This valve design is less bulky than its predecessors, and provides improved central laminar blood flow.

   a. **Bileaflet tilting-disk valve prosthesis** (Fig. 12.17). In 1977, a bileaflet St. Jude cardiac valve was introduced as a low-profile device to allow central blood flow through two semicircular disks that pivot on supporting struts. The St. Jude valve can be placed

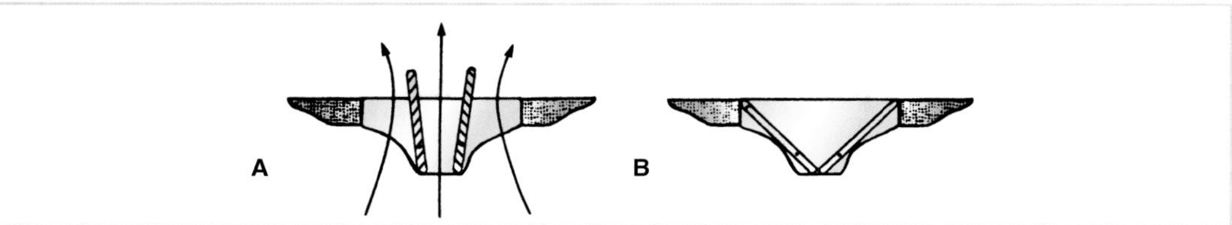

FIGURE 12.17 Bileaflet valve prosthesis showing disks in open **(A)** and closed **(B)** positions.

in the aortic, mitral, or tricuspid positions. These valves produce low resistance to blood flow and have a lower incidence of thromboembolic complications, though anticoagulation is still necessary. The most popular bileaflet tilting disc is still the St. Jude Medical. Other bileaflet tilting-disk valve prostheses include the CarboMedics, Edwards Tekna, Sorin Bicarbon, and Advancing the Standard (ATS).

2. **Bioprosthetic valves.** The Hancock porcine aortic bioprosthesis (now the Medtronic Hancock II stented porcine bioprosthesis) was introduced in 1970, followed by the Ionescu–Shiley bovine pericardial prosthesis in 1974, and the Carpentier–Edwards porcine aortic valve bioprosthesis in 1975. In contrast to modern mechanical prostheses, current bioprostheses are less durable, and also less thrombogenic. Long-term anticoagulation for a bioprosthetic valve is usually unnecessary. Bioprosthetic valves in the aortic position last longer than in the mitral position. Because durability is an issue, and because their lifespan is longer in older patients, bioprosthetic valves are usually used for patients older than 60 yrs and when anticoagulation is not a desirable option (e.g., when pregnancy is anticipated).
   a. Bioprosthetic valves fall into two types: Stented and nonstented. Stented bioprosthetic valves constructed from porcine aortic valves or bovine pericardium are placed on a polypropylene stent attached to a silicone sewing ring covered with dacron. These valves allow for improved central annular flow and less turbulence, but the stent does cause some obstruction to forward flow, thereby leading to a residual pressure gradient across the valve. Stented valves that can be found in clinical use today include the Carpentier–Edwards perimount (Fig. 12.18), Medtronic Mosaic, Carpentier–Edwards porcine, Hancock porcine, and Medtronic intact porcine.
   b. **Stentless bioprostheses.** Porcine valves fixed in a pressure-free glutaraldehyde solution and without the use of a stent make up the category of stentless bioprostheses.

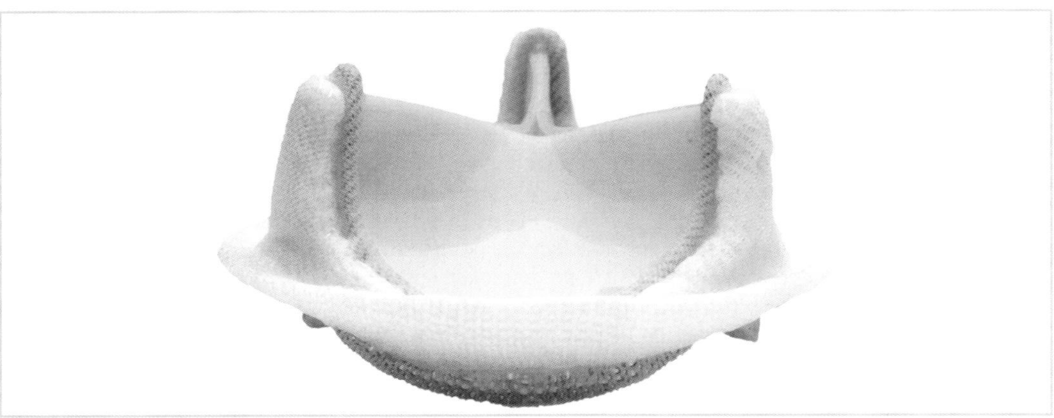

FIGURE 12.18 Carpentier–Edwards perimount RSR stented pericardial bioprosthetic aortic valve (Courtesy of Edwards Lifesciences, Irvine, California).

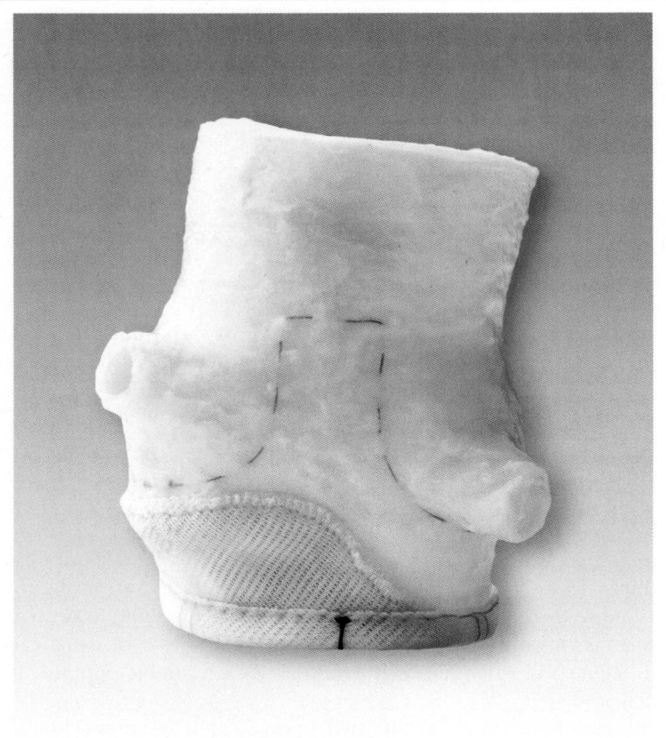

FIGURE 12.19 Edwards Prima Plus stentless bioprosthetic aortic valve (Courtesy of Edwards Lifesciences, Irvine, California).

The primary types of valves clinically encountered in this category include the St. Jude Medical Toronto SPV stentless porcine, Edwards Prima Plus stentless bioprosthesis (Fig. 12.19), and Medtronic Freestyle stentless porcine. Stentless bioprosthetic valves are used almost exclusively in the aortic position. They have excellent hemodynamic characteristics, but technically are more difficult to place. Modern stentless bioprosthetic valves are often used when aortic root replacement is also necessary.

3. **Human valves.** The first use of a bioprosthesis taken from a cadaver occurred in 1962. However, techniques such as irradiation or chemical treatment used to sterilize and preserve the early homografts for implantation led to a shortened life span. More recently, antibiotic solutions have been used to sterilize human valves, which then are frozen in liquid nitrogen until implantation. Using these techniques, weakness of the prosthesis leading to cusp rupture occurs infrequently, with more than 75% of prostheses lasting for longer than 10 yrs regardless of patient age. The incidence of prosthetic valve endocarditis and hemolysis resulting from blood flow through the homograft is very low. Anticoagulation is usually not required. Homografts are predominately used in the aortic position, especially when aortic root replacement is necessary, and for pulmonary valve replacement in the Ross procedure. Homografts may be most useful in patients younger than 35 and in patients with native valve endocarditis.

XVI. Prophylaxis of bacterial endocarditis

When an invasive procedure puts the patient with valvular heart disease at risk of bacteremia, precautions should be taken to prevent seeding of an abnormal or artificial valve with bacteria that, once present, are very hard to eradicate. Practically, this concern translates into (a) a strict aseptic

TABLE 12.16

	Agent	Adult dose (30–60 min before procedure)	Pediatric dose[a]
Standard general prophylaxis	Amoxicillin	2 g PO	50 mg/kg/PO
Patients unable to take oral medications	Ampicillin	2 g IV or IM	50 mg/kg IV or IM
Penicillin- and amoxicillin-allergic patients	Cephalexin[b] or Clindamycin or Azithromycin or Clarithromycin	2 g PO 600 mg PO 500 mg PO	50 mg/kg PO 20 mg/kg PO 15 mg/kg PO
Penicillin- and amoxicillin-allergic patients unable to take oral medications	Clindamycin or Cefazolin or Ceftriaxone	600 mg IV or IM 1g IV or IM	20 mg/kg IV or IM 50 mg/kg IV or IM

[a]Total pediatric dose should not exceed the adult dose.
[b]Cephalosporins should not be used in patients with immediate-type hypersensitivity reaction (urticaria, angioedema, or anaphylaxis) to penicillins.
Adapted from: Nishimura RA, Carabello BA, Faxon DP, et al. ACC/AHA 2008 Guideline update on valvular heart disease: focused update on infective endocarditis. *Circulation.* 2008;118:887–896.

technique for all procedures performed in patients with valvular heart disease, (b) elimination of existing sources of infection before implantation of a prosthetic valve, and (c) in selected cases, antibiotic prophylaxis. Guidelines from the American Heart Association on prevention of infective endocarditis limit antibiotic prophylaxis to cardiac conditions associated with the highest risk of infective endocarditis. These conditions include prosthetic cardiac valves or material used in heart valve repair, complex congenital heart diseases, prior infective endocarditis, and transplanted hearts with valvulopathy. Endocarditis prophylaxis is recommended only for "dental procedures that involve manipulation of gingival tissue or the periapical region of teeth or perforation of the oral mucosa." Endocarditis prophylaxis may be considered for invasive procedures of the respiratory tract involving incision or biopsy of respiratory mucosa, but not for simple bronchoscopy. Guidelines no longer recommend antibiotics solely for endocarditis prophylaxis for any gastrointestinal and genitourinary procedures. However, administration of antibiotics to prevent wound or urinary tract infection is reasonable [19]. Guidelines for antibiotic prophylaxis, to be begun 1 h prior to a procedure, are shown in Table 12.16.

REFERENCES

1. Otto CM, Bonow RO. Valvular heart disease. In: Bonow RO, Mann DL, Zipes DP, et al., eds. *Braunwald's Heart Disease: A Textbook of Cardiovascular Medicine.* 9th ed. St. Louis, MO: Elsevier; 2011:1468–1530.
2. Nikomo VT, Gardin JM, Skelton TN, et al. Burden of valvular heart disease: a population-based study. *Lancet.* 2006;368:1005–1011.
3. Cook DJ, Housmans PR, Rehfeldt KH. Valvular heart disease: replacement and repair. In: Kaplan JA, Reich DL, Savino JS, eds. *Kaplan's Cardiac Anesthesia: The Echo Era.* 6th ed. St Louis, MO: Elsevier Saunders; 2011:570–614.
4. Iung B, Baron G, Butchard EG, et al. A prospective survey of patients with valvular heart disease in Europe: the euro heart survey on valvular heart disease. *Eur Heart J.* 2003;24:1231–1243.
5. Otto CM. *Textbook of Clinical Echocardiography.* 4th ed. Philadelphia, PA: Elsevier Saunders; 2009:259–325.
6. Galderisi M, de Divitiis O. Risk factor induced cardiovascular remodeling and the effects of angiotensin-converting enzyme inhibitors. *J Cardiovasc Pharmacol.* 2008;51:523–531.
7. Roberts WC, Jong M, Ok BA. Frequency by decades of unicuspid, bicuspid, and tricuspid aortic valves in adults having isolated aortic valve replacement for aortic stenosis, with or without associated aortic regurgitation. *Circulation.* 2005;111:920–925.
8. Baumgartner H, Hung J, Bermejo J, et al. Echocardiographic assessment of valve stenosis: EAE/ASE recommendations for clinical practice. *J Am Soc Echocardiogr.* 2009;22:1–23.
9. Agricola E, Oppizzi M, Pisani M. Stress echocardiography in heart failure. *Cardiovasc Ultrasound.* 2004;2:11.
10. Maslow A, Casey P, Poppas A, et al. Aortic valve replacement with or without coronary bypass graft surgery: the risk of surgery in patients ≥80 years old. *J Cardiothorac Vasc Anesth.* 2010;24:18–24.
11. Webb JG, Altwegg L, Boone RH, et al. Transcatheter aortic valve implantation: Impact on clinical and valve-related outcomes. *Circulation.* 2009;119:3009–3016.
12. Boodhwani M, de Kerchove L, Glineure D. Repair oriented classification of aortic insufficiency: impact on surgical techniques and clinical outcomes. *J Thoracic Cardiovasc Surg.* 2009;137:286–294.

13. Sidebotham D, Legget ME, Sutton T. The mitral valve. In: Sidebotham D, Merry A, Legget M, et al., eds. *Practical Perioperative Transesophageal Echocardiography: With Critical Care Echocardiography.* 2nd ed. Philadelphia, PA: Elsevier Saunders; 2011:142–147.
14. Stewart WJ, Currie PJ, Salcedo EE, et al. Evaluation of mitral leaflet motion by echocardiography and jet direction by Doppler color flow mapping to determine the mechanisms of mitral regurgitation. *J Am Coll Cardiol.* 1992;20:1353–1361.
15. Bonow RO, Carabello BA, Chatterjee K, et al. ACC/AHA 2006 guidelines for the management of patients with valvular heart disease: a report of the American College of Cardiology/American Heart Association Task Force on Practice Guidelines. *J Am Coll Cardiol.* 2006;48(3):e1–e148.
16. Fattouch K, Guccione F, Sampognaro R, et al. POINT: Efficacy of adding mitral valve restrictive annuloplasty to coronary artery bypass grafting in patients with moderate ischemic mitral valve regurgitation: a randomized trial. *J Thorac Cardiovasc Surg.* 2009;138:278–285.
17. Denault AY, Lamarche Y, Couture P, et al. Inhaled milrinone: a new alternative in cardiac surgery? *Semin Cardiothorac Vasc Anesth.* 2006;10:346–360.
18. Rahimtoola SH. Choice of prosthetic heart valve in adults: an update. *J Amer Coll Cardiol.* 2010;55:2413–2426.
19. Nishimura RA, Carabello BA, Faxon DP, et al. ACC/AHA 2008 Guideline update on valvular heart disease: focused update on infective endocarditis. *Circulation.* 2008;118:887–896.

13 Alternative Approaches to Cardiac Surgery with and without Cardiopulmonary Bypass

James Y. Kim, James G. Ramsay, Michael G. Licina, and Anand R. Mehta

KEY POINTS

1. Off-pump coronary artery bypass grafting (OPCAB) challenges the anesthesiologist and surgeon to maintain hemodynamic stability while delicate coronary arterial anastomoses are performed on a beating heart.
2. OPCAB has not produced the expected reductions in neurologic and renal complications, although it has consistently reduced perioperative blood loss and transfusion.
3. Adept positioning of the heart during OPCAB minimizes hemodynamic disturbances from reduced venous return, especially while performing coronary anastomoses within the right coronary and left circumflex arterial distributions. Maintaining adequate intravascular volume is essential.
4. Adjuncts such as intracoronary shunts, ischemic and/or anesthetic preconditioning, and intra-aortic balloon pumps may help to minimize ischemia during OPCAB. Circulatory support with vasoconstrictors and/or inotropic drugs is often required.
5. Robotic-assisted minimally invasive techniques can be used for coronary artery bypass grafting (CABG) performed either on- or off-cardiopulmonary bypass (CPB).
6. Transesophageal echocardiography (TEE) monitoring during OPCAB can promptly identify acute ischemia, although transgastric views are often compromised by the cardiac positioning required for distal coronary anastomoses.
7. Anesthetic techniques compatible with fast-tracking are most often used for OPCAB, which typically involves a "balanced" technique utilizing a combination of inhalational anesthetic, modest

(continued)

amounts of opioid, and intermediate-duration muscle relaxation. Excessive use of benzodiazepines and long-acting medications is avoided.

8. Minimally invasive cardiac valve surgery most often requires CPB, but the incisions are smaller and sometimes off the midline, and cannulation for CPB often utilizes port-access technology. Robotic-assisted techniques can be used for minimally invasive mitral valve replacement or repair.
9. TEE is critical during minimally invasive valve surgery (MIVS) for CPB cannulation and assessment of valve structure and function.
10. Percutaneous approaches to mitral regurgitation (Mitraclip), mitral stenosis (balloon mitral valvuloplasty), and aortic stenosis (transcatheter aortic valve implantation [TAVI]) are rapidly growing in popularity. Each approach presents unique challenges to the anesthesiologist; these procedures can be performed either with sedation or general anesthesia, each with its own benefits and risks.
11. Percutaneous valve procedures often involve transient profound hypotension from obstruction (e.g., balloon mitral valvuloplasty and predilation for TAVI) and either incidental or intentional dysrhythmias (e.g., rapid ventricular pacing for TAVI).
12. Hybrid operating rooms allow for interventional cardiology or radiology procedures to be performed in conjunction with open cardiac surgery including the use of CPB.
13. Transmyocardial laser revascularization (TMLR) may provide relief from ischemia through neovascularization and sympathetic denervation, although the exact mechanism remains unclear.
14. Patients undergoing TMLR typically have severe coronary artery disease, poor left ventricular (LV) function, and multiple coexisting diseases, making intraoperative anesthetic management challenging.
15. Intraoperative TMLR complications include gas embolization, major hemorrhage, acute decrease in ventricular function, injury to the mitral valve apparatus or conduction system, and atrial and ventricular arrhythmias.

THE PAST TWO DECADES HAVE witnessed a major evolution in cardiac surgery in parallel with "minimally invasive" and laparoscopic developments in other surgical fields [1]. Two major objectives have been a reduction in the use of CPB for revascularization and a reduction in the invasiveness of the surgical approach. The overall goals are to preserve and enhance the quality of the procedure(s) while providing faster recovery, reduced procedural costs, and reduced morbidity and mortality. The contribution of the anesthesia care team is to facilitate cost-effective early recovery while providing safe, excellent operating conditions both for the patient and the surgeon. Anesthetic techniques and monitoring modalities have needed to evolve with changes in surgical practice. Anesthesiologists have learned more about how to support the circulation during cardiac manipulation and periods of coronary occlusion. We have been charged with monitoring and support while the surgeon operates with minimal exposure while at the same time facilitating early recovery and discharge. The surgical techniques and their anesthetic considerations discussed in this chapter include the following: CABG without the use of CPB (off-pump CABG [OPCAB] and minimally invasive direct coronary artery bypass [MIDCAB]); MIVS, including TAVI; computer-enhanced, endoscopic robotic-controlled CABG; and TMLR, as an alternative revascularization technique. Although not mentioned subsequently, we recommend the routine use of intra-arterial blood pressure monitoring for all of these procedures because of the rapidity and frequency of significant hemodynamic disturbances and the need for frequent assessment of labs (e.g., arterial blood gases, activated clotting times, coagulation studies, etc.).

I. Off-pump coronary artery bypass (OPCAB) and minimally invasive direct coronary artery bypass

A. Historical perspective

1. Early revascularization surgery

a. Early attempts at coronary artery surgery without the use of CPB included the Vineberg procedure in Canada (tunneling the internal mammary artery [IMA] into the ischemic myocardium) in the 1950s, and internal mammary to coronary anastomosis in the 1960s by Kolessov in Russia.

b. Sabiston from the United States and Favolaro from South America reported the use of the saphenous vein for aorta-to-coronary artery bypass grafts, performed without CPB, in the same period.

c. The introduction of CABG in the late 1960s expanded the indications for CPB, which had enabled congenital heart repairs and heart valve surgery since the 1950s. CPB with the use of cardioplegia became the standard of care in the 1970s, providing a motionless field and myocardial "protection" with asystole and hypothermia.

2. **Reports in the early 1990s**

a. South American surgeons with limited resources continued to develop techniques for surgery without CPB, publishing in North American journals in the 1980s and early 1990s. In 1991, Benetti et al. [2] reported on 700 CABG procedures without CPB performed over a 12-yr period with very low morbidity and mortality.

b. North American and European interest grew in the 1990s, fueled by a desire to make surgery more appealing (vs. angioplasty) as well as the need to reduce cost and length of stay. Alterative incisions were explored, and techniques and devices to facilitate surgery on the beating heart were developed. The terms "OPCAB" and "MIDCAB" were coined.

3. **Port-access (or "Heartport")**

a. Simultaneous with attempts to perform CABG without CPB, a group from Stanford University introduced a technique permitting surgery to be done with endoscopic instrumentation through small (1 to 2 cm) ports and a small thoracotomy incision. This was termed port-access surgery or by the trade name of Heartport (Johnson and Johnson, Inc., New Brunswick, NJ, USA). A motionless surgical field was required, necessitating CPB. Extensive use of TEE is required to assist in the placement of and to monitor the position of the various cannulae and the endoaortic balloon (see below).

b. Port-access cardiac surgery contributed new knowledge in two major areas: Percutaneous, endovascular instrumentation for CPB and instrumentation for performing surgery through a small thoracotomy incision. The latter techniques continue to be developed and modified to permit "minimally invasive" valve surgery through partial sternotomy or thoracotomy incisions.

4. **MIDCAB.** A number of alternative incisions to midline sternotomy have facilitated access to specific coronary artery distributions to allow CABG without CPB. **The most popular alternative approach is the left anterior thoracotomy, which allows IMA harvest and grafting to the left anterior descending (LAD) artery territory. This is the procedure usually referred to as MIDCAB.**

5. **North American/European experience after 1998**

a. Initially viewed by most as experimental, off-pump techniques are now established as an acceptable alternative to CABG with CPB. The reported use of OPCAB has been reported to be as high as 33% [3], but the range in practice is wide. Some surgeons perform virtually all revascularizations as OPCAB, which typically refers to a multivessel CABG performed through a median sternotomy without CPB. Most large cardiac surgery practices have at least one surgeon who performs a significant number of OPCAB procedures. The physiology and anesthetic management for OPCAB has been recently reviewed by Chassot et al. [4].

b. **MIDCAB procedures are more technically demanding than OPCAB because they require specialized instrumentation and operating through a small incision.** These procedures are done in a smaller number of institutions than OPCAB. Some surgeons harvest the IMA endoscopically before making the small incision to do the coronary anastomosis.

B. **Rationale for avoiding sternotomy and cardiopulmonary bypass for coronary artery surgery**

1. **Reduction in complications**

1 a. Sewing coronary vessels on the beating heart is technically challenging and not necessarily appropriate for all surgeons [5]. Whether or not there is a benefit of performing on-pump versus OPCAB is a topic of heated debate. Several published randomized trials [6–10] confirm reductions in enzyme release, bleeding, time to extubation, and length of

stay. While there are long-term follow-up studies suggesting similar rates of survival and graft patency between the two groups [11,12], other studies suggest that graft patency is lower in off-pump procedures [9,13], with one large randomized controlled trial finding a higher 1-yr mortality rate in the off-pump group [13]. Of note, the latter studies came from surgeons less experienced in the off-pump technique. Intraoperative conversion from off-pump to on-pump has been associated with an increase in mortality [14,15]. Although reduction in stroke has been one of the proposed benefits of the technique (due to avoidance of aortic cannulation and cross-clamping), studies do not demonstrate this benefit. 2 Similarly, reduction in renal dysfunction has been proposed but not proved in these studies and in one additional recent publication [16]. In August 2004, an updated guideline for CABG surgery was published by the American College of Cardiology and American Heart Association; this guideline recognizes the potential benefits for avoiding CPB but the need for further data with the lack of proved benefit in randomized controlled trials [17].

b. Avoidance of aortic manipulation and cannulation might reduce embolic complications such as stroke, yet a partial or side-biting aortic clamp may be necessary to perform proximal venous anastomoses in multivessel OPCAB. This can be avoided by using the IMA as the only proximal vessel with its origin intact or with the use of devices designed to avoid the use of a cross-clamp (e.g., the "Heartstring").

c. The whole body "inflammatory response" induced by extracorporeal circulation is avoided with MIDCAB and OPCAB. This approach should result in lower fluid requirements and less coagulopathy and is consistent with lesser volumes of blood loss and transfusion demonstrated in several comparisons of OPCAB to CABG with CPB.

2. Competition with angioplasty. Refinements in interventional cardiology and reductions in postprocedure restenosis have allowed an ever-increasing population of patients to have coronary lesions treated in the catheterization laboratory, although long-term outcomes in multivessel coronary disease are slightly better with CABG than with stents. However, patients will often choose the less invasive interventional cardiology approach over surgery if those results are nearly equivalent. Evolution of surgical techniques to provide excellent results with less physiologic trespass may be necessary for coronary artery surgery to survive.

3. Progress toward truly "minimally invasive" surgery

a. Avoidance of CPB is more physiologically important than avoidance of sternotomy, but postoperative recovery from sternotomy is foremost in patients' minds. The smaller the surgical scar, the better. The MIDCAB addresses this issue, but this approach can only access the LAD and its diagonal branches.

b. Cardiac surgeons have been slow to embrace endoscopic approaches partly because, until recently, existing technology did not provide the range of motion and control required for coronary artery anastomoses.

c. The port-access approach introduced endoscopic techniques to cardiac surgery; surgeons are now working with computer-assisted instruments to perform surgery on the beating heart (see later). Techniques developed for off-pump surgery are likely to contribute to the ability to perform such procedures endoscopically.

C. Refinement of surgical approach

1. Development of modern epicardial stabilizers

a. In early reports, compressive devices (e.g., metal extensions rigidly attached to the sternal retractor) were used to reduce the motion of the coronary vessel during the cardiac and respiratory cycles. These devices often interfered with cardiac function and were impossible to use for left circumflex coronary artery lesions.

b. Modern devices typically apply gentle pressure or epicardial suction, reducing the effect on myocardial function while providing better fixation of the area immediately surrounding the coronary artery anastomotic site. These devices also allow greater access to arteries on the inferior and posterior surfaces of the heart (Fig. 13.1).

2. Techniques to position the heart (through midline sternotomy)

a. Surgery on the anterior wall of the heart (LAD and diagonal branches) usually requires only mild repositioning, such as a laparotomy pad under the cardiac apex. This is associated with minimal effects on cardiac function.

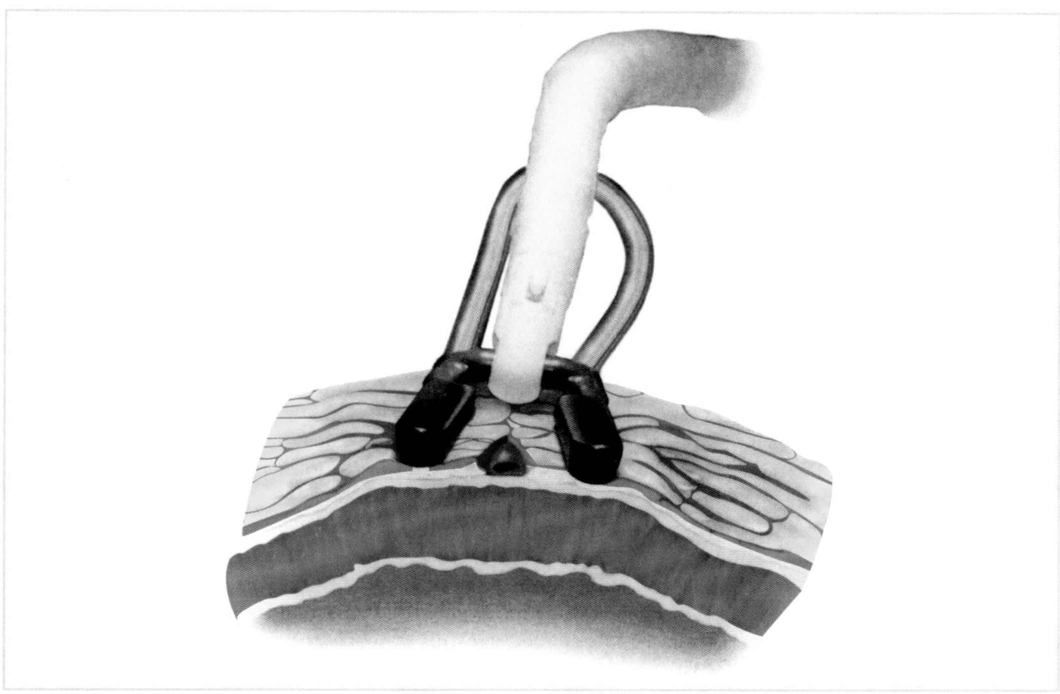

FIGURE 13.1 The Octopus 2 tissue stabilizer (Medtronic Inc., Minneapolis, MN, U.S.A.). Through gentle suction the device elevates and pulls the tissue taut, thereby immobilizing the target area. (Courtesy of Medtronic Inc.)

b. Surgery on the right coronary artery (RCA) or the circumflex artery and its marginal branches requires turning or twisting of the heart. To do this manually (i.e., by an assistant) is cumbersome and is associated with hemodynamic compromise.

c. Use of posterior pericardial traction stitches and a gentle retracting "sock" (web roll wrapped around the apex in a "sling" to pull the heart to either side) greatly improves the hemodynamic tolerance of these abnormal positions.

d. For circumflex vessel distribution surgery, dissection of the right pericardium to prevent the right ventricle (RV) from being compressed as it is being turned allows preservation of hemodynamic function.

3. **Surgical adjuncts to reduce ischemia**

a. Performing CABG surgery on the beating heart requires a mandatory period of coronary occlusion for each distal coronary artery anastomosis.

b. Intracoronary shunts can maintain coronary flow at the possible cost of trauma to the endothelium.

c. "Ischemic preconditioning" involves a brief (e.g., one to four 5-min periods) occlusion and then the same period of reperfusion before performing the anastomosis. In animal models of myocardial infarction, this technique reduces the area of necrosis. A nearly equivalent physiologic effect can be provided by 1 MAC end-tidal isoflurane [18] or other inhaled agents, which is termed anesthetic or pharmacologic preconditioning. Ischemic preconditioning for 7- to 10-min occlusions, such as those required for OPCAB and MIDCAB, probably does not provide the same benefit as one might see with longer periods of occlusion, but this technique is employed by some surgeons.

d. The proximal anastomosis of a vein graft can be performed first in order to allow immediate perfusion once the distal anastomosis is completed.

e. Regional hypothermia techniques have been described for use during coronary occlusion.

f. Preoperative insertion of an intra-aortic balloon pump (IABP) has been used for patients with reduced ventricular function requiring multivessel OPCAB.

D. Patient selection: High risk versus low risk

1. Early reports of OPCAB often described single-vessel or double-vessel bypass performed on low-risk patients. This was promoted as permitting early recovery and discharge.
2. **OPCAB is now promoted for multivessel bypass in patients with risk factors for adverse outcomes.** Elderly patients at risk for stroke, patients with severe lung disease, or patients with severe vascular disease and/or renal dysfunction are often selected. As mentioned earlier, scientific studies have not yet demonstrated reduced adverse outcomes with OPCAB in these populations.
3. Zenati et al. [19] and others have described combining MIDCAB (i.e., IMA to LAD) with angioplasty/stent to other vessels in high-risk patients.
4. As mentioned earlier, a small number of surgeons attempt to perform virtually all CABG procedures as OPCAB regardless of preoperative risk status.

E. Anesthetic management

1. **Preoperative assessment**
   a. The cardiac catheterization report should be reviewed and the procedure discussed with the surgeon, including the planned sequence of bypass grafts and the potential use of specific adjuncts (e.g., shunts or perfusion-assisted direct coronary artery bypass grafting, or PADCAB). This allows the anesthesiologist to predict the effect of each coronary occlusion, which requires knowledge of the coronary anatomy and its usual nomenclature (Fig. 13.2).
   b. The vessel, location, and degree of stenosis determine the functional response to intraoperative coronary occlusion. Even with a proximal stenosis, an important vessel (e.g., LAD) may supply adequate resting flow to a large area of myocardium. Acute loss of flow to this large area (with surgical occlusion) may cause ventricular failure.

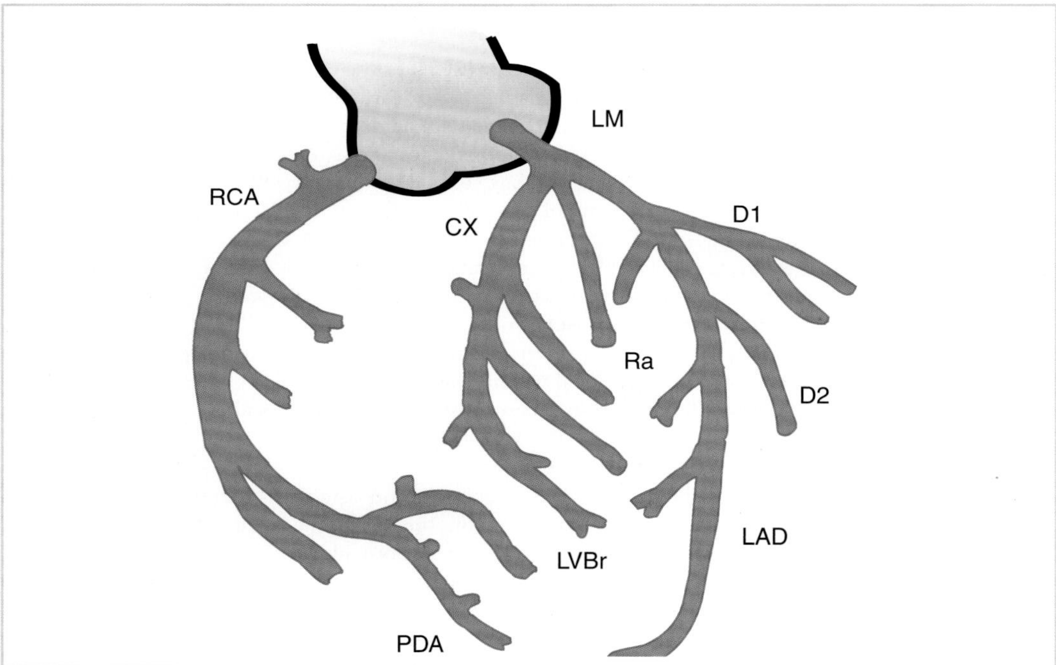

FIGURE 13.2 Coronary anatomy. The main branches from the circumflex artery (*CX*) are named "marginal" or "obtuse marginal" vessels. *D1*, first diagonal; *D2*, second diagonal; *LAD,* left anterior descending artery; *LM,* left main; *PDA,* posterior descending artery; *RCA,* right coronary artery; *LVBr,* LV branch; *Ra,* Ramus intermedius (<40% of individuals).

A stenosis further down the vessel may be less important for overall ventricular performance.

c. High-grade stenosis (e.g., 90%) is likely to be associated with some collateral blood flow from adjacent regions, as flow through the stenosis may be inadequate even at rest. A 10-min occlusion of such a vessel may have surprisingly little effect on regional function and hemodynamics because of the collateral flow. A lesser degree of stenosis (e.g., 75% to 80%) may not affect resting flow, hence there may be little or no collateral blood flow. Occlusion of such a vessel may cause severe myocardial dysfunction in the distribution of the vessel.

d. If incisions other than sternotomy are to be employed to access specific coronary regions, positioning of the arms and the body, the potential need for one lung anesthesia, and sites for vascular access need to be discuss. Some surgeons prefer one-lung anesthesia even for a median sternotomy approach to OPCAB.

2. **Measures to avoid hypothermia**

a. Unlike on-pump CABG, it is difficult to restore heat to a hypothermic OPCAB patient. In order to maintain hemostasis and facilitate early recovery, **prevention of heat loss needs to be planned before the patient enters the room**.

b. While in the preoperative area, the patient should be kept warm with blankets.

c. The operating room should be warmed to the greatest degree tolerated by the operating team (e.g., 75°F or higher). The temperature can be reduced once warming devices have been placed and the patient is fully draped.

d. The period and degree to which the patient remains uncovered for preoperative procedures (e.g., urinary catheter placement) and surgical skin preparation and draping should be minimized. This requires vigilance on the part of the anesthesiology team and frequent reminders to the surgical team.

e. Various adjuncts to preserve heat include heated mattress cover or insert; forced-air warming blankets, including sterile "lower body" blankets placed after vein harvesting; and circumferential heating tubes. A more expensive and possibly more effective option is the use of disposable surface-gel heating devices [20].

f. Fluid warmers should be used at least for the principal intravenous volume infusion "line," if not for all intravenous lines other than those used for intravenous drug infusions.

g. Low fresh-gas flows and circle/CO_2 reabsorption circuits will help prevent heat loss.

3. **Monitoring** (Table 13.1)

a. **Preoperative assessment of ventricular function**

(1) Preoperative LV function is a major determinant of the need for extensive monitoring. **Patients with normal or near-normal LV function are less likely to need diagnosis and therapy guided by invasive monitoring.**

(2) A patient with an elevated LV end-diastolic pressure (at cardiac catheterization) may have a "stiff" ventricle, or diastolic dysfunction. This commonly results from hypertrophy or ischemia. Filling pressures obtained intraoperatively must be interpreted in this context (i.e., the filling pressure may overestimate LV preload). Volumetric assessment of preload (by TEE) can be valuable in this situation.

(3) Patients with poor ventricular function may tolerate coronary occlusions poorly. Appropriate responses may be best guided by monitors of cardiac output (CO) and filling pressures, or TEE [21,22].

(4) Repeated occlusions in multiple regions of the myocardium (i.e., for multivessel OPCAB) are likely to result in a cumulative detrimental effect on hemodynamics. There may be a period of myocardial dysfunction requiring inotropic support even in patients with good underlying LV function. The combination of reduced ventricular function and the need for multiple bypass grafts is likely to result in a need for inotropic and/or vasopressor infusions guided by monitoring with a pulmonary artery catheter (PAC) and/or TEE.

TABLE 13.1 Monitoring approaches for OPCAB and MIDCAB

Monitor	Advantages	Disadvantages	Comment
ECG	• Universal • Simple • Inexpensive • Recognized criteria	• Insensitive • Position dependent (lead and heart) • Incision dependent • Loss of V4–5 (MIDCAB)	• Best if multilead • Should be calibrated • ST-segment trending helpful
Central venous pressure	• Simple • Inexpensive	• Pressure–volume relationship uncertain • Insensitive for LV dysfunction • No CO	• Important for drug infusions • Affected by position of heart and patient Use of "introducer" allows rapid insertion of PAC
PAC	• LV filling pressure • CO • Options may be helpful (mixed venous O_2 saturation, continuous CO, pacing)	• Pressure–volume relationship uncertain • Expensive • Insensitive for acute regional dysfunction	• Controversial monitor • May prolong ICU stay due to "abnormal numbers"
TEE	• Gold standard for acute ischemia • Verify restoration of function • Guide surgical cannula placement	• Expensive • User dependent • Distracting • May not have good view of heart	• Requires real-time interpretation
CO bioimpedance (BE); esophageal Doppler (ED); arterial waveform analysis (AW)	• Less invasive than PAC • AW gives stroke volume variation	• No measure of LV filling • ED positional • AW may vary with vascular tone	• BE and stroke volume variation (from AW) questionable with open chest • ED may interfere with TEE (or vice versa)

OPCAB, off-pump coronary artery bypass; ECG, electrocardiogram; MIDCAB, minimally invasive direct coronary artery bypass; LV, left ventricular; CO, cardiac output; PAC, pulmonary artery catheter; icu, intensive care unit; TEE, transesophageal echocardiography; ED, esophageal Doppler; AW, arterial waveform analysis.

(5) Preoperative placement of a PAC introducer, but with an obturator of some kind or a single- or double-lumen central venous catheter placed through it rather than a PAC may be a reasonable first approach in most patients. This avoids the use of the PAC in uncomplicated patients while allowing for rapid PAC placement should this be desired any time in the perioperative period.

b. Specific monitors

(1) Lead V_5 of the electrocardiogram (ECG) detects 75% of the ischemia found on all 12 leads. This lead should be monitored in all patients undergoing OPCAB or MIDCAB, as permitted by the surgical incision. Lead II gives clear P waves, but adds little to the sensitivity of ischemia detection.

(2) The PAC is variably useful during OPCAB. For single- or double-vessel bypass in patients with preserved LV function, there can be little justification for this monitor [23]. **The worse the ventricular function and the greater the number of planned bypass grafts, the more likely it is that information from the PAC will be useful.**

(3) Continuous CO from the PAC or other devices and continuous mixed venous oximetry may provide incremental benefit in assessing the adequacy of cardiac function. Use of these devices is often institution-specific or even surgeon/anesthesiologist-specific.

(4) **Monitoring with TEE can provide detailed information about the effects of coronary occlusion and recovery, and it provides the earliest, most specific**

6 **information during acute deterioration and interventions.** Acute ventricular dilatation and mitral regurgitation may occur when a large region of the myocardium becomes ischemic, and this is detected immediately with TEE. In addition, distortion of the mitral annulus due to abnormal positioning may cause mitral regurgitation [24]. Obtaining adequate images may be distracting to clinical care. With the heart in an unusual position, images may be difficult or impossible to obtain. A reversible wall-motion abnormality that resolves with restoration of flow is reassuring; however, this does not guarantee a good quality graft or anastomosis.

(5) Normal carbon dioxide (CO_2) elimination requires adequate CO. If ventilation is constant, an acute decline in CO will cause an acute decrease in end-tidal CO_2 concentration.

c. Monitoring for specific procedures

(1) For MIDCAB or other reduced-access procedures, provision must be made for transcutaneous defibrillation and pacing. An important consideration is the requirement to reinflate the lungs for defibrillation during closed-chest surgery to provide tissue (rather than air) for the current to traverse [25].

(2) For port-access surgery (Heartport or related procedures), TEE is required to guide and monitor cannula placement and function.

4. Anesthetic technique

a. Early recovery is usually desired. Extubation immediately or shortly after surgery should be the goal.

7 **b.** A vapor-based anesthetic technique facilitates early recovery. Keys to prevention of delayed awakening are as follows: Minimizing the dose of benzodiazepine; use of modest doses of opioids; and avoiding residual paralysis at the end of surgery. Some clinicians use very short-acting opioids such as remifentanil to facilitate early extubation, but this approach requires awareness of the need for effective longer-lasting analgesia at the time of extubation and thereafter. Use of bispectral index (BIS) monitoring can help guide administration of hypnotic agents.

c. Transfer of the intubated yet awakening patient to the intensive care unit (ICU), and early ICU care are facilitated by use of short-acting sedative drugs such as propofol or dexmedetomidine.

d. Thoracic epidural or lumbar spinal anesthetic and analgesic techniques have been promoted by some as suitable adjuncts to off-pump approaches. There are reports of OPCAB procedures done without general anesthesia. Most centers are reluctant to risk major neuraxial techniques immediately before full heparinization for CPB. Use of such techniques is unlikely to shorten postoperative length of stay and has not been shown to provide a measurable benefit.

e. For MIDCAB (thoracotomy), postoperative epidural analgesia [26], paravertebral block, or intercostal blockade may be useful for pain control.

5. Anticipation and management of ischemia

a. Knowledge of the coronary anatomy and surgical plan is essential. This allows appropriate timing of pharmacologic and other interventions before ischemia is induced. **Use of isoflurane (or other volatile inhalational agent) anesthesia can provide pharmacologic "preconditioning,"** as mentioned earlier. Avoidance of hemodynamic alterations associated with ischemia such as tachycardia (especially in the presence of hypotension) must be avoided. Intravenous β-adrenergic blockade may be beneficial; however, this must be balanced with the possibility of impaired myocardial performance during coronary occlusion.

b. Maintenance of adequate coronary artery perfusion pressure is of great importance in allowing collateral blood flow to ischemic regions. Volume loading and appropriate positioning (see following), alteration of the depth of anesthesia, and/or use of α-adrenergic agonists may all be indicated.

c. Prophylactic nitrate infusions may interfere with preload (see later).

d. Early experience without modern stabilizers suggested that bradycardia (to reduce motion) would aid the surgeon. This is no longer an issue. Grafting to the RCA territory (supplying the sinus and AV nodes) can be associated with bradycardia. Thus, although β-adrenergic blockade may be useful to prevent or treat tachycardia, epicardial pacing may be required for ischemia-induced bradycardia.

e. Anecdotally, patients with compromised ventricular function undergoing multivessel procedures may benefit from "prophylactic" administration of an inotropic medication.

6. **Intravascular volume loading**

3

a. **Positioning of the heart may kink or partially obstruct venous return and/or compress the RV. Intravascular volume loading and head-down (Trendelenburg) position can help reduce this effect** (Fig. 13.3) [27]. Close observation of the heart, filling pressures, and blood pressure to provide feedback to the surgeon is essential.

b. Intravenous vasodilators (e.g., nitrates) can exacerbate reductions in cardiac filling. More commonly, intravenous vasoconstrictors (phenylephrine, norepinephrine) will be required during abnormal cardiac positions.

7. **Surgery-anesthesiology interaction.** With all the above considerations, it should be clear that there must be excellent communication between the surgeon and the anesthesiologist for OPCAB or MIDCAB. Anticipation and planning for problems allow the anesthesiologist to intervene in a timely manner. The surgeon must say in advance what he is planning to do. Similarly, changes in cardiac performance and the need for intervention must be continuously communicated to the surgeon. The anesthesiologist must observe the surgical field, watching the procedure as well as the position, size, and function of the heart. An observant, communicative team with basic monitoring (ECG, blood pressure, and central venous pressure) is likely to produce better results than a team that communicates poorly, but uses extensive monitoring.

F. **Anticoagulation**

1. **Heparin management**

a. Heparin anticoagulation protocols are institution-specific. Similar to on-pump surgery, there are few data to recommend targeting specific activated clotting time (ACT) values.

b. Some surgeons request full heparinization similar to on-pump procedures (i.e., ACT target >400 s); others request lower doses of heparin such as would be used for noncardiac vascular procedures (ACT target typically >200 s), or something in between. Outcomes appear to be equivalent using either approach, which suggests that ACT targets as high as those used for CPB are unnecessary.

2. **Protamine reversal**

a. Extracorporeal circulation induces a postoperative multifactorial defect in coagulation that may reduce early graft thrombosis. When coagulation is reversed after OPCAB or MIDCAB, no such hypocoagulable state exists; indeed, there is evidence that the coagulation system is activated by the stress of surgery, similar to what has been showed for other major procedures [28].

b. In order to gradually return the coagulation to normal leaving perhaps a little residual heparin effect, reversal may be achieved with incremental doses of protamine. If "full" heparinization has been employed, administration of 50 mg of protamine may bring the ACT down to near 200 s, after which small increments (10 to 25 mg) can be given to achieve an ACT that is about 25% to 50% above control (i.e., 150 to 180 s).

c. If the patient is clinically bleeding with an elevated ACT, then heparin should be reversed completely. Even in the absence of clinical bleeding, some cardiac surgeons prefer complete reversal immediately after completion of the grafts.

d. Prolonged OPCAB procedures may be associated with extensive blood loss and therefore facilitated by the use of cell-saver devices (i.e., washing of salvaged blood so it is free of coagulation proteins and platelets). Over time, this may induce a dilutional coagulopathy similar to what is often seen after CPB.

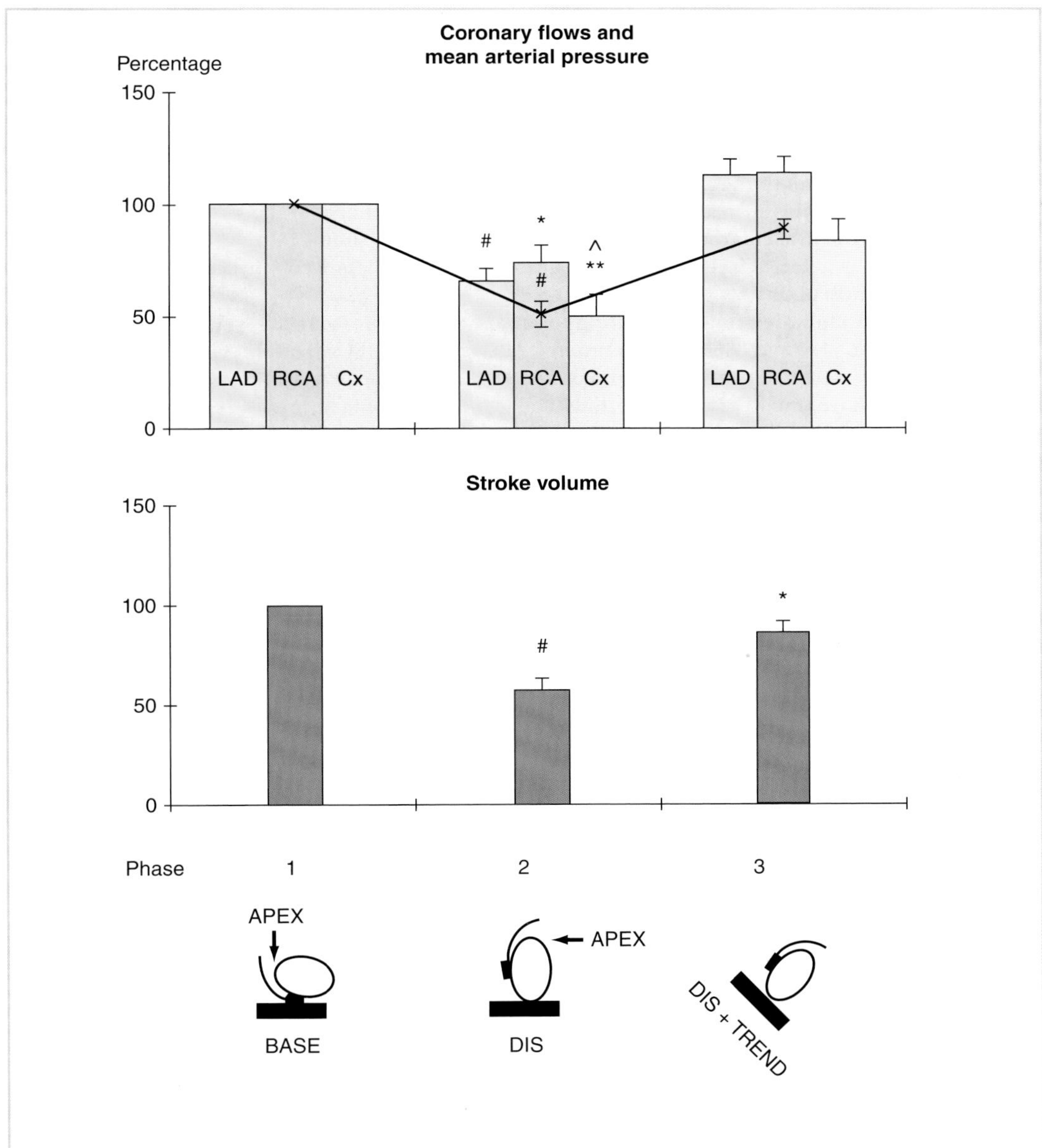

FIGURE 13.3 Relative changes in hemodynamic parameters during vertical displacement of the beating porcine heart by the Medtronic Octopus tissue stabilizer and the effect of head-down tilt. *BASE,* pericardial control position; *Cx,* circumflex coronary artery; *DIS,* displacement of the heart by the Octopus; *DIS + TREND,* Trendelenburg maneuver (20-degree head-down tilt while the heart remains retracted 90 degrees); *LAD,* left anterior descending artery; *RCA,* right coronary artery; x = mean arterial pressure. Statistical comparison with control values: $^*p < 0.05$; $^{**}p < 0.01$; $\#p < 0.001$; $^\wedge p = 0.046$ versus combined relative value of LAD and RCA flows. (From Grundeman PF, Borst C, van Herwaarden JA, et al. Vertical displacement of the beating heart by the Octopus tissue stabilizer: Influence on coronary flow. *Ann Thorac Surg.* 1998;65:1348–1352, with permission.)

3. **Antiplatelet therapy**
   a. Thrombosis at the site of vascular anastomoses is initiated by platelet aggregation and adhesion. Similar to strategies that are used in angioplasty/stent procedures, antiplatelet therapy may help reduce early graft thrombosis in CABG, whether done with or without CPB.

b. A common practice is to administer a dose of aspirin preoperatively. This can be achieved with a suppository if the patient is already anesthetized.
c. In on-pump CABG, administration of aspirin within 4 h after the procedure reduces graft thrombosis. This strategy should also be applied to OPCAB and MIDCAB.
d. There are no published data about the use of newer antiplatelet drugs in this setting. As with all such therapies (including aspirin), the concern for bleeding must be balanced with the desire to prevent graft thrombosis.

4. **Antifibrinolytic therapy.** Use of lysine analogs to inhibit fibrinolysis has become common practice with on-pump CABG, as they have been shown to reduce perioperative blood loss. Recent investigations now support the use of these agents during OPCAB as well [29].

G. **Recovery**

1. **Extubation in the operating room**
   a. For uncomplicated procedures, recovery from OPCAB or MIDCAB can be rapid without the requirement for postoperative ventilation or sedation.
   b. Normothermia, hemostasis, and hemodynamic stability must be assured.
   c. Residual anesthesia and paralysis from long-acting agents (e.g., pancuronium, large doses of morphine) must be avoided.
   d. Extra time spent in the operating room to achieve extubation may be more costly than a few hours of postoperative ventilation and sedation.
2. **ICU management**
   a. **For most patients, early postoperative management can employ the "fast track" technique where mechanical ventilation is withdrawn within a few hours of surgery, and patients are extubated and possibly mobilized at the bedside late in the day or during the evening of surgery.**
   b. ICU stay is driven by institutional practice, but for patients having straightforward, uncomplicated procedures, there may be no need for more than a few hours in a high-intensity nursing area (i.e., postanesthetic care unit or ICU).
   c. If length of stay is reduced, cost will almost certainly be reduced. If there is no significant reduction in stay, the cost of specialized retractor systems may exceed the cost of the disposables required for CPB.
   d. Some surgeons passionately believe that OPCAB is better for their patients; perhaps with time and additional randomized trials, the hoped-for reductions in neurologic events, renal dysfunction, and other adverse outcomes will become apparent.

II. Minimally invasive valve surgery (MIVS)

A. Introduction

The Society of Thoracic Surgeons National Database defines minimally invasive surgery as "any procedure that has not been performed with a full sternotomy and cardiopulmonary bypass support. All other procedures, on- or off-pump with a small incision or off-pump with a full sternotomy are also considered minimally invasive" [30]. Similar to MIDCAB, the premise of MIVS is that "smaller is better" for valve surgery as well. A partial sternotomy or small thoracotomy with port incisions may achieve some benefits when compared to standard median sternotomy. Similar to OPCAB, alternative approaches were explored in the late 1990s, with the first publication in 1998. Proposed [31,32] but unproved advantages to these approaches include the following:

1. Reduced hospital length of stay and costs
2. Quicker return to full activity
3. Less atrial fibrillation (26% vs. 38% in one report [33])
4. Less blood transfusion
5. Same results (mortality, valve function)
6. Less pain
7. Earlier ambulation

In addition, the surgical opinion is that reoperation should be easier after MIVS, as the pericardium is not opened over the RV outflow tract. These proposed benefits may be observed with specific surgeons in specific centers; however, there have been no rigorous or

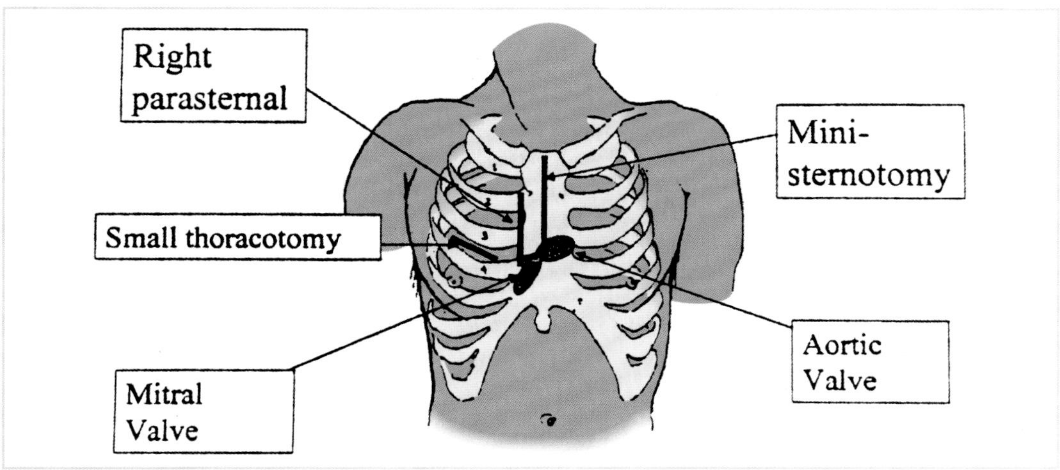

FIGURE 13.4 Incisions for MIVS. The most common approach is the "mini" sternotomy, which extends from the sternal notch part way to the xiphisternum but is diverted to the right at the level of the third or fourth interspace (for the aortic valve), leaving the lower sternum intact. The mitral valve can be accessed through the small right thoracotomy. (From Clements F, Glower DD. Minimally invasive valve surgery. In: Clements F, Shanewise J, eds. *Minimally Invasive Cardiac and Vascular Surgical Techniques. Society of Cardiovascular Anesthesiologists monograph.* Philadelphia, PA: Lippincott Williams & Wilkins; 2001:30.)

randomized studies. The limited data that exist suggest that acute postoperative pulmonary function impairment is not improved by the use of the limited incision. Minimally invasive reoperative aortic valve surgery is a new and successful technique, especially in patients who have had previous cardiac operations using a full sternotomy (e.g., prior CABG). This surgical approach does not disturb the vein grafts or the patent IMAs [34].

B. **Surgical approaches** (Fig. 13.4)

1. Port-access (Heartport): This approach involves direct surgical visualization and operation through small openings (ports) and a small right horizontal thoracotomy incision for access to the mitral valve or atrial septum. In order to avoid sternotomy, the port-access system uses alternative access sites and cannulae. The aorta is cannulated through a long femoral arterial catheter or a shorter transthoracic aortic catheter. These devices are advanced to the ascending aorta and include an "endo-aortic clamp" or inflatable balloon to achieve aortic occlusion ("cross-clamp") from within. They include a cardioplegia administration port. Venous cannulation is achieved with a long femoral venous catheter, supplemented as needed with a pulmonary artery vent. A coronary sinus catheter is used to administer cardioplegia. Placement of these catheters can be time-consuming and requires imaging with fluoroscopy and/or TEE. A limited number of institutions still use this approach to MIVS. Some reports have raised concerns about device-related aortic dissections as well as endoaortic balloon rupture and dislocation [35].
2. Video-assisted port-assisted (using the port-access cannulae and small incisions with video equipment to visualize and perform valve surgery). This is currently performed in a small number of institutions worldwide.
3. Robotic (see below). This is an evolving technique, particularly for mitral valve repair, with excellent results being reported.
4. Direct-access (small incision—many types: Anterolateral mini-thoracotomy, partial upper or lower sternotomy, right parasternal incision, and others). The right parasternal approach is preferred by some surgeons (especially for aortic valve access) because there is no sternal disruption and it is cosmetically pleasing. The avoidance of sternotomy bleeding into the pericardial sac with associated fibrinogen depletion may result in less perioperative bleeding and less pain that is easier to control, although the need to divide two or more

costochondral cartilages with the parasternal approach does induce considerable postoperative pain. As mentioned earlier, avoidance of opening the pericardium over the RV outflow tract may make future cardiac reoperation easier and safer. One problem with this approach is the sacrifice of the right IMA.

5. The current standard approach for aortic valve surgery using a minimally invasive approach is an "inverse L" shaped partial sternotomy extending to the third or fourth right intercostal space. In order to bring the entire heart more anteriorly, three to four retention stitches are passed through the pericardial rim and fixed to the skin incision. This may be associated with compression of the right atrium and a decrease in the venous return to the heart. The arterial cannula for CPB is placed in the ascending aorta. Venous return is established by direct cannulation of the right atrial appendage or by percutaneous femoral vein cannulation of the right atrium. With the latter cannulation technique, often a two-stage cannula is used with the distal tip placed at the junction of the SVC and RA as confirmed by TEE (bicaval view) [36].
6. Minimally invasive mitral valve surgery can use a right anterolateral minithoracotomy for which the patient is positioned supine with slight elevation of the right chest (often using a folded blanket) and extension of the right arm. Optimal visualization the heart requires deflation of the right lung, which is achieved most often by using a double-lumen endobronchial tube. CPB is established via the femoral vessels. The superior vena cava may also be cannulated percutaneously via the right internal jugular vein (IJV). A percutaneous transthoracic aortic cross-clamp is placed through a separate stab incision in the right posterior axillary line [35], and the mitral valve is accessed through the left atrium. Another approach is a right parasternal incision with mitral valve exposure via the right atrium and interatrial septum.
7. Reduced-size skin/soft tissue incision compared with full median sternotomy can give a more cosmetically pleasing result.

C. **Preoperative assessment.** In addition to understanding the valvular and associated cardiac disease, the anesthesiologist must have a good appreciation for the surgical plan. Nonsternotomy and port-access approaches require specific positioning, including having the arms extended or cephalad either suspended in a sling or resting on an "airplane" type of armrest, and will have implications for peripheral venous, central venous, and arterial catheter placement. Port-access procedures will require planning for fluoroscopic and TEE assistance to guide and monitor placement of catheters.

D. **Monitoring**

1. Central venous catheter versus PAC. Because of pericardial traction and/or compression of the right atrium, pulmonary artery, or RV outflow tract, the relationship between pressures recorded from central venous or PACs and chamber volumes may be changed. In addition, due to limited ability to palpate around the heart, there may be an increased risk of inadvertently including the PAC in surgical sutures. These considerations must be balanced with the potential need to guide fluid and inotropic therapy perioperatively.
2. TEE. There can be little doubt that TEE monitoring is an integral part of MIVS [36]. With such limited access, the surgeon cannot rely on visual cues about cardiac distension or volume status. Thus, TEE is used in the following ways:
   a. Pre-CPB to determine:
      (1) Valve dysfunction
      (2) Cardiac volume and function
      (3) Arterial cannulation site
      (4) Specialized cannula placement, especially for port access
   b. During CPB for port-access and robotic surgery, TEE is used to monitor appropriate placement of the endoaortic "clamp" and to detect intracardiac air, which can be extensive in MIVS cases.
   c. After CPB, TEE is used in the usual manner to assist with identification and management of new-onset ventricular dysfunction, which may occur in as much as 20% of MIVS patients. This is more frequent in patients with significant intracardiac air. TEE is also used to assess valve function and to look for aortic dissection.

E. **Specific anesthesiology concerns.** Regardless of the type of surgical access to MIVS, there are several common problems that require enhanced awareness:

1. Long surgical learning curve: Be prepared for anything during this period.
2. Limited surgical access (small incision)
   a. Urgent cardiac pacing and direct current cardioversion may need to be done transthoracically. Appropriate skin electrodes or patches must be placed before surgery is started.
   b. Big fingers, sponges, or instruments can compress vascular structures, causing large swings in hemodynamics.
   c. "Blind" suture placement can lead to bleeding from posterior sites which can be very difficult to control. Full median sternotomy is occasionally required to control the bleeding.
   d. Inadequate valve repair or replacement: Paravalvular leaks or valve dysfunction secondary to suture-induced valve leaflet sticking can occur.
   e. Errant suture placement may cause coronary artery compromise leading to myocardial ischemia, or may affect the conduction system leading to heart block or dysrhythmias.
   f. De-airing is very difficult, even when guided by TEE. Residual air may embolize to the coronary arteries resulting in acute cardiac decompensation. CO_2 gas is very commonly administered into the operating field to minimize this complication, with varying success.
   g. Tamponade: After chest closure, even a small amount of bleeding can lead to tamponade physiology in the mini-incision area.

F. **Postoperative management.** The goal is early recovery and extubation. As in MIDCAB and OPCAB, this is governed by a number of factors, including patient stability and temperature, duration of the procedure, and the use of short-acting agents. Extubation in the operating room is possible but uncommon. Certain incisions (i.e., thoracotomy) may lend themselves to the use of paravertebral or intercostal nerve blocks for postoperative pain relief.

G. **Percutaneous valve repair/replacement.** Percutaneous approaches to mitral regurgitation,
10 mitral stenosis, and aortic stenosis are rapidly growing in popularity. Each approach presents unique challenges to the anesthesiologist.

1. **MitraClip** [37,38]. A clip has been developed for mitral regurgitation which captures the free edges of both mitral valve leaflets, creating a double orifice valve similar to the Alfieri surgical repair. Under general anesthesia, the femoral vein is accessed, and with fluoroscopic and TEE guidance the device is advanced over a guidewire through the interatrial septum and through the regurgitant portion of the mitral valve, where it is deployed. Multiple clips may be used if necessary. Early studies suggest that though the procedure is safe, it may be most beneficial to high-risk surgical candidates with functional MR, as conventional surgical methods are more effective in reducing the severity of MR. Potential complications include hemopericardium leading to tamponade, damage to the mitral valve, device failure requiring surgical repair, device embolization, creation of mitral stenosis, and persistent interatrial shunt from the septal puncture. This procedure continues to be investigated.
2. **Percutaneous Balloon Mitral Valvuloplasty** [39]. Certain patients with symptomatic or severe mitral stenosis may be candidates for percutaneous balloon mitral valvuloplasty as an effective alternative to open surgical mitral commissurotomy. Prior to the procedure, TEE is performed to interrogate the left atrium and left atrial appendage for thrombus which may dislodge during the dilation and lead to systemic embolization. The procedure can be performed using local anesthesia with sedation or general anesthesia. Under fluoroscopic guidance, a guidewire is advanced through the femoral vein into the right atrium then through the interatrial septum. The balloon catheter is advanced along the guidewire and positioned in the mitral valve. Once properly positioned, the balloon is inflated, thereby dilating the valve. Repeated dilations are performed until there is an improvement of the pressure gradient between the left atrium and left ventricle, significant mitral regurgitation occurs, or echocardiographic assessment reveals adequate fracture of the commissures. Complications include damage to cardiac structures, hemopericardium leading to tamponade, emboli release, worsening or creation of mitral regurgitation, damage

to the subvalvular apparatus, and persistent interatrial shunt. Acute success rates and long-term restenosis rates are comparable to those for open surgical mitral commisurotomy.

3. **TAVI.** Although surgical replacement of the aortic valve is the treatment of choice for patients with severe aortic stenosis, some patients are at very high risk for mortality or major morbidity with surgery. TAVI is a less invasive alternative performed without CPB in which a bioprosthetic valve is implanted within the native aortic valve via a catheter introduced through a major artery or the apex of the left ventricle [40].
   a. There are two valves currently available:
      (1) Edwards SAPIEN valve (Edwards Lifesciences, Irvine, CA): Transfemoral or transapical deployment. This valve requires rapid ventricular pacing during deployment and is expanded with a balloon. Thus, the CO is zero during deployment.
      (2) CoreValve ReValving system (Medtronic, Minneapolis, MN): Transfemoral deployment. This valve is self-expanding and does not require rapid ventricular pacing to deploy. The left ventricle continues to eject during deployment.

      Both are available for use in Europe [41]. In the United States, only the SAPIEN valve is approved for nonsurgical candidates.
   b. **Contraindications.** Contraindications used in clinical trials to date include acute myocardial infarction within 1 month, congenital unicuspid or bicuspid valve, mixed aortic valve disease (stenosis and regurgitation), hypertrophic cardiomyopathy, LV ejection fraction below 20%, native aortic annulus size outside of the manufacturer's recommended range, severe vascular disease precluding safe placement of the introducer sheath (for the transfemoral approach), cerebrovascular event within 6 months, and need for emergency surgery.
   c. **Hybrid operating room** [42,43]. Cardiovascular hybrid surgery, which includes TAVI, is a rapidly evolving field where less invasive surgical approaches are combined with
12 interventional cardiology techniques in the same setting. Such procedures require a combination of high-quality imaging modalities found in a cardiac catheterization suite (fluoroscopy, navigation systems, post-processing capabilities, high-resolution invasive monitoring, intracardiac and intravascular ultrasound, echocardiography, etc.) in addition to the ability to perform open surgery under general anesthesia, including the use of CPB. These procedures require close collaboration and communication among multidisciplinary teams including interventional cardiologists, surgeons, anesthesiologists, perfusionists, technicians, and nursing staff, some of whom may be distant from the operating field. Thus, the presence of multiple monitor panels in areas visible to all and advanced communication systems are critical. Large amounts of space and careful planning of room layout are crucial for all of the equipment to be readily accessible and to allow unobstructed access to the patient. In addition, both the radiation safety requirements of the cardiac catheterization suite and the hygienic standards of the operating room must be met. These many demands have led to the creation of specialized hybrid operating rooms (Fig. 13.5).
   d. **Surgical approaches** (Fig. 13.6) [44–46]
      (1) **Retrograde or transfemoral approach**
         (a) The right femoral artery is accessed for device deployment. The left femoral artery and vein are accessed to provide for hemodynamic monitoring, transvenous pacing, contrast administration, and preparation for emergent CPB.
         (b) Heparin (100 to 150 units/kg) is given intravenously, titrating therapy to an ACT of about 300 s.
         (c) A guidewire is advanced across the aortic valve, and the balloon angioplasty catheter is advanced over the wire.
         (d) Ventricular pacing at about 200 beats/min (bpm) creates a low CO state (Fig. 13.7). In combination with apnea, a motionless field is obtained during inflation of the balloon, after which ventilation is resumed and pacing is terminated.
         (e) The valve catheter is positioned using fluoroscopy and TEE. Rapid ventricular pacing and apnea are used during valve deployment.

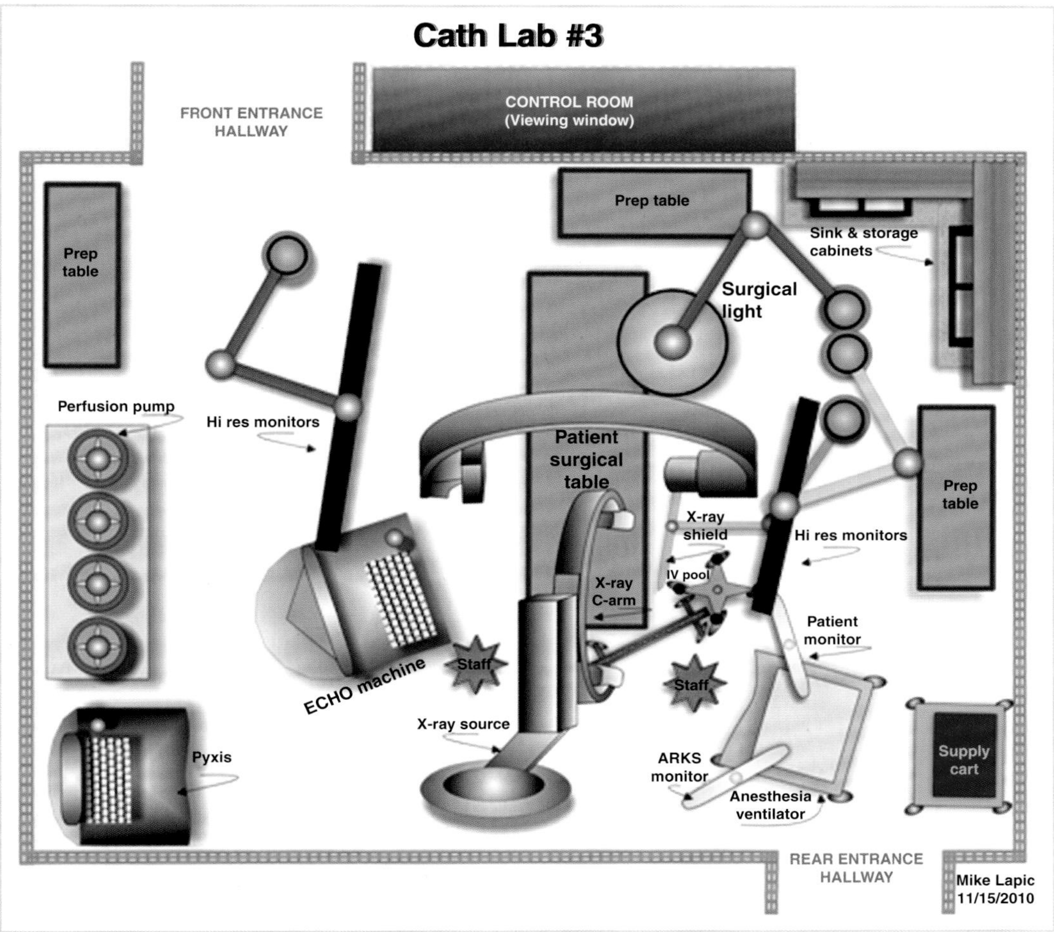

FIGURE 13.5 An example of a setup for a hybrid operating room; ARKS, anesthesia information system.

- **(f)** Fluoroscopy and TEE are used to assess valve position and function and to check for leak.

(2) Anterograde transapical approach

- **(a)** This more invasive approach is reserved for patients with peripheral arterial disease which would not accommodate the introducer and valve deployment systems.
- **(b)** The left femoral artery and vein are accessed as mentioned earlier.
- **(c)** The LV apex is exposed via left anterolateral thoracotomy. TEE may facilitate identification of the apex.
- **(d)** Heparin is given with the same ACT targets described earlier.
- **(e)** A needle is inserted through the LV apex, through which a guidewire is passed through the aortic valve under fluoroscopic and TEE guidance.
- **(f)** A balloon valvuloplasty catheter is introduced over the guidewire and positioned in the aortic valve. Similar to the retrograde approach, rapid ventricular pacing and apnea are initiated to create a motionless field during inflation.
- **(g)** The valvuloplasty sheath is then replaced by the device introducer sheath through which the prosthetic valve is deployed in a similar fashion.

Percutaneous aortic valve replacement

Percutaneous aortic valve replacement is done via a retrograde, antegrade, or transapical approach. Each has its challenges. In all three approaches, the positioning of the prosthetic valve is determined by the patient's native valvular structure and anatomy and is guided by fluoroscopic imaging, supra-aortic angiography, and transesophageal echocardiography. Current prosthetic valves are made from equine or bovine pericardial tissue.

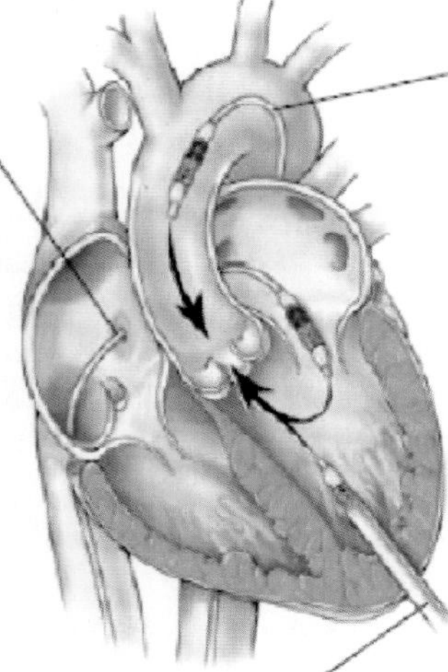

Antegrade technique

The catheter is advanced via the femoral vein, traversing the interatrial septum and the mitral valve, and is positioned within the diseased aortic valve.

Advantages

Femoral vein accommodates the large catheter sheath

Easy management of peripheral access site

Disadvantages

Risk of mitral valve injury and severe mitral valve regurgitation

Correctly positioning the prosthetic valve can be challenging

This technique is no longer in use.

Retrograde or transfemoral technique

The catheter is advanced to the stenotic aortic valve via the femoral artery.

Advantages

Faster, technically easier than antegrade approach

Disadvantages

Potential for injury to the aortofemoral vessels

Crossing the stenotic aortic valve can be challenging

Transapical technique

A valve delivery system is inserted via a small intercostal incision. The apex of the left ventricle is punctured, and the prosthetic valve is positioned within the stenotic aortic valve.

Advantages

Access to the stenotic valve is more direct

Avoids potential complications of a large peripheral access site

Disadvantages

Potential for complications related to puncture of the left ventricle

Requires general anesthesia and chest tubes

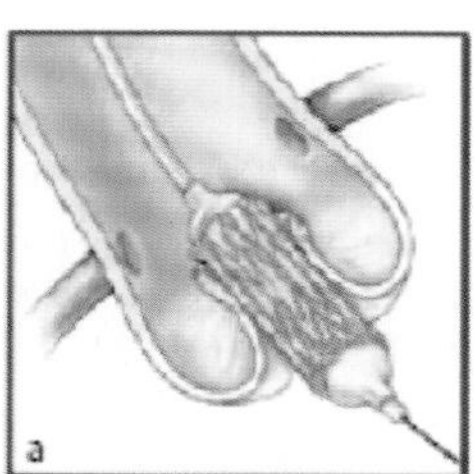

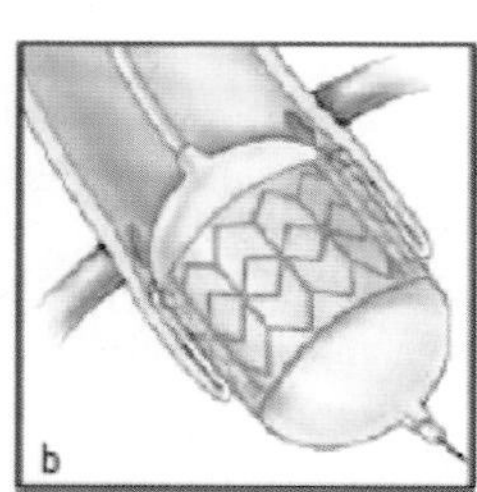

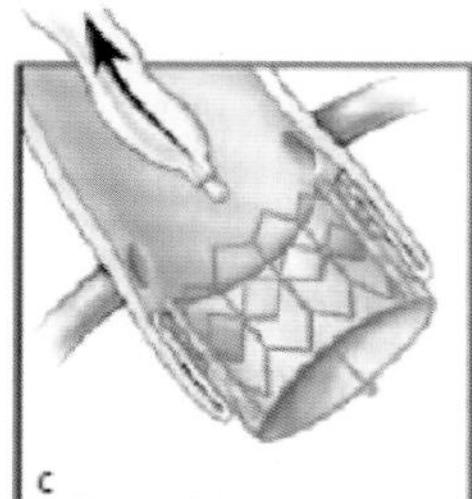

The aortic valve prosthesis is placed at mid-position in the patient's aortic valve so as not to impinge on the coronary ostia or to impede the motion of the anterior mitral leaflet (a). The prosthesis is deployed by inflating (b), rapidly deflating, and quickly withdrawing the delivery balloon (c).

FIGURE 13.6 Approaches to TAVI.

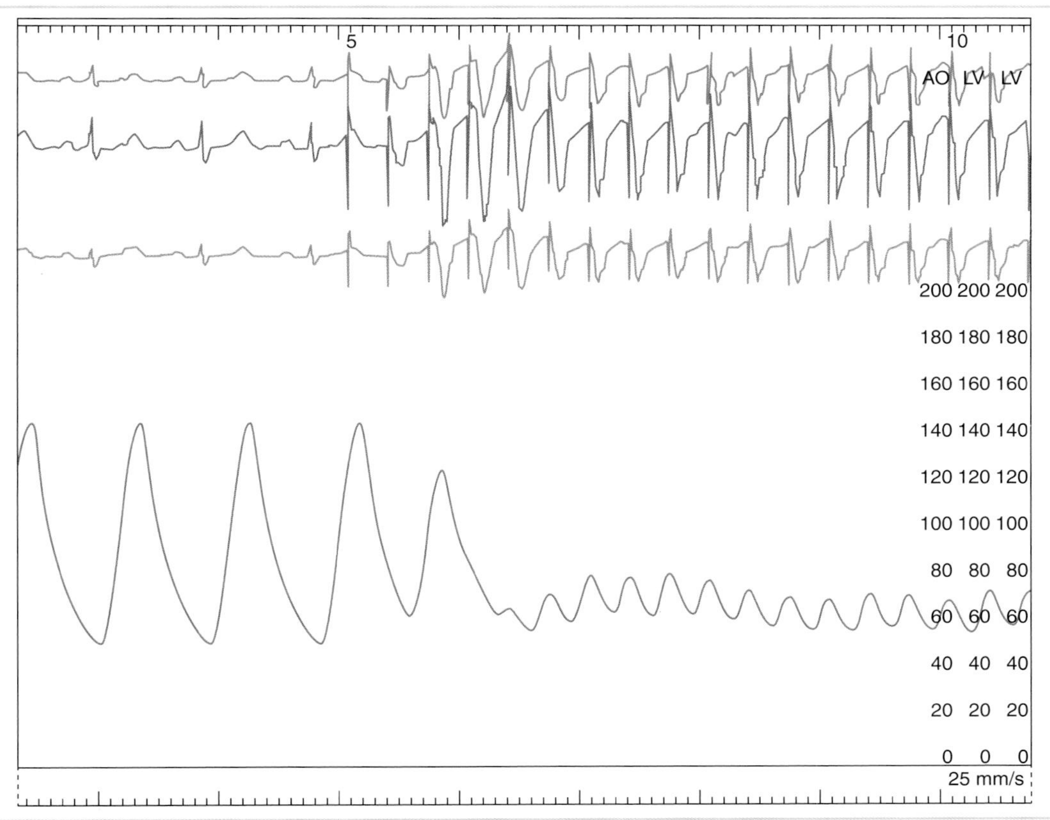

FIGURE 13.7 Hemodynamics during rapid ventricular pacing. The bottom waveform is taken from the arterial catheter.

(3) Other approaches

(a) Transsubclavian approach has been described as an alternative for patients with severe iliofemoral arterial disease [47]. Preoperative CT imaging is obtained to ensure that the vasculature is suitable for this approach. Access is obtained via surgical cutdown, and the valve is deployed similar to the retrograde (transfemoral) approach.

(b) Transaortic approach via ministernotomy has also been reported.

(c) Recently, a transcarotid approach has been used in patients not candidates for the other approaches.

e. Anesthetic considerations

(1) In addition to standard monitors, large-bore venous access and invasive blood pressure monitoring are essential. For the ongoing clinical trials, a PAC is usually placed; however, the catheter is withdrawn during the procedure itself as it interferes with the fluoroscopic image. TEE is helpful as a monitor and guide for valve placement, but transthoracic imaging or fluoroscopy alone may be used in patients having the procedure done via the retrograde transfemoral approach, using local anesthesia and sedation.

(2) Blood should be readily available, as massive hemorrhage from arterial injury can occur acutely.

(3) Radiolucent defibrillation pads should be placed prior to draping the patient in case the need arises for cardioversion or defibrillation.

(4) With the transapical approach, general anesthesia is necessary. Lung isolation may be helpful for surgical exposure, but it is not absolutely needed. For the retrograde approach, local or regional anesthesia with MAC may be adequate, but each patient should be assessed on an individual basis. The advantages of using local/regional anesthesia with sedation include the ability to assess neurologic status, avoidance of airway manipulation, and a more rapid early recovery. However, general anesthesia may be more comfortable for the patient, provide immobility during valve deployment, and provide a secure airway in the event of complications and the need for emergent CPB [48–50]. General anesthesia is especially helpful when TEE is used, and some clinicians see this as the "tipping point" for its selection. With either method of anesthesia, the goal is for the patient to recover rapidly. Shorter-acting anesthetic agents along with other adjuncts, such as intercostal nerve blocks performed under direct vision by the surgical team (transapical approach), will help accomplish this goal.

11 **(5)** During the procedure, there may be periods of acute hemodynamic instability as a result of the device occluding the already narrow valve, the creation of acute aortic regurgitation during valvuloplasty, massive bleeding from dissection of major vasculature, damage to the left ventricle or mitral valve, or acute occlusion of a coronary ostium. Arrhythmias are common during insertion of guidewires and catheters into the left ventricle. Clear communication with the surgical team is of utmost importance in order to treat appropriately and to avoid "overshooting" with vasopressors. Sometimes the solution is as simple as repositioning the catheter.

(6) Normothermia should be actively maintained with the use of forced air warming blankets and fluid warmers as needed.

(7) TEE is used to assess global cardiac function, measure the aortic root for sizing of valve, screen for aortic disease, facilitate proper valve positioning, and identify complications of the procedure such as paravalvular leak, tamponade, or coronary occlusion [41,51].

f. Complications [52,53]. Major complications of TAVI include stroke, vascular damage including dissection, rupture of the aortic root, occlusion of coronary ostia, cardiac conduction abnormalities, damage to other cardiac structures such as the mitral valve, embolization of the prosthesis requiring emergent surgical retrieval, and massive blood loss from vascular damage or rupture of the LV. Paravalvular leak is more common after TAVI than open surgery, probably because diseased, calcified tissue that may hinder optimal valve deployment is not removed. Paravalvular leaks may be treated with balloon reinflation to better appose the stented prosthesis to the aortic annulus.

g. Outcomes [40,54]. For nonsurgical candidates, TAVI has been associated with an improvement of symptoms and mortality at 1 yr as compared to medical management. In high-risk surgical candidates, TAVI and open surgery have similar 1-yr mortality rates. However, there appears to be a higher incidence of stroke and major vascular complications with TAVI. We look forward to more long-term outcome data as the procedure becomes more common.

III. Robotically enhanced cardiac surgery

A. Historical perspective

1. Use of robotics in surgery was initially considered for facilitation of surgical expertise at a site remote from the surgeon (e.g., battlefield, developing country).
2. Robotic enhancement of dexterity has been applied to endoscopic instruments, allowing on-site performance of complex tasks that were impossible using the endoscopic approach.
3. Computer-assisted, robotic cardiac surgery in patients was first reported by Loulmet et al. [55] and Reichenspurner et al. [56] in 1999.

5 4. Since then, a variety of procedures ranging from multivessel totally endoscopic coronary artery bypass grafting (TECAB), both on-pump and off-pump, to hybrid procedures involving robotic revascularization and PCI have evolved with promising results.

B. Overview

1. Taylor et al. [57] described the complementary capabilities of surgeon and machine.
   a. Surgeons are dextrous, adaptive, fast, and can execute motions over a large geometric scale; they develop judgment and experience. Limiting factors include geometric inaccuracy

and inexact exertion of directional force. Performance is compromised by confined spaces or bad exposure. Surgeons get tired, and with age can lose skills and vision.

b. Machines are precise and untiring. Computer-controlled instruments can be moved through an exactly defined trajectory with controlled forces, facilitating work in confined spaces.

2. Endoscopic surgery, by avoiding stress, pain, and cosmetic insult of open procedures, improves some outcomes and increases patient satisfaction. Laparoscopic cholecystectomy illustrates rapid adaptation of surgical practice to endoscopic techniques. In 1999, 85% of gall bladder surgeries (approximately 1,100,000 surgeries) were performed via this minimally invasive approach [58].
3. Many excisional or ablative procedures lend themselves to current endoscopic instrumentation. Reconstructive procedures (e.g., vascular anastomoses) are more difficult due to the requirement for multiple planes of fine motor activity.
4. Robotic enhancement of dexterity potentially allows the use of endoscopic techniques for complex surgery. For coronary artery bypass surgery, the goal is to avoid both sternotomy and CPB. Robotic devices permit construction of coronary artery grafts through endoscopic portals on the beating heart. This potentially allows surgical coronary bypass with a degree of invasiveness more comparable to angioplasty than to sternotomy [59].

C. Technologic advances permitting endoscopic surgery

1. Development of the charge-coupling device (CCD) allows high-resolution video images to be transmitted through optical scopes to the surgeon.
2. High-intensity xenon and halogen light sources improve visualization of the surgical field.
3. Improved hand instrumentation permit procedures that previously could only be performed through an open incision to be executed by less invasive methods [60].
4. The surgeon can now view digitally enhanced images that provide better visualization than direct viewing, due to magnification and illumination.
5. The major limitations of endoscopic instruments are the control of fine motor activity, surgery in a confined space, and a somewhat reduced sensory feedback of tissue resistance or firmness.
6. Placement of a microprocessor between the surgeon's hand and the tip of the surgical instrument dramatically enhances control and fine movement. Table 13.2 lists the ways in which computerized dexterity enhancement addresses limitations of conventional endoscopy.

TABLE 13.2 Endoscopic versus computer-enhanced instrumentation systems

Parameter	Conventional endoscopic instruments	Computer-enhanced systems
Degrees of freedom[a]	4	6
Tremor filter[b]	No	Yes
Motion transmission[c]	1:1	1:1 to 5:1
Hand–eye alignment[d]	Poor	Natural
Fulcrum effect[e]	Reversed motion	Not effective
Force ratio (hand/tip)[f]	Large/abnormal/not linear	Programmable/linear
Indexing[g]	Not possible	Possible
Ergonomics	Unfavorable	Favorable

[a]Number of different directions of movement. For instance, if something is capable of moving the *x*, *y*, and *z* directions, then it has three degrees of freedom. The da Vinci can probably move in the *x*, *y*, and *z* directions, plus it can rotate and act like forceps.
[b]Image filter that filters out camera vibrations or filters out surgeon tremors at the control station.
[c]Displacement amplifier to make finer movements possible. At the 5:1 setting, the robot moves 1 cm for every 5-cm movement of the surgeon at the control station.
[d]Assesses hand–eye coordination.
[e]Fulcrum is the point or support on which a lever turns. The conventional instrument is said to be reversed motion, meaning that if the surgeon moves in one direction, the actual motion of the instrument is in the opposite direction.
[f]Feedback physical force the surgeon feels at the control station when operating.
[g]Indexing denotes capability for manual dexterity enhancement.

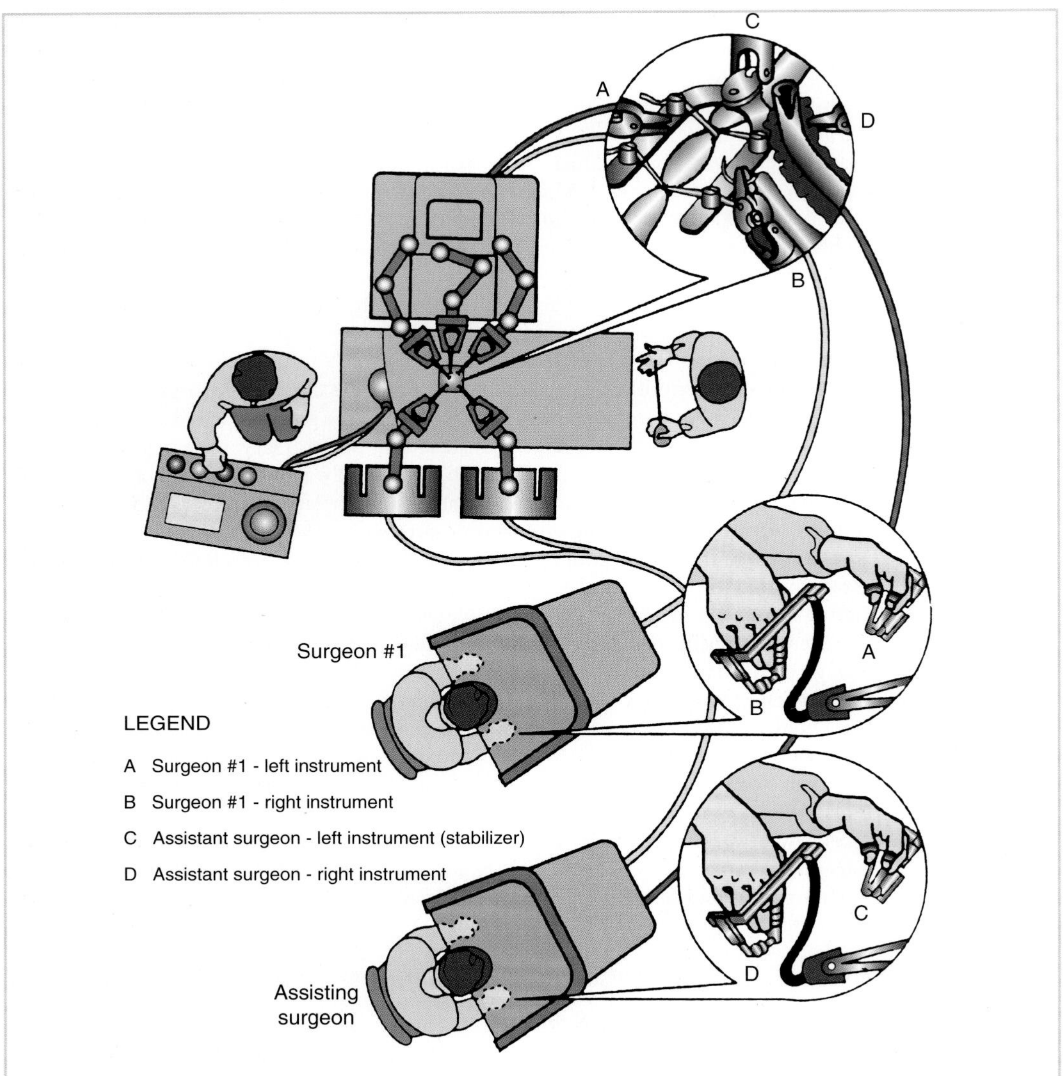

FIGURE 13.8 Schematic illustration of setup for endoscopic beating heart CABG using two consoles and five manipulator arms. The surgeon at the primary console manipulates two instruments and navigates the endoscope. The assisting surgeon directs the stabilizer and an assisting tool from a second console. *A,* left tool (primary surgeon); *B,* right tool (primary surgeon); *C,* stabilizer (left-hand assisting surgeon); *D,* assisting tool (right-hand assisting surgeon). (Adapted from Falk V, Fann JI, Grunenfelder J, et al. Endoscopic computer-enhanced beating heart coronary artery bypass surgery. *Ann Thorac Surg.* 2000;70:2029–2033, with permission.)

D. Endoscopic robotic-assisted systems

1. Robotic systems consist of three principal components (Fig. 13.8):
   a. A surgeon console. The surgeon sits at the console and grasps specially designed instrument handles. The surgeon's motions are relayed to a computer processor, which digitizes hand motions.
   b. A computer control system. The digitized information from the computer control system is related in real time to robotic manipulators, which are attached to the operating room table.

   c. Robotic manipulators. These manipulators hold the endoscopic instrument tips, which are inserted into the patient through small ports.
2. Currently, only one robotic system is commercially available: the da Vinci system (Intuitive Surgical, Mountain View, CA, USA).
3. A number of enhancements are required to move robotic systems toward more widespread acceptance.
   a. Development of endoscopic Doppler ultrasonography may aid in internal thoracic (mammary) artery harvesting, especially when the vessel is covered by fat or muscle.
   b. Although providing articulation, the endoscopic stabilizers need refinement to permit easier placement.
   c. Multimodal three-dimensional image visualization and manipulation systems may allow modeling of the range of motion of the robotic arms to individual patient data sets (computerized tomographic scan, ECG-gated magnetic resonance imaging). This may help optimize port placement and minimize the risk of collisions in the future.
   d. "Virtual" cardiac surgical planning platforms will allow the surgeon to examine the topology of a patient thorax for planning the port placement and the endoscopic procedure.

E. **Anesthetic considerations related to robotic surgery.** Robotic surgery requires the anesthesiologist to prospectively interact with the surgeon and machine to maintain ideal operating conditions, as well as stable hemodynamics and cardiac rhythm in an environment that may change rapidly from regional ischemia and cardiac manipulation. When the patient is fully instrumented and the robotic surgery is under way, direct access to the operative field is very limited and likely to be delayed. Anticipation and excellent communication are especially important where rapid surgical interventions are all but impossible.

1. Preoperative preparation
   a. Similar to OPCAB or MIDCAB, the anesthesiologist must discuss the procedure with the surgeon to understand the coronary anatomy, what is planned, and what special considerations might be involved (see above).
   b. Specific to robotic surgery are considerations that may be applicable to the robot (e.g., site of ports, location of manipulators, electrical interference).
2. Monitoring must take into account the patient's pathology (i.e., underlying ventricular function), the surgeon's familiarity with the robotic technique, anticipated problems, and duration of the procedure. As robotic procedures are still in the early stage of development, increased intensity of monitoring is probably warranted in most patients (i.e., use of PA catheters and/or TEE).
3. Induction and maintenance of anesthesia
   a. Specific anesthetic techniques are similar to other cardiac surgery where rapid emergence from anesthesia is desired ("fast track").
   b. Position is critical for appropriate location of ports and access for robotic manipulators. Typically this consists of the left arm stabilized beside the body, right arm up (i.e., suspended in a sling).
   c. Deflation of the left lung is required for visualization in robotic CABG surgery. This can be accomplished with a double-lumen endobronchial tube or bronchial blocker.
   d. Endoscopic robotic mitral valve surgery requires deflation of the right lung to facilitate access through the right fourth or fifth intercostal space.
   e. During robotic CABG surgery, CO_2 is insufflated into the left hemithorax during one-lung anesthesia. The insufflation pressure should be 6 to 8 mm Hg. This sustained positive intrathoracic pressure may mechanically decrease myocardial contractility and/or impair cardiac filling, which is rapidly reversible after the release of CO_2 from the chest cavity [61]. There may be sufficient absorption of CO_2 to induce respiratory acidosis and its attendant potential for tachycardia, dysrhythmias, and pulmonary hypertension.
   f. External defibrillator/pacing pads should be attached to the patient as surgical access to the heart for either of these functions is very limited and delayed.

g. Similar to OPCAB and MIDCAB, a multimodal approach should be taken to prevent heat loss. Although robotic procedures often reduce the extent of exposed intrathoracic surfaces as compared to OPCAB or CABG using CPB, the procedures can be lengthy, so the risk for hypothermia remains significant.

4. Anticoagulation and reversal. See discussion under "OPCAB and MIDCAB" in Section II. F.
5. Avoiding hemodynamic compromise. As in OPCAB, the heart may be positioned within the chest in a manner that compromises venous return or ventricular function.
   a. Keep preload high. Consider intravascular volume loading and the head-down (Trendelenburg) position.
   b. Tilt the operating table to the right or left as needed to facilitate surgical exposure.
   c. Maintain coronary perfusion pressure with α-adrenergic agonists if needed.
   d. Use epicardial pacing if bradycardia occurs.
   e. Closely watch insufflation pressure and monitor end-tidal CO_2 concentration as well as periodic arterial blood gases.
6. TEE. If the surgery is to be done on CPB, TEE guidance may be necessary to facilitate the placement of cannulas and endoaortic occlusion device, as described earlier (see MIVS section above).
7. Postoperative management
   a. Extubation in the operating room may be possible (see above for OPCAB and MIDCAB).
   b. If postoperative ventilation is anticipated, plan to change the double-lumen endobronchial tube to a single-lumen endotracheal tube.
   c. Postoperative pain management will depend on the size and number of port incisions. If a thoracotomy incision was made, intercostal, paravertebral, or epidural analgesia can be considered.

F. **Summary.** The field of robotically enhanced cardiac surgery will present a wide range of anesthetic challenges as it continues to develop. Anesthesiologists and surgeons alike must adapt to rapidly changing techniques in our continuing efforts to improve clinical outcomes.

IV. Transmyocardial laser revascularization

A. Historical perspective

1. TMLR is a procedure for the treatment of refractory angina pectoris that utilizes laser energy to create numerous channels in ischemic myocardium (Fig. 13.9).
2. TMLR was approved by the Food and Drug Administration (FDA) in 1998.
3. The concept dates back to 1933 when Wearn et al. [62] demonstrated direct vascular communication between the coronary arteries and the chambers of the heart via a sinusoidal network within the ventricular muscle. Beck's mobilization of omentum onto the heart in 1935 [63] and Vineberg's implantation of the IMA directly into the myocardium in 1954 [64] were attempts at indirect myocardial perfusion based on Wearn's description.
4. In 1965, Sen et al. [65] utilized acupuncture needles to create transmural channels through ischemic myocardium to direct blood into the myocardium from the ventricle. This concept was based on the reptile heart in which the LV is directly perfused via channels radiating from the LV.
5. In the 1980s, Mirhoseini et al. [66] utilized CO_2 laser energy to create transmyocardial channels.
6. Reports of prospective randomized clinical trials [67,68] led to the approval of CO_2 and holmium lasers for the treatment of refractory angina pectoris. In addition, the safety and efficacy of these lasers utilized as an adjunct to CABG has been evaluated [69].

B. Laser mechanism of injury

1. Three types of lasers are utilized for TMLR: CO_2, holmium:yttrium-aluminum-garnet (Ho:YAG), and XeCl excimer. CO_2 and holmium lasers operate in the infrared region, whereas excimer laser is in the ultraviolet region.
2. To create a channel through myocardium, tissue is ablated (chemical bonds between atoms are broken). The infrared lasers achieve ablation by vaporization of myocardium, which is followed by intense collagen deposition and scarring.

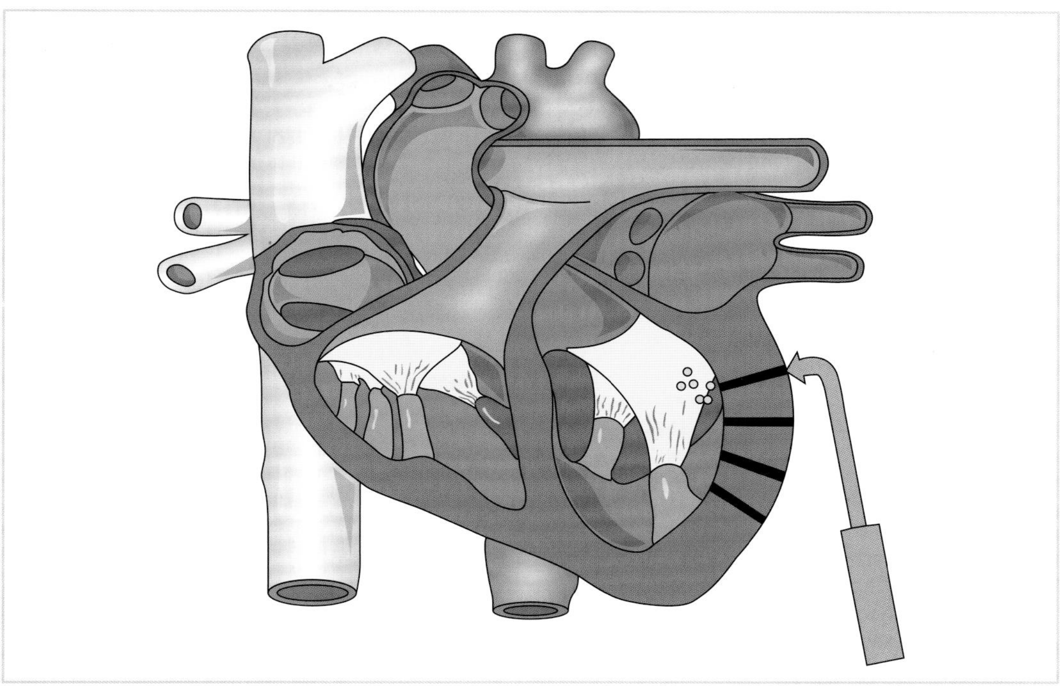

FIGURE 13.9 Illustration of transmyocardial laser and epicardial position of the laser device for creating channels. The device can be placed through a left thoracotomy incision (isolated procedure) or through a standard sternotomy (supplement to CABG). Full-thickness penetration is confirmed by transesophageal echocardiographic visualization of microbubbles in the LV cavity.

3. The ventricle should be filled with blood to act as beam stop and prevent perforation of the posterior ventricular wall or damage to the chordae tendineae of the mitral valve.
4. Infrared lasers tend to induce more thermal damage to the myocardium surrounding the channels than do ultraviolet lasers.
5. In addition to thermal injury, mechanical injury occurs through the production of vapor bubbles and the presence of shock waves [70,71].
6. Free radical molecules also form, which induce cellular injury.

C. **Mechanisms responsible for clinical benefit**

13

1. **The exact mechanism contributing to improved clinical outcome from TMLR remains controversial.**
2. Endothelialization of the channels has been proposed. However, histopathologic studies have failed to confirm this hypothesis.
3. Neovascularization in response to laser-induced tissue injury has also been proposed as a mechanism. TMLR may induce the production of vascular angiogenic growth factor–like molecules to result in neovascularization with improved regional collateral blood flow.
4. A placebo effect has been postulated, but is unlikely to account for the sustained relief of angina demonstrated in some studies.
5. Sympathetic afferent denervation has been postulated, especially to explain the immediate relief of angina experienced by some patients [72].
6. Although more studies are necessary, neovascularization and sympathetic denervation are the most likely mechanisms of benefit, and these may occur concurrently.

D. **Patient selection**

1. The largest use of TMLR is as an adjunct to conventional CABG, especially in reoperative CABG patients. TMLR is then used in anatomic regions where complete coronary artery revascularization is infeasible.

2. TMLR is also indicated in a select group of patients with severe diffuse coronary artery disease who are poor candidates for conventional angioplasty or coronary revascularization. These patients experience anginal symptoms that are either refractory to oral medical therapy or that cannot be weaned from intravenous antianginal medications. These patients must demonstrate reversible ischemia determined by myocardial perfusion scanning and possess an LV ejection fraction greater than 25%.
3. Additional candidates may include heart transplant recipients who develop severe coronary artery disease as a result of allograft rejection.
4. Contraindications to TMLR include severely depressed LV ejection fraction, ischemic mitral regurgitation, pre-existing ventricular arrhythmias, ventricular mural thrombus, long-term anticoagulant therapy, and severe chronic obstructive pulmonary disease.

E. Preoperative evaluation

1. Preoperative assessment of patients who present for TMLR is similar to that of patients who present for CABG.
2. Electrocardiography, exercise stress testing, and transthoracic echocardiography (with or without dobutamine stress) are performed to assess arrhythmias, valvular and ventricular function, or the presence of ventricular thrombus in low CO states. Multiple-gated scintigraphic angiography scanning may be utilized to assess ventricular function.
3. Coronary angiography is performed to determine if the vessels can be grafted, and to decide if TMLR will be performed as an isolated procedure or as an adjunct to CABG.
4. Myocardial perfusion scanning such as thallium scintigraphy or positron emission tomography is performed to identify areas of viable but ischemic myocardium. These tests also serve as a baseline for comparison of postoperative results.

F. Anesthetic considerations

1. **Laser safety**
   a. The operating room windows and outside doors must be marked with signs that indicate that a laser procedure is occurring.
   b. The patient's eyes must be protected with moist gauze. In addition, all operating room personnel must wear protective goggles.
2. **Preoperative preparation**

   a. Patients selected for TMLR present with severe coronary artery disease. In addition, there is a high incidence of coexisting diseases such as diabetes, lung disease, hypertension, prior myocardial infarction, and prior coronary bypass grafts. They require close hemodynamic control with focus on optimizing myocardial oxygen supply and consumption.
   b. Anticoagulant therapy should be discontinued prior to surgery. Antianginal, antiarrhythmic, and pulmonary medications should be continued the morning of surgery.
   c. Adequate venous access is essential as many patients have undergone previous cardiac surgery and bleeding is a significant risk.
   d. These patients are prone to acute ischemic events in the perioperative period. An ECG with computerized ST-segment analysis and trending is often utilized for ischemia detection. PACs are usually placed, as these patients often have poor ventricular function.
   e. The operating room should be warm, with every effort exercised to maintain patient normothermia.
3. **Induction and maintenance of anesthesia**
   a. The goals are to maintain hemodynamic stability, facilitate early extubation, and provide reliable postoperative analgesia.
   b. Isolated TMLR is typically performed off-bypass through a left anterior thoracotomy, in which case a double-lumen endobronchial tube or left bronchial blocker is placed to permit left lung collapse in order to avert pulmonary injury from the laser beams. In contrast, combined TMLR and CABG is performed through a median sternotomy on CPB.
   c. A TEE probe is inserted after induction to monitor ventricular function, mitral valve competence, and gaseous bubbles in the LV generated by transmyocardial laser strikes.

d. For isolated TMLR or repeat sternotomy, external defibrillation patches should be placed on the patient, and the groin should be exposed in preparation for emergency CPB or insertion of IABP.
e. During combined TMLR and CABG, TMLR is typically performed on the beating heart (e.g., early during CPB) that is relatively full in an attempt to minimize laser channel penetration across the ventricular chamber. TMLR may cause arrhythmias and ventricular distension, in which case the procedure may be delayed until after the administration of cardioplegia.
f. **The laser probe is positioned against the epicardium. The laser is synchronized to the electrocardiogram signal and fired at the peak of the R wave. The laser energy is absorbed by blood in the LV.**
g. Transmyocardial laser channels are confirmed by the detection of ventricular bubbles by TEE and the appearance of bright red blood from the channels.
h. It may be beneficial to avoid nitrous oxide with its attendant risk of bubble expansion during laser channel creation.

4. **Recovery**
   a. For isolated TMLR, the patient may be extubated in the operated room and transported to a telemetry area for postoperative monitoring [73,74].
   b. Recovery for combined TMLR and CABG is similar to CABG.
5. **Complications**

   a. Patients who present for isolated TMLR experience ongoing myocardial ischemia. There is no immediate physiologic benefit from the procedure; rather there may be ventricular failure, infarction, hypotension, arrhythmias, or hypoxemia related to anesthesia or myocardial manipulation. Laser vaporization can directly damage myocardium and further contribute to myocardial failure.
   b. Vasopressors, inotropes, an IABP, and CPB standby must be available to treat unexpected myocardial failure at any time in the perioperative period.
   c. **TMLR may induce atrial and ventricular arrhythmias.** This frequently occurs during surgical manipulation of the heart by the surgeon or the laser probe. Ventricular arrhythmias are common during the creation of transmyocardial channels. Gating of the laser to the cardiac cycle has decreased the incidence of ventricular arrhythmias. Direct injury to the Purkinje conduction system may further complicate these arrhythmias.
   d. **Direct laser injury to the mitral valve apparatus causing acute mitral regurgitation may precipitate heart failure.** This risk is reduced with the use of the holmium laser. A thorough intraoperative TEE exam must be performed following TMLR to diagnose this complication.
   e. Vaporization of myocardium generates bubbles in the LV cavity with a potential risk of stroke.
   f. Hemorrhage may occur secondary to surgical dissection in patients who have previously undergone CABG or from the transmyocardial laser channels. Bleeding from the laser channels can be controlled by digital pressure for isolated TMLR since systemic heparinization is not employed. However, if TMLR is performed during CPB, the risk of bleeding from the laser channels may increase.
6. **Outcome**
   a. Ongoing studies continue to examine the benefit from and indications for isolated TMLR and for combined TMLR/CABG [75,76].
   b. As compared to medical therapy in patients with angina refractory to medical treatment or inoperable coronary artery disease, TMLR is associated with symptomatic and functional improvement 12 months after the procedure.
   c. In a recent comparison of patients undergoing CABG alone with those undergoing CABG and TMLR, the latter group had a significantly higher preoperative incidence of diabetes, renal failure, peripheral vascular disease, previous CABG, three-vessel disease, and hyperlipidemia. Despite the increased risk associated with these

patients, the mortality rate was not significantly increased when TMLR was added to CABG [77].

7. **Future directions**
   a. Percutaneous laser revascularization involving creation of the laser channels from the inside of the heart is under investigation.
   b. Augmentation of the clinical benefits of TMLR by simultaneous delivery of growth factors, gene therapy, or stem cells is under investigation.

REFERENCES

OPCAB and MIDCAB

1. Clements F, Shanewise J, eds. *Minimally Invasive Cardiac and Vascular Surgical Techniques. Society of Cardiovascular Anesthesiologists Monograph.* Philadelphia, PA: Lippincott Williams & Wilkins; 2001.
2. Benetti FJ, Naselli G, Wood M, et al. Direct myocardial revascularization without extracorporeal circulation. *Chest.* 1991;100:312–316.
3. Mack M, Bachand D, Acuff T, et al. Improved outcomes in coronary artery bypass grafting with beating-heart techniques. *J Thorac Cardiovasc Surg.* 2002;124:598–607.
4. Chassot PG, van der Linden P, Zaugg M, et al. Off-pump coronary artery bypass surgery: physiology and anesthetic management. *Br J Anesth.* 2004;92:400–413.
5. Bonchek LI. Off pump coronary bypass: is it for everyone? *J Thorac Cardiovasc Surg.* 2002;124:431–434.
6. Angelini G, Taylor FC, Reeves BC, et al. Early and midterm outcome after off-pump and on-pump surgery in Beating Heart Against Cardioplegic Arrest Studies (BHACAS 1 and 2): a pooled analysis of two randomized controlled trials. *Lancet.* 2002;359:1194.
7. van Dijk D, Nierich AP, Jansen EWL, et al. Early outcome after off-pump versus on-pump coronary artery bypass. *Circulation.* 2001;104;1761–1766.
8. Puskas JD, Williams WH, Mahoney EM, et al. Off-pump vs conventional coronary artery bypass grafting: early and 1-year graft patency, cost, and quality-of-life outcomes: a randomized trial. *JAMA.* 2004;291:1795–1922.
9. Khan NE, De Souza A, Mister R, et al. A randomized comparison of off-pump and on-pump multivessel coronary artery bypass surgery. *N Engl J Med.* 2004;350:21–28.
10. Puskas JD, Williams WH, Duke PG, et al. Off-pump coronary artery bypass grafting provides complete revascularization with reduced myocardial injury, transfusion requirements, and length of stay: a prospective randomized comparison of two hundred unselected patients undergoing off-pump versus conventional coronary artery bypass grafting. *J Thorac Cardiovasc Surg.* 2003;125:797–808.
11. Hueb W, Lopes NH, Pereira AC, et al. Five-year follow-up of a randomized comparison between off-pump and on-pump stable multivessel coronary artery bypass grafting. *Circulation.* 2010;122(suppl 1):S48–S52.
12. Puskas JD, Williams WH, O'Donnell R, et al. Off-pump and on-pump coronary artery bypass grafting are associated with similar graft patency, myocardial ischemia, and freedom from reintervention: long-term follow-up of a randomized trial. *Ann Thorac Surg.* 2011;91:1836–1843.
13. Shroyer AL, Grover FL, Hattler B, et al. On-pump versus off-pump coronary-artery bypass surgery. *N Engl J Med.* 2009;361:1827–1837.
14. Legare JF, Buth KJ, Hirsch GM. Conversion to on pump from OPCAB is associated with increased mortality: results from a randomized controlled trial. *Eur J Cardiothorac Surg.* 2005;27:296–301.
15. Novitzky D, Baltz JH, Hattler B, et al. Outcomes after conversion in the veterans affairs randomized on versus off bypass trial. *Ann Thorac Surg.* 2011;92(suppl 6):2147–2154.
16. Schwann NM, Horrow JC, Strong MD III, et al. Does off-pump coronary artery bypass reduce the incidence of clinically evident renal dysfunction after multivessel myocardial revascularization? *Anesth Analg.* 2004;99:959–964.
17. Eagle KA, Guyton RA, Davidoff R, et al. ACC/AHA 2004 guideline update for coronary artery bypass graft surgery: summary article: a report of the ACC/AHA Task Force on Practice Guidelines (Committee to Update the 1999 Guidelines on CABG surgery). *Circulation.* 2004;100:1168–1176.
18. Cason BA, Gamperl AK, Slocum RE, et al. Anesthetic-induced preconditioning. *Anesthesiology.* 1997;87:1182–1190.
19. Zenati M, Cohen HA, Griffith BP. Alternative approach to multivessel coronary disease with integrated coronary revascularization. *J Thorac Cardiovasc Surg.* 1999;117:439–446.
20. Grocott HP, Mathew JP, Carver EH, et al. A randomized controlled trial of the Arctic Sun temperature management system versus conventional methods for preventing hypothermia during off-pump cardiac surgery. *Anesth Analg.* 2004;98:298–302.
21. Resano FG, Stamou SC, Lowery RC, et al. Complete myocardial revascularization on the beating heart with epicardial stabilization: anesthetic considerations. *J Cardiothorac Vasc Anesth.* 2000;14:534–539.
22. Moises VA, Mesquita CB, Campos O, et al. Importance of intraoperative transesophageal echocardiography during coronary surgery without cardiopulmonary bypass. *J Am Soc Echocardiogr.* 1998;11:1139–1144.
23. Djaiani G, Karski J, Yudin M, et al. Clinical outcomes in patients undergoing elective coronary artery bypass graft surgery with and without utilization of pulmonary artery catheter-generated data. *J Cardiothorac Vasc Anesth.* 2006;20:307–310.
24. George SJ, Al-Ruzzeh S, Amrani M. Mitral annulus distortion during beating hearty surgery: a potential cause for hemodynamic disturbance–a three-dimensional echocardiography reconstruction study. *Ann Thorac Surg.* 2002;73:1424–1430.
25. Hatton KW, Kilinski L, Ramiah C, et al. Multiple failed external defibrillation attempts during robot-assisted internal mammary harvest for myocardial revascularization. *Anesth Analg.* 2006;103:1113–1114.

26. Dhole S, Mehta Y, Saxena H, et al. Comparison of continuous thoracic epidural and paravertebral blocks for postoperative analgesia after minimally invasive direct coronary artery bypass surgery. *J Cardiothorac Vasc Anesth.* 2001;15:288–292.
27. Grundeman PF, Borst C, van Herwaarden JA, et al. Vertical displacement of the beating heart by the Octopus Tissue Stabilizer: influence on coronary flow. *Ann Thorac Surg.* 1998;65:1348–1352.
28. Mariani MA, Gu J, Boonstra P, et al. Procoagulant activity after off-pump coronary operation: is the current anticoagulation adequate? *Ann Thorac Surg.* 1999;67:1370–1375.
29. Murphy GJ, Mango E, Lucchetti V, et al. A randomized trial of tranexamic acid in combination with cell salvage plus a meta-analysis of randomized trials evaluating tranexamic acid in off-pump coronary artery bypass grafting. *J Thorac Cardiovasc Surg.* 2006;132:475–480.

Minimally Invasive Valve Surgery

30. Caffarelli AD, Robbins RC. Will minimally invasive valve replacement ever really be important? *Curr Op Cardiol.* 2004;19:123–127.
31. Cosgrove DM, Sabik JF, Navia JL. Minimally invasive valve operations. *Ann Thorac Surg.* 1998;65:1535–1539.
32. Swerc MF, Benckart DH, Savage EB, et al. Partial versus full sternotomy for aortic valve replacement. *Ann Thorac Surg.* 1999;68:2209–2213.
33. Asher CR, DiMengo JM, Weber MM, et al. Atrial fibrillation early postoperatively following minimally invasive cardiac valvular surgery. *Am J Cardiol.* 1999;84:744–747.
34. Byrne JG, Karavas AN, Filsoufi F, et al. Aortic valve surgery after previous coronary artery bypass grafting with functioning internal mammary artery grafts. *Ann Thorac Surg.* 2002;73:779–784.
35. Walther W, Volkmar F, Mohr F. Minimally invasive surgery for valve disease. *Curr Prob Cardiol.* 2006;31:399–437.
36. Secknus MA, Asher CR, Scalia GM, et al. Intraoperative transesophageal echocardiography in minimally invasive cardiac valve surgery. *J Am Soc Echocardiogr.* 1999;12:231–236.
37. Feldman T, Foster E, Glower D, et al. Percutaneous repair or surgery for mitral regurgitation. *N Engl J Med.* 2011;364:1395–1406.
38. Treede H, Schirmer J, Rudolph V, et al. A heart team's perspective on interventional mitral valve repair: percutaneous clip implantation as an important adjunct to a surgical mitral valve program for treatment of high-risk patients. *J Thorac Cardiovasc Surg.* 2012;143:78–84.
39. Nobuyoshi M, Arita T, Shirai S, et al. Percutaneous balloon mitral valvuloplasty: a review. *Circulation.* 2009;119:e211–e219.
40. Leon MB, Smith CR, Mack M, et al. Transcatheter aortic-valve implantation for aortic stenosis in patients who cannot undergo surgery. *N Engl J Med.* 2010;363:1597–1607.
41. Zamorano JL, Badano LP, Bruce C, et al. EAE/ASE recommendations for the use of echocardiography in new transcatheter interventions for valvular heart disease. *J Am Soc Echocardiogr.* 2011;24(suppl 9):937–965.
42. Kpodonu J. Hybrid cardiovascular suite: the operating room of the future. *J Card Surg.* 2010;25:704–709.
43. Kpodonu J, Raney A. The cardiovascular hybrid room a key component for hybrid interventions and image guided surgery in the emerging specialty of cardiovascular hybrid surgery. *Interact Cardiovasc Thorac Surg.* 2009;9:688–692.
44. Singh IM, Shishehbor MH, Christofferson RD, et al. Percutanous treatment of aortic valve stenosis. *Cleve Clin J Med.* 2008;75(suppl 11):805–812.
45. Billings FT, Kodali SK, Shanewise JS. Transcatheter aortic valve implantation: anesthetic considerations. *Anesth Analg.* 2009;108:1453–1462.
46. Heinze H, Sier H, Schäfer U, et al. Percutaneous aortic valve replacement: overview and suggestions for anesthetic management. *J Clin Anesth.* 2010;22:373–378.
47. Fraccaro C, Napodano M, Taratini G, et al. Expanding the eligibility for transcatheter aortic valve implantation. *JACC Cardiovasc Interv.* 2009;2(suppl 9):828–833.
48. Covello RD, Maj G, Landoni G, et al. Anesthetic management of aortic valve implantation: focus on challenges encountered and proposed solutions. *J Cardiothor Vasc Anesth.* 2009;23(suppl 3):280–285.
49. Dehedin B, Guinot PG, Ibrahim H, et al. Anesthesia and perioperative management of patients who undergo transfemoral transcatheter aortic valve implantation: an observational study of general versus local/regional anesthesia in 125 consecutive patients. *J Cardiothor Vasc Anesth.* 2011;25(suppl 6):1036–1043.
50. Covello RD, Ruggeri L, Landoni G, et al. Transcatheter implantation of an aortic valve: anesthesiological management. *Minerva Anesthesiol.* 2010;76:100–108.
51. Chin D. Echocardiography for transcatheter aortic valve implantation. *Eur J Echocardiogr.* 2009;10:21–29.
52. Krishnaswamy A, Tuczu EM, Kapadia SR. Update on transcatheter aortic valve implantation. *Curr Cardiol Rep.* 2010;12:393–403.
53. Abdel-Wahab M, Zahn R, Horack M, et al. Aortic regurgitation after transcatheter aortic valve implantation: incidence and early outcome. Results from the German transcatheter aortic valve interventions registry. *Heart.* 2011;97(suppl 11):899–906.
54. Smith CR, Leon MB, Mack MJ, et al. Transcatheter versus surgical aortic-valve replacement in high-risk patients. *N Engl J Med.* 2011;364:2187–2198.

Robotic Surgery

55. Loulmet D, Carpentier A, d'Attellis N, et al. Endoscopic coronary artery bypass grafting with the aid of robotic assisted instruments. *J Thorac Cardiovasc Surg.* 1999;118:4–10.
56. Reichenspurner H, Damiano RJ, Mack MJ, et al. Use of the voice-controlled and computer-assisted surgical system ZEUS for endoscopic coronary artery bypass grafting. *J Throac Cardiovasc Surg.* 1999;118:11–16.
57. Taylor, RH, Lavallee S, Burdea GC, et al. *Computer-Integrated Surgery: Technology and Clinical Applications.* Cambridge, MA: The MIT Press; 1996.
58. Mack MJ. Minimally invasive and robotic surgery. *JAMA.* 2001;285:568–572.

59. Damiano RJ. Endoscopic coronary artery bypass grafting–the first steps on a long journey [Editorial]. *J Thor Cardiovasc Surg.* 2000;120:806–807.
60. Mohr FW, Falk V, Digeler A, et al. Computer-enhanced 'robotic' cardiac surgery: experience in 148 patients. *J Thorac Cardiovasc Surg.* 2001;121:842–853.
61. Ohtsuka T, Imanaka K, Endsh M. Hemodynamic effects of carbon dioxide insufflation under single-lung ventilation during thoroscopy. *Ann Thorac Surg.* 1999;68:29–33.

Transmyocardial Laser Revascularization

62. Wearn JT, Mettier SR, Klump TG, et al. The nature of the vascular communications between the coronary arteries and the chambers of the heart. *Am Heart J.* 1933;9:143–170.
63. Beck CS. The development of a new blood supply to the heart by operation. *Ann Surg.* 1935;102:801–813.
64. Vineberg AM. Development of an anastomosis between the coronary vessels and a transplanted internal mammary artery. *Can Med Assoc J.* 1946;55:117–119.
65. Sen PK, Udwadia TE, Kinaire SG, et al. Transmyocardial acupuncture. *J Thorac Cardiovasc Surg.* 1950;50:181–189.
66. Mirhoseini M, Clayton MM. Revascularization of the heart by laser. *J Microsurg.* 1981;2:253–260.
67. Frazier OH, March RJ, Horvath KA. Transmyocardial revascularization with a carbon dioxide laser in patients with end stage coronary artery disease. *N Engl J Med.* 1999;341:1021–1028.
68. Allen KB, Dowling RD, Fudge TL, et al. Comparison of transmyocardial revascularization with medical therapy in patients with refractory angina. *N Engl J Med.* 1999;341:1029–1036.
69. Allen KB, Dowling RD, DelRossi AJ, et al. Transmyocardial laser revascularization combined with coronary artery bypass grafting: a multicenter, blinded, prospective, randomized, controlled trial. *J Thorac Cardiovasc Surg.* 2000;119:540–549.
70. Hartman RA, Whittaker P. The physics of transmyocardial laser revascularization. *J Clin Laser Med Surg.* 1997;15:255–259.
71. Shehada RE, Mansour HN, Grundfest WS. Laser tissue interaction in direct myocardial revascularization. *Semin Intervent Cardiol.* 2000;5:63–70.
72. Sola OM, Shi Q, Vernon RB, et al. Cardiac denervation after transmyocardial laser. *Ann Thorac Surg.* 2001;71:732.
73. Grocott HP, Newman MF, Lowe JE, et al. Transmyocardial laser revascularization: an anesthetic perspective. *J Cardiothorac Vasc Anesth.* 1997;11:206–210.
74. Thrush DN. Anesthesia for laser transmyocardial revascularization. *J Cardiothorac Vasc Anesth.* 1997;11:481–484.
75. Allen KB, Shaar CJ. Transmyocardial laser revascularization: surgical experience overview. *Semin Intervent Cardiol.* 2000;5: 75–81.
76. Kraatz EG, Misfeld M, Jungbluth B, et al. Survival after transmyocardial laser revascularization in relation to nonlasered perfused myocardial zones. *Ann Thorac Surg.* 2001;71:532–536.
77. Horvath KA, Ferguson Jr B, Guyton RA, et al. Impact of unstable angina on outcomes of transmyocardial laser revascularisation combined with coronary artery bypass grafting. *Ann Thorac Surg.* 2005;80:2082–2085.

14 Anesthetic Management for Patients with Congenital Heart Disease: The Pediatric Population

Laurie K. Davies, S. Adil Husain, and Nathaen S. Weitzel

KEY POINTS

1. Three important channels characteristic of the circulation in utero allow preferential shunting of blood to sustain fetal viability. These include the ductus venosus, foramen ovale, and ductus arteriosus. A thorough understanding of the fetal circulation and transition to the adult circulation is an important aspect in understanding congenital heart disease (CHD).
2. There are significant structural differences in the infant's heart compared to an adult heart that impact anesthetic management.
3. Most congenital cardiac defects can be assigned to one of three groups: Those resulting in increased pulmonary blood flow, decreased pulmonary blood flow, or obstruction to blood flow.
4. **Cyanosis** (associated with decreased pulmonary blood flow lesions) and **congestive heart failure (CHF)** (associated with increased pulmonary blood flow lesions and ventricular obstructive lesions) are the two major manifestations of CHD.
5. Neurologic sequelae remain one of the most common and potentially devastating complications of CHD and its repair.
6. All intravenous and monitoring tubing must be bubble-free whenever a potential shunt is present **regardless of shunt direction.** Intracardiac shunts can be bidirectional and shunt direction can be changed by anesthetic maneuvers such as positive-pressure ventilation.
7. For anesthetic induction and maintenance in children with CHD, the choice of drug(s) is not as important as an understanding of the lesion's pathophysiology. Of help is the development of hemodynamic goals for each patient in terms of heart rate, contractility, preload, SVR, and PVR.
8. There are two methods regarding carbon dioxide management during cardiopulmonary bypass (CPB) (alpha-stat and pH-stat) that have significant implications for pediatric cardiac surgery.
9. Many cardiac lesions can be categorized based on the manifestations of cyanosis or CHF. However, this division is somewhat arbitrary as some lesions may have elements of both manifestations (e.g., transposition of the great arteries).

I. Introduction

The care of children undergoing cardiovascular surgery provides a remarkable challenge to the anesthesiologist. In the last decade, improvements in diagnostic capability, CPB techniques, monitoring, and perioperative care have permitted more complicated procedures to be performed on smaller, sicker children with remarkable success. The environment is dynamic, because operative procedures and technology are being modified constantly in an effort to further improve the safety and outcome for these special children.

Each child presents a unique set of circumstances and pathophysiologic concerns. Much of the knowledge regarding appropriate management for adults undergoing cardiac surgery will not apply to these children. Anesthesiologists caring for these patients must be flexible and innovative. Rigid protocols are rarely appropriate; instead, an individualized plan for each patient is mandatory. Team effort and good communication are essential to the success of a pediatric cardiovascular surgical program. Being a part of a successful team effort and caring for these patients are among the most exciting and rewarding experiences in medicine today.

A. **Incidence.** CHD is relatively uncommon. It is estimated to occur in less than 1% of all live births (Table 14.1). The true incidence is probably quite a bit higher. Much fetal wastage is thought to occur because of the presence of congenital heart defects that are incompatible with life. Also, some heart lesions (e.g., bicuspid aortic valve and patent ductus arteriosus [PDA]) may be relatively asymptomatic early in life; thus, the true incidence of CHD is unknown.

Certain lesions are more likely to become manifest early in life than others. With these caveats in mind, **the lesions most likely to be encountered in the first year of life are ventricular septal defect (VSD), transposition of the great vessels (TGV), tetralogy of Fallot (TOF), coarctation of the aorta, and hypoplastic left heart syndrome.**

TABLE 14.1 Reported estimate of prevalence per 1,000 live births for specific congenital heart defects

Defect	Prevalence
VSD	0.38
Transposition	0.21
TOF	0.21
Coarctation of aorta	0.18
Hypoplastic left-sided heart syndrome	0.16
PDA	0.14
AV septal defect	0.12
Pulmonary stenosis	0.19
Pulmonary atresia	0.07
Secundum ASD	0.07
Total anomalous pulmonary venous drainage	0.06
Tricuspid atresia	0.06
Aortic stenosis	0.04
Double-outlet RV	0.03
Truncus arteriosus	0.03
Other	0.18

VSD, ventricular septal defect; TOF, tetralogy of Fallot; PDA, patent ductus arteriosus; AV, atrioventricular; ASD, atrial septal defect.
Modified from Daniels SR. Epidemiology. In: Long WA, ed. *Fetal and Neonatal Cardiology.* Philadelphia, PA: WB Saunders; 1990:430.

Different reference populations may demonstrate different patterns of CHD. For instance, infants who are premature and small for their gestational ages have an increased prevalence of CHD (especially VSD and PDA) compared to full-term newborns. Congenital heart defects are more common among infants of diabetic mothers than those of nondiabetic mothers. Infants with abnormal chromosomes have an increased frequency of congenital heart defects. About 23% to 56% of children with trisomy 21 have CHD [1]. The most common defects in children with Down syndrome appear to be VSD, atrial septal defect (ASD), PDA, and atrioventricular (AV) canal defects.

B. **Prognosis.** The outlook for these children today has improved considerably over that of previous years. A better understanding of the pathophysiology of individual lesions allows development of a rational treatment care plan. Earlier complete repairs are being performed successfully, often resulting in the avoidance of the long-term sequelae of unrepaired CHD. Cardiac transplantation also has become a viable option for some children whose lesions cannot be surgically repaired. For any of these options to be successful, the patient's care must be thoughtfully individualized with vigilance, anticipation, and meticulous attention to detail. Close communication with the surgeon preoperatively and intraoperatively will result in better anticipation and, hopefully, avoidance of potential problems or management of real issues in the perioperative period.

II. Physiologic considerations

A. *What is the difference between fetal and adult circulation?*

To develop an understanding of the clinical and anesthetic implications of CHD, one must be familiar with the fetal and the adult circulations. Three important channels characteristic of the
1 circulation in utero allow preferential shunting of blood: Ductus venosus, foramen ovale, and ductus arteriosus (Fig. 14.1).

1. **Ductus venosus.** Well-oxygenated blood from the placenta, with a partial pressure of oxygen of about 33 mm Hg, travels through the umbilical vein to enter the liver. The ductus venosus allows about one-half of this blood to be shunted from the liver directly into the inferior vena cava.

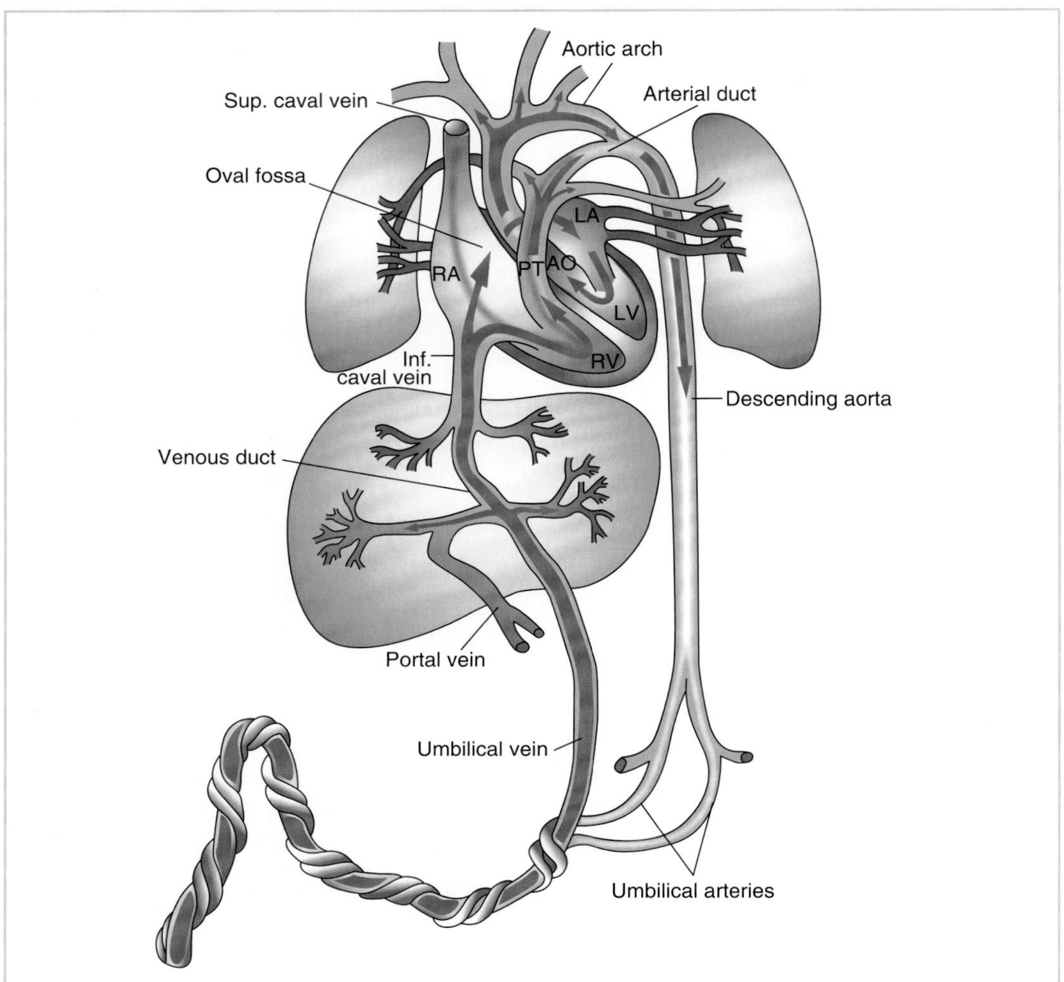

FIGURE 14.1 Course of fetal circulation. See text for description. Ao, aorta; DA, ductus arteriosus; DV, ductus venosus; LA, left atrium; PT, pulmonary trunk; RA, right atrium; RV, right ventricle. (From Hoffman JIE. The circulatory system. In: Rudolph AM, ed. *Pediatrics.* 17th ed. Norwalk, CT: Appleton & Lange; 1982:1232, with permission.)

2. **Foramen ovale.** About one-third of the blood entering the right atrium from the inferior vena cava is preferentially shunted across the foramen ovale into the left atrium. On the other hand, superior vena cava blood (which is poorly oxygenated) primarily enters the right ventricle (RV), with 2% to 3% crossing the foramen ovale.
3. **Ductus arteriosus.** RV blood is largely shunted across the ductus arteriosus into the descending aorta (rather than perfusing the high-resistance pulmonary circulation).
4. **Implications. The structure of the fetal circulation allows the well-oxygenated blood (which has a high glucose content) from the inferior vena cava to preferentially perfuse the brain, coronary circulation, and upper extremities.** The lower portion of the body receives blood with a low oxygen content from the ductus arteriosus. Hence, the systemic and pulmonary circulations in the fetus function in parallel, with each ventricle receiving only a portion of the systemic cardiac output (CO). The adult situation, in contrast, requires the two circulations to work in series, each processing the entire CO.

B. *What is the transitional circulation?*

At birth, remarkable changes occur rapidly in the circulation that allow the infant to adapt to the stresses of extrauterine life. A period of transition in the neonatal circulation occurs before permanent adaptation to the normal adult pattern takes place. This transitional stage is unstable and may exist for a few hours or for many weeks, depending on the stresses imposed. Factors contributing to the instability of the transitional circulation are the state of the ductus arteriosus, foramen ovale, and pulmonary vascular bed, as well as the immaturity of the neonatal heart. Conditions that may prolong the transitional circulation include hypoxia, hypothermia, acidosis, hypercarbia, sepsis, prematurity, and CHD.

1. **Closure of the ductus arteriosus.** Functional closure of the ductus arteriosus usually occurs within a few hours of birth, but anatomic closure may not occur for several weeks. During this period, the resistance to ductus arteriosus blood flow is responsive to changes in arterial Po_2 (P_ao_2); that is, increased P_ao_2 increases resistance, and decreased P_ao_2 decreases resistance. Prostaglandin E_1 (PGE_1) infusion relaxes the ductal musculature and increases ductal flow, which may be left-to-right, right-to-left, or bidirectional. Maintenance of ductal patency may be important for the infant with cyanotic heart disease until repair or palliative surgery can be performed.
2. **Closure of the foramen ovale and ductus venosus.** The foramen ovale functionally closes when the left atrial pressure exceeds right atrial pressure; this usually occurs within a few hours after birth. Anatomic closure does not occur for many months, and about 30% of adults demonstrate probe patency of the foramen ovale. Right-to-left intracardiac shunting may occur across this area with coughing or the Valsalva maneuver or if pulmonary hypertension develops. Umbilical arteries and veins close shortly after birth, as does the ductus venosus. The latter forms the ligamentum venosum.
3. **Pulmonary vascular resistance.** Pulmonary vascular resistance (PVR) is high in utero but declines rapidly after birth in the term infant. Usually, it is lower than systemic levels within 24 h of birth. Thereafter, it falls at a moderate rate for 5 to 6 wks and then more gradually for the next 2 to 3 yrs. During this period, a child's pulmonary vascular bed is more reactive than that of an adult, and a rise in pulmonary artery (PA) pressure can easily be produced by hypoxemia, hypercarbia, acidosis, or bronchospasm. If this reaction occurs shortly after birth, it may result in shunting across the ductus arteriosus or foramen ovale or other cardiac defects. Later in life, only a patent foramen ovale or cardiac defect remains as a possible shunt site.

2 **C. How is a child's heart structurally different from that of an adult?**

1. **Size.** At birth, both ventricles are approximately equal in size and wall thickness. With the changeover from the fetal circulation, the left ventricle (LV) must accommodate a greater pressure and volume workload; conversely, the pressure load of the RV is reduced, and its volume work is only slightly increased. The LV hypertrophies in response to the increased workload and becomes roughly twice as heavy as the RV by about age 6 mos.
2. **Ultrastructure.** The neonate's heart is ultrastructurally immature. Myofibrils are arranged in a disorderly fashion and have a smaller percentage of contractile proteins than those in the adult (30% vs. 60%). Autonomic innervation is incomplete at birth. The **sympathetic innervation to the heart is decreased,** as are cardiac catecholamine stores. In contrast, **the parasympathetic innervation of the neonatal heart is comparable to that of the adult heart**. These observations often are cited to explain the frequent **vagal predominance** that occurs in infants compared to adults. Sympathetic innervation also is immature in the peripheral vasculature. Therefore, control of vascular tone and myocardial contractility in infants depends largely on adrenal function and circulating or exogenously administered catecholamines. There are differences in myocardial calcium metabolism. In the mature myocardium, the sarcoplasmic reticulum is the predominant source of calcium ion for excitation–contraction coupling, but the sarcoplasmic reticulum is poorly developed in the immature heart. As the neonatal myocardial cell is deficient in T tubules that, in the mature myocardium, provide electrical coupling between the cell membrane and the sarcoplasmic reticulum, it

is incapable of internal release and reuptake of calcium for contraction and instead depends on transmembrane calcium transport for the development of tension. These **differences in calcium handling** by the cell provide some explanation for the clinical observation that newborns require **greater serum-ionized calcium levels for optimal myocardial contractility**.

3. **Compliance.** The immature heart has a functionally decreased compliance compared to the adult heart. This difference reflects, in part, the ultrastructure of the heart and the increased volume load that each ventricle must handle with the transition from a parallel fetal to an adult series circulation. The RV and LV are more intimately inter-related as a result of this decreased compliance and similarity in size. Dysfunction of one ventricle quickly leads to biventricular failure. Reduced compliance also means that the immature heart is more sensitive to volume overload. A neonate's ventricular function curve is shifted to the right and downward compared to that of an adult. Over the physiologic range of ventricular filling pressures, stroke volume changes are, in fact, small.

   This relatively fixed stroke volume makes a neonate highly dependent on heart rate and sinus rhythm for optimal CO. In comparison, the adult heart is much more responsive to changes in preload to effect a change in stroke volume and thereby change CO. Increases in pressure work are poorly tolerated by both the right and left sides of the immature heart. The neonate, therefore, responds poorly to either volume or pressure loading, because resting cardiac function is on or near the plateau of the cardiac function curve.

D. **How are congenital cardiac lesions meaningfully characterized?**

1. **Flow pattern.** Patients with congenital heart defects are a diverse group. Rather than memorize an approach to each lesion, one should group the many anatomic varieties into
3 a few understandable categories (Table 14.2). Most defects can be assigned to one of the three groups: (i) Those resulting in increased pulmonary blood flow, (ii) those resulting

TABLE 14.2 Flow characteristics of various congenital cardiac lesions

Increased pulmonary blood flow lesions	ASD
	VSD
	PDA
	Endocardial cushion defect (AV canal abnormality)
	Anomalous origin of coronary arteries
	TGA[a]
	Anomalous pulmonary venous drainage[a]
	Truncus arteriosus[a]
	Single ventricle[a]
Decreased pulmonary blood flow lesions	TOF
	Pulmonary atresia
	Tricuspid atresia
	Ebstein anomaly
	Truncus arteriosus[a]
	TGA[a]
	Single ventricle[a]
Obstructive lesions	Aortic stenosis
	Pulmonary stenosis
	Coarctation of the aorta
	Asymmetrical septal hypertrophy

[a]Systemic hypoxemia occurs as a result of the mixing of systemic and pulmonary venous returns. Classification as an increased or decreased pulmonary blood flow lesion depends on the absence or presence within the anatomic variation of obstruction to pulmonary blood flow.

ASD, atrial septal defect; VSD, ventricular septal defect; PDA, patent ductus arteriosis; AV, atrioventricular; TGA, transposition of the great arteries; TOF, tetralogy of Fallot.

Modified from Schwartz AJ, Campbell FW. Pathophysiological approach to congenital heart disease. In: Lake CL, ed. *Pediatric Cardiac Anesthesia*. Norwalk, CT: Appleton & Lange; 1988:9.

in decreased pulmonary blood flow, and (iii) those resulting in obstruction to blood flow. The first two groups feature an abnormal shunt pathway, whereas the third group has no shunting of blood. A fourth group could include lesions in which no pulmonary–systemic exchange of blood occurs (e.g., TGV). However, infants with TGV have either naturally occurring or artificially induced mixing of systemic and pulmonary venous returns and often can be classified into one of the first two groups, depending on whether obstruction to pulmonary blood flow is present.

4

2. **Clinical status: Cyanosis versus heart failure. Cyanosis and CHF are the major manifestations of CHD.** Thus, the pathophysiologic classification must be related to the clinical status. Cyanosis occurs most commonly with lesions in which pulmonary blood flow is anatomically decreased or functionally decreased as mixing of systemic and pulmonary venous blood occurs.

   CHF occurs most commonly in shunt lesions with excessively increased pulmonary blood flow or obstructive lesions that stress the ventricle beyond its capacity to pump effectively. Note that a child can be cyanotic but still fall into the category of having a lesion with increased pulmonary blood flow and may even manifest CHF. Two examples of such a situation are an infant with TGV and a large VSD or a child with truncus arteriosus. Even the most complex lesions usually fall into one of the three categories, even if they are characterized by mixed features (Table 14.2).

E. **When and why do patients become symptomatic?**

Many types of CHD may not be detected immediately after birth. The age at which heart defects become manifest depends on the type of lesion, its severity, and the state of the infant's transitional circulation. Increased pulmonary blood flow lesions typically become symptomatic as PVR decreases and shunt flow to the lungs increases. These changes may take days to weeks to occur. Also, if the defect is small, it may remain asymptomatic.

Decreased pulmonary blood flow lesions often are detected earlier, usually because they result in significant cyanosis. If obstruction to pulmonary blood flow is severe, patients with such lesions may be dependent on left-to-right flow across their PDA. As the PDA closes in the first few days of life, hypoxemia becomes even more pronounced and may be incompatible with survival.

Infants with TGV and inadequate intracardiac communication become extremely cyanotic as their PDA closes. On the other hand, if a large VSD or PDA is present, these patients may develop excessive pulmonary blood flow as PVR decreases during the first few weeks of extra-uterine life. Cyanosis will persist, however. Left untreated, hypertrophic vascular changes and pulmonary hypertension will occur.

Left-sided obstructive lesions cause pulmonary congestion without pulmonary volume overload. They impede flow from the pulmonary venous system to the systemic arterial system and can precipitate CHF. The symptomatology and age at presentation depend on the severity of the lesion. If the ductus arteriosus is patent, it allows right-to-left shunting of blood around the lesion, improving systemic perfusion but causing cyanosis.

III. Preoperative assessment

A. **What should the anesthesiologist look for?**

In developing an anesthetic plan for these children, one must understand the pathophysiology of the individual lesion and appreciate the degree of clinical symptomatology. As in any other assessment, taking a careful history and the physical examination probably are the most important parts of the preoperative evaluation. One must remember that the infant cannot relate the symptoms experienced, and the parents often fail to understand the significance of some of their observations.

1. **Age at presentation.** The age at presentation often provides a clue to the severity of the lesion. Infants with decreased pulmonary blood flow or inadequate mixing may be persistently cyanotic or may have intermittent episodes that often are associated with agitation, crying, or exercise. If a child is older, cyanotic episodes may be associated with "squatting" (which increases systemic vascular resistance [SVR] and promotes increased pulmonary blood flow). This change in pulmonary blood flow dynamics may

partially alleviate the cyanosis. However, particularly severe episodes can result in loss of consciousness or seizures.

2. **Frequency of episodes.** The frequency of episodes suggests the severity of the lesion. Knowledge that cyanotic episodes are intermittent confirms the dynamic nature of the shunt and should alert one to the fact that the same scenario is probable during anesthesia and surgical manipulations. Alterations in SVR and PVR may result in profound changes in the magnitude of the right-to-left shunt.
   a. **Cyanosis.** During the physical examination, an important consideration is that clinical cyanosis depends on the absolute concentration of deoxygenated hemoglobin in the blood rather than on the oxygen saturation. **More than 3 g/dL of deoxygenated arterial blood hemoglobin should make central cyanosis recognizable.** The oxyhemoglobin saturation at which central cyanosis becomes clinically apparent varies from about 62% when the hemoglobin level is 8 g/dL to about 88% in the polycythemic infant whose hemoglobin level is 24 g/dL. **Therefore, cyanosis is detected more easily when the infant's hematocrit (Hct) is elevated.** However, recognition of cyanosis is more difficult if a newborn has a significant proportion of fetal hemoglobin because it is more highly saturated at a given PO_2 (Fig. 14.2). Therefore, the newborn with a high proportion of fetal hemoglobin may have a large reduction in PO_2 before central cyanosis is clinically apparent.

      Infants with a preductal coarctation of the aorta may demonstrate cyanosis that is restricted to the lower half of the body, because the RV supplies the descending aorta with deoxygenated blood via the PDA.

3. **Respiration.** Infants with cyanotic heart disease often have an increased tidal volume. Clubbing of the fingers may occur but may not be evident early in life. Children with decreased pulmonary blood flow usually have exercise intolerance. These patients also have a blunted ventilatory response to hypoxia.

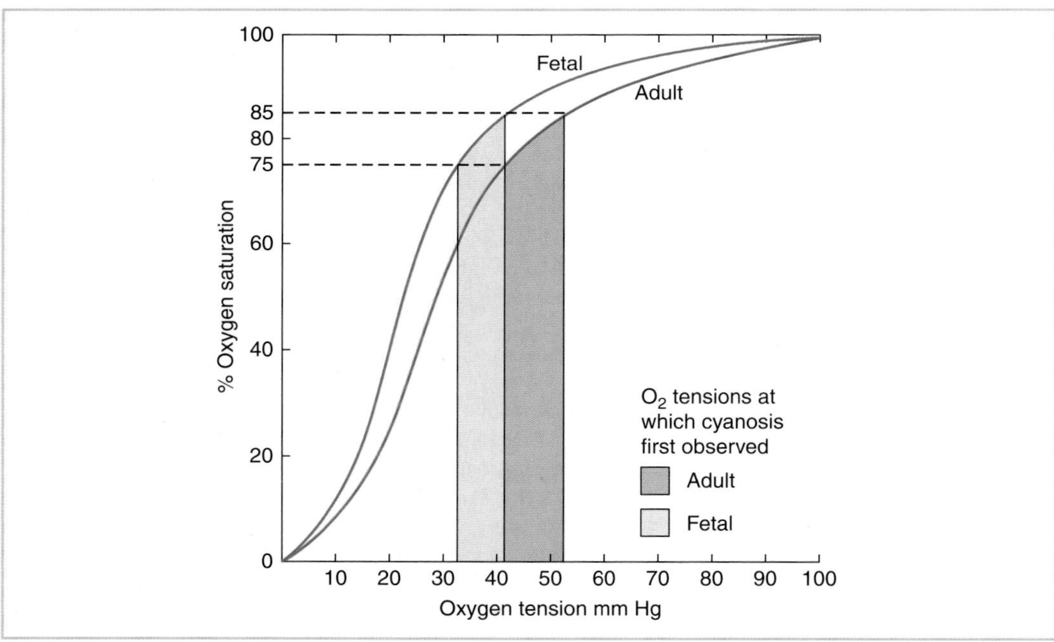

FIGURE 14.2 Hemoglobin–oxygen dissociation curves for fetal and adult hemoglobin. Note that an infant with a high proportion of fetal hemoglobin will have a low P_aO_2 (33 to 42 mm Hg) before cyanosis is observed. (From Lees MH, King DH. Heart disease in the newborn. In: Adams FH, Emmanouilides GC, Riemenschneider TA, eds. *Heart Disease in Infants, Children and Adolescents.* Baltimore, MD: Williams & Wilkins; 1989:844, with permission.)

4. **CHF.** Infants with too much pulmonary blood flow present with CHF early in infancy when PVR decreases. A history of feeding difficulties and failure to thrive are characteristics of CHF in infancy. Other features include tachypnea, tachycardia, irritability, inappropriate sweating (often with feeding), nasal flaring, sternal and intercostal retractions, cardiomegaly, and hepatomegaly. A history of wheezing, frequent respiratory infections, and pneumonia is common. The distinction between left-sided and right-sided heart failure in the newborn is less obvious than in the adult. Peripheral edema and rales are rarely present in the young infant. Systemic perfusion may be compromised, as evidenced by decreased pulses, pallor, and poor capillary refill. A severely compromised infant may be apathetic and have a weak cry and little spontaneous movement.

   Left-sided obstructive lesions may cause CHF with clinical manifestations that are similar to those of pulmonary volume overload. Note, however, that the symptoms are a result of pulmonary venous congestion without abnormal shunting. If the lesion is located so that LV *outflow* is obstructed, LV hypertrophy will develop. If the site of obstruction involves the *inflow* to the LV, LV hypertrophy does not occur, and LV end-diastolic pressure is normal.
5. **Associated anomalies.** Look carefully for associated congenital anomalies, because they are common in newborns with cardiac disease. Other problems peculiar to the newborn or premature infant include difficulty with temperature regulation, impaired nutrition, susceptibility to dehydration and hypoglycemia, respiratory difficulties, coagulation abnormalities, and central nervous system disorders.

B. **Which preoperative laboratory studies are helpful?**

Laboratory studies of particular interest include Hct, white blood cell count, coagulation profile, and electrolyte and serum glucose determinations. Sickle-cell screening and measurement of digoxin level should be included when applicable.

1. Hct. The Hct progressively rises as hypoxemia becomes more profound. In fact, periodic checks of the Hct provide a simple method to follow the patient's level of hypoxemia. Increasing Hct may serve as a cue for the appropriate timing of surgery for patients with complex cyanotic lesions. However, poor nutrition and iron deficiency in a hypoxemic child can prevent this increase in Hct and may mislead the clinician into thinking that the hypoxemia is less severe than it really is. A high Hct can result in increased blood viscosity, which can lead to spontaneous thrombosis and resultant cerebral, renal, or pulmonary infarctions. This process may be aggravated by the relative dehydration produced by a long period without oral intake. If the polycythemia is sufficiently severe (i.e., Hct is greater than 60% to 65%), phlebotomy may be required.
2. **White blood cell count.** Elevations in white blood cell count and a white blood cell shift in the differential should raise the suspicion of a systemic infection. Fever and upper respiratory infection must be ruled out. Children with elevated white blood cell counts should not be electively anesthetized, because immunologic function is compromised by CPB. Also, prosthetic material is frequently used in the surgical repair; if this material is inadvertently seeded by a bacteremia, the consequences may be disastrous.
3. **Coagulation studies.** Results of coagulation studies must be normal before CPB can be performed. A family history of bleeding tendencies should be sought. Unsuspected factor deficiencies have manifested and caused uncontrollable bleeding after surgery, when it may be difficult to identify the source of the problem. **Patients with cyanotic CHD are prone to develop coagulopathies because of platelet dysfunction and hypofibrinogenemia.**
4. **Electrolytes.** Electrolyte problems may be present in the newborn, especially if the child is receiving medication or total parenteral nutrition. Hypokalemia, hypomagnesemia, hypocalcemia, and hypoglycemia should be ruled out. Hypocalcemia is common in children with DiGeorge syndrome (a congenital disorder of the third and fourth branchial arches that is associated with thymic hypoplasia and congenital heart defects, especially aortic arch abnormalities or left-sided obstructive lesions).
5. **Glucose.** Hypoglycemia is especially common in infants with hypoplastic left-sided heart syndrome. The newborn's myocardium has an increased glucose dependence compared to the adult myocardium; thus, hypoglycemia may aggravate myocardial failure.

Hypoglycemia can occur because of reduced synthetic function, decreased glycogen stores, or reduced systemic perfusion, resulting in compromised hepatic function. Under anesthesia, hypoglycemia will be masked and may be missed unless the clinician looks for it. Conversely, these children often come to the operating room with concentrated dextrose in their hyperalimentation solution. Steroids are commonly administered on CPB, and this combination can result in significant hyperglycemia. Substantial literature exists, showing the detrimental effect of hyperglycemia during complete, incomplete, and focal cerebral ischemia in animals and adult humans. Specific data are lacking in children, although Steward et al. [2] suggested a worse neurologic outcome with hyperglycemia in a retrospective review of 34 children undergoing deep hypothermic circulatory arrest (DHCA). However, the Boston Circulatory Arrest Study suggested that normal blood glucose levels during reperfusion were associated with poorer neurologic outcome, whereas hyperglycemic levels appeared associated with better outcome [3]. It has been speculated that substrate deficiency in the immature brain may be an issue and that normal blood glucose levels during the reperfusion period after cerebral ischemia in infants may be insufficient for complete cerebral recovery.

6. **Digoxin.** Many children scheduled for heart surgery are receiving digoxin. After CPB, both a rebound increase in digoxin level and an increased sensitivity to the drug have been reported. Perioperative dysrhythmias are common and may be related to digoxin toxicity. Other factors may play a role in this enhanced toxicity, including hypokalemia, calcium fluxes, hypomagnesemia, and decreased creatinine clearance. Therefore, verify that the digoxin level is within the normal range and withhold digoxin preoperatively.
7. **Sickling test.** A sickling test should be performed in appropriate children. Hypothermia, acidosis, and anemia, as induced by CPB, decreased perfusion, and the bypass circuit itself enhance sickling if hemoglobin S is present. If the sickling test result is positive, hemoglobin electrophoresis should be performed to delineate the type of hemoglobinopathy. Depending on the type of defect, exchange transfusion may be indicated before or at the initiation of CPB.
8. **Electrocardiography.** The electrocardiogram shows great variability, especially during the first 24 h of life. In some instances, the electrocardiogram is diagnostically helpful. For example, extreme left- or right-axis deviation with counterclockwise frontal vector and RV hypertrophy suggests a form of endocardial cushion defect.
9. **Echocardiography and cardiac catheterization.** Two-dimensional echocardiography with quantitative Doppler and color flow mapping has revolutionized the diagnosis of CHD. In many institutions, the technology has become so refined that most surgical procedures are performed on the basis of this study alone. Cardiac catheterization may be used to confirm the diagnosis and to provide information concerning vascular resistance, the magnitude of shunts, and coronary anatomy. Cardiac catheterization may also be performed in conjunction with interventions such as device closures of septal defects.
10. **Chest radiography.** Chest radiography serves to evaluate the type and severity of the heart disease. It is also used to identify simulators of heart disease (e.g., meconium aspiration, mediastinal masses, pneumothorax, hyaline membrane disease, and diaphragmatic hernia) and to rule out significant pulmonary pathology.

C. What should the anesthesiologist tell the family about risk?

1. **Neurologic sequelae.** Morbidity and mortality vary with the lesion being repaired or palliated and with the institution involved. Ironically, as mortality has decreased, important
5 morbidities have become more prominent. **Neurologic sequelae remain one of the most common and potentially devastating complications of CHD and its repair.** Early postoperative neurologic dysfunction may occur in as many as 25% of these children, with seizures occurring in approximately 20% of neonates after CPB. The seizures are generally self-limited, and some early series reported no long-term adverse sequelae. However, the group from Boston was the first to prospectively study a relatively homogeneous group of infants with TGV undergoing repair using either a predominantly low-flow CPB or DHCA strategy. They demonstrated that seizures are an important prognostic indicator

of neurodevelopmental outcome [4]. The study also showed that there was a significantly higher incidence of seizures among infants randomized to circulatory arrest compared to those randomized to low-flow bypass. Follow-up of these children has shown a continuing important association between postoperative seizures and outcome, with an important decrement in cognitive and verbal skill assessments as well as motor skills [5]. Avoidance of circulatory arrest is not the entire solution to the problem, however, because the Boston group showed that there was a risk of seizures and suboptimal neurodevelopmental outcome even when continuous bypass was used.

Multiple factors contribute to the risk for neurodevelopmental sequelae. A complex interaction of preoperative, perioperative, and postoperative events can conspire to produce brain injury. Many children with CHD have pre-existing brain malformations. Multiple chromosomal anomalies with combined cardiac and neurologic features have been described, the best known being Down syndrome (trisomy 21) and the catch-22 spectrum of conditions associated with microdeletions in the 22q11 region of chromosome 22. Neurologic manifestations of the catch-22 spectrum may be subtle early in life but become more apparent over time. The potential impact of this chromosomal anomaly is enormous, because monosomy 22q11 has an estimated prevalence of 5% to 10% in the population of children with CHD. Brain injury also may be acquired in the preoperative period. Abnormal cardiovascular function may be associated with poor brain growth, embolic infarction, cerebrovascular thrombosis, and abscess formation. Hopefully, earlier repair of children with CHD will limit this mechanism of brain injury. Hypoxic–ischemic/reperfusion or embolic injury is thought to be the principal mechanism of brain injury occurring in the intraoperative period [6]. Injury also can occur in the postoperative period, during which unstable hemodynamics and increased cerebral energy needs may result in a mismatch of oxygen supply and demand to the brain. Intensive research is ongoing in this area of brain injury to try to prevent this devastating problem.

D. When should oral intake stop?

Nil per os (NPO) guidelines used for other infants and children generally can be used in patients with CHD. Recent evidence suggests that clear liquids can be continued until 2 to 4 h before surgery. In children with *cyanotic* heart disease, meticulous attention must be paid to the patient's state of hydration. Specifically, orders must be written to awaken the child 2 h before surgery to offer clear liquids. If uncertainty exists concerning the precise time of surgery, place an intravenous catheter and begin an infusion to prevent dehydration in patients with cyanotic heart disease.

E. Which sedation is appropriate?

The need for sedation must be individualized, but certain guidelines can be offered. A thorough explanation to the patient and family is in order, because the parents' anxiety often is transmitted to the child. Neonates and infants younger than 6 mos rarely require any sedation, because separation anxiety is not an issue. In older children, if intravenous access is already established and the child's parents are allowed to accompany him or her to the preoperative holding area, additional sedation may be unnecessary, because incremental intravenous agents can be titrated before transfer to the operating room.

Children between the ages of 1 and 5 yrs benefit most from judicious sedation. A variety of agents and routes can be used. The author prefers to avoid intramuscular injections and uses either intravenous or oral midazolam. If given intravenously, titrate in 0.1 to 0.25 mg increments; if given orally, the author gives 0.5 mg/kg. Patient acceptance is improved if the drug is offered in sweetened apple juice. An oral dose of 0.5 mg/kg typically results in easy separation from the parents at 15 to 30 min. If given intranasally, 0.2 mg/kg will be effective at about 10 to 15 min. These patients must be monitored when sedation is given. Pulse oximetry and careful observation are mandatory, because the hemodynamic status may be adversely and unpredictably affected if hypercarbia or hypoxemia occurs.

Some physicians routinely administer anticholinergics preoperatively. Others give atropine in the operating room only if clinically necessary. Keep in mind that slow heart rates often are not tolerated in infants whose stroke volume is relatively fixed.

F. When does the patient need intravenous infusions?

Children who require vasoactive infusions preoperatively come to the operating room with such access already available. For others, the timing of intravenous access is strictly up to the anesthesiologist involved. For many cases, a gentle inhalation induction with subsequent expeditious venous catheter placement before intubation is appropriate. Again, if the timing of surgery is uncertain, preoperative intravenous catheter placement is desirable to avoid dehydration, especially in children with cyanotic heart disease.

G. When is prostaglandin E_1 indicated?

PGE_1 is indicated whenever it is thought that maintaining, reopening, or enlarging an existing ductus arteriosus will benefit the neonate. Common situations in which it is used include the presence of (i) lesions with decreased pulmonary blood flow, (ii) TGV, and (iii) left-sided heart outflow obstruction.

With TGV, the response to PGE_1 is variable, but in some infants, mixing of systemic and pulmonary circulation improves sufficiently to reduce hypoxemia slightly and to relieve acidosis. With left-sided heart outflow obstruction (e.g., hypoplastic left-sided heart syndrome, coarctation), PGE_1 will open the ductus and allow right-to-left flow across it, improving systemic perfusion and perhaps even coronary blood flow. It may also dilate the pulmonary vascular bed.

Stabilization of the infant before surgical intervention and improved outcome often result from PGE_1 infusion. Side effects include apneic spells, seizures, systemic hypotension, inhibition of platelet aggregation, peripheral edema, and unexplained fever. Cortical proliferation in long bones can occur with chronic use. Because PGE_1 is metabolized rapidly, it must be infused continuously, usually at a dose of 0.05 to 0.1 μg/kg/min. As much as 80% of circulating PGE_1 is metabolized in one pass through the lungs; thus, the ductal response diminishes within minutes after its discontinuation.

IV. Equipment and infusions

A. What is required?

Care for an infant undergoing heart surgery demands meticulous attention to detail and extreme vigilance. A well-thought-out plan should be developed before induction so that all equipment needed is available and in working order (Table 14.3).

1. **Anesthetic and surgical considerations.** The anesthesia machine and circuit should be checked as for all procedures. Multiple sizes of endotracheal tubes, masks, and laryngoscope blades must be available. Appropriate equipment to keep the infant warm may be needed, including a heating/cooling blanket, radiant warming lights, a fluid warmer, and a heated humidifier. A working operating room table that allows optimal positioning to facilitate surgical exposure is required. A defibrillator with both nonsterile (external) and sterile (internal) paddles, a dual-chamber pacemaker generator, a CO computer, and a coagulation

TABLE 14.3 Equipment used during pediatric cardiac surgery

Equipment
Heating/cooling blanket
Radiant warming lights
Fluid warmer
Heated humidifier
Defibrillator (external, internal)
Pacemaker generator
CO computer
Coagulation analyzer
Fibrillator
Infusion pumps
Transesophageal echocardiography

CO, cardiac output

From Davies LK. Anesthesia for pediatric cardiovascular surgery. In: Kirby RR, Gravenstein N, Lobato EB, et al., eds. *Clinical Anesthesia Practice.* Philadelphia, PA: WB Saunders; 2002:1219, with permission.

analyzer must be operational. A fibrillator is frequently needed intraoperatively to induce ventricular fibrillation during open-chamber procedures.

2. **Monitoring.** Equipment needed to monitor the patient includes a pulse oximeter, a hemodynamic monitor, appropriate catheters for arterial and venous cannulation, transducers (zeroed and calibrated to mercury), a blood pressure cuff, a stethoscope, thermistors, and a mixed venous oxygen saturation monitor. Equipment used to monitor central nervous system function may include electroencephalography (EEG), transcranial Doppler (TCD), jugular venous saturation monitoring, and near-infrared spectroscopy. Transesophageal echocardiography has become an extraordinarily valuable tool for diagnostic purposes (confirmation and delineation of anatomy, detection of unsuspected defects or residual defects after repair) and for ventricular function and volume monitoring.
3. **Intravenous fluids.** Two intravenous fluid sets should be prepared, and all air bubbles should be removed from the tubing. This task is made easier if one begins with warm fluid; microbubble formation seems to occur less frequently than if cold fluid is allowed to warm when the room temperature is raised. All intravenous and monitoring tubing must be bubble-free whenever a potential shunt is present, because intracardiac shunts can be bidirectional and may become right-to-left during surgery. Air filters can be used, but the same amount of effort must be expended to remove air from intravenous tubing, because air filters cannot be relied on to trap all air. Another drawback of air filters is that they slow down intravenous infusions significantly and may make it difficult to keep up with volume replacement.

   A method to carefully control and limit intravenous fluid intake is important, because many patients have barely compensated excess pulmonary blood flow and volume. Infusion using a limited amount in a buret chamber and a minidripper, use of infusion pumps with set volumes, or administration of fluid via syringe in bolus increments are methods that can be used to limit intake. At least three infusion pumps that allow accurate titration of vasoactive drugs should be available.
4. **Preparation of infusions.** Appropriate intravenous solutions for mixing infusions (e.g., normal saline and 5% dextrose in water) and cassettes for the pumps should be on hand. Common infusions to be available on short notice include sodium nitroprusside, epinephrine, isoproterenol, dopamine, and milrinone. Some thought should be given to the appropriate concentrations for the patient's body size so that fluid overload can be minimized. Table 14.4 lists commonly used drugs and bolus doses or initial infusion rates.

   Children do not routinely require multiple vasoactive infusions postoperatively. I find it helpful to prepare commonly needed drugs in syringes so that a small bolus can be given if required. If needed repetitively, an infusion can be mixed. Table 14.5 lists drugs that should be available in syringes at the beginning of each pediatric cardiac surgical case. A narcotic, a benzodiazepine, and a muscle relaxant also should be on hand for ready use.
5. **Blood and blood products.** Blood products appropriate to the particular procedure and patient size should be readied in advance. Preparation may range from typing and screening for simple procedures to typing and cross-matching of multiple units of blood or platelets (or both) and fresh frozen plasma for complex pump cases. At the University of Florida, infants younger than 4 mos undergo typing and screening and then preferentially receive type O blood without a cross-match because the risk of transfusion reaction is low.

   Transfusion-acquired cytomegalovirus infection is generally a benign entity in immunocompetent patients who receive blood. However, immunologically immature patients (especially low-birth-weight infants) can become symptomatic if infected. Therefore, our routine is to use cytomegalovirus-negative blood products in children younger than 4 mos. For infants with aortic arch abnormalities, blood products should be irradiated, because these cardiac lesions may be associated with DiGeorge syndrome. Such patients may have an absent thymus and increased susceptibility to graft-versus-host disease after transfusion.

V. Anesthetic induction and maintenance

A. *Which monitors are needed before induction?*

No absolute rule exists for determining the amount of monitoring necessary before induction. In some patients, particularly if a "steal" induction is ideal, anesthesia can be started with just a

TABLE 14.4 Nonanesthetic drugs and dosages[a]

Drug	Dose
Inotropic infusions	
Epinephrine	0.01–0.1 μg/kg/min
Isoproterenol	0.01–0.1 μg/kg/min
Norepinephrine	0.01–0.1 μg/kg/min
Dopamine	2–10 μg/kg/min
Dobutamine	2–10 μg/kg/min
Amrinone[b]	2–2.5 mg/kg bolus divided over 30–60 min, followed by 5–20 μg/kg/min infusion
Milrinone	50 μg/kg bolus, followed by 0.4–0.8 μg/kg/min infusion
Vasodilator infusions	
Nitroglycerin	1–2 μg/kg/min
Nitroprusside	1–5 μg/kg/min
PGE_1	0.05–0.1 μg/kg/min
Labetalol	10–100 mg/h
Antiarrhythmic drugs	
Lidocaine	1 mg/kg bolus
Adenosine	0.03 mg/kg/min infusion
Procainamide	0.15 mg/kg bolus
Dilantin	2 mg/kg over 5 min
Bretylium	2–4 mg/kg over 5 min
Amiodarone	5 mg/kg bolus 5 mg/kg over 1 h, then 5 mg/kg over 12 h. Repeat as needed
β-Blocking drugs	
Propranolol	0.01–0.1 mg/kg
Esmolol	0.5–1 mg/kg bolus 100–300 μg/kg/min infusion
Others	
Calcium chloride	10–20 mg/kg
Sodium bicarbonate	1 mEq/kg (or as determined by base deficit)
Phenylephrine	1–10 μg/kg
Ephedrine	0.05–0.2 mg/kg
Heparin	≥3 mg/kg (300 U/kg)
Protamine	≥3 mg/kg

[a]The dose of each drug varies with the clinical context.
[b]Cannot be mixed in dextrose-containing solutions.
PGE_1, prostaglandin E_1.
From Davies LK. Anesthesia for pediatric cardiovascular surgery. In: Kirby RR, Gravenstein N, Lobato EB, et al., eds. *Clinical Anesthesia Practice*. Philadelphia, PA: WB Saunders; 2002:1220, with permission.

pulse oximeter and a precordial stethoscope. Then, as the patient is induced, electrocardiography and blood pressure monitoring can be quickly established. In others, it may be preferable to begin with all monitors (even invasive ones) in place. Generally, arterial and central venous catheters are placed after induction, although occasionally they may need to be placed before the procedure.

B. ***When does a patient need intravenous access before induction?***

The timing of intravenous access, as noted previously, often is a matter of personal preference. However, polycythemic patients must be well hydrated either by mouth or intravenously.

TABLE 14.5 Bolus drugs available in syringes

Drug	Syringe concentration	Bolus dose
Calcium chloride	100 mg/mL	10–20 mg/kg
Epinephrine	10 μg/mL 100 μg/mL	0.2–1 μg/kg (inotropy) 10–100 μg/kg (cardiac arrest)
Isoproterenol	20 μg/mL	1–10 μg
Phenylephrine	100 μg/mL	1–10 μg/kg
Lidocaine	20 mg/mL	1 mg/kg
Esmolol[a]	10 mg/mL	0.5–1 mg/kg
Heparin	1,000 U/mL	300 U/kg (CPB) 100 U/kg (vascular nonpump)
Atropine	0.4 mg/mL	0.01–0.02 mg/kg
Succinylcholine	20 mg/mL	1–2 mg/kg
Ephedrine	5 mg/mL	0.05–0.2 mg/kg
Pancuronium	1 mg/mL	0.1–0.15 mg/kg (intubation)

[a]Available for treatment of hypercyanotic spells in patients with tetralogy of Fallot.
CPB, cardiopulmonary bypass.
From Davies LK. Anesthesia for pediatric cardiovascular surgery. In: Kirby RR, Gravenstein N, Lobato EB, et al., eds. *Clinical Anesthesia Practice.* Philadelphia, PA: WB Saunders; 2002:1220, with permission.

Children with extremely poor cardiac function who require inotropes may not tolerate an inhalation induction; thus, an intravenous induction is preferred. Most other pediatric patients tolerate a judicious inhalation induction with subsequent placement of intravenous catheters.

If myocardial reserve is impaired, a high-dose inhalation technique cannot be used for long; once catheters are placed, a transition is made either to a completely intravenous narcotic technique or to a combination of intravenous and inhalation techniques. If the anesthesiologist is uncertain about his or her ability to place an intravenous catheter rapidly during an inhalation induction, it should be inserted before induction.

C. ***How does cardiac disease affect the rate of induction?***

1. **Inhalation agents.** Intracardiac shunting can alter the speed of induction with an inhalation anesthetic. The final effect on rate of induction depends on the size and direction of the shunt and the patient's CO. A right-to-left intracardiac shunt prolongs induction, because of a slower rate of rise in systemic arterial blood anesthetic partial pressure. This rate of rise is slowed because of the dilution of the pulmonary blood flow containing anesthetic by the blood passing through the right-to-left shunt to which no anesthetic has been added. If high concentrations of agents are used to speed induction and a relative anesthetic overdose occurs, it is difficult to remedy, because the inhalation agents are slow to be eliminated. A left-to-right shunt, generally, has a negligible effect on the speed of induction if the systemic perfusion is preserved at a normal level.
2. **Intravenous agents.** Response to intravenously administered drugs is faster with a right-to-left shunt because the dilution effect and the pulmonary transit time are reduced in proportion to the magnitude of the shunt. A left-to-right shunt has a minimal effect on the response to intravenous drugs if systemic perfusion is preserved.

D. What problems are likely to occur during induction?

Any number of untoward events can occur during induction of anesthesia in pediatric patients with heart disease.

1. **Airway obstruction.** Airway obstruction is poorly tolerated in these patients, especially small infants or those with cyanotic heart disease. The margin for error is extremely small and minor problems can quickly become life threatening. Airway obstruction that causes hypoxemia or hypercarbia increases PVR. A reversal of a left-to-right intracardiac shunt or aggravation of a right-to-left shunt may result, exacerbating the problem and creating a vicious cycle.

TABLE 14.6 Cardiac grid for common congenital heart diseases (desired hemodynamic changes)

	Preload	PVR	SVR	HR	Contractility
ASD	↑	↑	↓	N	N
VSD (right-to-left)	N	↓	↑	N	N
VSD (left-to-right)	↑	↑	↓	N	N
Idiopathic hypertrophic subaortic stenosis	↑	N	N–↑	↓[a]	↓[a]
PDA	↑	↑	↓	N	N
Coarctation	↑	N	↓	N	N
Valvular pulmonic stenosis	↑	↓	N	↓	↑
Infundibular pulmonary stenosis	↑	↓	N	↓	↓[a]
Aortic stenosis	↑	N	↑[a]	↓[a]	N–↑
Mitral stenosis	↑	N–↓	N	↓[a]	N–↑
Aortic regurgitation	↑	N	↓	N–↑	N–↑
Mitral regurgitation	↑	N–↓	↓	N–↑	N–↑

[a]An over-riding consideration.
PVR, pulmonary vascular resistance; SVR, systemic vascular resistance HR, heart rate; ASD, atrial septal defect; N, normal or no change; VSD, ventricular septal defect; PDA, Patent ductus arteriosus.
From Moore RA. Anesthesia for the pediatric congenital heart patient for noncardiac surgery. *Anesthesiol Rev.* 1981;8:27, with permission.

2. **Dysrhythmias.** The patient may become bradycardic or develop a nodal rhythm with induction. As stroke volume is relatively fixed, CO suffers in this context. Acidosis can occur quickly when perfusion is marginal; this further depresses myocardial contractility, increasing PVR and decreasing SVR.

   Dysrhythmias can result from many causes, including light anesthesia, hypoxemia, hypercarbia, drugs, and electrolyte abnormalities.

   Significant potential problems may occur during central venous access acquisition. The drapes or patient position may serve to kink the endotracheal tube as it warms to body temperature. Dysrhythmias during this phase are generally induced mechanically from the catheter or guidewire. Familiarity with the lengths of the catheter kit components makes insertion to excessive depth less likely. Mechanically induced dysrhythmias respond better to removal of the stimulus than to pharmacologic therapy.

7 **E. Which anesthetic technique should the anesthesiologist use?**

The choice of drug(s) is not as important as an understanding of the lesion's pathophysiology. Of help is the development of hemodynamic goals for each patient in terms of heart rate, contractility, preload, SVR, and PVR (Table 14.6). In several lesions, over-riding considerations dominate. An appropriate approach for a patient with aortic insufficiency may be completely different than that for a patient with TOF. Once the goals are defined, appropriate agents, dosages, and routes of administration can be selected. Many agents can be used so long as they are administered in a thoughtful fashion.

F. How should the patient be positioned?

Data are scarce regarding the safest way to position a patient for heart surgery.

Access to the patient's head is crucial for visual inspection to rule out superior vena cava syndrome, for pupil evaluation, and for airway manipulation. A piece of eggcrate foam can be placed under the patient's head to minimize the chance of pressure necrosis; many heart surgery cases are lengthy, and low perfusion pressure occurs during CPB. However, because infants have such large occiputs, elevation of the head in this way occasionally may result in encroachment on the surgical field.

VI. Monitoring

Anesthetic induction generally proceeds with noninvasive monitors. A five-lead electrocardiograph is used to facilitate detection of rhythm disturbances and myocardial ischemia. An esophageal lead also can be used to more easily diagnose dysrhythmias, especially when tachycardia is present. Lead V_5 can be placed in its normal position and covered with an adhesive drape to protect it from the surgical scrub solutions. The monitor mode of the electrocardiograph will minimize baseline drift, whereas the diagnostic mode allows better resolution of the P and T waves.

A. *When is an arterial catheter indicated?*

An indwelling arterial catheter is required whenever continuous monitoring of arterial pressure or frequent blood sampling is necessary. All procedures using CPB require placement of an arterial catheter, because noninvasive methods are not useful if no pulsatile flow is present. Most closed heart procedures also benefit from beat-to-beat monitoring of arterial pressure.

The arterial catheter is placed after intubation, preferably percutaneously in the nondominant radial artery. Other sites commonly used include the dorsalis pedis, posterior tibial, femoral, and, occasionally, temporal arteries. A surgical cutdown is used only as a last resort because of the disproportionately high incidence of thrombosis and infection. For coarctation repairs, the arterial catheter must be placed in the right radial artery; if this is unsuccessful, the catheter can be placed in a temporal artery. In patients with a Blalock–Taussig (BT) shunt, the catheter must be placed on the side opposite to the BT shunt or in a lower-extremity artery. A 22- or 24-gauge catheter is used, depending on the child's size.

B. When is central venous access needed?

1. **Central venous catheters.** Central venous access is established routinely when knowledge of right-sided heart filling pressure trends or the need to administer vasoactive drugs rapidly is desirable. Access to the central circulation also allows placement of PA or pacing catheters. The decision as to which type and size of catheter should be used depends on the type of operation performed and on the size and clinical status of the patient.

   A central venous catheter is used routinely in patients undergoing CPB. Monitoring superior vena caval pressure during extracorporeal circulation is useful for assessing adequacy of venous drainage, particularly when two venous cannulas are used. A central catheter with at least two lumens allows drug and fluid delivery via one lumen and uninterrupted central venous pressure (CVP) measurements via the other. Many centers avoid the use of SVC catheters in neonates because of the concern for venous thrombosis and SVC occlusion.

   My guidelines for catheter length and size are listed in Table 14.7. Follow-up verification of appropriate catheter position occurs on review of the postoperative chest film.

2. **PA catheters.** Monitoring of PA pressure is helpful when PVR is problematic. Placement of the PA catheter can be accomplished percutaneously or by the surgeon using a direct transthoracic approach. If the patient's size is too small to accept a balloon flotation catheter, a combined percutaneous and direct intraoperative approach can be used. In this scenario, the catheter is placed through a sterility sheath into the introducer and advanced into the superior vena cava. When the chest and heart are open, the surgeon can advance the catheter into the proximal PA. In complex cardiac anomalies with shunts, the surgeon

TABLE 14.7 Guidelines for central venous pressure catheter size and length in relationship to patient size

Patient weight (kg)	Internal jugular catheter size[a]	CVP catheter length (cm)
<2.5	3 Fr SL or 4 Fr DL	5
2.5–5	4 Fr DL or 5 Fr DL	5
5–10	5 Fr DL or 5 Fr introducer	8
10–20	5 Fr DL or 6 Fr introducer	8–12
>20	5–7 Fr DL or 6 Fr introducer	12–15

[a]Catheter size is also influenced by operative procedure. If significant blood loss is anticipated and peripheral venous access is limited, a larger-size CVP catheter may be preferred.
CVP, central venous pressure DL, double-lumen; Fr, French; SL, single-lumen.
From Davies LK. Anesthesia for pediatric cardiovascular surgery. In: Kirby RR, Gravenstein N, Lobato EB, et al., eds. *Clinical Anesthesia Practice.* Philadelphia, PA: WB Saunders; 2002:1222, with permission.

generally will thread the percutaneously placed PA catheter into position at the end of the surgical procedure, because the catheter often is in the field of repair.

Continuous mixed venous oximetry is available with selected PA catheters and may be helpful in titrating vasoactive infusions, in providing an early warning of deteriorating CO, and in assessing residual shunts. The patient's size must be large enough to accommodate a 5 to 6 Fr introducer to facilitate percutaneous placement of a PA catheter.

Smaller infants requiring PA pressure monitoring will have transthoracic PA catheters placed at the close of surgery. The PA catheter is also useful postoperatively to assess pressure gradients by carefully measuring pullback pressures upon its removal. Some PA catheters allow measurement of CO by thermodilution; however, this method is not used often in small children because of the significant fluid load it imposes on the patient.

3. **Left atrial catheters.** Left atrial pressure monitoring is commonly used in patients with CHD because disparities in left- and right-sided heart function often are present. This catheter is inserted by the surgeon at the end of repair, usually via the right superior pulmonary vein. One must be careful with its use; the risk of systemic embolization of clot or air is real because the catheter is in the left side of the heart. The risk of bleeding and cardiac tamponade is present when the catheter is removed.

C. Where should temperature be measured?

The optimal site for temperature monitoring during cardiac cases is controversial; remember that gradients exist between various sites (Fig. 14.3). Commonly used are the esophagus, nasopharynx, rectum, tympanic membrane, blood, and bladder. Temperature monitoring is important because the rate of cooling and rewarming appears to be important in the production of brain injury. Monitoring in at least two sites is advisable to ensure that the temperature gradient between inflow (blood temperature) and bladder or rectal temperature does not exceed 10°C and that uniform cooling and warming have occurred.

D. How do end-tidal and arterial carbon dioxide pressures correlate?

Monitoring of end-tidal carbon dioxide partial pressure ($P_{ET}CO_2$) is useful to corroborate tracheal intubation. The arterial to end-tidal carbon dioxide partial pressure difference ($P_{(a-ET)}CO_2$) can be increased in patients with cardiopulmonary disease. It may also be increased in small children, depending on the sampling site and ventilatory pattern. Patients with CHD have altered ventilation/perfusion ratios; this produces abnormalities of both the physiologic dead space to tidal volume ratio (VDS/VT) and venous admixture (Qs/Qt).

In patients with cyanotic heart disease, in which Qs/Qt can be large, $P_{ET}CO_2$ significantly underestimates P_aCO_2. As intracardiac shunting often is dynamic, the $P_{(a-ET)}CO_2$ is ever changing; thus, even $P_{ET}CO_2$ trends are not reliable in these patients. Periodic measurement of P_aCO_2 is necessary to document adequate ventilation. $P_{ET}CO_2$ monitoring during PA banding reflects the decrease in pulmonary blood flow. As the band is tightened, the $P_{(a-ET)}CO_2$ gradient increases.

E. How should blood gases be managed on cardiopulmonary bypass?

The strategy of management of the pH has received considerable attention over the past few
8 years. Blood gas management strategy may be more important in children because greater degrees of hypothermia are often used, resulting in more profound differences in blood carbon dioxide levels. Briefly, there are two schools of thought regarding carbon dioxide management. In the alpha-stat strategy, no carbon dioxide is added to the circuit, and electrochemical neutrality is maintained with the blood gas measurement not corrected to temperature (i.e., reported at 37°C). Enzymatic function is well maintained in this milieu. In contrast, with the pH-stat strategy, carbon dioxide is added to the system to maintain a constant pH over varying temperatures. Blood gases are temperature corrected and reported at actual body temperature. In this scenario, hydrogen ions accumulate, total carbon dioxide stores are elevated, and the microcirculatory pH becomes increasingly acidotic at deep hypothermic temperatures. It was initially believed that intracellular pH also became increasingly acidotic, but more recent data have shown that the intracellular pH changes only slightly [7].

Evidence in adults suggests that either carbon dioxide management on CPB does not matter or that an alpha-stat strategy is advantageous. Recently, randomized prospective studies of

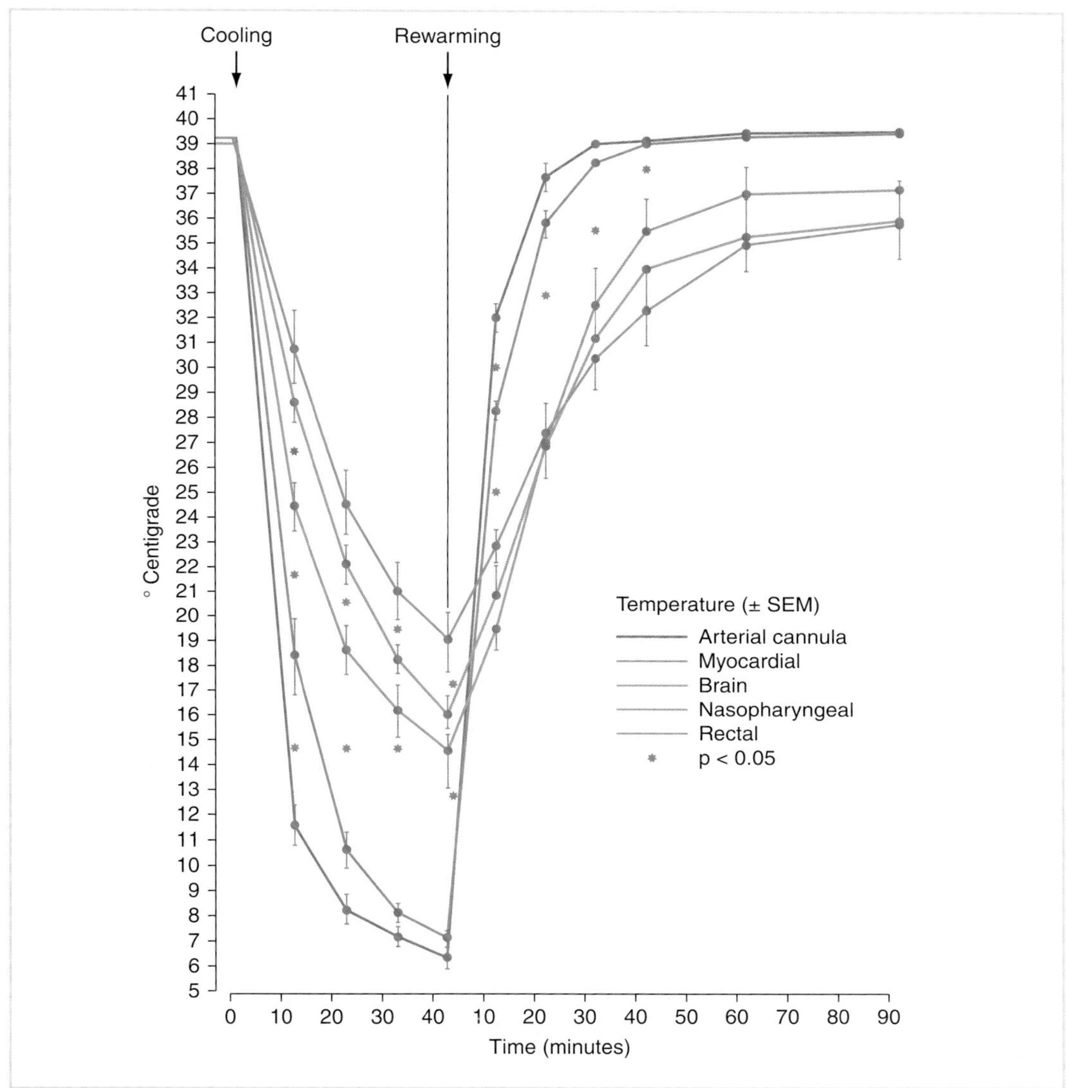

FIGURE 14.3 Average temperature (±SEM) of arterial cannula, myocardium, cerebral cortex, nasopharynx, and rectum during 40 min of cooling and 90 min of rewarming during CPB in six pigs. (From Stefaniszyn HJ, Novick RJ, Keith FM, et al. Is the brain adequately cooled during deep hypothermic cardiopulmonary bypass? *Curr Surg.* 1983;40:294, with permission.)

adults using moderate hypothermia showed that postoperative neurologic or neuropsychologic outcome is slightly, but consistently, better with alpha-stat management [8].

Although acid–base management is probably not so important when moderate hypothermic temperatures are used, it may be critical in the setting of deep hypothermia. Investigations have been performed to try to understand the correct acid–base management approach in children, but controversy remains. Proponents of the alpha-stat method suggest that the luxuriously high blood flows seen with pH-stat management may put the brain at risk for damage because of microemboli, cerebral edema, or high intracranial pressure, or it may predispose to an adverse redistribution of blood flow ("steal") away from marginally perfused areas in

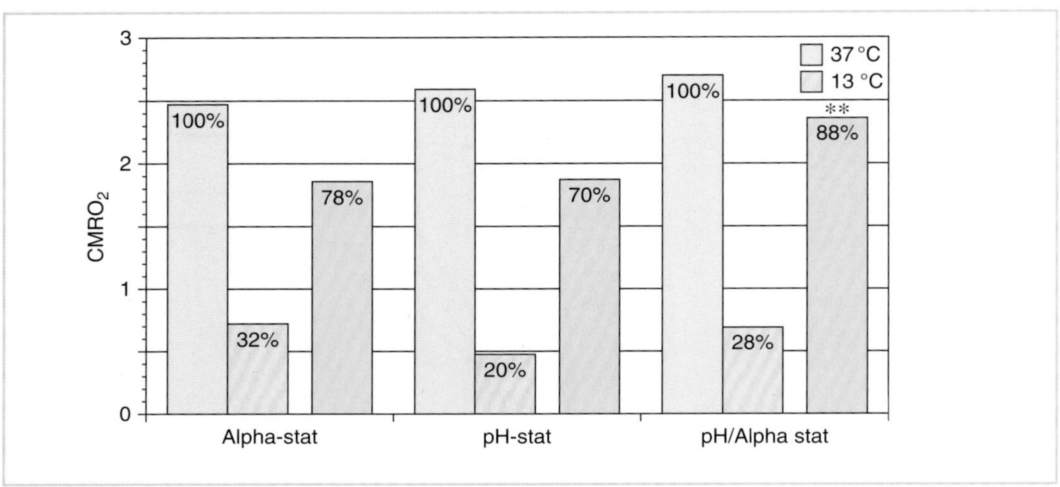

FIGURE 14.4 Effects of three different cooling strategies: alpha-stat, pH-stat, and a cross-over of pH-stat followed by alpha-stat on cerebral metabolic suppression before DHCA and recovery of cerebral metabolism after DHCA. The pH-stat strategy provides better metabolic suppression before DHCA than alpha-stat, but cerebral metabolic recovery after DHCA is poor. Initial cooling with a pH-stat strategy followed by conversion to alpha-stat before DHCA results in the greatest cerebral metabolic recovery after DHCA. *Yellow bar, 37°C; Pink bar, 13°C; Blue bar,* after DHCA. **Percent metabolic recovery significantly better for crossover strategy than either the alpha- or pH-stat strategy alone. (From Kern FH, Greeley WJ. pH-stat management of blood gases is not preferable to alpha-stat in patients undergoing brain cooling for cardiac surgery. *J Cardiothorac Vasc Anesth*. 1995;9:215, with permission.)

patients with cerebrovascular disease. On the other hand, proponents of the pH-stat strategy suggest that enhanced CBF may be helpful in improving cerebral cooling before the initiation of circulatory arrest. Total CBF is increased, global cerebral cooling is enhanced, and a redistribution of brain blood flow occurs during pH-stat management. An increased proportion of CBF is distributed to deep brain structures (thalamus, brainstem, and cerebellum) when pH-stat management is used [9]. However, other data suggest that cerebral metabolic recovery after circulatory arrest may be better with the alpha-stat method than with the pH-stat mode. This variation in results has led some authors to advocate a crossover strategy, that is, using a pH-stat approach during the first 10 min of cooling to provide maximal cerebral metabolic suppression followed by a change to alpha-stat strategy to remove the severe acidosis that accumulates during profound hypothermia with the use of pH-stat. This approach appears to offer maximal metabolic recovery in animals (Fig. 14.4) [10]. Choice of acid–base management may be particularly important in the subgroup of patients with aortopulmonary collaterals where cerebral cooling is problematic. It appears that addition of carbon dioxide during cooling enhances cerebral perfusion and improves cerebral metabolic recovery [11]. A randomized, single-center trial in human infants younger than 9 mos found that those managed with a pH-stat strategy generally had better outcomes than those in the alpha-stat group [12]. The pH-stat infants had a significantly shorter recovery time to first EEG activity and a tendency to fewer EEG-manifested seizures. In the subset of transposition babies, those assigned to pH-stat tended to have a higher cardiac index despite a lower requirement for inotropic agents, less-frequent acidosis and hypotension, and a shorter duration of mechanical ventilation and intensive care unit stay. The data suggest that pH-stat management may enhance systemic and cerebral protection in this group of patients.

Why the apparent difference in outcome between adults and children relative to pH management? It may be related to differences in the mechanism of brain injury on CPB. In adults, emboli appear to play a prominent role in adverse neurologic outcome. It is postulated that the decrease in CBF associated with alpha-stat management might be protective by limiting cerebral microemboli. On the other hand, the mechanism of injury in children may relate more to hypoperfusion or activation of excitotoxic pathways [13]. If a pH-stat strategy is used, the increase in CBF may be beneficial in ensuring complete brain cooling and slowing oxygen consumption, thus increasing the brain's tolerance for DHCA.

F. **How should the central nervous system be monitored?**

Central nervous system insults associated with cardiac surgery remain an unsolved problem. Brain damage can occur as a result of global hypoxia–ischemia or focal emboli. EEG has been used to try to provide a measure of cerebral electrical activity and function during cardiac surgery. Unfortunately, the EEG may not be reliable in predicting or preventing brain ischemia during CPB because of the effects of hypothermia and anesthetic agents and because of the likelihood of focal embolic injury. Newer, computerized, processed EEG monitors are less cumbersome and allow easier recognition of trends and abrupt changes. The advantage of EEG is that it can be obtained in patients of any age or size with no risk and may be effective in detecting catastrophic events causing global ischemia. EEG can also be useful for assessing adequacy of cerebral cooling by ensuring electrocerebral silence before circulatory arrest.

CBF has been measured using the Fick principle and xenon (Xe) 133 clearance. Unfortunately, this technique does not provide continuous measurement of CBF and is more applicable to the research setting rather than clinical care. TCD sonography uses the Doppler principle to detect shifts in frequency of reflected signals from blood in motion to calculate flow velocity. As it is thought that the diameters of the large cerebral arteries insonated are relatively constant, trends in flow velocity should pattern those of CBF. Thus, even though quantitative measurement of CBF cannot be made from TCD, qualitative inferences may be appropriate. TCD can provide an indirect measure of cerebral vascular resistance (which is increased with elevated intracranial pressure or markedly elevated CVP). TCD can be helpful in detecting suboptimally placed cannulae, because distortion of the superior vena cava can result in an impediment to cerebral venous drainage. TCD is also useful for detecting cerebral emboli. At present, the technology does not allow determination of emboli type (air vs. particulate) or size.

Cerebral metabolism has been estimated by monitoring jugular venous bulb saturation, the cerebral equivalent of "mixed venous" blood. A low saturation suggests an elevation in cerebral metabolism outstripping the cerebral oxygen provided. However, this blood is the effluent from many areas of the brain, and regional areas of cerebral hypoperfusion can easily be missed.

Challenges in monitoring the neonatal cardiac surgical patient while in the operating room are the result of an interplay between several ongoing variables. Metrics employed to assess CO, adequacy of CPB, changes in metabolic demand associated with temperature changes, and ongoing inflammatory responses all create significant difficulty in determining how to best monitor a patient undergoing surgical intervention. Many institutions and programs have begun to employ near infrared spectroscopy (NIRS) as a tool to best monitor cerebral and peripheral oxygenation [14]. Assessment of perfusion in the operating room setting has historically relied upon an indirect measurement of CO using parameters such as blood pressure, pulses, capillary refill, and urine output. While on CPB, perfusion pressure and the ability to control the patient's core temperature are often times the only sources of information regarding adequate CPB pump functionality. We have found that continuous monitoring of the regional oxygen saturation (rSO2) via NIRS allows for identification of acute changes in cerebral and systemic oxygen delivery and frequently precedes other indicators of decreased CO. Sensors are often placed on the forehead to look at cerebral oxygenation as well as over the kidney for a measure of somatic perfusion. This is helpful not only prior to and following the use of CPB, but also while the child is on CPB as a method of ensuring adequate cerebral perfusion as well as drainage. In addition, the postoperative patient can be expected to have lability with regard to CO, and the need for acute interventions should be anticipated because critical low-output syndrome may develop. Strategies for postoperative care are predicated upon optimizing rSO2 and CO. As such, an algorithmic and reproducible approach to initial medical management in the perioperative and immediate postoperative periods minimizes the potential for these predictable and necessary interventions to result in morbidity or mortality. Neurologic dysfunction can be a problem in patients with CHD. NIRS may provide data on cerebral oxygenation, and enthusiasm for this technology has increased with hopes of reducing neurologic dysfunction. Many centers have adopted NIRS as standard of care. Available data suggest that multimodality monitoring, including NIRS, may be a useful adjunct. However, the current literature on the use of NIRS alone does not conclusively demonstrate improvement in neurologic outcome. Data correlating NIRS findings with indirect measures of neurologic outcome or mortality are limited. **Although NIRS has promise for measuring regional tissue oxygen saturation, the lack of data demonstrating improved outcomes limits the support for wide-spread implementation** [15].

As neurologic morbidity is such an issue, I believe that neurologic monitoring will become more prevalent and techniques will be refined over the next decade. Anesthesiologists will become more skilled in "pattern recognition" of scenarios that require intervention.

G. What is the role of echocardiography?

Perioperative echocardiography is increasingly used in many centers for pediatric cardiac surgery. Both epicardial and, more recently, transesophageal studies have been performed to better define cardiac anatomy and assess surgical repair. Technologic improvements allow better imaging, smaller probe size, and multiplane capability, thereby substantially increasing the information provided by this modality. Several studies have demonstrated that two-dimensional and Doppler color-flow imaging can demonstrate previously unappreciated anatomic details and allow assessment of quality of repair and ventricular function after bypass. The ultimate role of echocardiography in the operating room and intensive care unit is still evolving and will hinge on demonstration of improvement in outcome in these patients.

VII. Cardiopulmonary bypass

A. How does it differ in children?

Although the physiology of extracorporeal circulation is similar in adults and children, significant differences exist in technique and physiologic sequelae (Table 14.8). Smaller cannulas are placed in children; however, they may still obstruct venous drainage into the heart or impede arterial outflow from the CPB circuit before institution of bypass or after its discontinuation. Almost all cardiac repairs in children necessitate the use of dual venous cannulas so that all venous blood can be diverted to the bypass circuit and the heart can be opened to allow repair of the intracardiac defect.

1. **Profound hypothermia and total circulatory arrest.** An alternative method used in very small children with complex heart disease is profound hypothermia and total circulatory arrest. This technique uses a single venous drainage cannula during the period of cooling. When a core temperature of about 18 to 20°C is reached, the pump is stopped and the venous cannula removed. The major advantage of this technique is that it provides excellent exposure without cannulas or blood in the operative field and is especially of benefit in the

TABLE 14.8 Differences in adult versus pediatric cardiopulmonary bypass

Parameter	Adult	Pediatric
Hypothermic temperature	Rarely below 25–32°C	Commonly 15–20°C
Use of total circulatory arrest	Rare	Common
Pump prime		200%–300%
Dilution effects on blood volume	25%–33%	
Additional additives in pediatric primes		Blood, albumin
Perfusion pressures	Typically 50–80 mm Hg	30–50 mm Hg
Influence of pH management strategy	Minimal at moderate hypothermia	Marked at deep hypothermia
Measured P_{aCO_2} differences	30–45 mm Hg	20–80 mm Hg
Glucose regulation		
Hypoglycemia	Rare; requires significant hepatic injury	Common; reduced hepatic glycogen stores
Hyperglycemia	Frequent; generally easily controlled with insulin	Less common; rebound hypoglycemia may occur

Modified from Kern FH, Schulman SR, Lawson DS, et al. Extracorporeal circulation and circulatory assist devices in the pediatric patient. In: Lake C, ed. *Pediatric Cardiac Anesthesia*. 3rd ed. Stamford, CT: Appleton & Lange; 1998:219–257.

small neonate. Deep hypothermia also enhances myocardial protection, decreases CPB time, and decreases blood trauma. The Boston Circulatory Arrest Study showed that the use of circulatory arrest is associated with a higher risk of seizures. There was a strong correlation between duration of circulatory arrest and the occurrence of seizures. Seizures in the perioperative period significantly increased the risk of both lower IQ scores and neurologic abnormalities [16]. On the basis of this study, most centers have minimized the use of DHCA; when it must be used, every effort is made to limit its duration to less than 35 to 40 min. As centers have become more advanced in their perfusion and protection techniques, many have begun to employ a strategy of low-flow cerebral perfusion, directed toward the innominate artery. This technique provides cerebral flow and protection while concurrently ceasing all pump flow to the remainder of the body.

2. **Venous drainage.** Venous drainage problems are more common in children. The inferior vena cava is quite short, and inadvertent cannulation of the hepatic veins is possible, resulting in marked engorgement of the splanchnic vessels and subsequent mesenteric ischemia. Problems with superior vena cava drainage are possible, especially if a left superior vena cava is present. Occlusion of this vessel may cause significant cerebral venous hypertension, and cerebral ischemia may result. Careful attention should be paid to superior vena cava pressure by frequent inspection of the head and monitoring of the CVP via an SVC catheter.
3. **Systemic-to-PA–shunt occlusion.** When CPB is first initiated, the surgeon must quickly occlude any systemic-to-PA shunts (e.g., PDA or BT shunt). These shunts are often constructed as palliative first-stage interventions for creation of a source of pulmonary blood flow. Lack of occlusion of these shunts with initiation of CPB can lead to underperfusion of the systemic circulation, possible hemorrhagic edema of the lungs, and continued pulmonary venous return with possible overdistention of the left side of the heart.
4. **Perfusion flow and pressure.** CPB flow rates are proportionately higher in infants and children than in adults, ranging from 80 to 150 mL/(kg min). Adult rates usually range from about 1.8 to 2.2 L/(min m^2) or about 50 mL/(kg min). Perfusion pressures tend to be lower in children (30 to 50 mm Hg) when adequate oxygenation and perfusion are apparent. The optimal pressure or flow is unclear, and significant interinstitutional variation exists. The use of NIRS has greatly enhanced the intraoperative monitoring and adjustments of perfusion flows and pressures.
5. **Moderate hypothermia and ventricular fibrillation.** Moderate hypothermia combined with ventricular fibrillation is occasionally employed in pediatric cardiac repair. With this technique, the patient is cooled to about 28 to 30°C, and the heart is fibrillated but continues to be perfused because an aortic cross-clamp is not placed. The surgeon can open the cardiac chambers without risking entrainment of air into the left side of the heart and subsequent ejection into the arterial circulation.

   Deliberate fibrillation is often used during work on the right side of the heart or for relatively simple repairs such as ASD closure. The advantages of deliberate fibrillation with moderate hypothermia include a favorable myocardial supply/demand ratio, decreased risk of air embolus to the brain, and avoidance of aortic cross-clamping and cardioplegia. However, surgical exposure is limited because of intracardiac blood and continued motion of the heart. Therefore, aortic cross-clamping and cardioplegic protection of the heart are necessary for more complex intracardiac repairs, especially in small children.
6. **Bypass circuit volume.** The bypass circuit volume is large relative to the blood volume in infants. In pediatric CPB circuits, the priming volume may be as much as 700 mL, whereas the estimated blood volume of a 3 kg neonate is 250 to 300 mL. Accordingly, the Hct is reduced by approximately 70%. In contrast, an adult CPB circuit is primed with 1,500 mL for a patient with an estimated blood volume of 5 L; a drop in Hct of less than 25% results. Small infants undergoing complex repairs often require transfusion of red blood cells, platelets, and fresh frozen plasma to offset the dilutional reduction of Hct and clotting factors. More recently, technologic improvements have allowed miniaturization of the circuit with priming volumes as low as 300 to 350 mL. The prime in these instances

often consists of reconstituted whole blood and allows for the employment of a blood cardioplegia system. Improvements in air filters have allowed for even miniaturized circuits to maintain a high level of safety despite the changes in the arteriovenous loop diameters. However, there may be significant tradeoffs in using these miniaturized systems. They often entail use of a closed system and may lack some of the usual safety features many practitioners consider standard like an air filter and blood cardioplegia system.

B. When should blood be added to the bypass circuit?

The optimal Hct during CPB is unknown. In general, moderate hemodilution during bypass is well tolerated, because microcirculatory perfusion is improved and metabolic needs are reduced by hypothermia. However, if the Hct is lowered too far, oxygen-carrying capacity is diminished and anaerobic metabolism results. Variation exists among surgical centers, but for most complex repairs, an Hct of 25% to 30% during CPB is used.

The CPB circuit must be primed. Each circuit has an obligatory volume that is required to fill the tubing, filters, pumps, and oxygenator. Therefore, it may be necessary to add red blood cells to the priming solution to reach the desired Hct. Calculation of the Hct on bypass is as follows.

1. Determine the patient's estimated blood volume.
2. Multiply the estimated blood volume by the measured Hct to yield the patient's red blood cell mass (RBCM).
3. Ask the perfusionist what the circuit priming volume is.
4. Add the estimated blood volume to the priming volume to obtain the total volume on bypass (CPBV).
5. Predicted Hct on bypass = RBCM/CPBV.
6. If the predicted Hct on bypass is less than desired, the quantity of red blood cells that must be added is calculated as follows:

$$\text{CPBV} \times \text{Desired hematocrit} = \text{Required RBCM}$$

$$\text{Required RBCM} - \text{Patient's RBCM} = \text{RBCM to be added}$$

C. How is anticoagulation managed?

Heparin is given to prevent initiation of the coagulation cascade by contact of blood with the bypass circuit. A dose of 300 units/kg is generally sufficient, although 400 units/kg is sometimes recommended for neonates. This dose is given through a central catheter after aspiration to verify blood return.

1. **Activated clotting time.** Measuring activated clotting time about 3 to 5 min after heparin administration can allow documentation of its effect. A value of about 400 s appears adequate to prevent clotting on bypass. Activated clotting time is relatively simple to determine and is reasonable to monitor, because occasionally a patient does exhibit marked heparin resistance. The activated clotting time also can signal a potentially catastrophic drug administration error when a substance other than heparin is injected. If the patient remains normothermic, the activated clotting time is generally rechecked every 20 to 30 min. With significant hypothermia, heparin effect is prolonged. Many centers advocate measuring actual heparin concentrations, especially during hypothermic CPB.

D. *Should antifibrinolytics be used?*

In an effort to minimize transfusion requirements, many groups have focused on preservation of platelet function and prevention of fibrinolysis, using drugs such as ε-aminocaproic acid (amicar®), tranexamic acid, and aprotinin. Although the data supporting the decreased transfusion requirement in redo operations in adults are fairly convincing, the data are not as clear as in infants. Some groups have reported dramatic decreases in blood loss, whereas others have shown no difference in donor exposures to banked blood [17,18]. The use of aprotinin in the pediatric population has been avoided since October of 2007 due to concerns raised by the Food and Drug Administration regarding its association with increased mortality in the cardiac surgical population. As such, most centers employ the use of amicar or tranexamic acid exclusively.

E. TEG and TEM

CPB induces derangements in the coagulation cascade and this often leads to challenges with immediate postoperative bleeding and the need for significant transfusion of blood and clotting products [19]. This is especially true and of significant challenge in the neonatal cyanotic patient undergoing surgical intervention [20]. Concerns regarding transfusions have historically been well documented and, in particular, can be of challenge in the congenital heart surgical patient population. Proactive detection of hemostatic abnormalities increases the ability to adequately plan treatment strategies and, as a result, minimizes the overall need for transfusion therapies. Due to issues of heparinization and dilution, routine coagulation assays may indeed not be appropriate for adequate assessment during operative intervention [21].

The use of TEM and TEG has gained favor as a tool for measuring coagulation profiles and parameters in the intra- and immediate postoperative management for congenital heart surgery. Both methods measure the viscoelastic properties of the fibrin clot but with somewhat different technology and terminology. The TEG analyzer examines whole blood as the clot forms, to measure the time it takes to reach certain levels of clot formation. It also measures the strength and contribution of key elements in the hemostasis system [21]. It is important to note that levels are not measured; rather, the functional contribution of these various components is assessed.

Several groups have described a reduction in the overall transfusion prevalence in pediatric cardiac surgical patients with use of TEM/TEG [22]. More specifically, red blood cell and plasma transfusion rates have decreased when intraoperative decisions have been guided by TEM or TEG data [21]. These findings are in concert with already well-described similar findings in the adult population.

F. How are patients weaned?

Success in weaning from bypass is critically dependent on the surgeon's ability to completely repair the defect. Residual shunts, obstruction, or valvular dysfunction are tolerated poorly after bypass. In addition, close communication between surgeon, anesthesiologist, and perfusionist is essential for a planned approach toward separation from the CPB circuit.

1. **Preparation.** Be certain that the patient is optimally prepared before attempting discontinuation of bypass (Table 14.9). Near the end of the surgical repair, gradual rewarming is begun. Temperature gradients are common; be sure that the patient is thoroughly and evenly rewarmed. The speed and method of rewarming may be critical. Postischemia hyperthermia is particularly deleterious in the setting of altered cerebral energy metabolism. In addition, it is known to be associated with an induction of tachyarrhythmias. On the other hand, mild degrees of hypothermia have been shown to be protective. Infusion of afterload-reducing agents, such as sodium nitroprusside, given during rewarming may be helpful to dilate the vascular bed and promote uniform rewarming. Allowing time for reperfusion of the heart after the cross-clamp is removed makes possible dissipation of "evil humors" (cardioplegia) and re-establishment of aerobic metabolism.

TABLE 14.9 Checklist for discontinuation of bypass

I.	Complete rewarming (core temperature ≥35°C)
II.	Complete reperfusion of heart after cardioplegia
III.	Sinus rhythm with appropriate heart rate
IV.	Evaluate ST changes
V.	Check electrolytes, blood gases, and Hct
VI.	Optimize pulmonary function
VII.	Check hemodynamic monitors
VIII.	Prepare vasodilator or inotropic drugs, if indicated
IX.	Prepare platelets and fresh frozen plasma, if indicated

Hct, hematocrit.
From Davies LK. Anesthesia for pediatric cardiovascular surgery. In: Kirby RR, Gravenstein N, Lobato EB, et al., eds. *Clinical Anesthesia Practice.* Philadelphia, PA: WB Saunders; 2002:1227, with permission.

2. **Heart rate and rhythm.** Sinus rhythm is essential, because ventricular function is typically impaired after bypass and ischemia. Optimal heart rate is also important in improving CO, because stroke volume may be less than ideal. A heart rate of 120 to 160 beats/min is desirable. The atrium may be paced if the patient has a slower sinus rate, or sequential AV pacing may be required if a rhythm other than sinus exists. New electrocardiographic ST changes may indicate the presence of air in the coronary arteries or ongoing myocardial ischemia. In these instances, a more patient and gradual wean from CPB and the focus upon higher perfusion pressures will promote clearance of this air and a return of appropriate ECG findings.
3. **Other monitored parameters.** Hemodynamic monitors should be rechecked and transducers rezeroed. The surgeon may elect to insert a left atrial pressure catheter to assess ventricular filling and function. Laboratory values, including Hct, potassium, ionized calcium, arterial blood gas partial pressures, and pH, should be rechecked after aortic cross-clamp release and before discontinuation of bypass is attempted.
4. **Vasoactive drugs.** Vasodilator and inotropic drugs should be available for infusion by calibrated pumps, especially after intracardiac repair. Significant hemodynamic compromise may result from hypoxic–ischemic reperfusion injury that is superimposed on marginal baseline ventricular function. Ventricular performance is usually readily improved by inotropic or combined inotropic and vasodilator support. Impaired postoperative cardiac performance is clearly associated with higher morbidity and mortality.
5. **Cardiovascular changes.** Arterial pressure may be normal or above normal regardless of CO. As such, the arterial pressure may not exclusively be helpful with regard to diagnosis of cardiac dysfunction. After CPB, SVR is generally high in both adults and children because of circulating catecholamines and antidiuretic hormone as well as other influences. In the neonate, this response may be amplified, leading to uninhibited vasoconstriction.
6. **Afterload reduction.** Children poorly tolerate an increased pressure workload. Therefore, afterload reduction (generally with sodium nitroprusside) may be useful to improve CO. If CO is still impaired after vasodilator therapy, a combination of afterload reduction, volume expansion, and inotropic support is warranted.

G. Measurement of blood pressure

If the blood pressure is low during attempted weaning from bypass, another method of blood pressure measurement must be available to check the accuracy of the peripheral data. The surgeon can easily place an exploring needle into the ascending aorta (often at the site of the previous cardioplegia infusion) and connect it to a pressure transducer. A noninvasive (cuff) blood pressure measurement also can be obtained.

In small children, a significant difference in blood pressure measurements often is present between central aortic and peripheral arterial sites. The reason for this discrepancy is not clear, but it usually resolves over time. Before starting administration of inotropes or vasopressors, be certain that the pressure measurement is accurate. If the discrepancy persists, placement of a femoral arterial catheter helps to guide therapy.

H. *How is increased pulmonary vascular resistance managed?*

Pulmonary function must be optimized before discontinuation of bypass is attempted. Increased PVR results from pulmonary edema, complement activation, catecholamines, and atelectasis.

1. **Lung expansion and oxygenation.** The lungs must be vigorously re-expanded to increase functional residual capacity (Fig. 14.5). The endotracheal tube is not routinely suctioned, as suctioning may precipitate bleeding in anticoagulated patients. Any wheezing is treated vigorously with inhaled bronchodilators. Albuterol 2.5 mg, administered via a nebulizer attached between the endotracheal tube and the circle system, can be quite beneficial. If secretions prevent appropriate deflation of the lungs, careful suctioning with a soft catheter is indicated.

   Vigorous hyperventilation without positive end-expiratory pressure (PEEP) is one of the most powerful tools available to decrease PVR. The pulmonary vascular responsiveness to hypercarbia is accentuated in the postbypass period; thus, even small increases in P_aCO_2 are

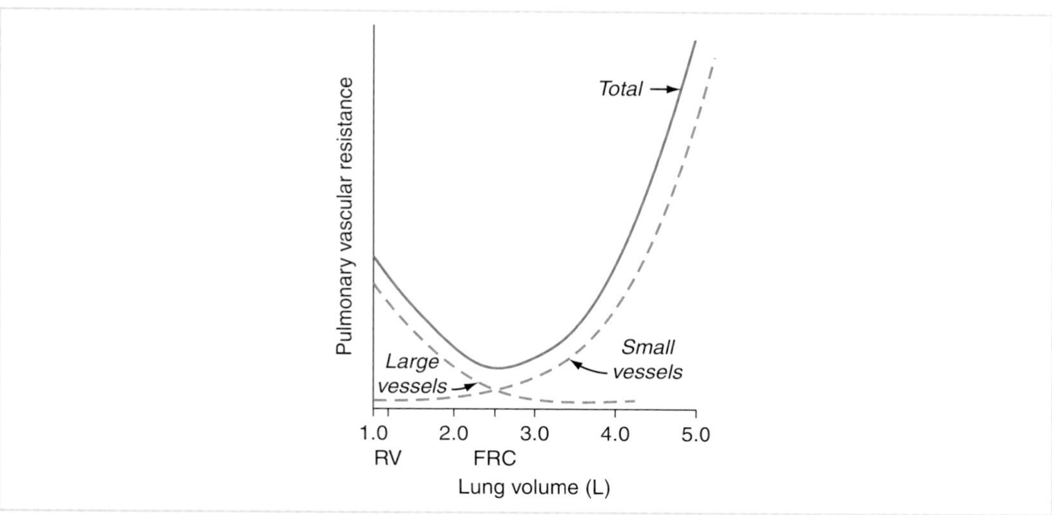

FIGURE 14.5 Asymmetrical U-shaped curve relates total PVR to lung volume. The trough of the curve occurs when lung volume equals function residual capacity (FRC). Total pulmonary resistance is the sum of resistance in small vessels (increased by increasing lung volume) and in large vessels (increased by decreasing lung volume). RV, residual volume. (From Benumof JL. Respiratory physiology and respiratory function during anesthesia. In: Miller RD, ed. *Anesthesia.* 2nd ed. New York, NY: Churchill Livingstone; 1986:1122, with permission.)

associated with significant increases in resistance. High inspired oxygen concentrations should be used, and metabolic acidosis should be avoided.

2. **Pharmacologic interventions.** α-Stimulation causes pulmonary vasoconstriction, whereas β-stimulation causes vasodilation. Many pharmacologic agents have been used with only marginal success in an attempt to selectively decrease PVR. The agents most commonly used include sodium nitroprusside, nitroglycerin, isoproterenol, aminophylline, milrinone, PGE_1, and perhaps adenosine. Inhaled nitric oxide offers promise as a truly selective pulmonary vasodilator, but its use is prohibitively expensive and it may not be readily available in all institutions. Inhaled prostanoid (Iloprost) is gaining popularity in some pediatric centers as a pulmonary vasodilator. Factors that increase or decrease PVR are summarized in Table 14.10.

TABLE 14.10 Alteration of pulmonary vascular resistance

Increase resistance	Decrease resistance
Hypoxia	Oxygen
Hypercarbia	Hypocarbia
Acidosis	Alkalosis
Hyperinflation	Normal functional residual capacity
Atelectasis	Blocking sympathetic stimulation
Sympathetic stimulation	Low Hct
Surgical constriction	MUF
High Hct	Nitric oxide Phosphodiesterase inhibitors

Hct, hematocrit; MUF, modified ultrafiltration.
Modified from Hickey PR, Wessel DL. Anesthesia for treatment of congenital heart disease. In: Kaplan JA, ed. *Cardiac Anesthesia.* 2nd ed. Orlando, FL: Grune & Stratton; 1987:656.

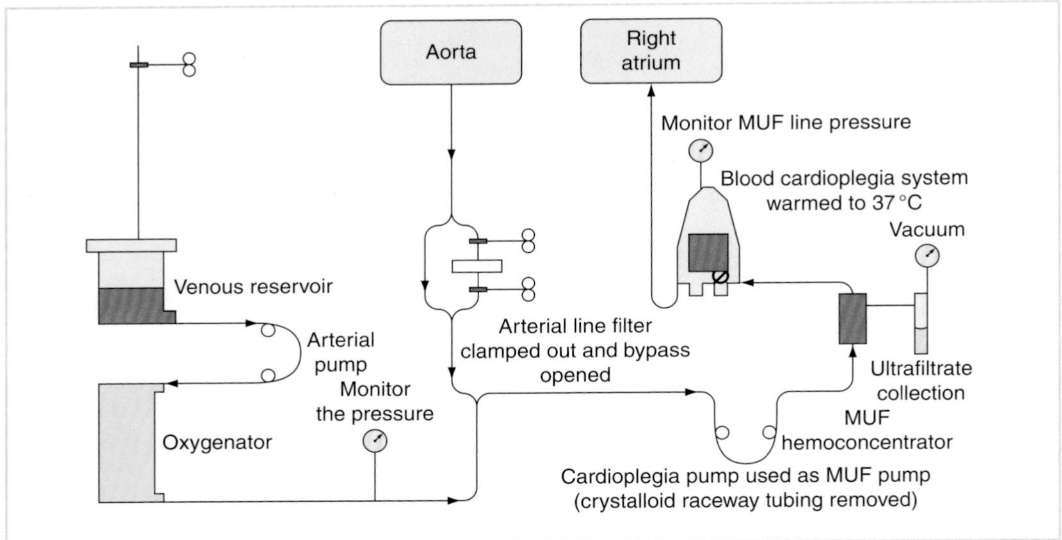

FIGURE 14.6 Diagram of an MUF system. After CPB, MUF proceeds using the blood cardioplegia roller pump from the CPB circuit. Blood is pumped from the aortic cannula through the ultrafilter and heat exchanger and is reinfused into the patient through the venous cannula. (From Kern FH, Shulman SR, Lawson DS, et al. Extracorporeal circulation and circulatory assist devices in the pediatric patient. In: Lake CL, ed. *Pediatric Cardiac Anesthesia.* 3rd ed. Stamford, CT: Appleton & Lange; 1998:219, with permission.)

VIII. Postbypass issues

A. What is modified ultrafiltration and when is it used?

The inflammatory response on bypass is significant and may be responsible for much of the morbidity seen in these children. Endothelial injury can cause an increase in total body water and increased capillary permeability, with resultant multiorgan failure. Conventional ultrafiltration on CPB has been used to try to prevent tissue edema, but its effectiveness has been limited. It is difficult to remove much volume during bypass, yet still maintain a safe reservoir volume. In 1993, the technique of modified ultrafiltration (MUF) performed in the immediate postbypass period was described [23]. The aortic cannula is left in place and approximately 10 to 30 mL/kg/min of blood is siphoned from the aorta, pumped through a hemoconcentrator (dialysis membrane), and returned to the right atrium (Fig. 14.6). Volume is infused from the reservoir as necessary to maintain hemodynamic stability. Once again, communication between surgeon, anesthesiologist, and perfusionist is critical during this period of time as hemodynamic monitoring often guides the extent to which MUF may be employed. Multiple studies have documented the effectiveness of MUF in ameliorating many of the adverse effects of CPB. MUF improves hemodynamics, reduces total body water, and decreases the need for blood transfusions compared with nonfiltered controls [24]. It is associated with significant increases in Hct, fibrinogen, and total plasma protein levels, but no change in platelet count [25]. MUF has been shown to improve intrinsic LV systolic function, improve diastolic compliance, increase blood pressure, and decrease inotropic drug use in the early postoperative period [26]. It has been shown to decrease levels of the lung vasoconstrictor endothelin-1, significantly decrease the pulmonary/systemic pressure ratio after CPB, and may help prevent pulmonary hypertensive crises [27]. It improves lung compliance, reduces cytokine levels, and removes activated complement (C3a and C5a) [28]. After DHCA, MUF also improves the brain's ability to use oxygen [29]. The data summarizing its beneficial effects are listed in Table 14.11.

TABLE 14.11 Summary of effects of modified ultrafiltration

Feature	Effect	Reports
Total body water accumulation	⇓	a
Hct	⇑	a,b,c
Blood loss	⇓	a,c,d
Blood transfusion requirement	⇓	a,c,d
Colloid osmotic pressure	⇑	b,e
CO	⇑	a,f
Heart rate	⇓	f
Arterial blood pressure	⇑	a,f
SVR	/	g
PVR	⇓	g,h
Diastolic compliance	⇑	f
Inotropic drug use	⇓	f
Renal function	/	a
Cerebral recovery from DHCA	⇑	b,i
Plasma endothelin-1	⇓	h
Lung compliance	⇑	j
Cytokine levels	⇓	k
Activated complement levels	⇓	l
Heparin concentration	⇑	m

[a]Naik SK, Knight A, Elliott MJ. A prospective randomized study of a modified technique of ultrafiltration during pediatric open-heart surgery. *Circulation.* 1991;84:III422–431.
[b]Daggett CW, Lodge AJ, Scarborough JE, et al. Modified ultrafiltration versus conventional ultrafiltration: A randomized prospective study in neonatal piglets. *J Thorac Cardiovasc Surg.* 1998;115:336–341.
[c]Draaisma AM, Hazekamp MG, Frank M, et al. Modified ultrafiltration after cardiopulmonary bypass in pediatric cardiac surgery. *Ann Thorac Surg.* 1997;64:521–525.
[d]Friesen RH, Campbell DN, Clarke DR, et al. Modified ultrafiltration attenuates dilutional coagulopathy in pediatric open heart operations. *Ann Thorac Surg.* 1997;64:1787–1789.
[e]Ad N, Snir E, Katz J, Birk E, et al. Use of the modified technique of ultrafiltration in pediatric open-heart surgery: A prospective study. *Isr J Med Sci.* 1996;32:1326–1331.
[f]Davies MJ, Nguyen K, Gaynor JW, et al. Modified ultrafiltration improves left ventricular systolic function in infants after cardiopulmonary bypass. *J Thorac Cardiovasc Surg.* 1998;115:361–369.
[g]Naik SK, Balaji S, Elliott MJ. Modified ultrafiltration improves haemodynamics after cardiopulmonary bypass in children. *J Am Coll Cardiol.* 1992;19:37A.
[h]Bando K, Vijay P, Turrentine MW, et al. Dilutional and modified ultrafiltration reduces pulmonary hypertension after operations for congenital heart disease: A prospective randomized study. *J Thorac Cardiovasc Surg.* 1998;115:517–525.
[i]Skaryak LA, Kirshbom P, DiBernardo LR, et al. Modified ultrafiltration improves cerebral metabolic recovery after circulatory arrest. *J Thorac Cardiovasc Surg.* 1995;109:744–752.
[j]Meliones JN, Gaynor JW, Wilson BG, et al. Modified ultrafiltration reduces airway pressure and improves lung compliance after congenital heart surgery. *J Am Coll Cardiol.* 1995;25:271A.
[k]Millar AB, Armstrong L, van der Linden J, et al. Cytokine production and hemofiltration in children undergoing cardiopulmonary bypass. *Ann Thorac Surg.* 1993;56:1499–1502.
[l]Andreasson S, Gothberg S, Berggren H, et al. Hemofiltration modifies complement activation after extracorporeal circulation in infants. *Ann Thorac Surg.* 1993;56:1515–1517.
[m]Williams GD, Ramamoorthy C, Totzek FR, et al. Comparison of the effects of red cell separation and ultrafiltration on heparin concentration during pediatric cardiac surgery. *J Cardiothorac Vasc Anesth.* 1997;11:840–844.
Modified from Elliott MJ. Recent advances in paediatric cardiopulmonary bypass. *Perfusion.* 1999;14:237–246.
Hct, hematocrit; CO, cardiac output; SVR, systemic vascular resistance; PVR, pulmonary vascular resistance; DHCA, deep hypothermic circulatory arrest.

B. *How should protamine be administered?*

Protamine is given after termination of CPB to neutralize the effects of heparin. It is not administered until MUF is complete and the venous cannula has been removed. Generally, a dose of 3 to 4.5 mg/kg (1 to 1.5 mg for every 100 units of heparin) is given. Satisfactory reversal of heparin is suggested by return of the activated clotting time to baseline value. Protamine can cause serious adverse reactions in some patients. These reactions include systemic hypotension, pulmonary hypertension, and allergic reactions. The mechanism for these events is not entirely clear, but it may involve antibody-mediated immune responses, complement activation, and histamine release.

Histamine release is provoked by rapid administration of large doses of protamine. Slow administration with a controlled infusion is effective in ameliorating this side effect. Pretreatment with antihistamine or administration into the left atrium also has been proposed. Catastrophic pulmonary hypertension is less common and probably occurs because of complement activation and thromboxane release. Allergic reactions to protamine can occur, usually in patients with prior exposure to protamine-containing insulin preparations.

Fortunately, serious reactions to protamine may be less common in neonates and children than in adults [30]. It appears that adverse reactions are more common in females than in males, although it is not clear why this difference exists. If the drug is administered slowly after removal of the venous cannula but with the aortic cannula still in place, CPB can be re-instituted quickly if a catastrophic reaction occurs.

C. What are the causes of low cardiac output?

Low CO can have many causes but is categorized according to its major determinants: Heart rate, rhythm, contractility, preload, and afterload.

1. **Heart rate.** Infants and children have a relatively fixed cardiac stroke volume and therefore modify CO by heart rate changes. Therefore, CO is considered to be rate dependent. Heart rates of atleast 120 beats/min should be sought in an effort to optimize CO. A lower heart rate should be treated either pharmacologically or by pacing via surgically placed temporary epicardial leads which are brought through the skin. Pacing is often preferred, because it has negligible side effects.
2. **Dysrhythmias.** Dysrhythmias after CPB are often tolerated poorly and may require electrical conversion. Sinus rhythm at a reasonable rate is crucial to maximize CO. Do not hesitate to use electrical pacing to optimize myocardial performance. Unfortunately, arrhythmias caused by abnormal automaticity may occur that are difficult to treat. Junctional ectopic tachycardia (JET) is an uncommon but life-threatening arrhythmia seen almost exclusively in neonates and infants after congenital heart surgery [31]. JET is of special significance for the anesthesiologist because it usually manifests intraoperatively or in the immediate postoperative period. JET remains among the more difficult tachycardias to control, leading to severe hemodynamic instability and death. It is thought to result from abnormal automaticity, with the focus of active discharge located at the AV node or the proximal bundle of His, yet the atrial tissue is not directly involved in the arrhythmia mechanism. Therefore, an important characteristic of this tachyarrhythmia is a lack of response to cardioversion, overdrive pacing, and conventional medications.

   JET is classically recognized as a narrow QRS tachycardia with AV dissociation and an atrial rate that is slower than the ventricular rate. Typically, peak JET rates range from 170 to 300 beats/min. The onset ("warmup") and termination are gradual (Fig. 14.7). Retrograde conduction and retrograde P waves can be seen on the ECG. Interestingly, a wide QRS may be seen if there is an associated bundle branch block that occurs either as a rate-dependent aberration or as a fixed abnormality due to surgical damage of the bundle branch.

   Postoperatively, JET has been generally refractory to most conventional antiarrhythmic drugs. Amiodarone has been used with some limited success. If the chest is still open, topical cooling with cold saline may be helpful. Remarkably, it usually resolves on its own within the first 3 days of presentation. Therapy should be directed toward decreasing the junctional rate to allow atrial pacing with AV synchrony to re-establish hemodynamic stability.
3. **Decreased contractility.** Poor contractility can occur due to surgical trauma (as from a ventriculotomy incision), pre-existing volume or pressure overload condition, injury or malperfusion of a coronary artery, residual effects of myocardial ischemia and reperfusion, metabolic and acid–base derangements, hypoxemia, and drug effects.

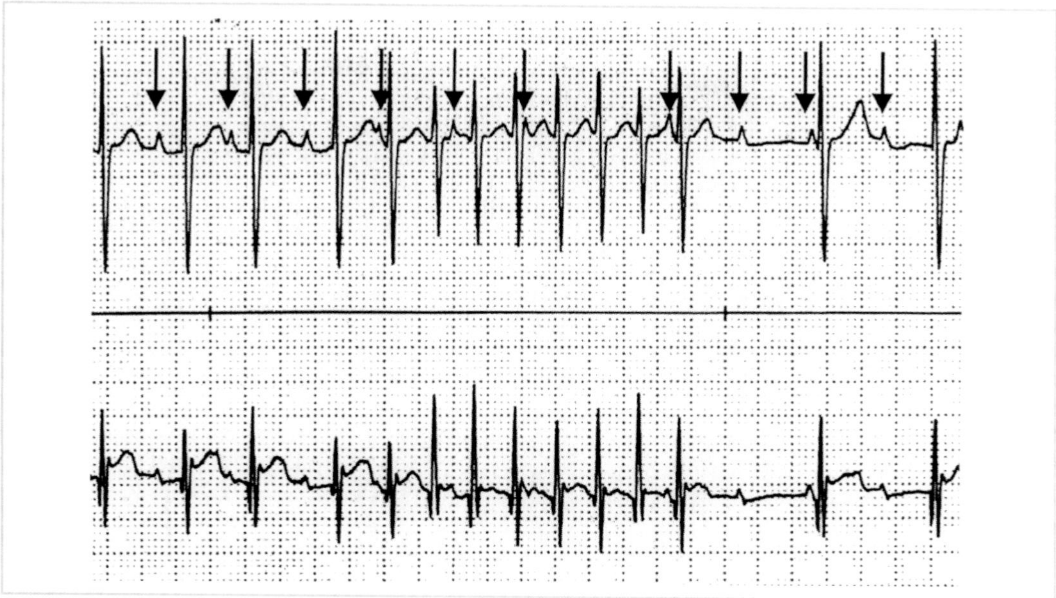

FIGURE 14.7 JET at 280 beats/min. Note AV dissociation as JET warms up with no change in atrial rate (*arrows*).

4. **Decreased preload.** Decreased preload may occur from hypovolemia, cardiac tamponade, positive airway pressure, and increased PVR that causes diminished return to the left side of the heart.
5. **Increased afterload.** Increased afterload can be a major problem for both the left and right sides of the heart. Many congenital lesions are associated with pulmonary vascular changes and pulmonary hypertension. Thus, control of RV function and afterload is crucial to maintain adequate CO.

D. **What are the causes and treatment of excessive bleeding?**

1. **Causes.** Most commonly, patients bleed postoperatively as a result of inadequate surgical hemostasis. Inadequate heparin neutralization also can be a factor. Thrombocytopenia or platelet dysfunction is the next most common cause. Platelets are sequestered in the bypass circuit and become dysfunctional because of surface exposure and hypothermia.

   Patients with cyanotic heart disease and significant polycythemia have a baseline abnormality of platelet function and clotting factors. They often demonstrate a decrease in factors II, V, VII, VIII, and IX, hypofibrinogenemia, and an increase of fibrin split products, all of which may lead to excessive bleeding.
2. **Treatment.** While a source of bleeding is sought, the patient must be aggressively treated with volume replacement. Crystalloid solutions are the mainstay of therapy, but their administration should be tempered by the knowledge that a total body inflammatory response after bypass leads to problems with increased vascular permeability and edema. Decreased colloid oncotic pressure can be a problem after CPB because of hemodilution and destruction of serum proteins. Judicious use of albumin-containing solutions may be warranted.

   If continuing red blood cell loss is a problem, packed red blood cell transfusion is indicated. Typically, an Hct 30% to 40% in acyanotic children and greater than 40% in cyanotic children seems reasonable. In young adults with good cardiac reserve after simple repairs, a lower Hct may be well tolerated. If no surgical source is found and the activated clotting time is normal, an empiric platelet transfusion is often used. Only after prolonged, deep hypothermic cases in small infants, transfusion with fresh frozen plasma should be necessary. Certainly, use of TEG or TEM technology can be helpful in delineating what blood products might be necessary to treat a developing coagulopathy.

E. What metabolic problems are likely?

1. **Potassium disorders.** Metabolic derangements are relatively common. Hyperkalemia and hypokalemia are the most common electrolyte abnormalities. Hyperkalemia is commonly seen immediately after the cross-clamp is removed if large amounts of cardioplegic solution have been used. If CO is poor, hyperkalemia may remain problematic. Typically, hypokalemia evolves because patients exhibit a marked kaliuresis after bypass. Unless the serum potassium value is at least 4.5 mEq/L or renal function is impaired, one should consider beginning a potassium chloride infusion of approximately 0.25 mEq/kg/h after CPB.
2. **Calcium abnormalities.** Hypocalcemia occurs frequently, especially after rapid transfusion of blood products. A decrease in the ionized fraction can lead to decreased myocardial contractility and decreased vascular smooth muscle tone. Infants diagnosed with, or suspected to have, Di George syndrome (22q11.2 deletion syndrome) are especially vulnerable to hypocalcemia. Infants with conotruncal malformations (TOF, Interrupted Aortic Arch with VSD and Persistent Truncus Arteriosus) have an increased risk for this genetic abnormality. This patient population often benefits from a calcium infusion following separation from CPB.
3. **Miscellaneous problems.** Hypomagnesemia can occur and can enhance ventricular irritability. Hyperglycemia is common after CPB and is relatively resistant to treatment with insulin. Although hyperglycemia occurs somewhat less frequently in children than in adults, maintenance of normoglycemia is often difficult. The increased use of preoperative steroid infusions employed to minimize the inflammatory response of the CPB circuit has led to an increase in the incidence of postoperative hyperglycemia. Sodium changes typically do not present a major problem after bypass, although hypernatremia can occur if large quantities of sodium bicarbonate have been given.

F. When should the patient be extubated?

Most patients undergoing complex repairs remain intubated and mechanically ventilated for several hours to days after surgery. This approach allows heavy sedation, recovery of myocardial function, and stabilization of hemodynamic status. For simple repairs (e.g., ASD, simple VSD, and coarctation), extubation may be considered at the end of the procedure if the patient is stable and awake and if bleeding is controlled. In addition, patients who are undergoing second- or third-stage palliation procedures for single ventricle physiology (Glenn or Fontan) benefit from earlier extubation. Positive-pressure ventilation is known to have deleterious effects on pulmonary blood flow in this patient population. Obviously, all normal criteria for extubation, including reversal of muscle relaxation, good spontaneous ventilation, and the ability to maintain and protect the airway, should be present.

IX. Specific lesions

The following section reviews some of the more common lesions encountered in practice. Although separated into categories based on manifestation of cyanosis or CHF, it is important to remember
9 that these divisions are arbitrary. For some lesions such as transposition of the great arteries (TGA), the patient may be cyanotic, may be in CHF, or both, depending on other associated lesions. The consequences of these lesions vary from patient to patient, so one must be careful to individualize care to each child.

A. Lesions likely to cause cyanosis

1. **TOF**

   a. General considerations

   (1) The four basic abnormalities are subvalvar, valvar, or supravalvar pulmonary stenosis, VSD, RV hypertrophy, and an over-riding aorta (Fig. 14.8).

   (2) Spectrum of disease ranges from "pink tet" (mild stenosis, large VSD with predominant left-to-right shunt) to pulmonary atresia with obliteration of the outflow tract and marked cyanosis.

   (3) Classic TOF will have decreased pulmonary blood flow and increased blood flow to the body. Variations in the physiology are dependent on the location and degree of pulmonary stenosis.

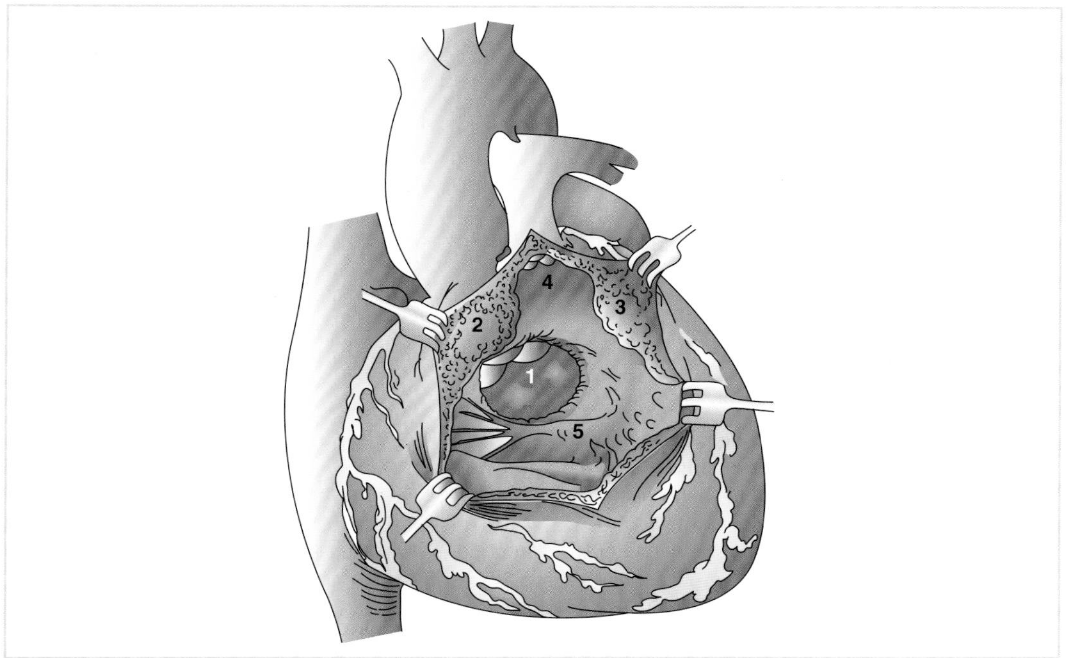

FIGURE 14.8 TOF showing VSD with over-riding aorta (*1*) and RV parietal (*2*) and septal (*3*) bands of myocardial hypertrophy. The infundibular septum (*4*) is hypoplastic and deviated anteriorly. The papillary muscle of the conus (*5*) inserts along the lower margin of the VSD. (From Arciniegas E, ed. *Pediatric Cardiac Surgery*. Chicago, IL: Year Book; 1985:204, with permission.)

(4) Occurs equally in males and females.

(5) In ~5% of patients with TOF, the left anterior descending coronary artery (LAD) arises from the right rather than the left coronary artery.

(6) Rarely overtly cyanotic at birth unless the RV outflow tract (RVOT) is atretic. Cyanosis may not develop for several months but then becomes progressively more severe.

(7) X-ray film shows decreased pulmonary markings. Right aortic arch occurs in about 25% of cases.

(8) Squatting increases SVR, helping to shunt more blood to the lungs.

(9) TOF spells are episodes of paroxysmal hyperpnea that occur in 20% to 70% of patients, with a peak frequency at age 2 to 3 mos. The spells are usually initiated by crying, feeding, or defecation. Although the etiology is uncertain, spells are probably initiated by events that result in increased oxygen demand associated with decreasing arterial P_aO_2 and pH and increasing P_aCO_2. As the hypoxia continues, SVR decreases further and the right-to-left shunt increases. Some suggest that the spells may be initiated or exacerbated by infundibular hypercontractility or "spasm." Transient cerebral ischemia can occur, leading to paleness, limpness, and unconsciousness.

b. Surgical procedures

(1) Complete repair

(a) Ligate previous BT shunt if present.

(b) Infundibular resection of excess muscle in RVOT.

(c) Patch closure of VSD.

(d) Patch the RVOT (subannular or transannular) to enlarge that area.

(e) RV to PA conduit may be necessary if the patient has pulmonary atresia or an anomalous LAD coursing across the RVOT.

(2) **Palliative** systemic to PA shunts. These procedures may be indicated to palliate cyanotic children who are not candidates for complete repair, such as small neonates, or patients in which one is hoping to achieve branch PA growth secondary to small PAs. The resulting increased pulmonary blood flow is thought to stimulate growth of small PAs, allowing subsequent complete repair.

(a) Subclavian artery to PA anastomosis (BT shunt), either native (division and swing-down of subclavian artery) or modified (use of a synthetic graft material)

(b) Central shunt: Anastomosis between aorta and PA with tube graft

(c) Waterston: Ascending aorta to right PA; no longer performed because of kinking of the right PA and difficulty controlling the amount of pulmonary blood flow

(d) Potts: Descending aorta to left PA; no longer performed because of difficult takedown at later surgery and difficulty in controlling shunt size

c. **Anesthetic considerations.** Knowing the patient's anatomy is crucial in developing a rational anesthetic plan. It is particularly critical to know whether there is antegrade flow across the RVOT or if the patient is totally dependent on a shunt for pulmonary circulation. Patients with antegrade flow across the RVOT have the potential for dynamic obstruction and the possibility for therapeutic interventions to change the caliber of the outflow tract.

(1) Preoperative. Preoperative evaluation should center around the assessment of degree of cyanosis. One should seek evidence of hypercyanotic spells and their frequency. A spot check of O_2 saturation may be helpful. It is also helpful to follow the Hct over time, because increasing cyanosis will provoke an increase in red blood cells in an attempt to maintain O_2-carrying capacity. Other laboratory values that may be useful are coagulation studies, because hypercyanotic patients often have a coexisting coagulopathy.

(a) NPO status. It is important to keep the patient with TOF well hydrated for two reasons.

(i) If the patient is polycythemic, a prolonged NPO period may put the patient at risk for dehydration with increased viscosity and sludging. If the degree of polycythemia is too extreme, preoperative phlebotomy may even be indicated.

(ii) Hypovolemia will exacerbate the RV outflow obstruction if the patient has infundibular stenosis. I would like to think of TOF as a right-sided version of idiopathic hypertrophic subaortic stenosis. Keeping the patient euvolemic or even a bit hypervolemic will help "stent open" the RVOT and improve pulmonary blood flow.

(b) Premedication. The goal in approaching the anesthetic is to have a calm, relaxed child. Good preoperative interactions with the parents and child are crucial. Premedication can be a valuable aid, but it is important that the patient not be sedated to the point of hypercarbia, which can increase PVR and precipitate increased right-to-left shunting. Intramuscular injections are best avoided, because the anxiety and stress they cause can lead to a TOF spell. Careful monitoring of S_pO_2 after premedication is indicated because the response may be variable.

(c) Subacute bacterial endocarditis (SBE) prophylaxis is essential. See American Heart Association guidelines for appropriate drugs and timing [32].

(2) Intraoperative. Choice of anesthetic should be individualized. Many different drugs have been used successfully. It is imperative to maintain or even augment intravascular volume. Hemodynamic goals are a deep anesthetic (to avoid sympathetic surges) with maintenance of normal-to-high SVR and low PVR. Meticulous

attention must be paid to airway management, because airway obstruction can quickly result in the triggering of a "TOF spell." Hypercarbia with a further decrease in oxygenation will cause an increase in PVR, triggering a vicious cycle of further desaturation and decreased pulmonary blood flow. Inhalational induction has been used successfully in children with TOF. Halothane (when it was available) was an ideal drug because it maintains SVR and relaxes the RV infundibulum, increasing pulmonary blood flow. Currently, sevoflurane is often used for inhalational induction. One must be cautious with inhalational induction, however, because the baseline decreased pulmonary blood flow results in a slow change in blood anesthetic tension. Induction of anesthesia may be slowed, but, more importantly, if a relative overdose of inhalation agent results, it is difficult to remove agent from the body because of the limited pulmonary blood flow. If intravenous induction is preferred, one should choose a technique that maintains SVR and minimizes PVR.

One should be watchful for problems with RV dysfunction after repair. Surgical repair mandates relief of RV outflow obstruction, and muscular resection is usually extensive. A ventriculotomy may be required. Annular or valvar stenosis may necessitate the placement of a patch across the annulus with significant regurgitation, though techniques are available to minimize this. Fortunately, these patients usually do not have baseline elevated PVR, because their preoperative situation is characterized by decreased pulmonary blood flow. However, the patient may have small PAs, which will exacerbate any RV dysfunction. If aortic cross-clamp time is prolonged, one might anticipate myocardial dysfunction. Therapeutic interventions should revolve around efforts to support RV function and decrease PVR. Afterload reduction and/or an inotrope may be beneficial, especially if a right ventriculotomy was performed.

(a) Problems and complications
- **(i)** Hemorrhage
- **(ii)** Residual RVOT obstruction
- **(iii)** RV failure (especially if RV/LV peak pressure is greater than 0.7 after repair)
- **(iv)** Heart block
- **(v)** Residual VSD
- **(vi)** Late arrhythmias and sudden death

2. TGA

a. General considerations

(1) **TGA is the most common severe congenital cardiac abnormality diagnosed during infancy.** Males predominate over females by a ratio of almost 3:1. Additional cardiac or noncardiac anomalies, other than a VSD, are rare. These infants usually are of normal birth weight.

(2) Left and right circulations are arranged in separate parallel circuits rather than the usual series configuration (Fig. 14.9). Thus, the aorta arises from the right side of the heart, which pumps deoxygenated blood to the body, which then returns back to the right atrium. The PA arises from the LV, which pumps oxygenated blood back to the lungs. After birth, the patient must retain some method that allows mixing of the pulmonary and systemic circulations to sustain life. Typically, an ASD, VSD, or PDA allows that mixing. If the patient does not have adequate mixing, a Rashkind balloon atrial septostomy is performed in the cardiac catheterization laboratory to improve the patient's clinical condition.

(3) Clinical presentation. The diagnosis of TGA is generally made shortly after birth. The patient will be cyanotic and, if mixing is inadequate, will develop marked metabolic acidosis. If the patient has an associated VSD, cyanosis will be less severe. The patient can develop pulmonary overload and signs of CHF if the VSD is large. If a patient has a PDA, differential cyanosis of the upper and the lower body may be

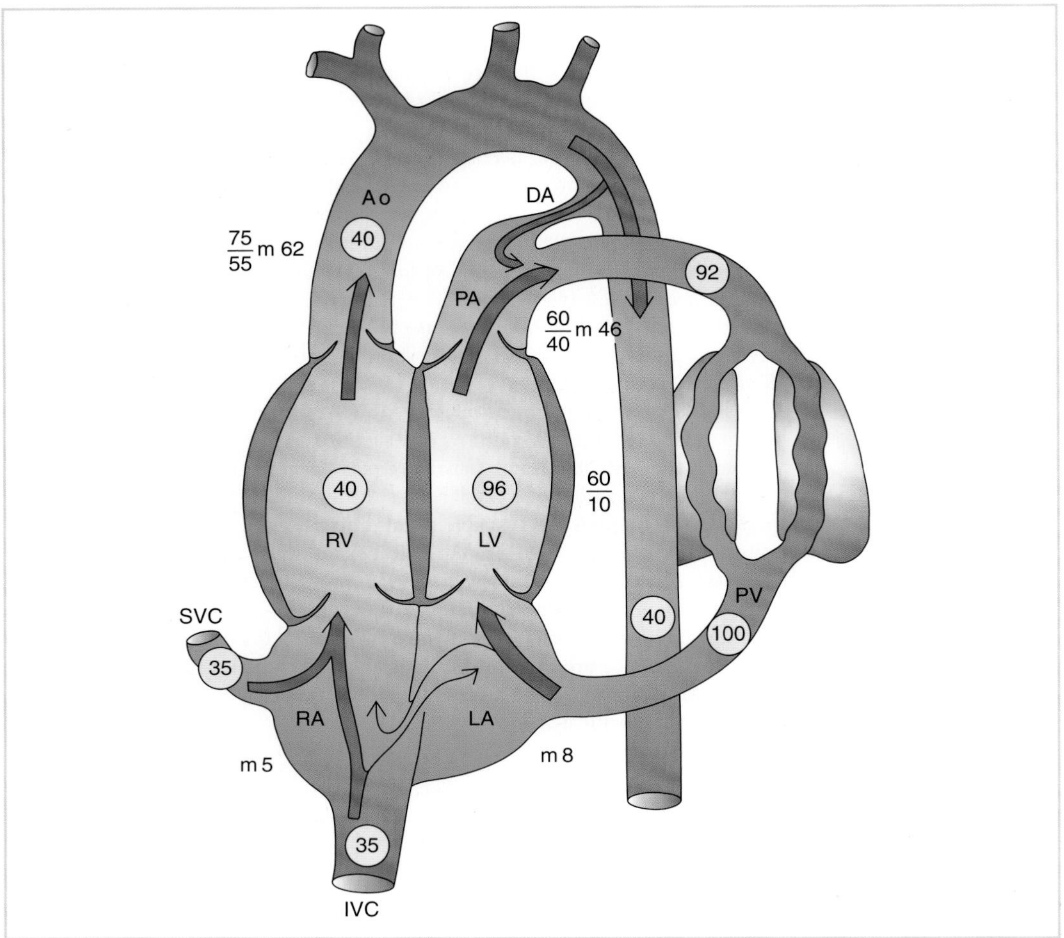

FIGURE 14.9 TGA. Systemic venous blood returns to the right heart and is pumped to the body through the transposed aorta. Similarly, left heart blood is pumped to the lungs. Survival after birth is possible only if mixing occurs between the two circulations (e.g., ASD, patent foramen ovale, VSD, PDA). Ao, aorta; DA, ductus arteriosus; IVC, inferior vena cava; LA, left atrium; PV, pulmonary vein; RA, right atrium; RV, right ventricle; SVC, superior vena cava. (From Rudolph AM. Aortopulmonary transposition. In: *Congenital Diseases of the Heart.* Chicago, IL: Year Book; 1974:475, with permission.)

observed. This occurs because oxygenated blood is pumped from the LV to the PA and ductus arteriosus into the descending aorta. In this situation, the upper part of the body will be more cyanotic than the trunk and lower extremities.

b. Surgical procedures

(1) Atrial switch operations (Senning and Mustard procedures) are designed to reroute the blood coming into the atrium using an intra-atrial baffle. Therefore, systemic venous blood (deoxygenated) goes to the LV (and then to the PA and the lungs), while the oxygenated pulmonary venous return is redirected to the RV (and then to the aorta and the systemic circulation). In the case of the Senning procedure, the baffle is configured using a right atrial flap, whereas the Mustard procedure uses a pericardial baffle. Both of these procedures result in a physiologic correction of the problem but not an anatomic correction, because the RV remains the ventricle that pumps to the systemic circulation. These palliative procedures are performed infrequently within the current surgical era.

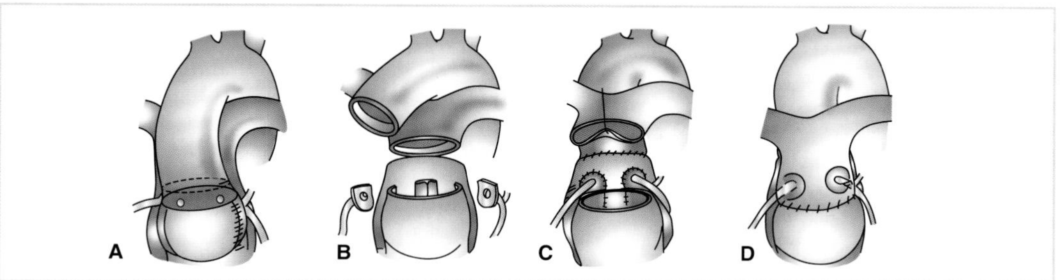

FIGURE 14.10 The arterial switch operation repairs TGA **(A)** by dividing the great arteries and excising the coronary ostial buttons **(B)**, transferring the coronary arteries to the neoascending aorta, and anastomosing the neoascending aorta to the distal ascending aorta **(C, D)** and the neomain PA to the distal main PA. (From Arciniegas E, ed. *Pediatric Cardiac Surgery.* Chicago, IL: Year Book; 1985:275, with permission.)

(2) Arterial switch operation (Jatene). The arterial switch operation has become the procedure of choice since it provides both a physiologic and anatomic correction of the problem (Fig. 14.10). The great vessels are transected above the valves and moved to their opposite ventricles. The origins of the left and right coronary arteries are dissected off as individual buttons that are rotated into place and reimplanted into the neoaorta. The new PA is reconstructed where the coronary artery buttons were removed. When the procedure is complete, the LV receives oxygenated blood from the lungs, which then pumps to the body. The RV pumps the systemic venous return to the lungs in the usual fashion.

(3) The Rastelli procedure may be an appropriate choice for patients with TGA, VSD, and LV outflow tract obstruction. In that situation, the VSD is closed so that LV blood is directed to the aorta and a conduit is created between the RV and the PAs.

c. Anesthetic considerations

(1) Preoperative. Medical management is initially used to stabilize the patient and improve perfusion. If mixing is inadequate, the patient will develop profound metabolic acidosis. PGE_1 can be infused to maintain or reopen the ductus arteriosus. The patient may require an emergent Rashkind atrial septostomy to facilitate adequate mixing. Cardiac catheterization may be helpful if there are concerns regarding variations of normal coronary artery anatomy.

The timing of surgical intervention is dictated by the patient's particular anatomy. If the child has TGA with intact ventricular septum, it is important to perform the Jatene procedure during the first weeks of life while the LV mass is still adequate. If surgery is delayed, the LV will decondition because it is working against the relatively low-resistance pulmonary circuit. On the other hand, if the patient has TGA with a VSD, the LV will remain "loaded" and the ventricular mass will not decrease. Thus, if necessary, surgery can be delayed to optimize the patient's condition.

(2) Intraoperative. These patients typically come to the operating room for their arterial switch operation with an intravenous catheter in place and PGE_1 infusing. It is critical that the PGE_1 infusion not be interrupted in order to maintain patency of the ductus arteriosus. Premedication is not necessary. An intravenous induction is usually used with a predominant narcotic technique. As the mixing occurs at the atrial level, few strategies exist to improve mixing if the patient becomes even more hypoxemic. Volume loading occasionally will improve the situation, and ensuring adequate depth of anesthesia may be helpful to decrease oxygen consumption. Neonates undergoing the Jatene procedure have the potential to manifest both left and right heart dysfunction. LV dysfunction can occur secondary to coronary artery insufficiency or prolonged cross-clamp time. During the Jatene procedure, the coronary arteries undergo significant dissection and manipulation. Careful attention must be paid to the ST-segment patterns, because myocardial ischemia can occur in these infants. A nitroglycerin infusion at a rate of about 1 to 2 μg/kg/min can aid in relaxation of these vessels. On occasion, surgical revision of one of the coronary artery implantations may be necessary if there is too much stretch or kinking of the vessel. Right heart dysfunction also can be a problem, because these children are typically operated on in the first few weeks of life. PVR during this time period is often high and dynamic. CPB during this time frame increases the PVR, putting an increased workload on the right heart. If the patient has been receiving PGE_1 for a prolonged period of time (more than 2 wks), it may be advisable to keep a low dose infusing after the repair and wean off it over about 3 days. Abrupt discontinuation of the drug may result in exacerbation of pulmonary hypertension. In addition, the Jatene procedure includes a reorientation of the PA via the LeCompte maneuver where the pulmonary outflow tract is reconstructed anterior to the aorta. As a result, an anatomic gradient may occur across the main PA which may exacerbate RV dysfunction.

d. Problems and complications

(1) Mustard or Senning operation

- **(a)** Arrhythmias, especially related to sinus node dysfunction
- **(b)** Caval obstruction, particularly the superior vena cava
- **(c)** Pulmonary vein obstruction
- **(d)** Tricuspid insufficiency
- **(e)** RV (systemic) failure
- **(f)** Residual atrial shunt

(2) Arterial switch (Jatene) operation

- **(a)** Hemorrhage
- **(b)** Coronary insufficiency
- **(c)** Myocardial infarction and LV failure
- **(d)** Narrowing of the reconstructed PA (late)

(3) Rastelli

- **(a)** Conduit narrowing or obstruction
- **(b)** Residual atrial shunt

3. Tricuspid atresia

a. General considerations. Tricuspid atresia is the third most common cyanotic lesion after TOF and TGA. There is an absence of the tricuspid valve with no direct communication between the right atrium and the RV. The right atrium is enlarged and thickened, and an obligatory right-to-left shunt at the atrial level, often a secundum ASD or stretched foramen ovale, is essential to maintain left heart filling. The left side of the heart becomes volume overloaded because it must accept both the systemic and pulmonary blood flow. The RV is generally severely hypoplastic and a VSD is present. Extracardiac anomalies are present in 20% of patients with tricuspid atresia.

Clinical presentation depends on the type of tricuspid atresia (Fig. 14.11). In the most common form, the great arteries are related normally and there is some degree of obstruction to pulmonary blood flow. Over time, the cyanosis will increase as the VSD closes or the infundibular obstruction increases. In about one-third of cases, the great arteries are transposed. In this situation, the patient may have normal or increased pulmonary blood flow and manifest signs of CHF. In addition, the VSD can become restrictive, resulting in significant subaortic obstruction.

b. Surgical procedures. The goal in caring for these patients is to optimize their physiologic state so that the Fontan operation can be performed by about age 2 to 4 yrs. Typically, these patients require a multistaged approach to accomplish this goal. Symptomatic neonates may require palliation for either severe cyanosis or CHF. Most commonly, the infant will have decreased pulmonary blood flow and require a systemic-to-PA shunt. On the other hand, about 10% to 15% of patients with tricuspid

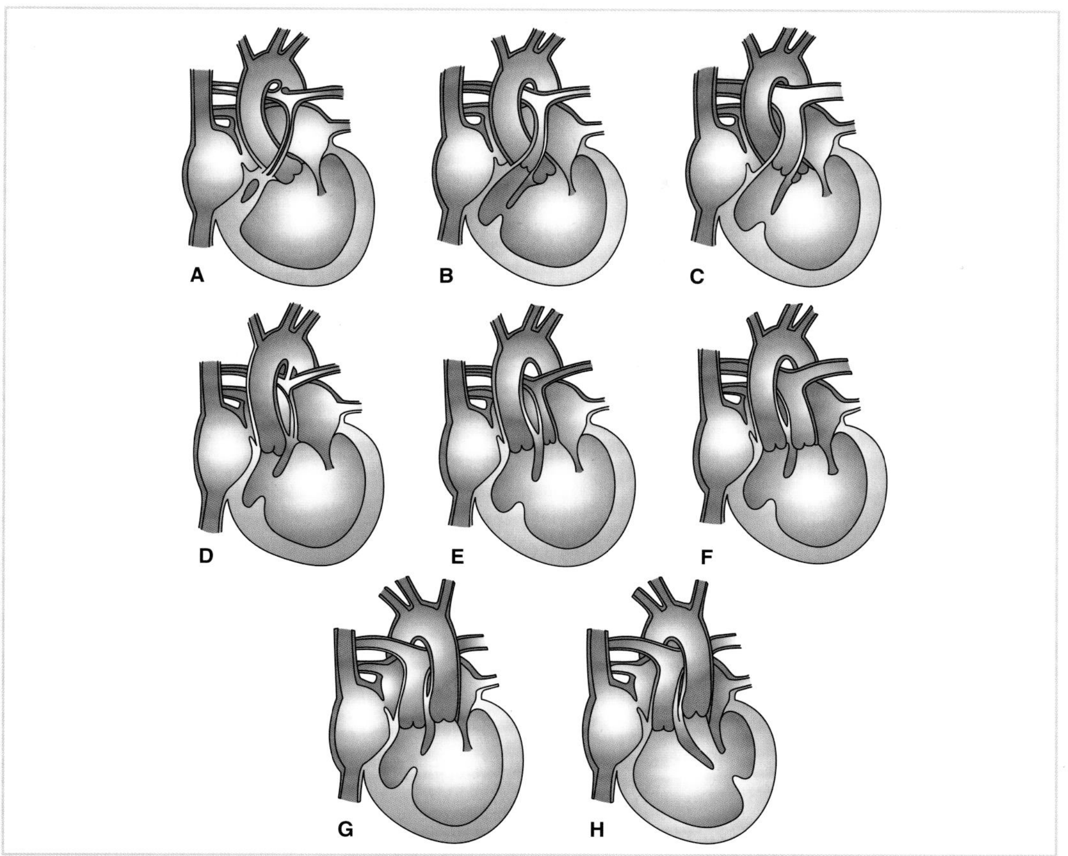

FIGURE 14.11 Type I tricuspid atresia, without TGA. **A:** Type Ia, pulmonary atresia with virtual absence of the RV. **B:** Type Ib, pulmonary hypoplasia with subpulmonary stenosis, diminutive right ventricle, and small VSD. **C:** Type Ic, no pulmonary hypoplasia. There is a diminutive right ventricle. Type II, tricuspid atresia, with D-transposition of the great arteries. **D:** Type IIa, pulmonary atresia, aorta arises from the right ventricle. **E:** Type IIb, pulmonary or subpulmonary stenosis. **F:** Type IIc, normal or enlarged PA. Type III, tricuspid atresia, with L-transposition of the great arteries. **G:** Type IIIa, pulmonary or subpulmonary stenosis. **H:** Type IIIb, subaortic stenosis. There is ventricular inversion. (From Arciniegas E, ed. *Pediatric Cardiac Surgery.* Chicago, IL: Year Book; 1985:298–300, with permission.)

atresia have markedly increased pulmonary blood flow and may require PA banding to protect the pulmonary vascular tree. If the ASD is restrictive, the patient will require a balloon atrial septostomy.

At about age 6 to 8 mos, a bidirectional cavopulmonary anastomosis is created by performing either a bidirectional Glenn procedure (Fig. 14.12) or a hemi-Fontan operation (Fig. 14.13). Both of these procedures result in the same physiologic outcome. Superior vena caval blood passes directly into the PA. These procedures will decrease the volume load on the heart and lower the PA pressures, making the patient a better candidate for the final operation, the Fontan procedure. Cavopulmonary anastomoses are usually not performed in the neonatal period because PVR is too high. As systemic venous return to the lungs is a passive process, resistance must be minimal or adequate flow will not occur.

At about age 2 to 4 yrs, the completion Fontan procedure is performed (Fig. 14.14). It is accomplished by channeling the remaining systemic venous return in the inferior vena cava to the PAs, often by using a lateral tunnel technique with a Gore-Tex tube graft in the extracardiac position. This technique is employed in patients who

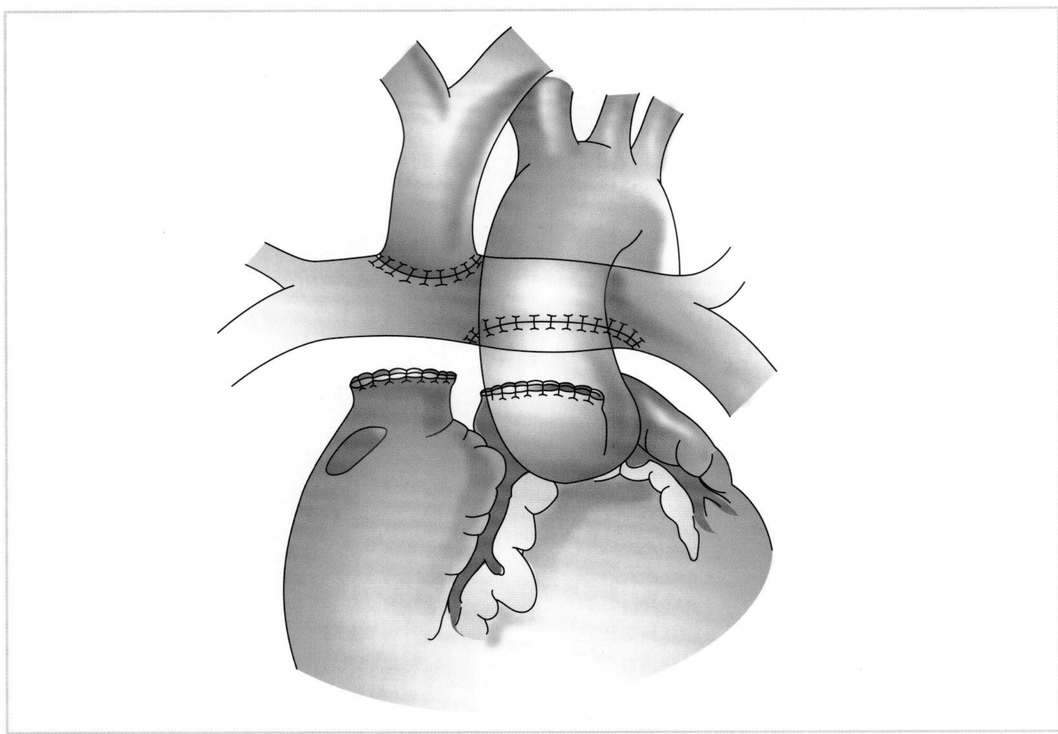

FIGURE 14.12 Bidirectional cavopulmonary anastomosis. The divided main PA is seen behind the aorta with patch closure of the distal main PA, and the proximal main PA is oversewn. The superior vena cava has been divided. The cardiac end is oversewn, whereas the cephalic end is sewn end-to-side to the right PA. Superior vena caval blood can flow bidirectionally into both the right and left PAs.

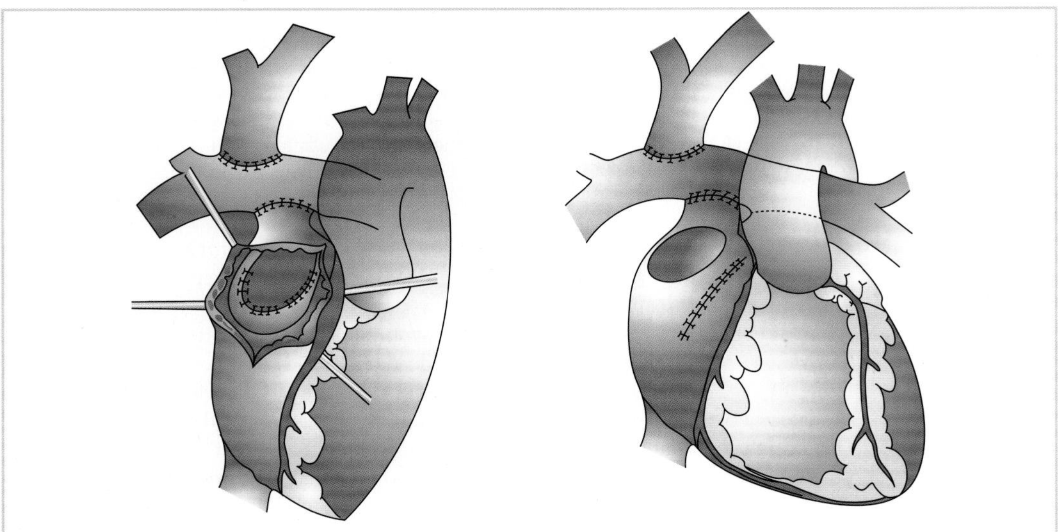

FIGURE 14.13 Hemi-Fontan operation. The superior vena cava is divided and each end is anastomosed to the right PA. The right atrium is opened, and a Gore-Tex patch is sewn over the orifice of the superior vena cava as it enters the right atrium. Physiologically, this repair is the same as the bidirectional cavopulmonary anastomosis (see Fig. 14.12). The hemi-Fontan simplifies subsequent surgery to complete the Fontan operation. To complete the Fontan procedure, the Gore-Tex patch is excised and a rectangular piece of Gore-Tex is used to fashion a tunnel from the inferior to the superior vena caval orifice (not shown).

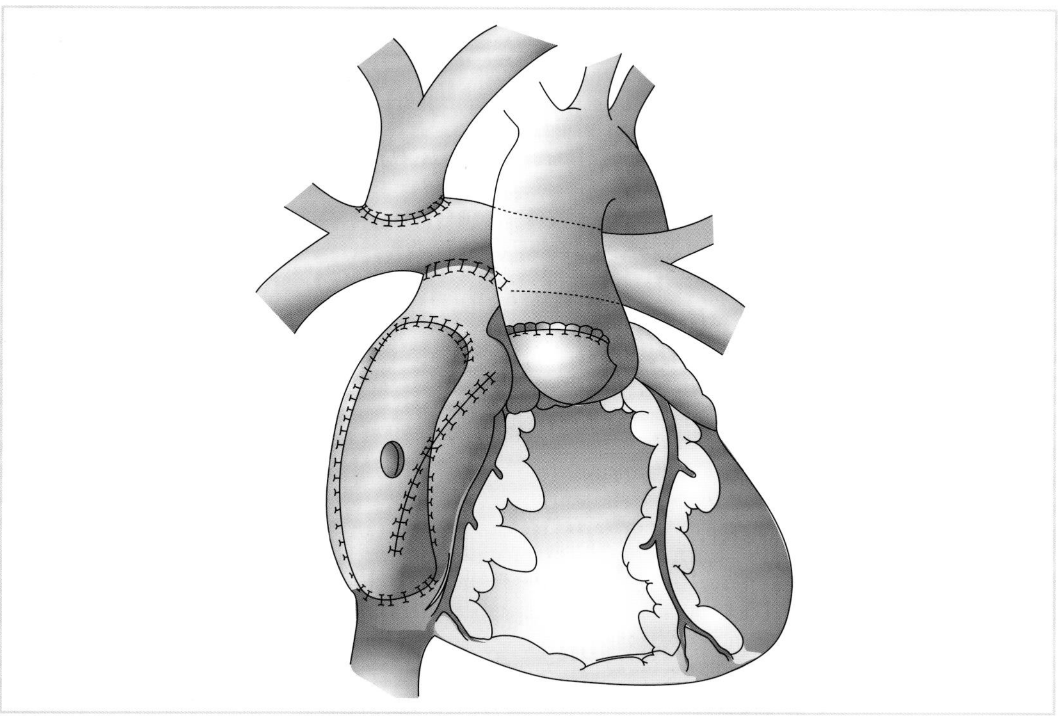

FIGURE 14.14 The fenestrated Fontan operation. The superior vena cava is divided and each end is sewn to the right PA. The right atrium is opened and a rectangular piece of Gore-Tex is used to fashion a tunnel (lateral baffle) to direct all the inferior vena caval blood flow to the superior vena caval orifice and into the pulmonary arteries. A fenestration (3 or 4 mm in diameter) is placed in the midportion of the Gore-Tex baffle.

underwent a bidirectional Glenn procedure. Patients who underwent a hemi-Fontan procedure will require placement of an intracardiac atrial baffle as their completion Fontan. Often a fenestration is also placed either in the extracardiac conduit or across the intra-atrial baffle, which allows some venous blood to shunt into the left atrium and improves left heart filling. However, this deoxygenated blood can cause some mild desaturation. The fenestration typically will close spontaneously in the first year postoperatively. If it does not close or hypoxemia becomes problematic, the patient can be taken to the cardiac catheterization laboratory and an ASD closure device can be used to resolve it.

Patient selection is extremely important in determining the success of the Fontan procedure. Ideally, PVR should be low (less than 4 Woods units) and the mean PA pressure less than 15 mm Hg. Adequately sized PAs, no systemic AV valve dysfunction, reliable sinus rhythm, and preserved LV function are also important.

c. **Anesthetic considerations**

(1) Preoperative. It is imperative to determine the patient's primary physiologic impairment by examining the chest x-ray, echocardiogram, and cardiac catheterization data. If a neonate has reduced pulmonary blood flow, PGE_1 is given to maintain ductal patency. A balloon atrial septostomy may be necessary if the ASD is small. If the patient has ventricular dysfunction on the basis of chronic volume overload, inotropic support may be needed. In the older patient undergoing a completion Fontan procedure, judicious use of premedication may be beneficial as long as hypoventilation is avoided. If the patient is polycythemic due to hypoxemia, care should be taken to avoid a prolonged NPO status.

(2) Intraoperative. Care of the patient undergoing either a systemic-to-PA shunt or a PA band is discussed elsewhere. In general, the goal in caring for children undergoing a bidirectional Glenn, hemi-Fontan, or Fontan procedure is to optimize PVR to promote pulmonary blood flow. An inhalational induction can be used as long as care is taken to maintain airway patency and minimize PVR. If the patient's pulmonary blood flow is ductal dependent, hypotension should be avoided because ductal flow depends on arterial pressure. If ventricular dysfunction is an issue, careful intravenous induction with agents with minimal depressant effects may be preferable.

After the repair, pulmonary blood flow becomes passive and depends on the caval pressure to be able to overcome PVR. Measurement of filling pressures on both the right and left sides of the heart can be helpful in optimizing therapy for patients after the Fontan procedure. **A right atrial pressure greater than 10 mm Hg more than the left atrial pressure (transpulmonary gradient) suggests obstruction to pulmonary blood flow, and therapy should be directed toward decreasing PVR.** These maneuvers include optimizing functional residual capacity, hyperventilation, increasing FIO_2, and avoiding acidosis. If the patient is bronchospastic, treatment with inhaled β-agonists may be beneficial. Nitric oxide at a dose of 10 to 40 ppm can be given. Typically, a CVP of about 12 to 15 mm Hg will be necessary to drive blood through the lungs. If a CVP greater than 20 mm Hg is necessary, the prognosis for survival is poor. Fenestrating the Fontan has become the norm, because blood which shunts right to left helps load the LV and preserve the CO. Patients generally tolerate the resultant mild hypoxemia well as long as CO is maintained.

The bidirectional Glenn or hemi-Fontan procedure is tolerated well because inferior vena caval blood continues to be connected to the systemic ventricle. This blood, even though it is desaturated, allows adequate filling of the ventricle, maintaining CO. Attention must be paid to minimizing PVR to ensure adequate pulmonary blood flow and oxygenation.

Increased intrathoracic pressure will limit pulmonary blood flow after a pre-Fontan or Fontan procedure. Spontaneous ventilation is preferable for optimizing flow. However, hypercarbia will increase PVR and counteract any positive effect of spontaneous ventilation. Ideally, it is best to have a limited time of positive-pressure ventilation and to tailor the anesthetic so that the patient can begin spontaneous ventilation and be extubated as soon as possible. Infusion of a short-acting narcotic after bypass may facilitate that goal.

d. Problems and complications

(1) Systemic venous hypertension (with resultant pleural or pericardial effusions, hepatomegaly, ascites, and peripheral edema)

(2) Decreased CO

(3) Atrial arrhythmias

(4) Hypoxemia secondary to residual right-to-left shunt

(5) Thrombosis along the conduit

(6) Pulmonary arteriovenous fistulas (late)

4. Total anomalous pulmonary venous return (TAPVR)

a. General considerations. In this lesion, all of the pulmonary venous blood drains into the right atrium either directly or indirectly. There is an obligatory interatrial communication by which mixed systemic and pulmonary venous blood enters the left atrium and then the LV and aorta. There are four basic types of TAPVR (Fig. 14.15): (i) *Supracardiac*—the common pulmonary vein drains through a vertical vein into either a left or right superior vena cava; (ii) *intracardiac*—the common pulmonary vein drains into the coronary sinus and then into the right atrium; (iii) *infracardiac*—the pulmonary venous blood drains into a descending vein, which traverses the diaphragm and enters the inferior vena cava, portal vein, or ductus venosus; (iv) *mixed type*—the different pulmonary segments drain to separate sites in the systemic venous system.

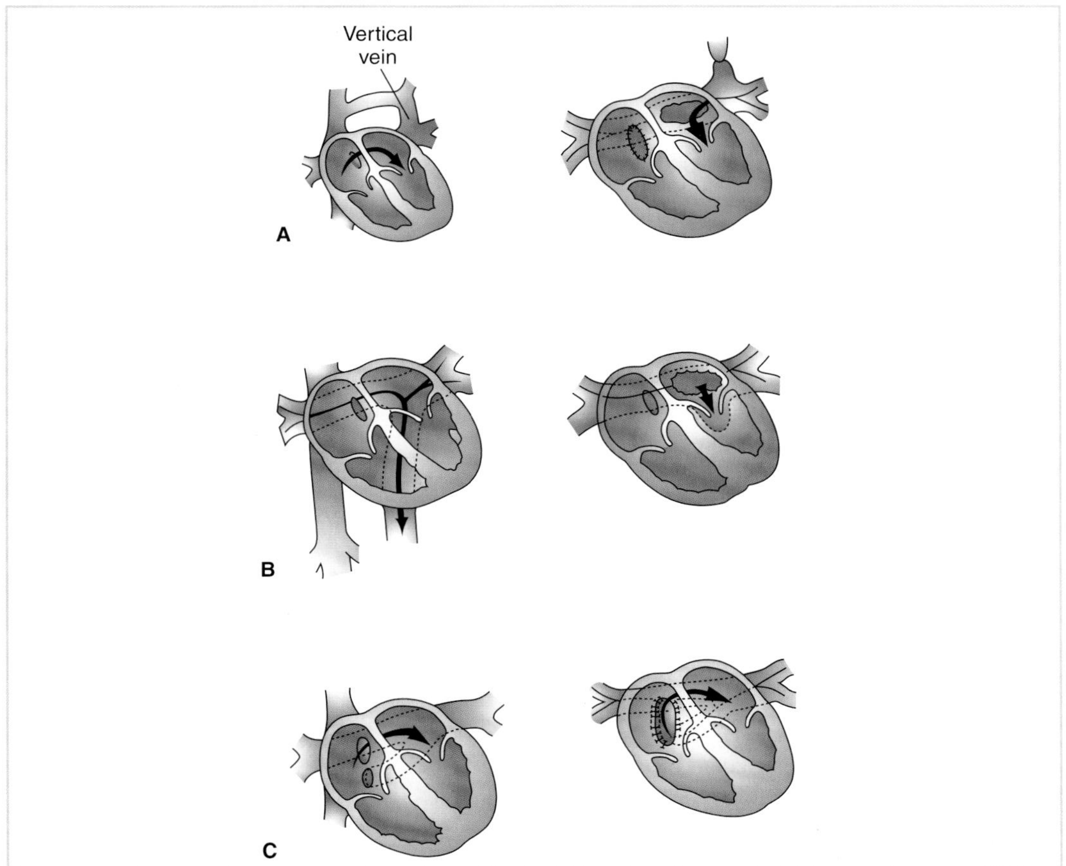

FIGURE 14.15 TAPVR. **A:** Supracardiac type **(left)** and surgical correction **(right)**. **B:** Infra-cardiac type **(left)** and surgical correction **(right)**. **C:** Intracardiac type **(left)** and surgical correction **(right)**. (From Waldhausen JA, Pierce WS, eds. *Johnson's Surgery of the Chest.* 5th ed. Chicago, IL: Year Book; 1985:355, 357, 359, with permission.)

The most important factor in evaluating these patients is whether or not there is any obstruction to the pulmonary venous drainage. The presence or absence of obstruction is the main determinant of the patient's clinical presentation and prognosis. It should be noted that TAPVR is associated with other complex cardiac lesions in a significant percentage of patients.

The patient with obstruction to drainage will be severely symptomatic in the first hours to days of life. The patient will be markedly cyanotic with respiratory distress. The chest x-ray is remarkable for a nearly normal heart size but shows a pulmonary interstitial pattern characteristic of pulmonary venous obstruction. Severe obstruction is most likely in patients with the infracardiac type but can occur in patients with any of the types of TAPVR. Infants with severe obstruction have severe pulmonary hypertension and require surgical intervention within the first few hours to days of life.

Patients without pulmonary venous obstruction will have a much more subtle clinical presentation. In this scenario, the patient may be relatively asymptomatic early but has pulmonary overcirculation of both systemic and pulmonary venous return. Mild cyanosis with oxygen saturation of about 85% to 90% may be difficult to appreciate. These patients are at risk for early development of pulmonary vascular obstructive disease.

b. **Surgical procedures.** Patients with TAPVR with obstruction must be surgically repaired expeditiously because medical management is not effective. Their condition can rapidly deteriorate and lead to death. The goal of correction is to connect the pulmonary venous system back into the left atrium, eliminate the anomalous connection to the systemic venous system, and close the ASD. Hypothermic CPB with circulatory arrest is commonly used. In the supracardiac type, the common pulmonary trunk is connected directly to the posterior left atrium, the ASD is closed, and the vertical vein is ligated. With the intracardiac type, the coronary sinus is "unroofed" and a patch is used to divert the pulmonary venous return (and the coronary sinus blood) into the left atrium across the ASD. For the infracardiac type, the common pulmonary vein is directly anastomosed to the left atrium, the descending vein is ligated, and the ASD is closed.

c. Anesthetic considerations

(1) Preoperative. Neonates with TAPVR and obstruction represent a true surgical emergency. The only therapy that may be considered preoperatively would be a balloon or blade atrial septostomy in the cardiac catheterization laboratory if the ASD is restrictive. This intervention will increase flow into the left atrium and potentially improve systemic perfusion. This is only a temporizing measure, and surgical intervention should occur as soon as possible. These neonates typically present with severe pulmonary hypertension, cyanosis, metabolic acidosis, and poor perfusion. They are often already intubated and receiving inotropic support. PGE_1 may decompress a hypertensive PA system and even open a ductus venosus, relieving a degree of pulmonary venous obstruction.

(2) Intraoperative. A technique should be used to minimize myocardial depression, typically with intravenous narcotics and paralytics. Inhalational anesthetics are generally not tolerated in the sick neonate but may be acceptable in the older child without obstruction and minimal symptoms.

Two issues arise when planning therapy for separation from CPB. First, these children have reactive pulmonary vascular beds, and efforts must center around decreasing PVR to improve right heart function. Therefore, high oxygen levels, hyperventilation, alkalosis, nitrates, isoproterenol, PGE_1, and nitric oxide may be considered. Second, because the left heart has been chronically underloaded, it may be relatively hypoplastic, noncompliant, and poorly functional. Inotropes and vasodilators may be helpful in improving systemic perfusion. Thus, these patients are at risk for significant dysfunction of both the LV and the RV.

d. **Problems and complications**

(1) Pulmonary venous obstruction
(2) Pulmonary hypertension and increased reactivity
(3) RV failure
(4) LV failure
(5) Arrhythmias, predominantly supraventricular

5. **Truncus arteriosus**

a. **General considerations.** These patients have a single arterial vessel, the truncus, arising from the base of the heart (Fig. 14.16). A high VSD is invariably present under the truncal valve. PAs arise either from a common stem (90% of the time) or separately from the truncus. A right aortic arch occurs in about 25% of cases. The truncal valve usually consists of three or four cusps, although this can vary from two to six cusps. In about half of patients, the valve is dysplastic and insufficient. Extracardiac anomalies are common. Fortunately, this defect is relatively uncommon.

These patients are symptomatic early in infancy, with a picture of CHF. These infants have markedly increased pulmonary blood flow, and arterial saturation is dependent on the ratio of pulmonary blood flow to systemic blood flow. Even though mixing of the two circulations occurs, cyanosis may be only minimal. Because of the degree of pulmonary overcirculation, damage to the pulmonary vascular bed occurs early. Untreated, the majority of children will die in the first 6 mos of life.

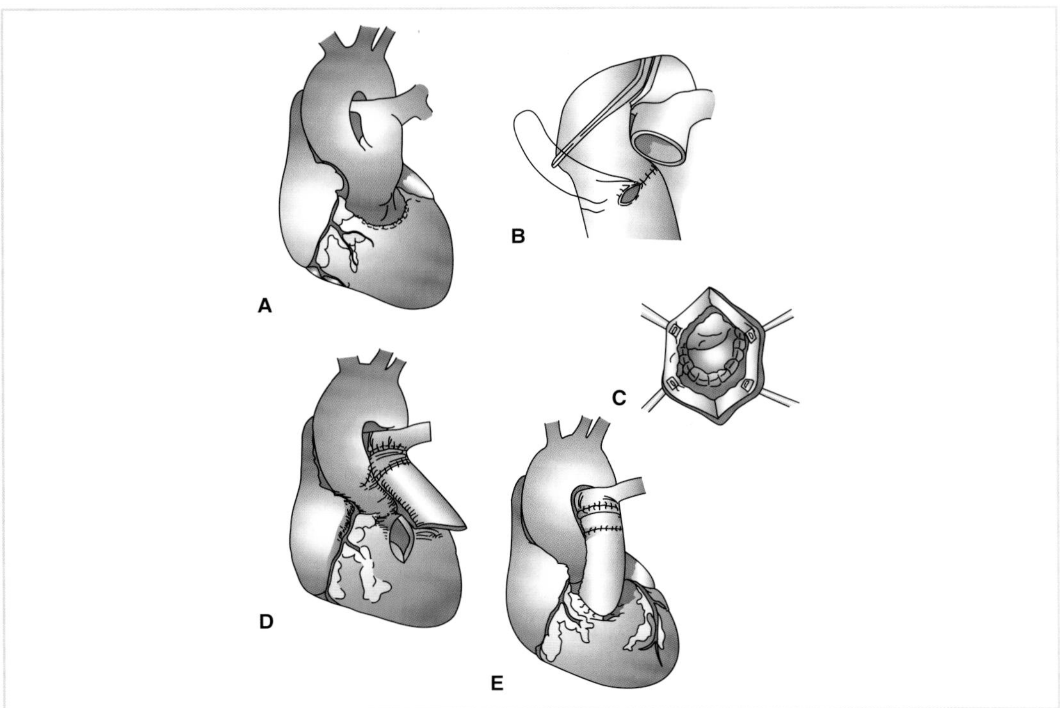

FIGURE 14.16 **A:** Truncus arteriosus. **B:** The pulmonary trunk is separated. **C:** The VSD is closed with a prosthetic patch. **D:** A valved conduit (usually pulmonary allograft) is used to establish RV to PA continuity. **E:** The complete repair. (From Waldhausen JA, Pierce WS, eds. *Johnson's Surgery of the Chest.* 5th ed. Chicago, IL: Year Book; 1985:397, with permission.)

b. **Surgical procedures.** Palliation with PA banding can be done, but it is not effective and is associated with a high mortality. More commonly, complete repair is performed in infants younger than 6 mos. In this procedure, the VSD is patched so as to direct blood from the LV out of the aorta (truncus). The PAs are disconnected from the truncus, unifocalized, and an RV-to-PA conduit is placed to the PA confluence. If the truncal valve is severely insufficient, it must be repaired or replaced.

c. **Anesthetic considerations**

(1) Preoperative. Care of these patients is similar to any other critically ill neonate. Preoperative sedation is not necessary. These patients may already be intubated on positive-pressure ventilation. If CHF is severe, they may be receiving positive inotropic drugs.

Some of these patients have DiGeorge syndrome with absent thymus and immunologic deficiency. If so, they are susceptible to graft-versus-host disease and require irradiated blood products. They are also prone to infection and require regular antibiotic prophylaxis. Until the diagnosis is known with certainty, one should assume the worst and take appropriate precautions. If a thymus is found at operation, then the diagnosis has been excluded.

(2) Intraoperative. The anesthetic technique must account for the fact that the child is in a tenuous hemodynamic state. The goal should be to preserve systemic blood flow while minimizing pulmonary blood flow. High-dose narcotics are used most often. One must take care not to hyperventilate the patient, as the resultant decrease in PVR will induce further pulmonary overcirculation. **Maneuvers to try to limit pulmonary blood flow include limiting inspired oxygen concentration,**

maintaining normocarbia or even hypercarbia, and using PEEP. The surgeon also can put a tourniquet around the PAs to constrict flow. This is especially important during CPB to ensure that systemic perfusion is adequate. One must be careful not to lower SVR too much, especially if the truncal valve is insufficient. In that case, diastolic pressure may already be low, which predisposes the baby to coronary insufficiency.

After the repair, therapy should be directed toward increasing pulmonary blood flow. These children have an incredibly reactive pulmonary vasculature and often benefit from sedation and possibly nitric oxide for several days postoperatively to minimize pulmonary vascular crises. Inotropic therapy is usually necessary for separation from bypass.

d. Problems and complications

(1) LV dysfunction

(2) Pulmonary hypertensive crises and RV failure

(3) Truncal valve regurgitation

(4) Heart block

(5) Conduit stenosis due to growth (late)

6. Hypoplastic left heart syndrome

a. General considerations. Hypoplastic left heart syndrome is a term used to describe a spectrum of diseases, with the common denominator being underdevelopment of the left-sided heart structures (Fig. 14.17). The patient may have mitral atresia, aortic atresia, and/or a hypoplastic aortic arch. With all of these lesions, the LV is small. All blood flow returning to the heart from the lungs passes from the left atrium to the right atrium, where it mixes with the systemic venous return. The RV then becomes the pumping chamber for both the pulmonary and systemic circulations. Blood entering the PA goes to the lungs and across the PDA to the systemic circulation. Perfusion to the cerebral and coronary circulation is dependent on retrograde flow through the hypoplastic aortic arch.

These infants often may appear healthy at birth as long as the ductus arteriosus is widely patent. Within a few hours to a few days, the patient's condition rapidly deteriorates as the ductus arteriosus begins to close and systemic perfusion becomes inadequate. These infants manifest tachypnea, tachycardia, cardiomegaly, poor peripheral pulses, and what has been termed **"gray cyanosis" (a result of both systemic desaturation and low CO).** Without therapy, the average age at death is 4 to 5 days. Extracardiac anomalies (usually minor genitourinary malformations) occur in about 15% to 25% of cases.

b. Surgical procedures. There are basically two surgical options for these infants. They can undergo either orthotopic cardiac transplantation or a staged reconstructive procedure as first described by Norwood. Although transplantation is an attractive option, it is not generally performed, primarily because of limited availability of donor organs. The Norwood procedure has been refined over the years, but it still consists of the following important components (Fig. 14.17B–F): (i) Atrial septectomy, (ii) anastomosis of the proximal PA to the diminutive aorta, with homograft augmentation of the aorta and aortic arch, and (iii) the establishment of a reliable pathway for blood flow to the lungs (either an aortopulmonary shunt or an RV to PA conduit [Sano shunt]). The first stage of a Norwood procedure is a palliative operation whose purpose is to create a more stable physiology. By augmenting the aorta and anastomosing it to the PA, systemic perfusion then comes directly from the RV and is no longer dependent on the PDA. The main pulmonary trunk is disconnected from the PAs, and pulmonary blood flow is provided via the aortopulmonary shunt, or, more recently, the Sano shunt [33]. The Norwood procedure is generally performed in the first month of life. Then, at about 6 mos, the child undergoes the second stage of palliation, either a bidirectional Glenn shunt or a hemi-Fontan. This interim procedure is necessary in order to take some of the volume load off the RV, which allows remodeling and helps preserve its function. Later, at about 24 to 36 mos, the completion Fontan is performed.

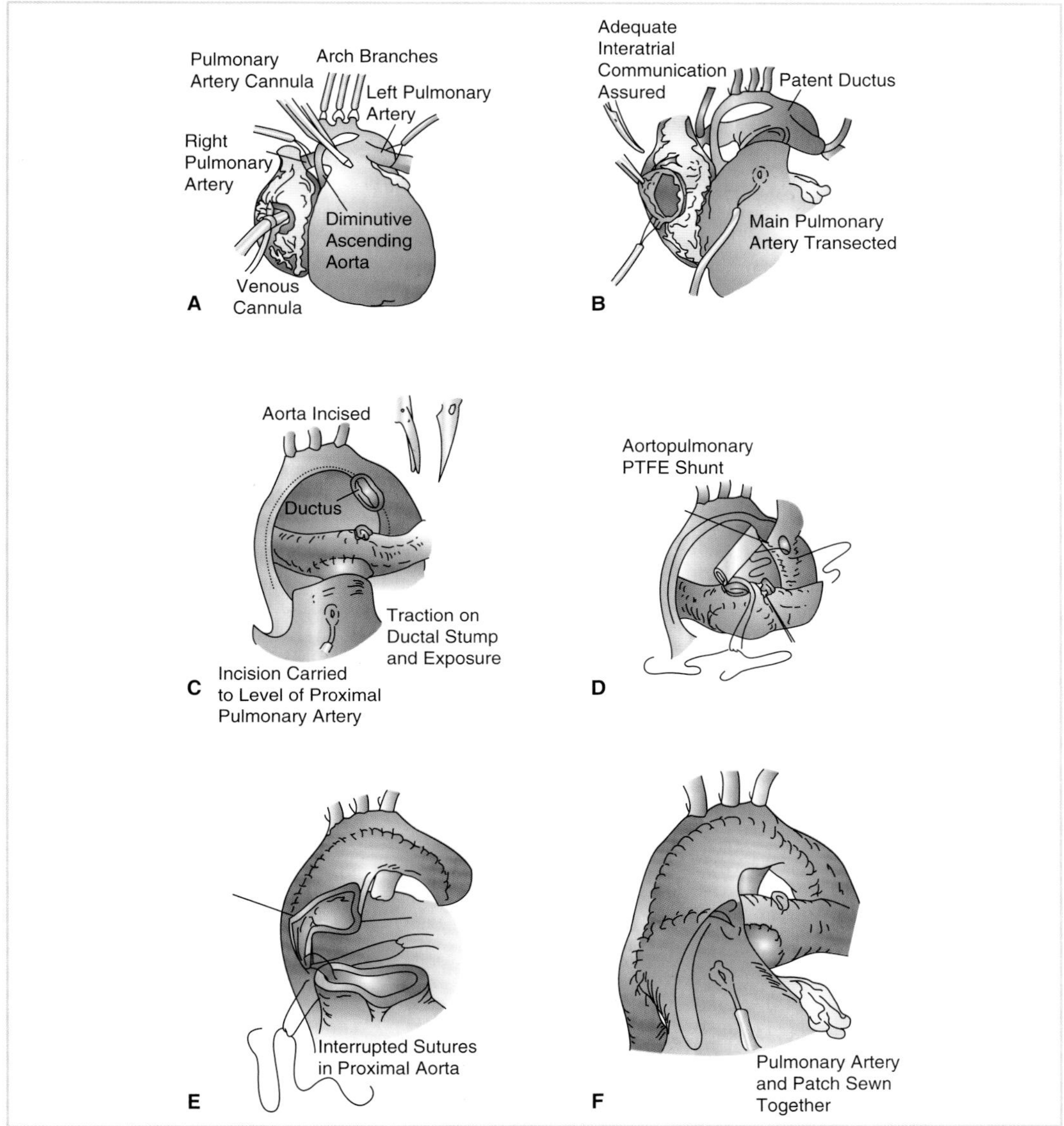

FIGURE 14.17 **A:** Hypoplastic left heart anatomy. **B:** Atrial septectomy and division of main PA. **C:** Patch closure of distal main PA, ligation, and division of PDA. **D:** Incision of the entire hypoplastic aortic arch and homograft patch enlargement and central aortopulmonary shunt. **E:** Anastomosis of proximal main PA and reconstructed aortic arch. **F:** Completed repair. (From Edwards LH, Norwood W, eds. *Atlas of Cardiothoracic Surgery*. Philadelphia, PA: Lea & Febiger; 1989, with permission.)

c. **Anesthetic considerations.** The following discussion centers on care of the infant undergoing the first stage of the Norwood procedure. Anesthetic considerations for stage 2 (cavopulmonary connection) or stage 3 (Fontan) have been covered elsewhere.

(1) Preoperative. **There are two major goals that must be accomplished to successfully care for these critically ill neonates.** First, the **PDA must be kept patent to allow systemic perfusion.** Second, **the balance between SVR and PVR must be maintained in order to optimize blood flow to each circuit.** PGE_1 is infused to maintain patency of the ductus arteriosus. These neonates typically present with profound metabolic acidosis at the time of diagnosis. This abnormality should be

aggressively treated to improve cardiac function. The children are typically intubated and sedated to minimize oxygen consumption. Mild hypercarbia (Pco_2 45 to 55 mm Hg), low oxygen concentrations, and PEEP are helpful in restricting pulmonary blood flow. It is important to remember that oxygen is a powerful pulmonary vasodilator and can cause excessive pulmonary blood flow and inadequate systemic perfusion. These children are commonly maintained on room air. If PVR is too low, a mildly hypoxic (Fio_2 18%) mixture also can be considered. **When the pulmonary and systemic circuits are well balanced, one would expect to see S_pO_2 values of about 75% to 80%.** Higher values imply inadequate systemic perfusion and pulmonary overload. Transfusion is often necessary to keep the Hct about 45% to ensure adequate oxygen delivery to the tissues. The children may require inotropic support, and dopamine may be advantageous if PVR is low.

(2) Intraoperative. All of the preoperative strategies must be continued in the operating room. Anesthesia is usually accomplished with narcotics to minimize myocardial depression. Inotropic agents may be required to maintain stability during dissection. After repair, individual management is dictated by how large the pulmonary shunt is and how much pulmonary blood flow results. The same physiology exists after repair, with emphasis on balancing the systemic and pulmonary blood flows. One must aggressively expand the lungs to avoid atelectasis. The degree of ventilation and the oxygen concentration employed depends on the patient's oxygen saturation. Some centers advocate adding CO_2 to the circuit to allow vigorous ventilation and maintenance of functional residual capacity without causing respiratory alkalosis. As previously mentioned, one would expect to see a S_pO_2 of about 75% to 80% when the pulmonary and systemic flows are ideally matched. These children may benefit from heavy postoperative sedation to avoid pulmonary hypertensive crises.

d. Problems and complications

(1) Too much or too little pulmonary blood flow
(2) Inadequate systemic perfusion
(3) Myocardial dysfunction
(4) AV valvular regurgitation
(5) Myocardial ischemia
(6) Pulmonary hypertensive crisis

B. Lesions likely to cause CHF

1. VSD

a. General considerations. VSD occurs commonly, either in conjunction with other cardiac defects or as an isolated lesion. VSDs can be categorized into four types (Fig. 14.18): (i) *Supracristal defect* just under the pulmonary valve, (ii) *infracristal perimembranous defect,* the most common type, (iii) *canal or inlet-type defect,* a form of partial AV canal, and (iv) *muscular defects* in the trabecular portion of the ventricular septum. The size of the defect and the PVR determine the amount of blood flow that passes left to right to the pulmonary bed. A small VSD, termed "restrictive," will often cause minimal symptoms and may close spontaneously in the first 5 yrs of life. Large defects are nearly equal in cross-sectional area to the area of the aortic annulus and allow free communication between the two ventricles. The pressures in both ventricles will be equal and, because PVR is usually about one-sixth of SVR, pulmonary blood flow will be greater than systemic blood flow. This excess flow will cause dilation of the left atrium, LV, and usually the RV. If the defect is large, the patient will develop symptoms of CHF at about age 1 mo as the PVR falls. The child generally manifests tachypnea, tachycardia, failure to thrive, and frequent respiratory infections. The child may have mild cyanosis if he or she has a respiratory infection or pulmonary overload, but this hypoxemia improves with oxygen. **If a large VSD remains unrepaired, the high pressure and flow to the lungs will result in irreversible pulmonary vascular damage.** As this situation develops, the patient will become less symptomatic as

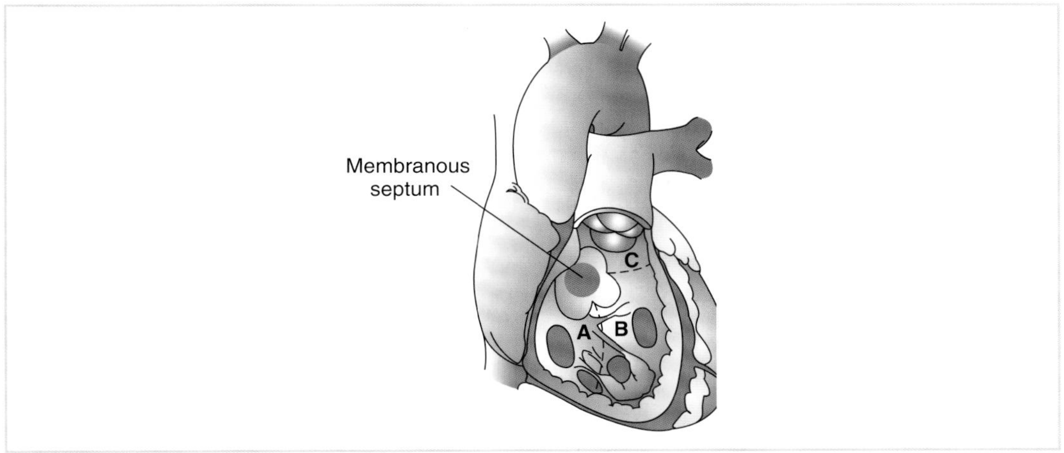

FIGURE 14.18 The location of VSDs in the membranous inlet (*A*), trabecular (*B*), and infundibular (*C*) septa. (From Waldhausen JA, Pierce WS, eds. *Johnson's Surgery of the Chest.* 5th ed. Chicago, IL: Year Book; 1985:335, with permission.)

the pulmonary blood flow decreases. The terminal stage of this process results in a reversal of the shunt so that the flow becomes right to left, the so-called "Eisenmenger complex." If the process has advanced to this point, surgical repair can no longer be performed. The time course for the development of this pulmonary vascular damage is variable. **Because of this problem, most centers plan repair of large defects within the first year of life.**

b. Surgical procedures

(1) Complete repair using CPB is typically the operation of choice for most patients. Patch closure of the defect is usually accomplished by approaching it through the right atrium and tricuspid valve. On occasion, a right ventriculotomy may be necessary to visualize defects in the ventricular apex or RVOT.

(2) PA banding was formerly the procedure of choice for infants in order to limit the excessive pulmonary blood flow and allow growth, then complete repair was performed in a delayed fashion. Today a one-stage complete repair is done more commonly, even in infancy. However, PA banding may still play a role in patients with multiple muscular VSDs or other complex lesions associated with VSD and excess pulmonary perfusion.

c. Anesthetic considerations

(1) Preoperative. Children who require surgery early in life have large VSDs and excessive pulmonary blood flow. Initial medical management may include afterload reduction, diuretics, and often antibiotics (because the children typically present with respiratory infections). The choice of whether or not premedication is indicated depends on the age of the child and the degree of ventricular dysfunction. Most children younger than about 10 mos will not need any preoperative sedation. On the other hand, an older child may benefit from judicious sedation, keeping in mind the importance of avoiding hypercarbia so that pulmonary hypertension is not exacerbated.

(2) Intraoperative. Choice of anesthetic agents depends on the clinical status of the patient. If the patient has limited cardiac reserve, a primary narcotic technique may be beneficial. If the child is less symptomatic, inhalational induction can be used, with a switch toward a balanced technique when intravenous access is secured.

One must be meticulous in deairing the intravenous fluids whenever there is an abnormal connection between the left and right sides of the heart. Even when the patient has a predominant left-to-right shunt, the direction of flow can easily change at any time. If air ends up on the left side of the heart, it can be pumped to the brain and cause a cerebrovascular event.

If the VSD is nonrestrictive, care must be taken not to overventilate the child after intubation. Hypocarbia and hyperoxia will lower PVR and make the left-to-right shunt even more profound, often at the expense of systemic perfusion. Using a lower inspired oxygen concentration and normocarbia can help to balance the circulations. Application of 5 to 10 cm H_2O PEEP can help limit the excessive pulmonary flow by diverting more to the body.

Separation from CPB is generally straightforward for most patients. However, if the patient has pre-existing pulmonary vascular disease, RV dysfunction can be problematic. In that case, efforts should be directed toward decreasing PVR and optimizing CO. A combination of vasodilators and inotropes often can be beneficial. Phosphodiesterase inhibitors may be particularly helpful because of their pulmonary vasodilatory properties.

d. Problems and complications

(1) Pulmonary hypertension and RV dysfunction
(2) Residual left-to-right shunt
(3) LV dysfunction, especially if the cross-clamp time is prolonged
(4) Heart block, usually due to swelling along the patch suture line. Usually, it resolves over several days; however, it can be permanent if the conduction system is inadvertently damaged during the repair.
(5) Respiratory insufficiency and slow weaning from the ventilator if the patient had increased lung water preoperatively
(6) Aortic insufficiency only occurs rarely if the VSD was supracristal and sutures distort the septal cusp.

2. ASD

a. General considerations. There are three types of ASDs (Fig. 14.19): (i) *Ostium secundum* (the most common type) is located centrally at the area of the fossa ovalis; (ii) *sinus venosus type* occurs at the junction of the superior vena cava and right atrium and is usually associated with partial anomalous pulmonary venous return; (iii) *ostium primum defect* occurs low in the septum and is often associated with a cleft mitral valve. Ostium primum defects are sometimes referred to as partial AV canals, and the patient may have some associated mitral insufficiency. These defects also form the atrial component of a complete AV canal defect. ASDs occur more commonly in females than in males.

ASDs will result in an atrial-level left-to-right shunt causing increased volume to the right side of the heart. **The size of the defect and the ratio of LV and RV compliance**

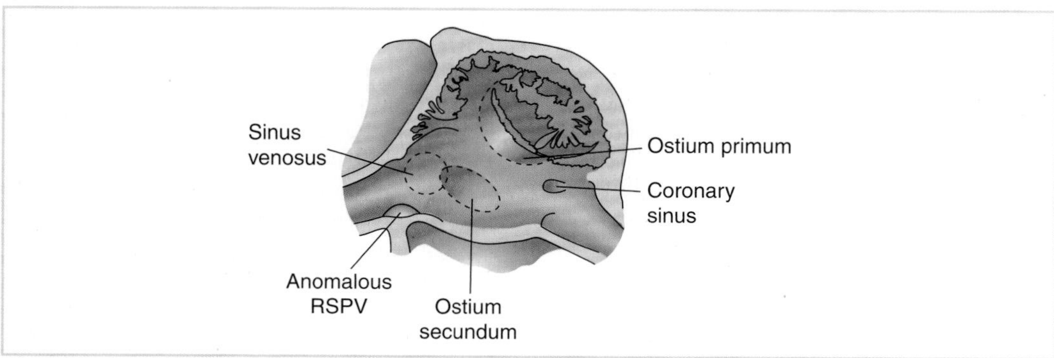

FIGURE 14.19 Artist's depiction of the opened right atrium showing the anatomic location of ASDs. RSPV, right superior pulmonary vein. (From Doty DB. *Cardiac Surgery.* Chicago, IL: Year Book; 1985:1, with permission.)

determine the amount of flow. These defects often can be large and the pulmonary blood flow can be three to four times the systemic blood flow. Patients are usually asymptomatic, especially if it is a secundum defect. If CHF symptoms occur early in infancy, one should be suspicious that the patient has another coexisting defect. PVR changes do not develop early, and the Eisenmenger physiology usually does not occur until after the second decade of life, if at all. It is not unusual for a patient to reach the fourth decade of life and have an undiagnosed ASD. Patients may first come to medical attention due to occurrence of a stroke or because of development of symptomatology during pregnancy. Closure of ASDs is typically recommended in order to prevent paradoxical emboli and pulmonary vascular disease.

b. Surgical procedures. Repair, most commonly, is performed with CPB and mild hypothermia. The procedure can be done using fibrillation, or the aorta can be cross-clamped. The defect is visualized through a right atriotomy. If it is a secundum defect, it often can be closed primarily. If it is large, a patch may be necessary. For a sinus venosus defect, a patch is positioned to redirect flow from the partial anomalous pulmonary venous return to the left atrium. If the pulmonary veins enter the superior vena cava, a rather elongated patch may be necessary to tunnel the veins over to the left atrium. Repair of an ostium primum defect requires a patch and attention to the cleft mitral valve. If necessary, sutures are used to restore competency to the mitral valve, taking care not to make it stenotic. Because the AV conduction system runs right along the inferior rim of the defect, particular attention must be paid to the placement of these stitches in order to avoid heart block.

Device closure of ASDs in the cardiac catheterization laboratory may be an option for some patients, depending on the size and location of the defect. This form of intervention is limited to those patients with a secundum-type ASD and for those who have adequate rims or borders surrounding the defect. As more experience is gained and the technology of the device improves, transcatheter ASD closure may become more common, thus obviating the need for surgery in some patients.

c. Anesthetic considerations. These children are typically healthy and usually undergo surgery at about age 4 to 5 yrs. Just about any anesthetic technique can be used successfully. Premedication is often helpful to facilitate separation from their parents and a smooth induction. Typically, the CPB time is relatively short and weaning from bypass is uneventful. The anesthetic technique should be tailored toward a goal of extubation at the end of the procedure if no complications arise. Therefore, we usually limit the amount of narcotics used and rely more heavily on inhaled anesthetics. As with any lesion involving an intracardiac communication, one must be sure to avoid any air in the intravenous catheters.

One interesting thing to keep in mind is that CVP in these patients can be misleading postoperatively. The right atrium has become accustomed to handling a high volume and often is dilated and compliant. Subsequently, when the ASD is closed, the volume in the right atrium decreases acutely. If one relies on the CVP measurement with a goal of replacing volume to a "normal" value of 8 to 10 mm Hg, it is likely that the patient will be markedly overhydrated and liable to fall off the back of the Frank–Starling curve. It is much better to visually inspect the surgical field to determine adequacy of volume replacement.

d. Problems and complications

(1) Atrial arrhythmias, especially atrial fibrillation or paroxysmal atrial tachycardia
(2) Complete heart block in ostium primum repairs
(3) Mitral insufficiency or stenosis after cleft repair with ostium primum defects
(4) Persistent left-to-right shunt
(5) Pulmonary edema if patient is overtransfused

3. AV canal defects

a. General considerations. This defect, also known as endocardial cushion defect, represents a spectrum of disease resulting from failure of the endocardial cushions, which

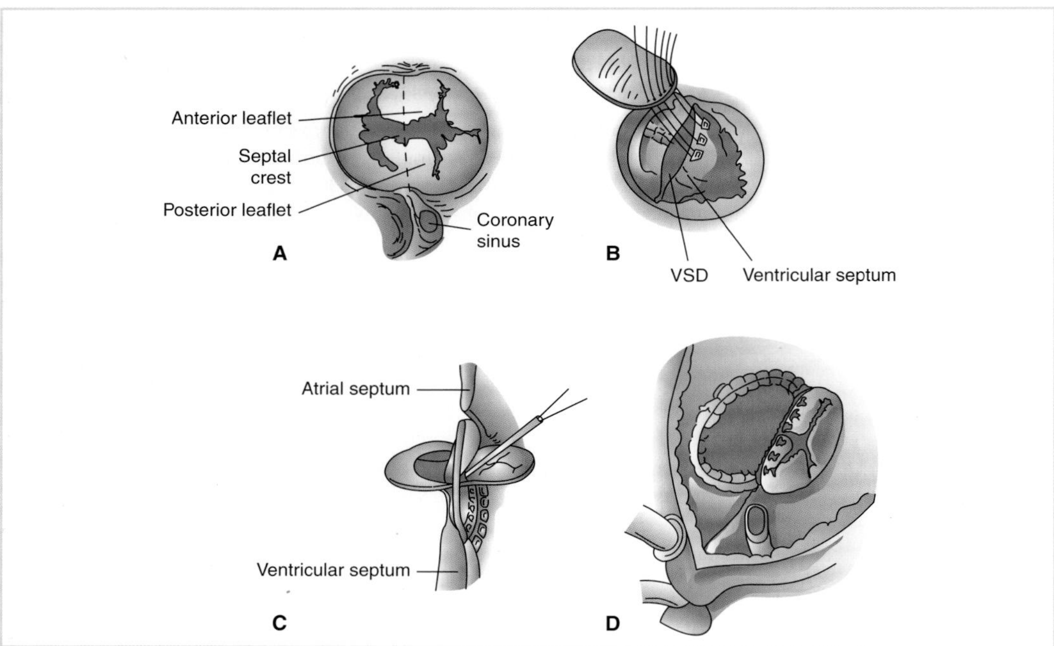

FIGURE 14.20 **A:** Artist's depiction of complete AV canal as viewed from above. **B:** The pericardial patch is attached to the rightward aspect of the ventricular septum. VSD. **C:** The valve leaflets are attached to the pericardial patch. **D:** The completed repair from the right atrial view. (From Waldhausen JA, Pierce WS, eds. *Johnson's Surgery of the Chest.* 5th ed. Chicago, IL: Year Book; 1985:349, with permission.)

form the central part of the heart, to develop and fuse properly. The result is a defect in lower atrial and upper ventricular septae and deficiencies in the mitral and tricuspid valves (Fig. 14.20). The defect can be partial or complete. In the partial type, there may be just an interatrial communication (an ostium primum defect) or just an interventricular communication. A cleft in the mitral valve is usually present, causing varying degrees of mitral valve insufficiency. In the complete type of AV canal, the entire central portion of the cardiac septum is absent and there is a single AV valve with free communication among the four cardiac chambers. The common AV valve may be relatively competent or freely insufficient. This lesion occurs with equal frequency in males and females. It is the most common cardiac anomaly seen in children with Down syndrome.

The patient's clinical condition depends on the anatomic variation present. In general, AV canal physiology results from a large left-to-right shunt with pulmonary overload and CHF. These children normally manifest symptoms early in life, with the typical features of excessive pulmonary blood flow. Generally, the larger the ventricular defect and the greater the mitral insufficiency, the sicker the infant. Cyanosis is rare, unless the child has superimposed pulmonary stenosis, a respiratory infection, or high PVR. Some patients with AV canal have LV outlet tract obstruction, which alters their prognosis.

Infants with complete AV canal develop irreversible pulmonary vascular disease early in life. Therefore, most centers plan surgical repair within the first 6 mos of life.

b. Surgical procedures. The practice of PA banding as a palliative step before complete repair has largely been abandoned, except in infants with complex anatomy that precludes complete repair at an early age. Results from PA banding have been disappointing, and the results of early complete repair have steadily improved. PA banding still may be indicated in patients with an unbalanced AV canal and in those infants who will undergo a single ventricle pathway in order to limit the pulmonary blood flow and protect the vasculature for future interventions.

Complete repair is accomplished using CPB with moderate hypothermia or occasionally DHCA. The defects are visualized through a right atriotomy. Careful inspection of the defects must be carried out, because there is significant variability among patients. The septal defects are closed with either one or two patches and the AV valves are reconstructed and attached to the patch(es). When reconstructing the AV valves, it is important to make them as competent as possible without creating AV valve stenosis. Extreme care must be taken when suturing the VSD and ASD patch(es) to avoid the conduction system, which lies close to the defect and near the coronary sinus.

c. Anesthetic considerations

(1) Preoperative. Infants with complete AV canal generally have been managed medically with afterload reduction and diuretics before surgery. It is important to check for electrolyte abnormalities. In patients being treated with digitalis, one may consider holding the morning dose on day of surgery. These infants typically do not require preoperative sedation, especially if they have Down syndrome.

(2) Intraoperative. Choice of anesthetic agents depends on the patient's clinical condition. If the child has severe CHF, intravenous induction with predominantly narcotics may be advisable. With lesser degrees of symptomatology, an inhalational technique may be appropriate. The goals in managing these patients are to minimize myocardial depression and to maintain or even slightly increase PVR while preventing increases in SVR. One must be careful to keep the patient normocapnic after intubation, with consideration for decreasing inspired oxygen concentration and perhaps using PEEP to limit pulmonary blood flow.

Complete repair of an AV canal requires a lengthy period of CPB. One should anticipate difficulty with elevated PVR as well as ventricular dysfunction and possibly AV valve insufficiency upon separation from bypass. Transesophageal echocardiography has proven of great value in these patients as an excellent tool for intraoperative anatomic evaluation of surgical repair. Typically, both inotropic and vasodilator therapies are required. Because of the dysplastic nature of the AV valves, early inotropic support is begun in an effort to allow the heart to operate more efficiently at a lower filling pressure. The goal is to avoid ventricular distention and annular dilation, which are likely to exacerbate AV valve insufficiency. Thus, it is ideal to try to keep the left atrial pressure around 10 to 12 mm Hg or lower. If AV conduction problems occur, AV pacing may be necessary. Because of the reactivity of these infants' pulmonary vasculature, they typically are deeply sedated and ventilated for a variable period of time postoperatively to facilitate their recovery.

d. Problems and complications

(1) Pulmonary hypertension and RV failure
(2) LV dysfunction and low systemic output
(3) Mitral and/or tricuspid insufficiency
(4) Heart block
(5) Ventricular and atrial arrhythmias
(6) Residual shunt

4. PDA

a. General considerations. This lesion is one of the more common lesions encountered, especially in conjunction with other cardiac anomalies. The ductus arteriosus is a normal fetal vessel between the aorta and the left PA, which serves in utero to allow most of the blood from the RV to bypass the nonaerated lungs. Normally, this vessel functionally closes within hours after birth. Patency beyond the first few days of life can occur and may result in significant hemodynamic consequences if the lumen is large and the PVR is low. Rubella, prematurity, and hypoxemia are known risk factors associated with nonclosure of the ductus arteriosus.

Typically, the clinician is likely to encounter two distinct populations with isolated PDA. It is noted commonly in the premature neonatal intensive care unit group, often causing pulmonary overload with respiratory distress and inability to wean from the ventilator. These children often can be successfully medically treated with indomethacin to promote closure of the PDA. However, on occasion, surgical therapy may be necessary if indomethacin is contraindicated or not successful. Older children, often asymptomatic, represent the other group of patients in whom a heart murmur is detected on their routine physical examination before school. The degree of symptomatology depends on the amount of flow to the lungs. One would expect to see a wide pulse pressure with bounding pulses and a continuous murmur heard both on the front and back of the chest. Of course, one must remember that PDA commonly occurs in association with other more complex lesions and, in those cases, the manifestations will be more dependent on the associated anatomy.

b. Surgical procedures. The classic surgical approach for repair involves a limited left thoracotomy. The vessel is located and can be ligated with suture or clamped with vascular clips. In the older infants, many surgeons doubly ligate and divide the vessel to ensure that it will not recanalize. Recently, some centers have advocated a thoracoscopic approach to the procedure. In addition, many interventional cardiologists perform catheter closure of PDAs, using a variety of closure devices. These have included disk devices, coils, and buttons. Although there is a learning curve to all of the newer procedures, improvement in the design of the equipment has resulted in excellent results with minimal complications. For the neonatal population, surgical ligation at the NICU bedside remains the technical procedure of choice.

c. Anesthetic considerations. Most of the patients will be tiny premature infants. In addition to the usual considerations for these types of children, one must pay particular attention to respiratory care, temperature, and fluid management. Because of the increased pulmonary blood flow, these neonates usually will come to surgery already intubated. They may benefit from the judicious application of continuous positive airway pressure to help improve oxygenation and manage the excess lung water. During the thoracotomy, the nondependent lung will be compressed and not ventilated, and hypoxemia can become an issue. One must balance the need to ventilate aggressively enough to maintain oxygenation while trying to avoid using airway pressures that may injure these immature lungs. It is important and can be a challenge to keep these children warm, especially if the infant must be transported to the operating room for the procedure. One should try to restrict the fluids administered, because these neonates already are fluid overloaded and in CHF.

Management of the older child is straightforward. The surgical procedure is short, and invasive monitoring is generally not required. It is important to be sure to obtain adequate venous access because there is a chance of significant blood loss, although this complication is rare. These patients may benefit from preoperative sedation to facilitate separation from their parents. Any anesthetic technique is acceptable, tailoring it toward a goal of extubation at the end. The pain from a thoracotomy is significant, so judicious use of intravenous, intrathoracic, or epidural narcotics is advisable.

In all patient populations, intraoperative monitoring of lower-extremity noninvasive blood pressures or continuous pulse oximetry is helpful to ensure that surgical ligation does not adversely impact systemic blood flow via the descending thoracic aorta.

d. Problems and complications

(1) Ligation of the incorrect vessel (descending aorta or left PA) can cause systemic hypoperfusion or hypoxemia

(2) Recurrent laryngeal nerve damage

(3) Ductal recanalization (late)

(4) LV dysfunction caused by the acute increase in afterload due to removal of the low-resistance pulmonary circuit

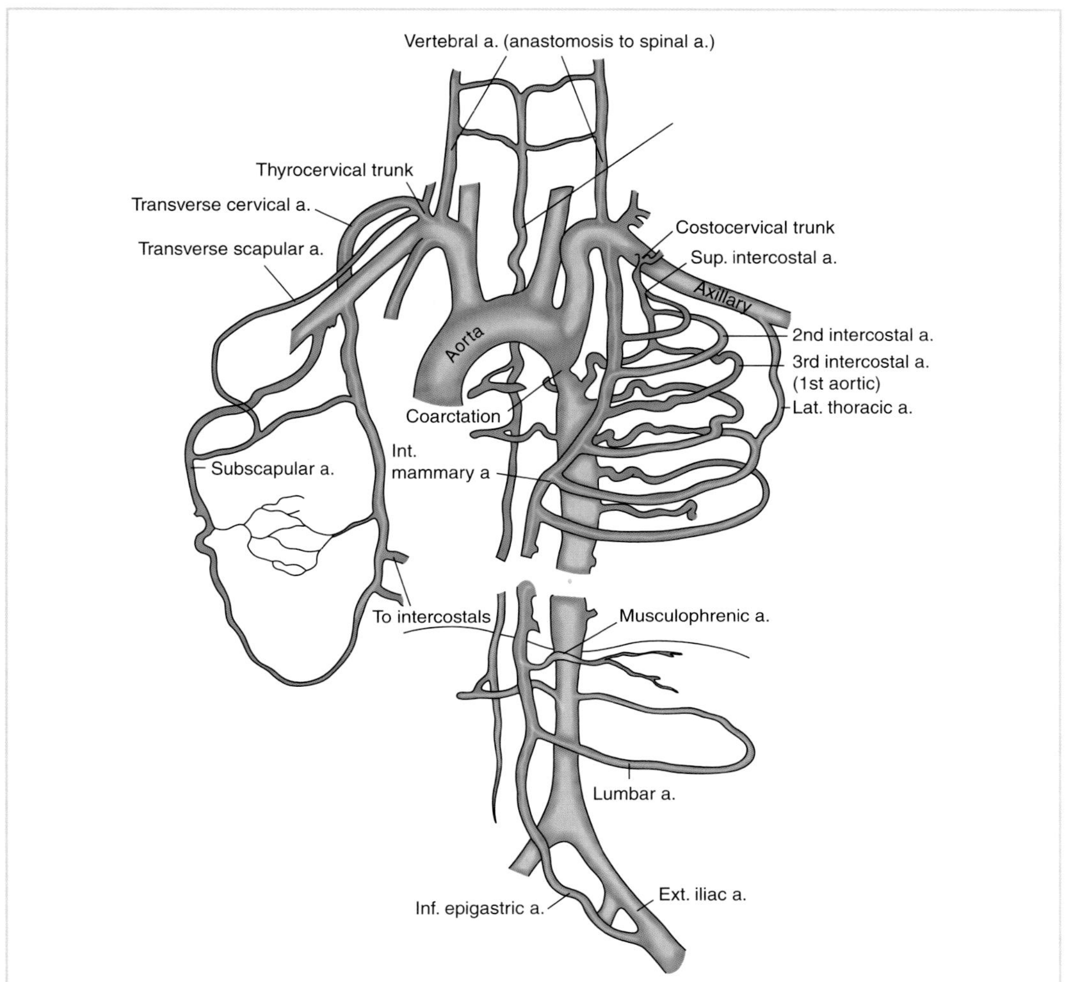

FIGURE 14.21 Coarctation of the aorta. Depiction of the course of collateral circulation in patients with coarctation of the aorta. (From Edwards JE, et al. The collateral circulation in coarctation of the aorta. *Mayo Clin Proc.* 1948;23:334, with permission.)

5. **Coarctation of the aorta**
   a. **General considerations.** The typical aortic coarctation is a localized narrowing of the aorta just distal to the left subclavian artery and just proximal, opposite, or distal to the insertion of the ductus arteriosus. This lesion is likely to become symptomatic during two periods of life. Infants with severe obstruction can develop symptoms of CHF early in life. Others remain asymptomatic until adolescence or adulthood. Often the lesion is discovered at a routine physical examination because of a heart murmur, with diminished distal pulses and a pressure gradient between the upper and lower limbs. These children often exhibit upper-extremity hypertension, and rib notching on chest x-ray film occurs after about age 8 yrs due to the development of collateral circulation (Fig. 14.21).

   The symptomatic neonate with coarctation demonstrates LV failure, with distal hypoperfusion and metabolic acidosis. If the child has a preductal coarctation and pulmonary hypertension, flow across the ductus can be right to left, causing "differential cyanosis" of the upper (pink) and lower (blue) body. In the first few days of life, the discrepancy in pressures in the upper versus lower extremities may be difficult to appreciate, especially if the ductus is open and ventricular function is poor. Maintenance of patency of the ductus is very helpful in improving systemic perfusion. Many neonates with this lesion require preoperative inotropic support.

Associated cardiovascular malformations are common, especially bicuspid aortic valve (occurring in about 50% of patients as a coexisting lesion). In the extreme form of aortic isthmus narrowing, complete interruption of the aorta may occur. In that case, a large VSD is present almost invariably. The lower part of the body is then perfused by the ductus arteriosus.

b. **Surgical procedures.** Surgical repair is through a left thoracotomy. Several different surgical techniques have been used. For infants, a subclavian flap reconstruction may be employed; however, the procedure of choice remains an extended end-to-end reconstruction. In older children, the affected area is resected and an end-to-end anastomosis is performed. Occasionally, interposition grafts are required if the coarctation segment is long. Patch augmentation of the aorta has generated concern because of the high incidence of aneurysm formation at the site of repair. Balloon angioplasty of the coarctation is another option, but its use has been associated with a high incidence of residual or recurrent stenosis. There may be a place for its use, however, in situations of recurrent stenosis after surgical repair.

c. **Anesthetic considerations.** Although the surgical approach is similar, anesthetic technique will be markedly different between an infant with coarctation and CHF and an older child with relatively asymptomatic coarctation. The critically ill neonate typically will come to the operating room with PGE_1 infusing to allow postductal flow. This infant will require a high-dose narcotic technique to minimize hemodynamic embarrassment. The older child typically has LV hypertrophy and hypertension and can benefit from volatile anesthetics that provide some myocardial depression. Either an inhalational technique or an intravenous induction is acceptable in the older child. Both groups require antibiotic prophylaxis.

The site for monitoring blood pressure is important. A right radial arterial catheter should be placed. The left arm is avoided, because the subclavian artery often must be clamped or ligated to facilitate repair. When the aorta is cross-clamped, the upper-body blood pressure will rise. One must be careful not to try to lower this pressure back to "normal," because spinal cord perfusion is critically dependent on this pressure head. Inadequate perfusion to the spinal cord can result in paraplegia. Some centers monitor the spinal cord with somatosensory evoked potentials. If so, one must design a plan to provide a steady-state anesthetic with agents that only minimally affect the evoked potentials. A continuous infusion of narcotics with a low concentration of volatile agent works well. Other strategies which may be employed for spinal cord protection include steroids, hypothermia, and mannitol. After removal of the cross-clamp, aggressive control of the blood pressure is indicated. The neonates typically do not manifest hypertension, but the older patients often exhibit a paradoxical increase in blood pressure to levels even higher than beginning levels. Initial control can be obtained with sodium nitroprusside, but prolonged use of this drug is associated with tachyphylaxis. Combination agents such as labetalol, which provide both α- and β-blockade, are ideal. It can be initially infused intravenously and later switched to oral use when the patient is taking fluids by mouth.

Adequate pain control can help to control postoperative hypertension. Thoracic epidural infusions of local anesthetics and narcotics are effective and well tolerated. Intravenous patient-controlled analgesia is another alternative in the older population. Intercostal nerve blocks may not be a good choice because of the prominent collateral vessels in that area, which increase the potential for significant bleeding.

In the older group, extubation at the end of the surgical procedure is desirable. Early extubation aids in blood pressure control. It also allows one to perform a thorough neurologic examination. The neonatal population usually benefits from short-term continued intubation, ventilation, and diuresis.

d. **Problems and complications**
   (1) Paraplegia, although rare (a reported incidence of 0.4%), occurs unpredictably. It seems to be associated with poor collateralization and prolonged distal hypotension.
   (2) Hemorrhage
   (3) Paradoxical hypertension, often requiring treatment for weeks to months
   (4) Mesenteric arteritis with abdominal pain, thought to be secondary to reactive vasoconstriction and ischemia
   (5) Damage to adjacent structures, including the left recurrent laryngeal nerve (resulting in vocal cord paralysis), phrenic nerve (causing diaphragm paralysis), sympathetic trunk (causing Horner syndrome), and thoracic duct (causing a chylothorax)

C. Miscellaneous procedures

1. **Vascular rings**
   a. **General considerations.** Although the specific anatomy can vary, these anomalies of the aortic arch and its branches result in the presence of a blood vessel on each side of the trachea and esophagus. Encirclement of these structures generally causes significant symptoms that appear in infancy. These children may present with severe inspiratory stridor, dyspnea, wheezing, dysphagia, and a cough. Frequent respiratory infections are common, resulting from airway obstruction and aspiration from esophageal compression. Three types of vascular rings are likely (Fig. 14.22): (i) *Double aortic arch* (from persistence of the primitive double arch), (ii) *right aortic arch with left ductus arteriosus,* and (iii) *retroesophageal right subclavian artery* (resulting in an incomplete ring). PA sling is a rarer type of vascular ring that occurs when the left PA comes off the right PA and encircles the right main stem bronchus and distal trachea before going to the left lung.
   b. **Surgical procedures.** The surgical approach depends on the particular vascular anatomy. Repair is usually performed through a left thoracotomy. It is important to define the anatomy carefully to determine which vessel of the rings is expendable. This vessel is ligated and divided, and the ductus or ligamentum is divided to provide as much mobility as possible. Repair of a PA sling usually requires a median sternotomy and may require CPB. The left PA is divided from the right PA and reimplanted into the main PA anterior to the trachea. Many of these children will have complete tracheal rings and will require tracheoplasty.
   c. **Anesthetic considerations.** These children typically are small, with varying degrees of respiratory distress. Careful airway management is critical. Vascular rings can behave similar to an anterior mediastinal mass, with tracheal compression during induction of anesthesia. An inhalational induction is preferred, with neuromuscular blocking agents given only after the airway is secured. Multiple sizes of endotracheal tubes should be available.

      Monitoring should include an arterial line; in some cases, a central line may be advisable. Adequate venous access is mandatory, because significant bleeding occasionally occurs during this type of procedure. In infants with this lesion, intraoperative transesophageal echocardiography is probably contraindicated. It contributes little to the management of these patients, and limited space within the vascular ring may precipitate an airway crisis with probe placement.

      Many of these children have tracheomalacia from the vascular ring, and the condition often persists even after the ring is released. They often have significant secretions in their airways, because their cough has been ineffective due to the ring. In small children with preoperative respiratory distress, one should anticipate postoperative mechanical ventilation.

      Older children with incomplete rings and minimal symptoms often can be extubated at the end of the procedure. Effective pain management with either an epidural or patient-controlled analgesia can help facilitate postoperative management.
   d. **Problems and complications**
      (1) Hemorrhage

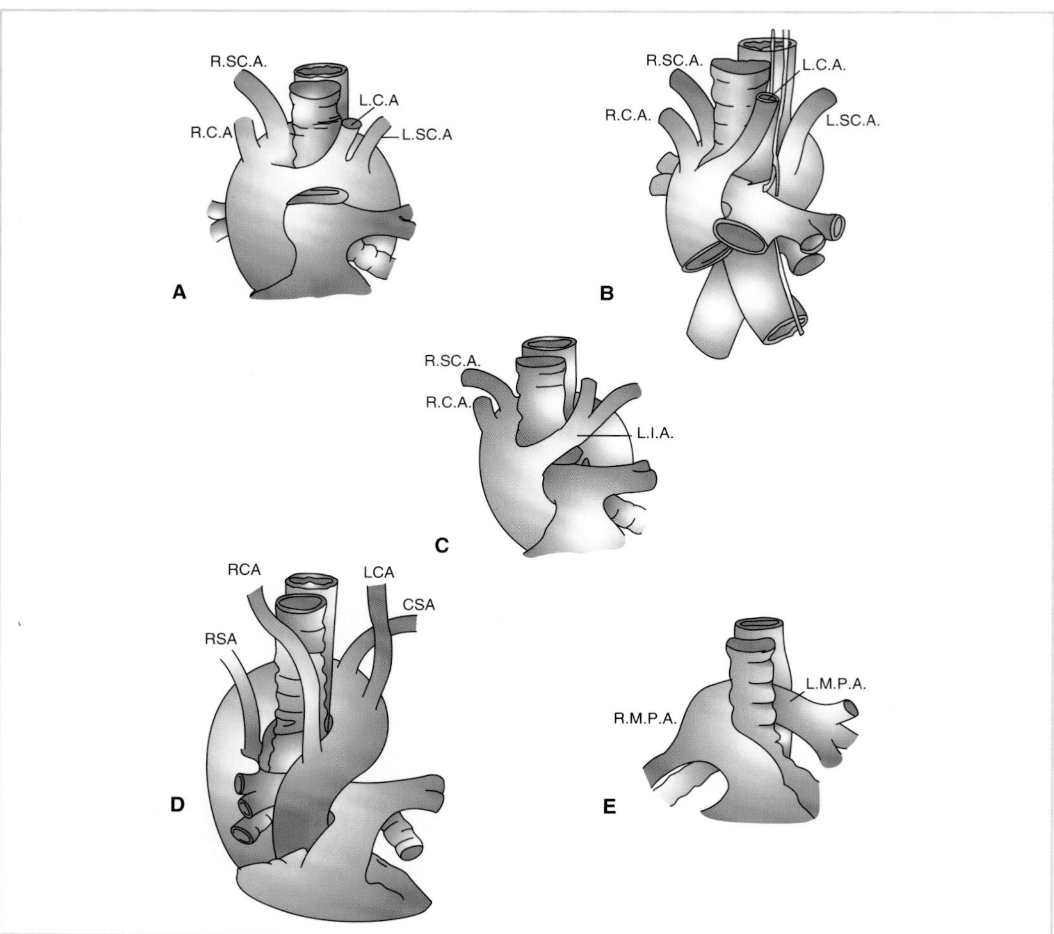

FIGURE 14.22 **A:** Double aortic arch. **B:** Right aortic arch with retroesophageal left subclavian artery. **C:** Right aortic arch with mirror-image branching and left ligamentum arteriosum. **D:** Left aortic arch with retroesophageal right subclavian artery and right ligamentum arteriosum. **E:** Anomalous left PA from right PA. LCA, left carotid artery; LMPA, left main PA; LSCA (LSA), left subclavian artery; RCA, right carotid artery; RMPA, right main PA; RSCA (RSA), right subclavian artery. (From Arciniegas E, ed. *Pediatric Cardiac Surgery.* Chicago, IL: Year Book; 1985:119, 122, 123, with permission.)

(2) Injuries to adjacent structures (phrenic nerve, recurrent laryngeal nerve, thoracic duct)

(3) Prolonged respiratory support

2. PA banding

a. General considerations. PA banding is performed when an infant has a cardiac lesion causing excessive pulmonary blood flow and pressures that is not amenable to primary repair. PA banding is now rarely performed, but it still has a place for patients in whom total repair is not technically feasible. It is important to palliate the situation with a PA band so that the lungs are not subjected to high flow and pressure for a long period, thus preventing permanent damage to the vasculature. The child can undergo a more definitive repair of the lesion at a later time. Infants scheduled for PA banding may have a wide variety of lesions, but the objective is the same: To limit PA flow and avoid irreversible PA hypertension. Application of the band will decrease some of the left-to-right shunt (without causing it to flow right to left) and improve systemic perfusion.

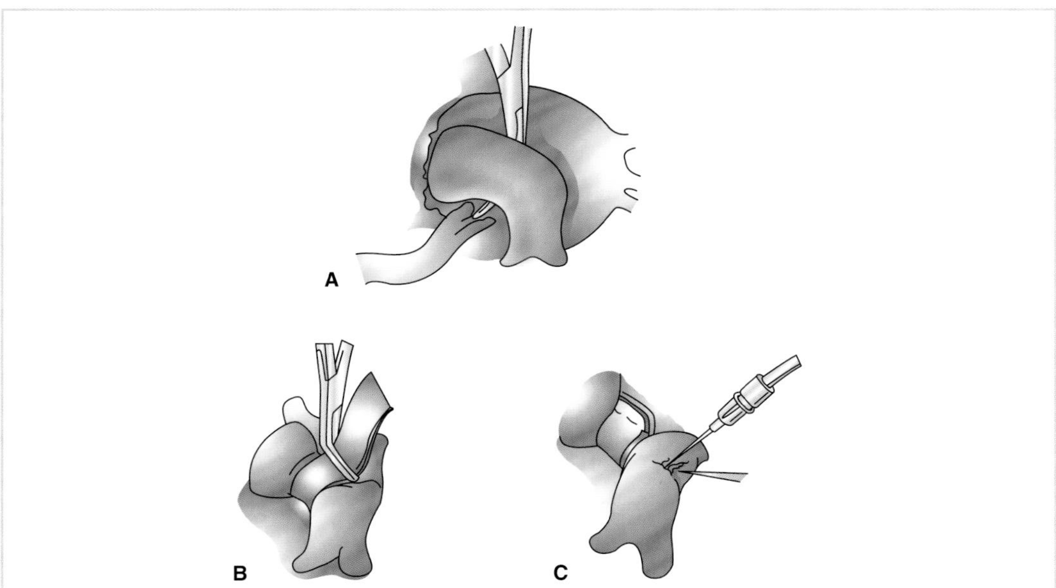

FIGURE 14.23 PA banding. The band is passed around the main PA **(A)** and is snugged down **(B)**. PA pressure measurements are obtained **(C)** to verify proper "tightness" of the band. (From Waldhausen JA, Pierce WS, eds. *Johnson's Surgery of the Chest*. Chicago, IL: Year Book; 1985:345, with permission.)

b. **Surgical procedure.** PA banding may be performed through a small left anterior thoracotomy or median sternotomy. A Silastic band is passed around the main PA and then a clip is used to tighten the band (Fig. 14.23). The goal is to limit the flow without causing hypoxemia. We generally measure pressures distal to the band and progressively tighten the band until the pressure distally is half the systemic pressure. As the band is tightened, one would expect to see an increase in systemic pressure as more blood is diverted from the lungs to the body.

c. **Anesthetic considerations.** This procedure is usually performed in infants with failure to thrive and complex cardiac anatomy. Premedication is usually not necessary. Both inhalational and intravenous inductions have been used successfully. The goals of therapy include keeping PVR high and SVR low, and minimizing myocardial depression. It is a good idea to avoid hyperoxia and hyperventilation to prevent pulmonary blood flow from increasing even more than baseline. The procedure is typically short, and if the child was not in respiratory distress preoperatively, extubation at the end of the case often can be accomplished.

   Careful attention must be paid to pulse oximetry and capnography during the banding. **Typically, the patient's saturation decreases, but rarely below 85%. A significant drop in end-tidal CO_2 can be an early warning sign that the band is too tight.**

d. **Problems and complications**
   (1) Inappropriate sizing of the band, either too loose or too tight
   (2) Migration of the band causing interference with blood flow to the right or left lung
   (3) Distortion and possible stenosis of the branch PAs

3. **Systemic-to-PA shunts**

a. **General considerations.** Children who are cyanotic because of inadequate pulmonary blood flow can be palliated with systemic-to-PA shunts. The partially saturated systemic arterial blood picks up more oxygen on its second pass through the lungs but then mixes with desaturated systemic venous return before being ejected into the systemic circulation. The resulting systemic saturation depends on the ratio of pulmonary-to-systemic

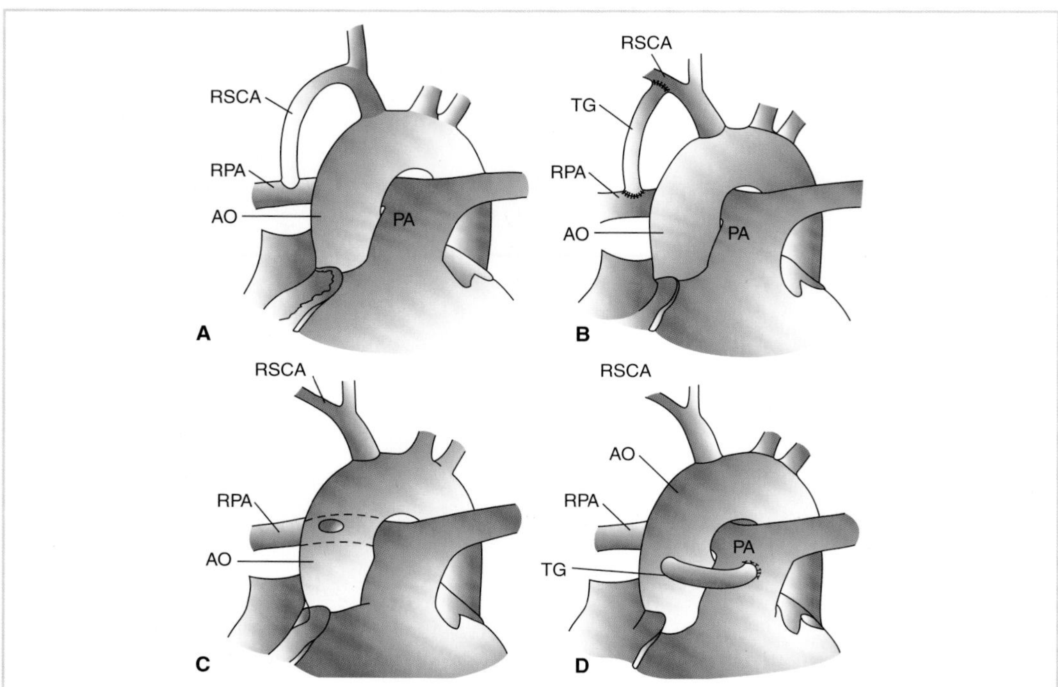

FIGURE 14.24 Types of systemic-to-PA anastomoses. **A:** Classic BT anastomosis. **B:** Modified BT shunt using prosthetic graft. **C:** Direct aortopulmonary (Waterston) anastomosis. **D:** Central aortopulmonary shunt with prosthetic graft. AO, aorta; RPA, right PA; RSCA, right subclavian artery; TG, tube graft. (From Hickey PR, Wessel DL. Anesthesia for treatment of congenital heart disease. In: Kaplan JA, ed. *Cardiac Anesthesia.* 2nd ed. Philadelphia, PA: Grune & Stratton; 1987:683, with permission.)

blood flow and the degree of desaturation of the mixed venous blood. In addition to improving systemic oxygen saturation, these shunts are often used to stimulate PA growth in children whose PAs are too small for definitive repair.

As the pulmonary blood flow exceeds the systemic blood flow, ventricular volume overload can result. The shunt size must be chosen carefully to prevent excessive pulmonary blood flow and systemic hypoperfusion. Long-term systemic-to-PA shunts can cause pulmonary vascular obstructive changes.

b. Surgical procedures. There are several different surgical procedures that have been used to deliver more blood to the lungs in children with inadequate pulmonary blood flow (Fig. 14.24). These include the BT shunt, the modified BT shunt, Potts, Waterston, and central shunt. The BT shunt (or the modified shunt) is used most commonly. The surgical approach is through a thoracotomy, usually on the side opposite to the aortic arch. In this procedure, the subclavian artery is identified, ligated, and anastomosed to the PA. In the modified version, the subclavian artery is left *in situ,* and a tube graft is sewn from the subclavian artery to the PA. Various shunts and their connections are listed in Table 14.12.

c. Anesthetic considerations. Some of these infants have pulmonary blood flow that is totally ductal dependent (e.g., pulmonary atresia) and come to the operating room on PGE_1. Clearly it is important to ensure that infusion is not interrupted. Others will have more dynamic obstruction (e.g., TOF) and may benefit from judicious sedation to prevent anxiety and crying. Oral midazolam at a dose of approximately 0.5 mg/kg works well. Inhalational induction is usually well tolerated and may help to relax the dynamic infundibular obstruction, if present.

TABLE 14.12 Systemic-to-pulmonary shunts

Shunt	Anastomosis	Complications
Classic BT	Right subclavian artery to right PA (with left aortic arch)	Kinking of right PA, right arm ischemia, excessive pulmonary flow
Modified BT	Tube graft from right (or left) subclavian artery to right (or left) PA	Kinking of right PA, tube graft does not allow for growth, chylothorax
Waterston	Ascending aorta to right PA	Kinking of right PA, amount of blood flow difficult to control
Potts	Descending aorta to left PA	Rarely used, difficult to control shunt size, and difficult takedown at later repair
Central (aortic–pulmonary shunt)	Anastomosis between aorta and PA with tube graft	Distortion of main PA, excessive pulmonary flow
Glenn	Superior vena cava to right PA	Thrombosis, superior vena cava syndrome, insufficient pulmonary blood flow, pulmonary arteriovenous fistula

BT, Blalock–Taussig; PA, pulmonary artery.

One should use maneuvers to try to decrease PVR and promote pulmonary blood flow. High oxygen concentration, hyperventilation, and avoidance of metabolic acidosis are helpful. One must recognize that end-tidal CO_2 will underestimate arterial P_aCO_2 during this procedure because the branch PA is clamped and not perfused. Measurement of arterial blood gases can be helpful in guiding management. The arterial catheter must be placed in the arm opposite to the surgical procedure during a BT shunt because the subclavian artery will be clamped.

After the shunt is complete and open, the lung should be re-expanded and ventilated. The shunt size can be assessed by temporarily clamping and unclamping the shunt and watching the hemodynamics. One should expect to see a drop in systemic blood pressure when the shunt is open. **A decrease in mean arterial blood pressure of more than 10 mm Hg suggests that the shunt is too large.** Excessive pulmonary blood flow can cause systemic hypoperfusion, pulmonary edema, and metabolic acidosis. Difficulty weaning from the ventilator might occur. On the other hand, one would like to use a shunt as large as the child can tolerate in order to promote PA growth. Getting the right balance is critical.

It may be feasible to extubate older infants at the end of the procedure. Smaller neonates may benefit from overnight mechanical ventilation and diuresis.

d. Problems and complications

(1) Inappropriate size shunt, either too large or too small

(2) Problems specific to the type of shunt used (listed in Table 14.12)

X. Noncardiac surgery

The care of patients with CHD undergoing noncardiac surgery often is more challenging than caring for them during corrective repair. Likely scenarios for which these patients will require an anesthetic include the following:

A. Diagnostic workup before planned cardiac repair. These children may require an anesthetic for cardiac catheterization, magnetic resonance imaging, or transesophageal echocardiography. It is ideal to provide an anesthetic that replicates their baseline condition as closely as possible so that measurements of pressures and resistances will be representative. It is particularly important to deliver an inspired oxygen concentration close to room air with a normal P_aCO_2. A retrospective review of cardiac catheterizations in infants and children showed a significant incidence (9.3%) of adverse incidents, especially in children less than 1 yr of age undergoing therapeutic interventions [34].

B. Dental procedures before planned cardiac repair. Removal of carious or infected teeth with dental restoration may be indicated before cardiac surgery in order to remove a potential source of infection. This may be particularly important if synthetic material is to be implanted during the cardiac repair.

C. After surgical palliation or correction for elective noncardiac surgery. In this situation, it is imperative that the team has access to the old records and cardiology follow-up to ensure that the patient's condition is optimized. Knowing the patient's physiology and anatomy is necessary to develop a rational anesthetic plan. Not all patients are left with a perfect cardiac surgical repair, and one must understand what residual problems exist. Occasionally it is appropriate to delay elective surgery until further cardiac surgery is performed.

D. Emergent noncardiac surgery. This situation is particularly problematic because there may be no time to obtain old medical records or ensure that the patient is in optimal condition.

E. Pregnancy with labor and delivery or cesarean section. As more children have undergone successful cardiac repair, many of them are reaching childbearing age. Understanding their particular physiology allows one to individualize their care. See the following chapter for a more complete discussion of care of the adult patient with CHD.

F. Surgery for the patient with inoperable cardiac disease. Occasionally patients with this problem (for example, intracardiac shunt with pulmonary vascular disease and Eisenmenger physiology) will present for noncardiac surgery. The risks in this scenario are tremendous, and the patient and family should be informed of the prognosis and participate in the decision-making process as to whether the surgery should go forward. Careful monitoring and postoperative management are required for even the most superficial cases.

Preoperative testing before noncardiac surgery is somewhat dependent on the type and extent of the planned procedure. A Hct and coagulation profile is particularly important in patients who are cyanotic. Echocardiographic and cardiac catheterization data should be reviewed to assess the (a) type and severity of the lesion, (b) ventricular function, (c) status of the pulmonary vasculature, and (d) response to pulmonary vasodilators. Many patients will require bacterial endocarditis prophylaxis as dictated by the American Heart Association [32] One issue of concern regarding monitoring is that the end-tidal CO_2 measurement often is inaccurate as an estimate of P_aCO_2, particularly in cyanotic children. The extremity in which the blood pressure is taken also may be important. One should avoid the arm on the side of a BT shunt, because the subclavian artery is no longer supplying blood to that arm. In a patient with coarctation of the aorta, blood pressure should be measured in the right arm, since the other extremities may be distal to the obstruction. The patient with supravalvar aortic stenosis will have an artifactually elevated right arm blood pressure.

Care of the patient undergoing noncardiac surgery should be similar to that provided during cardiac surgery. It is critically important to understand the patient's individual physiology and to develop hemodynamic goals for the particular lesion.

REFERENCES

1. Hoffman JIE. Incidence of congenital heart disease: I. Postnatal incidence. *Pediatr Cardiol.* 1995;16:103–113.
2. Steward DJ, DaSilva CA, Flegel T. Elevated glucose levels may increase the danger of neurological deficit following profoundly hypothermic cardiac arrest. *Anesthesiology.* 1988;68:653.
3. Burrows FA. Neurologic protection in pediatric cardiac surgery. In: Society of Cardiovascular Anesthesiologists 20th Annual Meeting 1998 Workshops, Seattle, WA, April 25–29, 1998.
4. Newburger JW, Jonas RA, Wernovsky G, et al. A comparison of the perioperative neurologic effects of hypothermic circulatory arrest versus low flow cardiopulmonary bypass in infant heart surgery. *N Engl J Med.* 1993;329:1057–1064.
5. Bellinger DC, Wypij D, Kuban KCK, et al. Developmental and neurological status of children at 4 years of age after heart surgery with hypothermic circulatory arrest or low-flow cardiopulmonary bypass. *Circulation.* 1999;100:526–532.
6. DuPlessis AJ. Mechanisms of brain injury during infant cardiac surgery. *Semin Pediatr Neurol.* 1999;6:32–47.
7. Swain JA, McDonald TJ, Robbins RC, et al. Relationship of cerebral and myocardial intracellular pH to blood pH during hypothermia. *Am J Physiol.* 1991;260:H1640–H1644.
8. Murkin JM, Martzke JS, Buchan AM, et al. A randomized study of the influence of perfusion technique and pH management strategy in 316 patients undergoing coronary artery bypass surgery. II. Neurologic and cognitive outcomes. *J Thorac Cardiovasc Surg.* 1995;110:349–362.
9. Aoki M, Nomura F, Stromski ME, et al. Effects of pH on brain energetics after hypothermic circulatory arrest. *Ann Thorac Surg.* 1993;55:1093–1103.

10. Skaryak LA, Chai PJ, Kern FH, et al. Blood gas management and degree of cooling: Effects on cerebral metabolism before and after circulatory arrest. *J Thorac Cardiovasc Surg.* 1995;110:1649–1657.
11. Kirshbom PM, Skaryak LA, DiBernardo LR, et al. pH-stat cooling improves cerebral metabolic recovery after circulatory arrest in a piglet model of aorto-pulmonary collaterals. *J Thorac Cardiovasc Surg.* 1996;111:147–157.
12. DuPlessis AJ, Jonas RA, Wypij D, et al. Perioperative effects of alpha-stat versus pH-stat strategies for deep hypothermic cardiopulmonary bypass in infants. *J Thorac Cardiovasc Surg.* 1997;114:990–1001.
13. Vannucci RC. Mechanisms of perinatal ischemic brain damage. In: Jonas RA, Newburger JW, Volpe JJ, eds. *Brain Injury and Pediatric Cardiac Surgery.* Boston, MA: Butterworth-Heinemann; 1996:201–214.
14. Tweddell JS, Hoffman GM. Postoperative management in patients with complex congenital heart disease. *Semin Thorac Cardiovasc Surg Pediatr Card Surg Annu.* 2002;5:187–205.
15. Hirsch JH, Charpie JR, Ohye RG, et al. Near infrared spectroscopy (NIRS) should not be standard of care for postoperative management. *Semin Thorac Cardiovasc Surg Pediatr Card Surg Annu.* 2010;13(1):51–54.
16. Jonas R. Neurological protection during cardiopulmonary bypass/deep hypothermia. *Pediatr Cardiol.* 1998;19:321–330.
17. Boldt J, Knothe C, Zickmann B, et al. Comparison of two aprotinin dosage regimens in pediatric patients having cardiac operations: Influence on platelet function and blood loss. *J Thorac Cardiovasc Surg.* 1993;105:705–711.
18. D'Errico CC, Shayevitz JR, Martindale SJ, et al. The efficacy and cost of aprotinin in children undergoing reoperative open heart surgery. *Anesth Analg.* 1996;83:1193–1199.
19. Paparella D, Brister SJ, Buchannan MR. Coagulation disorders of cardiopulmonary bypass: A review. *Intensive Care Med.* 2004;30:1873–1881.
20. Osthaus WA, Boethig D, Johanning K, et al. Whole blood coagulation measured by modified thrombelastography (ROTEM) is impaired in infants with congenital heart diseases. *Blood Coagul Fibrinolysis.* 2008;19:220–225.
21. Romlin BS, Wahlander H, Berggren H, et al. Intraoperative thromboelastometry is associated with reduced transfusion prevalence in pediatric cardiac surgery. *Anesth Analg.* 2011;112:30–36.
22. Moganasudndram S, Hunt BJ, Sykes K, et al. The relationship among thromboelastography, hemostatic variables and bleeding after cardiopulmonary bypass surgery in children. *Anesth Analg.* 2010;110:995–1002.
23. Elliott MJ. Ultrafiltration and modified ultrafiltration in pediatric open-heart operations. *Ann Thorac Surg.* 1993;56:1518–1522.
24. Naik SK, Knight A, Elliott MJ. A prospective randomized study of a modified technique of ultrafiltration during pediatric open-heart surgery. *Circulation.* 1991;84:III-422–III-431.
25. Friesen RH, Campbell DN, Clarke DR, et al. Modified ultrafiltration attenuates dilutional coagulopathy in pediatric open-heart operations. *Ann Thorac Surg.* 1997;64:1787–1789.
26. Davies MJ, Nguyen K, Gaynor JW, et al. Modified ultrafiltration improves left ventricular systolic function in infants after cardiopulmonary bypass. *J Thorac Cardiovasc Surg.* 1998;115:361–370.
27. Bando K, Vijay P, Turrentine MW, et al. Dilutional and modified ultrafiltration reduces pulmonary hypertension after operations for congenital heart disease: A prospective randomized study. *J Thorac Cardiovasc Surg.* 1998;115:517–527.
28. Andreasson S, Gothberg S, Berggren H, et al. Hemofiltration modifies complement activation after extracorporeal circulation in infants. *Ann Thorac Surg.* 1993;56:1515–1517.
29. Skaryak LA, Kirshbom P, DiBernardo LR, et al. Modified ultrafiltration improves cerebral metabolic recovery after circulatory arrest. *J Thorac Cardiovasc Surg.* 1995;109:744–752.
30. Seifert HA, Jobes DR, Ten Have T, et al. Adverse events after protamine administration following cardiopulmonary bypass in infants and children. *Anesth Analg.* 2003;97:383–389.
31. Botero M, Davies LK. Diagnosis and management of arrhythmias in children after cardiac surgery. *Semin Cardiothorac Vasc Anesth.* 2001;5:122–133.
32. Wilson W, Taubert KA, Gewitz M, et al. Prevention of infective endocarditis. Guidelines from the American Heart Association. A guideline from the American Heart Association Rheumatic Fever, Endocarditis, and Kawasaki Disease Committee, Council on Cardiovascular Disease in the Young, and the Council on Clinical Cardiology, Council on Cardiovascular Surgery and Anesthesia, and the Quality of Care and Outcomes Research Interdisciplinary Working Group. *Circulation.* 2007;106:1–19.
33. Sano S, Ishino K, Kado H, et al. Outcome of right ventricle-to-pulmonary artery shunt in first-stage palliation of hypoplastic left heart syndrome: A multi-institutional study. *Ann Thorac Surg.* 2004;78:1951–1958.
34. Bennett D, Marcus R, Stokes M. Incidents and complications during pediatric cardiac catheterization. *Paediatr Anaesth.* 2005;15:1083–1088.

15

Anesthetic Management for Patients with Congenital Heart Disease: The Adult Population

Nathaen S. Weitzel, S. Adil Husain, and Laurie K. Davies

KEY POINTS

1. In adult CHD, a clinically relevant classification of lesions into three categories is useful: (1) Complete surgical correction, (2) partial surgical correction or palliation, and (iii) uncorrected CHD.
2. Over 1 million patients with congenital heart disease have reached adulthood in the United States.
3. Improvements in surgical techniques have allowed 90% of children with CHD to survive to adulthood with relatively normal functionality.
4. Ventricular and atrial arrhythmias are extremely common in adult CHD, accounting for nearly 50% of emergency hospitalizations.
5. Adult CHD patients have an incidence of pulmonary artery hypertension (PAH) as high as 10%.
6. Patients with PAH have a high surgical mortality rate (4% to 24%).
7. For both cyanotic (right-to-left shunts) and left-to-right shunts, there are general principles that impact anesthetic management.
8. Patients with complicated residual lesions requiring medium- to high-risk surgery should be managed at centers of excellence with physicians and staff trained in adult congenital disease.

I. Introduction

In 1938, Robert Gross performed the first ligation of a patent ductus arteriosus (PDA), thus initiating a major advance in congenital heart surgery and paving the way for development of modern surgical techniques [1]. Major improvements followed, with significant improvements in mortality throughout the 70s and 80s, leading to a greater survival. In 2000, the 32nd Bethesda Conference report generated from the American College of Cardiology indicated that approximately 85% of patients operated on with congenital heart disease (CHD) survive to adulthood [2]. It was estimated that 800,000 patients with adult congenital heart disease (ACHD) were in the United States in 2000. This report highlighted the importance of an emerging problem in our health care system. The issue is how to develop a model for seamless transition of care of patients presently cared for at pediatric heart centers who now must move into the adult population and adult hospitals. There has been a widespread call for an increased number of physicians capable of providing continuity of care for these patients in an outpatient setting, as well as during the perioperative period. This section will focus on the specific issues facing the patient with ACHD as they enter the perioperative period as it relates to the anesthesiologist.

II. Epidemiology

A. Defining ACHD: Attempts to establish prevalence and even mortality data for ACHD depend on the defining characteristics of which patients to include. A strict definition of ACHD was proposed by Mitchell et al., "a gross structural abnormality of the heart or intrathoracic great vessels that is actually or possibly of functional significance" [3]. This definition excludes persistent left-sided vena cava, abnormalities of major arteries, and in addition excludes bicuspid aortic valve (AV) disease, mitral valve prolapse, and the like [4].

B. Classification: A pathologic categorization scheme divides patients into categories of great complexity, moderate complexity, and simple CHD [5,6] (Table 15.1). These categories are particularly helpful in neonatal disease, as well as to establish prevalence data. In ACHD, a
1 different categorization approach may be more clinically relevant and will be utilized later in this section. These three categories are listed below [7]:

1. **Complete surgical correction**
   a. Examples include repaired atrial septal defect (ASD), ventricular septal defect (VSD), and PDA without hemodynamic sequelae.
2. **Partial surgical correction or palliation**
   a. Examples include palliative repairs such as Fontan, tetrology of Fallot (ToF), and transposition of great arteries (TGA) (Mustard repair), leaving hemodynamic or physiologic compromise.

TABLE 15.1 Adult congenital heart disease classification [7]

Simple	Moderate complexity	Great complexity

• Minor ASD
• Minor VSD
• Mild PS
• Congenital valve disease
• Aortic or mitral
	• Anomalous pulmonary venous drainage
	• AV canal defects
	• Tetralogy of Fallot
	• Ebstein's anomaly
	• Coarctation of aorta
	• Right ventricular outflow obstruction
	• ASD
	  • Ostium primum
	  • Sinus venosus
	• Persistent PDA
	• PV disease
	  • Stenotic or regurgitant lesions
	• Fistula:
	  • Aorto–LV
	  • Sinus of valsalva
	• VSD associated with the following:
	  • Valve abnormality (mitral, tricuspid)
	  • Aortic insufficiency
	  • RVOTO
	  • Stenotic lesions (AV, RVOT)
	• AV disease
	• Subaortic stenosis
	• Supra-aortic stenosis
		• Single ventricle lesions and Fontan physiology
		  • TA
		  • Mitral atresia
		• Eisenmenger's physiology
		• Cyanotic CHD
		• Existence of conduits—either with valve or without
		• Presence of intracardiac baffles
		• TGV
		  • Jatene procedure
		  • Mustard procedure
		• Truncus arteriosus/hemitruncus

ASD, adult atrial septal defect; VSD, ventricular septal defect; AV, aortic valve; TA, tricuspid atresia; PS, pulmonary stenosis; CHD, congenital heart disease; TGV, transposition of the great vessels; PV, pulmonary valve; LV, left ventricle; RVOTO, right ventricular outflow tract obstruction.

Adapted with permission from Warnes CA, Williams RG, Bashore TM, et al. ACC/AHA 2008 Guidelines for the management of adults with congenital heart disease: Executive summary: A report of the American College of Cardiology/American Heart Association Task Force on Practice Guidelines. *Circulation.* 2008;118:2395–2451.

3. **Uncorrected CHD**
   a. Examples include minor ASD, minor VSD, Ebstein's anomaly, or undiagnosed ACHD due to limited health care access as child.

C. **Prevalence**

2 1. The actual number of adult patients with congenital heart defects is difficult to obtain; however, recent estimates suggest that over 1 million patients have reached adulthood in the United States, with an additional 8,500 corrected each year [4,8]. Significant
3 improvements in surgical techniques have allowed many patients (>90% of children with CHD) to survive to adulthood, and maintain relatively normal function [2,4,8].

2. **Select populations**
   a. A recent estimate from Canada reported 11.89 cases per 1,000 children and 4.09 cases per 1,000 adults with CHD. Selecting out patients with complex ACHD (Table 15.1) reduces these estimates to 1.45 per 1,000 children and 0.38 per 1,000 adult cases.
   b. ACHD becomes a significant issue in certain populations such as obstetrics where patients with CHD now represent the majority (60% to 80%) of obstetric patients with cardiac disease. This population is in general young and healthy, so it makes sense that as patients with CHD reach childbearing age, they begin to represent a higher proportion of patients in this group with cardiac disease.

3. **Survival data**
   a. It is estimated that 96% of newborns who survive the first year will reach the age of 16 [4].
   b. Median expected survival has increased significantly since 2000, with current estimates placing the median age of death for ACHD at 57 yrs [4].

D. **Health care system considerations**

1. The ACC/AHA 2008 guidelines for ACHD highlight the fact that the pediatric cardiology centers have significant infrastructure to support patients with CHD, but that this is largely lacking in the adult health care system. This includes access to physicians with training in ACHD, as well as advanced practice nursing, case management, and social workers familiar with the needs of these patients [9]. These guidelines echo the recommendations made by the Bethesda Conference, as well as the Canadian Cardiovascular Society Consensus Conference statements from 2010 [2,10–15].
2. Overall recommendations taken from these reports suggest a focus on improvement in ACHD health care delivery through the following:
   a. Improved transition clinics for adolescents approaching adulthood
   b. Outreach programs to educate patients and families of key issues related to their disease
   c. Enhanced education of adult caregivers trained in ACHD management
   d. Coordination of health care delivery through regional centers of excellence
   e. Development of primary-care physicians with ready referral access to these regional centers of excellence
3. Centers of excellence
   a. The services and provider requirements for such centers are summarized in Table 15.2, taken from the 2008 ACC/AHA guidelines. Key areas with physicians specializing in ACHD are indicated.

III. What are the key anesthetic considerations in ACHD?

To evaluate the ACHD patient prior to surgery, the anesthesiologist must gain an understanding of the patient's medical history, current functional status, state of surgical repair, and overall health. Key items are discussed below.

A. **History:** Obtaining a thorough and accurate surgical and medical history is critical, however challenging, as only half of patients with ACHD are able to correctly describe their diagnosis [16]. Patients with ACHD have varying functional capacities which may make evaluation of true cardiac capacity more challenging.

B. **Signs and symptoms of ACHD:** Some generalized exam findings that may indicate ACHD include the following [17]:

1. Continuous heart murmurs: There are relatively few acquired cardiac diseases producing a continuous type of murmur.
2. Right bundle branch block (RBBB): This can occur in the general population; however, if found in conjunction with a continuous murmur, this may indicate a congenital defect.
3. Evidence of cyanosis without existing pulmonary disease
4. The above findings should trigger an echocardiographic study prior to surgical care.

C. **How can you assess the perioperative risk for ACHD patients?**

Anesthetic evaluation should focus on predicting risk of surgery in this patient population. Some key prognostic indicators for outcomes in ACHD surgery (both cardiac and noncardiac) include the presence of the below-listed factors [7,9,16,18] (Table 15.3):

1. Pulmonary arterial hypertension (PAH)
2. Cyanosis or residual VSD
3. Need for reoperation (cardiac surgery)
4. Arrhythmias
5. Ventricular dysfunction
6. Single ventricle physiology or a systemic right ventricle

IV. What common sequelae are associated with ACHD?

In contrast to the neonate with CHD, ACHD patients begin to acquire additional medical comorbidities that should be considered in management planning. Common comorbidities in this patient population are listed in Table 15.3, and preoperative evaluation should take these into account. Cardiac arrhythmias, pulmonary hypertension, ventricular dysfunction, cyanosis (or residual VSD), valve abnormalities, and aneurysms represent some of the key comorbid conditions commonly associated with ACHD that have serious management considerations and result in

TABLE 15.2 Summary of qualifications for regional centers of excellence in adult congenital heart disease

Cardiologist specializing in ACHD	One or several 24/7
Congenital cardiac surgeon	Two or several 24/7
Nurse/physician assistant/nurse practitioner	One or several
Cardiac anesthesiologist	Several 24/7
Echocardiography[a] • **Includes TEE, intraoperative TEE**	Two or several 24/7
Diagnostic catheterization[a]	Yes, 24/7
Noncoronary interventional catheterization[a]	Yes, 24/7
Electrophysiology/pacing/AICD implantation[a]	One or several
Exercise testing	• Echocardiography • Radionuclide • Cardiopulmonary • Metabolic
Cardiac imaging/radiology[a]	• Cardiac MRI • CT scanning • Nuclear medicine
Multidisciplinary teams	• High-risk obstetrics • Pulmonary hypertension • Heart failure/transplant • Genetics • Neurology • Nephrology • Cardiac pathology • Rehabilitation services • Social services • Vocational services • Financial counselors
Information technology	• Data collection • Database support • Quality assessment review/protocols

[a]These modalities must be supervised/performed and interpreted by physicians with expertise and training in CHD.
ACHD, adult congenital heart disease; 24/7, availability 24 h/day, 7 days/wk; TEE, transesophageal echocardiography; AICD, automatic implantable cardioverter defibrillator; MRI, magnetic resonance imaging; CT, computed tomography.
Reproduced from Warnes, CA, Williams RG, Bashore TM, et al. ACC/AHA 2008 Guidelines for the management of adults with congenital heart disease: Executive summary: A report of the American College of Cardiology/American Heart Association Task Force on Practice Guidelines. *Circulation.* 2008;118(23): 2395–2451, with permission.

overall increased perioperative risk [4]. Obtaining a detailed history on the degree of involvement of these issues will enable adequate planning in management. Two of the most common and critical areas (arrhythmias and pulmonary hypertension) will be addressed here.

A. **Arrhythmias: Ventricular and atrial arrhythmias are extremely common in ACHD**
4 **patients accounting for nearly 50% of emergency hospitalizations** [7]. The type of rhythm disturbance depends primarily on the lesion and method of surgical repair. Tables 15.4 and 15.5 divide the bradyarrhythmias from tachyarrhythmias by lesion type.

1. In general, patients who fall in the moderate to complex categories are at higher risk for arrhythmias. **Tetralogy of Fallot** (Fig. 15.1) **and Fontan lesions carry an extremely high arrhythmia burden** [19,20]. **In addition, any patient with a ventricular repair or patch is at high risk for ventricular rhythm disturbances, while those patients with atrial repairs, atrial baffles, etc., are likely to develop atrial arrhythmias** [20].
2. Patients with right-sided lesions have a higher likelihood of developing arrhythmias, although the morbidity/mortality results are similar between right- and left-sided lesions [21].

TABLE 15.3 Common medical concerns in patients with ACHD [16]

Comorbidities associated with ACHD: • Cardiac arrhythmias • Pulmonary hypertension • Ventricular dysfunction • Cyanosis • Valve abnormalities • Aneurysm	**Common non–ACHD-related comorbidities:** • Systemic hypertension • Coronary artery disease • Diabetes mellitus • Renal insufficiency • Chronic lung disease • Cholelithiasis • Nephrolithiasis

Complications related to ACHD:
• Erythrocytosis
• Developmental delay
• Central nervous system defects
  • Previous ischemic/embolic events
  • Seizures
  • Intracranial abscesses
• Endocarditis
	Conditions associated with elevated surgical risk:
	• PAH
	• Cyanosis or residual VSD
	• Need for repeat sternotomy
	• Arrhythmias
	• Ventricular dysfunction
	• Single ventricle physiology or a systemic right ventricle

ACHD, adult congenital heart disease; PAH, pulmonary arterial hypertension; VSD, ventricular septal defect.

3. Patients with either ASD or VSD can have interruption in the normal conduction pathways or abnormal variants such as duplicate AV nodes (Fig. 15.2), leading to re-entrant arrhythmias [20].
4. **Management**
   a. **Antiarrhythmic** medical therapy remains the mainstay for most patients, although results are often suboptimal in many cases such as intra-atrial re-entrant tachycardia (IART), despite the use of potent agents such as amiodarone [20].
   b. **Ablative procedures:** Recent advances in electrophysiology have allowed significant improvements in management of these rhythm disturbances. Electrophysiologists are able to map out the conduction pathways in the heart, and ablate malignant tracts

TABLE 15.4 Tachyarrhythmias associated with ACHD [4,7,20]

Lesion[a]	VT	IART	AF	WPW
Tetralogy of Fallot				
• **Repaired**	++	++	+	–
• **Native**	+		–	–
Ebstein's anomaly	+	+	–	++
TGA				
• **Mustard/Senning**	++	++	–	–
• **Jatene**	–	–		–
• **cc**	+			+
Single ventricle Fontan	–	++	+	–
Congenital AV stenosis	+	–	+	–
LVOT obstruction	++	–	+	–
ASD	–	–	+	–
• **Sinus venosus**	–	–	+	–
VSD	+	–	–	–
AVSD	+	–	–	–

[a]All lesions listed are considered to have surgical correction or palliation unless noted as native and listed in order of degree of arrhythmia burden. – denotes rare manifestations. + denotes common occurrence. ++ denotes frequent occurrence.
ACHD, adult congenital heart disease; VT, ventricular tachycardia; IART, intra-atrial reentrant tachycardia; AF, atrial fibrillation; WPW, Wolff–Parkinson–White syndrome; TGA, transposition of great arteries; cc, congenitally corrected; LVOT, left ventricular outflow tract; ASD, atrial septal defect; VSD, ventricular septal defect; AVSD, atrioventricular septal defect.

TABLE 15.5 Bradyarrhythmias associated with ACHD [4,7,20]

Bradyarrhythmias associated with ACHD [4,7,20]	
Sinus node dysfunction	**AV block**
• Single ventricle lesions (Fontan physiology)[a]	• VSD
• ccTGA	• AVSD
	• LVOT obstruction
	• TGA (Senning/Mustard)

ccTGA, congenitally corrected; LVOT, left ventricular outflow tract; ASD, Atrial Septal Defect; VSD, Ventricular Septal Defect; AVSD, atrioventricular septal defect.

(Figs. 15.1 and 15.3). This is most useful for atrial arrhythmias, with short-term success rates nearing 90% [20]. Long-term outcomes following ablation are less promising and not widely reported. de Groot et al. reported a 59% recurrence after the initial ablation, with the location of the recurrent pathway being different for all but one patient. At 5 yrs, 58% of patients were in sinus rhythm and 33% of the initial population were maintained on antiarrhythmic drug therapy [22]. Electrophysiologic testing and ablative procedures are considered a Class I recommendation for patients with known rhythm disturbances [9].

c. **Implantable devices:** For patients at risk for ventricular arrhythmias, automatic implantable cardiac defibrillators (AICD) can offer a life-saving modality and are a class II recommendation for ACHD patients [9]. **While ventricular tachycardia (VT) is rare in the first and second decades, it becomes increasingly prevalent as the patient ages, with those patients with a history of ventricular intervention being at highest risk** [20]. VT circuits can develop a macro–re-entrant characteristic similar to the atrial IART (Fig. 15.3). ToF patients have a high risk, and a careful history should be obtained, inquiring about symptoms and any outpatient studies. Patients at risk for

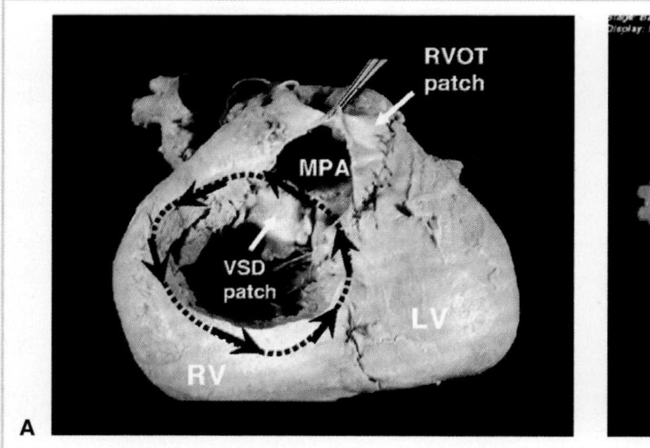

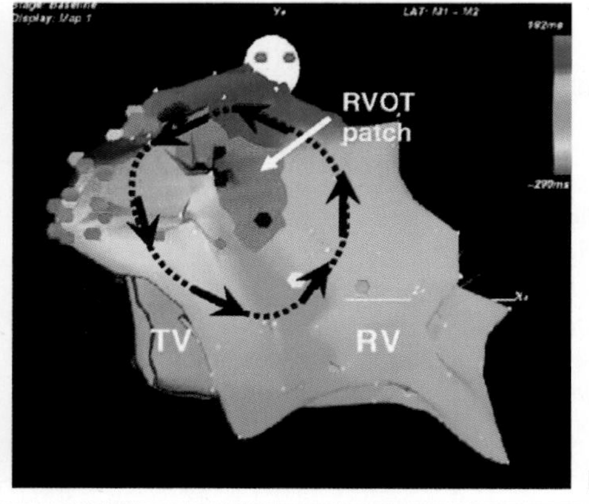

FIGURE 15.1 Macro–re-entrant VT in tetralogy of Fallot. **A:** An autopsy specimen of repaired tetralogy with the anterior RV surface opened to reveal the VSD patch and the patch-augmented RVOT (the outflow patch in this case is transannular). A hypothetical re-entry circuit is traced onto this image (*black arrows*), with the superior portion of the loop traveling through the conal septum (upper rim of the VSD). **B:** Actual electroanatomic map of sustained VT from an adult tetralogy patient, showing a nearly identical circuit. The propagation pattern is shown by the *black arrows* and is reflected by the color scheme (red > yellow > green > blue > purple). A narrow conduction channel was found between the rightward edge of the outflow patch scar (*gray area*) and the superior rim of the tricuspid valve. A cluster of radiofrequency applications at this site (*pink dots*) closed off the channel and permanently eliminated this VT circuit. LV, left ventricle; MPA, main pulmonary artery; TV, tricuspid valve. (Reused with permission from Walsh EP, Cecchin F. Congenital heart disease for the adult cardiologist: Arrhythmias in adult patients with congenital heart disease. *Circulation.* 2007;115:534–545.)

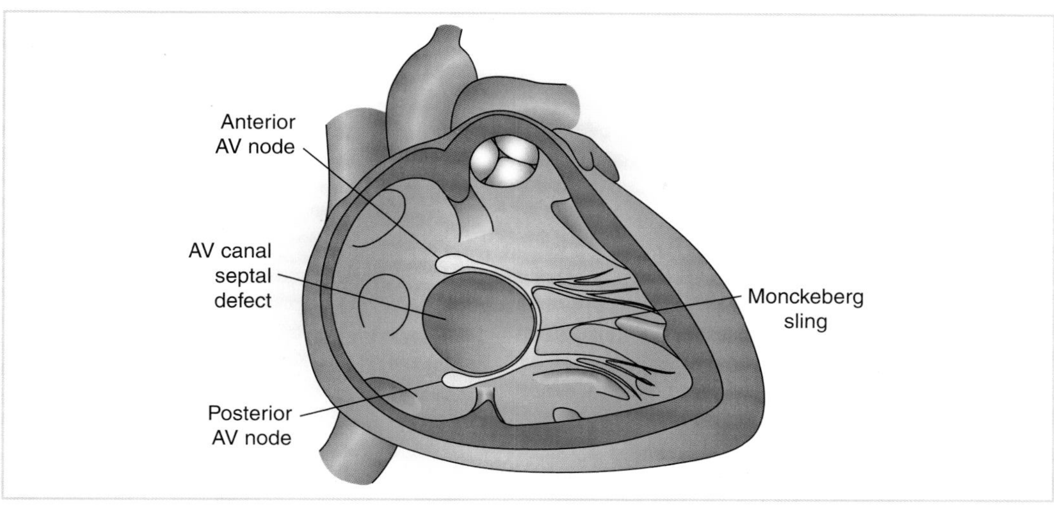

FIGURE 15.2 Representation of twin AV nodes with a Mönckeberg sling. The cardiac anatomy in this sketch includes a large septal defect in the AV canal region, shown in a right anterior oblique projection. Both an anterior and a posterior AV node are depicted (each with its own His bundle) along with a connecting "sling" between the two systems. This conduction arrangement can produce two distinct non–pre-excited QRS morphologies (depending on which AV node is engaged earliest by the atrial activation wave front), and a variety of re-entrant tachycardias. (Redrawn from Walsh EP, Cecchin F. Congenital heart disease for the adult cardiologist: Arrhythmias in adult patients with congenital heart disease. *Circulation*. 2007;115:534–545.)

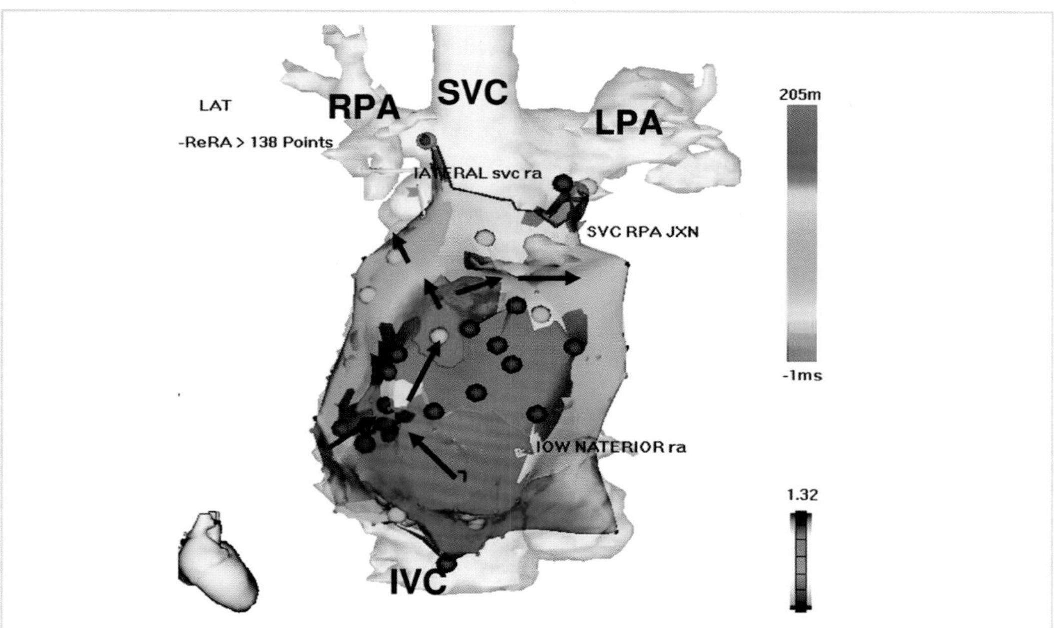

FIGURE 15.3 Electroanatomic map of an IART circuit involving the anterolateral surface of the right atrium in a patient with a previous Fontan operation (cavopulmonary connection). A detailed anatomic shell was generated for the ablation procedure by merging high-resolution computed tomography data with real-time data gathered from the 3D mapping catheter. The propagation pattern for the IART circuit is shown by *black arrows* and is also reflected by the color scheme (red > yellow > green > blue > purple). The critical component of the circuit appeared to be a narrow conduction channel through a region of scar (*central gray area*). A cluster of radiofrequency applications (*maroon dots*) was placed at the entrance zone to this narrow channel and permanently eliminated this IART circuit. LPA, left pulmonary artery; RPA, right pulmonary artery; RA, right atrium; JXN, junction; LAT, lateral. (Reused with permission from Walsh EP, Cecchin F. Congenital heart disease for the adult cardiologist: Arrhythmias in adult patients with congenital heart disease. *Circulation*. 2007;115:534–545.)

bradyarrhythmias often will have a pacemaker in place, which should be interrogated and sensitivity limits adjusted for the surgical procedure [18].

(1) **Anesthetic management:** The most recent practice advisory (2011) for patients with implanted cardiac devices recommends that AICD's be disabled prior to surgery to prevent inadvertent defibrillation due to electrocautery; however, this is specific to procedures where electromagnetic interference is likely [18]. If the AICD is disabled, it is imperative that the patient be placed on continuous monitoring, with external defibrillation pads in place, and that the device be enabled again in the PACU.

(2) **Complex patients:** Actual placement of AICD leads into the heart in patients with complex lesions is often difficult, if not impossible [20]. Presence of abnormal venous return, surgically created shunts or baffles, as well as scarring from previous surgery can make adequate placement challenging. Occasionally, patients will require an open surgical approach to place epicardial pacing/defibrillation leads, although this procedure often carries risk as well due to scarring and reoperative concerns (see Section IX below).

B. **Pulmonary Arterial Hypertension (PAH): PAH is defined as a mean pulmonary pres-**
5 **sure greater than 25 mm Hg at rest or 30 during exercise** [23]. ACHD patients have an incidence of PAH in up to 10% of patients, with Eisenmenger's syndrome (ES) being present in approximately 1% [4]. The etiology of the PAH typically falls in the World Health Organization category I or II. Group I is PAH due to primary PAH but includes congenital shunts, and group II is due to pulmonary venous hypertension (i.e., disease due to valve disorders, volume excess, and LV dysfunction).

6 1. **Surgical risk: PAH patients are high-risk surgical candidates. Published series demonstrate a range of surgical mortalities from a low of 4% to a high of 24% depending on disease severity and surgical procedure** [24]. Surgical and anesthetic risk should be clearly stated to the patient, especially for an elective case. Patients with ES should be considered higher-risk candidates and extreme care should be taken in managing these cases. See Section XII.B.2.

    a. **Hemodynamic spiral:** Acute deterioration is possible as RV failure causes reduced pulmonary blood flow, leading to hypoxia which subsequently increases the pulmonary vascular resistance (PVR). The elevated PVR ultimately leads to increased strain on the RV. This initiates a **catastrophic hemodynamic chain of events** where the decreased RV stroke volume decreases LV output, and coronary blood flow to both the LV and RV decreases. The already failing RV may not be able to recover from this insult, resulting in cardiac arrest. **This "death spiral" is always a potential in PAH patients; the anesthesia provider should be aware of it and take steps to prevent it** [23].

2. **How do you treat RV failure in the setting of PAH?** Treatment of acute RV failure should focus on reducing PVR (see Section IV.B.3 below), while utilizing β-stimulating inotropic agents such as dobutamine and/or phosphodiesterase-inhibiting agents such as milrinone, as these provide inotropic support with moderate reductions in PVR (and systemic vascular resistance [SVR]). Consider using a vasopressor such as norepinephrine in the setting of systemic hypotension to increase the coronary perfusion pressure. In severe scenarios, an intra-aortic balloon pump can also be used to increase coronary perfusion pressure, thus supporting the RV [8].

3. **What are some treatment modalities during surgery to reduce PVR acutely** [7]**?**

    a. Consider moderate hyperventilation ($Paco_2$ ~25 to 30 mm Hg) while administering 100% oxygen.

    b. Use low-pressure ventilation if possible as high intrathoracic pressure can mechanically compress extra-alveolar vessels and reduce CO.

    c. Utilize nitric oxide for acute reductions in PVR.

    d. Consider inhaled prostanoid (iloprost) if available.

    e. Intravenous (IV) magnesium sulfate may provide temporary reductions in PVR.

C. **What are some general hemodynamic goals for patients with PAH** [23]**?**

Anesthetic and hemodynamic goals for pulmonary hypertension

1. **Avoid elevations in PVR:** Prevent hypoxemia, acidosis, hypercarbia, and pain. Provide supplemental oxygen at all times. Consider inhaled nitric oxide (iNO) to acutely decrease PVR.
2. **Maintain SVR:** Decreased SVR dramatically reduces CO due to "fixed" PVR.
3. **Avoid myocardial depressants and maintain myocardial contractility.**
4. **Maintain chronic prostaglandin therapy without altering dosage.**
5. **Utilize low-pressure mechanical ventilation when possible.**

V. What laboratory and imaging studies are needed?

The overall goal in preoperative laboratory and imaging studies is to assist the physicians in understanding the degree of involvement of any comorbid disease.

A. Preoperative laboratory and imaging testing should be guided by degree of severity of disease. Patients with normal functional status can be treated as any adult presenting for surgery, whereas the patient with severe functional limitation due to cardiac disease warrants additional evaluation. Lab evaluation may include complete blood count, coagulation studies, and basic metabolic studies.

B. Cardiac catheterization and/or echocardiography studies are particularly helpful in symptomatic patients by providing information on structural status of the heart, functional status of the ventricles, and degree of PAH. Many patients will also have either magnetic resonance imaging (MRI) or computed tomography (CT) reconstructive imaging as part of standard surveillance, and these can add tremendous information to the history.

C. EKG should be obtained at baseline as there are often abnormalities present. This can also alert the practitioner to the presence of a pacemaker or other abnormal rhythm disturbances.

D. Chest radiography: It can be helpful to determine degree of heart and lung disease at baseline.

VI. What monitors should be used in ACHD surgery?

A. Standard ASA monitors should be employed for every case. In addition, most cases involving moderate to complex ACHD patients will utilize some degree of invasive monitoring. Some key considerations here include the following [25]:

1. Location of arterial line, if needed, should consider previous surgical procedures such as Blalock–Taussig shunts using the subclavian artery, which compromise blood flow to the ipsilateral upper extremity.
2. Central venous catheters should be reserved for the most symptomatic patients as risk of thrombus and stroke is higher.
3. Pulmonary artery (PA) catheters are often anatomically difficult or impossible to place and are seldom helpful in patients with cyanotic cardiac lesions.
4. **Transesophageal echocardiography (TEE)** may be the most useful real-time monitor of cardiovascular status, especially when using general anesthesia, and should strongly be considered for patients with reduced functional status for all medium- and high-risk procedures.
5. Near-infrared spectroscopy (NIRS) has been suggested as a tool to monitor both cerebral and peripheral oxygenation. The concept is that this technology helps identify changes in oxygen delivery and may be more sensitive to changes in cardiac output. See the discussion in the previous chapter on pediatric CHD.

VII. What are some general intraoperative anesthetic considerations for patients with ACHD?

While the pathologic categorization (simple, moderate, and complex) of CHD is useful, a more clinically based approach may be more useful in intraoperative planning. One scheme would be to consider patients based on surgical correction such as the following:

A. **Complete surgical correction** (i.e., repaired ASD, VSD, and PDA). Patients with surgically corrected lesions, as well as palliated lesions with good functional results, typically demonstrate hemodynamic stability and normal physiology. As such, these can be assumed to be very low-risk patients and managed as an otherwise healthy adult patient.

B. **Partial surgical correction** or **palliation** (i.e., Fontan, ToF, and TGA [Mustard or Senning repair]). Palliated patients with complex disease and reduced functional capacity due to the type of lesion should be managed with more concern and will be the main focus below.

C. **Uncorrected lesions** (i.e., minor ASD, minor VSD, and Ebstein's anomaly). Uncorrected patients warrant thorough examination into type of lesion and current functional state, as often these are minor lesions if they have not caused any medical or functional issues into adulthood.

D. **General approach:** For both cyanotic lesions (right-to-left shunts) and left-to-right shunts, there are general concepts that will aid in careful anesthetic planning.

7

1. **Cyanotic lesions** [25]
   a. Cyanotic lesions have some element of right-to-left shunt, often even after surgical repair. The degree of this shunt determines the level of cyanosis present. Caution should be taken with sedative medicines, as lowering ventilation can increase PVR and exacerbate cyanosis by increasing right-to-left shunt.
   b. Right-to-left shunting reduces the uptake of inhalational anesthetics and can prolong inhalation induction. Conversely, the onset of IV induction may be hastened.
   c. Nitrous oxide may elevate PA pressure and should be used cautiously.
   d. **Air embolus:** Take extreme care to avoid an air embolus. All IV lines should be aggressively deaired and monitored during medication administration. Epidural catheter placement should use saline for loss of resistance, not air, because air into an epidural vein can cross into the systemic circulation.
   e. **SVR:** Changes in SVR disrupt the balance between pulmonary and systemic circulations to change the shunt. All anesthetic medications should be slowly titrated to prevent rapid changes. This holds true for both regional and general anesthetics.
   f. Single-shot spinal anesthetic techniques are generally contraindicated, as quick onset of spinal sympathectomy is poorly tolerated.
   g. Administration of antibiotics (vancomycin), if given quickly, may reduce SVR and become clinically relevant.
   h. Choice of anesthetic induction drug is not as important as the manner and vigilance used by the anesthesiologist in managing hemodynamics.
   i. Clinical endpoints that might decrease PVR, such as increases in mixed venous O_2 (typically via high FiO_2) and modest degrees of respiratory alkalosis, are encouraged.
2. **Chronic left-to-right shunting:** Balance between SVR and PVR determines the shunt fraction and the direction of shunting. Chronic left-to-right shunting causes the following:
   a. Excessive pulmonary blood flow leading to pulmonary edema or pulmonary hypertension. The increased pulmonary flow causes PVR increases over time, reducing left-to-right shunting, and eventually equilibration of left and right ventricular pressures. Eventually, this process results in conversion of the left-to-right shunt into a right-to-left shunt, the so-called Eisenmenger's physiology or syndrome.
   b. Once ES develops, cyanosis ensues along with variable degrees of heart failure which places patients in the **highest-risk** category for surgical procedures.
   c. Even without Eisenmenger's complex, these patients may experience heart failure as a result of the high RV and pulmonary blood flow, which may be as much as four times systemic blood flow.
   d. **SVR:** Acute changes in SVR from anesthetic administration or pain can result in alteration or reversal of the shunt, leading to heart failure or cyanosis, depending upon where the patient is in her evolution from large left-to-right shunt into the right-to-left shunting of Eisenmenger's physiology. Overall anesthetic goals should be to maintain the balance that the patient has and avoid abrupt alterations.
   e. High levels of supplemental oxygen may allow for reduced PVR and worsening of the left-to-right shunt. On the other hand, hypoxemia should be prevented as this may shift the shunt to right-to-left and result in cyanosis. A fine balance must be struck when managing oxygenation for these patients.
   f. **Air embolus:** As in cyanotic lesions, take extreme care to avoid an **air embolus**. Even predominant left-to-right shunts can become bidirectional, putting the patient at risk for a systemic air embolus.
   g. **Single-shot spinal anesthesia is** contraindicated for patients who have or are approaching Eisenmenger's physiology. Spinal anesthesia is theoretically beneficial for

patients with large left-to-right shunts and normal or only slightly elevated PVR that remains far below SVR.

h. **Inhalational agents:** Uptake should not be affected by left-to-right shunting. Right-to-left shunting prolongs inhalation inductions, but this is rarely clinically relevant.

VIII. What is the ideal approach to postoperative management for ACHD patients?

Postoperative management should take into account all the risk factors described above in the anesthetic planning, and one should attempt to maintain the patient in the hemodynamic state to which he/she has adapted.

A. **Pain management:** Patients with palliated lesions often have some degree of residual shunt, or even single ventricle physiology. As such, overall cardiac performance depends to a large degree on the PVR. Attempts should be made to minimize impairment of ventilation in these patients as hypercarbia will increase PVR and potentially worsen cyanosis or increase ventricular failure in susceptible patients.

   1. **Regional anesthesia** may be ideal for patients with significant anticipated postoperative pain as this can greatly reduce the level of systemic opioid use, thus reducing risk of respiratory complications. Laboratory evaluation of coagulation status should be obtained in any patient with a history of anticoagulant therapy prior to neuraxial interventions.

B. **Arrhythmias:** For patients at elevated risk (Tables 15.4 and 15.5), perioperative monitoring in a telemetry bed may be indicated if there is not an AICD in place. For patients with AICDs or pacemakers, consider postoperative interrogation of the device if there was significant electrical interference during the surgery, or if the device had a magnet applied. Additionally, if the AICD was disabled for the procedure, it is imperative that defibrillation equipment be immediately available until the device is turned back on.

C. **Volume considerations:** Many ACHD patients with palliated lesions have a narrow margin of error in fluid management. They can easily be pushed into heart failure with too aggressive fluid management, and conversely may develop significant reductions in cardiac output with a minimalist approach. There is not an ideal volume strategy that fits all patients, but management must be closely tailored to each patient's physiologic status. As discussed above, invasive monitoring may not be possible in many of these patients or may not accurately reflect actual volume status, so management can be complicated. TEE use intraoperatively along with close monitoring of urine output may be the best approach in complex patients.

IX. What is the approach for patients presenting for repeat sternotomy?

A. What are the key surgical considerations in preparation for repeat sternotomy?

In patients with ACHD, the need for repeat sternotomy is often encountered as the initial challenge regarding surgical intervention. Often these patients have had multiple prior chest surgeries, increasing the degree of scarring in the pericardial space and thus making the surgical approach more demanding. Overall mortality increases with repeat sternotomy and is reported to be in the range of 3% to 6%. Re-entrant injury has been reported to greatly increase the risk in certain series and may approach 18% to 25%. However, other reports indicate no increase in mortality but a significant increase in duration of surgery [26–29]. **The risk appears to correlate to increased number of sternotomies, presence of single ventricle diagnosis, and presence of an RV–PA conduit.**

   1. **Preoperative preparation:** Several preoperative variables are of importance and can prove to be quite valuable in planning a repeat sternotomy. A PA and lateral chest radiograph can be quite helpful and should always be examined prior to operative intervention. The radiographs can supply important information regarding number of sternal wires in place and their condition as well as the lateral film in particular providing clues as to the degree of distance between the posterior sternal table and the heart itself. In addition, many patients have had preoperative cardiac catheterization studies. It is always quite helpful to assess this study and the lateral images in particular to obtain an anatomic roadmap as to areas of concern regarding the repeat sternotomy. These pictures can provide much data as to what portion of the sternum may be more impacted by adhesions to cardiac structures and which sternal wires are in closest approximation to these areas of concern.

2. **Cannulation options:** Should there be any significant concern regarding repeat sternotomy and a high index of suspicion for injury, femoral cannulation should be considered. Preoperative discussions with the perfusion and anesthesia teams is critical to planning alternative strategies for cannulation and the decision to begin use of the CPB circuit before completing the repeat sternotomy.
3. **Specifics of repeat sternotomy:** Several techniques are of importance when pursuing a repeat sternotomy. Manipulation of the surgical table with anesthesia assistance can be critical in obtaining better visualization of the posterior table of the sternum as one pursues the repeat entry from below. In addition, use of specified retractors can also be of great assistance (mammary retractor) to allow for slow and sequential separation and elevation of the sternum. The goal of this portion of re-entry should be to obtain safe removal of previously placed sternal wires and separation of the sternum.
4. **Lysis of adhesions:** Once the repeat sternotomy is accomplished, significant lysis of adhesions is undertaken. Good communication with the team is critical during this process. The surgical goals should be to define and separate from scar tissue areas of cannulation (assuming the patient was not cannulated via femoral access before initiating the repeat sternotomy). These areas include the ascending aorta, right atrium (in single venous cannulation), and/or the superior vena cava (SVC) and inferior vena cava (IVC) (in cases of bicaval cannulation). Further dissection of the heart and possible previously placed shunts may be more safely accomplished once cannulae are in place for initiation of CPB.
5. **Initiation of CPB:** It is important to have all systemic to PA conduits/shunts adequately isolated and secured prior to initiation of CPB. Once bypass is begun, these connections must be ligated so that the circuit will not induce pulmonary overcirculation and systemic undercirculation.

B. What are the key anesthetic considerations in preparation for repeat sternotomy?

The majority of ACHD patients requiring cardiac intervention will require repeat sternotomy. Often these patients have had multiple prior chest surgeries, increasing the degree of scarring in the pericardial space, thus making the surgical approach more demanding. Key anesthetic considerations for repeat sternotomy revolve around preparation for possible re-entrant injury as well as increased transfusion requirements.

1. **Large-bore IV** access is critical in the event of re-entrant injury. Consider the patient's vascular anatomy and evaluate any possible central venous clots/strictures as these patients may have had multiple central lines in the past. Ultrasound guidance is recommended during line placement to help evaluate vasculature. A large-bore central venous catheter (8.5 Fr introducer) in addition to one to two large-bore peripheral IV's attached to a high-flow fluid warmer may be prudent.
2. **Placement of external defibrillator patches since access to an open chest for internal defibrillation may be delayed.**
3. Type-specific blood products should be available and double-checked in a cooler in the OR at incision. Many patients will have had multiple transfusions in the past, and thus may have unique antibody profiles, which can delay the type and cross process. Typically, one should have 6 to 10 units of PRBCs available.
4. Ventilation management during re-entry should be discussed with the surgical team. There is suggestion that slight hyperinflation of the lungs, using a recruitment maneuver during sternal spreading, can actually minimize re-entrant injury as it reduces venous return through the increased intrathoracic pressure, decreasing the size of the RV and reducing the risk of re-entrant injury [30].
5. Full discussion of risk should be undertaken with the surgical team before surgery. On the basis of this discussion, the surgical team may elect to cannulate the femoral vessels or perform axillary cannulation to enable emergent institution of cardiopulmonary bypass in the event of re-entrant injury.

C. What is the role of antifibrinolytic therapy?

Fibrinolysis is known to occur during cardiopulmonary bypass and is associated with increased blood loss and need for transfusions in cardiac surgery. Due to this, antifibrinolytics have been recommended in the Society of Thoracic Surgeons and Society of Cardiovascular Anesthesiologists (STS/SCA) guidelines recently updated for 2011 [31]. Aprotinin was withdrawn from the world market in 2008 due to concerns for increased mortality despite reduction in blood loss which was demonstrated in various trials [31,32]. Current STS/SCA recommendations include routine use of either aminocaproic acid or tranexamic acid for all cardiac surgeries with a typical regimen being to initiate the infusion prior to skin incision and continue throughout the operation [32–36].

X. When should ACHD patients be listed for transplantation and what are the outcomes?

A. Heart and lung transplant can be a life-saving measure for the patient who has developed severe heart failure. ACHD patients most commonly listed for transplant include patients with uncorrectable or partially palliated lesions such as those listed below [9]:

1. Single ventricle physiology with pulmonary vascular disease (heart/lung transplant)
2. Lesions associated with LV dysfunction due to pulmonary vascular disease (heart/lung or isolated lung transplant)
3. Isolated heart failure without significant pulmonary vascular disease (more common in single ventricle physiology, or transposition of the great vessels [TGV] patients treated by atrial switch procedures) (heart transplant).
4. Patients who clinically meet the metrics for transplant should have a thorough pretransplant evaluation assessing the anatomy of the patient, as well as PVR. Longstanding elevations in PVR can easily lead to right heart failure in the donor heart and must be anticipated in these patients.
   a. For cases involving elevated PVR, it is recommended to take steps to avoid acute right heart failure in the transplanted donor heart. This often involves a combination of iNO and vasoactive infusions (dobutamine, milrinone) to provide inotropic support along with pulmonary vasodilation. See chapter on heart transplantation for full discussion.

B. **What are the outcomes of transplant?** ACHD patients make up nearly 3% of the total number of patients listed for cardiac transplantation [37]. Davies et al. investigated patients listed for transplant from 1995 to 2009. This study indicated that the ACHD patients who went on to obtain a heart transplant had a higher early mortality, possibly due to increased repeat sternotomy incidence in this group, but an equivalent long-term mortality as non-CHD patients (53% 10-yr survival in both groups).

XI. What are the specific details for managing patients with partially corrected or palliative repairs?

A. **Fontan repair:** Fontan palliation has been the primary surgical approach for complex lesions such as tricuspid atresia (TA), hypoplastic left heart, double inlet LV, double-outlet RV, severe AV defects, and heterotaxy syndrome [38]. Management of these lesions in both the neonate, and the adult patient, is one of the biggest challenges in anesthetic practice [39]. Survival rates are now approximately 90% at 10 yrs following palliation; thus, more and more Fontan patients may present for adult surgery [40]. This lesion is described in detail for the neonate previously, but key aspects pertaining to adult management are presented below.

1. **Pathophysiology:** TA creates a situation where blood must pass from the right atrium to the left atrium via an ASD, where it mixes with pulmonary venous return. Blood flow is then directed to both the PA and the aorta by various routes. Regardless of type of repair, blood flow depends entirely on the left ventricle for cardiac output [25,38]. For a more detailed review, please see the extensive discussion of adult Fontan physiology provided by Drs. Eagle and Daves in 2011 [38].
2. **Surgical correction.** The Fontan procedure is the definitive palliative surgical approach that creates a univentricular circulation via a cavopulmonary anastamosis. The Fontan procedure consists of creation of a classical or bidirectional Glenn shunt (SVC to PA connection), closure of the ASD, ligation of the proximal PA, and creation of a right atrial or IVC to PA connection. Multiple variations to the Fontan procedure exist (Fig. 15.4); however, the same general physiologic principles apply to most situations [25].

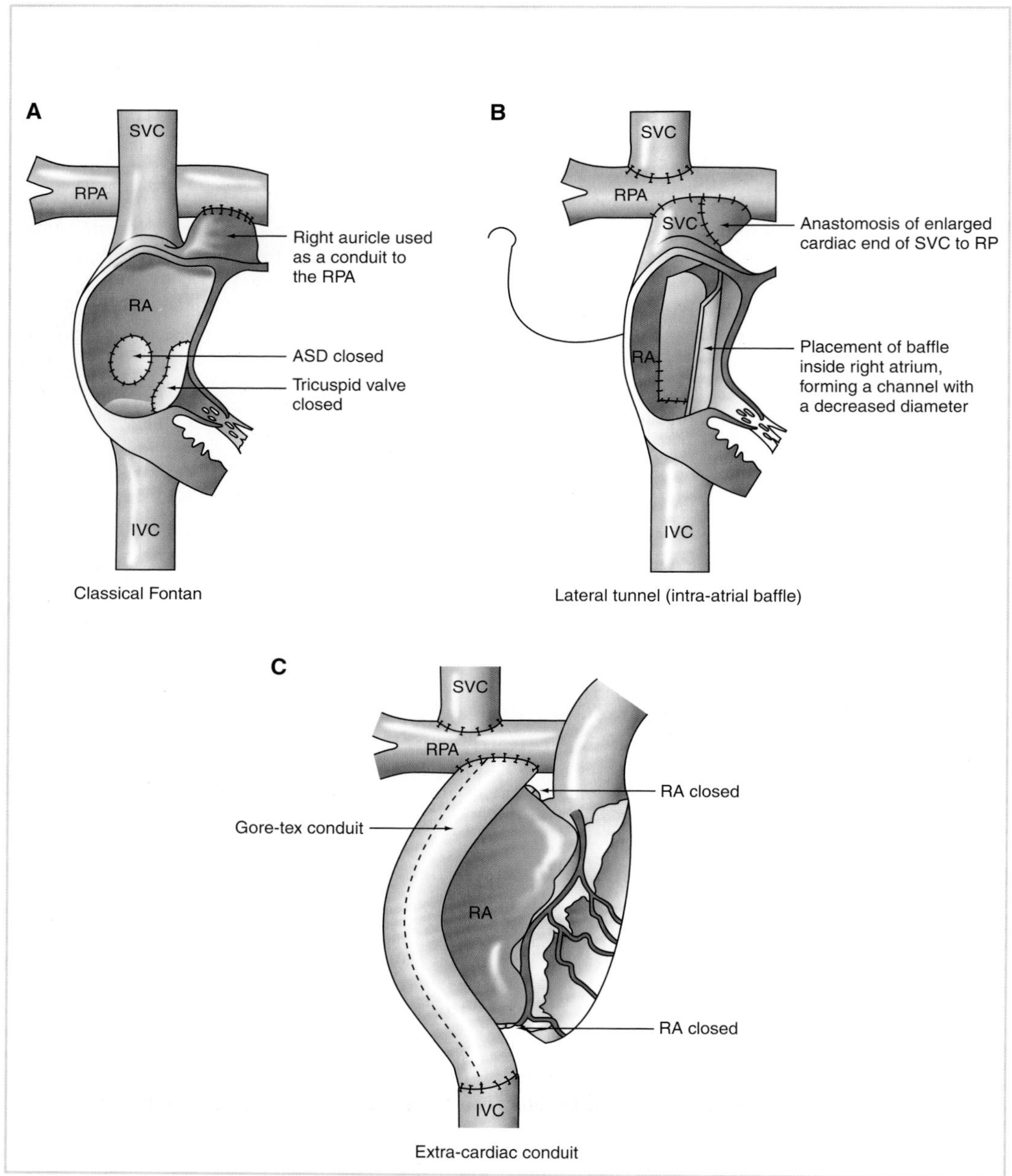

FIGURE 15.4 Fontan surgical techniques: Classical atriopulmonary connection **(A)**, lateral tunnel **(B)**, and extracardiac conduit **(C)**. (Redrawn from d'Udekem, Iyengar AJ, Cochrane AD, et al. The Fontan procedure: Contemporary techniques have improved long-term outcomes. *Circulation.* 2007;116:I-157–I-164.)

3. **What are the key physiologic and anesthetic management considerations?**
   a. **Blood flow to the PAs is passive.** Elevations in PVR will therefore reduce pulmonary flow, and hence decrease cardiac output, by reducing the gradient between the vena cava and the PA.
   b. **Hemodynamic stability is highly dependent upon maintaining appropriately high systemic venous pressures and right atrial preload.** Decreased right atrial

preload causes dramatic declines in pulmonary blood flow and cardiac output. Peripheral edema often results from the high systemic venous pressures.

c. Spontaneous respiration assists forward flow by keeping PVR low. Any compromise in pulmonary function can be detrimental by increasing PVR. Preoperative sedation should be used carefully due to risk of increasing hypercapnia and elevation in PVR. **If positive pressure ventilation is necessary, use the lowest pressure possible to achieve adequate ventilation.**

d. The single ventricle is prone to failure leading to pulmonary edema. The atrial contribution to flow is significant, but arrhythmias are common and poorly tolerated.

e. Progressive hepatic failure is widely prevalent due to altered hepatic circulation from increased systemic venous pressures. This can present as a bleeding tendency, a clotting tendency, or as a mixed picture. Pulmonary embolism and stroke are common late complications.

f. Invasive monitoring can be problematic and may be unnecessary except for hemodynamically unstable patients.

(1) Central venous catheter placement probably carries a higher risk of thromboembolic events but may nevertheless be appropriate for short-term use. CVPs as high as 25 to 30 mm Hg are not unexpected and may be essential to drive blood through the pulmonary circulation. Attempts to place PA catheters are not advised.

(2) Arterial line monitoring is advised, but must take into account surgical shunts regarding location of arterial access.

(3) TEE should be strongly considered for intraoperative monitoring during general anesthesia.

g. General anesthesia: A careful selection of induction agents that will provide a smooth hemodynamic profile is preferred.

(1) Etomidate and ketamine are excellent induction agents, and moderate doses of an opioid such as fentanyl, sufentanil, or remifentanil will reduce the stress response.

(2) A muscle relaxant with minimal hemodynamic effects (e.g., succinylcholine or rocuronium) is desirable.

h. Regional anesthesia may be employed for appropriate surgical cases. However, titrated epidural anesthesia may be preferable to single-shot spinal as abrupt reductions in sympathetic tone may not be well tolerated.

Anesthetic and hemodynamic goals for patients with Fontan physiology

1. **Maintain preload.** Avoid aortocaval compression.
2. **Avoid elevation in PVR** by preventing acidosis, hypoxemia, and hypercarbia.
3. **Maintain sinus rhythm.**
4. **Maintain spontaneous respiration when possible.**
5. **Avoid myocardial depressants.**

B. ToF—"Blue baby syndrome": ToF is characterized by existence of a VSD, pulmonic stenosis/right ventricular outflow tract obstruction (RVOTO), over-riding aorta, and right ventricular hypertrophy. There is great variability in the extent of these defects ranging from small VSD and over-riding aorta with minimal pulmonary stenosis (PS) to severe PS and large VSD. Outcomes with current surgical repair techniques are excellent and there is a 36-yr survival of nearly 86% [41].

1. **Palliative shunts** (Blalock–Taussig, Waterston, or Potts) were the initial solution, which involve systemic arterial (aorta or subclavian artery) to PA anastomoses. They provided temporary relief of symptoms, but often had long-term sequelae [25].
2. **Definitive surgical repair** involves closure of the VSD and relief of RVOTO using resection and reconstruction with Gore-Tex patch grafting across the RVOTO or conduits to bypass the RVOTO (Fig. 15.5).
3. Common reasons for reoperation include residual VSD or recurrence of the VSD (10% to 20%), residual RVOTO or stenosis (10%) leading to right heart failure, and rarely RV failure caused by pulmonic insufficiency (PI) from the RVOT patch.

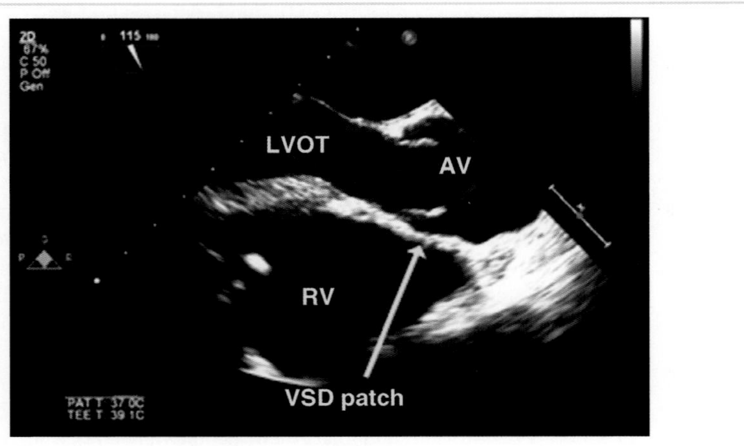

FIGURE 15.5 Transesophageal echocardiographic image of the VSD patch repair typically visualized in adult patients with previous ToF repair. This is the midesophageal long-axis view demonstrating the over-riding aorta with the *in situ* patch. Image provided by Bryan Ahlgren DO, University of Colorado Denver.

4. Additional concerns include a higher risk of sudden cardiac death compared with age-matched controls, elevated risk of arrhythmias (especially atrial fibrillation), right bundle branch block, pulmonary regurgitation, and right ventricular aneurysms.
5. Patients with PS or significant pulmonic valvular regurgitation are more likely to develop right heart failure. Avoidance of elevated PVR and maintenance of high-normal filling pressures are critical in patients with pulmonic valvular regurgitation [39]. See discussion for RV–PA conduits below.
6. **General anesthesia:** Choice of induction agents should be tailored to achieve the hemodynamic goals below and based on the underlying cardiac function.
   a. If an arterial catheter is placed, patients with Blalock–Taussig shunts will require cannulation in the contralateral arm, or in either leg.
   b. TEE should be considered during general anesthesia.
7. **Regional anesthesia** may be employed for appropriate surgical cases. However, titrated epidural anesthesia may be preferable to single-shot spinal for certain ToF patients depending on the degree of palliation and current symptoms.

   Anesthetic and Hemodynamic goals in ToF
   1. **Avoid changes (especially decreases) in SVR** to prevent altering existing shunt.
   2. **Avoid increases in PVR** by preventing hypoxia, hypercarbia, acidosis, and providing supplemental oxygen.
   3. Maintain normal to elevated cardiac filling pressures, especially in patients with right ventricular impairment. Avoid aortocaval compression.
   4. Continuous EKG monitoring is advisable due to high incidence of both atrial and ventricular arrhythmias.
   5. Tachycardia and increases in myocardial contractility should be avoided in situations where there is residual RVOTO, as this may exacerbate the obstruction and cause right-to-left shunting.

C. **Right (pulmonary) ventricle to pulmonary artery conduits:** The RV–PA conduit is a surgical technique used in the palliation of multiple lesions including pulmonary atresia, ToF, truncus arteriosus, TGA, PS, and forms of double-outlet RV [42]. Various types of conduits have been employed for initial repair ranging from aortic homografts (Ross procedure), pulmonary homografts, pericardial patches/reconstructions, to a variety of valved or nonvalved artificial conduits (Dacron, Gore-Tex, etc.). For this section, it is useful to discuss the ventricle as either the pulmonary ventricle or the systemic ventricle.

1. **Risk factors leading to reoperation:** Conduit failure is thought to occur in roughly 50% of patients at 10 yrs and 70% of patients at 20 yrs. Conduit failure, typically, is due to patient growth, thus resulting in a functionally "small" conduit, development of pulmonary valve (PV) insufficiency, and/or various degrees of calcification. Conduit failure is defined by a variety of methods depending on the type of conduit, but in general include the following [41–44]:
   a. Symptomatic patients (dyspnea, fatigue, chest pain, palpitations, presyncope, and decreased exercise tolerance) demonstrating signs of RV failure with elevated PV peak gradients >40 mm Hg.
   b. Asymptomatic patients with pulmonary ventricular pressures approaching systemic pressures, increasing pulmonary ventricular size with increasing PV insufficiency and/or tricuspid insufficiency.
   c. Patients with severe PI and NYHA functional class II or III symptoms should be considered for PV replacement ± conduit repair [44].
   d. Deterioration in exercise testing or functional capacity.
   e. Patients who are very young at the time of conduit placement, those with small-diameter conduits, those with diagnosis of truncus arteriosis or TGA, and those receiving homografts are at elevated risk of failure.
2. **What are the key anesthetic concerns for pulmonary ventricle–pulmonary artery conduit replacements?**
   a. These are repeat sternotomy procedures, so all the considerations outlined in Section IX should be followed. The pulmonary ventricle–PA conduit is an anterior structure, so has greater risk of injury on re-entry sternotomy.
   b. Hemodynamic considerations should take into account current physiologic and functional status of the patient. The majority of these patients will be suffering from degrees of right heart failure, so careful control of the PVR should be of utmost concern. In addition, PI is common and often in the moderate to severe range. This leads to overdistension of the RV with the potential to worsen RV failure.
   c. Patients with residual VSD are at risk for alterations in the shunt fraction if there are significant changes to either PVR or SVR, which can worsen right heart function or create cyanosis.
   d. As with PAH, the right ventricle is susceptible to failure which leads to reduced pulmonary blood flow, hypoxia, and subsequent increases in PVR. This in turn initiates a **catastrophic hemodynamic chain of events** where the decreased RV stroke volume decreases LV output and coronary blood flow to both the LV and RV decreases.
3. **What are the hemodynamic goals for patients with RV–conduit failure?**
   Management should be based on the etiology of the conduit failure, which generally falls into two basic categories: stenosis versus insufficiency. Stenotic lesions are discussed in the next section (XI.D) on PV stenosis. PI is frequently caused by balloon valvuloplasty to treat pulmonic stenosis. It is also common after successful repair of the RVOTO associated with ToF [45]. For patients with PI, there are some basic hemodynamic suggestions that will assist in developing the anesthetic plan.
   a. Overall goals for management are a relative tachycardia (heart rate 80 to 90), with overall reduction in PVR. This will help reduce the regurgitant fraction and promote increased forward flow.
   b. In patients with elements of RV failure, avoid agents with direct myocardial depressant effects such as propofol. Etomidate may be an ideal choice.
   c. Consider early inotropic support for patients with RV failure. Dobutamine is a good option given the relative tachycardia coupled with reduction in PVR/SVR associated with this β-adrenergic agent. Guidelines provided for PAH also apply to these patients (see Section IV.C) regarding management of PVR.

D. **Pulmonary Valve abnormalities:** PV abnormalities are associated with approximately 12% of ACHD lesions [43]. The causes of PS range from valve-specific abnormalities to problems with the development of the RV itself (see Table 15.6), and are almost exclusively due to congenital lesions. These lesions may be found in patients with palliated disease (i.e., ToF following

TABLE 15.6 Causes of RV outflow tract obstruction in adult patients

Unoperated
Valvular
Dome-shaped PV
Dysplastic PV
Unicuspid or bicuspid PV
Infundibular stenosis, usually associated with tetralogy of Fallot
Hypertrophic infundibular stenosis
Associated with PS, hypertrophic cardiomyopathy
Infundibular obstruction
Tricuspid valve tissue
Fibrous tags from inferior vena cava or coronary sinus
Aneurysm of the sinus of valsalva
Aneurysm of the membranous septum
Subinfundibular obstruction
Double-chambered RV
Supravalvular stenosis
Hourglass deformity at valve
PA membrane
PA stenosis
PA aneurysm
Peripheral PA stenosis
Associations: Rubella, Alagille, Williams, Keutel syndromes
Operated
Valvular
Native valve restenosis
Prosthetic valve stenosis
Conduit stenosis
Double-chambered RV restenosis
Peripheral or branch PS
At insertion site of prior systemic-to-pulmonary shunt
After other complex surgical repair
Infundibular stenosis after tunnel repair of double-outlet RV

Reproduced from Bashore TM. Adult congenital heart disease: Right ventricular outflow tract lesions. *Circulation.* 2007;115(14): 1933–1947, with permission.

repair), or may represent an unrepaired lesion, but are discussed here due to association with RV–conduit abnormalities.

1. **How is PS diagnosed and what are typical symptoms?** Clinical symptoms for patients with severe PS are generally related to shortness of breath and functional limitation to exercise. Diagnosis is generally made following echocardiographic exam, and in isolated PV disease, cardiac catheterization is rarely needed.
2. **How is PS categorized?**
   - **a.** Trivial PS = peak gradient < 25 mm Hg.
   - **b.** Mild PS = peak gradient of 25 to 49 mm Hg.
   - **c.** Moderate PS = peak gradient of 50 to 79 mm Hg.
   - **d.** Severe PS = peak gradient > 80 mm Hg.
3. **What are the available therapeutic options for PS?** Patients with trivial or mild PS can expect a 96% and 77% 10-yr surgery-free survival, respectively, based on existing outcome studies. These patients are typically followed by echocardiography every 5 to 10 yrs for progression, or more frequently based on symptom development [44].
   - **a. Balloon valvuloplasty** is the treatment of choice (Class I recommendation) for patients with PS with gradients >50 mm Hg and less than that of mild PI, or any patient with exertional dyspnea and gradients in the 30 to 40 mm Hg range. It is not recommended for patients with dysplastic valve disease (characterized by poorly mobile valve

without commissural fusion), for gradients <30 mm Hg or in patients with moderate to severe PI. Both short- and long-term results are quite good with balloon valvuloplasty with restenosis rates <5% [46,47], and these results are essentially equivalent to surgical management with commissurotomy.

b. Surgical intervention is also effective and carried out under direct visualization for patients deemed poor candidates for balloon valvuloplasty. There is typically some residual PI following surgical commissurotomy, and depending on the valve morphology, occasionally PV replacement is required. Bioprosthetic valves carry a long life span in the pulmonic position and are the replacement valve of choice [44,45].

4. What are the key anesthetic management concerns for patients with PS? Patients with PS tend to follow a similar course as a patient with aortic stenosis. Over time, the increased RV systolic pressure required to overcome the obstructive lesion leads to RV hypertrophy, and, if left untreated, to RV failure. Ideally, these lesions should be treated before the onset of RV failure for best outcomes. **Hemodynamic considerations** during anesthetic management should follow the guidelines for any stenotic lesion.

a. Relative bradycardia (heart rate in the 60 to 80 range) is preferred to allow time for complete ventricular ejection. Slower heart rates will also allow for increased coronary perfusion time.

b. PS represents a fixed obstruction to outflow, so alterations in PVR will not change the obstruction. Preload should be maintained to promote forward flow.

c. SVR should be maintained in the patient's normal range, as reductions in diastolic pressure will decrease coronary perfusion pressure, leading to RV ischemia. Normally, the RV receives blood flow during both diastole and systole; however, with RV hypertrophy this is shifted primarily to the diastolic phase.

E. Transposition of great vessels

TGV is relatively rare, representing 1% to 5% of congenital heart defects. Two main types are congenitally corrected TGV (L-TGV) and complete TGV (D-TGV). Without surgical intervention, survival to 6 mos in D-TGV is less than 10% [7,9,25]. L-TGV allows survival, albeit typically at the cost of early adult heart failure.

1. How is D-TGV palliated and what are the physiologic sequelae?

D-TGV is described as blood flow in a parallel system, such that systemic venous return flows to the right atrium and right ventricle, which then ejects blood into the aorta [8,25]. Pulmonary venous blood flow proceeds to the left atrium, left ventricle, and then into the PA. Without additional communication from septal defects or a PDA, there is no connection between blood oxygenated in the lungs and systemic arteries, and therefore survival is impossible.

a. Atrial switch operations such as the Mustard or Senning procedure create an atrial baffle that causes venous blood to cross at the atrial level into the appropriate ventricle. Since the morphologic right ventricle then continues to eject blood into the aorta, these patients experience a higher risk of heart failure as a result of that ventricle's impaired capacity to chronically pump against systemic arterial pressures [7].

b. The arterial switch, known as the Jatene procedure, switches the PA and aorta with reimplantation of the coronary vessels. This requires the left ventricle of sufficient size to provide systemic flows. These patients often have relatively normal physiology following surgical repair and should be considered in the surgically corrected category [7]. There are **two long-term complications** to be aware of, which include **development of aortic insufficiency on the neoaortic valve (occurring in 25% of patients), and coronary ostial lesions leading to increased risk of myocardial ischemia** [7].

2. What are the key anesthetic considerations for patients with TGV?

a. Patients with D-TGV who have been treated with the arterial switch (Jatene) will typically have normal cardiac function, so management should focus on any coexisting medical issues. Contrary to this, those patients managed with the Mustard or Senning approach (atrial switch) are at higher risk of developing heart failure due to the systemic right ventricle, as well as the atrial baffle which occasionally results in obstructive flow.

b. As mentioned above, L-TGV patients are also at increased risk of heart failure, so evaluation should focus on determining functional status and symptoms of heart failure.
c. Arrhythmias are very common in patients treated with Mustard or Senning repairs. Ventricular tachycardia and IART are the most common (Table 15.3).
d. Invasive monitors should be used selectively. Central venous catheters may be useful for vascular access and monitoring in patients with heart failure, but PA catheters are probably ill-advised in patients who have undergone atrial switch procedures. Preoperative information from recent echocardiograms can be invaluable for symptomatic patients.

3. **How should induction of general anesthesia be managed?**
Induction should focus on the degree of heart failure present in the patient. Choose induction agents with minimal myocardial depressant effects; etomidate, midazolam, or fentanyl may be ideal choices. Additional effects of inhaled agents in moderate doses are generally well tolerated as the afterload reduction improves forward flow.
Anesthetic and hemodynamic goals for TGV
1. Consider an arterial catheter and/or CVP catheter and avoid excessive fluids in patients with evidence of heart failure.
2. Avoid negative inotropic agents.
3. Monitor for arrhythmias and treat as indicated.

4. **Should regional anesthesia be utilized in patients with TGV?** As with general anesthesia, the afterload reduction following the sympathetic blockade from neuraxial anesthesia will improve forward flow in patients with mild to moderate degrees of heart failure. Care should be taken for patients with severe heart failure symptoms and single-shot spinal techniques may not be tolerated due to the rapid changes in hemodynamics. Consider using epidural techniques with a slow titration of local anesthetic agents.

XII. What are the key details for patients with uncorrected CHD?

Uncorrected lesions presenting in the adult patient represent a group of diagnoses that are typically on the mild end of the spectrum, given that these patients remain largely symptom-free into adulthood. Examples include ASD, VSD, Ebstein's anomaly, or undiagnosed ACHD due to limited health care access as child. Those patients with more complex disease states that are unrepaired due to health care access should be managed according to the existing lesion, and will represent a more complex situation. This section will focus primarily on the septal defects presenting in the adult patient.

A. Adult Atrial Septal Defect (ASD)

ASDs account for nearly one-third of adult congenital heart defects and are found in women more commonly than in men [48]. Small defects (less than 5 mm) are hemodynamically insignificant, but large defects (greater than 20 mm) can lead to significant shunting and eventual RV overload or failure [25,49]. ASDs do not typically close spontaneously and are commonly associated with additional cardiac defects. The anatomy of septal defects in the adult is typically the same as described for the child (Fig. 15.6). Common defects include ostium primum, ostium secundum, sinus venosus, and patent foramen ovale. These defects are often linked to more complex CHD, which should be considered during initial workup. Ostium primum defects are frequently associated with a mitral cleft or other atrioventricular valve abnormalities, while sinus venosus defects are associated with partial anomalous pulmonary venous return. Hemodynamic consequences of ASD follows that of a left-to-right shunt as described above, the severity of which depends on the shunt fraction (Qp:Qs ratio).

1. **What are the clinical symptoms for adult ASDs?**
The natural course of unrepaired ASD is that as the patient ages and LV diastolic dysfunction develops, the increased LV end-diastolic pressure tends to worsen the left-to-right shunt. This leads to increased shunt fraction, RV dilation, and development of clinical symptoms, often in the fourth or fifth decade of life [49]. Typical clinical symptoms include the following:
a. Dyspnea with exertion, possibly due to chronic preload reduction of the LV along with overloaded pulmonary system. This symptom typically is improved with ASD closure.

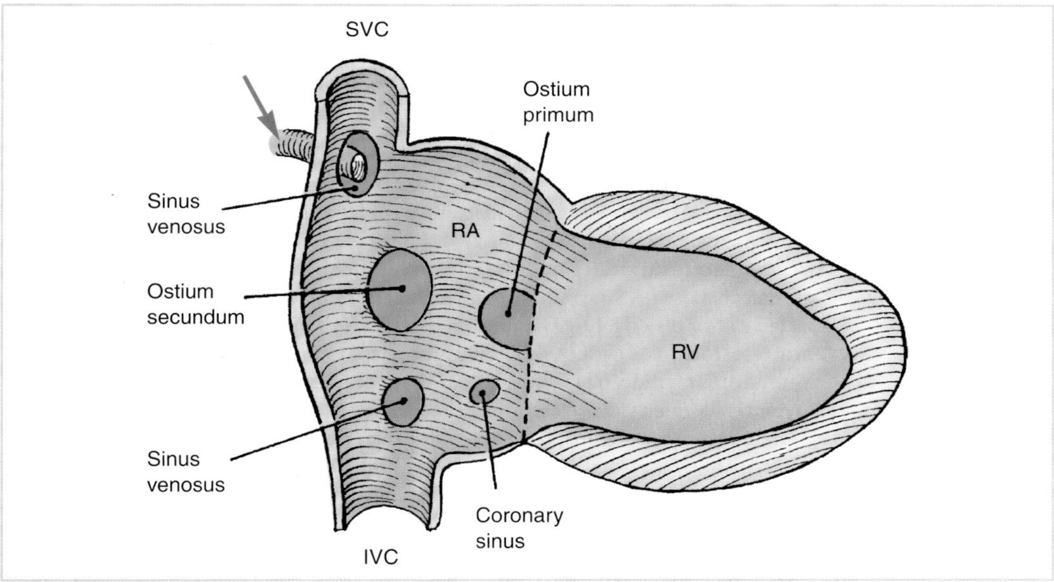

FIGURE 15.6 Location of ASDs. (Reproduced from Rouine-Rapp K, Miller–Hance WC. Transesophageal echocardiography for congenital heart disease in the adult. In: Perrino AC Jr, Reeves ST, eds. *A Practical Approach to Transesophageal Echocardiography*. 2nd ed. Philadelphia, PA: Lippincott Williams & Wilkins; 2008: 372, with permission.)

   b. Cardiac arrhythmias (atrial fibrillation) due to atrial enlargement and stretching of conduction system. Atrial volumes tend to remain elevated in the adult following repair, and thus arrhythmias tend to persist after repair.
   c. Embolic stroke—typically due to paradoxical embolism.

2. **What are the indications for repair** [48,49]**?** A combination of echocardiographic and catheterization-based diagnostic testing is generally used to determine eligibility for repair. Outcomes with repair (either surgical or transcatheter) seem to indicate a benefit in overall survival as 10-yr survival rates for adult patients following repair exceed 95%, while those treated with medical management alone have a 10-yr survival of 84% [50]. Outcomes appear to be better for patients repaired at earlier ages (before fourth decade) and medical management may be better later in life [50,51]. Indications for repair include the following:
   a. Adult patients with a pulmonary-to-systemic shunt (Qp:Qs) ratio >1.5:1.0
   b. Echocardiographic evidence of RV volume overload
   c. Development of arrhythmia due to atrial enlargement
   d. Exercise-induced cyanosis without existing pulmonary hypertension
3. **How does pulmonary hypertension relate to ASD? PAH is rarely caused by an ASD, is found in less than 10% of patients with ASD, and if PAH is not diagnosed by adulthood in the presence of an ASD, it rarely develops.** In addition, Eisenmenger's physiology rarely develops due to ASD. There is debate regarding the mechanism of PAH associated with ASD, but many consider ASD a marker of PAH, and not a causative agent [49,50]. Regardless, there are important considerations for patients with ASD and moderate to severe PAH. The presence of an ASD allows for blood to flow from right to left, bypassing the high-resistance pulmonary bed in PAH, and thus decompressing the RV. This reduces the classic heart failure symptoms, at the cost of cyanosis, and these patients should not have the ASD closed. Occasionally, creation of an ASD is a temporary measure used to bridge patients with severe PAH to transplant. **In fact, presence of PAH with PVR >14 Woods units is a contraindication for ASD closure.**
4. **Should surgical repair or transcatheter closure be used to repair the ASD?** Surgical closure of ASD is a safe and effective operation, with mortality rates at surgery below 1.5%,

and long-term survival >95% as mentioned above [50]. Recent advances in transcatheter approaches have shown excellent outcomes, equivalent to surgical repair, with the obvious avoidance of the morbidity associated with sternotomy [50–54]. Typically, transcatheter closure is associated with shorter hospital stays, less overall complications, and reduced cost.

5. **What characteristics of the lesion increase difficulty with transcatheter repair?** Once the indications for closure listed previously are established, certain anatomic characteristics must be considered for adequate transcatheter closure. Key anatomic features include the following:
   a. **Size of defect:** ASD <26 mm is considered normal size, with >26 mm considered a large defect. Large ASD is not a contraindication for device closure, but there is an elevated risk of dislodgement or erosion when using large devices [50].
   b. **Central lesions,** i.e., ostium secundum defects, are the most amenable to treatment. Ostium primum and sinus venosus lesions are often not anatomically suited to transcatheter techniques and are recommended to be repaired surgically [9].
      (1) **Lesions with deficient anterior-superior rim:** This deficiency is common in large ASDs, and makes placement of the device more technically challenging. Despite this, complications such as dislodgement or erosion are well below 1% in multiple studies [50], and seem to be most related to oversizing of devices. As such, device sizing should be limited to 1.5× the diameter of the ASD by TEE.
      (2) **Lesions with deficient posterior-inferior rim:** This lesion is even more technically challenging than deficient anterior-superior rim. However, the incidence is also lower and thus there are insufficient data to determine overall complications in these lesions.
   c. **Multiple lesions/fenestrated defects:** This type of abnormality is also a technical challenge. Approaches vary between balloon atrial septostomy to create a single ASD versus placement of multiple smaller occlusion devices.
   d. **Atrial septal aneurysms:** The aneurysmal septal wall creates difficulty with device closure using standard devices that rely to some degree on the septal structure. Patch or double disc devices are more appropriate, and again this type of lesion is more technically challenging.
6. **What are the typical devices used in the catheterization laboratory?**
   Currently, two main devices have become the standard following multiple studies using many different devices. In the United States, Amplatzer (AGA Medical Corp) and Helex (W.L. Gore) are the two devices with current FDA approval. Three-dimensional (3D) TEE imaging of an Amplatzer device in place is seen in Figure 15.7.
7. **What are the anesthetic considerations for device closure in ASD?** General considerations for patients with shunts are discussed in Section VII.D, which all apply to these patients. Typically, adult patients presenting for ASD closure are hemodynamically stable even in the setting of the clinical symptoms discussed above. On the basis of preoperative evaluation, specifically current functional status, the anesthesiologist can anticipate a relatively normal induction plan aiming for overall smooth hemodynamics. Some key aspects of this procedure to anticipate in anesthetic planning are listed below.
   a. Discuss the procedure plans with the cardiology team, as many times the interventional cardiologist will want to place right heart catheters while the patient is spontaneously ventilating to obtain catheter-based measurements of RA, RV, and PA pressures. Typically, this portion of the procedure will be carried out under mild sedation and on room air to avoid any changes to the PVR due to oxygen supplementation.
   b. Device closure is typically carried out using both echocardiography and X-ray imaging in the catheterization suite. Total procedural time can range in duration, but typically will take 1 to 4 h. Due to the length of the procedure along with need for prolonged TEE evaluation, general anesthesia is typically employed. Standard ASA monitors are usually all that is needed. However, for patients with severe hemodynamic compromise, invasive blood pressure monitoring may be utilized.

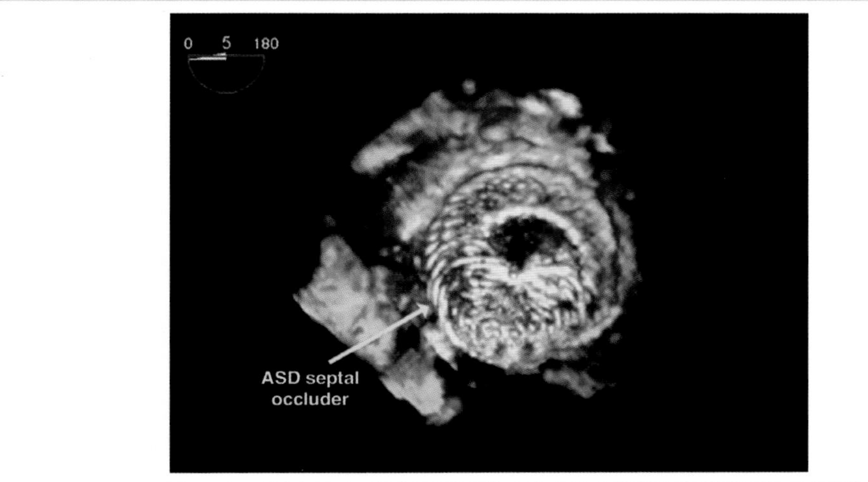

FIGURE 15.7 Three-dimensional TEE view of an Amplatzer device placed in a large centrally located ASD. Image by Nathaen Weitzel, MD, University of Colorado Denver.

c. General anesthesia can be safely induced with various approaches in nearly all patients and agents such as propofol or etomidate are acceptable. Heparin is typically given during the procedure to maintain an ACT >250 s.

d. **Key point: Patients with septal defects are at risk for embolic events to the brain. All IV lines should be aggressively deaired, and extreme care should be taken to avoid any injection of air through IV lines.**

B. **Ventricular Septal Defects:** VSD is the most common congenital heart lesion in children, although nearly 90% close spontaneously by age 10 [48,49]. Those patients with large lesions who are symptomatic at birth will usually be surgically corrected, while asymptomatic patients will often be closely monitored for evidence of spontaneous closure. Surgical closure often involves a right atriotomy or ventricular incision, and this carries a significant risk of interventricular and even atrioventricular conduction abnormalities. VSDs can present in multiple areas of the septum, with 80% being in the perimembranous region (Fig. 15.8), the muscular septum the next highest frequency, and the subarterial or double committed outlet being rather rare. **In contrast to ASD, unrepaired VSDs can have significant consequences and may lead to development of Eisenmenger's physiology if left untreated.**

1. **Can transcatheter closure be utilized to treat VSD?** This question is not as clearly answered as for ASD closure. However, advances over the past decade have led to significant improvements in device closure for VSD. Outcome data seem to favor this approach, with the most common associated complication being arrhythmias. Placement success is more than 95% in multiple studies, and 6-yr follow-up demonstrates more than 85% freedom from event rates [55–60]. The considerations for device closure in ASD will apply here as well, with the biggest issue being establishing good communication with the cardiology team before the procedure to discuss specific diagnostic planning that may impact anesthetic planning.

2. **What if ES is present? ES represents the most common cyanotic cardiac defect in adults** [61]. Chronic left-to-right shunting results in right ventricular hypertrophy, elevated PVR, and significant ventricular and arterial remodeling on the right side. ES carries a maternal mortality ranging from 30% to 70% along with high incidence of fetal demise, so patients are usually **counseled against pregnancy** [61], and considered extremely high risk for surgery. Sudden death is common and may be due to stroke, arrhythmia, abscess, or heart failure. Twenty-five–yr survival after diagnosis of ES is reported to be 42% in the absence of pregnancy [48].

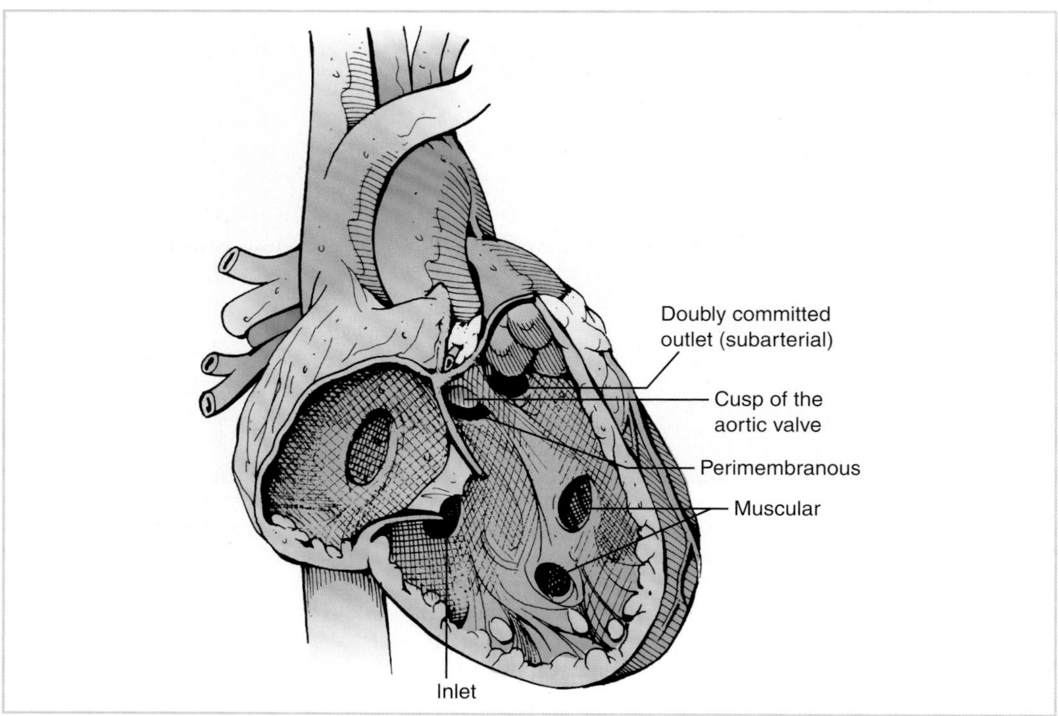

FIGURE 15.8 Common locations for VSDs. (Reproduced from Rouine-Rapp K, Miller-Hance WC. Transesophageal echocardiography for congenital heart disease in the adult. In: Perrino AC Jr, Reeves ST, eds. *A Practical Approach to Transesophageal Echocardiography*. 2nd ed. Philadelphia, PA: Lippincott Williams & Wilkins; 2008: 377, with permission.)

a. **Pathophysiology:** ES is defined by a PVR greater than 800 dyn·s/cm^5 along with right-to-left or bidirectional shunt flow. Correction of the shunt may resolve the pulmonary hypertension, but once pulmonary arteriolar remodeling (i.e., medial hypertrophy) develops, the elevated PVR is **irreversible,** differentiating ES from primary pulmonary hypertension.
b. Symptoms: Fatigue, dyspnea, cyanosis, edema, clubbing, and polycythemia.
c. The underlying right-to-left shunt, hyperviscosity from polycythemia, and the development of heart failure promote thrombus formation and may elevate stroke risk.

3. **Anesthetic management in ES:** Historically, regional anesthesia was thought to be contraindicated and general anesthesia was the standard. A review of cases of noncardiac surgery including labor and cesarean section in ES indicates that regional anesthesia is indeed safe for these patients [62]. Martin and colleagues state that mortality is related to type of surgical procedure, independent of choice of anesthetic. Despite this, anesthetic delivery requires utmost vigilance to maintain the above hemodynamic goals with any type of anesthesia.
   a. **Regional anesthesia:** Slow titration of local anesthetic with aggressive treatment for any reduction in SVR (i.e., systemic hypotension) using phenylephrine is effective. Maintenance of intravascular volume status using careful fluid boluses along with the use of phenylephrine for decreased SVR should be used to prevent onset or exacerbation of cyanosis. Single-shot spinal anesthesia should not be used and is considered contraindicated. Avoidance of elevations in PVR is critical; thus, additional sedative medications should be used cautiously as reductions in ventilation will lead to hypercarbia and elevation of PVR.

b. **For general anesthesia,** slow titration of induction agents is preferred as rapid sequence inductions carry high risk of SVR alterations and subsequent hemodynamic collapse. This places the patient at increased risk of aspiration, so strict NPO guidelines, use of pharmacologic prophylaxis against aspiration (sodium citrate, H_2 blockade, etc.), and mask ventilation using cricoid pressure should be considered. Ketamine and etomidate are probably the best options for induction agents, whereas propofol and thiopental should be avoided due to marked reductions in SVR or cardiac output. Inhalational agents should be used with caution because of their propensity to decrease SVR. Nitrous oxide should be avoided because of its propensity to increase PVR. Maintenance of anesthesia may be accomplished using careful titration of IV agents such as nondepolarizing neuromuscular blockers, opioids, and sedative-hypnotic agents such as midazolam or ketamine, "topping off" with potent inhalational agents being used at concentrations of less than 0.5 MAC.

c. **Monitors: Pulse oximetry** may be the most important monitor as changes in saturation directly correlate with alterations in shunt flow [25]. **Intra-arterial monitoring** is generally employed to closely follow blood pressure. Central venous catheters are controversial. CVP catheter placement carries a risk of air embolus, thrombus, and pneumothorax, which can be devastating in these patients, although information regarding cardiac filling pressures can be useful. **PA catheters are relatively contraindicated** in patients with ES for a number of reasons [25]. The anatomic abnormality causing ES typically renders flow-directed flotation of PA catheters difficult or impossible, and the risk of arrhythmia, PA rupture, and thromboembolism are elevated. Cardiac output measurements will be inaccurate due to the large shunt. TEE may provide the best real-time monitor of cardiac preload and of the status of right-to-left shunting.

Anesthetic and hemodynamic goals for ES

1. **Avoid elevations in PVR:** Prevent hypoxemia, acidosis, hypercarbia, and pain. Provide supplemental oxygen at all times.
2. **Maintain SVR:** Reductions in SVR will increase right-to-left shunting.
3. **Avoid myocardial depressants and maintain myocardial contractility.**
4. **Maintain preload and sinus rhythm.**

4. **Can iNO be employed in ES?** iNO is a direct-acting pulmonary vasodilator that avoids systemic vasodilation, thus reducing shunt flow and hypoxia. Evidence for the use of iNO for labor in Eisenmenger patients is limited, but several case reports indicate improvement in oxygenation and reduced pulmonary pressures [63]. Therapy with IV pulmonary vasodilators may be required postoperatively to prevent rebound elevation in pulmonary pressures.

XIII. What are the antibiotic prophylactic considerations for patients with ACHD?

Infective endocarditis carries high morbidity and mortality, and as such has led to previous recommendations regarding antibiotic prophylaxis regimens for patients with heart defects. Current recommendations center around the concept that most exposures to infectious agents occur during daily activities, and suggest maintaining a high index of suspicion for signs of endocarditis in susceptible patients [64]. Good oral hygiene is critical for these patients to help prevent infection and antibiotic prophylaxis is recommended only in select lesions listed in Table 15.7.

XIV. Conclusions

ACHD encompasses a wide range of patients with variable presentations, symptoms, and degree of illness. Some of the key and most common presentations have been addressed in this chapter; however, due to the huge range of presentations, variations in all of these lesions are likely to be found, and many other diagnoses have not been covered. The underlying concept found throughout management of ACHD is to obtain as much information as possible about the patient's medical and surgical history, along with current functional capacity as this will give the greatest information about current level of heart failure. On the basis of this information, consider the lesion based on the classifications discussed above, and develop an anesthetic management plan based on individualized physiology for your patient. Consultation with congenital cardiologists or cardiothoracic surgeons can be invaluable.
8 Patients with complicated residual lesions requiring medium- to high-risk surgery should be handled at centers of excellence with physicians and nursing staff trained in adult congenital disease.

TABLE 15.7 Cardiac conditions associated with highest risk of adverse outcomes from endocarditis for which prophylaxis with dental procedures is reasonable

Condition	Congenital specific condition[a]
• Previous infective endocarditis • Prosthetic cardiac valve or prosthetic material used for cardiac valve repair	• Unrepaired cyanotic CHD, including palliative shunts and conduits • Completely repaired congenital heart defect with prosthetic material or device, whether placed by surgery or by catheter intervention, during the first 6 mos after the procedure[b] • Repaired CHD with residual defects at the site or adjacent to the site of a prosthetic patch or prosthetic device that inhibit endothelialization • Cardiac transplant recipients who develop cardiac valvulopathy

[a]Except for the conditions listed above, antibiotic prophylaxis is no longer recommended for any other form of CHD.
[b]Prophylaxis is reasonable because endothelialization of prosthetic material occurs within 6 mos after the procedure.
CHD, congenital heart disease.
Modified with permission to include footnotes from Wilson W, Taubert KA, Gewitz M, et al. Prevention of infective endocarditis: Guidelines from the American Heart Association: A guideline from the American Heart Association Rheumatic Fever, Endocarditis, and Kawasaki Disease Committee, Council on Cardiovascular Disease in the Young, and the Council on Clinical Cardiology, Council on Cardiovascular Surgery and Anesthesia, and the Quality of Care and Outcomes Research Interdisciplinary Working Group. *Circulation.* 2007;116:1736–1754.

REFERENCES

1. Kaemmerer H, Meisner H, Hess J, et al. Surgical treatment of patent ductus arteriosus: A new historical perspective. *Am J Cardiol.* 2004;94:1153–1154.
2. Webb GD, Williams RG. 32nd Bethesda Conference: "Care of the adult with congenital heart disease". *J Am Coll Cardiol.* 2001;37:1162.
3. Mitchell SC, Korones SB, Berendes HW. Congenital heart disease in 56,109 births. Incidence and natural history. *Circulation.* 1971;43:323–332.
4. van der Bom T, Zomer AC, Zwinderman AH, et al. The changing epidemiology of congenital heart disease. *Nat Rev Cardiol.* 2011;8:50–60.
5. Connelly MS, Webb GD, Somerville J, et al. Canadian Consensus Conference on Congenital Heart Defects in the Adult 1996. *Can J Cardiol.* 1998;14:533–597.
6. Connelly MS, Webb GD, Somerville J, et al. Canadian Consensus Conference on Adult Congenital Heart Disease 1996. *Can J Cardiol.* 1998;14:395–452.
7. Warnes CA, Williams RG, Bashore TM, et al. ACC/AHA 2008 Guidelines for the Management of Adults with Congenital Heart Disease: Executive Summary: A report of the American College of Cardiology/American Heart Association Task Force on Practice Guidelines (writing committee to develop guidelines for the management of adults with congenital heart disease). *Circulation.* 2008;118:2395–2451.
8. Chassot PG, Bettex DA. Anesthesia and adult congenital heart disease. *J Cardiothorac Vasc Anesth.* 2006;20:414–437.
9. Williams RG, Pearson GD, Barst RJ, et al. Report of the National Heart, Lung, and Blood Institute Working Group on research in adult congenital heart disease. *J Am Coll Cardiol.* 2006;47:701–707.
10. Silversides CK, Dore A, Poirier N, et al. Canadian Cardiovascular Society 2009 Consensus Conference on the management of adults with congenital heart disease: Shunt lesions. *Can J Cardiol.* 2010;26:e70–e79.
11. Silversides CK, Kiess M, Beauchesne L, et al. Canadian Cardiovascular Society 2009 Consensus Conference on the management of adults with congenital heart disease: Outflow tract obstruction, coarctation of the aorta, tetralogy of Fallot, Ebstein anomaly and Marfan's syndrome. *Can J Cardiol.* 2010;26:e80–e97.
12. Silversides CK, Marelli A, Beauchesne L, et al. Canadian Cardiovascular Society 2009 Consensus Conference on the management of adults with congenital heart disease: Executive summary. *Can J Cardiol.* 2010;26:143–150.
13. Silversides CK, Salehian O, Oechslin E, et al. Canadian Cardiovascular Society 2009 Consensus Conference on the management of adults with congenital heart disease: Complex congenital cardiac lesions. *Can J Cardiol.* 2010;26:e98–e117.
14. Sable C, Foster E, Uzark K, et al. Best practices in managing transition to adulthood for adolescents with congenital heart disease: The transition process and medical and psychosocial issues: A scientific statement from the American Heart Association. *Circulation.* 2011;123:1454–1485.
15. Karamlou T, Diggs BS, Ungerleider RM, et al. Adults or big kids: What is the ideal clinical environment for management of grown-up patients with congenital heart disease? *Ann Thorac Surg.* 2010;90:573–579.
16. Seal R. Adult congenital heart disease. *Paediatr Anaesth.* 2011;21:615–622.
17. Ashley EA, Niebauer J. *Cardiology Explained.* London: Remedica Pub Ltd; 2004.
18. Gallagher M, David Hayes M, Jane EH. Practice advisory for the perioperative management of patients with cardiac implantable electronic devices: Pacemakers and implantable cardioverter-defibrillators. *Anesthesiology.* 2011;114:247.
19. Khairy P, Aboulhosn J, Gurvitz MZ, et al. Arrhythmia burden in adults with surgically repaired tetralogy of Fallot: A multi-institutional study. *Circulation.* 2010;122:868–875.

20. Walsh EP, Cecchin F. Arrhythmias in adult patients with congenital heart disease. *Circulation.* 2007;115:534–545.
21. Bernier M, Marelli AJ, Pilote L, et al. Atrial arrhythmias in adult patients with right- versus left-sided congenital heart disease anomalies. *Am J Cardiol.* 2010;106:547–551.
22. de Groot NM, Atary JZ, Blom NA, et al. Long-term outcome after ablative therapy of postoperative atrial tachyarrhythmia in patients with congenital heart disease and characteristics of atrial tachyarrhythmia recurrences. *Circ Arrhythm Electrophysiol.* 2010;3:148–154.
23. Weitzel N. Pulmonary hypertension. In: Chu L, Fuller A, eds. *Manual of Clinical Anesthesiology.* 1st ed. Philadelphia, PA: Lippincott Williams & Wilkins; 2012:447–452.
24. Blaise G, Langleben D, Hubert B. Pulmonary arterial hypertension: Pathophysiology and anesthetic approach. *Anesthesiology.* 2003;99:1415–1432.
25. Weitzel N, Gravlee G. Cardiac disease in the obstetric patient. In: Bucklin B, Gambling D, Wlody D, eds. *A Practical Approach to Obstetric Anesthesia.* 1st ed. Philadelphia, PA: Lippincott Williams & Wilkins; 2009:403–434.
26. Holst KA, Dearani JA, Burkhart HM, et al. Risk factors and early outcomes of multiple reoperations in adults with congenital heart disease. *Ann Thorac Surg.* 2011;92:122–130.
27. Kirshbom PM, Myung RJ, Simsic JM, et al. One thousand repeat sternotomies for congenital cardiac surgery: Risk factors for reentry injury. *Ann Thorac Surg.* 2009;88:158–161.
28. Park CB, Suri RM, Burkhart HM, et al. Identifying patients at particular risk of injury during repeat sternotomy: Analysis of 2555 cardiac reoperations. *J Thorac Cardiovasc Surg.* 2010;140:1028–1035.
29. Elahi M, Dhannapuneni R, Firmin R, et al. Direct complications of repeat median sternotomy in adults. *Asian Cardiovasc Thorac Ann.* 2005;13:135–138.
30. Asghar Nawaz M, Patni R, Chan KM, et al. Hyperinflation of lungs during redo-sternotomy, a safer technique. *Heart Lung Circ.* 2011;20:722–723.
31. Ferraris VA, Brown JR, Despotis GJ, et al. 2011 update to the Society of Thoracic Surgeons and the Society of Cardiovascular anesthesiologists blood conservation clinical practice guidelines. *Ann Thorac Surg.* 2011;91:944–982.
32. Fergusson DA, Hebert PC, Mazer CD, et al. A comparison of aprotinin and lysine analogues in high-risk cardiac surgery. *N Engl J Med.* 2008;358:2319–2331.
33. Henry DA, Carless PA, Moxey AJ, et al. Anti-fibrinolytic use for minimising perioperative allogeneic blood transfusion. *Cochrane Database Syst Rev.* 2011:CD001886.
34. Henry DA, Carless PA, Moxey AJ, et al. Anti-fibrinolytic use for minimising perioperative allogeneic blood transfusion. *Cochrane Database Syst Rev.* 2007:CD001886.
35. Karkouti K, Beattie WS, Dattilo KM, et al. A propensity score case-control comparison of aprotinin and tranexamic acid in high-transfusion-risk cardiac surgery. *Transfusion.* 2006;46:327–338.
36. Ranucci M, Castelvecchio S, Romitti F, et al. Living without aprotinin: The results of a 5-year blood saving program in cardiac surgery. *Acta Anaesthesiol Scand.* 2009;53:573–580.
37. Davies RR, Russo MJ, Yang J, et al. Listing and transplanting adults with congenital heart disease. *Circulation.* 2011;123:759–767.
38. Eagle SS, Daves SM. The adult with Fontan physiology: Systematic approach to perioperative management for noncardiac surgery. *J Cardiothorac Vasc Anesth.* 2011;25:320–334.
39. Heggie J, Karski J. The anesthesiologist's role in adults with congenital heart disease. *Cardiol Clin.* 2006;24:571–585, vi.
40. d'Udekem Y, Iyengar AJ, Cochrane AD, et al. The Fontan procedure: Contemporary techniques have improved long-term outcomes. *Circulation.* 2007;116:I157–I164.
41. Nollert G, Fischlein T, Bouterwek S, et al. Long-term survival in patients with repair of tetralogy of Fallot: 36-year follow-up of 490 survivors of the first year after surgical repair. *J Am Coll Cardiol.* 1997;30:1374–1383.
42. Dearani JA, Danielson GK, Puga FJ, et al. Late follow-up of 1095 patients undergoing operation for complex congenital heart disease utilizing pulmonary ventricle to pulmonary artery conduits. *Ann Thorac Surg.* 2003;75:399–410; discussion 1.
43. Rodefeld MD, Ruzmetov M, Turrentine MW, et al. Reoperative right ventricular outflow tract conduit reconstruction: Risk analyses at follow up. *J Heart Valve Dis.* 2008;17:119–126; discussion 26.
44. Bashore TM. Adult congenital heart disease: Right ventricular outflow tract lesions. *Circulation.* 2007;115:1933–1947.
45. Bonow RO, Carabello BA, Chatterjee K, et al. 2008 Focused update incorporated into the ACC/AHA 2006 guidelines for the management of patients with valvular heart disease: A report of the American College of Cardiology/American Heart Association Task Force on Practice Guidelines (Writing Committee to Revise the 1998 Guidelines for the Management of Patients With Valvular Heart Disease): Endorsed by the Society of Cardiovascular Anesthesiologists, Society for Cardiovascular Angiography and Interventions, and Society of Thoracic Surgeons. *Circulation.* 2008;118:e523–e661.
46. Jarrar M, Betbout F, Farhat MB, et al. Long-term invasive and noninvasive results of percutaneous balloon pulmonary valvuloplasty in children, adolescents, and adults. *Am Heart J.* 1999;138:950–954.
47. Chen CR, Cheng TO, Huang T, et al. Percutaneous balloon valvuloplasty for pulmonic stenosis in adolescents and adults. *N Engl J Med.* 1996;335:21–25.
48. Brickner ME, Hillis LD, Lange RA. Congenital heart disease in adults. First of two parts. *N Engl J Med.* 2000;342:256–263.
49. Sommer RJ, Hijazi ZM, Rhodes JF, Jr. Pathophysiology of congenital heart disease in the adult: part I: Shunt lesions. *Circulation.* 2008;117:1090–1099.
50. Rao PS. When and how should atrial septal defects be closed in adults? *J Invasive Cardiol.* 2009;21:76–82.
51. Calvert PA, Rana BS, Kydd AC, et al. Patent foramen ovale: Anatomy, outcomes, and closure. *Nat Rev Cardiol.* 2011;8:148–160.
52. Tomar M, Khatri S, Radhakrishnan S, et al. Intermediate and long-term followup of percutaneous device closure of fossa ovalis atrial septal defect by the Amplatzer septal occluder in a cohort of 529 patients. *Ann Pediatr Cardiol.* 2011;4:22–27.
53. Kretschmar O, Sglimbea A, Corti R, et al. Shunt reduction with a fenestrated Amplatzer device. *Catheter Cardiovasc Interv.* 2010;76:564–571.

54. Sadiq M, Kazmi T, Rehman AU, et al. Device closure of atrial septal defect: Medium-term outcome with special reference to complications. *Cardiol Young.* 2011:1–8 [Epub ahead of print July 11].
55. Zeinaloo A, Macuil B, Zanjani KS, et al. Transcatheter patch occlusion of ventricular septal defect in Down syndrome. *Am J Cardiol.* 2011;107:1838–1840.
56. Yang R, Sheng Y, Cao K, et al. Transcatheter closure of perimembranous ventricular septal defect in children: Safety and efficiency with symmetric and asymmetric occluders. *Catheter Cardiovasc Interv.* 2011;77:84–90.
57. Wei Y, Wang X, Zhang S, et al. Transcatheter closure of perimembranous ventricular septal defects (VSD) with VSD occluder: Early and mid-term results. *Heart Vessels.* 2011. [Epub ahead of print May 27]
58. Ramakrishnan S, Saxena A, Choudhary SK. Residual VSD closure with an ADO II device in an infant. *Congen Heart Dis.* 2011;6:60–63.
59. Li X, Li L, Wang X, et al. Clinical analysis of transcatheter closure of perimembranous ventricular septal defects with occluders made in China. *Chin Med J (Engl).* 2011;124:2117–2122.
60. Gu M, You X, Zhao X, et al. Transcatheter device closure of intracristal ventricular septal defects. *Am J Cardiol.* 2011;107: 110–113.
61. Lovell AT. Anaesthetic implications of grown-up congenital heart disease. *Br J Anaesth.* 2004;93:129–139.
62. Martin JT, Tautz TJ, Antognini JF. Safety of regional anesthesia in Eisenmenger's syndrome. *Reg Anesth Pain Med.* 2002;27:509–513.
63. Ray P, Murphy GJ, Shutt LE. Recognition and management of maternal cardiac disease in pregnancy. *Br J Anaesth.* 2004;93:428–439.
64. Wilson W, Taubert KA, Gewitz M, et al. Prevention of infective endocarditis. Guidelines from the American Heart Association. A guideline from the American Heart Association Rheumatic Fever, Endocarditis, and Kawasaki Disease Committee, Council on Cardiovascular Disease in the Young, and the Council on Clinical Cardiology, Council on Cardiovascular Surgery and Anesthesia, and the Quality of Care and Outcomes Research Interdisciplinary Working Group. *Circulation.* 2007;116:1736–1754.

16 Anesthetic Management of Cardiac Transplantation

Kishan Dwarakanath, Anne L. Rother, and Charles D. Collard

KEY POINTS

1. Nonischemic cardiomyopathy (53%) is the most common pretransplant diagnosis worldwide.
2. Nearly 70% of recipients in the United States require some form of life support prior to cardiac transplantation. For example, in the United States, the number of pretransplant patients with ventricular assist devices has risen dramatically over the recent years.

(continued)

3. Increased preoperative pulmonary vascular resistance in the recipient is predictive of early graft dysfunction and increased mortality related to an increased incidence of right heart dysfunction.
4. Because of intact spinal reflexes, transplant donors may exhibit hypertension, tachycardia, and muscles movement. These responses do not indicate cerebral function or pain perception.
5. During orthotopic cardiac transplantation, the cardiac autonomic plexus is transected, leaving the transplanted heart without autonomic innervation. Inotropes are utilized in the postbypass period.
6. Right ventricular failure is a significant cause of early morbidity and mortality accounting for nearly 20% of early deaths after transplantation. RV failure and increased pulmonary vascular resistance in the postbypass period can be often challenging for the cardiac anesthesiologist to manage.
7. Cardiac allograft vasculopathy (CAV) is a form of graft failure. Unlike atherosclerotic CAD, CAV is characterized by diffuse intimal hyperplasia.
8. In contrast to the non-transplanted patient, where increases in cardiac output can be quickly achieved through a sympathetically mediated increase in heart rate, the cardiac transplanted patient, whose sympathetic innervation to the heart will be interrupted, tends to require an increase in preload in order to increase cardiac output.
9. Autonomic denervation of the heart alters the pharmacodynamic response of many drugs (Table 16.8). Drugs that act directly on the heart are effective.
10. Regional or general anesthesia has been successfully utilized in the postcardiac transplant patient for surgical procedures. For any selected anesthetic technique, maintenance of preload is essential (see keypoint 8 above).

ALTHOUGH "DESTINATION THERAPY" USING MECHANICAL circulatory support (MCS) devices has increasingly become a viable option, cardiac transplantation remains the gold standard for the treatment of heart failure (HF) refractory to medical therapy [1]. Since the first human cardiac transplant by Christiaan Barnard in 1967, over 89,000 cardiac transplants have been performed worldwide [2]. Currently, approximately 3,500 cardiac transplants are performed per annum, with approximately 2,200 occurring in the United States [2]. Despite an increasingly high-risk patient population, survival rates continue to improve due to advances in immunosuppression, surgical technique, perioperative management, and the diagnosis and treatment of allograft rejection [3]. In the United States, cardiac transplantation is limited to member centers of the United Network for Organ Sharing (UNOS). UNOS, in turn, administers the Organ Procurement and Transplantation Network (OPTN) which maintains the only national patient transplant waiting list in the United States.

I. Heart failure

More than 5 million American adults carry a diagnosis of HF, with an incidence of 670,000 per year [4]. The American College of Cardiology (ACC) and the American Heart Association (AHA) define HF as a clinical syndrome that can result from any structural or functional cardiac disorder that impairs the ability of the ventricle to fill with, or eject blood. The majority of patients with HF owe their symptoms to impairment of left ventricular (LV) myocardial function [5]. Because volume overload is not necessarily present, the term "HF" is now preferred to the older term "congestive HF."

The New York Heart Association (NYHA) scale is used to quantify the degree of functional limitation imposed by HF. Most patients with HF, however, do not show an uninterrupted and inexorable progression along the NYHA scale [5]. In 2005, the ACC/AHA created a staging scheme reflective of the fact that HF has established risk factors, a clear progression, and specific treatments at each stage that can reduce morbidity and mortality (Fig. 16.1). Patients presenting for heart transplantation invariably present in Stage D, refractory HF.

A. Etiology

1 **Nonischemic cardiomyopathy (53%) is the most common pretransplant diagnosis worldwide** [2]. Ischemic cardiomyopathy accounts for 38%, with valvular cardiomyopathy, retransplantation, and congenital heart disease accounting for the remaining percentage of adult heart transplant recipients.

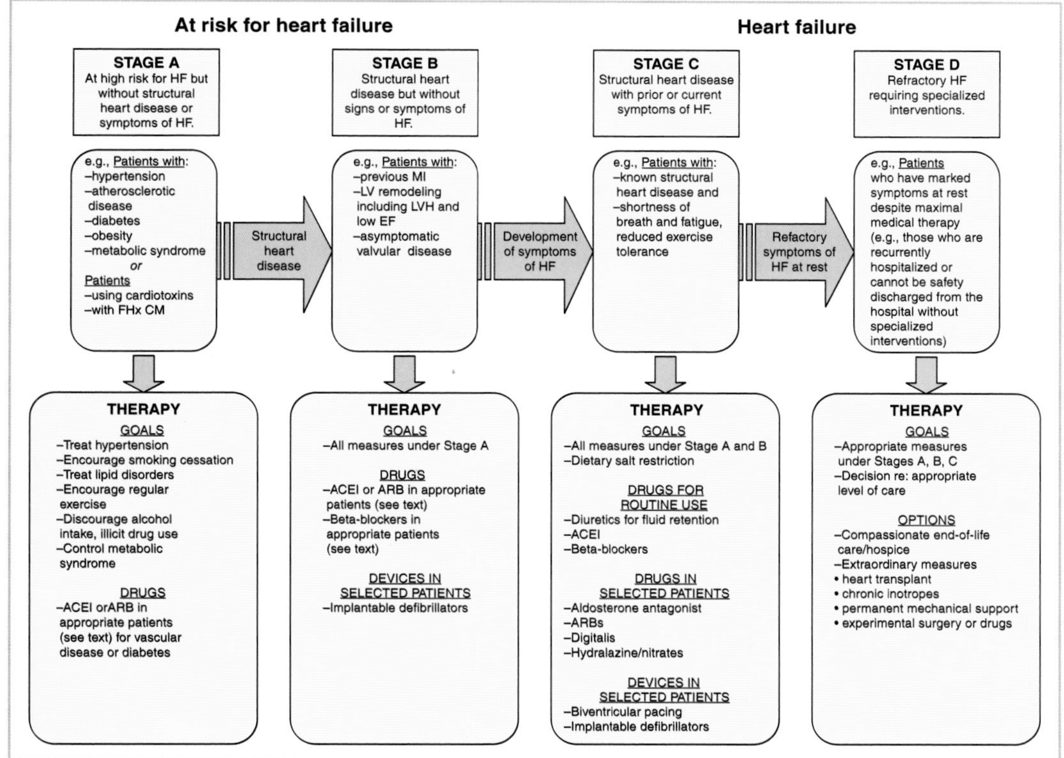

FIGURE 16.1 Stages in the development of HF and recommended therapy. (From Jessup M, Abraham WT, Casey DE, et al. Focused update incorporated into the ACC/AHA 2005 guidelines for the diagnosis and management of heart failure in adults. *Circulation.* 2009;119:e391–e479.)

B. Pathophysiology

The neurohormonal model portrays HF as a progressive disorder initiated by an index event, which either damages the myocardium directly or disrupts the ability of the myocardium to generate force [6]. HF progression is characterized by declining ventricular function and activation of compensatory adrenergic, and salt and water retention pathways. Ejection fraction (EF) is initially maintained by increases in LV end-diastolic volume, myocardial fiber length, and adrenergically mediated increases in myocardial contractility. LV remodeling takes place during this time, and while initially adaptive, may independently contribute to HF progression [6]. The chronic overexpression of molecular mediators of compensation (e.g., norepinephrine, angiotensin II, endothelin, natriuretic peptides, aldosterone, and tumor necrosis factor) may lead to deleterious effects on cardiac myocytes and their extracellular matrix [6,7]. The result is progressive LV dilation, as well as decreasing EF and cardiac output (CO). Fatigue, dyspnea, and signs of fluid retention develop. Other organ systems such as the liver and kidneys become compromised by persistent decreases in CO and elevated venous pressures. With continued progression of HF, stroke volume (SV) becomes unresponsive to increases in preload, and increases in afterload are poorly tolerated (Fig. 16.2). Chronic exposure to circulating catecholamines may result in downregulation of myocardial β_1-adrenergic receptors, making the heart less responsive to inotropic therapy.

C. Medical management of HF

1. Therapeutic goals

The therapeutic goal for HF management is to slow or halt the progression from Stage A to D. Lifestyle modifications and selected pharmacotherapy are the mainstays of therapy

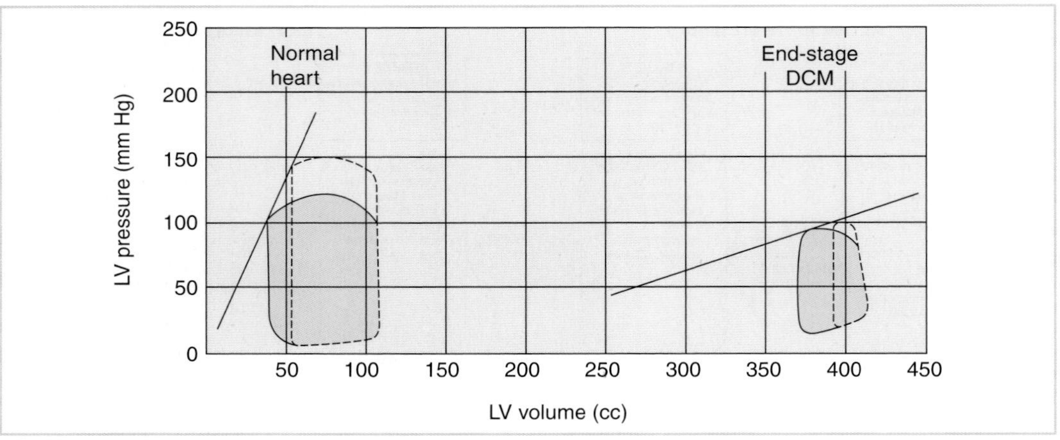

FIGURE 16.2 Pressure–volume (P–V) relationships in a normal heart and a heart with end-stage dilated cardiomyopathy (DCM). Shown are the LV P–V loops (*dotted lines*) obtained from a normal heart and a heart with end-stage DCM following an increase in afterload. The slope depicts the LV end-systolic P–V relationship. Note that the myopathic heart SV is markedly decreased by increases in afterload. (From Clark NJ, Martin RD. Anesthetic considerations for patients undergoing cardiac transplantation. *J Cardiothorac Anesth.* 1988;2:519–542, with permission.)

for Stages A and B. When Stage C is reached, combination pharmacotherapy includes diuresis, interruption of the renin–angiotensin axis, and β-blockade. Selective use of direct vasodilators and inotropes is also indicated. Utilization of cardiac resynchronization therapy (CRT) and/or an implantable defibrillator may be recommended. Despite optimum medical management, some patients will progress to Stage D, refractory HF. Chronic intravenous (IV) inotropes, mechanical support devices, and heart transplantation are the only measures available for palliation or treatment.

a. Inotropes

Inotropic agents commonly used to treat cardiac failure include digitalis, catecholamines, and phosphodiesterase-III (PDE) inhibitors. Digitalis, in combination with β-blockers, is effective in treating HF complicated by atrial fibrillation, but does not confer increased survival [5]. Administered orally, digitalis exerts a positive inotropic effect by inhibiting the myocardial cell sodium pump and increasing cytosolic calcium concentrations. Digitalis also prolongs atrioventricular conduction time, leading to a decrease in heart rate. Digitalis blood levels should be monitored as significant side effects including atrial and ventricular arrhythmias can occur, particularly in the presence of hypokalemia.

Myocardial β_1-adrenergic receptor stimulation by IV administration of catecholamines, such as epinephrine, norepinephrine, dobutamine, or dopamine, is often used to improve cardiac performance, diuresis, and clinical stability. PDE inhibitors, such as milrinone, may also be used. PDE inhibitors combine both positive inotropic and vasodilatory activity by inhibiting cyclic adenosine monophosphate (cAMP) metabolism. Occasionally, patients may not be weaned from IV inotropic support despite repeated attempts. At such times, an indwelling IV cannula may be placed to allow for the continuous infusion of an inotrope for patients awaiting transplantation, or to facilitate home palliation. However, the use of chronic inotrope has not been shown to increase survival [5].

b. Diuretics

Diuretics provide symptomatic relief to HF patients more quickly than any other class of drug, and are the only class of drug used in HF that can adequately control fluid retention. Classes of diuretics used include the loop diuretics (e.g., furosemide, bumetanide, torsemide) and the thiazide diuretics (e.g., hydrochlorothiazide, metolazone). Adverse diuretic effects include electrolyte disturbances (particularly of potassium and magnesium), hypotension, intravascular volume depletion, and azotemia.

c. **Renin–angiotensin–aldosterone system inhibitors**
The renin–angiotensin–aldosterone system may be inhibited by angiotensin converting enzyme inhibitors (ACEIs), angiotensin receptor blockers (ARBs), or the aldosterone receptor. In combination with β_1-antagonists, ACEIs have been shown to reduce HF progression by interfering with the neurohormonal pathways that modulate LV remodeling; ACEIs alleviate symptoms, enhance the overall sense of well-being, and reduce the risk of hospitalization and death in patients with HF [5]. Adverse effects of ACEIs include hypotension, worsening renal function, and hyperkalemia. If the adverse effects of ACEIs cannot be tolerated, ARBs may be considered as an alternative. The propensity of ARBs to increase serum potassium levels limits their usage in patients with impaired renal function. Aldosterone exerts an adverse effect on heart structure and function independent of angiotensin II [5]. Spironolactone is the most widely used aldosterone antagonist in HF patients, although eplerenone has been studied in HF after myocardial infarction.

d. **Vasodilators**
Vasodilators are used in the acute treatment of HF to reduce myocardial preload and afterload, thereby reducing myocardial work and oxygen demand. Nitrates (e.g., nitroglycerine and sodium nitroprusside) may also be useful for relieving the symptoms of pulmonary edema by reducing ventricular filling pressures and afterload. β-Type natriuretic peptide (nesiritide) is used effectively for the medical management of decompensated HF [5]. Nesiritide, an arterial and venous dilator, acts by increasing cyclic guanosylmonophosphate (cGMP) [8]. In hospitalized patients, the use of nesiritide was associated with a dose-dependent reduction of pulmonary capillary wedge pressure (PCWP), right atrial pressure, and mean pulmonary artery (PA) pressure, along with improvements in cardiac index and clinical outcome [9]. However, a clear benefit in terms of morbidity and mortality has not been demonstrated for the use of nesiritide in acute or chronic HF [5].

e. **β-Adrenergic receptor blockade**
In combination with interruption of the renin–angiotensin–aldosterone axis and diuresis, β-adrenergic receptor blockade is the standard treatment for HF. Carvedilol, bisoprolol, and sustained release metoprolol have been demonstrated to be effective in reducing mortality in patients with chronic HF [5]. **Chronic adrenergic stimulation is initially supportive to the failing heart, but may lead to progression of HF through neurohormonally mediated LV remodeling.** β-Blockers likely exert their benefit through attenuation of this influence. Adverse reactions to β-blockers in patients with HF include fluid retention, fatigue, bradycardia, heart block, and hypotension.

f. **Anticoagulants**
Patients with HF are at increased risk of thromboembolism as a result of low CO and a high incidence of coexistent atrial fibrillation. Long-term prophylactic anticoagulation with agents such as coumadin is common and may contribute to perioperative bleeding at the time of cardiac transplantation.

g. **Cardiac implantable electronic devices (CIEDs)**
CIEDs broadly consist of devices that seek to manage bradyarrhythmias (pacemakers), tachyarrhythmias (implantable cardiac defibrillators), and ventricular dyssynchrony (biventricular pacing/CRT). These devices are used to slow HF progression and reduce the incidence of sudden death [5,10]. Their presence may complicate the placement of central venous catheters and require the involvement of an electrophysiology team for interrogation and reprogramming [11].

D. **Mechanical circulatory support (MCS) devices**

2 Nearly 70% of recipients in the United States require some form of life support prior to heart transplantation [12]. These include IV medications, mechanical ventilation, intra-aortic balloon

pumps (IABPs), extracorporeal life support (ELS), total artificial hearts (TAH), and ventricular assist devices (VADs). IV medications, IABPs, ELS, and extracorporeal VADs are useful in temporizing a hospitalized patient with cardiogenic shock. Intracorporeal MCS devices offer the potential for discharge to home and may yield the greatest potential improvement in quality of life for patients with Class D HF who are awaiting heart transplant.

In the United States, the number of patients undergoing heart transplantation with a preexistent VAD has risen dramatically (16% in 1999 vs. 29% in 2008) [12]. The increased use of VADs has resulted in an increase in the number of outpatients being transplanted (39% to 48%), and has in part contributed to a decline in the heart transplant waiting list mortality secondary to their use as a bridge to transplantation [12]. Six-month survival while being supported on a VAD approaches 75% [13]. However, the influence of VADs on post–heart-transplant survival is controversial, with some studies suggesting an increased 6-mo mortality after transplant, while more recent studies suggest no increase in mortality [14–17]. Confounding the task of answering these questions is the rapid evolution of the devices being used, and problems inherent in applying results from earlier pulsatile devices to more recent continuous-flow devices.

II. Cardiac transplant recipient characteristics

Between 1999 and 2008, the number of active transplant candidates in the United States declined by 32%, despite an increase of 20% between 2007 and 2008 [12]. The decline has taken place despite an increasing number of patients with Stage D HF. In 1999, UNOS modified its listing system to be two-tiered (Table 16.1), and in 2006, UNOS modified the allocation of donor hearts to expand organ sharing within geographic regions. In 2007, the median time to transplantation was 113 days. Among adults, there was an increase in the number of candidates >65 yrs (9% in 1999 vs. 14% in 2008) [12]. Among all age groups, there was an increase in congenital heart disease as a primary diagnosis (4.4% in 1999 vs. 8.9% in 2008), and a decrease in coronary artery disease (CAD) as a primary diagnosis (47% in 1999 vs. 40% in 2008) [12]. Finally, the percentage of patients classified as 1A or 1B has increased dramatically (18% in 1999 vs. 46% in 2008) [12]. The reduction in waiting list mortality and increases in Category 1A and 1B candidates may be in part due to the impact of VADs.

A. Cardiac transplantation indications

Indications for heart transplantation are listed in Table 16.2 [5,18]. Potential cardiac transplant candidates must have all reversible causes of HF excluded, and their medical management optimized.

B. Cardiac transplantation contraindications

There has been a gradual relaxation in the cardiac transplantation exclusion criteria as experience with increasingly complex cases has grown [2]. Absolute exclusion criteria have been simplified (Table 16.3) [18].

TABLE 16.1 UNOS listing criteria for heart transplantation

1A. Admitted to the listing transplant center hospital with *at least one* of the following:
- **a.** Assisted MCS for acute hemodynamic decompensation
- **b.** Assisted MCS with significant device-related complications
- **c.** Continuous mechanical ventilation
- **d.** Continuous infusion of a single high-dose IV inotrope or multiple inotropes, in addition to continuous hemodynamic monitoring of LV filling pressures

1B. Has at least one of the following devices or therapies in place:
- **a.** Left and/or right VAD implanted
- **b.** Continuous infusion of IV inotrope

2. A patient who does not meet the criteria for Status 1A or 1B

3. Considered temporarily unsuitable to receive a thoracic organ transplant

MCS, mechanical circulatory support; VAD, ventricular assist device; IV, intravenous.
From OPTN policy 3.7.3 at http://optn.transplant.hrsa.gov/policiesandbylaws2/policies/pdfs/policy_9.pdf. Accessed 15 July, 2011.

TABLE 16.2 Indications for heart transplantation

Cardiogenic shock requiring either continuous IV inotropic support or MCS
Persistent NYHA Class IV HF symptoms refractory to maximal medical therapy (LVEF < 20%; peak VO_2 < 10–12 mL/kg/min)
Intractable or severe anginal symptoms in patients with CAD not amenable to percutaneous or surgical revascularization
Intractable life-threatening arrhythmias unresponsive to medical therapy, catheter ablation, and/or implantation of a intracardiac defibrillator

IV, intravenous; MCS, mechanical circulatory support; NYHA, The New York Heart Association; LVEF, left ventricular ejection fraction; HF, heart failure; CAD, coronary artery disease.
From Mancini D, Lietz K. Selection of cardiac transplantation candidates in 2010. *Circulation.* 2010;122:173–183.

Increased preoperative pulmonary vascular resistance (PVR) is predictive of early graft dysfunction and increased mortality because of an increased incidence of right heart dysfunction [18]. Methods used to quantify the severity of pulmonary HTN include calculation of PVR and the transpulmonary gradient (mean PA pressure – PCWP). At most centers, patients are not considered orthotopic cardiac transplant candidates if they demonstrate a PVR >6 Wood units or transpulmonary gradient >15 mm Hg without evidence of pharmacologic reversibility [18]. The reversibility of pulmonary HTN can be evaluated by vasodilator administration, including IV sodium nitroprusside, inhaled nitric oxide (iNO), and inhaled epoprostenol (PGI_2).

TABLE 16.3 Contraindications to heart transplantation

Absolute contraindications
Systemic illness with a life expectancy <2 yrs despite transplant, including the following:
Active or recent solid organ or blood malignancy within 5 yrs
AIDS with frequent opportunistic infections
Systemic lupus erythematosus, sarcoid, or amyloidosis that has multisystem involvement and is still active
Irreversible renal or hepatic dysfunction in patients considered only for heart transplant
Significant obstructive pulmonary disease (Forced expiratory volume in 1 second [FEV_1] <1 L/min)
Fixed pulmonary hypertension
PA systolic pressure >60 mm Hg
Mean transpulmonary gradient >15 mm Hg
Pulmonary vascular resistance >6 Wood units
Relative contraindications
Age >72 yrs
An active infection excepting device-related infection in patients with VAD
Severe peripheral vascular or cerebrovascular disease
Symptomatic carotid stenosis
Uncorrected abdominal aortic aneurysm > 6 cm
Severe diabetes mellitus with end-organ damage (neuropathy, nephropathy, or retinopathy)
Peripheral vascular disease not amenable to percutaneous or surgical therapy
Morbid obesity (BMI >35 kg/m^2)
Recent pulmonary infarction (6–8 wks)
Irreversible neurological or neuromuscular disorder
Drug, tobacco, or alcohol abuse within 6 mos
Active mental illness or psychosocial instability
Difficult-to-control hypertension
Active peptic ulcer disease
Heparin-induced thrombocytopenia within 100 days
Creatinine >2.5 mg/dL or creatinine clearance <25 mL/min
Bilirubin >2.5 mg/dL, serum transaminases >3×, INR >1.5 off Coumadin

PA, pulmonary artery; ventricular assist device; BMI, body mass index; VAD, ventricular assist device; INR, international normalized ratio.
From Mancini D, Lietz K. Selection of cardiac transplantation candidates in 2010. *Circulation.* 2010;122:173–183.

In patients who receive VADs, "fixed" elevated PVR may be reduced and thus improve post-transplant outcome, or qualify a previously excluded patient for heart transplant [18–22]. **The only transplant options for patients with severe irreversible pulmonary HTN include heterotopic cardiac or combined heart–lung transplantation (HLT).**

III. The cardiac transplant donor

A. Donor selection

The primary factor limiting cardiac transplantation is a shortage of donors. Standard criteria for donors, first outlined in the 1980s, resulted in a paucity of donor organs relative to the number of patients who could benefit from heart transplantation. In an attempt to increase donor numbers, the criteria for cardiac organ donation have been relaxed. The so-called "marginal donor" hearts may be transplanted into borderline heart transplant candidates with good results when compared to their expected prognosis without transplantation [18,23–25]. Characteristics of marginal donors include older age (>55 yrs), the presence of CAD, donor–recipient size mismatch, history of donor drug abuse, increased ischemic times, and donor seropositivity for viral hepatitis [18,23–25]. Nonetheless, the risk of failed transplantation increases with donor age and the presence of concomitant disease [2]. Contraindications to heart donation are listed in Table 16.4.

Before a donor heart may be harvested, permission for donation must be obtained, the suitability of the heart for donation must be ascertained, and the diagnosis of brain death must be made. Initial functional and structural evaluation of the potential heart donor is made with electrocardiography and transthoracic echocardiography. Normal LV function is predictive of suitability for heart transplantation, and subsequent management of the donor may be guided by other invasive monitors such as PA catheters or serial echocardiography [24,25]. Coronary angiography may be performed on patients ≥40 yrs [26]. Donor–recipient factors such as size, ABO compatibility, and antihuman leukocyte antigen (HLA)–antibody compatibility are also be assessed. Logistic factors, including ischemic organ time, must be considered. Finally, the harvesting surgeon will directly inspect the donor heart [26].

B. Determination of brain death

In the United States, The Uniform Determination of Death Act defines death as either (1) the irreversible cessation of circulatory and respiratory functions or (2) irreversible cessation of all functions of the entire brain, including the brain stem. The determination of death must be made in accordance with accepted medical standards. For the diagnosis of brain death to be made, the patient's core body temperature must be >32.5°C, and no drug with the potential to alter neurologic or neuromuscular function should be present.

C. Pathophysiology of brain death

When brain death results from severe brain injury, increased intracranial pressure results in progressive herniation and ischemia of the brain stem. Subsequent hemodynamic instability,

TABLE 16.4 Contraindications to heart donation

Contraindications
Absolute contraindications
Positive serology for syphilis, HTLV-4, and HIV
Presence of malignancy with extracranial metastatic potential
LVEF of < 40%
Significant valvular abnormality
Significant CAD
Relative contraindications
Sepsis
Hepatitis B surface antigen positive
Hepatitis C antibody positive
Repeated need for cardiopulmonary resuscitation
High-dose inotropic support exceeding 24 h

HTLV, human T-lymphotropic virus; HIV, human immunodeficiency virus; CAD, coronary artery disease.

TABLE 16.5 Incidence of pathophysiologic changes after brain stem death

Hypotension	81%
DI	65%
Disseminated intravascular coagulation	28%
Cardiac arrhythmias	25%
Pulmonary edema	18%
Metabolic acidosis	11%

DI, diabetes insipidus.
From Smith M. Physiologic changes during brain stem death – Lessons for management of the organ donor. *J Heart Lung Transplant*. 2004;23:S217–S222.

endocrine, and metabolic disturbances disrupt homeostasis, and may render organs unsuitable for transplantation (Table 16.5).

1. **Cardiovascular function**
   In an attempt to maintain cerebral blood flow to the increasingly ischemic brain stem, blood pressure (BP) and heart rate rise. While usually transient, this adrenergically mediated "sympathetic storm" may precipitate electrocardiographic and echocardiographic findings consistent with myocardial ischemia [27–29]. Occasionally, severe systemic hypertension may persist and require management [28]. Hypotension will affect most brain-dead patients and may be refractory to pressors [28]. Hypotension may result from hypovolemia caused by traumatic blood loss, central diabetes insipidus (DI), or osmotic therapy for management of elevated intracranial pressure. Loss of sympathetic tone resulting in blunted vasomotor reflexes, vasodilatation, and impaired myocardial contractility also contributes to hypotension [28]. Noxious stimuli may induce exaggerated hypertensive responses mediated by intact spinal sympathetic reflexes that are no longer inhibited by descending pathways. Despite optimal donor support, terminal cardiac arrhythmias may occur within 48 to 72 h of brain death.
2. **Endocrine dysfunction**
   Dysfunction of the posterior pituitary gland occurs in a majority of brain-dead organ donors. The loss of antidiuretic hormone (ADH) results in DI, which is manifested by polyuria, hypovolemia, and hypernatremia [28]. Derangements in other electrolytes including potassium, magnesium, and calcium may also occur as a result of DI. Dysfunction of the anterior pituitary has been inconsistently described, with hemodynamic and electrolyte disturbances attributable in part to loss of thyroid-stimulating hormone (TSH), growth hormone (GH), and adrenocorticotropic hormone (ACTH) [28,29]. Plasma concentrations of glucose may become variable (most often elevated) due to changes in serum cortisol levels, the use of catecholamine therapy, progressive insulin resistance, and the administration of glucose-containing fluids [29].
3. **Pulmonary function**
   Hypoxemia resulting from lung trauma, infection, or pulmonary edema may occur following brain death. Pulmonary edema in this setting may be neurogenic, cardiogenic, or inflammatory in origin [28].
4. **Temperature regulation**
   Thermoregulation by the hypothalamus is lost after brain death. Increased heat loss occurs as a result of an inability to vasoconstrict, along with a reduction in metabolic activity, puts brain-dead organ donors at risk for hypothermia. Adverse consequences of hypothermia include cardiac dysfunction, arrhythmias, decreased tissue oxygen delivery, coagulopathy, and cold-induced diuresis [28].
5. **Coagulation**
   Coagulopathy may result from hypothermia, and dilution of clotting factors following massive transfusion and fluid resuscitation. For reasons that are not fully understood, disseminated intravascular coagulation occurs in approximately 28% of brain dead donors [28,29].

D. Management of the cardiac transplant donor

Post-transplant graft function is in part dependent on donor care prior to organ harvesting. Strategies for managing the brain-dead organ donors seek to stabilize the donor's physiology so that the functional integrity of potentially transplantable organs is maintained [29].

1. Cardiovascular function

Donor systemic BP and central venous pressure (CVP) should be monitored continuously using arterial and central venous catheters [28]. Goals include a mean arterial pressure >60 mm Hg, a CVP of 6 to 10 mm Hg, urinary output >1 mL/kg/h, and a left ventricular ejection fraction (LVEF) >45% [28,30]. The initial treatment step in maintaining hemodynamic stability is aggressive replacement of intravascular volume with crystalloids, colloids, and packed red blood cells (PRBCs) if the hemoglobin concentration is less than 10 g/dL or the hematocrit is less than 30% [28,30].

If hemodynamic stability is not restored with fluid resuscitation, placement of a PA catheter, echocardiography, or continuous CO monitoring should be used to assess right- and left-sided intracardiac pressures, CO, and systemic vascular resistance (SVR) [28,30]. Use of inotropes and pressors should be guided by these additional diagnostics. Dopamine, epinephrine, and norepinephrine are commonly used for donor cardiovascular support. However, prolonged use of catecholamines at high doses should be avoided due to potential downregulation of β-receptors on the donor heart, and the negative impact this may have on graft function after cardiac transplant [27,28]. High-dose α-adrenergic receptor agonists should be used cautiously, as peripheral and splanchnic vasoconstriction may result in decreased perfusion of other potential donor organs and metabolic acidosis. An infusion of vasopressin has catecholamine-sparing effects without impairing graft function [28,30].

Brain-dead donors with hemodynamic instability refractory to fluids, catecholamines, and vasopressin have higher rates of organ procurement when hormonal therapy is added [28,30]. Thyroid hormone and methylprednisolone are part of the UNOS standard donor management protocol [30].

2. Fluid and electrolytes

Hypernatremia in the donor has been associated with higher rates of primary graft failure [28]. Aggressive treatment of DI with 1-desamino-8-D-arginine vasopressin (DDAVP) is indicated. IV fluids should be given to replace urinary losses and to maintain urine output [28]. Euglycemia (80 to 150 mg/dL) should be achieved through the use of dextrose-containing fluids or an insulin infusion [28]. Metabolic acidosis and respiratory alkalosis should be corrected, with a goal pH of 7.40 to 7.45 [28,30].

3. Pulmonary function

If lung procurement is also being considered, management of the brain-dead donor may become more complicated. The management from the standpoint of maximizing heart graft viability calls for aggressive fluid resuscitation, whereas a minimal volume strategy improves lung graft function after transplant, and recommendations for precise hemodynamic goals are different [28]. Management described here is from the standpoint of maximizing procurement of the heart.

In the absence of metabolic acidosis or alkalosis, minute ventilation should be adjusted to target a P_aCO_2 of 30 to 35 mm Hg [30]. The inspired oxygen concentration (F_iO_2) should be titrated to a P_aO_2 >80 mm Hg [30]. Efforts to prevent pulmonary aspiration, atelectasis, and infection are warranted. Pulmonary edema should be managed with positive end-expiratory pressure (PEEP) and diuresis.

4. Temperature

Monitoring of core temperature is mandatory as hypothermia adversely affects coagulation, cardiac rhythm, and oxygen delivery. Use of heated IV fluids, blankets, and humidifiers may prevent hypothermia.

5. Coagulation

Different transplant centers have individual guidelines for blood component therapy for management of coagulopathy. In general, component therapy should be guided by repeated donor platelet and clotting factor measurements. Generally accepted goals include an international normalized ratio (INR) of <1.5 and a platelet count of >50,000/mm^3

[28]. Antifibrinolytics to control donor bleeding are not recommended due to the risk of microvascular thromboses.

E. Anesthetic management of the donor

Anesthetic management of the donor during organ harvesting is an extension of preoperative management. An F_iO_2 of 1 is optimal for organ viability unless the lungs are to be harvested. To decrease the possibility of oxygen toxicity in the case of donor lung harvest, the minimum F_iO_2 that will maintain a P_aO_2/F_iO_2 gradient of at least 300 mm Hg should be used [28]. **Although**
4 **intact spinal reflexes may result in hypertension, tachycardia, and muscle movement, these signs do not indicate cerebral function or pain perception.** Nondepolarizing muscle relaxants may be used to prevent spinal reflex-mediated muscle movement.

F. Organ harvest technique

After initial dissection, the patient is fully heparinized. The perfusion-sensitive organs (i.e., kidneys and liver) are removed prior to cardiectomy. The donor heart is excised *en bloc* via median sternotomy after dissection of the pericardial attachments. The superior and inferior venae cavae are ligated first, allowing exsanguination. The aorta is cross-clamped and cold cardioplegia administered. The aorta and pulmonary arteries are transected, leaving the native donor arterial segments as long in length as possible. Finally, the pulmonary veins are individually divided after lifting the donor organ out of the thoracic cavity. Most donor hearts are currently preserved with specialized cold colloid solutions (e.g., University of Wisconsin solution) and placed in cold storage at 2°C [26]. When this technique is used, optimal myocardial function after transplantation is achieved when the donor heart ischemic time is less than 4 h [26].

IV. Surgical techniques for cardiac transplantation

A. Orthotopic cardiac transplantation

Over 98% of cardiac transplants performed are orthotopic. The recipient is placed on standard cardiopulmonary bypass (CPB) and, if present, the PA catheter withdrawn into the superior vena cava. The femoral vessels are often selected for arterial and venous CPB cannulation in patients undergoing repeat sternotomy. Otherwise, the distal ascending aorta is cannulated and bicaval cannulae with snares placed, completely excluding the heart from the native circulation. The aorta and pulmonary arteries are then clamped and divided. Depending on the implantation technique (Fig. 16.3), either both native atria or a single left atrial cuff containing the pulmonary veins is preserved. The native atrial appendages are discarded because of the risk of postoperative thrombus formation.

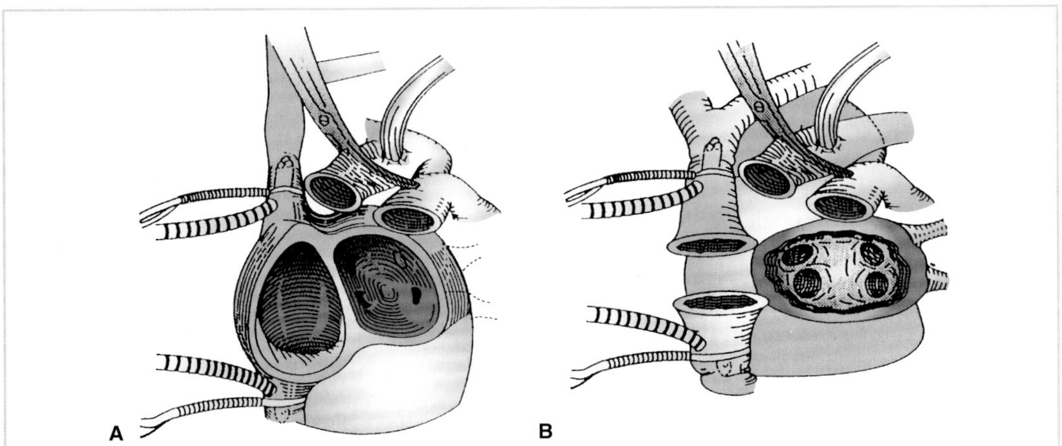

FIGURE 16.3 Surgical techniques for cardiac transplantation. **A:** Biatrial technique. The donor heart is anastomosed to the main bulk of the recipient's native right and left atria. **B:** Bicaval technique. The donor heart left atrium is anastomosed to a single left atrial cuff, including the pulmonary veins, in the recipient. (From Aziz TM, Burgess MI, El Gamel A, et al. Orthotopic cardiac transplantation technique: A survey of current practice. *Ann Thorac Surg.* 1999;68:1242–1246, with permission.)

The donor heart is inspected for the presence of a patent foramen ovale. If patent, it is surgically closed, as right-to-left interatrial shunting and hypoxemia may occur in the presence of elevated right-sided pressures following transplantation. The donor and recipient left atria are anastomosed first, followed by the right atria, or cavae when a bicaval anastomotic technique is chosen. The subsequent order of anastomoses varies depending on the donor heart ischemic time and the experience of the surgeon. The donor and recipient aortas are joined and the aortic cross-clamp removed with the patient in Trendelenburg to decrease air embolism. After completion of the PA anastomosis and placement of temporary epicardial pacing wires, the heart is deaired and the patient weaned from CPB.

1. **Biatrial implantation**

   Biatrial implantation is the technique originally described by Barnard. It preserves portions of the recipient's native atria to create two atrial anastomoses (Fig. 16.3, Panel A). Biatrial orthotopic heart transplantation has been performed successfully for over four decades and has the advantage of being relatively simple, and possibly faster to perform [31]. It is, however, falling out of favor with a decreasing percentage of heart transplants being performed this way (34.7% in 2007) [31]. The biatrial technique puts the sinoatrial node at risk of injury, redundant atrial tissue may contribute to atrial dysrhythmias, and distortion of the right atrium may contribute to a higher risk for tricuspid regurgitation [31]. Although patients receiving biatrial transplant require a higher incidence of permanent pacemakers, no definitive difference in long-term survival has been demonstrated [31,32].

2. **Bicaval implantation**

   The bicaval implantation technique is a modification of the biatrial technique. Only a single, small left atrial cuff containing the pulmonary veins is preserved in the recipient. Bicaval and left atrial anastomoses are performed (Fig. 16.3, Panel B). The bicaval technique is growing in popularity, particularly at higher volume transplant centers [31]. **Demonstrated advantages of the bicaval technique include a higher incidence of postoperative sinus rhythm, lower right atrial pressures, and a reduced need for permanent pacemaker** [31,32]**. A decreased risk of perioperative mortality may exist** [31,32]**.**

B. Heterotopic cardiac transplantation

Heterotopic transplantation accounts for less than 1% to 2% of cardiac transplantation procedures per annum. In this technique, the recipient's heart is not excised. Instead, the donor heart is placed within the right anterior thorax, and anastomosed to the recipient's native heart such that a parallel circulation is established. The recipient and donor atria are anastomosed, followed by the aortas. An artificial conduit usually joins the pulmonary arteries, with the native and donor right ventricles ejecting into the native PA. Similarly, both the native and donor left ventricles eject into the native aorta. Thus, the recipient's RV, which is conditioned to eject against elevated PA pressures, will provide most of the right-sided ventricular output, whereas the healthy donor LV will make the major contribution to left-sided ventricular output. Situations in which heterotopic cardiac transplantation may be advantageous include recipients with severe pulmonary HTN, a small donor-to-recipient size ratio, and a marginal donor heart [33]. Disadvantages of heterotopic cardiac transplantation include relatively high operative mortality, a requirement for continued medical treatment of the failing native heart, the potential for the native heart to be a thromboembolic source, and compromised pulmonary function due to placement of donor heart in the right chest [33].

V. Preoperative management of the cardiac transplant patient

A. Timing and coordination

Important considerations when planning the timing of the operation include the time required for donor organ transport, and potential for failure to complete recipient cannulation in a timely fashion (e.g., repeat sternotomy) [34]. Since the timing of heart transplants is dictated by donor availability, transplantation can take place at any hour of the day. Ideally, to minimize ischemic time, anesthetic induction of the recipient should be timed so that the recipient is already on CPB when the donor heart arrives. However, since the attendant risks of general anesthesia are magnified in the recipient, who by definition has advanced HF, induction of anesthesia ought to be delayed until a definitive "go" is received from the harvesting team.

B. Preoperative evaluation

The anesthesiologist usually has limited time for preoperative assessment of the cardiac transplant recipient. Furthermore, the use of VADs has increased the number of outpatient recipients, further reducing the available time [2,12]. These recipients will have been under the care of a medical team experienced in the management of HF, and their medical therapy is likely to have already been optimized. When the recipient is already admitted to the intensive care unit (ICU), all aspects of their ongoing care should be reviewed, including pulmonary status and ventilation settings, presence of invasive monitors and existing venous access, use of inotropes and/or pressors, and the use of MCS devices. In any case, the preoperative anesthetic evaluation should include a thorough history, physical examination, and review of the patient's medical record. The electrocardiogram (ECG), echocardiogram, chest x-ray, and cardiac catheterization results should be noted, and all hematological, renal, and liver function tests reviewed.

1. Concomitant organ dysfunction

Chronic systemic hypoperfusion and venous congestion in the recipient may produce reversible hepatic and renal dysfunction. Mild-to-moderate elevations of hepatic enzymes, bilirubin, and prolongation of prothrombin time are common. Preoperative hepatic dysfunction and anticoagulant medication may also contribute to the abnormal coagulation profile frequently observed in cardiac transplant recipients. Blood urea nitrogen is commonly elevated in patients with end-stage heart disease due to chronic hypoperfusion and the concomitant prerenal effects of high-dose diuretics.

2. Preoperative medications

Preoperative inotropic support should be continued throughout the pre-CPB period. Patients receiving digitalis and diuretics have an increased risk of dysrhythmias in the presence of hypokalemia. Anticoagulants such as coumadin, heparin, and aspirin may increase the need for perioperative blood product administration.

3. Preoperative monitoring

The position, function, and duration of invasive monitoring catheters should be noted. The function and settings of IABPs and VADs should be reviewed. If a CIED is present, it should be interrogated and the antitachyarrhythmia functions suspended in the operating room after external defibrillation pads have been applied [11]. Patients with invasive monitoring and/or MCS require extra personnel and vigilance to ensure safe transport from the ICU to the operating room.

4. The combined heart–lung recipient

The combined heart–lung transplant recipient often requires special preoperative evaluation. Recipients with cystic fibrosis should first have an otolaryngologic evaluation before being placed on a waiting list. Many of these patients will require endoscopic maxillary antrostomies for sinus access and monthly antibiotic irrigation. This measure has decreased the incidence of serious post-transplant bacterial infections in this patient population. Ex-smokers must undergo screening to exclude malignancy. A negative sputum cytology, thoracic computed tomography (CT) scan, bronchoscopy, and otolaryngologic evaluation are required. Additionally, left heart catheterization, coronary angiography, and a carotid duplex scan may be performed in previous smokers.

VI. Anesthetic management of the cardiac transplant recipient

A. Premedication

The HF patient has elevated levels of circulating catecholamines and is preload-dependent. Even a small dose of sedative medication may result in vasodilatation and hemodynamic decompensation. Supplemental oxygen should be given, and sedative avoided or carefully titrated.

Patients presenting for cardiac transplantation should be considered as having a "full stomach" as most present with short notice. If oral cyclosporine or azathioprine is started preoperatively, gastric emptying is delayed. Oral sodium citrate and/or IV metoclopramide may be useful in raising gastric pH and reducing gastric volumes.

B. Importance of aseptic technique

Perioperative immunosuppressive therapy places the cardiac transplant recipient at increased risk of infection. All invasive procedures should be done under aseptic or sterile conditions.

C. Monitoring

Noninvasive monitoring should include a standard five-lead ECG, noninvasive BP measurement, pulse oximetry, capnography, nasopharyngeal temperature, and urinary output. If not already *in situ,* large-bore peripheral and central venous access should be obtained. Invasive monitoring should include systemic arterial as well as central venous and/or PA pressures. Intraoperative transesophageal echocardiography (TEE) is commonly used. A PA catheter may be helpful in the post-CPB period, allowing monitoring of CO, ventricular filling pressures, and calculation of SVR and PVR. Traditionally, catheterization of the right internal jugular vein has been avoided to preserve this route for the endomyocardial biopsies (EMBs) routinely performed to screen for myocardial rejection. Nonetheless, difficulty with EMB by alternative routes has not been reported in circumstances where the right internal jugular vein was used for central access.

D. Considerations for repeat sternotomy

Many cardiac transplant recipients will have undergone previous cardiac surgery and are at increased risk of inadvertent trauma to the great vessels or pre-existing coronary artery bypass grafts during sternotomy. Patients having repeat sternotomy should have external defibrillation pads placed before induction, and cross-matched, irradiated PRBCs available in the operating room prior to sternotomy. If the recipient has had previous sternotomy, additional time for surgical dissection may be required and should be accounted for in planning the timing for the induction of general anesthesia. Other considerations for repeat sternotomy include the potential for bleeding and the need for femoral or axillary CPB cannulation.

E. Anesthetic induction

1. **Hemodynamic goals**

   Cardiac transplant recipients typically have hypokinetic, noncompliant ventricles sensitive to alterations in myocardial preload and afterload. Hemodynamic goals for anesthetic induction are to maintain HR and contractility, avoid acute changes in preload and afterload, and prevent increases in PVR. Inotropic support is often required during anesthetic induction and throughout the pre-CPB period.

2. **Aspiration precautions**

   Rapid sequence induction with maintenance of cricoid pressure should be considered.

3. **Anesthetic agents**

   Due to the slow circulation time in patients with end-stage HF, a delayed response to administered anesthetic agents on induction is common. IV anesthetics commonly used for anesthetic induction of the cardiac transplant recipient include etomidate (0.2 to 0.3 mg/kg) in combination with fentanyl (5 to 10 μg/kg) or sufentanil (5 to 8 μg/kg). High-dose narcotic regimens have also been used successfully. Bradycardia occurring in response to high-dose narcotics should be treated promptly, as CO in patients with end-stage heart disease is HR-dependent. Small doses of midazolam, ketamine, or scopolamine help ensure amnesia, but should be used cautiously as they may synergistically lower SVR and induce hypotension.

4. **Muscle relaxants**

   Due to its vagolytic and mild sympathomimetic properties, pancuronium is commonly used to counteract narcotic-induced bradycardia. Muscle relaxants with minimal cardiovascular effects (e.g., cisatracurium or vecuronium) may be more appropriate for patients who present with tachycardia secondary to preoperative inotropic support.

F. Anesthetic maintenance

During the pre-CPB period, anesthetic goals include maintenance of hemodynamic stability and end-organ perfusion. Most anesthetic maintenance regimens are narcotic-based, with supplemental inhalational agents and benzodiazepines. Although most inhalational agents have negative inotropic effects, low concentrations of these agents are usually well tolerated and decrease the risk of awareness. Anesthetic depth can be difficult to assess in this patient population as the sympathetic response to light planes of anesthesia is often blunted. The use of narcotic-based anesthetic regimens may also increase the risk of awareness during anesthesia.

Antifibrinolytics such as tranexamic acid, or ε-aminocaproic acid may be administered following anesthetic induction to reduce bleeding.

G. Cardiopulmonary bypass

CPB for cardiac transplantation is similar to that employed for routine cardiac surgical procedures. Femoral venous and arterial cannulation sites are frequently chosen in patients undergoing repeat sternotomy. Moderate hypothermia (28 to 30°C) is commonly used during CPB to improve myocardial protection. Hemofiltration and/or mannitol administration is common during CPB as patients with CHF often have a large intravascular blood volume and coexistent renal impairment. Although immunosuppressive regimens vary amongst transplantation centers, high-dose IV glucocorticoids such as methylprednisolone are frequently administered prior to aortic cross-clamp release to reduce the likelihood of hyperacute rejection. Immunosuppressive induction therapy with an interleukin-2 receptor (IL2R) antagonist, or a polyclonal antilymphocyte antibody, occurred in 54% of heart transplant recipients in 2009 [2]. The availability and timing of immunosuppressive medications should be discussed with the transplant team ahead of time.

VII. Postcardiopulmonary bypass

Prior to CPB termination, the patient should be normothermic and have all electrolyte and acid–base abnormalities corrected. Complete deairing of the heart prior to aortic cross-clamp removal is essential. TEE may be particularly useful for assessing the efficacy of cardiac deairing maneuvers. Inotropic agents should be commenced prior to CPB termination. A HR of 90 to 110 beats/min, a mean systemic arterial BP >65 mm Hg, and ventricular filling pressures of approximately 12 to 16 mm Hg (CVP) and 14 to 18 mm Hg (PCWP) are often required in the immediate post-CPB period. Although inotropic support is usually required for several days, patients are often extubated within 24 h and discharged from the ICU by third postoperative day. Clinical considerations in the immediate postoperative period include the following:

A. Autonomic denervation of the transplanted heart

5 During orthotopic cardiac transplantation, the cardiac autonomic plexus is transected, leaving the transplanted heart without autonomic innervation. The transplanted heart thus does not respond to direct autonomic nervous system stimulation or to drugs that act indirectly through the autonomic nervous system (e.g., atropine). The denervated, transplanted heart responds to direct-acting agents such as catecholamines. Transient bradycardia and slow nodal rhythms are common following aortic cross-clamp release. An infusion of direct-acting β-adrenergic receptor agonist such as isoproterenol is frequently started prior to CPB termination, and titrated to achieve a HR around 100 beats/min. Newly transplanted hearts unresponsive to pharmacological stimulation may require temporary epicardial pacing. Although most initial dysrhythmias resolve, some cardiac transplant recipients require placement of a permanent pacemaker.

B. RV dysfunction

6 **RV failure is a significant cause of early morbidity and mortality, accounting for nearly 20% of early deaths after heart transplantation** [26]. Acute RV failure following cardiac transplantation may be due to prolonged donor heart ischemic time, mechanical obstruction at the level of the PA anastomosis, pre-existing pulmonary HTN, protamine-induced pulmonary HTN, donor–recipient size mismatch, and acute rejection [35]. RV distension and hypokinesis may be diagnosed by TEE or direct observation of the surgical field. Other findings suggesting RV failure include elevations in the CVP, PA pressure, or the transpulmonary gradient (>15 mm Hg).

The goal of managing RV dysfunction is to maintain systemic BP, while minimizing RV dilation. Maintaining atrioventricular synchrony is especially important in optimizing RV preload. Correction of electrolyte and acid–base disturbances, and the use of inotropic support may improve RV function. Minimizing blood transfusions, optimizing ventilator settings, and the use of inhaled pulmonary vasodilators may reduce RV afterload [35]. Useful inotropes include epinephrine, dobutamine, and milrinone, as these may also cause a degree of relaxation in the pulmonary vasculature [35]. Inhaled pulmonary vasodilators include prostacyclin (PGI_2), prostaglandin E_1 (PGE_1), and NO [26,34,35]. NO selectively reduces PVR by activating guanylate cyclase in vascular smooth muscle cells, producing an increase in cGMP and smooth muscle relaxation. Little systemic effect is seen as it is inactivated by hemoglobin and has a 5- to 10-s half-life. NO administration results in the formation of the toxic metabolites nitrogen dioxide and methemoglobin. In the presence of severe LV dysfunction, selective dilation of the pulmonary vasculature by NO may lead to an increase in PCWP and pulmonary edema. PGI_2 is an arachidonic acid derivative with a half-life of 3 to 6 min. It binds to a prostanoid receptor and affects an increase in intracellular cAMP and, consequently, vasodilation. PGI_2 is equivalent to NO in reducing PA pressures [36]. Relative to NO, PGI_2 is less costly, easier to administer, and does not create toxic metabolites. It may, however, cause a degree of systemic hypotension due to its longer half-life, and may be implicated in increased bleeding due to inhibition of platelet function [36]. RV failure refractory to medical treatment may require insertion of a right VAD or institution of extracorporeal circulation.

C. LV dysfunction

Post-CPB LV dysfunction may be a result of a prolonged donor heart ischemic time, inadequate myocardial perfusion, intracoronary embolization of intracavitary air, or surgical manipulation. The incidence of post-CPB LV dysfunction is greater in donors requiring prolonged, high-dose inotropic support prior to organ harvest. Continued postoperative inotropic support with dobutamine, epinephrine, or norepinephrine may be required.

D. Coagulation

Coagulopathy following cardiac transplantation is common, and perioperative bleeding should be treated early and aggressively. Potential etiologies include hepatic dysfunction secondary to chronic hepatic venous congestion, preoperative anticoagulation, CPB-induced platelet dysfunction, hypothermia, and hemodilution of clotting factors. After ruling out surgical bleeding, blood product administration should be guided by repeated measurements of platelet count and clotting factors. Due to an increased risk of infection and graft-versus-host disease, all administered blood products should be cytomegalovirus (CMV)-negative, and irradiated or leukocyte-depleted. RBC and platelets should be administered through leukocyte filters. The efficacy of DDAVP for the treatment of postoperative bleeding has not been proven.

E. Renal dysfunction

Renal dysfunction, as evidenced by increased serum creatinine and oliguria, is common in the immediate postoperative period. Contributing factors include pre-existing renal impairment, cyclosporine-associated renal toxicity, perioperative hypotension, and CPB. Treatment of renal dysfunction includes optimization of CO and systemic BP, and the use of diuretics.

F. Pulmonary dysfunction

Postoperative pulmonary complications such as atelectasis, pleural effusion, and pneumonia are common and may be reduced by PEEP ventilation, regular endobronchial suctioning, and chest physiotherapy. Bronchoscopy to clear pulmonary secretions is often useful. Pulmonary infection in the immunosuppressed recipient should be treated early and aggressively.

G. Hyperacute allograft rejection

Cardiac allograft hyperacute rejection is caused by preformed HLA antibodies present in the recipient [37]. There are several explanations for the pre-existing antibodies that initiate hyperacute rejection. First, prior recipients of blood transfusions may develop antibodies to major histocompatibility complex (MHC) antigens in the transfused blood. Multiple pregnancies may also expose females to fetal paternal antigens, resulting in antibody formation. Finally, prior transplant recipients may have already formed antibodies to other MHC antigens, so that they may be present at the time of a second transplant. Although extremely rare, hyperacute rejection results in severe cardiac dysfunction and death within hours of transplantation. Assisted MCS until cardiac retransplantation is the only therapeutic option.

VIII. The role of intraoperative TEE

Intraoperative TEE is a valuable tool for the evaluation and management of the cardiac transplant recipient. In addition to monitoring ventricular function, TEE in the pre-CPB period may be used to identify intracavitary thrombus, estimate recipient PA pressures, and evaluate the aortic cannulation and cross-clamp sites for the presence of atherosclerotic disease. TEE may also be used in the post-CPB period to evaluate the efficacy of cardiac deairing, cardiac function, and surgical anastomoses. The caval veins, left atrium, and pulmonary vein anastomoses should be evaluated for any evidence of obstruction or distortion [38]. Stenosis of the main PA should also be excluded by continuous-wave Doppler measurement of the pressure gradient across the anastomosis. After orthotopic cardiac transplantation, the long axis of the left atrium often appears larger than usual because of the joining of donor and recipient left atria. Occasionally, excess donor atrial tissue may obstruct the mitral valve orifice resulting in pulmonary HTN and RV failure. TEE findings in the immediate post-CPB period frequently include impaired ventricular contractility, decreased diastolic compliance, septal dyskinesia, and acute mild-to-moderate tricuspid, pulmonic, and mitral valve regurgitation. Although LV size and function are typically normal on long-term echocardiographic follow-up of healthy cardiac transplant recipients, RV enlargement and tricuspid valve regurgitation persists in up to 33% of patients. Persistent tricuspid valve regurgitation may result from geometrical alterations of the right atrium or ventricle, asynchronous contraction of the donor and recipient atria, or valvular damage occurring during EMB.

IX. Cardiac transplantation survival and complications

Survival following cardiac transplantation in the United States in 2008 was 93%, 89%, 75%, and 56% at 3 mos, 1, 5, and 10 yrs, respectively [12]. These figures are consistent across the adult range of ages, except for recipients aged 65 or older (10-yr survival of 46%) [12]. At all time points, survival in women is lower by 2% to 3%, and long-term survival in African-Americans is lower than in other ethnic/racial groups (10-yr survival of 43%) [12]. Overall, however, survival after heart transplantation has continued to improve since 1982 (Fig. 16.4). Important causes of morbidity and mortality are infection, acute rejection, graft failure and cardiac allograft vasculopathy (CAV), renal insufficiency (RI), and malignancy. Other long-term morbidity after transplantation is due to hypertension, diabetes mellitus, and hyperlipidemia (prevalence at 5 yrs of 90%, 39%, and 91%, respectively) [2].

A. Infection

Infections in the early postoperative period (<30 days) are mainly nosocomial and bacterial in nature, and account for 11% of deaths [2,3]. With the routine use of bacterial and viral prophylaxis, there has been a significant reduction in pneumocystis pneumonia infection and herpesviridae (including CMV) [3]. Beyond 30 days, infection remains an important cause of mortality, reaching its peak as a primary cause of death (29%) at 31 days to 1 yr post-transplant [2].

B. Acute rejection

Improvements in management have rendered acute rejection of the transplanted heart as a less common cause of death (<11%) [2]. However, up to 30% of recipients may experience rejection

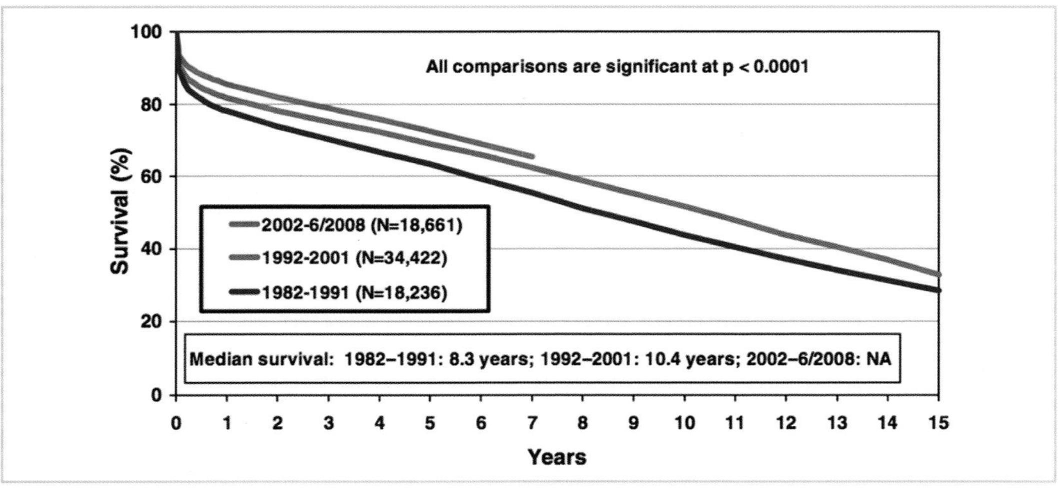

FIGURE 16.4 Survival for adult heart transplants performed between January 1982 and June 2008, stratified by era of transplant. (From Stehlik J, Edwards LB, Kucheryavaya AY, et al. The Registry of the International Society for Heart and Lung Transplantation: Twenty-seventh official a dult heart transplant report – 2010. *J Heart Lung Transplant.* 2010;29: 1089–1103.)

within the first year [2]. Female recipients are at higher risk than males, and the risk of rejection decreases with increasing age of the recipient [2]. EMB remains the gold standard for confirming acute allograft rejection [3]. Repeated EMB is associated with an increased incidence of tricuspid valve regurgitation.

C. Graft failure and Cardiac allograft vasculopathy (CAV)

Graft failure, presumably due to primary graft failure, is the leading cause of death in the first 30 days after transplant (39% of deaths) [2]. After 30 days, chronic processes such as antibody-mediated rejection and CAV are more likely causes of graft failure. Graft failures continue to be a significant cause of death after 1 yr, accounting for 16% to 24% of deaths [2]. Graft failures due to CAV become prominent between 1 and 3 yrs after transplant, and account for 10% to 15% of deaths [2]. The prevalence of CAV is 30% at 5 yrs and >50% at 10 yrs [2]. Significant CAV
7 is defined angiographically by a stenosis of at least 50%. **Unlike atherosclerotic CAD, CAV is characterized by a diffuse intimal hyperplasia** [3]. Nonimmune risk factors for CAV include hypertension, hyperlipidemia, diabetes mellitus, explosive (e.g., gunshot to the head) cause of donor brain death, hyperhomocysteinemia, and increased donor age [3]. Immune risk factors include HLA donor–recipient mismatch, recurrent cellular rejection, and antibody-mediated rejection [3]. Aggressive management of risk factors is the primary strategy for preventing CAV. The diffuse nature of the vasculopathy defies percutaneous or surgical revascularization strategies [3].

D. Renal Insufficiency (RI)

RI is a strong predictor of survival after transplant. Defined as a serum creatinine >2.5 mg/dL, or necessitating dialysis or kidney transplant, severe RI is identified as the primary cause of death in a significant number of patients [2]. Risks for early RI, developing within 1 yr of transplant, are increased donor and recipient age, increased recipient serum creatinine at the time of transplant, presence of a VAD, female recipient, rapamycin use at discharge, and IL2R-antagonist induction [2]. Fortunately, the incidence of impaired renal function after heart transplant is decreasing, with 82% of patients transplanted between 2001 and 2008 being free of severe renal dysfunction at 5 yrs [2].

E. Malignancy

Presumably as a consequence of the effects of long-term immunosuppression, the risk of malignancy in the solid-organ transplant recipient is elevated compared to the general population [2]. Skin cancer is the most common malignancy in heart transplant recipients, with incidence at 1, 5, 10, and 14 yrs of 1%, 10%, 20%, and 29%, respectively [2]. Lymphoproliferative malignancies occur less frequently than do malignancies of the skin, but their treatments are much less likely to be curative [2]. Incidence at 1, 5, 10, and 14 yrs are 1%, 2%, 4%, and 5%, respectively [2]. Mortality attributed to malignancy depends on time after transplant and is as high as 23% after 10 yrs [2].

F. Immunosuppressive drug side effects

Cardiac transplant recipients require life-long immunosuppression. Protocols vary among transplant centers; however, most regimens include triple therapy with corticosteroids, a calcineurin inhibitor, and an antiproliferative agent [3]. Immunosuppressants increase the risk of infection and are associated with numerous side effects (Table 16.6) [39]. Furthermore, chronic immunosuppression increases the risk of malignancies including skin cancers, lymphoproliferative malignancies, various adenocarcinomas, cancers of the lung, bladder, renal, breast, and colon, and Kaposis sarcoma.

X. Pediatric cardiac transplantation

In the United States in 2008, cardiac transplantation in children accounted for 17% of cardiac transplants [12]. The primary indications for pediatric cardiac transplantation are complex congenital heart disease and cardiomyopathy [12]. At present, the majority of pediatric heart transplants take place in children >1 yr of age at highly specialized pediatric centers [12]. Survival rates for transplant recipients are lowest in infants, and higher than adults when aged 6 to 17 yrs [12]. Similar to adult programs, pediatric cardiac transplant programs face a severe donor heart shortage. The use of implantable VADs for bridge to transplantation is limited by the small body size of most pediatric transplant candidates [12].

TABLE 16.6 Immunosuppressive agents

Agent	Mechanism of action	Side effects
Cyclosporine	Inhibits T-cell proliferation. Inhibits interleukin-2 expression	Nephrotoxicity, hypertension, tremors, headache, paresthesias, hyperkalemia, hypomagnesemia, hepatotoxicity, gingival hyperplasia
Azathioprine	Inhibits DNA synthesis. Inhibits lymphocyte proliferation	Leukopenia, thrombocytopenia, anemia, infection, hepatotoxicity, pancreatitis, nausea, vomiting, diarrhea
Corticosteroids	Decreases T-cell activation. Inhibit cytokine production. Inhibits leukocyte chemotaxis	Infection, hyperglycemia, hypertension, osteoporosis, adrenal suppression, myopathy, peptic ulcer disease, hyperlipidemia, psychological disturbances
Mycophenolate mofetil	Inhibits DNA synthesis. Inhibits lymphocyte proliferation	Nausea, abdominal cramps, diarrhea, neutropenia, rarely hepatic and bone marrow toxicity
Tacrolimus (FK506)	Inhibits T-cell activation	Nephrotoxicity, anemia, hyperkalemia, hyperglycemia, hypertension, nausea, vomiting
OKT3	Opsonizes and lyses T-cells	Fever, chills, hypotension, bronchospasm, pulmonary edema, aseptic meningitis, seizures, nausea, vomiting, diarrhea
Antilymphocyte globulin	Opsonizes and lyses T-cells	Anaphylaxis, leukopenia, thrombocytopenia, hypotension, infection, fever, chills, hepatitis, serum sickness
Rapamycin	Promotes T-cell apoptosis	Abdominal pain, weakness, back pain, headache, upset stomach, swelling of the hands, feet, ankles, or lower legs, joint pain insomnia, tremor, rash, fever
Basiliximab or Daclizumab	IL2R blocker inhibits IL2-dependent T-cell activation	Anaphylaxis, abdominal pain, back pain, fever or chills, loss of energy or weakness, sore throat, vomiting, white patches in the mouth or throat, tremor

ILTR, interleukin-2 receptor.

XI. Combined heart lung transplant (HLT)

During 2007 and 2008, only 58 HLTs were done in the United States [12]. Thirty-three percent carried the diagnosis of Eisenmenger's syndrome and 24% had idiopathic pulmonary HTN [12]. Approximate survival rates at 3 mos, 1, 5, and 10 yrs were 86%, 81%, 45%, and 29%, respectively. Donor procurement is of critical importance to the success of the operation, especially with respect to lung preservation. However, current techniques have led to safe procurement with ischemic times up to 6 h.

The operation is performed using a double- or single-lumen endotracheal tube with the patient in the supine position. The surgical approach is generally performed through a median sternotomy, with particular emphasis on preservation of the phrenic, vagal, and recurrent laryngeal nerves [40]. After fully heparinizing the recipient, the ascending aorta is cannulated near the base of the innominate artery, and the venae cavae are individually cannulated laterally and snared. CPB with systemic cooling to 28 to 30°C is instituted, and the heart is excised at the midatrial level. The aorta is divided just above the aortic valve, and the PA is divided at its bifurcation. The left atrial remnant is then divided vertically at a point halfway between the right and left pulmonary veins. Following division of the pulmonary ligament, the left lung is moved into the field, allowing full dissection of the posterior aspect of the left hilum, being careful to avoid the vagus nerve posteriorly. After this is completed, the left main PA is divided, and the left main bronchus is stapled and divided. The same technique of hilar dissection and division is repeated on the right side, and both lungs removed from the chest. Meticulous hemostasis of the bronchial vessels is necessary, as this area of the dissection is obscured once graft implantation is completed. Once absolute hemostasis is achieved, the trachea is divided at the carina.

The donor heart–lung block is removed from its transport container, prepared, and then lowered into the chest, passing the right lung beneath the right phrenic nerve pedicle. The left lung is then gently manipulated under the left phrenic nerve pedicle. The tracheal anastomosis is then performed, and the lungs ventilated with room air at half-normal tidal volumes to inflate the lungs and reduce atelectasis. The heart is then anastomosed as previously described. After separation from CPB, the patient is usually ventilated with an F_iO_2 of 40% and PEEP at 3 to 5 cm H_2O, being very careful to avoid high inspiratory pressures that may disrupt the tracheal anastomoses.

XII. Anesthesia for the previously transplanted patient

Many heart transplant recipients will undergo additional surgical procedures in their lifetime [41]. Common surgical procedures following cardiac transplantation are listed in Table 16.7. Many of these subsequent surgical procedures are attributable to sequelae of the transplant surgery itself, atherosclerosis, and immunosuppression. Understanding the physiologic and pharmacologic features of the previously transplanted patient is essential to ensure optimal anesthetic management.

A. Physiology of the previously transplanted patient

During orthotopic cardiac transplantation, the cardiac autonomic plexus is transected, leaving the transplanted heart without autonomic innervation [42]. Due to the absence of parasympathetic innervation of the sinoatrial node, the transplanted heart will exhibit a resting HR of 90 to 110 beats/min. In addition, reflex bradycardia does not occur. Increases in HR and SV in response to stress are blunted as they depend on circulating adrenal hormones. In the normal heart, the **immediate** response to stress is to increase CO by **increasing heart rate** through
8 an intact sympathetic nervous system. The **transplant patient** lacking that response is **dependent on maintenance or increase in SV**. Thus, any drop in preload during anesthetic interventions, regardless of technique, will not be well tolerated. Although most transplanted hearts have near-normal contractility at rest, stress may reveal a reduction in functional reserve. The Starling volume–pressure relationship, however, tends to remain intact.

A higher rate of dysrhythmia is seen due to the absence of parasympathetic tone coupled with conduction abnormalities. First-degree atrioventricular block is common, and 30% of patients will have right bundle branch block [42].

TABLE 16.7 Common surgical procedures following cardiac transplantation

Re-exploration for mediastinal bleeding
Infectious complications
Laparotomy
Craniotomy
Thoracotomy
Abscess drainage
Bronchoscopy
Steroid-related complications
Hip arthroplasty or pinning
Laparotomy for perforated viscus
Cataract excision
Vitrectomy
Scleral buckle
Aortic or peripheral vascular surgery and amputation
Pancreatic and biliary tract surgery
Retransplantation

Modified from Wyner J, Finch EL. Heart and heart-lung transplantation. In: Gelman S, ed. *Anesthesia and Organ Transplantation*. Philadelphia, PA: WB Saunders; 1987:111–137.

TABLE 16.8 Drug effects on the denervated heart

Drug	Action	Heart rate	Blood pressure
Atropine	Indirect	—	—
Digoxin	Direct	—/↓	—
Dopamine	Indirect and direct	↑	↑
Ephedrine	Indirect and direct	—/↑	—/↑
Fentanyl	Indirect	—	—
Isoproterenol	Direct	↑	—/↑
Neostigmine	Indirect	—/↓	—
Norepinephrine	Direct	↑	↑
Pancuronium	Indirect	—	—
Phenylephrine	Direct	—	↑
Verapamil	Direct	↓	↓

↑, increased; ↓, decreased; —, no effect.

B. Pharmacology of the previously transplanted patient

9 Autonomic denervation of the transplanted heart alters the pharmacodynamic activity of many drugs (Table 16.8). Drugs that mediate their actions through the autonomic nervous system are ineffective in altering HR and contractility. In contrast, drugs that act directly on the heart are effective. The β-adrenergic response of the transplanted heart to direct-acting catecholamines such as epinephrine is often increased. Reflex bradycardia or tachycardia in response to changes in systemic arterial BP is absent. Narcotic-induced decreases in HR are frequently diminished in the transplanted heart. Drugs with mixed activity (e.g., dopamine and ephedrine) will mediate an effect only through their direct actions. Parasympathomimetics such as atropine and glycopyrrolate will not alter HR, although their peripheral anticholinergic activity remains unaffected. Anticholinergic coadministration with reversal of neuromuscular blockade is still warranted to counteract the noncardiac muscarinic effects.

C. Preoperative evaluation

A thorough medical history, physical examination, and review of the medical record should be undertaken. Current medications should be noted. Particular attention should be paid to determining cardiac allograft function, evidence of rejection or infection, complications of immunosuppression, and end-organ disease. Systemic HTN is common and a significant proportion of patients will have CAV within 1 yr of cardiac transplantation. The absence of angina pectoris does not exclude significant CAD, because the transplanted heart is denervated. The patient's activity level and exercise tolerance are good indicators of allograft function. Symptoms of dyspnea and CHF suggest significant CAD or myocardial rejection. The presentation of infection may be atypical in immunosuppressed patients, with fever and leukocytosis often absent. Soft tissue changes in the patient's airway may occur due to lymphoproliferative disease and corticosteroid administration. Cyclosporine may cause gingival hyperplasia and friability. Hematocrit, coagulation profile, electrolytes, and creatinine should be checked, because immunosuppressive therapy is commonly associated with anemia, thrombocytopenia, electrolyte disturbances, and renal dysfunction. Recent chest x-rays, ECGs, and coronary angiograms should be reviewed. More than one P wave may be seen on the ECG in patients in whom cardiac transplantation was performed using a biatrial technique (Fig. 16.5). Although seen on the ECG, the P wave originating in the native atria does not conduct impulses across the anastomotic line.

D. Anesthesia management

1. Clinical implications of immunosuppressive therapy

All cardiac transplant patients are immunosuppressed and consequently at higher risk of infection. All vascular access procedures should be carried out using aseptic or sterile technique. Antibiotic prophylaxis should be considered for any procedure with

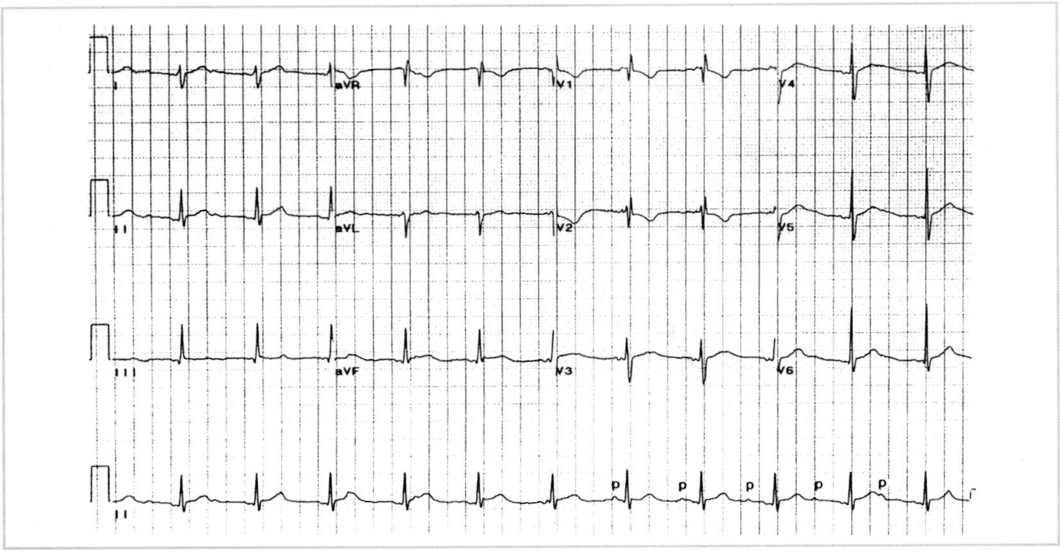

FIGURE 16.5 Transplanted heart ECG. The transplanted heart ECG is commonly characterized by two sets of P waves, right-axis deviation, and incomplete right bundle branch block. The donor heart P waves are small and precede the QRS complex, whereas P waves originating from the recipient's atria (labeled as *p*) are unrelated to the QRS complex. (From Fowler NO. *Clinical Electrocardiographic Diagnosis.* Philadelphia, PA: Lippincott Williams & Wilkins; 2000:225, with permission.)

the potential to produce bacteremia. Oral immunosuppressive medication should be continued without interruption or given intravenously to maintain blood levels within the therapeutic range. IV and oral doses of azathioprine are approximately equivalent. Administration of large volumes of IV fluids will decrease blood levels of immunosuppressants, and therefore levels should be checked daily. Immunosuppressant nephrotoxicity may be exacerbated by coadministration of other potentially renal toxic medications such as nonsteroidal anti-inflammatory agents or gentamicin. Chronic corticosteroid therapy to prevent allograft rejection may result in adrenal suppression. Supplemental "stress" steroids should thus be administered to critically ill patients or patients undergoing major surgical procedures.

2. **Monitoring**

Standard anesthetic monitors should be used, including five-lead ECG to detect ischemia and dysrhythmias. Cardiac transplant patients frequently have fragile skin and osteoporotic bones secondary to chronic corticosteroid administration. Care with tape, automated BP cuffs, and patient positioning is essential to avoid skin and musculoskeletal trauma. As for all patients undergoing anesthesia, invasive monitoring should only be considered for situations in which the benefits outweigh the risks. Importantly, cardiac transplant patients have an increased risk of developing catheter-related infections with a high associated morbidity and mortality. Intraoperative TEE permits rapid evaluation of volume status, cardiac function, and ischemia, and may be a useful substitute for invasive monitoring. Should central venous access be required, alternatives to the right internal jugular vein should be considered to preserve its use for EMB. Careful monitoring of neuromuscular blockade with a peripheral nerve stimulator is recommended in the previously transplanted patient as cyclosporine may prolong neuromuscular blockade following administration of nondepolarizing neuromuscular blocking agents. In contrast, an attenuated response to nondepolarizing muscle relaxants may be seen in patients receiving azathioprine.

3. **Anesthesia techniques**

10 Both general and regional anesthesia techniques have been used safely in cardiac transplant patients. In the absence of significant cardiorespiratory, renal, or hepatic dysfunction, there is no absolute contraindication to any anesthetic technique. **For any selected anesthetic technique, maintenance of ventricular filling pressures is essential as the transplanted heart increases CO primarily by increasing SV.**

a. **General anesthesia**

General anesthesia is frequently preferred over regional anesthesia for cardiac transplant patients as alterations in myocardial preload and afterload may be more predictable. Cyclosporine and tacrolimus decrease renal blood flow and glomerular filtration via thromboxane-mediated renal vasoconstriction. Thus, renally excreted anesthetics and muscle relaxants should be used with caution in patients receiving these medications. Cyclosporine and tacrolimus also lower the seizure threshold, and hyperventilation should be avoided. **Elevations in the resting HR and a delayed sympathetic response to noxious stimuli in cardiac transplant recipients may make anesthetic depth difficult to assess.**

b. **Regional anesthesia**

Many immunosuppressants cause thrombocytopenia and alter the coagulation profile. Both the platelet count and coagulation profile should be within normal limits if spinal or epidural regional anesthesia is planned. Ventricular filling pressures should be maintained following induction of central neural axis blockade to prevent hypotension caused by the delayed response of the denervated, transplanted heart to a rapid decrease in sympathetic tone. Volume loading, ventricular filling pressure monitoring, and careful titration of local anesthetic agents may avoid hemodynamic instability. Hypotension should be treated with vasopressors that directly stimulate their target receptors.

4. **Blood transfusion**

The cardiac transplant recipient is at increased risk for blood product transfusion complications. Adverse reactions include infection, graft-versus-host disease, and immunomodulation. Use of irradiated, leukocyte-depleted, CMV-negative blood products, and white blood cell filters for blood product administration reduces the incidence of adverse transfusion reactions. The blood bank should receive early notification if the use of blood products is anticipated, because the presence of reactive antibodies delaying cross-match is not infrequent.

E. Pregnancy following cardiac transplantation

Despite an increased incidence of pre-eclampsia and preterm labor, increasing numbers of cardiac transplant recipients are successfully carrying pregnancies to term. In general, the transplanted heart is able to adapt to the physiological changes of pregnancy. Due to an increased sensitivity to the β-adrenergic effects of tocolytics such as terbutaline and ritodrine, use of alternative drugs such as magnesium and nifedipine may be considered. Although pregnancy does not adversely affect cardiac allografts, the risk of acute cardiac allograft rejection may be increased postpartum. All immunosuppressive drugs used to prevent cardiac allograft rejection cross the placenta, though most are not thought to be teratogenic.

XIII. Future directions

As medical management of HF continues to improve, a patient's need for definitive therapy with heart transplantation may become delayed or diminished. On the basis of trends over the previous decade, it is to be expected that patients who do present for heart transplant will have an increasing number and severity of comorbidities [2]. The emerging role of MCS devices for destination therapy will also affect future developments in heart transplantation [1]. Intensive investigation into the use of stem cells and bioengineered organs may someday obviate the current organ shortage. Continuing advances in our understanding of mechanisms of rejection are likely to improve immunomodulation and delay graft failure. Improvements in surveillance, such as intravascular ultrasound, may eliminate the need for routine EMB. For the immediate future, however, heart transplantation continues to offer patients with advanced HF their best opportunity for a better quality and length of life.

REFERENCES

1. Lietz K. Destination therapy: Patient selection and current outcomes. *J Card Surg.* 2010;25:462–471.
2. Stehlik J, Edwards LB, Kucheryavaya AY, et al. The registry of the International Society for Heart and Lung Transplantation: Twenty-seventh official adult heart transplant report – 2010. *J Heart Lung Transplant.* 2010;29:1089–1103.
3. Hunt SA, Haddad F. The changing face of heart transplantation. *J Am Coll Cardiol.* 2008;52:587–598.
4. Roger VL, Go AS, Lloyd-Jones DM, et al. Heart disease and stroke statistics – 2011 update: A report from the American Heart Association. *Circulation.* 2011;123:e18–e209.
5. Jessup M, Abraham WT, Casey DE, et al. 2009 Focused update incorporated into the ACC/AHA 2005 guidelines for the diagnosis and management of heart failure in adults. *Circulation.* 2009;119:e391–e479.
6. Mann DL, Bristow MR. Mechanisms and models in heart failure, the biomechanical model and beyond. *Circulation.* 2005;111:2837–2849.
7. Neubauer S. The failing heart – An engine out of fuel. *N Engl J Med.* 2007;356:1140–1151.
8. Sinha AM, Breithardt OA, Schmid M, et al. Brain natriuretic peptide release in cardiac surgery patients. *Thorac Cardiovasc Surg.* 2005;53:138–143.
9. Colucci WS, Elkayam U, Horton DP, et al. Intravenous nesiritide, a natriuretic peptide, in the treatment of decompensated congestive heart failure. *N Engl J Med.* 2000;343:246–253.
10. Epstein AE, DiMarco JP, Ellenbogen KA, et al. ACC/AHA/HRS 2008 guidelines for device-based therapy of cardiac rhythm abnormalities: A report of the American College of Cardiology/American Heart Association Task Force on Practice Guidelines (Writing Committee to Revise the ACC/AHA/NASPE 2002 guideline update for implantation of cardiac pacemakers and antiarrhythmia devices) developed in collaboration with the American Association for Thoracic Surgery and Society of Thoracic Surgeons. *J Am Coll Cardiol.* 2008;51:e1–e62.
11. American Society of Anesthesiologists. Practice advisory for the perioperative management of patients with cardiac implantable electronic devices: Pacemakers and implantable cardioverter-defibrillators. An updated report by the American Society of Anesthesiologists Task Force on perioperative management of patients with cardiac implantable electronic devices. *Anesthesiology.* 2011;114:247–261.
12. Johnson MR, Meyer KH, Haft J, et al. Heart transplantation in the United States, 1999–2008. *Am J Transplant.* 2010;10:1035–1046.
13. Kirlin JK, Naftel DC. Mechanical circulatory support, registering a therapy in evolution. *Circ Heart Fail.* 2008;1:200–205.
14. Patlolla V, Patten RD, DeNofrio D, et al. The effect of ventricular assist devices on post-transplant mortality, an analysis of the United network for organ sharing thoracic registry. *J Am Coll Cardiol.* 2009;53:264–271.
15. Shuhaiber JH, Hur K, Gibbons R. The influence of preoperative use of ventricular assist devices on survival after heart transplantation: Propensity score matched analysis. *BMJ.* 2010;340:c392.
16. John R, Pagani FD, Naka Y, et al. Post-cardiac transplant survival after support with a continuous-flow left ventricular assist device: Impact of duration of left ventricular device support and other variables. *J Thorac Cardiovasc Surg.* 2010;140:174–181.
17. Shah KB, Parameshwar J. Advances in heart transplantation: The year in review. *J Heart Lung Transplant.* 2011;30:241–246.
18. Mancini D, Lietz K. Selection of cardiac transplantation candidates in 2010. *Circulation.* 2010;122:173–183.
19. Zimpfer D, Zrunek P, Roethy W, et al. Left ventricular assist devices decrease fixed pulmonary hypertension in cardiac transplant candidates. *J Thorac Cardiovasc Surg.* 2007;133:689–695.
20. Etz CD, Welp HA, Tjan TD, et al. Medically refractory pulmonary hypertension: Treatment with nonpulsatile left ventricular assist devices. *Ann Thorac Surg.* 2007;83:1697–1706.
21. Beyersdorf F, Schlensak C, Berchtold-Herz M, et al. Regression of "fixed" pulmonary vascular resistance in heart transplant candidates after unloading with ventricular assist devices. *J Thorac Cardiovasc Surg.* 2010;140:747–749.
22. Alba AC, Rao V, Ross HJ, et al. Impact of fixed pulmonary hypertension on post-heart transplant outcomes in bridge-to-transplant patients. *J Heart Lung Transplant.* 2010;29:1253–1258.
23. Wittwer T, Wahlers T. Marginal donor grafts in heart transplantation: Lessons learned from 25 years of experience. *Transpl Int.* 2008;21:113–125.
24. Russo MJ, Davies RR, Hong KN, et al. Matching high-risk recipients with marginal donor hearts is a clinically effective strategy. *Ann Thorac Surg.* 2009;87:1066–1071.
25. Venkateswaran RV, Townend JN, Wilson IC, et al. Echocardiography in the potential heart donor. *Transplantation.* 2010;89:894–901.
26. Daneshmand MA, Milano CA. Surgical treatments for advanced heart failure. *Surg Clin North Am.* 2009;89:967–999.
27. Apostolakis E, Parissis H, Dougenis D. Brain death and donor heart dysfunction: Implications in cardiac transplantation. *J Card Surg.* 2010;25:98–106.
28. Dictus C, Vienenkoetter B, Esmaeilzadeh M. Critical care management of potential organ donors: Our current standard. *Clin Transplant.* 2009;23(suppl 21):2–9.
29. Smith M. Physiologic changes during brain stem death – Lessons for management of the organ donor. *J Heart Lung Transplant.* 2004;23:S217–S222.
30. Zaroff JF, Rosengard BR, Armstrong WF, et al. Consensus conference report: Maximizing use of organs recovered from the cadaveric donor: Cardiac recommendations: March 28–29, 2001, Crystal City, VA. *Circulation.* 2002;106:836–841.
31. Davis RR, Russo MJ, Morgan JA, et al. Standard versus bicaval techniques for orthotopic heart transplantation: An analysis of the United Network for Organ Sharing database. *J Thorac Cardiovasc Surg.* 2010;140:700–708.
32. Schnoor M, Schäfer T, Lühmann D, et al. Bicaval versus standard technique in orthotopic heart transplantation: A systematic review and meta-analysis. *J Thorac Cardiovasc Surg.* 2007;134:1322–1331.
33. Newcomb AE, Esmore DS, Rosenfeldt FL, et al. Heterotopic heart transplantation: An expanding role in the twenty-first century? *Ann Thorac Surg.* 2004;78;1345–1351.

34. Shanwise J. Cardiac transplantation. *Anesthesiol Clin North America.* 2004;22:753–765.
35. Haddad F, Couture P, Tousignant C, et al. The right ventricle in cardiac surgery, a perioperative perspective: II. pathophysiology, clinical importance, and management. *Anesth Analg.* 2009;108:422–433.
36. Khan TA, Schnickel G, Ross D, et al. A prospective, randomized, crossover pilot study of inhaled nitric oxide versus inhaled prostacyclin in heart transplant and lung transplant recipients. *J Thorac Cardiovasc Surg.* 2009;138:1417–1427.
37. Stewart S, Winters GL, Fishbein MC, et al. Revision of the 1990 working formulation for the standardization of nomenclature in the diagnosis of heart rejection. *J Heart Lung Transplant.* 2005;24:1710–1720.
38. Asante-Korang A. Echocardiographic evaluation before and after cardiac transplantation. *Cardiol Young.* 2004;14:88–92.
39. Page RL, Miller GG, Lindenfeld J. Drug therapy in the heart transplant recipient: Part IV: Drug-drug interactions. *Circulation.* 2005;111:230–239.
40. Roselli EE, Smedira NG. Surgical advances in heart and lung transplantation. *Anesthesiol Clin North America.* 2004;22: 789–807.
41. Rothenburger M, Hulsken G, Stypmann J, et al. Cardiothoracic surgery after heart and heart-lung transplantation. *Thorac Cardiovasc Surg.* 2005;53:85–92.
42. Blasco LM, Parameshwar J, Vuylsteke A. Anaesthesia for noncardiac surgery in the heart transplant recipient. *Curr Opin Anaesthesiol.* 2009;22:109–113.

17 Arrhythmia, Rhythm Management Devices, and Catheter and Surgical Ablation

Soraya M. Samii and Jerry C. Luck, Jr.

KEY POINTS

1. Patients with moderate to severe left ventricular dysfunction are at a higher risk for sustained monomorphic VT than those with preserved left ventricular function.
2. VT more commonly causes syncope and when it is associated with structural heart disease it is also associated with a high risk of sudden cardiac death.
3. Symptomatic patients with SND or evidence of conduction disease such as second- or third-degree AV block almost always need a permanent pacemaker preoperatively.
4. For VT, IV amiodarone is the initial drug of choice, but lidocaine is also considered especially if there is concern for ongoing ischemia. For torsades de pointes, management includes eliminating offending drugs in the setting of the long QT syndromes. Correcting electrolyte deficiencies with IV magnesium and potassium are particularly helpful in correcting the prolonged QT interval, as possibly stopping medications contributing to bradycardia. Amiodarone in the setting of torsades de pointes can prolong the QT interval and make the problem worse.
5. Bifascicular block with periodic third-degree AV block and syncope is associated with an increased incidence of sudden death. Prophylactic permanent pacing is indicated in this circumstance.
6. The requirement for temporary pacing with acute MI by itself does not constitute an indication for permanent pacing.
7. Sensor-driven tachycardia may occur with adaptive-rate devices that sense vibration, impedance changes, or the QT interval if they sense mechanical or physiologic interference, which leads to inappropriate high-rate pacing. Thus, it is advised that ARP be disabled in perioperative settings.
8. Because of the unpredictable interaction between the MRI and CIEDs, MRIs are generally contraindicated in individuals with CIEDs. There is now an approved compatible pacemaker generator and lead system for individuals likely to need MRI.
9. Most contemporary pacemaker devices respond to magnet application by a device-specific single- or dual-chamber asynchronous pacing mode. Adaptive-rate response is generally suspended with magnet mode as well. With asynchronous pacing, the pacemaker will no longer be inhibited by sensed activity and instead pace at a fixed rate regardless of underlying rhythm.

10. Some manufacturers, Biotronik, St. Jude Medical, and Boston Scientific devices, have a programmable magnet mode that may make response to magnet application different than anticipated. Although rarely used, this feature may be programmed to save patient-activated rhythm recordings with magnet application rather than revert the pacemaker to asynchronous pacing.
11. EMI signals between 5 and 100 Hz are not filtered, because these overlap the frequency range of intracardiac signals. Therefore, EMI in this frequency range may be interpreted as intracardiac signals, giving rise to abnormal behavior. Possible responses include (i) inappropriate inhibition or triggering of stimulation, (ii) asynchronous pacing (Fig. 17.5), (iii) mode resetting, (iv) direct damage to the pulse generator circuitry, and (v) triggering of unnecessary ICD shocks.
12. Treatment options for VT include antitachycardia pacing, cardioversion, or defibrillation. Up to 90% of monomorphic VTs can be terminated by a critical pacing sequence, reducing the need for painful shocks and conserving battery life. With antitachycardia pacing, trains of stimuli are delivered at a fixed percentage of the VT cycle length.
13. Acute MI, severe acute acid–base or electrolyte imbalance, or hypoxia may increase defibrillation thresholds, leading to ineffective shocks. Any of these also could affect the rate or morphology of VT and the ability to diagnose VT.
14. Response of an ICD to magnet application [8]. Magnet application does not interfere with bradycardia pacing and does not trigger asynchronous pacing in an ICD. Magnet application in contemporary ICDs causes inhibition of tachycardia sensing and delivery of shock only. All current ICDs remain inhibited as long as the magnet remains in stable contact with the ICD. Once the magnet is removed, the ICD reverts to the programmed tachyarrhythmia settings.
15. Baseline information about the surgery is needed by the CIED team (cardiologist, electrophysiologist, and pacemaker clinic staff managing the device) such as (i) type and location of the procedure, (ii) body position at surgery, (iii) electrosurgery needed and site of use, (iv) potential need for DC cardioversion or defibrillation, and (v) other EMI sources.
16. For pacemaker-dependent patients: These patients are at particular risk of asystole in the presence of EMI. If EMI is likely (e.g., unipolar cautery in the vicinity of the pulse generator or leads and surgery above the umbilicus), then the device should be programmed to an asynchronous mode. In the case of pacemakers, this can be done with magnet application in most situations, which will also inactivate the rate-responsive pacing.
17. In cases where the pacemaker-dependent patient has an ICD or the location of surgery precludes placement of a magnet, consideration of programming the device to asynchronous mode with the proprietary programmer is recommended. The other alternative if reprogramming is not an option is to limit the EMI to short bursts while watching the response of pacing and minimize episodes of asystole. For patients with adaptive-rate pacemakers (including some ICDs), this capability should be programmed off if EMI causes inappropriate rate response.
18. Use of a magnet eliminates the complexity of reprogramming the CIED in the operating room. The magnet can be easily removed when competing rhythms develop with asynchronous pacing.
19. In a situation with an ICD and no device information, a magnet should not be placed over the ICD pulse generator unless EMI is unavoidable. If EMI is unavoidable, then the patient needs to be placed on cardiac monitor and a magnet will need to be placed on (and kept on) the ICD generator during cautery or RF therapy.

ANY DISTURBANCE OF RHYTHM OR conduction, or arrhythmia that destabilizes hemodynamics perioperatively will need to be addressed. Treatment with antiarrhythmic agents has been the standard approach to manage symptomatic arrhythmias acutely. More recently, electrical therapies have gained wider acceptance in rhythm management. They presently play a premiere role in patients undergoing cardiac surgery and greatly impact a growing number of noncardiac surgery cases. The emphasis in this chapter is on perioperative management of patients with implanted devices. Concepts of arrhythmogenesis, antiarrhythmic action, and drug selection are discussed only briefly. The reader is referred to Chapter 2 for discussion of specific antiarrhythmic drugs and their pharmacology and to Chapter 1 for a discussion of arrhythmogenesis.

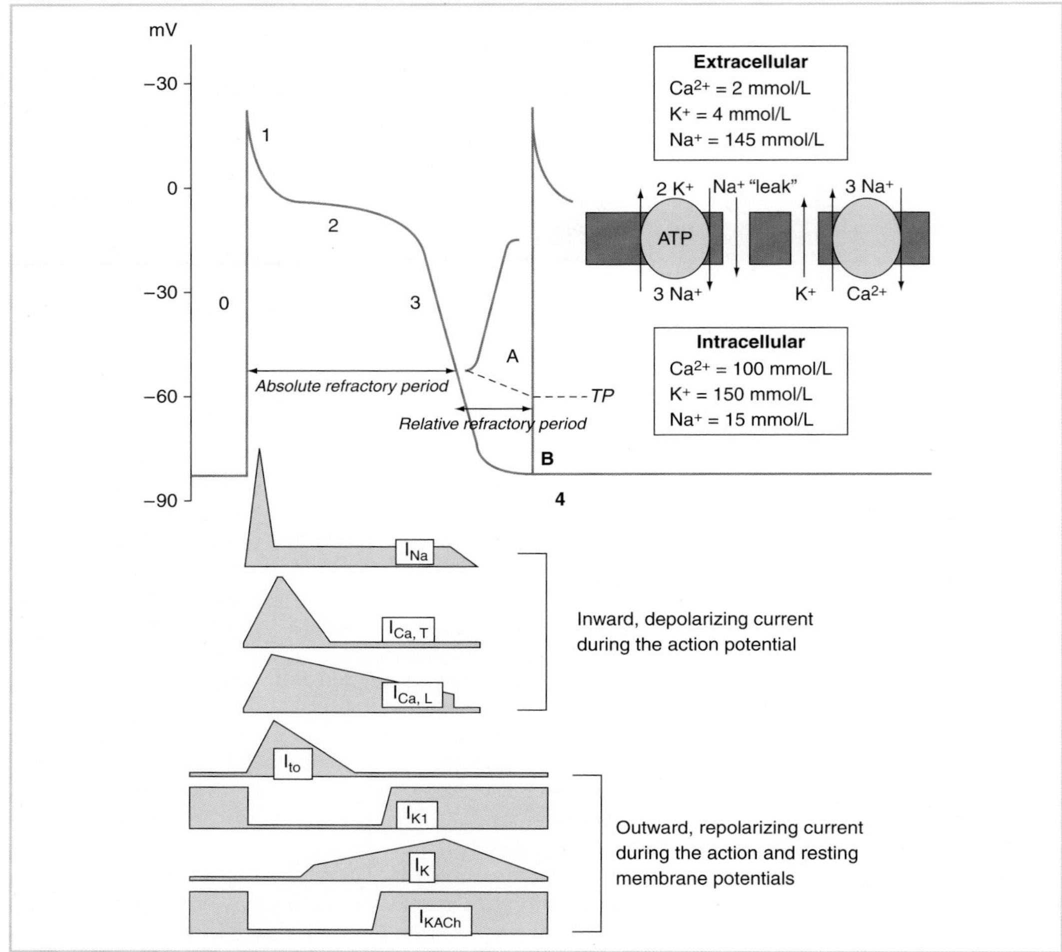

FIGURE 17.1 Action potential (AP) and resting membrane potential (RMP) of a quiescent Purkinje fiber. Extracellular and intracellular ion concentrations during Phase 4, and the active and passive ion exchangers that restore intracellular ion concentrations during Phase 4 are shown to the right of the AP. Inward depolarizing and outward repolarizing currents are shown below the AP. The adenosine triphosphate (ATP)-dependent Na/K pump maintains steep outwardly and inwardly directed gradients (*arrows*) for K^+ and Na^+, respectively, and generates small net outward current. The passive Na/Ca exchanger generates small net inward current. A small, inward "leak" of Na^+ keeps the RMP slightly positive to the K equilibrium potential (−96 mV). AP Phase 0 is the upstroke, Phase 1 is initial rapid repolarization, Phase 2 is the plateau, and Phase 3 is final repolarization. The cell is unresponsive to propagating AP or external stimuli during the absolute refractory period. A small electrotonic potential **(A)** occurs in response to a propagating AP or external stimulus during the relative refractory period (RRP). It is incapable of self-propagation. A normal AP is generated at the end of the RRP **(B)**, when the Na channels have fully recovered from inactivation. It is capable of propagation. Note that threshold potential (TP) for excitation is more positive during the RRP.

I. Concepts of arrhythmogenesis

A. Basic electrophysiology

1. **Action potential (AP).** A ventricular muscle cell's AP has five phases caused by changes in the cell membrane's permeability to sodium, potassium, and calcium (Fig. 17.1). Phase 0 represents depolarization and is characterized by a rapid upstroke as sodium rapidly enters the cell. There is a rapid drop in the cell's impedance from a resting state at −80 to −85 mV. Phase 1 is an early rapid repolarization period caused by potassium egress from the cell.

Phase 2 is a plateau phase representing a slow recovery phase: The slow inward calcium current is counterbalanced by outward potassium current. Phase 3 is a rapid repolarization phase as a result of accelerated potassium efflux. The diastolic interval between APs is termed Phase 4 and is a cell's resting membrane state in atrial and ventricular muscle.

2. **Ion channels.** Electrical activation of cardiac cells is the result of membrane currents crossing the hydrophobic lipid membranes through their specific protein channel. Opening and closing of gates in these channels are determined by the membrane potential (voltage dependence) and by the time elapsed after changes in potential (time dependence). Membrane channels cycle through the "activated," "inactivated," and "recovery" stages with each AP. Inward currents of sodium and calcium ions enter the cell using this gating mechanism. On the surface electrocardiogram (ECG), rapid-acting sodium currents contribute to the "P" and the "QRS" complexes. Depolarization of the sinoatrial (SA) node and the atrioventricular (AV) node, in contrast, occurs as a result of the slower-opening calcium-dependent channels. The slowly conducting calcium channel in the AV node creates the delay in the node and is responsible for nearly two-thirds of the PR interval during normal conduction. A group of potassium channels are responsible for repolarization and the "T" wave on the electrocardiogram (ECG).

   Cardiac arrhythmias occur when abnormal channel proteins are substituted for the normal protein and the ion channel is altered. For example, QT prolongation may be inherited as a result of encoding an altered gene or it may be acquired as a consequence of an antiarrhythmic agent inhibiting a specific ion channel [1].

3. **Excitability.** Reducing the cell's transmembrane potential to a critical level will initiate a propagated response and this level is termed the threshold potential. There are two mechanisms by which a propagated AP is developed: (i) a natural electrical stimulus and (ii) an applied electrical current. For an applied stimulus, threshold of a tissue is defined as the minimum amount of energy that will elicit a response. When external electrodes are used, only that part of the stimulus which penetrates the cell membrane contributes to excitation. The size of the stimulating electrode is critical to threshold. Reducing the size of the stimulating electrode (from 3 mm to 0.5 mm) will increase the current density over a smaller area and decrease the amount of energy needed to achieve threshold. It is common practice in pacing to use a small stimulating electrode and a larger indifferent electrode to reduce threshold and facilitate excitation.

4. **Conduction.** There are regions of cells with specialized conduction characteristics within the heart that propagate conduction in a preferential direction, spreading to adjacent areas faster though the preferential sites. This allows for a more organized direction of conduction so that, for example, both atria are depolarized prior to the stimulus reaching the AV node to depolarize the ventricles. In the sinus and AV nodes, L- and T-type calcium channels are the source of the propagated current [2]. In the Purkinje fiber the sodium channel is the source of the conducted current. Conduction velocity is much slower at about 0.2 m/s in the node versus 2 m/s in the Purkinje cells. These different characteristics explain the effects of certain antiarrhythmic medications. For instance, blocking the sodium channel with a Class I antiarrhythmic agent will preferentially reduce the conduction velocity in the Purkinje cells compared to the AV node because of this agent's primary effect on sodium channels.

B. Mechanism of arrhythmia (Table 17.1)

1. **Automaticity.** Automaticity is a unique property of an excitable cell allowing spontaneous depolarization and initiation of electrical impulse in the absence of external electrical stimulation. The SA node serves as the primary automatic pacemaker for the heart. Subsidiary pacemakers exhibiting automaticity are also found along the crista terminalis, the coronary sinus ostium, within the AV junction and in the ventricular His–Purkinje system. They may assume control of the heart if the SA node falters. Automaticity is either normal or abnormal. Alterations in automaticity due to changes in the ionic currents normally involved in impulse initiation are considered normal. Examples of normal automaticity include sinus tachycardia and junctional tachycardia during catecholamine states that increase current through the T-type calcium channels in the nodal cells.

TABLE 17.1 Confirmed or postulated electrophysiologic mechanisms for clinical arrhythmias

Mechanism	Arrhythmias
Altered normal automaticity	Sinus bradycardia and tachycardia; wandering atrial pacemaker; AV junctional and ventricular escape rhythms
Abnormal automaticity	Slow monomorphic VT, junctional or idioventricular rhythms in acute MI; some ectopic atrial tachycardia
Triggered activity (DAD)	VT in first 24 hrs of acute MI; atrial or VT with digitalis toxicity; catecholamine-mediated VT
Triggered activity (EAD)	Long QT interval with polymorphic VT (i.e., torsades de pointes)
Anatomic re-entry	Paroxysmal SVT due to re-entry involving the sinoatrial node, atria, AV node, or accessory AV pathways; VT with healed infarction; atrial flutter
Functional re-entry	Atrial fibrillation; monomorphic or polymorphic VT with acute MI; VF

AV, atrioventricular; DAD, delayed after depolarization; VT, ventricular tachycardia; MI, myocardial infarction; EAD, early after depolarization; SVT, supraventricular tachycardia.

Abnormal automaticity occurs when ionic currents not normally involved in impulse initiation cause spontaneous depolarizations in atrial and ventricular muscle cells that normally do not have pacemaker activity. An example of abnormal automaticity occurs during ischemic injury causing muscle cells to shift their maximum diastolic potential to a more positive resting level and thus facilitate spontaneous depolarization [3].

2. **Triggered activity.** Triggered activity is the result of abnormal oscillations in membrane potential reaching the threshold to induce another AP following a normal AP depolarization. These after depolarizations can occur before full repolarization has occurred, known as early after depolarizations (EADs), or late after repolarization has occurred, known as delayed after depolarization (DAD). Oscillations of either type of after depolarizations that exceed the threshold potential may trigger an abnormal tachycardia.

   EADs occur most frequently with delays in repolarization and prolongation of the QT interval. Acquired and congenital QT prolongation syndromes are predisposed to EADs and can result in torsades de pointes sometimes known as polymorphic ventricular tachycardia (VT) and sudden death. The torsades de pointes, triggered in prolonged QT syndromes, is facilitated by bradycardia and adrenaline. Examples of inherited predisposition to triggered initiation include defects in genes encoding Na and K ion channels that produce a net reduction in outward positive current during repolarization resulting in prolongation of the QT interval. Acquired prolongation of the QT interval from hypokalemia, pharmacologic agents including class IA and III antiarrhythmics, antibiotics such as erythromycin and antifungal agents, antihistamines, and the phenothiazine piperidine class can cause EADs.

   Delayed after depolarization potentials cause arrhythmias related to calcium overload. Digoxin toxicity is the most common agent causing DAD, and triggered activity is the common mechanism for digitalis-induced accelerated junctional rhythm and bidirectional VT. Catecholamines facilitate calcium loading and the development of DADs.

3. **Re-entry.** For either anatomical or functional re-entrant excitation to occur, the electrical wave front must circle around a core of inexcitable tissue at a rate that preserves an excitable gap. For initiation, there must be (i) an area of unidirectional conduction block, (ii) two conduction pathways that are connected at each end, and (iii) an area of slow conduction. Anatomical re-entrant circuits are common to several supraventricular tachycardias (SVTs) including Wolff–Parkinson–White syndrome, with an accessory AV pathway, and typical and atypical AV nodal re-entrant tachycardia. Classic atrial flutter has an anatomical right atrial loop classically involving the area of slow conduction known as the cavotricuspid isthmus. Pathologic sustained monomorphic VT is commonly due to anatomic re-entry from and is frequently associated with scarring from a prior myocardial infarction or fibrosis associated with dilated nonischemic cardiomyopathy.

   A functional re-entrant loop involves a small circuit around an area of tissue with an inexcitable core. Functional re-entry may occur with some forms of atrial tachycardia and is a mechanism for the multiple wavelet theory of atrial fibrillation.

C. Anatomical substrates and triggers

1. **Supraventricular.** The highly complex atria have a heterogeneous branching network of subendocardial muscle bundles that create functional areas of block as well as preferential planes of excitation. Longitudinal connected myocardial fibers conduct faster than fibers connected along transverse or parallel lines (so-called anisotropic conduction). In the right atrium, the crista terminalis and Eustachian ridge tend to act as anatomical barriers that help to facilitate a single re-entrant loop during atrial flutter. An area of slow conduction can usually be found in the isthmus of atrial tissue between the tricuspid annulus and the inferior vena cava. This is a frequent anatomical area for ablation of both clockwise and counterclockwise atrial flutter. The ostia of the pulmonary veins are frequently the sites of the initiation of atrial fibrillation. This chaotic atrial rhythm can be triggered by a single focus frequently localized to a pulmonary vein. Once initiated by a premature depolarization, the multiple wavelets are facilitated by the complex nature of the atria.
2. **Ventricular.** Myocardial ischemia and infarction can create both acute and chronic substrates for VT and fibrillation. As discussed above, scar from previous infarction can create an anatomic re-entrant circuit providing the substrate for re-entrant VT. In the acute events such as acute coronary occlusion, metabolic derangements occur including local hyperkalemia, hypoxia, acidosis and an increase in adrenergic tone increasing the likelihood for automaticity, triggered activity, and functional re-entry. With acute coronary occlusion, ventricular fibrillation (VF) is common and is directly related to an increase in sympathetic tone. Accelerated idiopathic ventricular rhythm is frequently seen with acute myocardial infarction and is attributed to abnormal automaticity. In the chronic phase, the infarct becomes mottled and over several weeks islands of viable muscle cells are surrounded by electrically inert barriers of scar tissue. Slow conduction is present and allows for unidirectional block. These factors are conducive to re-entry which is the mechanism for sustained monomorphic VT in about 6% to 8% of survivors of myocardial infarction. Myocardial remodeling as a consequence of infarction provides a classic substrate for
1 arrhythmias. Patients with moderate to severe left ventricular dysfunction are at a higher risk for sustained monomorphic VT than those with preserved left ventricular function.

D. Neural control of arrhythmias

1. ***β*-Adrenergic modulation.** Increased sympathetic tone increases the susceptibility to VF in the early stage of myocardial infarction. In the chronic phase it facilitates initiation of sustained monomorphic VT. *β*-Adrenergic blocking drugs, propranolol, metoprolol, and nadolol significantly reduce the incidence of VF during acute infarction and reduce the risk of sudden death later. Also, *β*-blockers do not prevent reperfusion arrhythmias.
2. **Parasympathetic activation.** During acute infarction, vagal activation exerts a protective effect against VF. Bradycardia appears necessary for this protective effect. Increasing heart rate by pacing will negate this protective effect. Vagal stimulation does little to protect against reperfusion arrhythmias.

E. Clinical approach to arrhythmias

1. **Syncope** is defined as the loss of consciousness and muscle tone with spontaneous resolution. It may occur in up to 40% of the general population. The most common is vasovagal or neurally mediated syncope which is quite common in the young. This type of syncope is not associated with increased risk of death. Syncope occurs at an annual rate of 6% in patients 75 yrs old or older, but in only 0.7% of those below age 45. The goal is to determine if syncope is of the benign vasovagal variety or of the more dangerous cardiac type [4]. The 1-yr mortality from syncope of a cardiac cause can range from 18% to 33% while the noncardiac group has 0% to 6% mortality. Patients with vasovagal mediated syncope do not die from syncope. The anatomical cardiac causes of syncope result in obstruction to cardiac output, such as aortic stenosis and outflow obstruction in hypertrophic cardiomyopathy. Arrhythmias that suddenly reduce cardiac output and profoundly affect blood pressure can cause syncope. Sinus node dysfunction (SND) and AV block are common causes of bradyarrhythmias that
2 can cause syncope. SVT causes syncope less often. VT more commonly causes syncope and when it is associated with structural heart disease it is also associated with a high risk of sudden cardiac death. In patients with syncope, check the ECG for arrhythmias such as

atrial fibrillation, evidence of myocardial infarction, or conduction disease such as bundle branch block. Other important features to evaluate include pre-excitation (delta waves), the QT interval, and ectopy. Any of these abnormalities may predict a greater risk of mortality and a need for further evaluation.

2. **Bradycardia.** Heart rates less than 60 bpm are considered bradycardic. Slow heart rhythms become an issue generally in older patients who may be asymptomatic. Resting slow heart rates in young patients are most likely a result of high vagal tone and are not pathologic. Heart rates greater than 50 tend to be hemodynamically stable while those less than 40 bpm while the patient is awake often are not. If the asymptomatic bradycardic patient has no evidence of conduction disease (normal QRS morphology) and a chronotropic response to exercise, atropine or Isoproterenol, a pacemaker is rarely indicated. On the other hand, symptomatic patients with SND or evidence of conduction disease
3 such as second- or third-degree AV block almost always need a permanent pacemaker preoperatively. Bradycardia secondary to neurocardiogenic syncope, medications, or increased vagal tone will not generally require a pacemaker. Simply removing the offending medicine or treating the inciting condition will be sufficient.
3. **Tachycardia.** Heart rates above 100 bpm are termed "tachycardia." These can be sinus, a pathologic SVT, or VT. Sinus tachycardia rarely exceeds 140 bpm at rest unless the patient is in distress, shock, acute respiratory failure, or thyroid storm. In adults not in distress, a narrow, regular QRS tachycardia at rates above 150 bpm is rarely sinus. Regular and narrow QRS tachycardia at these rapid rates are frequently paroxysmal supraventricular tachycardia (PSVT) or atrial flutter with 2 to 1 conduction. Irregular SVTs are either the more common atrial fibrillation or multifocal atrial tachycardia. The later is seen in elderly patients with severe chronic pulmonary disease.

   Wide QRS tachycardia may be ventricular or supraventricular in origin. In general, if the patient has underlying heart disease, the mechanism of the wide complex tachycardia is VT until proven otherwise. However, there are several conditions in which the mechanism may be SVT including (i) SVT with an underlying or functional bundle branch block, (ii) SVT with nonspecific intraventricular conduction delay, or (iii) pre-excitation syndrome. The ECG diagnosis of VT hinges on seeing AV dissociation or fusion or capture beats. Intraventricular conduction delay can occur with the use of Class I antiarrhythmic agents or in the setting of extreme hyperkalemia. Wolff–Parkinson–White syndrome should be considered in a young healthy individual presenting with atrial fibrillation and a wide QRS rhythm. Functional bundle branch block is seen in the young and rarely in the elderly.

II. Treatment modalities

A. Pharmacologic treatment. Algorithms are now in place for acute treatment of SVTs. SVT is usually treated with intravenous (IV) adenosine acutely in the symptomatic patient. For atrial fibrillation the initial focus is on rate control. Agents that are effective acutely include IV diltiazem and the β-blockers metoprolol and esmolol. Esmolol has an extremely short half-life. Digoxin is of little use acutely and is very unpredictable. IV amiodarone is now being used more frequently in the acute management of patients with poor ventricular function and atrial fibrillation with rapid ventricular rates. This medication should be infused through a central line given the risk for tissue necrosis with extravasation. The pharmacologic treatment of ventricular arrhythmias in the hemodynamically stable patient involves treating the underlying causes.
4 For VT, IV amiodarone is the initial drug of choice, but lidocaine is also considered especially if there is concern for ongoing ischemia. For torsades de pointes, management includes eliminating offending drugs in the setting of the long QT syndromes. Correcting electrolyte deficiencies with IV magnesium and potassium are particularly helpful in correcting the prolonged QT interval, as possibly stopping medications contributing to bradycardia. Amiodarone in the setting of torsades de pointes can prolong the QT interval and make the problem worse. For the hemodynamically unstable patient with sustained ventricular arrhythmias, pharmacologic management would follow the current advanced cardiac life support (ACLS) protocols.

Proarrhythmia. Although drugs have proved safe and effective in the normal heart, their safety and efficacy have proved worrisome in the structurally abnormal heart. Chronic drug therapy for arrhythmias in patients with structural heart disease is associated with increased mortality due to proarrhythmic effects. Class IA antiarrhythmic agents are contraindicated in individuals with congestive heart failure and poor left ventricular function (ejection fraction below 0.30). Class IC agents should be avoided in individuals with a prior myocardial infarction because of the increased risk of sudden death [5]. Class III agents will prolong the QT interval and increase the risk of torsades de pointes.

B. **Nonpharmacologic treatments.** The emphasis on the chronic treatment for arrhythmias, especially ventricular arrhythmias in patients with structural heart disease, has moved from drugs to electricity. Because of technologic advances, cardiac implantable electrical devices (CIEDs) have become smaller and increasingly complex. This complexity has greatly expanded therapeutic options, but it has greatly increased the potential for malfunction in the perioperative setting. Except in infants and small children, a formal thoracotomy is no longer used for implantation of a CIED. Contemporary devices are small enough to be suitable for pectoral implantation.

1. **External cardioversion and defibrillation.** External direct-current (DC) cardioversion differs from defibrillation only in that the former incorporates a time delay circuit for shock synchronization to the QRS complex of the surface ECG. Current devices employ universal use of biphasic shocks, which lower shock current requirements for DC cardioversion and defibrillation. Automated external defibrillators self-analyze and give instructions for defibrillation [6].
   a. **Indications:** Synchronized shocks are used for most pathologic hemodynamically unstable tachycardias, except VF or VT when the QRS complex cannot be distinguished from T waves. Automatic rhythm disturbances (e.g., accelerated AV junctional or accelerated idioventricular rhythms) are not amenable to DC cardioversion.
   b. **Procedure:** Synchronized **cardioversion** with the largest R or S wave on the ECG will prevent inadvertent triggering of VF. Improper synchronization may occur when there is bundle branch block with a wide R wave, when the T wave is highly peaked, and with pacing artifacts from a malfunctioning pacemaker (i.e., failure to capture). Synchronization should be checked after each discharge. Electrodes are placed in an anterior-lateral, posterior-lateral, or an anteroposterior (AP) position. Current should pass though the heart's long axis, depolarize the bulk of myocardium, and minimize flow through high-impedance bony tissue. Electrode paste or gel is used to reduce transthoracic impedance. Bridging of the electrodes by conductive paste or gel should be avoided, because this will reduce the amount of energy delivered to the heart. Present-day units automatically boot to an energy setting of 200 J. This is the starting energy dosage for defibrillating adults. For cardioversion, energy titration (initially use only the lowest possible energies) reduces both energy use and complications. Initial settings of 20 to 50 J may be successful for terminating typical atrial flutter or stable monomorphic VT. DC cardioversion is extremely painful. Patients must be sedated for DC cardioversion at any power setting. Generally, an anesthesiologist or nurse anesthetist will administer a short-acting sedative such as IV propofol or etomidate. The combination of midazolam and fentanyl can be an alternative but is not ideal due to the prolonged duration of action.
   c. **CIEDs and cardioversion.** Older and especially unipolar devices could be easily affected by DC cardioversion. Transient loss of capture and electrical reset were not uncommon. This interference does not happen with modern bipolar and well-protected devices. Using the anterior–posterior pads position and the anterior pad location at least 8 cm from the CIED will prevent malfunction or damage to the device. Directly applied currents of 10 to 30 J to the ventricles during cardiac surgery on occasion can cause reset of the pulse generator.
2. **Temporary pacing.** Compared to drugs for treating cardiac rhythm disturbances, temporary pacing has several advantages. The effect is immediate, control is precise, and there is reduced risk of untoward effects and proarrhythmia.
   a. **Indications.** Temporary pacing is indicated for rate support in patients with symptomatic bradycardia or escape rhythms. Prophylactic or stand-by pacing is indicated for patients at increased risk for sudden high-degree AV heart block. Temporary

TABLE 17.2 Usual and less-established indications for temporary cardiac pacing

Usual indications	Less-established indications
• Sinus bradycardia or escape rhythm with symptoms or hemodynamic compromise • As bridge to permanent pacing with advanced second- or third-degree AV heart block, regardless of etiology • During AMI: asystole; new bifascicular block with first-degree AV heart block; alternating BBB with disadvantageous bradycardia not responsive to drugs; or Type II, second-degree AV heart block • Bradycardia-dependent tachyarrhythmias (e.g., torsades de pointes with LQTS)	• During AMI: New or age-indeterminate right BBB with LAFB, LPFB, or first-degree AV heart block, or with left BBB; recurrent sinus pauses refractory to atropine; overdrive pacing for incessant VT • During AMI: New or age-indeterminate bifascicular block or isolated right BBB • Heart surgery: (i) to overdrive hemodynamically disadvantageous AV junctional and ventricular rhythms; (ii) to terminate re-entrant SVT or VT; (iii) to prevent pause- or bradycardia-dependent tachydysrhythmias; (iv) insertion of pulmonary artery catheter with left BBB

AMI, acute myocardial infarction; AV, atrio-ventricular; BBB, bundle branch block; LAFB, left anterior fascicular block; LPFB, left posterior fascicular block; LQTS, long QT syndrome.

pacing can be used to overdrive or terminate atrial flutter and some sustained monomorphic VT. More specific established and emerging indications for temporary pacing are shown in Table 17.2. The endpoint for temporary pacing is resolution of the indication or implantation of a permanent pacemaker for a continuing indication.

b. Technology. Transvenous endocardial or epicardial leads are usually used for temporary pacing. Temporary endocardial bipolar active fixation wires are available for both atrial and ventricular pacing. Single- or dual-chamber pacing can be achieved. Transvenous leads are passed from above using the internal jugular or subclavian approaches or from below using a femoral vein. Epicardial leads are routinely used in patients having cardiac surgery. The noninvasive transcutaneous and transesophageal routes are also available. Transcutaneous pacing is uncomfortable and used in emergency situations. In the operating room it is for transient backup pacing only. It produces ventricular capture and does not preserve optimal hemodynamics in patients with intact AV conduction. With available technology for transesophageal pacing, only atrial pacing is reliable. Thus, the method is not suitable for patients with advanced AV block or atrial fibrillation.

3. **Permanent pacing.** Permanent pacemakers are no longer prescribed simply for rate support. They have become an integral part of treatment, along with drugs and other measures, to prevent arrhythmias and improve quality of life in patients with heart failure [7].

a. Indications. The presence or absence of symptoms directly attributable to bradycardia has an important influence on the decision to implant a permanent pacemaker. There is increasing interest in multisite pacing as part of the management for patients with structural heart disease and heart failure. In the past, pacemakers were prescribed to treat re-entrant tachyarrhythmias. Today, this capability can be programmed for either the atrium or ventricle as part of "tiered therapies" with an **internal cardioverter–defibrillator** (ICD).

(1) AV block. Patients may be asymptomatic or have symptoms related to bradycardia, ventricular arrhythmias, or both. There is little evidence that pacing improves survival with isolated first-degree AV block. With Type I, second-degree AV block due to AV nodal-conduction delay, progression to higher-degree block is unlikely. Pacing is usually not indicated unless the patient has symptoms. With Type II, second-degree AV block within or below the His bundle, symptoms are frequent, prognosis is poor, and progression to third-degree AV block is common. Pacing is recommended for chronic Type II second-degree AV block. It is recommended for Type I second-degree AV block in the presence of symptoms such as syncope. Pacing improves survival in both types of second-degree AV block. Nonrandomized studies strongly suggest that pacing improves survival in patients with third-degree AV block.

(2) Bifascicular and trifascicular block. Although third-degree AV block is commonly preceded by bifascicular block, the rate of progression is slow (years). Further, there is no credible evidence for acute progression to third-degree AV block

5 during anesthesia and surgery. Bifascicular block with periodic third-degree AV block and syncope is associated with an increased incidence of sudden death. Pro-
6 phylactic permanent pacing is indicated in this circumstance.

(3) **AV block after acute MI.** The requirement for temporary pacing with acute MI by itself does not constitute an indication for permanent pacing. The long-term prognosis for survivors of acute MI is related primarily to the extent of myocardial injury and nature of intraventricular conduction defects, rather than to AV block itself. Acute MI patients with intraventricular conduction disturbances have unfavorable short- and long-term prognoses, with increased risk of sudden death. This prognosis is not necessarily due to the development of high-grade AV block, although the incidence of such block is higher in these patients.

(4) **SND.** SND may manifest as sinus bradycardia, pause or arrest, or SA block, with or without escape rhythms. It often occurs in association with atrial fibrillation or atrial flutter (tachycardia–bradycardia syndrome). Patients with SND may have symptoms due to bradycardia, tachycardia, or both. Correlation of symptoms with arrhythmias is essential and is established by ambulatory monitoring. SND also presents as chronotropic incompetence (inability to increase rate appropriately). An adaptive-rate pacemaker may benefit these patients by restoring more physiologic heart rates. Although symptomatic SND is the primary indication for a pacemaker, pacing does not necessarily improve survival, but it can improve the quality of life.

(5) **Hypersensitive carotid sinus syndrome or neurally mediated syndrome.** Hypersensitive carotid sinus syndrome is manifest by syncope due to an exaggerated response to carotid sinus stimulation. It is an uncommon cause of syncope. If purely cardioinhibitory (asystole, heart block) and without vasodepressor components (vasodilatation), then a pacemaker can be prescribed. A hyperactive response is defined as asystole for longer than 3 s due to sinus arrest or heart block and an abrupt decrease in blood pressure. With the more common neurally mediated mixed response, attention to both components is essential for effective therapy. Neurally mediated (vasovagal) syncope accounts for nearly 25% of all syncope. The role of permanent pacing is controversial but probably limited.

(6) **Pacing in children and adolescents.** Indications for pacing are similar in children and adults, but there are additional considerations. For example, what is the optimal heart rate for the patient's age? Further, what is optimal given ventricular dysfunction or altered circulatory physiology? Hence, pacing indications are based more on correlation of symptoms with bradycardia, rather than arbitrary rate criteria, and include the following:

   (a) Bradycardia only after other causes (e.g., seizures, breath holding, apnea or neurally mediated mechanisms) are excluded.
   (b) Symptomatic congenital third-degree AV block
   (c) Persistent advanced second- or third-degree AV block after cardiac surgery. However, for patients with residual bifascicular block and intermittent AV block, the need is less certain.
   (d) Use along with β-blockers in patients with congenital long QT syndrome, especially with pause-dependent VT.

(7) **Miscellaneous pacing indications**

   (a) A dual-chamber pacemaker with short AV delay reduces left ventricular outflow tract obstruction, alleviates symptoms in **obstructive hypertrophic cardiomyopathy** in some cases, and may improve functional status. Permanent pacing does not reduce mortality or prevent sudden death in this disease.
   (b) **Bradyarrhythmias after cardiac transplantation** are mostly due to SND. Cardiac transplantation today preserves the sinus node so SND is much less likely. Most patients with bradycardia show improvement by 1 yr so that long-term pacing is unnecessary.

(c) A combination of pacing and β-blockers may be used for **prophylaxis for tachyarrhythmias** in congenital long QT syndrome. Pacing therapy alone is not recommended. Backup dual-chamber defibrillator therapy is now preferred.

b. Technology. Contemporary single- and dual-chamber pacemakers are sophisticated devices, with multiple programmable features, including automatic mode switching, rate adaptive pacing, automatic threshold pacing, and programmable lead configuration. Pacemakers are powered by lithium iodide batteries, with an expected service life of 5 to 12 yrs, depending on device capabilities, need for pacing, and programmed stimulus parameters. Most systems use transvenous leads. Lead configuration is programmable. With the unipolar configuration, the pacemaker housing (can) serves as anode (+) and the distal electrode of the bipolar pacing lead as cathode (–). With the bipolar configuration, proximal and distal lead electrodes serve as anode and cathode, respectively. The ability to program unipolar pacing is necessary if lead insulation or conductor failure occurs in a bipolar lead system. Also, it permits exploitation of either configuration while minimizing its disadvantages (e.g., oversensing with unipolar leads). A dual-chamber pacemaker with automatic mode switching is optimal for patients with AV block and susceptibility to paroxysmal atrial fibrillation. Algorithms detect fast, nonphysiologic atrial rates and automatically switch the pacing mode to one that excludes atrial tracking and the associated risk of upper-rate ventricular pacing.

4. Implantable cardioverter—defibrillator. Contemporary ICDs are multiprogrammable, are longer lived, use transvenous leads, and may incorporate **all** capabilities of a modern dual-chamber pacemaker. ICDs are powered by combination of both batteries and capacitors. Many current models also have wireless technology that allows patients to have remote follow-up via their home phone lines for routine ICD evaluations limiting the in-person visits to the pacer clinic or doctor's office to annual or bi-annual evaluations. Additionally, ICDs have multiple tachycardia detection zones, with programmable detection criteria and "tiered therapy" for each (antitachycardia pacing → cardioversion shocks → defibrillatory shocks if necessary). ICDs also store arrhythmia event records and treatment results. Future devices will be tailored to meet all nonpharmacologic aspects of cardiac rhythm management for individual patients. Finally, ICDs have undergone significant downsizing (50 mL or smaller) and nearly all are prepectoral implants.

a. Indications. ICDs are used for **secondary or primary prevention** of sudden death.

(1) Secondary prevention. ICDs are used for **secondary prevention** in patients who have survived a cardiac arrest from sustained ventricular arrhythmias. Most commonly these are patients with heart failure and reduced left ventricular systolic function. Of this population, coronary artery disease and ischemic cardiomyopathy are the most common etiologies of the heart failure. Secondary prevention indications for ICDs also include individuals with structural heart disease who have documented sustained ventricular tachyarrhythmias or inducible sustained ventricular tachyarrhythmias by electrophysiologic testing. ICDs are widely accepted for improving outcomes in these patients by preventing sudden cardiac death. Other indications for secondary prevention include patients with long QT syndrome and recurrent syncope, sustained ventricular arrhythmias, or sudden cardiac arrest despite drug therapy. ICD plus Class IA drugs are prescribed for patients with idiopathic VF and Brugada syndrome with recurrent ventricular arrhythmias. Other indications are (i) sudden death survivors with hypertrophic cardiomyopathy; (ii) prophylaxis for syncope and sudden death with drug-refractory arrhythmogenic right ventricular dysplasia; and (iii) children with malignant tachyarrhythmias or sudden death and congenital heart disease, cardiomyopathies, or primary electrical disease (e.g., long QT syndrome).

(2) Primary prevention. ICDs are used for **primary prevention** of sudden death in patients who are at high risk for sudden cardiac death. This population mainly includes those with systolic heart failure with ejection fractions ≤35% that has not improved despite medical therapy. The cause of heart failure may be from coronary artery disease or of nonischemic origin. Other indications for primary prevention ICDs include patients with high risk features with inherited or acquired conditions that place them at increased risk for life-threatening ventricular arrhythmias including long QT syndrome, hypertrophic cardiomyopathy, arrhythmogenic right ventricular dysplasia, cardiac sarcoid, Brugada syndrome, and congenital heart disease.

b. Technology. The ICD pulse generator is a self-powered minicomputer with one or two (in series) batteries that power the pulse generator, circuitry, and aluminum electrolytic capacitors. The batteries may be lithium–silver vanadium oxide or evolving hybrid technology and vary between the manufacturers. A major challenge in ICD design is the large range of voltages within a very small package. Intracardiac signals may be as low as 100 μV, and therapeutic shocks approach 750 V. Further, ICD batteries contain up to 20,000 J, and a potential hazard exists if the charging and firing circuits were to electrically or thermally unload all this energy into the patient in a brief time period. The number of shocks delivered during treatment is usually limited to five or six per arrhythmia. The expected service life is 5 to 8 yrs.

III. Device function, malfunction, and interference [8]

A. Pacemakers. A single-chamber pacemaker stimulates the atria or ventricles at programmed timing intervals. Sensing spontaneous atrial or ventricular depolarizations inhibit the device from delivering unnecessary or inappropriate stimuli. Dual-chamber devices time the delivery of ventricular stimuli relative to sensed atrial depolarizations to maintain proper AV synchrony. Figure 17.2 illustrates how a pacemaker might be configured to pace in patients with SND or atrioventricular heart block (AVHB).

In Figure 17.2 and throughout this chapter, the North American Society for Pacing and Electrophysiology–British Pacing and Electrophysiology Group (NASPE/BPEG) pacemaker code (also known as the NBG code) is used as a short-hand to describe pacing modes (Table 17.3).

1. Function. Today, most US pacemakers are dual-chamber (DDD or DDDR) devices with rate-adaptive features (rate response) that can be activated if clinically indicated. Single-chamber pacemakers may pace either the atrium or ventricle depending on lead placement and also may have rate-adaptive features turned on. Dual-chamber pacemakers may also be programmed to act like a single-chamber pacer activating either the atrial or ventricular lead through the use of the proprietary programmer. For example, in individuals with normal conduction and sinus node function, dual-chamber pacemakers may operate as a single-chamber device in the AAI (AAIR, AAI) or VVI (VVIR) modes (Fig. 17.2).

TABLE 17.3 NASPE/BPEG (NBG) pacemaker code used as shorthand to designate pacing modes

I	II	III	IV	V
Chamber paced	Chamber sensed	Response to sensed event	Programmability/ rate response[a]	Antitachycardia functions[b]
O = none	O = none	O = none	O = none	O = none
A = atrium	A = atrium	I = inhibit	R = adaptive rate	P = ATP
V = ventricle	V = ventricle	T = triggered		S = shock
D = dual (A & V)	D = dual (A & V)	D = dual (I & T)		D = dual (P + S)
S = single[c]	S = single[c]			

[a]In current terminology, only the adaptive rate response (R) is indicated by the fourth position. All current pacemakers have full programming and communicating capability; therefore, the letters P (programmable), M (multiprogrammable), and C (communicating) are no longer used.
[b]Implantable cardioverter–defibrillator with antibradycardia and antitachycardia pacing capabilities.
[c]Single-chamber device that paces either the atrium or ventricle.
ATP, antitachycardia pacing.
From Bernstein AD, Daubert JC, Fletcher RD, et al. The revised NASPE/BPEG generic code for antibradycardia, adaptive-rate, and multisite pacing. North American Society of Pacing and Electrophysiology/British Pacing and Electrophysiology Group. *Pacing Clin Electrophysiol.* 2002;25:260–264.

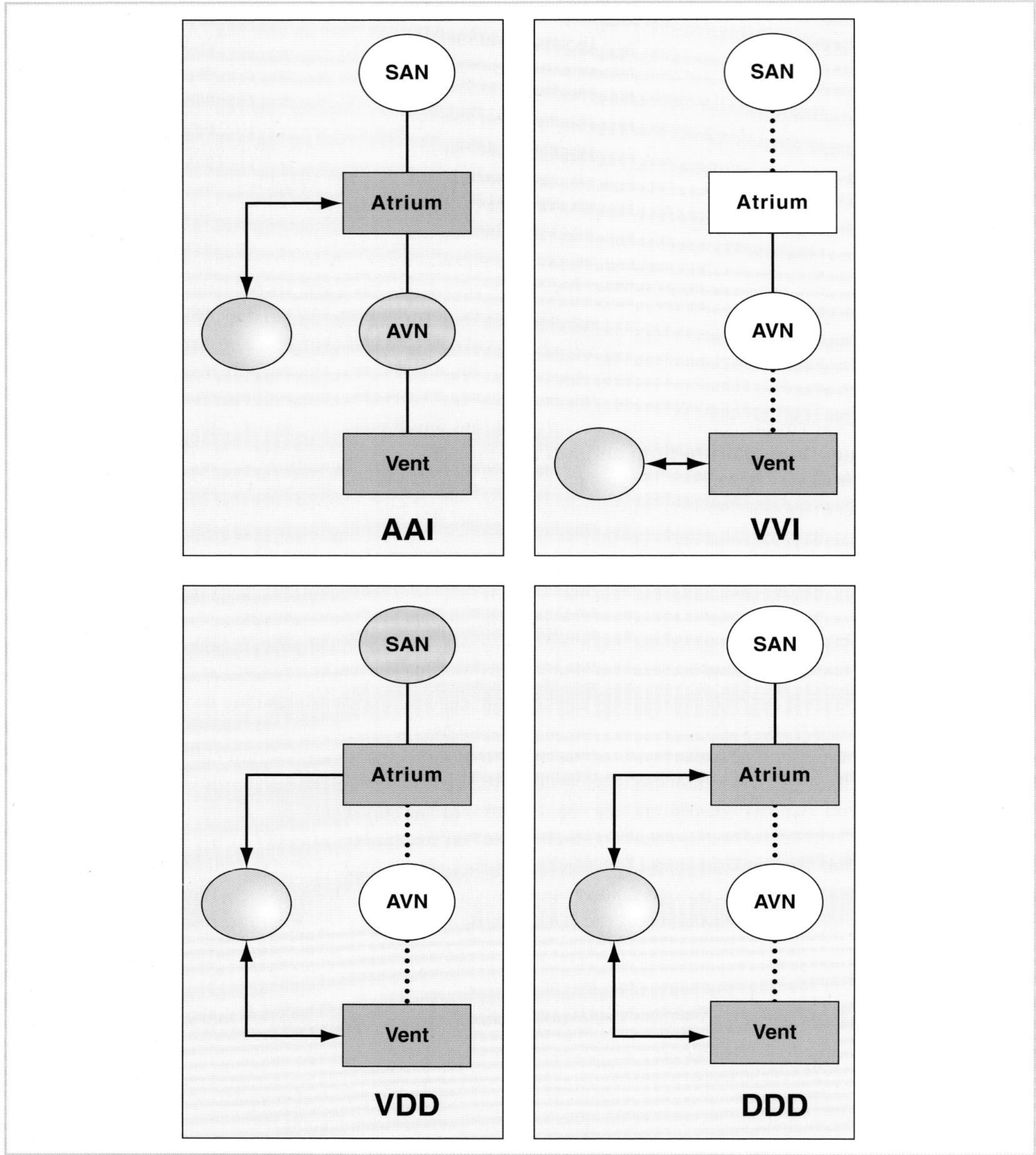

FIGURE 17.2 Bradycardia pacing modes. A dysfunctional sinoatrial node (SAN), atrium, or atrioventricular node (AVN) is indicated by *white circles* or *rectangles.* Normal impulse transmission between these structures and the ventricles (*VENT*) is indicated by *solid lines,* with blocked or ineffective conduction indicated by *hashed lines.* An *arrow* pointing toward the pulse generator (blue) indicates sensing, whereas one pointing toward the atrium or ventricle indicates pacing in that chamber. **Top left:** AAI pacing for sinus arrest or bradycardia. There is a single atrial lead for both sensing and pacing. Atrial pacing occurs unless inhibited by a sensed spontaneous atrial depolarization. **Top right:** VVI pacing for AV heart block with atrial fibrillation. There is a single ventricular lead for both sensing and pacing. Ventricular pacing occurs unless inhibited by a sensed spontaneous ventricular depolarization. **Bottom left:** VDD pacing for AV heart block with normal SAN and atrial function. The atrial lead is for sensing only, and the ventricular lead is for both pacing and sensing. After a sensed atrial depolarization, the ventricle is paced after the programmed AV interval (i.e., atrial-triggered ventricular pacing [VAT]), unless first inhibited by a sensed ventricular depolarization (i.e., the VVI component of the VDD mode). **Bottom right:** Dual-chamber sequential or AV universal (DDD) pacing for sinus bradycardia with AV heart block. Both atrial and ventricular leads are for sensing and pacing. This mode incorporates all of the preceding pacing capabilities (AAI, VVI, and VAT).

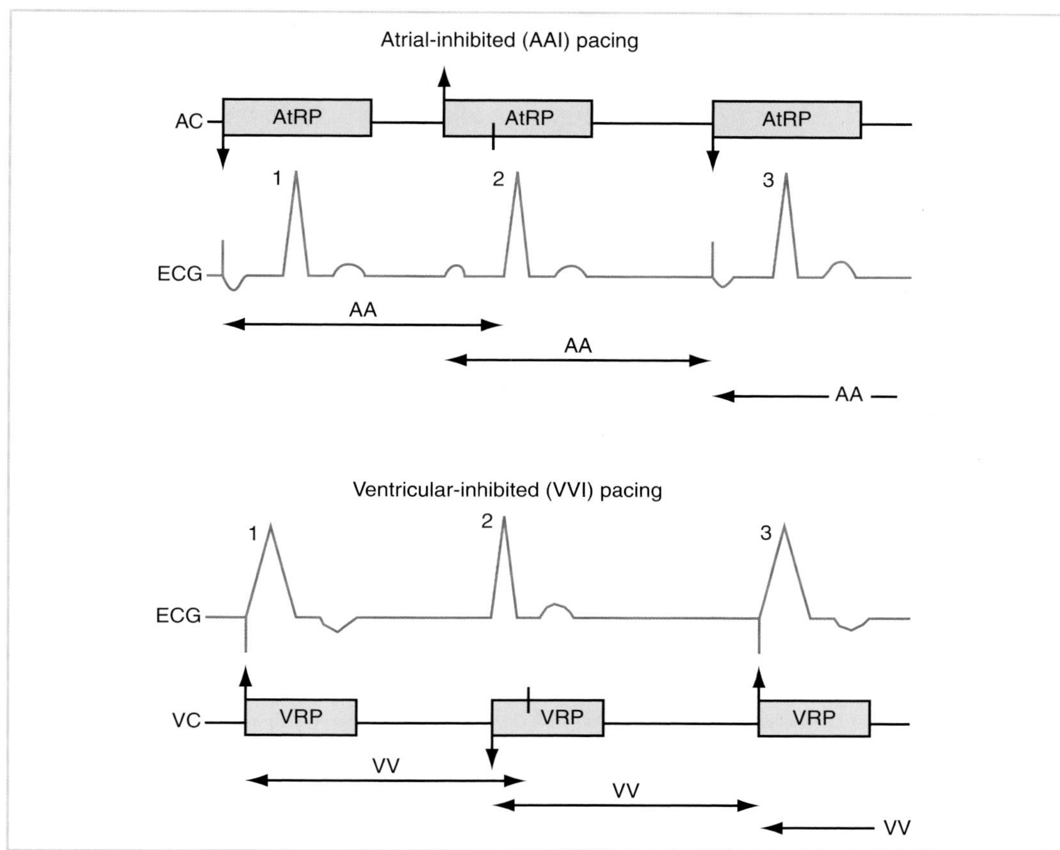

FIGURE 17.3 **Top:** AAI pacing, as for a patient with sinus bradycardia and intact AV conduction. The atrium is paced (beats 1 and 3)—*arrow* pointing toward the ECG in the atrial channel (*AC*) timing diagram—unless inhibited by sensed spontaneous atrial depolarization (beat 2)—*arrow* pointing away from the ECG in the AC timing diagram. The atrial refractory period (AtRP) prevents R and T waves from being sensed by the AC and inappropriately resetting the atrial escape timing (AA interval). Note that spontaneous atrial depolarization (beat 2) occurs before the AA interval times out, resetting the AA interval. The *short vertical line* in the AC timing diagram above beat 2 shows where the stimulus would have occurred had the previous AA interval timed out. In the absence of subsequent spontaneous atrial depolarization (beat 3), the AA interval times out with delivery of a stimulus. **Bottom:** VVI pacing, as for a patient with atrial fibrillation and AV heart block. Beats 1 and 3 are paced, and beat 2 is spontaneous. The latter resets the ventricular escape interval (VV), which otherwise would have timed out with delivery of a stimulus, indicated by the *short vertical line* in the ventricular channel (VC) timing diagram above beat 2. The new VV interval times out with stimulus delivery (beat 3), because there is no sensed ventricular depolarization to reset the timing. VRP, ventricular refractory period.

a. **Single-chamber pacemaker.** These devices have a single timing interval, the atrial or ventricular escape interval, between successive stimuli in the absence of sensed depolarization. In the AAI or VVI mode (Fig. 17.3), pacing occurs at the end of the programmed atrial or ventricular escape interval unless a spontaneous atrial or ventricular depolarization is sensed first, resetting these intervals. If the device has rate hysteresis as a programmable option, then the atrial or ventricular escape interval after a sensed depolarization is programmed longer than that after a paced depolarization to encourage emergence of intrinsic rhythm and prolong battery life.
b. **Dual-chamber pacemaker.** A DDD ("AV universal") pacemaker can pace and sense in both the atrium and the ventricle. It has two basic timing intervals whose sum is the pacing cycle duration (Fig. 17.4). The first is the AV interval, which is the programmed

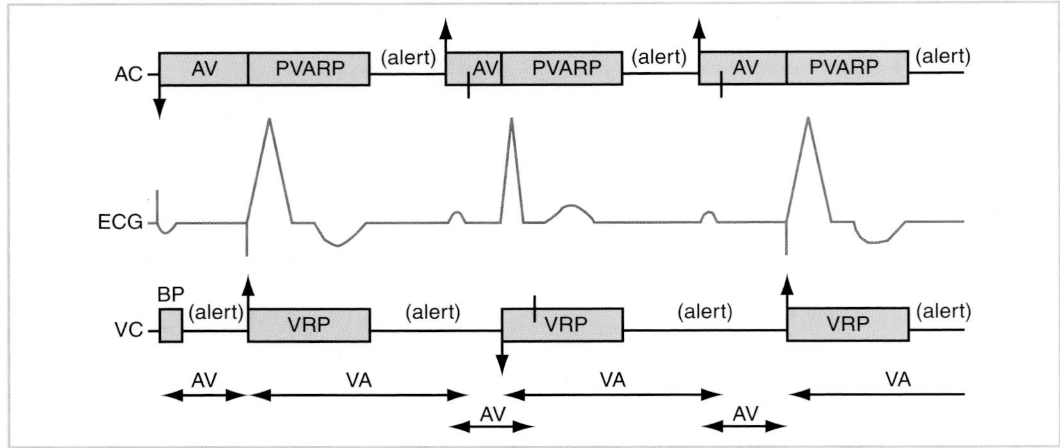

FIGURE 17.4 AV universal (DDD) pacing, as for a patient with sinus node dysfunction and atrio-ventricular (AV) heart block. The atrium is paced (beat 1)—*arrow* pointing toward the ECG in the atrial channel (AC) timing diagram above beat 1—unless inhibited by sensed atrial depolarization (beats 2 and 3)—*arrows* pointing away from the ECG in the AC timing diagram. The AC is refractory during the AV interval and from delivery of the ventricular stimulus until the end of the post-ventricular atrial refractory period (PVARP). This prevents atrial sensing from resetting the escape timing (i.e., AV interval). The ventricular channel (VC) blanking period (BP) prevents sensing of the atrial pacing stimulus, thereby resetting the AV interval and delaying ventricular stimulus delivery. However, sensed ventricular depolarization or noise (e.g., electrocautery) in the alert period (VC) after the blanking period also could inhibit ventricular stimulation. As shown, this does not occur, so the AV interval times out with delivery of a ventricular stimulus. The ventricular refractory period (VRP) prevents sensed T waves from inappropriately resetting the ventriculo-atrial (VA) interval. However, sensing during the alert periods after the PVARP or VRP will reset basic timing, initiating new AV and VA intervals, respectively. Since the first beat is fully paced, it is an example of asynchronous AV sequential pacing (i.e., DOO). With the second beat, a sensed spontaneous atrial depolarization initiates a new AV interval, inhibiting the atrial stimulus that would have occurred, indicated by the *short vertical line* in the AC timing diagram. Subsequently, there is spontaneous ventricular depolarization before the AV interval times out. The ventricular stimulus that otherwise would have occurred at the end of the AV interval is indicated by the *short vertical line* in the VC timing diagram below beat 2. The third beat begins with a sensed atrial depolarization. As with beat 2, this also occurs before the VA interval times out. In the absence of sensed ventricular depolarization (beat 3), the new AV interval times out with ventricular stimulus delivery. Beat 3 is an example of atrial-inhibited, ventricular-triggered pacing (i.e., VDD).

interval from a paced or sensed atrial depolarization to ensuing ventricular stimulation. Some devices offer the option of programmable AV interval hysteresis. If so, the AV interval after paced atrial depolarization is longer than that after sensed depolarization to maintain greater uniformity between atrial and ventricular depolarizations. The second interval is the VA interval, the interval between sensed or paced ventricular depolarization and the next atrial stimulus. During atrial and ventricular refractory periods (Fig. 17.4), sensed events do not reset the device escape timing. During the ventricular channel blanking period (Fig. 17.4), ventricular sensing is disabled to avoid overloading of the ventricular sense amplifier by voltage generated by the atrial stimulus, thereby inappropriately resetting the VA interval. Sensing during the alert periods outside the ventricular blanking and postventricular atrial and ventricular refractory periods initiates new AV or VA intervals (Fig. 17.4). Operationally, depending on sensing patterns, a DDD pacemaker can provide atrial, ventricular, dual-chamber sequential, or no pacing (Fig. 17.4).

c. **Adaptive-rate pacing (ARP).** ARP is a programmable feature in nearly all implanted devices (both pacemakers and ICDs) in service today. In patients with chronotropic incompetence, ARP has been shown to improve exercise capacity and quality of life. Activity-based sensors are used most commonly to determine the paced heart rate. These are piezoelectric crystals that sense vibration (up-and-down motion) or acceleration (forward–backward movement) as an index of physical activity. However, they do not provide feedback proportional to physiologic need. A better alternative is the QT interval, in which a QT-sensing device measures the stimulus to T wave interval during ventricular pacing. However, this measure is affected by changes in heart rate and catecholamines. Minute ventilation sensors measure changes in transthoracic impedance with respiration (i.e., increase with inspiration and decrease with expiration) and provide an estimate of metabolic need that is more proportional to exercise. However, they increase current drain on the device. Other sensors in use or under development measure O_2 saturation, pH, stroke volume, or temperature. Finally, because ARP sensors may have a disproportionate response time at the beginning of exercise versus steady-state exercise, a dual-sensor ARP device may provide a more proportional response. Obviously, such complexity and the use of multiple physiologic sensors increase the potential for device malfunction in the perioperative setting.

2. **Malfunction.** Primary pacemaker malfunction is rare (less than 2% of all device-related problems). Pacing malfunction can occur with ICDs, because all ICDs today include a pacing function which can pace at least the ventricle. Some devices have programmed behavior that simulates malfunction, termed pseudomalfunction. For example, failure to pace may be misdiagnosed with programmed rate hysteresis. Also, apparent device malfunction in response to electromagnetic interference (EMI) may be normal device operation, as described later in this chapter.

   Pacemaker malfunction is classified as failure to pace, failure to capture, pacing at abnormal rates, failure to sense, oversensing, and malfunction unique to dual-chamber devices (Table 17.4). Among the causes for failure to capture are drugs or conditions that affect pacing thresholds (Table 17.5). To diagnose malfunction, it is necessary to obtain a 12-lead ECG and chest X-ray film and to interrogate the device for pacing and sensing thresholds, lead impedances, battery voltage, and magnet rate.

TABLE 17.4 Categories of pacemaker malfunction, ECG appearance, and likely cause for malfunction

Category of malfunction	ECG appearance	Cause for malfunction
Failure to pace	For one or both chambers, either no pacing artifacts will be present on the ECG, or artifacts will be present for one but not the other chamber	Oversensing; battery failure; open circuit due to mechanical problems with leads or system component malfunction; fibrosis at electrode–tissue interface; lead dislodgment; recording artifact
Failure to capture	Atrial and/or ventricular pacing stimuli are present, with persistent or intermittent failure to capture	Fibrosis at electrode–tissue interface; drugs or conditions that increase pacing thresholds (Table 17.5)
Pacing at abnormal rates	I. Rapid pacing rate (upper-rate behavior) II. Slow pacing rate (below lower rate interval) III. No stimulus artifact; intrinsic rate below lower rate interval	I. Adaptive-rate pacing; tracking atrial tachycardia; pacemaker-mediated tachycardia; oversensing II. Programmed rate hysteresis, or rest or sleep rates; oversensing III. Power source failure; lead disruption; oversensing
Failure to sense	Pacing artifacts in middle of normal P waves or QRS complexes	Inadequate intracardiac signal strength; component malfunction; battery depletion; misinterpretation of normal device function
Oversensing	Abnormal pacing rates with pauses (regular or random)	Far-field sensing with inappropriate device inhibition or triggering; intermittent contact between pacing system conducting elements
Malfunction unique to dual-chamber devices	Rapid pacing rate (i.e., upper-rate behavior)	Cross-talk inhibition; pacemaker-mediated tachycardia (see text)

TABLE 17.5 Drugs and conditions that affect or have no proven effect on pacing thresholds

Effect	Drugs	Conditions
Increase pacing threshold	Bretylium, encainide, flecainide, moricizine, propafenone, sotalol	Myocardial ischemia and infarction; progression of cardiomyopathy; hyperkalemia; severe acidosis or alkalosis; hypoxemia; hypothermia; irradiation; after cardioversion or defibrillation (implantable cardioverter–defibrillator or external)
Possibly increase pacing threshold	β-Blockers, lidocaine, procainamide, quinidine, verapamil	Myxedema; hyperglycemia
Possibly decrease pacing threshold	Atropine, catecholamines, glucocorticoids	Pheochromocytoma; hyperthyroid or other hypermetabolic states
No proven effect on pacing threshold	Amiodarone; anesthetic drugs, both inhalation and intravenous	Hyperthermia

Malfunctions unique to dual-chamber devices are crosstalk inhibition and pacemaker-mediated tachycardia (PMT).

a. Crosstalk inhibition. Crosstalk refers to the oversensing of atrial signals from atrial stimulation on the ventricular sense channel or circuit of a dual-chamber pacemaker. This oversensing has the potential of inhibiting ventricular output. Crosstalk is prevented by increasing the ventricular sensing threshold, decreasing atrial stimulus output, or programming a longer ventricular blanking period (Fig. 17.4), so long as these provide adequate safety margins for atrial capture and ventricular sensing. If crosstalk cannot be prevented, many dual-chamber devices have a feature referred to as nonphysiologic AV delay or ventricular safety pacing. Whenever the ventricular channel senses anything early during the AV interval, a ventricular stimulus is triggered after an abbreviated AV interval. This either will depolarize ventricular myocardium or will fail to do so if myocardium is refractory due to spontaneous depolarization. The premature timing of the triggered ventricular stimulus prevents it from occurring during the vulnerable period of the T wave.

b. Pacemaker-mediated tachycardia (PMT). PMT is undesired rapid pacing caused by the device or its interaction with the patient. PMT includes sensor-driven tachycardia, tachycardia during magnetic resonance imaging (MRI), tachycardia due to tracking of myopotentials or atrial tachyarrhythmias, pacemaker re-entrant tachycardia, and runaway pacemaker.

7 **Sensor-driven tachycardia** may occur with adaptive-rate devices that sense vibration, impedance changes, or the QT interval if they sense mechanical or physiologic interference, which leads to inappropriate high-rate pacing. Thus, it is advised that ARP be disabled in perioperative settings.

MRI. Powerful forces exist in the MRI suite, including static and gradient magnetic fields, and radiofrequency (RF) fields. The static magnetic field may exert a torque effect on the pulse generator or close the magnetic reed switch to cause asynchronous pacing. The gradient magnetic field may induce voltage large enough to inhibit a demand pacemaker but is unlikely to cause pacing. The RF field may generate enough current in the
8 leads to cause pacing at the frequency of the pulsed energy (60 to 300 bpm). Because of the unpredictable interaction between the MRI and CIEDs, MRIs are generally contraindicated in individuals with CIEDs. There is now an approved compatible pacemaker generator and lead system for individuals likely to need MRI.

Tachycardia due to myopotential tracking occurs in a dual-chamber device when the atrial sense channel is programmed unipolar and the device programmed to VAT, VDD, or DDD modes. Sensed myopotentials from pectoral muscle beneath the pulse generator can trigger ventricular pacing up to the maximum atrial tracking rate.

Tachycardia due to **tracking atrial tachyarrhythmias** has a similar explanation. Medication to suppress the arrhythmia (often atrial fibrillation) or cardioversion may be necessary. Placing a magnet over the pulse generator to disable sensing in most instances (see response to magnet, later) will terminate high-rate atrial tracking. Newer dual-chamber devices with automatic mode switching detect fast, nonphysiologic atrial tachycardia and automatically switch the device to a nontracking mode.

Finally, **pacemaker-re-entrant tachycardia** can occur in a device programmed to an atrial tracking mode. Up to 50% of patients with dual-chamber devices are susceptible to PRT because they have retrograde (VA) conduction via the AVN or an accessory AV pathway. PRT occurs when spontaneous or paced ventricular beats are conducted back to the atria to trigger ventricular pacing. To prevent PRT, a longer postventricular atrial refractory period is programmed (Fig. 17.4). Also, placing a magnet over the pulse generator will terminate PRT in most devices by disabling sensing. However, PRT may recur after the magnet is removed.

3. **Response of pacemaker to magnet application.** Most contemporary pacemaker devices
9 respond to magnet application by a device-specific single- or dual-chamber asynchronous pacing mode. Adaptive-rate response is generally suspended with magnet mode as well. With asynchronous pacing, the pacemaker will no longer be inhibited by sensed activity and instead pace at a fixed rate regardless of underlying rhythm. The first few magnet-triggered beats may occur at a rate and output other than that seen later. Pacing amplitudes remain constant at the programmed output in Biotronik, Boston Scientific, and Medtronic pacemakers. The pacing amplitude with magnet application in ELA/Sorin and St. Jude pacemakers may be higher than the programmed output settings. The response to a magnet should be determined prior to an anticipated surgical procedure and is predicted by the brand of the pacemaker in most circumstances. However, some manufacturers,
10 Biotronik, St. Jude Medical, and Boston Scientific devices, have a programmable magnet mode that may make response to magnet application different than anticipated. Although rarely used, this feature may be programmed to save patient-activated rhythm recordings with magnet application rather than revert the pacemaker to asynchronous pacing. To confirm that the typical magnet response is "'on," place magnet on the device and evaluate if there is a change to asynchronous pacing on telemetry. The magnet-triggered rate and the duration of pacing do vary based on manufacturer and battery status. For example, Biotronik pacemakers have a magnet rate at 90 bpm for 10 beats only while all other manufacturers pace asynchronously as long as the magnet is in contact with the pacemaker. The fixed magnet rate for Boston Scientific pacemakers is 100 bpm; St. Jude is 98.6 bpm; ELA/Sorin is 96 bpm. Medtronic pacemakers are triggered for three beats at 100 bpm then default to 85 bpm. However, with impending power source depletion, the magnet rate will approach the programmed rate of the end-of-life (EOL) or elective replacement indicator (ERI) and is usually a slower pacing interval than the standard magnet rate (Table 17.6).

   In a patient whose intrinsic rhythm inhibits the device, magnet application may serve to identify the programmed mode when the correct programmer is not available for telemetry. Also, with device malfunction due to malsensing, magnet-initiated asynchronous pacing may temporarily correct the problem, confirming the presence of far-field sensing, crosstalk inhibition, T-wave sensing, or PMT. Finally, in pacemaker-dependent patients, magnet application may ensure pacing if EMI inhibits output (e.g., surgical electrocautery).
4. **Interference.** CIEDs are subject to interference from nonbiologic electromagnetic sources. In general, devices in service today are effectively shielded against EMI. Increasing

TABLE 17.6 Elective replacement indicators that may affect the nominal rate of pacing

- **Stepwise change in pacing rate:** Pacing rate changes to some predetermined fixed rate or some percentage decrease from the programmed rate
- **Stepwise change in magnet rate:** Magnet-pacing rate decreases in a stepwise fashion related to the remaining battery life
- **Pacing mode change:** DDD and DDDR pulse generators may automatically revert to another mode, such as VVI or VOO, to reduce current drain and extend battery life

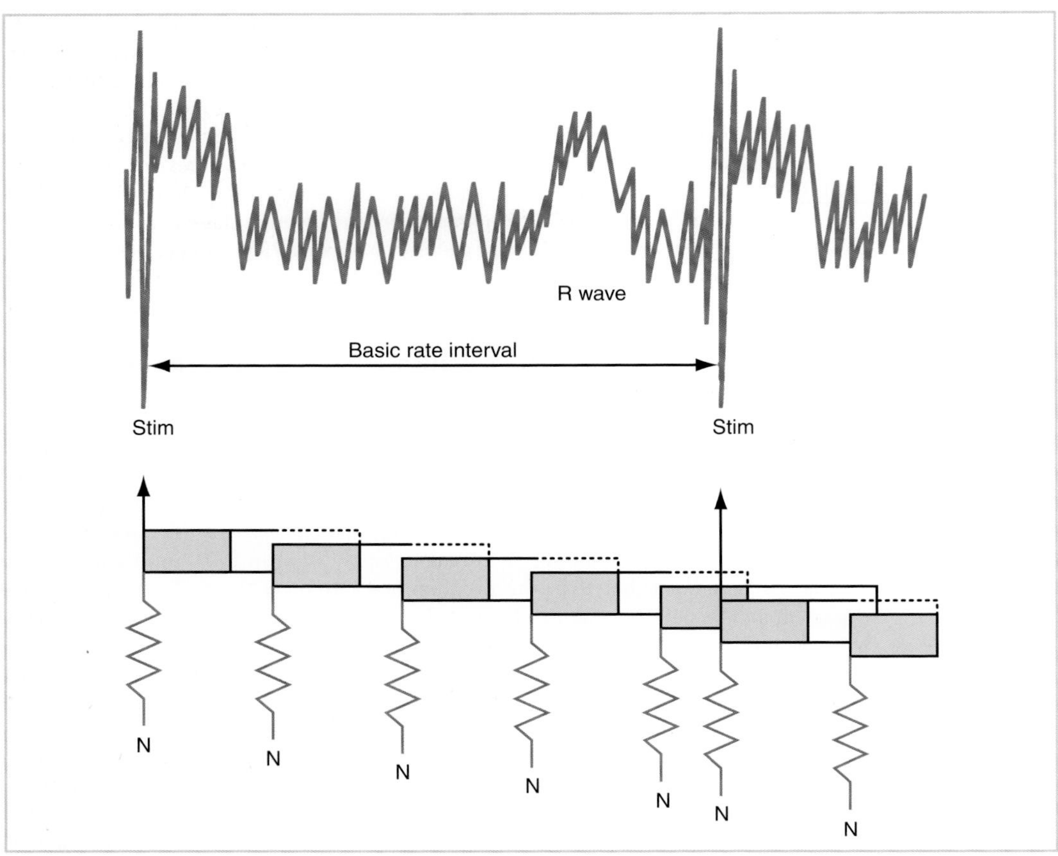

FIGURE 17.5 VVI pacemaker to continuous EMI. Temporary asynchronous pacing stimulation (*Stim*) occurs at the programmed basic rate interval. The ventricular refractory period (*rectangles*) begins with the noise (*N*) sampling period (*blue rectangles*), during which time there is no sensing. During the remainder of this refractory period, repeated noise (N) sensing above a specified minimal frequency (e.g., 7 Hz) is interpreted as EMI. This restarts the ventricular refractory period. Portions of the previous refractory period pre-empted by the newly initiated ventricular refractory period are indicated by *hashed rectangles*. Therefore, so long as interference persists, the pacemaker remains refractory and escape timing is determined entirely by the programmed basic rate interval. In this example, the second paced *R* wave falls in the noise sampling period. It is not sensed, but it initiates a new ventricular refractory period. The spontaneous R wave is not sensed and does not affect escape timing.

use of bipolar sensing has further reduced the problem. EMI frequencies above 10^9 Hz (i.e., infrared, visible light, ultraviolet, X-rays, and gamma rays) do not interfere with pacemakers or ICDs, because the wavelengths are much shorter than the device or lead dimensions. High-intensity therapeutic X-rays and irradiation can directly damage circuitry. EMI enters a device by conduction (direct contact) or radiation (leads acting as an antenna). Devices are protected from EMI by (i) shielding the circuitry, (ii) using a bipolar versus unipolar lead configuration for sensing to minimize the antenna, and (iii) filtering incoming signals to exclude noncardiac signals. If EMI does enter the pulse generator, noise protection algorithms in the timing circuit help reduce its effect on the patient. However, EMI signals between 5 and 100 Hz are not filtered, because these overlap the frequency range of intracardiac signals. Therefore, EMI in this frequency range may be interpreted as intracardiac signals, giving rise
11 to abnormal behavior. Possible responses include (i) inappropriate inhibition or triggering of stimulation, (ii) asynchronous pacing (Fig. 17.5), (iii) mode resetting, (iv) direct damage to the pulse generator circuitry, and (v) triggering of unnecessary ICD shocks (Table 17.7).

TABLE 17.7 Perioperative EMI sources and their potential effects on implanted pacemakers or implantable cardioverter–defibrillators

EMI source	Generator damage	Complete inhibition	One-beat inhibition	Asynchronous pacing	Rate increase	Spurious shocks
Electrocautery	Yes	Yes	Yes	Yes	Yes[a,b]	Yes
External DC/DF	Yes	No	No	Yes	Yes	No
Magnetic resonance imaging scanner	Possible	No	Yes	Yes	Yes	Yes
Lithotripsy	Yes[b]	Yes[c]	Yes[c]	Yes[c]	Yes[d]	Yes
Radiofrequency ablation	Yes	Yes	No	No	Yes	Yes
Electroconvulsive therapy	No	Yes	Yes	Yes	Yes[b]	Yes
Transcutaneous electrical nerve stimulation	No	Yes	No	Yes	Yes	Unlikely
Radiation therapy	Yes	No	No	No	Yes	Yes
Diagnostic radiation	No	No	No	No	Yes	No

[a]Impedance-based adaptive-rate (AR) pulse generators.
[b]Piezoelectric crystal-based AR pulse generators.
[c]Remote potential for interference.
[d]DDD mode only.
DC/DF, direct-current cardioversion or defibrillation; EMI, electromagnetic interference.

Finally, with EMI and inappropriate device behavior, it is widely assumed that placing a magnet over a pulse generator invariably will cause asynchronous pacing as long as the magnet remains in place. However, this is not always the case. Although used rarely, some devices (see above in Section III.A.3.) may have programmed magnet response off. In contrast to pacemakers, magnet application on ICDs will not alter the pacing mode and will not change the mode to asynchronous pacing (see below). Thus, if possible, one should determine before EMI exposure what pulse generator is present and what must be done to provide protection. If this is not possible preoperatively, then one must observe the magnet response during EMI to ascertain whether there is protection from EMI sensing. For example, if a pacemaker-dependent patient has inappropriate inhibition or triggering of output during electrosurgery even with magnet application, then electrosurgery must be limited to short bursts.

B. **ICD.** An ICD consists of a pulse generator and leads for tachyarrhythmia detection and therapy. Modern ICDs use transvenous lead systems for sensing, pacing, and biphasic shock delivery. Epicardial leads are still used in infants and small children. Use of biphasic compared to monophasic shocks has greatly lowered defibrillation energy requirements and has led to development of smaller ICDs.

1. **Sensing ventricular depolarizations.** Reliable sensing is essential. The sense amplifier must respond quickly and accurately to rates of 30 to 360 bpm or greater, and to the varying amplitude and morphology of intracardiac signals during VT or VF. Unfiltered intracardiac electrograms are sent to the sense amplifier. This has a band-pass filter to reject low-frequency T waves and high-frequency noise. There is automatic gain control (auto-gain), a rectifier to eliminate polarity dependency, and a fixed or auto-adjusting threshold event detector. The sense amplifier produces a set of R–R intervals for the VT/VF detection algorithms to use.
2. **VF detection.** ICDs use rate criteria as the sole method for detecting VF. Due to the circumstances of VF, the detection algorithms must have high sensitivity and low specificity. If criteria for detection are too aggressive, the ICD likely will oversense T waves during sinus rhythm, leading to spurious shocks. If too conservative, it likely will undersense some VF but work very well during sinus rhythm. An ICD *X/Y* detector triggers when *X* of the previous *Y* sensed ventricular intervals are shorter than the VF detection interval. Typically, this is 70% to 80% of intervals in a sliding window of 10 to 24. This approach is very good at ignoring the effect of a small number of undersensed events due to the small amplitude of VF intracardiac

signals. Any tachycardia with a cycle length less than the VF detection interval will initiate VF therapy. After capacitor charging but before shock delivery, an algorithm confirms the presence of VF. After shock delivery, redetection and episode-termination algorithms determine whether VF has terminated, continued, or changed.

3. **Tachycardia detection and discrimination (single-chamber ICD).** Most VT algorithms require a programmable number of consecutive R–R intervals shorter than the VT detection interval. A longer R–R interval, as might occur during atrial fibrillation, would reset the VT counters. In patients with both supraventricular and ventricular tachyarrhythmias, up to 45% of ICD discharges may be inappropriate if rate is used as the sole criterion for VT therapy.

   To increase specificity, VT detection algorithm enhancements are programmed for one or more VT zones in single-chamber ICDs, including criteria for stability of rate, suddenness of onset, and intracardiac QRS morphology.

   a. The **rate stability criterion** is used to distinguish sustained monomorphic VT with little cycle length variation from atrial fibrillation with much greater cycle length variation. Such enhancement criteria are not available in the VF zone, where maximum sensitivity is required. Also, they are programmed only in rate zones that correspond to VT hemodynamically tolerated by the patient.
   b. The **suddenness of onset criterion** is used to distinguish sinus tachycardia from VT, because VT has a more sudden rate increase.
   c. Finally, **morphology algorithms** discriminate VT from SVT based on morphology of intracardiac electrograms.

4. **Tachycardia detection and discrimination (dual-chamber ICD).** Inadequate specificity of VT detection algorithms, despite enhancements, has been a significant problem with single-chamber ICDs. Dual-chamber ICDs use an atrial lead, which is used for bradycardia pacing and sensing for tachycardia discrimination. Detection algorithms use atrial and ventricular timing data to discriminate SVT from VT. For example, the algorithm in devices of one manufacturer has several key elements: (i) the pattern of atrial and ventricular events; (ii) atrial and ventricular rates; (iii) regularity of R–R intervals; (iv) presence or absence of AV dissociation; and (v) atrial and ventricular pattern analysis.

12 5. **Tiered therapy.** Treatment options for VT include antitachycardia pacing, cardioversion, or defibrillation. Up to 90% of monomorphic VTs can be terminated by a critical pacing sequence, reducing the need for painful shocks and conserving battery life. With antitachycardia pacing, trains of stimuli are delivered at a fixed percentage of the VT cycle length. Repeated and more aggressive trains result either in termination of VT or progression to cardioversion or defibrillation.

6. **ICD malfunction.** Malfunctions specific to ICD include inappropriate shock delivery, failure to deliver therapy, ineffective shocks, and interactions with drugs or devices affecting the efficacy of therapy. There is potential for pacing malfunction as well since all ICDs have a pacemaker function.

   a. **Inappropriate delivery of shocks.** Artifacts created by lead-related malfunction may be interpreted as tachycardia, with inappropriate shock delivery. Electrocautery artifact may be similarly misinterpreted. Rapid SVT or nonsustained VT may be misdiagnosed as sustained VT or VF, especially if rate-only criteria are used for diagnosis. R- and T-wave oversensing, causing double counting during bradycardia pacing, has led to inappropriate shocks.
   b. **Failure to deliver therapy or ineffective shocks.** Especially after repeated shocks for VF, tachyarrhythmias may be undersensed with failure to deliver therapy. Exposure to diagnostic X-rays or computed tomographic scans does not adversely affect shock delivery. Acute MI, severe acute acid–base or electrolyte imbalance, or hypoxia may
13 increase defibrillation thresholds, leading to ineffective shocks. Any of these also could affect the rate or morphology of VT and the ability to diagnose VT. Finally, isoflurane and propofol do not affect defibrillation thresholds. The effect of other anesthetics or drugs used to supplement anesthesia is unknown.

c. **Drug–device interactions affecting efficacy of ICD therapy.** Antiarrhythmic drugs are used along with ICD to suppress (i) recurring sustained VT and the need for shocks; (ii) nonsustained VT that triggers unnecessary shocks; and (iii) atrial fibrillation with inappropriate shocks. Also, they may be used to slow VT to make it better tolerated or more amenable to termination by antitachycardia pacing and to slow AV nodal conduction with atrial fibrillation.

Possible adverse effects of combined drug and ICD therapy are (i) slowing of VT to below the programmed rate-detection threshold; (ii) proarrhythmia, increasing the need for shocks; (iii) increased defibrillation thresholds; (iv) reduced hemodynamic tolerance of VT; (v) increase in PR, QRS, or QT intervals, causing multiple counting and spurious shocks; and (vi) altered morphology or reduced amplitude of intracardiac electrograms and failure to detect VT/VF. Lidocaine, chronic amiodarone, Class IC drugs (e.g., flecainide), and phenytoin can increase defibrillation thresholds. Class IA drugs (e.g., quinidine) generally do not affect defibrillation thresholds.

d. **Device–device interactions affecting efficacy of therapy.** In the past, pacemakers were used for bradycardia and antitachycardia pacing in ICD patients. Today, ICD incorporates both pacing capabilities, but still there may be occasional patients with an ICD and a pacemaker. More common today may be the consideration of brain or nerve stimulators in a patient with an ICD or pacemaker. Regardless of the type of pulse stimulators, possible adverse interactions between two devices include (i) sensed pacing artifacts or depolarizations that may lead to multiple counting, misdiagnosis as VT/VF, and spurious shocks; and (ii) ICD shocks that may reprogram a pacemaker or cause failure to capture or sense. The use of only bipolar pacing from the other device will minimize such interference, but must be fully evaluated prior to permanent implantation.

7. **Response of an ICD to magnet application [8].** Magnet application does not interfere with bradycardia pacing and does not trigger asynchronous pacing in an ICD. Magnet application in contemporary ICDs causes inhibition of tachycardia sensing and delivery of shock only. All current ICDs remain inhibited as long as the magnet remains in stable contact with the ICD. Once the magnet is removed, the ICD reverts to the programmed tachyarrhythmia settings. One deviation from this is in some Biotronik ICD platforms where a magnet placed in direct contact with the ICD will inhibit continuously up to 8 hrs. After 8 hrs, the programmed tachycardia therapy will be reactivated even with the magnet is still in contact. This universal response to magnet across all manufacturers has not always been the case and has caused confusion on how to deal with ICDs in the operative setting. Older platforms manufactured by Boston Scientific/Guidant Corp. had a programmable response to magnet application, most commonly programmed to Magnet Use Enable, but there were exceptions. Most of these device platforms are no longer in service.

   With an appropriately placed magnet, Boston Scientific (Guidant) ICDs have R-synchronous beeping followed by a continuous sound that indicates inactivation of tachyarrhythmia function. Medtronic devices emit a continuous sound for 20 to 30 s to indicate inactivation of tachyarrhythmia sensing. ICDs by St. Jude Medical, Biotronik, and ELA/Sorin do not emit sounds in the presence of a magnet. These different audible responses to magnets may continue to be a source of confusion. Regardless of the audible response, all ICDs turn off tachycardiac sensing and therapy when a magnet remains applied to the generator.

8. **Interference and ICD.** Reports of inappropriate ICD shocks due to EMI oversensing are infrequent. EMI initially might be misinterpreted as VF, but spurious shocks will not occur unless it continues beyond the capacitor charging period (see Section III.A.4 and Table 17.7). Magnet application does not interfere with bradycardia pacing and does not trigger asynchronous pacing in an ICD.

IV. Perioperative considerations for the patient with a CIED [8]

A. **Preoperative patient evaluation.** Patients with pacemakers or ICDs, especially the latter, often have serious cardiac functional impairment. Many have debilitating coexisting systemic disease as well. Special attention is paid to progression of disease and functional status, current

medications, and compliance with treatment. No special testing is required just because the patient has an implanted device. However, baseline information about the surgery is needed
15 by the CIED team (cardiologist, electrophysiologist, and pacemaker clinic staff managing the device) such as (i) type and location of the procedure, (ii) body position at surgery, (iii) electrosurgery needed and site of use, (iv) potential need for DC cardioversion or defibrillation, and (v) other EMI sources.

B. **CIED team evaluation.** Most surgical facilities today have an onsite CIED clinic or service (or access to one) that should be consulted to provide preoperative consultation on the management of the device. If not, the next best strategy is to identify the device and contact the manufacturer for advice. All patients should carry a card that identifies the model and serial numbers of the device, the date of implantation, and the implanting physician or clinic. Unless the planned surgery is truly emergent or poses little risk of EMI-related device malfunction (e.g., bipolar cautery will be used; the surgical field is far removed from the device, leads and grounding plate), it is imperative to (i) identify the device (manufacturer, model, leads, battery status), (ii) determine the date and indication(s) for its implantation, and (iii) to check its function. If a recent device check (for pacemakers <12 mos and for ICDs <6 mos) is not available, then the CIED team should perform a check. The data to be provided by this interrogation are (i) type of device (single, dual, biventricular), (ii) programmed mode, (iii) programmed rates, energy, sensing, tachyarrhythmia settings for an ICD, (iv) pacemaker-dependent status, (v) underlying rhythm, (vi) specifics about magnet response, and (vii) pacing safety margin and battery longevity. If the CIED has no recent device check data and it cannot be interrogated, then obtain (i) a 12-lead ECG (for pacemakers, with and without a magnet) and (ii) an X-ray film of the pulse generator area which **may** reveal a unique radiopaque code ("signature") that identifies the manufacturer and model of the device (Table 17.8). If the surgery is truly **emergent** and it is not possible to identify the device, the basic function of most suppressed pacemakers is confirmed by placing a magnet over the pulse generator to establish the asynchronous pacing rate, provided the magnet function has not been programmed off. Cholinergic stimulation (e.g., Valsalva maneuver, carotid sinus massage, adenosine, or edrophonium) might be useful to slow the intrinsic rate sufficiently to show the presence of pacing stimuli.

C. **Device management.** A qualified physician with device expertise must supervise the recommended preoperative prescription for device management. The prescription should not be provided by industry-employed representatives.

For pacemaker-dependent patients: These patients are at particular risk of asystole in the
16 presence of EMI. If EMI is likely (e.g., unipolar cautery in the vicinity of the pulse generator or leads and surgery above the umbilicus), then the device should be programmed to an asynchronous mode. In the case of pacemakers, this can be done with magnet application in most situations, which will also inactivate the rate-responsive pacing, but confirmation of the

TABLE 17.8 North American manufacturers of pacemakers and implantable cardioverter–defibrillators

Biotronik, Inc. 6024 Jean Road Lake Oswego, OR 97035–5369 1-800-547-9001 (24-hr hotline) 1-503-635-9936 (fax) *www.biotronik.com*	Medtronic Corporation 7000 Central Avenue NE Minneapolis, MN 55432 1-800-328-2518 (24-hr hotline) 1-800-824-2362 (fax) *www.medtronic.com*
Boston Scientific CRM (Guidant, CPI, Intermedics)[a] 4100 Hamline Avenue North St. Paul, MN 55112–5798 (CPI, Intermedics) 1-800-227-3422 (24-hr hotline) 1-800-582-4166 (fax) *www.bostonscientific.com*	St. Jude Medical[a] Cardiac Rhythm Management Division (Pacesetter, Ventritex)[a] 15900 Valley View Court Sylmar, CA 91342 1-800-777-2237 (24-hr hotline) 1-800-756-7223 (fax) *www.sjm.com*

[a]Recently acquired or merged companies by parent company.

magnet response is recommended prior to the surgical procedure if possible. In cases where the pacemaker-dependent patient has an ICD or the location of surgery precludes placement of a magnet, consideration of programming the device to asynchronous mode with the propri-
17 etary programmer is recommended. The other alternative if reprogramming is not an option is to limit the EMI to short bursts while watching the response of pacing and minimize episodes of asystole. For patients with adaptive-rate pacemakers (including some ICDs), this capability should be programmed off if EMI causes inappropriate rate response. As stated above, for pacemakers, magnet application will inactivate this feature, but ICDs will need to be reprogrammed (Table 17.7). In ICDs, tachycardia sensing and therapy should be turned off. This can be accomplished with magnet application or with reprogramming. If any reprogramming is planned, then patients must stay on monitored telemetry until the CIED is reprogrammed back to baseline settings.

In an emergency, if the patient is 100% pacing on the 12-lead ECG and on telemetry, then the assumption is that the patient is pacemaker dependent. In this situation, there needs to be continuous hemodynamic monitoring that will not be distorted with EMI such as a pulse wave form from an arterial line or plethysmography. A form of backup pacing should also be considered such as anterior–posterior transcutaneous pacing pads.

If intrinsic conduction (i.e., no pacing) is seen on the 12-lead ECG, then proceed with surgery and have a magnet available.

Magnet versus reprogramming: If the CIED is reprogrammed then continuous monitoring is mandated. In the operating room, it is difficult to reverse reprogramming. If spontaneous heart rates exceed the asynchronous programmed pacing rate then both deleterious hemodynamic and arrhythmia events may develop. Likewise, post procedure, the ICD antitachyarrhythmia therapies must be reactivated. This does not always occur and is a possible source of medical error. Use of a magnet eliminates the complexity of reprogramming the CIED in the
18 operating room. The magnet can be easily removed when competing rhythms develop with asynchronous pacing. However, the magnet behavior of the specific CIED needs to be known preoperatively.

D. Precautions: Surgery unrelated to device. The chief concern is to reduce risk of hemodynamic instability due to inappropriate inhibition or triggering of output (pacing stimuli or shocks), or upper-rate pacing behavior (adaptive-rate devices). If EMI is likely to cause device malfunction and the patient does not have an adequate intrinsic rhythm, a pacemaker should be programmed to an asynchronous mode and tachycardia sensing disabled for ICD. If the device features ARP, this should be programmed off. If ICD sensing is disabled, continuous cardiac monitoring must be maintained and an external cardioverter–defibrillator must be available.

1. **Surgical sources for EMI.** Technology has provided a variety of new surgical tools to assist in a variety of procedures. Many of these new technologies create EMI. It is this EMI that can cause erratic behavior in pacemakers and ICDs. Any tool that uses electricity or uses a magnet field can emit interfering signals when close to the device or heart. Locating the grounding plate as far as possible from the cautery tool reduces EMI from unipolar cautery. The pulse generator and leads should not be between the Bovie tool and grounding plate (i.e., in the current pathway). Pacing function is confirmed by monitoring heart sounds or the pulse waveform. Only the lowest possible energies and brief bursts of electrocautery or other sources of EMI such as RF should be used, especially with instability due to device malfunction. If cautery must be used in the vicinity (less than 15 cm) of the pulse generator or leads and there is significant hemodynamic instability due to EMI, then it is reasonable to place a magnet directly over the pulse generator of a pacemaker. This will cause most devices to pace asynchronously until the magnet is removed, unless the magnet mode has
19 been programmed off. In a situation with an ICD and no device information, a magnet should **not** be placed over the ICD pulse generator unless EMI is unavoidable. If EMI is unavoidable, then the patient needs to be placed on cardiac monitor and a magnet will need to be placed on (and kept on) the ICD generator during cautery or RF therapy. In this case, EMI has a potential to trigger antitachycardia pacing or shocks that may destabilize the patient. By placing the magnet over the generator, the device will no longer sense or

treat tachyarrhythmias. It will not react to EMI or to a real tachyarrhythmia. However, as discussed above, the magnet will not affect the pacing programming including rate response of the ICD.

2. **External cardioversion or defibrillation.** Shocks probably will not cause temporary inhibition or transient loss of capture. Today's devices are better shielded and nearly all have a backup bradycardia pacing capability and a reset mode. Pulse generator damage is related to the distance of the external paddles from the pulse generator. All device manufacturers recommend the AP paddle configuration, with the paddles located at least 10 cm from the pulse generator. Further, it is advised that the lowest possible energies be used for cardioversion or defibrillation. After cardioversion or defibrillation, the device must be interrogated to assure proper function.

E. **Management for system implantation or revision.** Except in infants and small children, in whom epicardial leads are widely used, most CIED systems use transvenous leads. The pulse generator and leads are often implanted using local anesthesia and sedation. For epicardial lead placement with a thoracotomy, general anesthesia is needed. General anesthesia or monitored anesthesia care with heavy sedation may be requested for some pacer and ICD system implants especially if the patient has significant advanced comorbidities.

1. Lead extraction [9]—General anesthesia is often recommended for cases involving lead extractions especially in leads that are more than 10 yrs old. Cases involving lead extraction are often more prolonged procedures and carry additional procedural risk, the most concerning being catastrophic bleeding. Indications for lead extraction have expanded with recent updates in the HRS Guidelines. Class I indications for lead extraction mainly involve infected pacemaker and ICD systems and symptomatic occlusion of central veins. Other important indications involve removing nonfunctional leads to avoid future complications of superior vena cava syndrome, especially in young patients. In the case of device infection, these patients may have sepsis and are certainly at risk of becoming septic during the lead extraction. The potential bleeding sites include tearing of the superior vena cava and intracardiac perforation or avulsion. This type of procedure also involves the use of large-bore central venous sheaths up to 18F in size that may be used from both the subclavian and femoral venous sites. The prolonged procedure time involving large sheaths also places the patients at risk for pulmonary embolism or stroke caused by either air or clot. Fortunately, enhanced tools have been devised that improve patient safety and ease of extraction, including Eximer laser tools and cutting sheaths. Even with these enhanced tools, the risk of life-threatening bleeding is real and requires immediate recognition and action. Cardiothoracic surgeons and facilities need to be available within minutes if there are complications. In these situations there is an emergent need for thoracotomy and surgical repair. Tools for pericardiocentesis and chest tube insertion must be in arms reach. In addition, these cases may be further complicated by the patient being pacemaker dependent. This situation will require the use of temporary pacing that may become dislodged during the intracardiac manipulation of the leads. Because of the potential complications that can occur in lead extraction it is imperative to have continuous hemodynamic monitoring. A sudden drop in blood pressure may be the only warning signs to alert clinicians of pending circulatory collapse due to a complication from lead extraction.

2. For all procedures requiring general anesthesia or monitored anesthesia care, consider the following:
   a. Most patients with symptomatic bradycardia will have temporary pacing. Otherwise, chronotropic drugs with backup external pacing should be available. Sedation may make an escape rhythm due to conduction disease worse.
   b. Have reliable plethysmography waveform or direct arterial blood pressure monitoring.
   c. Select the best surface ECG leads for P waves (II, V1) and for ischemia diagnosis (V5).
   d. Pulmonary artery catheters are seldom used or needed today. They may interfere with ICD lead positioning.
   e. An external cardioverter–defibrillator must be available and functioning. Defibrillator patches should be applied to the patient in the anterior–posterior configuration.

f. With an ICD, tachycardia sensing should be disabled by a magnet or with reprogramming when unipolar electrosurgery is used.

g. Contemporary inhalation and IV anesthetics are not known to increase defibrillation thresholds and are selected more with a view to hemodynamic tolerance. Inhalation agents and propofol may affect the morphology of sensed intracardiac electrograms and inducibility of tachyarrhythmias, which is a consideration during EP testing. Contemporary inhalation anesthetics (sevoflurane, desflurane) and small amounts of lidocaine for vascular access are not known to affect defibrillation thresholds.

h. Paralytic agents must be used with caution during lead implant procedures. It is customary to assure that lead placement does not cause diaphragmatic or chest wall stimulation during pacing. This avoidable extracardiac stimulation will be inhibited by paralytic agents. If extracardiac stimulation occurs, the pacemaker lead usually requires repositioning.

V. Catheter or surgical modification of arrhythmia substrates. RF catheter ablation has replaced antiarrhythmic drug therapy for treatment of many types of chronic or recurring cardiac tachyarrhythmias. Tachyarrhythmias amenable to this form of treatment include those shown at EP study to have a focal origin (triggered or automatic) or are sustained by fixed, defined re-entry circuits. Surgical ablation may be performed for these same arrhythmias if catheter ablation has failed or is not feasible. In addition, a catheter or surgical maze procedure may be used to interrupt multiple re-entry circuits associated with atrial fibrillation [10].

A. **RF catheter ablation** [11]. RF catheter ablation procedures are performed in an EP laboratory using conscious sedation (generally with midazolam, fentanyl, and/or propofol). Usually, both tachyarrhythmia diagnosis and RF ablation can be performed in a single session. Three to five electrode catheters are inserted percutaneously into the femoral, internal jugular, or subclavian vein, or via a retrograde aortic or transseptal approach, and positioned within the heart to allow pacing and recording at key sites. The efficacy of RF catheter ablation depends on accurate identification of the site of origin of the arrhythmia. Once this site has been identified and the electrode catheter is positioned in direct contact with the site, RF energy is delivered through the catheter to eliminate the source or circuit of the arrhythmia. Arrhythmias that can be "cured" by RF catheter ablation and the success rates are listed in Table 17.9. RF ablation of the AV node is effective in controlling the ventricular rate in severely symptomatic patients with

TABLE 17.9 Tachyarrhythmias that can be "cured" by catheter RF ablation

- Paroxysmal SVT due to AV nodal re-entry (success rate for fast or slow pathway ablation 82%–96% and 98%–100%, respectively)
- Paroxysmal SVT due to orthodromic AV reciprocation[a] (success rate 85%–100%)
- Paroxysmal SVT arising in the atria and due to re-entry, abnormal automaticity, or triggered activity (success rate ≥92%)
- Paroxysmal SVT due to orthodromic or antidromic[b] AV reciprocation in WPW syndrome (success rate ≥95%)
- Type I atrial flutter[c] (success rate >90%)
- Focal atrial fibrillation with triggered focus in pulmonary veins or right atrium (success rate unknown, author's experience >80%)
- Idiopathic, monomorphic VT arising in the right ventricular outflow tract or verapamil-responsive left VT (success rate >90%)
- Monomorphic VT in patients with coronary artery disease to reduce need for drugs or as adjunct to ICD to reduce shocks (success rate 67%–96%[d])
- Miscellaneous tachyarrhythmias: Nonphysiologic sinus tachycardia (success rate for relief of symptoms 90%); automatic junctional tachycardia (success rate 82%); bundle branch re-entry, wide QRS tachycardia (nearly 100% without associated myocardial VT)

[a]Atrioventricular (AV) node serves as the anterograde limb of the re-entry circuit, and a concealed accessory pathway (i.e., does not manifest as delta wave during normal sinus rhythm) as the retrograde limb.
[b]Manifest accessory pathway serves as the anterograde limb (causing a pre-excited, wide QRS tachycardia), and the AV node serves as the retrograde limb of the re-entry circuit.
[c]Atrial rate <340 bpm.
[d]Particular ventricular tachycardia (VT) targeted for ablation.
ICD, implantable cardioverter–defibrillator; RF, radiofrequency; SVT, supraventricular tachycardia; WPW, Wolff–Parkinson–White.

atrial fibrillation or multifocal atrial tachycardia when drug therapy has failed or is poorly tolerated. After AV nodal ablation all patients require a permanent pacemaker because of AV block. Pulmonary vein isolation with RF energy or cryoablation with transvenous catheters is used generally for younger patients with recurrent paroxysmal and persistent atrial fibrillation [12].

For CIED patients undergoing RF catheter ablation, RF energy may cause electrical reset, reprogramming, over- or undersensing, and inappropriate inhibition. Rarely does RF energy lead to reset or damage at the lead–tissue interface.

B. **Arrhythmia surgery [13].** The potential morbidity of open chest surgery, as well as associated high costs, length of hospitalization, and delayed functional recovery, fostered the development of percutaneous catheter ablation. Nonetheless, direct surgical approaches continue to have an important role for patients with arrhythmogenic conditions refractory to catheter ablation or with associated surgical abnormalities. Surgical procedures have been designed for almost all supraventricular tachyarrhythmias but today have application primarily to the treatment of atrial fibrillation.

1. **Surgical approaches to therapy of atrial fibrillation** [14]. To maintain atrial contraction and AV synchrony, preserve sinus node function, and provide symptomatic relief, Cox et al. devised the surgical **MAZE procedure.** With this procedure, both atrial appendages are excised and a pattern of incisions is made in the right and left atria. The maze procedure (i) eliminates most opportunities for re-entry, (ii) reduces the likelihood of fibrillation in any remaining tissue segment due to myocardial mass reduction, (iii) allows the sinus impulse to be conducted to the AV node in proper sequence via tissue strips joining adjacent segments (i.e., preserves atrial transport function), and (iv) eliminates blood stasis to reduce the risk of thromboembolism. As an isolated procedure for treating atrial fibrillation, the maze procedure has the limitation of requiring cardiopulmonary bypass and cardioplegic circulatory arrest. However, it has been used in conjunction with other cardiac operations, notably mitral valve surgery. The most recent modification of the procedure uses minimally invasive surgery and either RF current or cryoablation, resulting in fewer atriotomies.
2. **Accessory AV pathway.** There are essentially two surgical approaches to division of accessory AV pathways: The endocardial and epicardial approaches. Both require a median sternotomy. With the aid of multiple-electrode recording, EP mapping of the pathways is accomplished off cardiopulmonary bypass. This is particularly attractive when the epicardial approach is to be used for division of the accessory pathway, because this technique is feasible off pump. The **endocardial approach** involves a supra-annular incision within the left atrium for left-sided pathways (requires aortic cross-clamping and cold cardioplegia) and from within the right atrium for pathways crossing the tricuspid annulus (requires only cardiopulmonary bypass). Accessory pathways are divided using sharp dissection. The **epicardial approach** does not require opening the atria. It is carried out on a normothermic beating heart without cardiopulmonary bypass. Lesions are created by cryoablation. No clear-cut superiority has been demonstrated for the endocardial or epicardial approach, at least in terms of clinical results.
3. **Other supraventricular and ventricular arrhythmias.** For other **supraventricular arrhythmias** amenable to cure by focal ablation, surgery is reserved for patients with associated cardiac surgical abnormalities, intractable arrhythmias after failed RF catheter ablation, or arrhythmias not amenable to RF catheter ablation [15]. For patients with **ventricular arrhythmias**, the role of surgery must be reconsidered in view of the dramatic advances in ICD technology. Nonetheless, in selected circumstances, surgical ablation may lead to the best quality of life (e.g., spurious shocks with ICD). Patients with preserved left ventricular function have the lowest surgical risk but also good long-term survival, whatever the therapy. The surgical technique is a compromise between preservation of cardiac function and neutralization of the current or future arrhythmogenic substrates. It is based on two surgical concepts: Exclusion and ablation. **Exclusion** is aimed at isolating the arrhythmogenic mechanism from the rest of heart. **Ablation** is aimed at neutralizing the arrhythmogenic foci. Surgical techniques include ventriculotomy, transmural resection, endocardial resection, cryoablation, and laser photocoagulation. The latter two methods

produce a well-demarcated mass of neutralized tissue that accomplishes the treatment goal without undue myocardial functional impairment. Cryosurgery is enhanced by cold cardioplegia, whereas laser photocoagulation can be accomplished on the normothermic, beating heart. Another surgical issue is the value of intraoperative mapping which can lead to inordinately prolonged pump times.

4. **Perioperative considerations.** Whether arrhythmia surgery is performed on or off pump, the requirement for cardioplegic circulatory arrest is dictated by the surgical procedure. Arrhythmia surgery can be accomplished safely with total IV anesthesia, obviating the need for volatile inhalation anesthetics that might modify arrhythmia substrates or the results of EP testing during the surgical procedure.

REFERENCES

1. Yang P, Kanki H, Drolet B, et al. Allelic variants in long-QT disease genes in patients with drug-associated torsades de pointes. *Circulation.* 2002;105:1943–1948.
2. Schram G, Pourrier M, Melnyk P, et al. Differential distribution of cardiac ion channels as a basis for regional specialization in electrical function. *Circ Res.* 2002;90:939–950.
3. Janse MJ, Wit AL. Electrophysiological mechanisms of ventricular arrhythmias resulting from myocardial ischemia and infarction. *Physiol Rev.* 1989;69:1049–1169.
4. Moya A, Sutton R, Ammirati F, et al. Guidelines for the diagnosis and management of syncope (version 2009). *Eur Heart J.* 2009;30(21):2631–2671.
5. Echt DS, Liebson PR, Mitchell LB, et al. Mortality and morbidity in patients receiving encainide, flecainide, or placebo. The Cardiac Arrhythmia Suppression Trial. *N Engl J Med.* 1991;324:781–788.
6. Field JM, Hazinski MF, Sayre MR, et al. Part 1: Executive summary: 2010 American Heart Association Guidelines for Cardiopulmonary Resuscitation and Emergency Cardiovascular Care. *Circulation.* 2010;112:s640.
7. Epstein AE, DiMarco JP, Ellenbogen KA, et al. ACC/AHA/HRS 2008 Guidelines for device-based therapy of cardiac rhythm abnormalities. *Heart Rhythm.* 2008;5:e1–e62.
8. Crossley GH, Poole JE, Rozner MA, et al. HRS/Expert consensus statement on the perioperative management of patients with implantable defibrillators, pacemakers and arrhythmia monitors: Facilities and patient management. *Heart Rhythm.* 2011;8:1114–1152.
9. Wilkoff BL, Love CJ, Byrd CL, et al. Transvenous lead extraction: Heart Rhythm Society expert consensus on facilities, training, indications and patient management. *Heart Rhythm.* 2009;6:1086–1104.
10. Pappone C, Oreto G, Lamberti F, et al. Catheter ablation of paroxysmal atrial fibrillation using a 3D mapping system. *Circulation.* 1999;100:1203–1208.
11. Morady F. Radio-frequency ablation as treatment for cardiac arrhythmia. *N Engl J Med.* 1999;340:534–544.
12. Falk RH. Atrial fibrillation. *N Engl J Med.* 2001;344:1067–1078.
13. Page PL. Surgery for atrial fibrillation and other supraventricular tachyarrhythmias. In: Zipes DP, Jalife J, eds. *Cardiac Electrophysiology.* 2nd ed. Philadelphia, PA: WB Saunders; 2000:1065–1077.
14. Cox JL, Schussler RB, D'Agostino HJ Jr, et al. The surgical treatment of atrial fibrillation. III. Development of a definitive surgical procedure. *J Thorac Cardiovasc Surg.* 1991;101:569–583.
15. Guiraudon GM, Klein GJ, Guiraudon CM, et al. Surgical treatment of ventricular tachycardias. In: Zipes DP, Jalife J, eds. *Cardiac Electrophysiology.* 2nd ed. Philadelphia, PA: WB Saunders; 2000:1078–1086.

18 Blood Transfusion

Colleen G. Koch

KEY POINTS

1. Both anemia and transfusion carry significant risks. Balancing these risks is the key to appropriate blood transfusion decisions.
2. Despite published guidelines about transfusion, clinical transfusion practice still varies substantially among clinicians and centers and often falls outside recommended guidelines.
3. In addition to well-established acute immunologic and infection transmission complications, RBC transfusion in cardiac surgical patients has more recently been associated with increased mortality and infectious complications.
4. Transfusion-related acute lung injury (TRALI) is the most frequent cause of mortality complicating blood transfusion. Among blood components, fresh frozen plasma (FFP) may carry the highest risk for TRALI.
5. RBC storage duration has been associated with increased morbidity and mortality in cardiac surgery.
6. One retrospective study associated platelet transfusion with increased morbidity and mortality in cardiac surgery, but several other studies did not.
7. FFP transfusion alone has been associated with increased risk for perioperative mortality, infection, multiorgan failure, and acute respiratory distress syndrome.

"**BLOOD TRANSFUSION IS LIKE MARRIAGE:** ***it should not be entered upon lightly, unadvisedly or wantonly or more often than is absolutely necessary.***"

—*R. Beale R* [1]

I. Background

Competing risks form the core of perioperative transfusion. We are faced with tangible risks of patient complications from low hemoglobin values, yet we face different but equally real risks when we expose patients to red blood cell (RBC) transfusion. **The risks of both anemia and transfusion vary with patient comorbidities, degree of and ability to tolerate anemia, and surgical procedure.** In the dynamic milieu of the operating rooms, clinicians caring for cardiovascular surgical patients face challenging transfusion decisions daily. There are no measures that can definitively direct RBC transfusion decisions, rather clinical judgment using the balance of perceived risk versus benefit guides individual transfusion decisions. Given this background, the substantial variability of RBC transfusion even within a single institution becomes understandable [2,3].

1

2 A. **Variability in practice patterns** often serves as the impetus for evidence-based guidelines that are intended to reconcile disparate evidence. **Recent work highlights the low level of practitioner adoption of published transfusion practice guidelines.** Although a number of factors contributed to low physician adoption, the authors principally attributed it to the low level of evidence provided to support guideline recommendations [4]. Others have also reported limited evidence basis for use of RBC transfusion [5].

B. **The reports on complications of RBC transfusion** have increased scrutiny of transfusion practices in the last decade; however, economics and anticipated changes in population demographics have also driven change. A population-based cross-sectional study projected a growing gap between future demand and donation of blood with substantial increases in blood demand related to the changes in population demographics [6]. A recent editorial noted that 55% to 60% of the blood products transfused in the United States are given to the patients over 65 yrs old, and projected that this population will increase by 36% in the next 10 yrs, whereas the principal blood donor population will only increase by 5% over the same period. These demographic changes will influence medical practices and surgical procedures while increasing demand for blood products [7].

II. Red Blood Cell Transfusion and Adverse Outcomes

RBC units contain red cells separated from whole blood by centrifugation or by apheresis [8] (Table 18.1). **Isbister and colleagues reported on the abundance of data supporting morbidity risk associated with transfusion, yet noted transfusion remains "ingrained" in current medical practice almost as a "default" position** [9]. Furthermore, establishing causation between RBC transfusion and morbidity is difficult because of the potential for confounding in cohort study designs. Some argue that the etiology of poor outcomes relates to the "sicker" patient who receives a transfusion rather than the RBC product itself. Although it is difficult to discern whether morbidity is patient or transfusion related, either way RBC transfusion remains a significant risk factor for poor outcome [9].

A. Morbidity and Mortality Risk

3 1. **RBC transfusion has been associated with a number of immunologic complications such as hemolytic, anaphylactoid and febrile transfusion reactions, graft-versus-host disease, and transfusion of viral and bacterial contaminants** [8]. RBC transfusion has been associated with an increased risk for a number of complications following surgery. In an isolated coronary artery bypass grafting (CABG) population of over 11,000 patients, RBC transfusion was associated with a dose-dependent increased risk for morbidity: More postoperative cardiac complications, prolonged postoperative ventilator support, more infectious complications, renal failure, and higher in-hospital mortality (Fig 18.1). Following risk adjustment for known confounders, RBC transfusion remained a significant risk factor for

TABLE 18.1 Fast facts: red blood cells from American Red Cross compendium[8]

Fast facts: RBC units	
Concentrated from whole blood	By centrifugation or collected by apheresis
Hematocrit	55%–65% or 65%–80%
Plasma content	20–100 mL plasma
Typical volume	300–400 mL
Volume of hemoglobin	42.5–80 g
Iron content	**Approximately 250 mg**
1 unit RBC transfusion	Increases hematocrit by 3%
Perioperative/Peri-procedural/Critically ill indications for RBC transfusion	**When hemoglobin less than 6 g/dL in young healthy patient; in critically ill patients, when hemoglobin is less than 7 g/dL**
Indication intermediate 6–10 g/dL	Based on patient comorbidity, ongoing bleeding, or organ ischemia

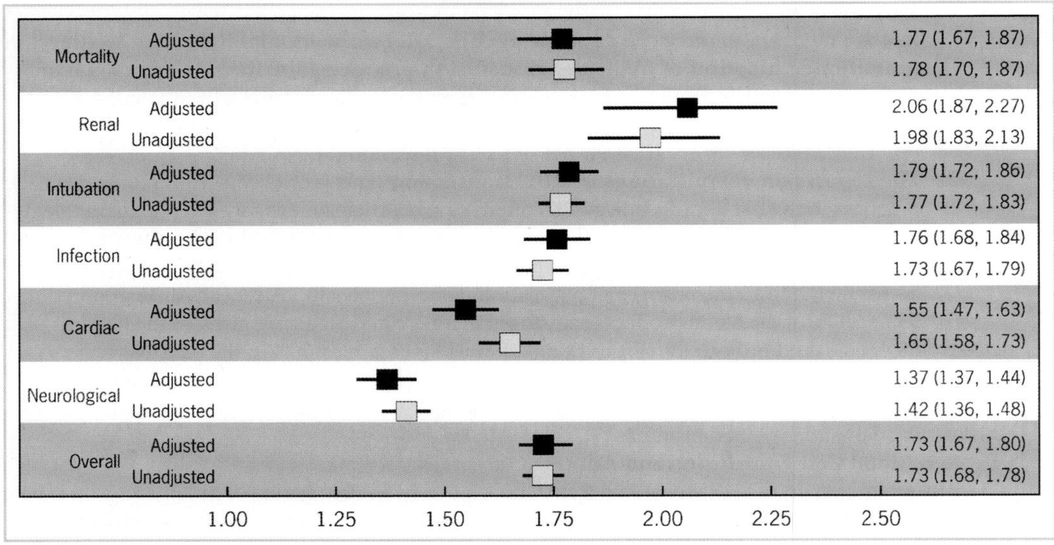

FIGURE 18.1 Forest plot displays the unadjusted and adjusted odds ratios and their 95% confidence limits for seven postoperative morbid outcomes when comparing patients undergoing cardiac surgery who did and did not receive an RBC transfusion. (Reproduced with permission from Koch CG, Li L, Duncan AI, et al. Morbidity and mortality risk associated with red blood cell and blood-component transfusion in isolated coronary artery bypass grafting. *Crit Care Med.* 2006;34:1608–1616.)

poor clinical outcomes. **The effect of transfusion on morbidity was dose-dependent,** that is, more RBC units transfused incrementally increased risk (Fig. 18.2). A number of factors were related to patients' need for transfusion: Demographics such as older age, history of peripheral vascular disease and chronic obstructive pulmonary disease, clinical presentation such as emergency surgery, and surgical factors such as reoperation and prolonged aortic clamp time [10].

2. Kudivalli and colleagues examined the effect of RBC transfusion on 30-day and 1-yr mortality in cardiac surgical patients. Risk-adjusted mortality at 30 days and 1 yr was significantly higher for patients who were transfused. Risk factors for RBC transfusion were lower hemoglobin, lower body mass index, female gender, renal dysfunction, reoperation and use of cardiopulmonary bypass [11]. **An investigation of long-term survival in over 10,000 isolated CABG patients reported a risk-adjusted reduction in survival both early and late to 10 yrs for patients who received perioperative RBCs. This relationship was dose dependent and was sustained after adjustment for confounding variables known to increase mortality risk following isolated CABG** [12].
3. A recent investigation examined over 9,000 patients who underwent cardiac surgical procedures and who were and were not exposed to 1 to 2 unit RBC transfusion. Patients who received RBCs had a 16% increased hazard for reduced survival 6 mos following the cardiac surgery. The authors emphasized the decision to transfuse even these small volumes of RBCs placed patients at significant risk for mortality [13]. Others have also reported reduced survival in cardiac surgical patients receiving RBC transfusions [14].
4. Murphy and colleagues examined outcomes after RBC transfusion in over 8,500 cardiac surgical patients. There was a strong association between transfusion and postoperative infectious complications, early and late mortality, length of stay, and overall hospital costs. The authors reported a significant risk for composite ischemic outcome noting this was somewhat counterintuitive as transfusion is intended to restore tissue oxygenation [15].
5. Banbury and colleagues identified risk factors for the occurrence of postoperative infectious complications following cardiac surgery in a population of over 15,000 patients in which

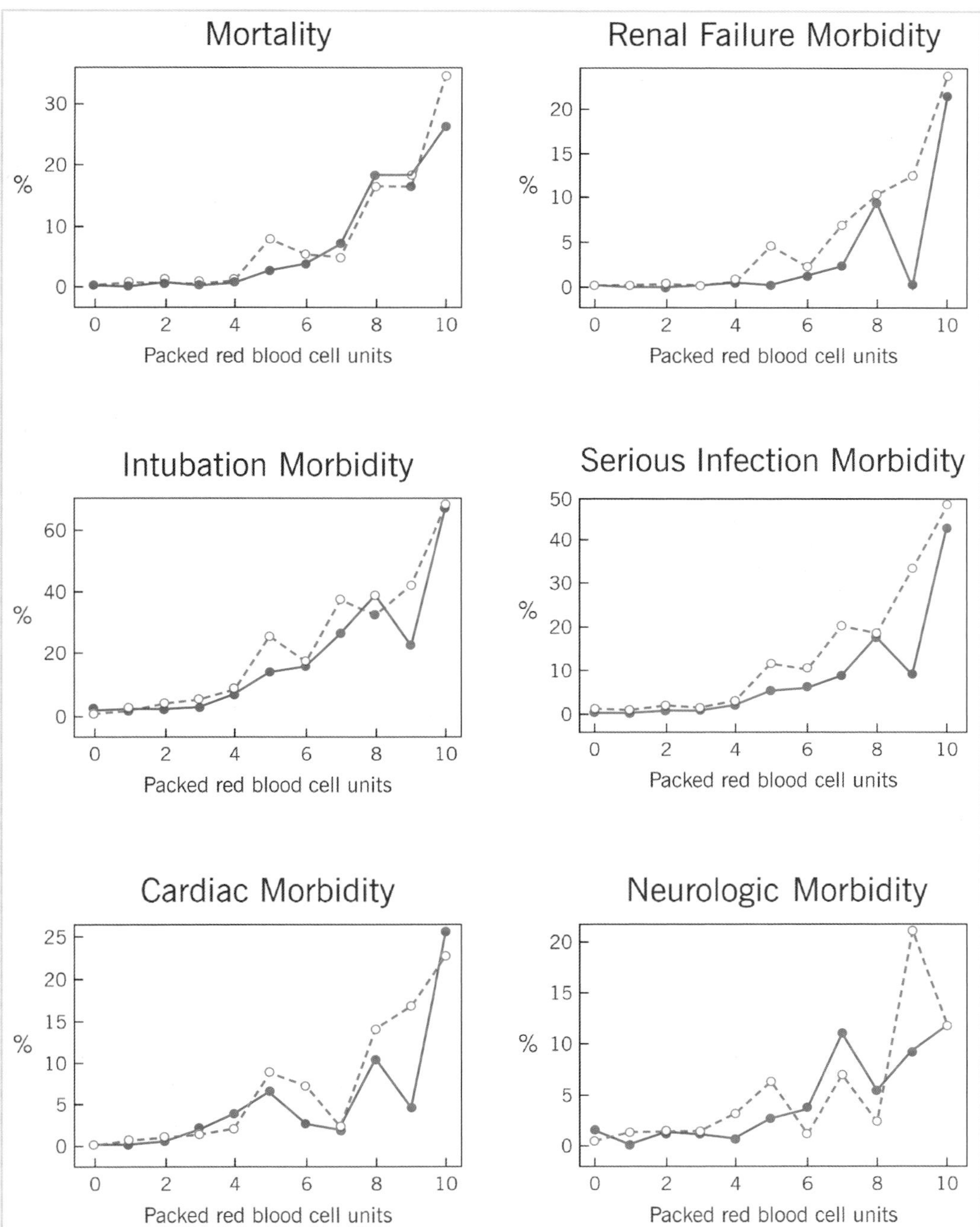

FIGURE 18.2 Panel of six morbidity outcomes displays the dose–response relationship between increasing number of RBC units transfused and risk for postoperative morbidity outcomes. The dashed lines represent the patient who received only RBC transfusion; the solid lines represent those patients who received platelet transfusion as well. (Koch CG, Li L, Duncan AI, et al. Morbidity and mortality risk associated with red blood cell and blood-component transfusion in isolated coronary artery bypass grafting. *Crit Care Med.* 2006;34:1608–1616.)

over 50% of patients were transfused. There was a dose-dependent effect of increasing RBC transfusion and increased prevalence of postoperative septicemia/bacteremia and superficial and deep sternal wound infections. These authors appropriately noted that transfusion occurred in patients who were the sickest; yet, even following risk adjustment, transfusion contributed to postoperative infectious risk [16].

6. Transfusion of RBCs plays a role in augmenting the inflammatory response to cardiac surgery. Development of atrial fibrillation is a common and costly complication following cardiac surgery that links partially an inflammatory mechanism. In a population of 5,841 cardiac surgical patients, transfusion of RBCs increased the prevalence of postoperative atrial fibrillation. The analysis was risk-adjusted for traditional risk factors associated with development of atrial fibrillation such as demographics, history of atrial fibrillation, preoperative medications, and perioperative variables. RBC transfusion increased risk for postoperative atrial fibrillation in both on- and off-cardiopulmonary bypass procedures [17].
7. A recent publication by Tuinman and colleagues related complications of transfusion during cardiac surgery to activation of pulmonary inflammation and coagulation [18].
8. **The Food and Drug Administration's (FDA) summary of fatalities related to transfusion for fiscal year 2009 listed transfusion-related acute lung injury (TRALI) and transfusion-associated circulatory overload (TACO) among the more common**
4 **complications associated with transfusion** (Fig. 18.3). **TRALI has consistently been one of the most common causes of death associated with transfusion** [19]. TRALI, which is primarily a clinical diagnosis, can vary from mild to severe. It is defined by presence of hypoxemia and specific X-ray findings that occur within a certain time following transfusion. The purported mechanism for TRALI involves activation of neutrophils with endothelial injury and resultant pulmonary edema [20–22].

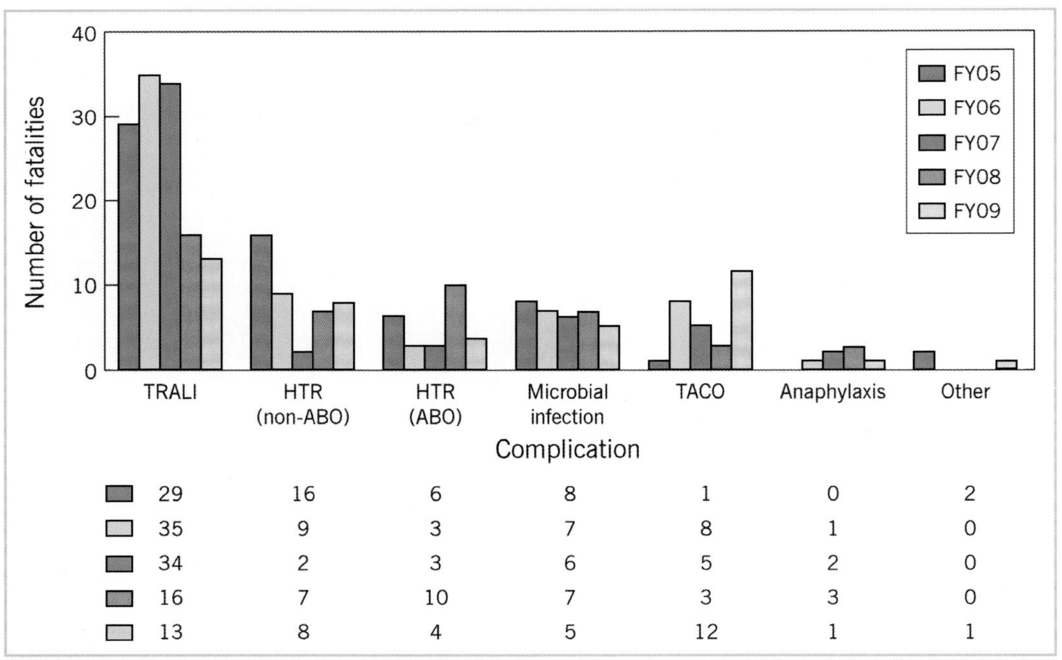

	TRALI	HTR (non-ABO)	HTR (ABO)	Microbial infection	TACO	Anaphylaxis	Other
FY05	29	16	6	8	1	0	2
FY06	35	9	3	7	8	1	0
FY07	34	2	3	6	5	2	0
FY08	16	7	10	7	3	3	0
FY09	13	8	4	5	12	1	1

FIGURE 18.3 A report from the Food and Drug Administration illustrates the transfusion-related fatalities by complication for fiscal years 2005–2009. For each year TRALI represents the most frequently reported cause of transfusion-related mortality [19]. TRALI, transfusion-related acute lung injury; HTR (non-ABO), hemolytic transfusion reactions unrelated to ABO incompatibility; HTR (ABO), hemolytic transfusion reactions related to ABO incompatibility; TACO, transfusion-associated circulatory overload; FY05, Fiscal Year 2005 (similarly for other FYs).

9. A recent investigation noted that TRALI, a diagnosis of exclusion, can be difficult to diagnose in patients undergoing cardiac surgery. The authors reported greater pulmonary morbidity in the postoperative period for patients transfused with RBCs and FFP; this pulmonary morbidity may have been related to TRALI, TACO, or both. Nevertheless, **transfusion of either RBCs or FFP was independently associated with pulmonary morbidity in the postoperative period** [23].
10. Stokes and colleagues recently examined the influence of bleeding-related complications, use of blood products, and costs in a population of inpatient surgical services. They recognized that inadequate surgical hemostasis leads to bleeding complications as well as to transfusion. The authors were able to rank incremental cost per hospitalization associated with bleeding-related complications and adjusted for covariates. Their findings support further need for implementation of blood conservation strategies [24].
11. Bleeding complications and the associated need for reoperation in cardiac surgery are associated with increased morbidity. Recent work attempted to delineate whether increased morbidity risk for reoperation was related to the reoperation, blood transfusion, or both. The patients who underwent reoperation had greater subsequent morbidity, increased resource utilization, and higher in-hospital mortality even after risk adjustment [25] (Fig. 18.4).
12. **A recent investigation in non-cardiac thoracic surgical patients reported worse postoperative outcomes in patients who received 1 to 2 unit RBC transfusions.** The negative effect of transfusion was dose dependent and was associated with increased morbidity and resource utilization. The authors urged clinicians to be cautious in transfusing patients for mild degrees of anemia [26].
13. Grimshaw and colleagues emphasize that the use of RBCs has not been scrutinized using current methods for assessing efficacy and safety, and that mechanisms for the observed complications are not well understood. They suggest that RBC transfusion-associated inflammation and thrombosis may be related to RBC storage [27].

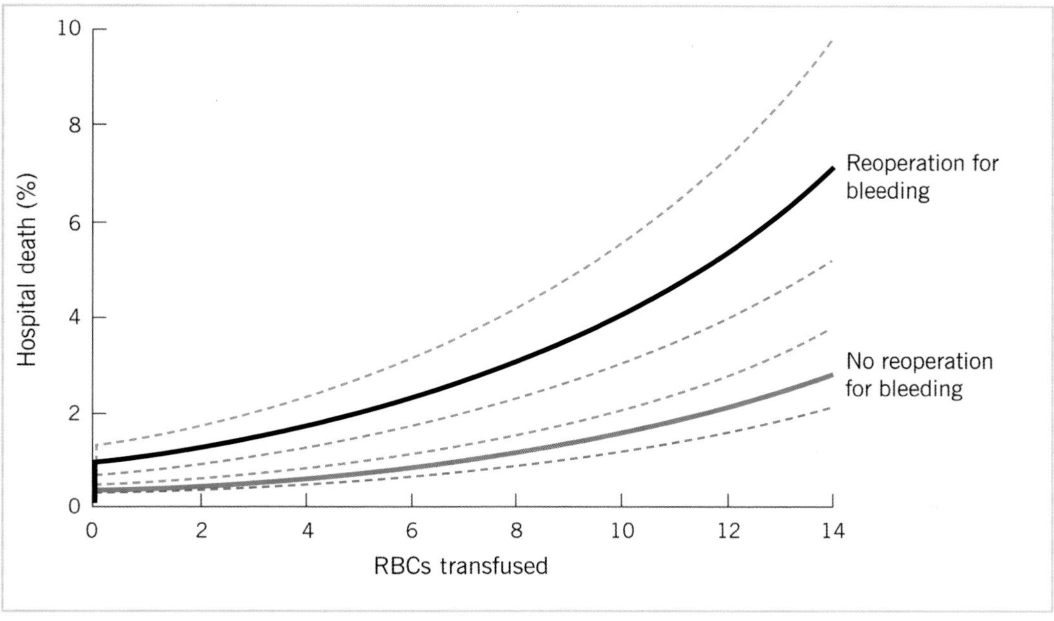

FIGURE 18.4 Predicted probability of operative mortality stratified on reoperation for bleeding and RBC transfusion. RBC transfusion and reoperation for bleeding were associated with increased mortality. (Reproduced with permission from Vivacqua A, Koch CG, Yousuf AM, et al. Morbidity of bleeding after cardiac surgery: Is it blood transfusion, reoperation for bleeding, or both? *Ann Thorac Surg.* 2011;91:1780–1790.)

B. Red Blood Cell Storage Duration

Changes in RBC product with increasing storage are well described and include alterations in RBC structural shape and in biochemical properties. Implications of these time-dependent changes may contribute to adverse clinical outcomes associated with RBC transfusion. However, clinical and experimental animal studies have reported inconsistent findings [28–30].

1. A group of investigators examined age of RBC products at the time of transfusion to gain an understanding of the age of RBC products used. Approximately one-third of RBC units transfused were stored longer than 3 wks storage duration, and for blood groups AB negative and A negative, more than 60% of total number of units transfused were older than 3 wks storage duration [31].
2. Survival of red cells following transfusion is an important variable as it relates to the ability of red cells to perform their intended use. The FDA currently allows donor RBCs stored in ADSOL to have a shelf life of 42 days. The set time limit relates to a requirement for 75% of RBCs to remain in circulation 24 hrs after transfusion, without regard to their functional state. With fresh blood, RBC survival is approximately 90% 24 hrs post-transfusion. As storage duration increases, 24-hr survival (i.e., circulatory retention) rate decreases; however, it must be at least 75% during the approved life of the product [32,33].
3. **Laboratory Investigation**
   a. **As storage time increases, RBCs degrade in structural shape, aggregability, and metabolic function. The entire host of changes is referred to as the "storage lesion,"** which contributes to limited post-transfusion RBC survival and potentially to impaired oxygen delivery via the microcirculation. The storage lesion may contribute to the morbidity associated with RBC transfusion [34,35].
   b. A number of biochemical changes that occur over time in stored RBCs product have been well described. S-nitrosothiol (SNOs) levels change 2 to 3 hrs after collection; changes occurring after several days of storage progressive increases in lactate, potassium, and free hemoglobin and a decrease in pH [35]. Storage-induced reduction in RBC membrane structural integrity (reduced deformability and increased fragility) is thought to be related to intra-RBC energy source depletion. Release of cell-free hemoglobin and microparticles (MPs) can lead to increased consumption of nitric oxide (NO) [36]. Some investigators have proposed insufficient NO bioavailability as an explanation for the increased morbidity and mortality observed after transfusion [37,38].
   c. **Relevy and colleagues showed that routine cold storage damaged RBC membranes to increase stiffness, thereby potentially impairing flow properties.** A continuous reduction in deformability was noted, ultimately producing rigid cells at the end of the storage period. The percentage of undeformable cells increased continuously starting as early as 2 wks after RBC collection. Increased RBC adherence was also noted. These findings suggest that transfusion of rheologically impaired RBCs might introduce morbidity risk, perhaps particularly to patients with cardiovascular disease [39].
   d. In an animal model, Rigamonti and colleagues suggested that stored blood has a reduced capacity to deliver oxygen to brain tissue. They reported that fresh blood better restores cerebral oxygen delivery and tissue oxygen tension than stored blood does [40]. **Recent studies suggest that stored RBCs may contribute to reported morbidity complications via release of RBC-derived MPs, which may facilitate thrombosis and lung injury** [41–43].
4. **Clinical Investigation**

   Clinical studies examining the role of RBC storage duration on patient outcomes report inconsistent findings, yet many have small sample size with heterogeneous patient populations. **A large investigation in cardiac surgery reported an increased risk of
5 postoperative complications and higher mortality in patients who were transfused RBCs with prolonged storage.** In total 2,800 patients received RBCs with 14 days storage

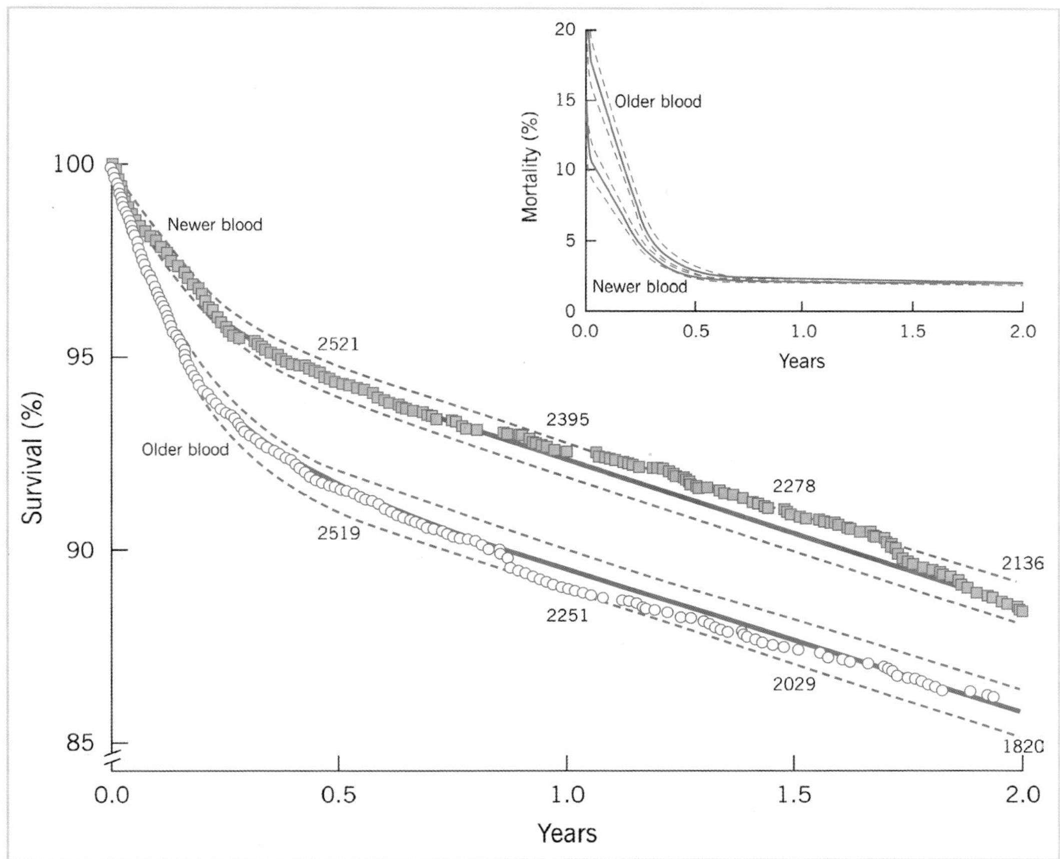

FIGURE 18.5 Kaplan–Meier estimates of survival and death for patients given exclusively newer blood (stored for 14 days or less; *squares*) and patients given exclusively older blood (stored more than 14 days; *circles*). Survival was lower for patients who received older blood as compared to those receiving newer blood, especially during the initial follow-up period. Inset shows the same data presented as mortality at each time interval rather than cumulative survival. (Reproduced with permission from Koch CG, Li L, Sessler DI, et al. Duration of red-cell storage and complications after cardiac surgery. *N Engl J Med.* 2008;358:1229–1239.)

or less and 3,130 patients received RBC units with greater than 14 days storage. Risks for mortality, postoperative ventilatory support beyond 72 hrs, renal failure, sepsis, and composite adverse outcome were all higher in patients receiving older blood. Following risk adjustment, composite adverse outcome and lower survival were still found in patients who received "older" RBCs [30] (Fig. 18.5). A recent investigation in cardiac surgery reported a higher prevalence of new renal complications and length of hospital stay in patients receiving older RBCs [44].

a. **In trauma settings, transfusion of older RBCs is associated with increased incidences of infection** [45], **deep vein thrombosis, death** [46,47], **and multisystem organ failure** [48]. In cohorts of critically ill intensive care unit (ICU) patients, exposure to older RBCs was independently associated with increased mortality, and this response may be proportionate to the number of units transfused [49–52].
b. Of note, there are investigations reporting similar patient outcomes with fresh blood and with blood of increasing storage duration. Findings from Walsh and colleagues did not support the use of fresh RBCs in critically ill ICU patients. They reported transfusion of stored leukodepleted RBCs had no adverse effects on gastric tonometry or

global indexes of tissue oxygenation [53]. In a group of 897 patients, Leal-Noval and colleagues reported that prolonged storage did not increase overall morbidity risk in cardiac surgery, but RBCs stored longer than 28 days might increase the risk for pneumonia [54]. An exceedingly small investigation recently reported that the number of RBC units, but not the storage duration, was associated with poor outcomes. Only 68 patients received RBCs with 14 days storage or less and none had a mortality event or prolonged ventilation beyond 72 hrs [55]. Others have also reported no effect of RBC storage duration on patient morbidity [29,56].

c. Even if one should accept that prolonged RBC storage duration indisputably increases risk, in the absence of a change in the acceptable "shelf life" of collected RBCs there is little that practicing clinicians can do to address this risk.

III. Component Therapy

A. Restrictive RBC transfusion practices have become a standard of care; yet, evidence-based indications for the use of blood component therapy such as FFP and platelet concentrate transfusion have been more limited [57]. Following donation, whole blood is separated into components, which are stored at different temperatures. While RBCs can be stored up to 42 days at 1 to 6°C , platelets are stored at room temperature with a shorter storage duration of 5 days. Plasma and cryoprecipitate can be stored frozen for 1 yr [58].

Use of predetermined ratios of component therapy to RBCs has gained increased attention as a result of recent research in military and civilian trauma resuscitation. These investigations focus on earlier and increased use of component therapy (i.e., ratios of 1:1:1 of RBC to FFP to platelets). This strategy is thought to prevent dilutional and traumatic coagulopathy [59]. Liumbruno and colleagues provided detailed recommendations for transfusion of FFP and platelets in a number of clinical settings [60]. Mitra et al. found an increased initial survival in association with higher FFP/RBC ratios. However, those authors also noted that this association is difficult to interpret because of an inherent survival bias [61].

Sperry and colleagues associated the FFP to RBC ratios ≥1:1.5 with lower mortality after massive transfusion. In a population of patients with serious blunt injury and who required greater than or equal to 8 units of RBCs, survival was better; yet, the risk of acute respiratory distress syndrome was higher [62]. **While there is retrospective evidence to support increased survival with more aggressive use of plasma and platelets in massive transfusion, the efficacy of such practice has not been established with prospective, randomized studies** [63,64].

B **Platelet Therapy (Table 18.2)**

Platelets are stored at 20 to 24°C and have a shelf life limited to 5 days [58]. General recommendations for platelet therapy stress that platelet transfusion cannot be based simply on platelet count. In general, for major surgical procedures or during massive transfusion (e.g., one or more blood volumes has been replaced) a platelet count of at least 50,000/μL is recommended [60]. A standard dose of platelets for adults is approximately one unit per 10 kg body weight. In general, transfusion of six units of platelets harvested from whole blood increases the platelet count by approximately 30,000/μL [65] (Table 18.2). This platelet "dose" corresponds roughly with that provided by a single-donor plateletpheresis.

1. **Specific morbidity associated with platelet transfusion remains unclear.** TRALI
6 [19] has been associated with platelet transfusion more than other morbidities. In a large investigation of over 11,000 patients, Karkouti and colleagues reported no increased risk for adverse outcomes in cardiac surgical patients who received platelet transfusions [66]. Similarly, McGrath and colleagues studied over 30,000 cardiac surgical patients and found no association between platelet transfusion and patient morbidity. Analysis was performed on patients with and without concomitant RBC transfusion and the results were similar. The patients who received platelet transfusions were considered higher risk based on comorbidity, but even after risk adjustment they experienced similar outcomes as the patients who did not receive platelet transfusion. The authors concluded that platelet transfusion in the setting of microvascular bleeding did not increase morbidity [67].

TABLE 18.2 Fast facts: platelets from American Red Cross compendium[8]

Fast facts: platelets	
Derived from whole blood	5.5×10^{10} platelets per bag
Plasma content (whole blood derived)	40–70 mL
Apheresis platelets	3.0×10^{11} platelets per bag
Plasma content (apheresis derived)	100–500 mL
Platelet count increase on average (70 kg) adult per each random donor platelet transfusion	5,000–10,000/μL
In general, appropriate indication for transfusion	Platelet count less than 50,000/μL, active bleeding or procedures/surgery
In cardiac surgery, appropriate indication for transfusion	Plasma coagulation testing not significantly abnormal in setting with count less than 100,000/μL and microvascular bleeding

2. One retrospective investigation of cardiac surgical patients associated higher stroke risk and mortality with platelet transfusion. These data were extracted from a clinical trial on aprotinin [68].
3. **Similar to RBCs, storage leads to changes in platelet structural and biochemical properties over time.** A recent study found no increase in short-term adverse outcomes with increasing platelet storage time [69]. These authors and others reviewed current challenges of maintaining adequate platelet inventory with the limit of 5 days storage and also described the platelet storage lesion and the interesting controversy surrounding the proposed extension of platelet storage to 7 days (e.g., the increased risk for bacterial contamination over time is well described) [69–74].

C. **Fresh Frozen Plasma (Table 18.3)**

FFP is human donor plasma and refers to plasma that is separated and frozen at temperatures of −18°C within 8 hrs of collection; frozen plasma-24 (FP-24) refers to plasma separated and frozen at −18°C within 24 hrs of collection. FFP from a collection of whole blood has a volume of ~300 mL and can be stored up to 1 yr. Both products contain necessary plasma coagulation factors which are maintained after thawing and storage at 1 to 6°C for up to 5 days. In general, the dose of FFP is 10 to 20 mL/kg [58,60,75]. FFP should be ABO-compatible but does not require crossmatching [76].

1. **Excessive blood loss, coagulation factor consumption, and specific deficiencies in coagulation factors are among a number of factors that can lead to inadequate hemostasis and the need for an FFP transfusion, particularly when a concentrate**

TABLE 18.3 Fast facts: fresh plasma from American Red Cross compendium[8]

Fast facts: FFP	
Non-cellular portion of blood	From whole blood or apheresis
Volume of 1 unit (approximate)	250 mL
Frozen at −18°C	Within 6–8 hrs of collection
Contains all coagulation factors	
Thawed and used or stored at 1–6°C for 24 hrs	
Transfusion should be guided by coagulation testing	Prothrombin time >1.5× normal, activated partial thromboplastin time >1.5× normal, or factor assay <25%
Dose	10–20 mL/kg
Selected indications	Massive transfusion with coagulopathic bleeding, active bleeding due to coagulation multiple factor deficiency, severe bleeding due to warfarin therapy

TABLE 18.4 Fast facts: cryoprecipitate, from American Red Cross compendium[8]

Fast facts: Cryoprecipitate	
Unit is prepared from 1 unit of FFP at 1–6°C	Recovering cold insoluble precipitate
Refrozen within 1 hr	
Contains concentrated levels of	Fibrinogen, Factor VIII:C, Factor VIII:vWF, Factor XIII, and fibronectin
Each unit contains	At least 80 IU of Factor VIII:C
Each unit contains	150 mg of fibrinogen
Plasma volume of 1 unit	5–20 mL
Dose and response 1 pool (5 bags)	Fibrinogen increases by approximately 50 mg/dL for average adult
Selected indications	Bleeding associated with fibrinogen deficiencies; massive transfusion when fibrinogen <100 mg/dL

is unavailable [76]. In the setting of massive transfusion, it is well recognized that the use of crystalloids, colloids, and RBCs can lead to a dilutional coagulopathy, and that these conditions can potentially lead to disseminated intravascular coagulation [60,77]. A number of publications address limited adherence to published guidelines for FFP transfusion [78,79]. **In the setting of excessive surgical bleeding, it has been suggested that clinicians guide their FFP use and dosing by point-of-care testing coagulation studies rather than by preset formulas** (see also Chapter X) [79].

2. Interestingly, in patients with minimally prolonged international normalized ratio (INR) (less than 1.6), Holland and Brooks reported that FFP transfusion failed to change the INR; INR decreased only with the treatment of the disease causing the increase in INR [78]. Prophylactic use of FFP is not supported by evidence from good quality randomized controlled trials (RCTs). **The strongest RCT evidence indicates that prophylactic plasma for transfusion is not effective across a range of clinical settings** [80].

7

3. In addition to the risk for TRALI, FFP transfusion carries the risk for other morbidities. Bilgin and colleagues analyzed data from two RCTs about the effects of platelet and FFP transfusion on postoperative infections, length of ICU stay, and all-cause mortality. Perioperative FFP transfusion was associated with all-cause mortality [81]. Similarly, Watson and colleagues reported greater risk for multisystem organ failure and acute respiratory distress syndrome with FFP transfusion in the trauma setting [82]. Others also have associated an increase in adverse patient outcomes with FFP administration [83].

D. Cryoprecipitate (Table 18.4)

One bag of cryoprecipitate contains 10 to 15 mL of insoluble protein. When FFP is thawed for 24 hrs at 1 to 6°C, high molecular weight proteins separate out from the plasma; this can be frozen at −18°C for up to 1 yr. Cryoprecipitate contains Factors I (fibrinogen), VIII, XIII, von Willebrand Factor, fibronectin, and platelet MPs. It is most commonly used as a concentrated source of fibrinogen. A common indication is hypofibrinogenemia in the setting of hemorrhage, yet its role in management of hemostasis remains unclear. Depending upon the weight of the recipient, 10 bags of cryoprecipitate will increase plasma fibrinogen by 70 to 100 mg/dL [58,75,76,84].

IV. Conclusion

While transfusion is a necessary treatment strategy for selected patients, it is associated with a number of morbidity risks (as is anemia). Recent work suggests moving from the current blood banking, "supply-centric" perspective to a "patient-centric" approach [9]. Implementation of institutional blood management protocols enhances practitioner knowledgebase and the consistency of transfusion practices (see Chapter 19) while inducing a more conservative approach to blood product usage.

REFERENCES

1. Beale RJ. The rational use of blood. *Aust N Z J Surg.* 1976;46:309–313.
2. Bennett-Guerrero E, Zhao Y, O'Brien SM, et al. Variation in use of blood transfusion in coronary artery bypass graft surgery. *JAMA.* 2010;304:1568–1575.
3. Karkouti K, Wijeysundera DN, Beattie WS, et al. Variability and predictability of large-volume red blood cell transfusion in cardiac surgery: a multicenter study. *Transfusion.* 2007;47:2081–2088.
4. Likosky DS, FitzGerald DC, Groom RC, et al. Effect of the perioperative blood transfusion and blood conservation in cardiac surgery clinical practice guidelines of the Society of Thoracic Surgeons and the Society of Cardiovascular Anesthesiologists upon clinical practices. *Anesth Analg.* 2010;111:316–323.
5. Wilkinson KL, Brunskill SJ, Doree C, et al. The clinical effects of red blood cell transfusions: an overview of the randomized controlled trials evidence base. *Transfusion Med Rev.* 2011;25:145–155 e2.
6. Greinacher A, Fendrich K, Brzenska R, et al. Implications of demographics on future blood supply: a population-based cross-sectional study. *Transfusion.* 2011;51:702–709.
7. Benjamin RJ, Whitaker BI. Boom or bust? Estimating blood demand and supply as the baby boomers age. *Transfusion.* 2011;51:670–673.
8. American Red Cross. *A Compendium of Transfusion Practice Guidelines.* 1st ed. 2010:1–112.
9. Isbister JP, Shander A, Spahn DR, et al. Adverse blood transfusion outcomes: establishing causation. *Transfusion Med Rev.* 2011;25:89–101.
10. Koch CG, Li L, Duncan AI, et al. Morbidity and mortality risk associated with red blood cell and blood-component transfusion in isolated coronary artery bypass grafting. *Crit Care Med.* 2006;34:1608–1616.
11. Kuduvalli M, Oo AY, Newall N, et al. Effect of peri-operative red blood cell transfusion on 30-day and 1-year mortality following coronary artery bypass surgery. *Eur J Cardiothorac Surg.* 2005;27:592–598.
12. Koch CG, Li L, Duncan AI, et al. Transfusion in coronary artery bypass grafting is associated with reduced long-term survival. *Ann Thorac Surg.* 2006;81:1650–1657.
13. Surgenor SD, Kramer RS, Olmstead EM, et al. The association of perioperative red blood cell transfusions and decreased long-term survival after cardiac surgery. *Anesth Analg.* 2009;108:1741–1746.
14. Engoren MC, Habib RH, Zacharias A, et al. Effect of blood transfusion on long-term survival after cardiac operation. *Ann Thorac Surg.* 2002;74:1180–1186.
15. Murphy GJ, Reeves BC, Rogers CA, et al. Increased mortality, postoperative morbidity, and cost after red blood cell transfusion in patients having cardiac surgery. *Circulation.* 2007;116:2544–2552.
16. Banbury MK, Brizzio ME, Rajeswaran J, et al. Transfusion increases the risk of postoperative infection after cardiovascular surgery. *J Am Coll Surg.* 2006;202:131–138.
17. Koch CG, Li L, Van Wagoner DR, et al. Red cell transfusion is associated with an increased risk for postoperative atrial fibrillation. *Ann Thorac Surg.* 2006;82:1747–1756.
18. Tuinman PR, Vlaar AP, Cornet AD, et al. Blood transfusion during cardiac surgery is associated with inflammation and coagulation in the lung: a case control study. *Crit Care.* 2011;15:R59.
19. FDA. *Fatalities Reported to the FDA Following Blood Collection and Transfusion: Annual Summary for Fiscal Year 2009.* 2009.
20. Toy P, Lowell C. TRALI – definition, mechanisms, incidence and clinical relevance. *Best Pract Res.* 2007;21:183–193.
21. Gilliss B, Looney MR. Experimental models of transfusion-related acute lung injury. *Transfusion Med Rev.* 2011;25(suppl 1): 1–11.
22. Khan SY, Kelher MR, Heal JM, et al. Soluble CD40 ligand accumulates in stored blood components, primes neutrophils through CD40, and is a potential cofactor in the development of transfusion-related acute lung injury. *Blood.* 2006;108:2455–2462.
23. Koch C, Li L, Figueroa P, et al. Transfusion and pulmonary morbidity after cardiac surgery. *Ann Thorac Surg.* 2009;88:1410–1418.
24. Stokes ME, Ye X, Shah M, et al. Impact of bleeding-related complications and/or blood product transfusions on hospital costs in inpatient surgical patients. *BMC Health Serv Res.* 2011;11:135.
25. Vivacqua A, Koch CG, Yousuf AM, et al. Morbidity of bleeding after cardiac surgery: is it blood transfusion, reoperation for bleeding, or both? *Ann Thorac Surg.* 2011;91:1780–1790.
26. Ferraris VA, Davenport DL, Saha SP, et al. Intraoperative transfusion of small amounts of blood heralds worse postoperative outcome in patients having noncardiac thoracic operations. *Ann Thorac Surg.* 2011;91:1674–1680.
27. Grimshaw K, Sahler J, Spinelli SL, et al. New frontiers in transfusion biology: identification and significance of mediators of morbidity and mortality in stored red blood cells. *Transfusion.* 2011;51:874–880.
28. Raat NJ, Ince C. Oxygenating the microcirculation: the perspective from blood transfusion and blood storage. *Vox Sang.* 2007;93:12–18.
29. Yap CH, Lau L, Krishnaswamy M, et al. Age of transfused red cells and early outcomes after cardiac surgery. *Ann Thorac Surg.* 2008;86:554–559.
30. Koch CG, Li L, Sessler DI, et al. Duration of red-cell storage and complications after cardiac surgery. *N Engl J Med.* 2008;358:1229–1239.
31. Raat NJ, Verhoeven AJ, Mik EG, et al. The effect of storage time of human red cells on intestinal microcirculatory oxygenation in a rat isovolemic exchange model. *Crit Care Med.* 2005;33:39–45; discussion 238–239.
32. Simon E. Adenine in Blood banking. *Tranfusion.* 1997;17:317–325.
33. Hamasaki N, Yamamoto M. Red blood cell function and blood storage. *Vox Sang.* 2000;79:191–197.
34. Chin-Yee IH, Arya N, d' Almeida M. The Red cell storage lesion and its implication for transfusion. *Transfus Sci.* 1997;18:447–458.

35. Bennett-Guerrero E, Veldman TH, Doctor A, et al. Evolution of adverse changes in stored RBCs. *Proc Natl Acad Sci USA.* 2007;104:17063–17068.
36. Kim-Shapiro DB, Lee J, Gladwin MT. Storage lesion: role of red blood cell breakdown. *Transfusion.* 2011;51:844–851.
37. Roback JD, Neuman RB, Quyyumi A, et al. Insufficient nitric oxide bioavailability: a hypothesis to explain adverse effects of red blood cell transfusion. *Transfusion.* 2011;51:859–866.
38. Weinberg JA, Barnum SR, Patel RP. Red blood cell age and potentiation of transfusion-related pathology in trauma patients. *Transfusion.* 2011;51:867–873.
39. Relevy H, Koshkaryev A, Manny N, et al. Blood banking-induced alteration of red blood cell flow properties. *Transfusion.* 2008;48:136–146.
40. Rigamonti A, McLaren AT, Mazer CD, et al. Storage of strain-specific rat blood limits cerebral tissue oxygen delivery during acute fluid resuscitation. *Br J Anaesth.* 2008;100:357–364.
41. Jy W, Ricci M, Shariatmadar S, et al. Microparticles in stored red blood cells as potential mediators of transfusion complications. *Transfusion.* 2011;51:886–893.
42. Sweeney J, Kouttab N, Kurtis J. Stored red blood cell supernatant facilitates thrombin generation. *Transfusion.* 2009;49:1569–1579.
43. Ho J, Sibbald WJ, Chin-Yee IH. Effects of storage on efficacy of red cell transfusion: when is it not safe? *Crit Care Med.* 2003;31:S687–S697.
44. Sanders J, Patel S, Cooper J, et al. Red blood cell storage is associated with length of stay and renal complications after cardiac surgery. *Transfusion.* 2011;51:2286–2294.
45. Offner PJ, Moore EE, Biffl WL, et al. Increased rate of infection associated with transfusion of old blood after severe injury. *Arch Surg.* 2002;137:711–716; discussion 6–7.
46. Spinella PC, Carroll CL, Staff I, et al. Duration of red blood cell storage is associated with increased incidence of deep vein thrombosis and in hospital mortality in patients with traumatic injuries. *Crit Care.* 2009;13:R151.
47. Weinberg JA, McGwin G, Jr., Griffin RL, et al. Age of transfused blood: an independent predictor of mortality despite universal leukoreduction. *J Trauma.* 2008;65:279–282; discussion 82–84.
48. Zallen G, Offner PJ, Moore EE, et al. Age of transfused blood is an independent risk factor for postinjury multiple organ failure. *Am J Surg.* 1999;178:570–572.
49. Pettila V, Westbrook AJ, Nichol AD, et al. Age of red blood cells and mortality in the critically ill. *Crit Care.* 2011;15:R116.
50. Gauvin F, Spinella PC, Lacroix J, et al. Association between length of storage of transfused red blood cells and multiple organ dysfunction syndrome in pediatric intensive care patients. *Transfusion.* 2010;50:1902–1913.
51. Eikelboom JW, Cook RJ, Liu Y, et al. Duration of red cell storage before transfusion and in-hospital mortality. *Am Heart J.* 2010;159:737–743 e1.
52. Pettila V, Westbrook AJ, Nichol AD, et al. Age of red blood cells and mortality in the critically ill. *Crit Care.* 2011;15:R116.
53. Walsh TS, McArdle F, McLellan SA, et al. Does the storage time of transfused red blood cells influence regional or global indexes of tissue oxygenation in anemic critically ill patients? *Crit Care Med.* 2004;32:364–371.
54. Leal-Noval SR, Jara-Lopez I, Garcia-Garmendia JL, et al. Influence of erythrocyte concentrate storage time on postsurgical morbidity in cardiac surgery patients. *Anesthesiology.* 2003;98:815–822.
55. McKenny M, Ryan T, Tate H, et al. Age of transfused blood is not associated with increased postoperative adverse outcome after cardiac surgery. *Br J Anaesth.* 2011;106:643–649.
56. van de Watering L, Lorinser J, Versteegh M, et al. Effects of storage time of red blood cell transfusions on the prognosis of coronary artery bypass graft patients. *Transfusion.* 2006;46:1712–1718.
57. Gajic O, Dzik WH, Toy P. Fresh frozen plasma and platelet transfusion for nonbleeding patients in the intensive care unit: benefit or harm? *Crit Care Med.* 2006;34:S170–S173.
58. Silvergleid A, Kleinman S, Landaw S. Preparation of Blood Components. UpToDate 2011; www.uptodate.com/contents/preparation-of-blood-components.
59. Jansen JO, Thomas R, Loudon MA, et al. Damage control resuscitation for patients with major trauma. *BMJ.* 2009;338:b1778.
60. Liumbruno G, Bennardello F, Lattanzio A, et al. Recommendations for the transfusion of plasma and platelets. *Blood Transfus.* 2009;7:132–150.
61. Mitra B, Mori A, Cameron PA, et al. Fresh frozen plasma (FFP) use during massive blood transfusion in trauma resuscitation. *Injury.* 2010;41:35–39.
62. Sperry JL, Ochoa JB, Gunn SR, et al. An FFP:PRBC transfusion ratio >/ = 1:1.5 is associated with a lower risk of mortality after massive transfusion. *J Trauma.* 2008;65:986–993.
63. Phan HH, Wisner DH. Should we increase the ratio of plasma/platelets to red blood cells in massive transfusion: what is the evidence? *Vox Sang.* 2010;98:395–402.
64. Stansbury LG, Dutton RP, Stein DM, et al. Controversy in trauma resuscitation: do ratios of plasma to red blood cells matter? *Transfusion Med Rev.* 2009;23:255–265.
65. Yuan S, Goldfinger D, Silvergleid A, et al. Clinical and Laboratory Aspects of Platelet Transfusion Therapy. UpToDate 2011; www.uptodate.com/contents/clinical-and-laboratory-aspects-of-platelet-transfusion.
66. Karkouti K, Wijeysundera DN, Yau TM, et al. Platelet transfusions are not associated with increased morbidity or mortality in cardiac surgery. *Can J Anaesth.* 2006;53:279–287.
67. McGrath T, Koch CG, Xu M, et al. Platelet transfusion in cardiac surgery does not confer increased risk for adverse morbid outcomes. *Ann Thorac Surg.* 2008;86:543–553.
68. Spiess BD, Royston D, Levy JH, et al. Platelet transfusions during coronary artery bypass graft surgery are associated with serious adverse outcomes. *Transfusion.* 2004;44:1143–1148.
69. Welsby IJ, Lockhart E, Phillips-Bute B, et al. Storage age of transfused platelets and outcomes after cardiac surgery. *Transfusion.* 2010;50:2311–2317.

70. Seghatchian J, Krailadsiri P. The platelet storage lesion. *Transfusion Med Rev.* 1997;11:130–144.
71. Cauwenberghs S, van Pampus E, Curvers J, et al. Hemostatic and signaling functions of transfused platelets. *Transfusion Med Rev.* 2007;21:287–294.
72. Holme S. Storage and quality assessment of platelets. *Vox Sang.* 1998;74(suppl 2):207–216.
73. Kleinman S, Dumont LJ, Tomasulo P, et al. The impact of discontinuation of 7-day storage of apheresis platelets (PASSPORT) on recipient safety: an illustration of the need for proper risk assessments. *Transfusion.* 2009;49:903–912.
74. Eder AF, Moroff G. Platelet storage and adverse transfusion outcomes: old platelets? *Transfusion.* 2010;50:2288–2291.
75. Stanworth S. The evidence-based use of FFP and cryoprecipitate for abnormalities of coagulation tests and clinical coagulopathy. *Hematology.* 2007:179–186.
76. May A, Manaker S, Wilson K. Use of Blood Products in the Critically Ill. UpToDate 2011;www.uptodate.com/contents/use-of-blood-products-in-the-critically-ill.
77. Hellstern P, Muntean W, Schramm W, et al. Practical guidelines for the clinical use of plasma. *Thromb Res.* 2002;107(suppl 1): S53–S57.
78. Holland LL, Brooks JP. Toward rational fresh frozen plasma transfusion: The effect of plasma transfusion on coagulation test results. *Am J Clin Pathol.* 2006;126:133–139.
79. O'Shaughnessy DF, Atterbury C, Bolton Maggs P, et al. Guidelines for the use of fresh-frozen plasma, cryoprecipitate and cryosupernatant. *Br J Haematol.* 2004;126:11–28.
80. Verghese SG. Elective fresh frozen plasma in the critically ill: what is the evidence? *Crit Care Resusc.* 2008;10:264–268.
81. Bilgin YM, van de Watering LM, Versteegh MI, et al. Postoperative complications associated with transfusion of platelets and plasma in cardiac surgery. *Transfusion.* 2011;51(12):2603–2610.
82. Watson GA, Sperry JL, Rosengart MR, et al. Fresh frozen plasma is independently associated with a higher risk of multiple organ failure and acute respiratory distress syndrome. *J Trauma.* 2009;67:221–227; discussion 8–30.
83. Bochicchio GV, Napolitano L, Joshi M, et al. Outcome analysis of blood product transfusion in trauma patients: a prospective, risk-adjusted study. *World J Surg.* 2008;32:2185–2189.
84. Callum JL, Karkouti K, Lin Y. Cryoprecipitate: the current state of knowledge. *Transfus Med Rev.* 2009;23:177–188.

19 Coagulation Management During and After Cardiopulmonary Bypass

Linda Shore-Lesserson, S. Nini Malayaman, Jay C. Horrow, and Glenn P. Gravlee

KEY POINTS

1. Previous concepts of independent intrinsic and extrinsic plasma coagulation pathways, a cell-free final common pathway, and platelet clotting have given way to an integrated concept of cell-based coagulation occurring on the platelet surface as depicted in Figure 19.2.
2. In the absence of a history suggesting a preoperative bleeding disorder (e.g., von Willebrand's Disease, warfarin therapy), routine hemostatic screening for patients undergoing cardiac surgery is not cost-effective at predicting excessive perioperative bleeding.
3. Unfractionated heparin (UFH) is a hydrophilic macromolecular glycosaminoglycan of varying chain lengths which anticoagulates principally by potentiating antithrombin III (AT III)-induced inactivation of factors IIa (thrombin) and Xa.
4. Intravenously administered heparin typically peaks within 1 min, redistributes only slightly, and has a dose-related half-life that reaches approximately 2 hrs in the large doses used for cardiopulmonary bypass (CPB). Heparin bolus administration decreases systemic vascular resistance by 10% to 20%.
5. The usual initial heparin dose is 300 to 350 units/kg to achieve an Activated Clotting Time (ACT) exceeding 400 s for safe initiation and maintenance of CPB. Heparin 5,000 to 10,000 units should be added to CPB priming solution.
6. Heparin is most often monitored using ACT, but ACT precision is suboptimal at the heparin concentrations required for CPB, and it is also subject to prolongation from hemodilution and hypothermia. As a result, some practitioners choose to monitor and maintain a target whole blood heparin concentration (typically 3 to 4 units/mL) in addition to exceeding a target ACT during CPB.
7. Resistance to heparin-induced anticoagulation has a variety of causes, but therapy with either AT III concentrates or fresh frozen plasma (FFP) nearly always resolves it regardless of its cause.
8. Heparin-induced thrombocytopenia (HIT) produces a severe procoagulant state that may occur after 5 or more continuous days of heparin administration. Diagnosis requires the combination of an appropriate clinical context and a complex variety of laboratory tests.

9. Documented presence of HIT in a patient who must urgently undergo cardiac surgery requiring CPB is possibly best managed by using bivalirudin for anticoagulation.
10. Protamine neutralizes heparin stoichiometrically as a result of a strong cation (protamine)-to-anion (heparin) interaction.
11. A variety of protamine dosing methods are used clinically. Most often 60 to 80 mg of protamine per 100 units of heparin administered prior to CPB (including heparin placed in the CPB priming solution if residual CPB volume is to be reinfused unaltered by hemoconcentration or cell washing) suffices to neutralize heparin. Excessive protamine administration impairs blood clotting.
12. In order to avoid hypotension, protamine should be administered slowly, ideally by a continuous intravenous infusion over 5 to 10 min.
13. Protamine can induce severe anaphylactic or anaphylactoid reactions.
14. Post-CPB clotting abnormalities are best managed using a systematic approach. Post-CPB bleeding algorithms reduce bleeding and transfusion.

IN ESSENCE, CPB CREATES a blood "detour" to permit surgery on the heart. This detour must route the blood through an artificial heart and lung while maintaining its fluidity. Historically, fluidity represented the final frontier in the development of cardiac surgery because effective mechanisms for blood gas exchange and for propelling the blood had been established more than a decade before surmounting the fluidity challenge. The challenge was to find a therapeutic approach that would inhibit blood's natural propensity to clot when it contacts foreign surfaces. Since the restoration of normal coagulation was desirable at the end of the surgical procedure, this clotting inhibition needed to be reversible, like turning a spigot on and off. The long-awaited solution was monumental: **anticoagulation with heparin followed by neutralization with protamine. This fundamental approach to establishing and reversing blood fluidity remains unchanged after almost 50 yrs,** although much fine-tuning has occurred. This chapter reviews anticoagulation and the restoration of coagulation in the patients undergoing CPB.

I. Physiology of Coagulation

A. Mechanisms of hemostasis

1. Plasma coagulation. Figure 19.1 depicts the plasma coagulation pathway. Blood contact with foreign surfaces classically was thought to activate the intrinsic pathway, whereas vascular injury or disruption was thought to activate the extrinsic pathway. These definitions seem counterintuitive because vascular disruption should be intrinsic and foreign bodies extrinsic, but logic has held little sway in coagulation pathway nomenclature. Thankfully, distinctions between the intrinsic and extrinsic pathways have become less important because both the activants and the pathways overlap (e.g., connection between VIIa and IXa). The coagulation factor numbering system was defined in order of discovery rather than use, which explains the illogic numerical progression through the pathways [1].
   a. Intrinsic pathway. Contact activation involves binding of factor XII to negatively charged surfaces, which leads to the common pathway through factors XI, IX, platelet factor 3, cofactor VIII, and calcium. Kallikrein is also formed in this reaction and serves as a positive feedback mechanism and as an initiator of fibrinolysis (a negative feedback mechanism) and inflammation. For cardiac surgery, this pathway's clinical importance lies more in the access it provides for heparin monitoring and neutralization than in its role in normal hemostasis.
   b. Extrinsic pathway. Tissue factor (TF) initiates the extrinsic pathway, which proceeds to activate factor IX and rapidly stimulates the common pathway with the aid of factor VII and calcium.
   c. Common pathway. Beginning with the assisted activation of factor X, this pathway proceeds to convert prothrombin (factor II) to thrombin and fibrinogen (factor I) to fibrin monomer, which initiates the actual substance of the clot. Fibrin monomer then cross-links to form a more stable clot with the aid of calcium and factor XIII. **Rather than thinking of the common pathway as the result of activation of two**

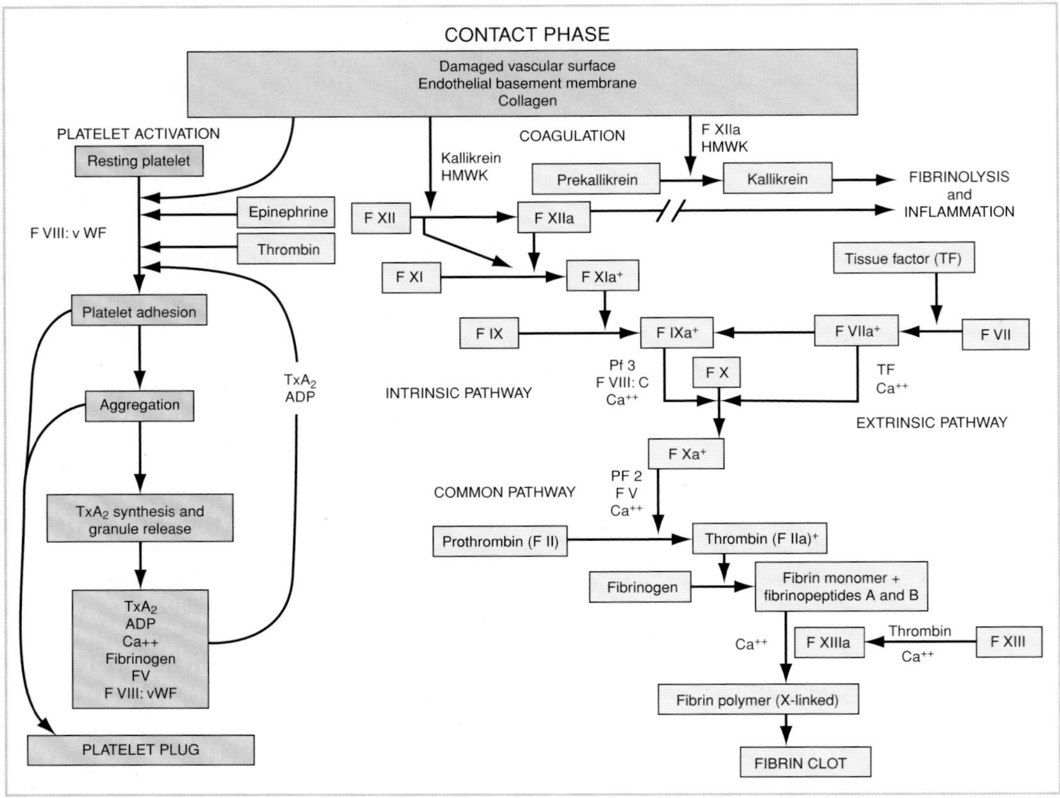

FIGURE 19.1 Schematic representation of the hemostatic system depicting the vascular, platelet, and coagulation components. F, factor; HMWK, high-molecular weight kininogen; vWF, von Willebrand's factor; Ca^{++}; ionized calcium; VIII:C, factor VIII coagulation component; TxA_2, thromboxane A_2; ADP, adenosine diphosphate.

independent paths, the concept of cell-based coagulation has been adapted to better explain the hemostatic mechanisms that occur simultaneously in the body (Fig. 19.2). When tissue injury occurs, TF is expressed on the surface of TF-bearing cells. Presentation of TF to its ligand factor VII causes the activation of factors IX and X on the TF-bearing cell. This is called "Initiation." The activation of factor X causes thrombin formation which then incites further protease activation. These reactions occur on the phospholipid surface of the platelet and are called "Amplification." The final stage of clot formation is known as "Propagation."

Activated factor X also initiates platelet-surface clotting activity as depicted in Figure 19.2. This platelet-surface activity greatly speeds the overall formation of clot and should be considered as a vital component of the clotting cascade.

d. Thrombin is the most important enzyme in the pathway because (in addition to activating fibrinogen) it

(1) Provides positive feedback by activating cofactors V and VIII

(2) Accelerates cross-linking of fibrinogen by activating factor XIII

(3) Strongly stimulates platelet adhesion and aggregation

(4) Facilitates clot resorption by releasing tissue plasminogen activator (tPA) from endothelial cells

(5) Activates protein C, which provides negative feedback by inactivating factors Va and VIIIa

2. Platelet activation. As shown in Figure 19.1, a variety of stimuli initiate platelet activation, and thrombin is an especially potent one. This sets off a cascade of events that initiates

1

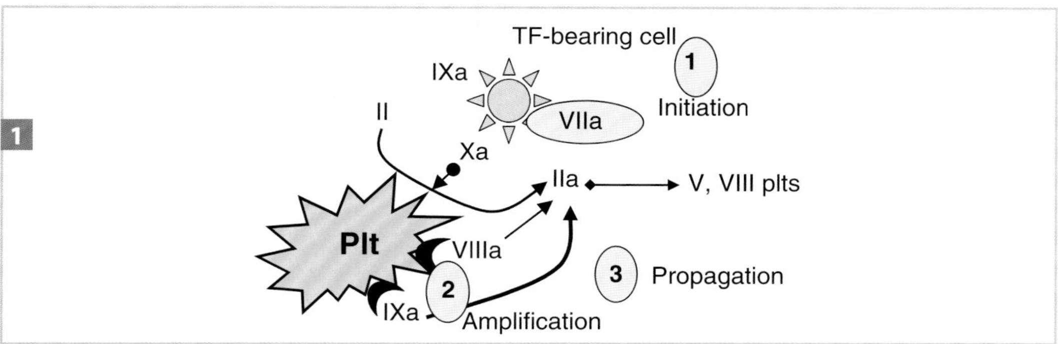

FIGURE 19.2 Cell-based model of hemostasis. Cellular hemostasis is thought to occur in three stages: Initiation, amplification, and propagation. The initiation stage (*1*) takes place on TF-bearing cells (cells such as monocytes that can bind TF and present it to a ligand), which come into play when endothelial injury occurs and TF is exposed. The initiation stage is characterized by presentation of TF to its ligand factor VII and the subsequent activation of factors IX and X on the TF-bearing cell. The activation of factor X to Xa causes thrombin production and activation. Once generated, thrombin feeds back to activate factors VIII, V, and platelets. The amplification stage (*2*) then occurs on the surface of the activated platelet, which exposes surface phospholipids that act as receptors for the activated factors VIIIa and IXa. The platelet surface allows for further thrombin formation and hence the amplification of coagulation. Continued generation and activation of thrombin causes further positive feedback mechanisms (*3*) to occur that ultimately ensure the formation of a stable clot, including cleavage of fibrinogen to fibrin, release and activation of factor XIII for fibrin cross-linkage, and the release of a thrombin-activatable fibrinolysis inhibitor.

platelet adhesion to endogenous or extracorporeal surfaces, followed by platelet aggregation and formation of a primary platelet plug. Fibrin clots and platelet plugs form simultaneously and mesh together, yielding a product more tenacious and difficult to dissolve than either alone. Whereas formerly plasma-based and platelet-based clotting were often thought to represent independent pathways, more recent accounts show that **the plasma coagulation pathway evolves mainly on the platelet surface,** such that the plasma and platelet clotting processes are more interdependent than independent.

   a. Von Willebrand factor (vWF) is an important ligand for platelet adhesion at low shear stress, and for aggregation at higher shear rates. Fibrinogen is the major ligand for platelet aggregation.

   b. Products released from platelet storage granules (adenosine diphosphate [ADP], epinephrine, calcium, thromboxane A_2, factor V, and vWF) serve to perpetuate platelet activation and the plasma coagulation cascade.

3. Nature's system of checks and balances demands counterbalancing forces to discourage runaway clot formation and to dissolve clots. These counterbalances include the following:

   a. Proteins C and S, which inactivate factors Va and VIIIa

   b. ATIII, antithrombin, or AT, which inhibits thrombin as well as factors XIa, IXa, XIIa, and Xa

   c. TF inhibitor, which inhibits the initiation of the extrinsic pathway

   d. tPA, which is released from endothelium and converts plasminogen to plasmin, which in turn breaks down fibrin. Plasminogen activator inhibitor 1 in turn inhibits tPA to prevent uncontrolled fibrinolysis.

B. Tests of hemostatic function

1. Table 19.1 lists commonly used tests of hemostatic function [1]. These tests may be used to detect hemostatic abnormalities preoperatively or after CPB. With the exception of the ACT, typically they are not used during CPB except under extenuating circumstances, because most of them will be abnormal as a result of hemodilution, anticoagulation, and sometimes hypothermia.

2 **a. Most studies suggest that routine preoperative hemostatic screening is not helpful in predicting patients who will bleed excessively during surgery.** If the patient's clinical history (e.g., nosebleeds; prolonged bleeding with small cuts, dental work, or

TABLE 19.1 Common clinical tests of hemostatic function

Test	Normal values	Comment
Platelets		
Platelet count	150,000–400,000/μL	
Bleeding time (IVY)	<8 min	Controversial clinical test of platelet function; inconvenient; arms must be exposed
Coagulation system		
Whole blood clotting time (WBCT; Lee–White CT)	2.5–6 min	Prolonged by marked deficiencies in intrinsic system or final common pathway; formerly used to monitor heparin therapy
Activated clotting time (ACT)	Manual = 90–110 s Automated = 90–130 s[a] = 100–140 s[b]	Modified WBCT: commonly performed to monitor heparin in the operating room because of convenience
Prothrombin time (PT)	12–15 s; compare to control INR 1.0–1.5	Tests extrinsic system and final common pathway; used to monitor warfarin anticoagulation
Activated partial thromboplastin time (aPTT)	35–45 s; compare to control	Tests intrinsic system and final common pathway; used to monitor heparin anticoagulation
Thrombin time	<14 s; compare to control	Tests final common pathway; prolonged by heparin, fibrinogen ≤100 mg/dL, abnormal fibrinogen and increased fibrin split products
Fibrinogen	250–500 mg/dL	Decreased in disseminated intravascular coagulation (DIC)
Fibrinolytic system		
Fibrin(ogen) split (degradation) products	<10 μg/mL	Increased during fibrinolysis (normal clot lysis process) or fibrinogenolysis (pathologic process that compromises clotting)
D-Dimer	<0.5 μg/mL	Increased during fibrinolysis; specific assay of cross-linked fibrin degradation

[a]Hemochron, International Technidyne, Edison, NJ, USA.
[b]Medtronic, HemoTec, Minneapolis, MN, USA.
INR, international normalized ratio.

surgery; easy bruising; strong family history of pathologic bleeding) suggests the need for hemostatic screening, selective use of these and other tests is appropriate. Similarly, when the patient is taking medications that alter hemostatic function, specific hemostatic function tests may be indicated. Examples include the following:

(1) Heparin: Activated partial thromboplastin time (aPTT) or ACT

(2) Low-molecular-weight heparin (LMWH), including the pentasaccharide fondaparinux: No test or anti-Xa plasma activity

(3) Warfarin: Prothrombin time (PT) and/or international normalized ratio (INR)

(4) Platelet inhibitors including aspirin: No testing, bleeding time, or specific platelet function tests. Preliminary data suggests that specific platelet function tests in patients taking thienopyridine agents may correlate with postoperative bleeding risk.

II. Heparin anticoagulation

A. Heparin pharmacology [2]

Structure. As drugs go, UFH might be described as impure. Heparin resides physiologically in mast cells, and it is commercially derived most often from the lungs of cattle (bovine lung heparin) or the intestines of pigs (porcine mucosal heparin). Commercial preparations used for CPB typically include a range of molecular weights from 3,000 to 40,000 Da, with a mean molecular weight of approximately 15,000 Da. Each molecule is a heavily sulfated glycosaminoglycan polymer, so heparin is a strong biologic acid that is negatively charged at physiologic pH.

a. Porcine mucosal and bovine lung heparin both are satisfactory for CPB and both have been widely used.

3 1. **1.** Action. A specific pentasaccharide sequence that binds to ATIII is present on approximately 30% of heparin molecules. This binding potentiates the action of ATIII more than 1,000-fold, thereby allowing heparin to inhibit thrombin and factor Xa most importantly, but also factors IXa, XIa, and XIIa.

   a. Inhibition of thrombin requires simultaneous binding of heparin to both ATIII and thrombin, whereas inhibition of factor Xa requires only that heparin binds to ATIII. The former reaction limits thrombin inhibition to longer saccharide chains (18 or more saccharide units); hence, shorter chains can selectively inhibit Xa. This is the primary principle underlying therapy with LMWH and with the "ultimate" LMWH fondaparinux, which contains just the critical pentasaccharide sequence needed for binding ATIII, hence it induces virtually exclusive Xa inhibition.

      (1) Because thrombin inhibition appears pivotal for CPB anticoagulation and also because LMWH and heparinoids have a long half-life and are poorly neutralized by protamine, LMWH (including fondaparinux) is inadvisable as a CPB anticoagulant. Fondaparinux lasts even longer than traditional LMWHs and is even less neutralized by protamine.

   b. Heparin binds and activates cofactor II, a non–ATIII-dependent thrombin inhibitor. This may explain why heparin-induced anticoagulation can be effective even in the presence of marked ATIII deficiency, although the primary mechanism of anticoagulant action is ATIII inhibition.

2. Potency. Heparin potency is tested by measuring the anticoagulation effect in animal plasma. The United States Pharmacopoeia (USP) defines 1 unit of activity as the amount of heparin that maintains the fluidity of 1 mL of citrated sheep plasma for 1 hr after recalcification.

   a. Heparin dosing is best recorded in USP units, because commercial preparations vary in the number of USP units per milligram. The most common concentration is 100 units/mg (1,000 units/mL) [3].

4 **3.** Pharmacokinetics. **After central venous administration, heparin's effect peaks within 1 min, and there is a small rapid redistribution that most often is clinically insignificant** [4,5].

   a. Heparin's large molecular size and its polarity restrict its distribution mainly to the intravascular space and endothelial cells.

   b. The onset of CPB increases circulating blood volume by approximately 1,000 to 1,500 mL; hence, plasma heparin concentration drops proportionately with the onset of CPB unless heparin is added to the CPB priming solution.

   c. Heparin is eliminated by the kidneys or by metabolism in the reticuloendothelial system.

   d. Elimination half-life has been determined only by bioassay, that is, by the time course of clotting time prolongation. By this standard, heparin's elimination time is dose dependent [6]. At lower doses, such as 100 to 150 USP units/kg, elimination half-time is approximately 1 hr. At CPB doses of 300 to 400 USP units/kg, elimination half-time is 2 or more hours; hence, clinically significant anticoagulation might persist for 4 to 6 hrs in the absence of neutralization by protamine. Hypothermia and probably CPB itself prolong elimination.

4. Side effects. Heparin's actions on the hemostatic system extend beyond its primary anticoagulant mechanism to include activation of tPA, platelet activation, and enhancement of TF pathway inhibitor.

   a. Lipoprotein lipase activation influences plasma lipid concentrations, which indirectly affects the plasma concentrations of lipid-soluble drugs.

   b. Heparin boluses decrease systemic vascular resistance. Typically this effect is small (10% to 20%), but rarely it can be more impressive and may merit treatment with a vasopressor or calcium chloride.

   c. Anaphylaxis rarely occurs.

   d. HIT is covered elsewhere in this chapter.

5 **B. Dosing and monitoring**

1. Dosing. **The most common initial dose for CPB is 300 to 350 USP U/kg.** Some centers choose an initial dose of 400 U/kg or base the initial dose on a bedside ex vivo heparin dose-response titration.
   a. Since heparin distributes primarily into the plasma compartment, increasing the dose with increasing body weight assumes that plasma volume increases in direct proportion to body weight. This is not the case, because fat does not increase blood volume in proportion to weight. Consequently, there is seldom reason to exceed an initial dose of 35,000 to 40,000 units, even in patients weighing more than 100 kg, as lean body mass tends to peak at 90 kg for females and 110 kg for males.
   b. Heparin dosing for coronary revascularization procedures performed without CPB is controversial. Published doses range from 100 to 300 U/kg, but most centers use 100 to 150 units/kg and set minimum acceptable ACT values at 200 to 300 s.
   c. **The CPB priming solution should contain heparin at approximately the same concentration as that of the patient's bloodstream at the onset of CPB.** Since this most often would be 3 to 4 U/mL, a priming volume of 1,500 mL should contain at least 5,000 units of heparin. CPB priming solutions commonly contain 5,000 to 10,000 units of heparin.
   d. Supplemental heparin doses typically are guided by monitoring of anticoagulation.
2. Monitoring. Until the late 1970s, heparin dosing was guided by experiential practices and varied a great deal from hospital to hospital. Using ACT, a variation on the Lee–White clotting time, **Bull et al. [7] identified rather staggering variations in the approach to heparin dosing and in both the initial anticoagulant response and the time course of anticoagulation in response to a fixed dose of heparin.** This landmark work rapidly led to the realization that the anticoagulant response to heparin should be monitored, although a few centers continue to dose heparin empirically.
3. Approaches to anticoagulation monitoring for CPB. **The ACT is the most widely used test,** although some centers monitor blood heparin concentration as well.
   a. ACT uses an activant such as celite or kaolin to activate clotting, then measures the clotting time in a test tube. Heparin prolongs ACT with a roughly linear dose-response pattern (Fig. 19.3). Normal ACT depends upon such factors as the specific activant and device, prewarming (vs. room temperature) of test tubes, and operator technique, but generally falls between 110 and 140 s.

      Although originally described as a manual test, most centers use one of the two automated approaches to ACT (International Technidyne, Edison, NJ, U.S.A., or Medtronic HemoTec, Fridley, MN, U.S.A.). These two automated approaches yield slightly different values both at baseline and with anticoagulation because of different activators and endpoint detection techniques.

      ACT is prolonged by hypothermia and hemodilution; hence, conditions often imposed by CPB alter the ACT-heparin dose-response relationship [8]. Some see this as risking underanticoagulation, although hemodilution and hypothermia legitimately enhance anticoagulation. Overreliance on hypothermic enhancement of ACT prolongation risks underanticoagulation upon rewarming. Also, at temperatures below 25°C, ACT prolongation becomes so profound that alternative tests such as whole blood heparin concentration measurement may be advisable.

      The target ACT level for CPB is controversial. There are studies supporting the safety of ACT values as low as 300 s, inside and outside of the context of heparin-coated surfaces, yet most centers accept only values exceeding 400 to 480 s. In addition, different devices and tests yield different dose-response relationships for heparin concentration versus ACT, as well as different sensitivities to hypothermia and hemodilution.

      (1) **As a clotting test, ACT is somewhat crude and may vary as much as 10%**
6 **on repeated testing at heparin concentrations used for CPB [9], so it seems reasonable to build in a safety margin by accepting 400 s as a minimum safe threshold for sustained CPB.**

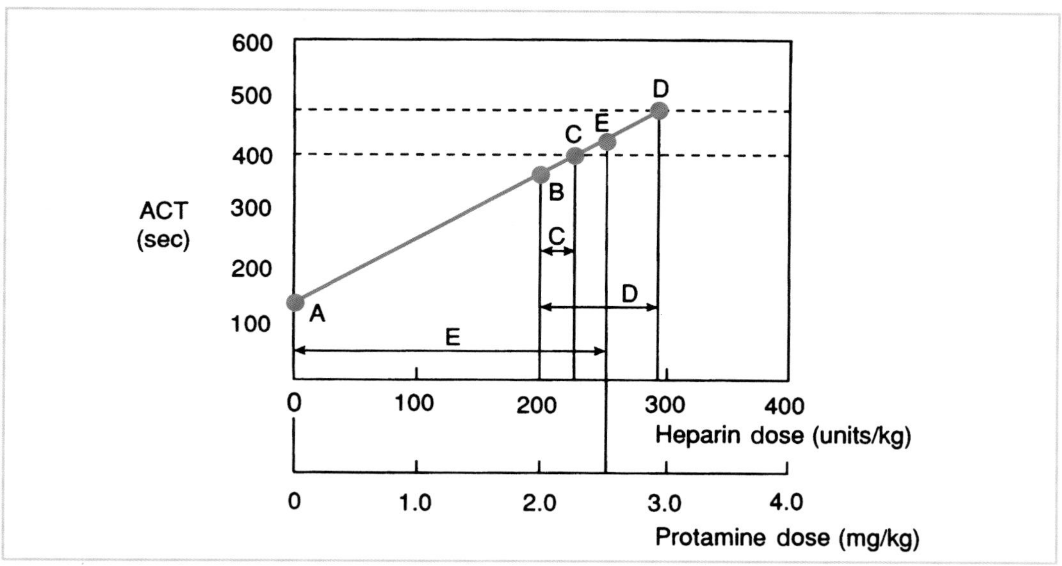

FIGURE 19.3 Graph of a heparin (and protamine) dosing algorithm. In the graph, the control *ACT* is shown as *point A* and the ACT resulting from an initial heparin bolus of 200 units/kg is shown in *point B*. The line connecting *A* and *B* then is extrapolated and a desired ACT is selected. *Point C* represents the intersection between this line and a target ACT of 400 s, theoretically requiring an additional heparin dose represented by the difference between points *C* and *B* on the *horizontal axis* (*arrow C*). Similarly, to achieve an ACT of 480 s (*higher horizontal dotted line* intersecting the ACT versus heparin dose line at *point D*), one would administer the additional heparin dose represented by *arrow D*. To estimate heparin concentration and calculate protamine dose at the time of heparin neutralization, the most recently measured ACT value is plotted on the dose-response line (*point E* in the example). The whole blood heparin concentration present theoretically is represented by the difference between *point E* and *point A* on the *horizontal axis* (*arrow E*). The protamine dose required to neutralize the remaining heparin then may be calculated. Protamine 1.0 mg/kg is administered for every 100 units/kg of heparin present. (Modified from Bull BS, Huse WM, Brauer FS, et al. Heparin therapy during extracorporeal circulation: II. The use of a dose-response curve to individualize heparin and protamine dosage. *J Thorac Cardiovasc Surg.* 1975;69:686; and Gravlee GP. Anticoagulation for cardiopulmonary bypass. In: Gravlee GP, Davis RF, Kurusz M, et al., eds. *Cardiopulmonary Bypass: Principles and Practice,* 2nd ed. Philadelphia, PA: Lippincott Williams & Wilkins; 2000:435–472, with permission.)

(2) Aprotinin, which is now used rarely in clinical practice, complicates the use of ACT monitoring, as a result of marked prolongation of celite ACTs in the presence of heparin and aprotinin. This may represent enhanced anticoagulation to some degree, but in the presence of aprotinin it is probably wise to titrate heparin to a celite ACT level exceeding 750 s or to use a kaolin ACT instead. Kaolin ACT minimum levels do not have to be adjusted in the presence of aprotinin.

b. Whole blood heparin concentrations can be measured during CPB. The most commonly used technique is automated protamine titration (Medtronic HemoTec, Fridley, MN). Advocates of this monitoring technique argue that CPB-induced distortion of the ACT-heparin dose-response relationship mandates maintenance of the heparin concentration originally needed before CPB to achieve the target ACT level [10]. **Heparin dosing based upon concentration alone substantially increases the amount of heparin given during CPB,** which enhances suppression of thrombin formation. This benefit may accrue at the expense of heparin rebound, if not monitored, and more profound platelet activation that may aggravate and prolong platelet dysfunction after CPB. The distortion of the ACT-heparin sensitivity relationship can be partly overcome using plasma-modified ACT testing [11] or by maximal activation of the ACT test sample, as is done in a Thromboelastograph (TEG) modification of the ACT [12]. Whole blood point-of-care measurement of heparin concentration can also be performed with the HepTest POC-Hi (Americana Diagnostica, Stamford, CT). This test correlates well with heparin concentrations during CPB and more closely approximates the trend in plasma anti-Xa levels than does the standard ACT [13].

(1) **Whole blood heparin concentrations of 3.0 to 4.0 U/mL most often are sufficient for CPB.** Plasma heparin concentrations (typically anti-Xa concentrations) are higher because circulating heparin resides in the plasma compartment.

(2) Patients can vary widely in their sensitivity to heparin-induced anticoagulation; therefore, **isolated use of heparin concentration could lead to dangerous underanticoagulation.** If this technique is chosen, simultaneous use of ACT or another clotting time is strongly advised.

(3) Heparin concentration monitoring may be a useful adjunct to ACT monitoring both in the presence of aprotinin and during periods of hypothermia below 25°C.

(4) Heparin concentration monitoring may be advantageous in selecting a protamine dose, because the dose will be chosen in relation to approximate actual blood heparin concentration. The weakness of this technique is its dependence on a calculated blood volume determination at a time when blood volume may vary substantially.

c. **Other monitors of anticoagulation.** Neither ACT nor heparin concentration is perfect, so other tests have been evaluated or are under investigation. The aPTT and traditional thrombin time are typically so sensitive to heparin that those tests are not useful at the heparin concentrations needed for CPB. The high-dose thrombin time (HiTT, International Technidyne) offers a linear dose-response in the usual heparin concentration range used for CPB. The heparin management test (HMT, Helena, Beaumont, TX) offers another platform for ACT monitoring and can be used to monitor heparin at high (cardiac surgery) and low (vascular surgery) concentration ranges. Clotting times have also been successfully monitored using viscoelastic tests—the Sonoclot (SkACT, Sienco, Arvada, CO) [14] and the TEG.

C. **Heparin resistance.** Heparin resistance is loosely defined as the need for greater than expected heparin doses to achieve the target ACT for CPB. As noted earlier, ACT prolongation in response to heparin varies greatly. A number of factors that may decrease the ACT response to heparin are listed in Table 19.2 [2]. ATIII deficiency is cited most often for heparin resistance, but overall the

TABLE 19.2 Potential causes of heparin resistance

Hypercoagulable states
Antithrombin III deficiency
Familial
Acquired
Arteriosclerotic disease
Unstable angina pectoris
Septicemia
Bacterial endocarditis
Pregnancy
HIT
Thrombocytosis
Drugs
Heparin
Nitroglycerin[a]
Protein binding
Acid glycoprotein
Histidine-rich glycoprotein
Immunoglobulins
Others
Neonates
Elderly patients

[a]Controversial cause. Probably not clinically significant.

correlation between ATIII concentrations and anticoagulant response to a bolus of heparin has been weak and inconsistent, perhaps because heparin resistance often is multifactorial.

Clinical approach. **Most often heparin resistance can be managed by simply giving more heparin.** It is reasonable to consider administering supplemental ATIII if more than
7 600 USP units/kg has been required to reach the target ACT level. In some circumstances (e.g., urgent need to initiate CPB, minimal ACT prolongation after 300 U/kg), a lower intervention threshold seems reasonable. Similarly, if maintaining the target ACT during CPB requires administering more than 100 USP units/kg per 30 min of CPB, supplemental ATIII seems reasonable.

- **a. ATIII can be provided in the form of FFP, liquid plasma, and ATIII concentrates (human or recombinant).**
  - **(1)** FFP or liquid plasma dose typically is 2 to 4 units in adults.
  - **(2)** For ATIII concentrates, an initial dose of 500–1,000 units is usually sufficient.

1. Prediction of heparin resistance. Medtronic HemoTec's HMS Plus Hemostasis Management System and International Technidyne's Hemochron RxDx system each provide an in vitro opportunity to titrate the patient's whole blood to predetermined heparin concentrations and hence to predict the initial heparin dose required to achieve a particular target ACT. Some centers use one of these devices to predict heparin resistance prior to heparin administration. This approach allows "customization" of initial heparin dosing as well as advance preparation for anticipated heparin resistance, for example, ordering ATIII concentrate or FFP.

D. Heparin-induced thrombocytopenia (HIT)

1. Benign Thrombocytopenia from heparin's proaggregatory effect on platelets develops in 5% to 28% of patients.

- **a.** This mild decrease in platelet count typically occurs within 1 to 2 days of heparin administration without thrombosis or immune response. This response was formerly called HIT type I, and it is not considered pathologic. However, thrombocytopenia occurring within 1 to 2 days of heparin administration can be pathologic immune-mediated HIT if the patient's plasma retains heparin antibodies from a previous exposure. This latter situation is most likely to occur in a patient who has experienced clinical HIT within the past several weeks.
- **b. HIT is a severe condition that most often occurs after 5 continuous days of heparin administration** (average onset time, 9 days), and is immune mediated. Antibody binding to the complex formed between heparin and platelet factor 4 (PF4) is responsible for the syndrome. Antibody binding to platelets and endothelial cells causes platelet activation, endothelial injury, and complement activation. The platelet clots formed are referred to, in lay terms, as "white clots." This syndrome is highly morbid and can
8 be fatal as a result of thromboembolic phenomena.
  - **(1) Among patients who develop HIT II, the incidence of thrombosis approximates 20%, the mortality of which can be as high as 40%.**
  - **(2)** Diagnosis: thrombocytopenia (usually defined as platelet count <100,000/uL, but this is complicated for several days by post-CPB hemodilution), demonstration of heparin/PF4 antibody plus (ideally) documentation of heparin-induced aggregation of platelets.
    - **(a)** Heparin-induced serotonin release assay: a functional test, often considered the gold standard.
    - **(b)** Heparin-induced platelet activation assay (HIPAA): a functional test, may be nonspecific.
    - **(c)** Enzyme-linked immunosorbent assay (ELISA) specific for the heparin/PF4 complex or for PF4 alone: patients with a positive antibody test do *not* always develop thrombosis. Antibodies to the heparin/PF4 complex are associated with adverse outcomes after cardiac surgery [15]. Whether the antibody is causative of outcome or merely a marker for a more critically ill patient has not yet been determined. Antibodies associated with HIT often become

undetectable 50 to 85 days after discontinuing heparin. After 100 days of heparin discontinuation, one can be confident that short-term re-exposure to heparin (as for CPB) will not result in antibody formation [16]. Continued heparin re-exposure is not recommended even though the clinical syndrome does not always recur upon reexposure to the drug. Sometimes the syndrome resolves despite continued heparin therapy. HIT can be associated with heparin resistance and thus should be part of the differential diagnosis.

(3) Treatments for HIT and alternative anticoagulant sources

(a) In HIT, changing tissue source of heparin, LMWH, heparinoids, and ancrod have been used but are no longer recommended. Cross-reactivity with other heparins does exist (see Section E).

(b) Plasmapheresis can be used to remove the antibody, but may be insufficient therapy by itself. Heparin plus platelet inhibitors can be combined to reduce the aggregability of platelets. Hirudin, bivalirudin, and argatroban are direct thrombin inhibitors.

E. Alternatives to unfractionated heparin

1. LMWH (shorter-chain heparin molecules, including fondaparinux). Intravenously administered LMWH has a half-life at least twice as long as that of UFH and possibly several times as long for some LMWH compounds. Problems in CPB arise from the fact that protamine neutralization only reverses the factor IIa inhibition and leaves the predominant factor Xa inhibition intact. LMWH therapy also complicates heparin monitoring because aPTT (and presumably ACT) is much less sensitive to Xa inhibition and will not accurately measure the full anticoagulant effect. Factor Xa inhibition can be measured directly in plasma and with a plasma-modified whole blood test, but there is no simple point-of-care test available. LMWHs are not recommended for use in HIT patients because of cross-reactivity of the antibody, although some reports suggest that fondaparinux may be safe because it is too small to bind antibodies.

2. Heparinoids. Two glycosaminoglycans with heparin-like properties may be available for clinical use: Dermatan sulfate and danaparoid. They are referred to as heparinoids because they represent a class of synthetic or naturally occurring heparin analogs. Danaparoid is a natural composite of heparan sulfate (80%), dermatan sulfate (20%), and chondroitin sulfates. Case reports document that they have been used successfully in CPB when heparin use was contraindicated, but cross-reactivity and bleeding complications preclude their current use in HIT patients [17]. Since 2002, Danaparoid has not been available in the United States but is still available in some other countries.

3. Hirudin [18]

a. Thrombin inhibitor isolated from the salivary glands of the medicinal leech (*Hirudo medicinalis*).

b. Independent of ATIII and inhibits clot-bound thrombin.

c. Inhibits thrombin activation of protein C.

d. Hirudin is a small molecule (molecular weight 7 kDa) that is eliminated by the kidney and is easily filtered at the end of CPB. Half-life is 40 min.

e. r-Hirudin dose: 0.25 mg/kg bolus and an infusion to maintain the hirudin concentration at 2.5 μg/mL as determined by ecarin clotting time.

f. Ecarin clotting time: not clinically available at this time [19].

g. r-Hirudin-treated patients maintain platelet counts and hemoglobin levels and have few bleeding complications, if renal function is normal.

4. Bivalirudin

a. Synthetic polypeptide that directly inhibits thrombin by binding simultaneously to its active catalytic site and its substrate recognition site.

9 **b.** Half-life is 24 min. Elimination is primarily by proteolysis and, to a smaller degree, renal elimination. **Even though this half-life is shorter than heparin's, the absence of a reversal agent and the profound degree of anticoagulation used for CPB may cause coagulopathy for 2 or more hours following CPB.**

c. Dose during interventional procedures: 0.75 mg/kg bolus followed by a 1.75 mg/kg/hour infusion, yielding a median ACT of 346 s.

d. Dose for CPB: 1.0 mg/kg bolus followed by a 2.5 mg/kg/hr infusion. **A recirculation limb and avoidance of circuit (and saphenous vein graft) stasis is necessary.**

e. Studies in interventional procedures suggest lower bleeding rates than UFH and similar efficacy.

5. Argatroban. A direct thrombin inhibitor that is approved by the U.S. Food and Drug Administration (FDA) for anticoagulation in HIT patients but not yet approved for use in CPB. Argatroban undergoes hepatic metabolism with a half-life 39 to 51 min.

III. Neutralization of heparin

A. Proof of concept. Protamine, commercially prepared from fish sperm, first found clinical utility in its combination with insulin to delay insulin's absorption and prolong its effect. Combination of protamine with heparin, intended to achieve a similar prolongation of heparin's effect, resulted instead in inactivation of heparin. Combining the strongly cationic protamine
10 with strongly anionic heparin produces a stable complex devoid of anticoagulant activity.

1. Heparin and protamine combine in proportion to weight. One milligram of protamine neutralizes 1 mg (typically 100 U) of heparin [20].

B. Protamine dose. Since protamine appears to distribute within the circulatory system as heparin does, the protamine dose required to neutralize a given dose of heparin equals the number of milligrams of heparin remaining in the patient's circulation at the time of neutralization. Thus, clinical protocols to determine the initial dose of protamine first estimate the blood heparin concentration and blood volume. Direct assay of heparin concentration is difficult and unnecessary. Indirect assay using protamine effect in vitro is more accurate than ratio-based estimates and is easily performed. Three different methods of choosing an initial protamine dose are commonly used:

1. Empiric ratio. Most clinicians choose a dose of protamine based on the total number of units of heparin administered, giving between 0.6 and 1.3 mg of protamine for every 100 units of heparin administered. **Clinical efficacy has been documented using a ratio
11 as low as 0.6 mg protamine to 100 units of heparin administered.** Initial doses using this ratio result in a mild-to-moderate protamine excess relative to heparin that ensures total neutralization and minimizes the likelihood of subsequent heparin rebound. Ratios exceeding 1 mg/100 units tend to be excessive.

Example: A patient receives 25,000 units of heparin before CPB, with no subsequent heparin required, and 5,000 units in the bypass pump prime. A ratio of 1 mg:100 units yields a 300 mg protamine neutralizing dose. A ratio of 0.6 mg:100 units would result in 180 mg of protamine as the neutralizing dose. The former dose applies best when the patient receives all pump blood, unwashed, prior to protamine administration; the latter dose makes most sense for prolonged bypass during which heparin had ample opportunity for metabolism and excretion.

2. Estimated from a heparin dose-response curve. This method depends upon construction of a heparin dose-response curve prior to or during bypass (see Fig. 19.3). The technique then estimates the blood concentration of heparin at the time of neutralization. See Fig. 19.3 legend for details. Assumptions include (i) linearity of the heparin dose–ACT response relationship; (ii) potential extrapolation beyond actual data collected; (iii) constancy of the volume of distribution of heparin and protamine. Most often, clinicians choose the arbitrary ratio of 1 mg of protamine to 100 units of heparin to calculate the protamine dose.

3. Calculated from in vitro protamine effect, by measuring ACT both with and without protamine added to blood at the time of neutralization. The HMS system from Medtronic HemoTec automates this technique to calculate protamine dose. These curves assume a linear dose-response and extrapolate to a baseline ACT in calculating the initial protamine dose. These devices also calculate blood volume based on patient height and weight rather than on any definitive measurement, which can be a source of error. The same protamine titration curve can be performed using the TEG, but this assay has not become fully automated.

C. Protamine administration. Always administer protamine slowly. The rate of administration is more important than the route of administration in preventing adverse hemodynamic

effects (see Section **III.E.1**). One can either use a syringe or dilute the drug in a small volume of intravenous fluid and infuse by gravity or calibrated pump. Because the
12 syringe technique results in multiple boluses, restricting its use to doses less than 1 mg/kg, or 20 mg in any 60-s period, appears advisable. **We recommend a continuous infusion technique rather than hand-operated syringe administration,** because this reduces the natural tendency to administer the protamine too quickly and it frees our hands for other important patient care activities (e.g., vasoactive drug titration, echocardiography examination) that coincide with protamine administration.

1. The injected dose of protamine cannot neutralize heparin bound to plasma proteins or within endothelial cells. Release of heparin from these stored areas after initial protamine administration may result in reappearance of heparin anticoagulant effect (heparin rebound). Small additional doses of protamine will provide neutralization when repeat testing (e.g., ACT initially normalizes to 110 s but 30 min later is 140 s) shows a heparin effect in a bleeding patient.
2. Protamine does not remain long in the vascular system following administration. Therefore, administration of heparinized blood, such as that remaining in the CPB machine without washing, following completion of the neutralizing protamine infusion, will likely result in renewed anticoagulation to a small extent. An additional small dose of protamine, about 1 mg/20 mL of transfused pump blood, should address this contingency.

D. **Monitoring heparin neutralization**

1. ACT. After protamine administration, the ACT test should return a value no more than 10% above the value before heparin administration. If more prolonged, residual heparin activity is likely. An ACT value that remains prolonged despite additional protamine suggests a technical error or, less commonly, some other hemostatic abnormality.
2. Protamine titration. This test utilizes a series of tubes with increasing amounts of added protamine, beginning with none. One adds patient blood to each tube and determines which tube clots first. Because protamine has anticoagulant properties in vitro, it prolongs the coagulation time of normal blood in test tubes. Knowing which tube clots first allows identification of unneutralized heparin as well as estimation of the additional amount of protamine needed to achieve complete neutralization. This test can be performed manually or by using an automated device (Medtronic HemoTec).

E. **Adverse effects** [21].

1. **Hypotension from rapid administration. Administration of a neutralizing dose of**
13 **protamine (about 3 mg/kg) over 3 or fewer minutes decreases both systemic and pulmonary arterial pressures as well as venous return.** This predictable response may be blunted, but not predictably avoided, by volume loading. Release of vasoactive compounds from mast cells or other sites may be responsible for this adverse response.
2. Anaphylactoid reactions. Although protamine is a foreign protein, immune responses occur infrequently following exposure so that true allergy to protamine is uncommon. Table 19.3 lists those patients at potential risk.

TABLE 19.3 Patients at potential risk for true allergy to protamine

Condition	Risk increase
Prior reaction to protamine	189-fold
Allergy to true (vertebrate) fish	24.5-fold
Exposure to neutral protamine Hagedorn (NPH) insulin	8.2-fold
Allergy to any drug	3.0-fold
Prior exposure to protamine	No increase!

Adapted from Kimmel SE, Sekeres MA, Berlin JA, et al. Risk factors for clinically important adverse events after protamine administration following cardiopulmonary bypass. *J Am Coll Card.* 1998;32:1916.

3. Pulmonary vasoconstriction. Occasionally protamine increases pulmonary arterial pressure, resulting in right ventricular failure, decreased cardiac output, and systemic hypotension. Formation of large heparin–protamine complexes may stimulate production of thromboxane by pulmonary macrophages, causing vasoconstriction. In some animal models, the probability of experiencing this response is increased by faster rates of protamine administration.
4. Antihemostatic effects. Protamine activates thrombin receptors on platelets, causing partial activation and subsequent impairment of platelet aggregation. Transient thrombocytopenia also occurs in the first hour after a full neutralizing dose of protamine. Inhibition of plasma coagulation can also occur.
5. **Treatment of adverse protamine reactions.** Systemic hypotension within 10 min of protamine administration suggests protamine as the cause, but other causes such as hypovolemia and left ventricular dysfunction should be considered. Specific treatment depends on other hemodynamic events.
   a. Normal or low pulmonary artery pressures suggest either rapid administration or an anaphylactoid reaction. Rapid fluid administration alone often suffices to treat the former, whereas the latter cause usually requires aggressive volume resuscitation, large doses of epinephrine, and possibly other vasoactive compounds and inhaled bronchodilators. Refer to other sources for the treatment of acute anaphylaxis, including use of systemic steroids.
   b. High pulmonary artery pressures suggest a pulmonary vasoconstriction reaction. Inotropes with pulmonary dilating properties, such as isoproterenol or milrinone, will support the failing heart while facilitating movement of blood across the pulmonary circulation. Nitric oxide may also be useful. With extreme hemodynamic deterioration, reinstitution of CPB may be necessary. In this case, give a full heparin dose (at least 300 U/kg). Occasionally, heparin alone will correct the pulmonary hypertension (presumably by breaking up large heparin–protamine complexes, the putative stimulant to thromboxane production) such that reinstitution of CPB no longer becomes necessary.
6. **Prevention of adverse responses**
   a. **Rate of administration. Always administer fully neutralizing doses of protamine slowly (minimum duration 3 min, with a target of 10 min recommended).** Rather than depend on volume loading to prevent hypotension, simply dilute the drug and give it slowly. Place the calculated dose in 50 mL or more of clear fluid and connect a small-drop (approximately 60 drops/mL) administration set to limit the infusion rate or use an infusion pump connected either to a 50 mL syringe or a 50 mL (or greater) fluid bag containing protamine. Some clinicians advocate a protamine "test dose," such as 1 mg intravenously, prior to protamine administration. Our view is that slow initiation of a continuous protamine infusion accomplishes the same end, after which the infusion rate can be increased as tolerated down to a minimum infusion time as above.
   b. Route of administration. The preponderance of evidence suggests that peripheral vein infusion offers no benefit over central venous infusion as long as the infusion is dilute and not rapid. Injection directly into the aorta provides no reliable protection and risks introduction of embolic material, such as small bubbles, pieces of rubber stopper, or glass.
   c. High-risk subgroups. Patients without previous exposure to protamine, including those with diabetes or prior vasectomy, require no special measures before initial exposure. **Even patients who have received protamine-containing insulin preparations rarely develop an adverse response.** Only patients with a prior history of an adverse response to protamine warrant special treatment. See Table 19.3 for the relative risks of protamine administration to these subgroups.
   d. Prior protamine reaction. Prepare a special, dilute protamine solution of about 1 mg in 100 mL and administer over 10 min. If no adverse response occurs, administer the fully neutralizing dose as described earlier. Skin tests taken before giving protamine provide little predictive value and frequently are falsely positive. Special immunologic tests for protamine allergy, such as radioallergosorbent test (RAST) and ELISA, also demonstrate many false-positive results.

F. Alternatives to protamine administration

1. Allow heparin's effect to dissipate. This approach results in continued hemorrhage with substantial transfusion requirements and bouts of hypovolemia and the potential for consumptive coagulopathy. Although this may be the only option available, ideally it should be avoided.
2. Platelet concentrates. Platelet factor 4 (PF4) is released from activated platelets. It combines with and neutralizes heparin. However, platelet concentrates do not effectively restore coagulation following CPB. A recombinant form of PF4 failed in clinical trials as a protamine alternative.
3. Hexadimethrine. This synthetic polycation, no longer readily available in the United States because of renal toxicity, can avoid true allergic reactions to protamine. However, like protamine, it forms complexes with heparin that can incite pulmonary vasoconstriction if administered quickly.
4. Methylene blue. Even large doses do not effectively restore the ACT. However, inhibition of nitric oxide synthetase can incite pulmonary hypertension, making this approach potentially hazardous.
5. Investigational substances. Heparinase I, an enzyme produced by harmless soil bacteria, failed in clinical trials as a protamine alternative. Virus-like particles, engineered from bacteriophage Qβ coat protein, have shown consistent neutralization of heparin with less variability than protamine in plasma from heparin-treated patients [22]. Cationically modified chitosan binds to heparin to form complexes similar to those formed by protamine [23].
6. With no alternative to protamine immediately available, or even under active clinical investigation, alternatives to heparin (see Section II.E) assume greater importance in the management of patients with demonstrated severe adverse responses to protamine.

IV. Hemostatic abnormalities in the cardiac surgical patient [1,24]

A. Management of the patient taking preoperative antithrombotic drugs. Table 19.4 lists commonly used antithrombotic drugs and their mechanisms of action.

1. Anticoagulant therapy. Patients receiving warfarin anticoagulant medications should be advised to discontinue the medication 3 to 5 days before the anticipated cardiac surgery. Generally an INR value less than 2 reflects an acceptable recovery of vitamin K-dependent clotting factors. In fact, some residual inhibition of the extrinsic coagulation pathway advantageously accentuates anticoagulation for CPB. If anticoagulation is so vitally important that it must be maintained until the time of surgery, an intravenous infusion of heparin may be started preoperatively. Heparin may be discontinued a few hours before surgery or continued into the operative period.
   a. In urgent or semi-urgent surgery, the effects of warfarin may need rapid reversal which can be accomplished by giving FFP until INR correction occurs [25].
   b. In clinical studies, prothrombin complex concentrate was found more effective with quicker time to INR correction and no volume overload observed compared to FFP [26].
2. Antiplatelet therapy
   a. Aspirin. Many studies support the use of aspirin in the prevention of thrombosis in coronary and cerebral vascular disease. The patients taking aspirin therapy who are undergoing cardiac surgery have a propensity for increased bleeding postoperatively; however, the benefits of aspirin therapy, weighed against a potential for bleeding, often lead to preoperative continuation of aspirin therapy. Most patients do not bleed excessively with this approach. An increase in bleeding, if it exists, is not necessarily accompanied by an increase in transfusion requirements due to blood conservation strategies in use.
   b. Glycoprotein IIb/IIIa (GPIIb/IIIa) inhibitors. The GPIIb/IIIa receptor is the platelet fibrinogen receptor, which causes fibrinogen bridging of adjacent platelets and subsequent platelet aggregation. GPIIb/IIIa inhibitors inhibit platelet aggregation and have been increasingly used during interventional cardiology procedures. Their beneficial effects include reductions in mortality and cardiac events after angioplasty and stent procedures. However, there is strong potential for hemorrhagic complications if these patients present for emergent cardiac surgery. Currently, the three intravenous

TABLE 19.4 Common antithrombotic drugs

Drug	Mechanism	Clinical uses
Plasma coagulation inhibitors	All are parenteral agents unless otherwise stated	
Heparin	Antithrombin III agonist, anti-Xa and anti-IIa	Deep vein thrombosis, atrial fibrillation, unstable angina, surgical, extracorporeal circulation, heart valve, shunts
Low-molecular-weight heparin (includes fondaparinux)	Antithrombin III agonist, anti-Xa primarily	Deep vein thrombosis, pulmonary embolus, unstable angina
Bivalirudin	Direct thrombin inhibitor (2 site inhibition)	Percutaneous coronary intervention, acute coronary syndrome
Warfarin	Inhibit production of vitamin K-dependent coagulation factors	Deep vein thrombosis, atrial fibrillation, heart valve
Dabigatran	Oral direct thrombin inhibitor	Deep vein thrombosis, atrial fibrillation
Apixaban and Rivaroxaban	Oral anti-Xa agents	Deep vein thrombosis, atrial fibrillation
Platelet Inhibitors	(all are oral agents)	
Acetylsalicylic acid (aspirin)	Inhibit cyclooxygenase, inhibit thromboxane, prevent platelet activation	Atherosclerotic cardiovascular disease, cerebrovascular disease, percutaneous coronary intervention
Dipyridamole	Adenosine enhancing, inhibit thromboxane	Peripheral vascular disease
Abciximab	Glycoprotein IIb/IIIa receptor antagonist (monoclonal antibody)	Percutaneous coronary intervention/stent
Eptifibatide	Glycoprotein IIb/IIIa receptor antagonist (small peptide)	Percutaneous coronary intervention/stent
Tirofiban	Glycoprotein IIb/IIIa receptor antagonist (nonpeptide)	Percutaneous coronary intervention/stent
Ticlopidine	Thienopyridine, ADP receptor antagonist	Percutaneous coronary intervention/stent, cerebrovascular disease
Clopidogrel	Thienopyridine, ADP receptor antagonist	Percutaneous coronary intervention/stent, acute coronary syndrome, acute myocardial infarction
Prasugrel and Ticagrelor	Thienopyridine, P2Y12 ADP receptor inhibitors	Percutaneous coronary intervention/stent, acute coronary syndrome

ADP, adenosine diphosphate.

GPIIb/IIIa inhibitors in clinical use are abciximab, tirofiban, and eptifibatide. Abciximab is a monoclonal antibody to the GPIIb/IIIa receptor that inhibits fibrinogen binding and covalently alters the GPIIb/IIIa receptor. Tirofiban and eptifibatide are smaller competitive receptor blockers whose effects are reversible after discontinuation of therapy. Their short duration of action may mitigate some perioperative bleeding complications [26] and may actually provide some platelet protection during CPB.

c. ADP receptor inhibitors. The thienopyridine derivatives ticlopidine, clopidogrel, and prasugrel noncompetitively antagonize at a platelet ADP receptor known as the P2Y12 receptor. Blockade of this receptor by one of these agents elevates cyclic adenosine monophosphate levels to induce profound and rapid platelet disaggregation. Clopidogrel use in conjunction with percutaneous coronary intervention or in acute coronary syndromes reduces the occurrence of adverse ischemic events [27]. Antiplatelet activity is permanent for the life span of the platelet because the P2Y12 receptor is permanently altered. Clopidogrel is a pro-drug that is metabolized by cytochrome P450 (2C19 and

TABLE 19.5 Causes of platelet dysfunction in cardiac surgery

CPB-related causes
Hypothermia
Materials-induced activation
Trauma-induced activation (cardiotomy suction)
Fibrinolysis
Glycoprotein Ib receptor downregulation
Glycoprotein IIb/IIIa receptor downregulation/destruction
Thrombin receptor downregulation/destruction
Drug-related causes
Heparin
Nitrates
Phosphodiesterase inhibitors
Protamine
Platelet antagonists preoperatively

3A4) to its active metabolite. The combination of clopidogrel and aspirin is synergistic. Meta-analyses of comparative trials demonstrate that clopidogrel pre-treatment is associated with more bleeding than that observed in non-exposed patients [28].

B. Abnormalities acquired during cardiac surgery

1. Endothelial dysfunction. Contact of blood with extracorporeal surfaces initiates a "total body inflammatory response" characterized by activation of coagulation, fibrinolysis, and inflammation. This leads to an abnormal cellular–endothelial interaction.
2. Persistent heparin effect. This is uncommon because most clinicians fully neutralize the administered heparin, although **heparin rebound (resumption of heparin effect after complete neutralization) is relatively common within the first 2 hrs following CPB, and usually responds well to small (e.g., 25 mg) incremental doses of protamine.**
3. Platelet abnormalities (Table 19.5)
   a. Thrombocytopenia occurs frequently after CPB due to dilution of the blood volume with extracorporeal circuit volume and to platelet consumption or sequestration. This thrombocytopenia can be severe (<50,000/μL) but, in the absence of other hemostasis abnormalities, often does not lead to excessive bleeding. With modern techniques, platelet counts after CPB most often exceed 100,000/μL.
   b. Platelet dysfunction. **The most prevalent yet elusive cause of hemostatic abnormalities after CPB is platelet dysfunction.** Platelets are rendered inactive by contact activation from the extracorporeal surfaces, hypothermia, receptor downregulation, and by heparin and protamine. Heparin activates platelets to render them less functional after CPB, and protamine also depresses platelet function. The use of antithrombotic drugs preoperatively leads to an even greater degree of platelet dysfunction after CPB.
4. Coagulopathy. Hemodilution and consumption of coagulation factors by microvascular coagulation combine to cause the deficiencies of coagulation seen after CPB. Despite the use of large doses of heparin, contact activation causes microvascular activation of factor XII and initiates the intrinsic pathway of coagulation.
5. Fibrinolysis. Fibrinolysis can be primary or secondary during CPB (Fig. 19.4). Primary fibrinolysis occurs from release of endothelial plasminogen activators. Secondary fibrinolysis describes activation of plasmin as a result of a feedback response to fibrin formation. Circulating plasmin degradation products adversely affect platelet function.
6. Pharmacology. As noted earlier, heparin and protamine impair platelet function. Other drugs commonly used during CPB (milrinone, nitroglycerin, nitroprusside) adversely affect platelet function in vitro, but in vivo their effects appear to be clinically undetectable.
7. Hypothermia. Hypothermia impairs the enzymatic cascades of the coagulation pathway. Platelets are activated during mild hypothermia and are depressed during moderate-to-severe hypothermia.

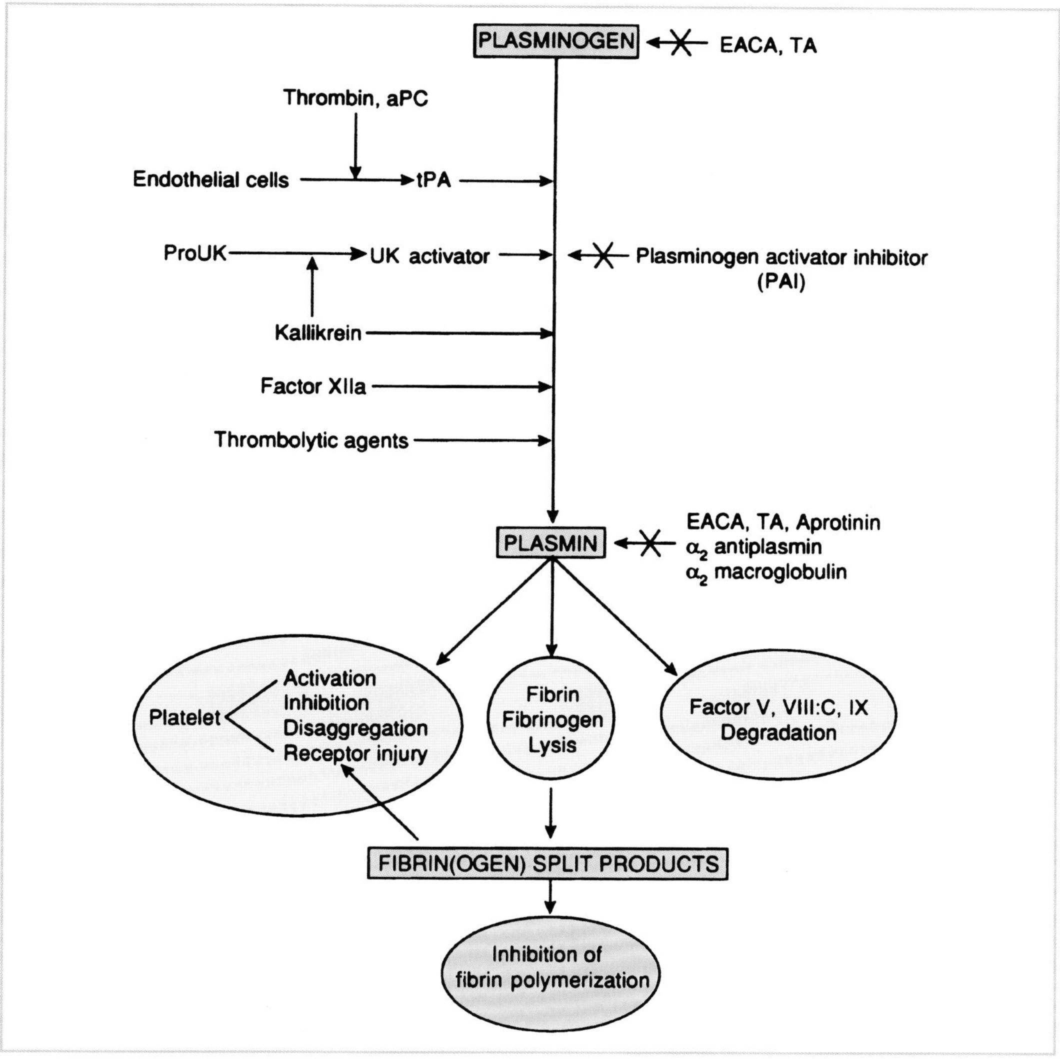

FIGURE 19.4 Schematic diagram of the fibrinolytic system displaying endogenous and exogenous activators and inhibitors of fibrinolysis. The antihemostatic actions of plasmin and fibrin(ogen) split products (FSPs) are illustrated. *aPC*, activated protein C; *EACA*, ε-aminocaproic acid; *TA*, tranexamic acid; *tPA*, tissue plasminogen activator; *UK*, urokinase.

C. Pharmacologic and protective prophylaxis

1. Platelet protection
   a. Antifibrinolytic agents. See IV.C.2.
   b. Coated surfaces. Heparin-bonded circuits attenuate the inflammatory response to CPB and may confer some platelet protective properties.
   c. Antiplatelet agents that are active during CPB may confer some platelet protection so long as they are short-acting. Patients who have emergency surgery after having been exposed to tirofiban or eptifibatide do not experience excessive postoperative bleeding and receive equivalent or reduced transfusion volumes.
2. Antifibrinolytic agents [29]
   a. Synthetic antifibrinolytic agents: ε-aminocaproic acid (EACA) and tranexamic acid (TA). EACA and TA act as lysine analogs that bind to the lysine-binding sites of

plasmin and plasminogen (Fig. 19.4). TA is a more potent analog of EACA that has a higher affinity for plasminogen than does EACA. Fibrin degradation products inhibit platelet function. Thus, plasmin inhibition may protect platelets. **The benefits of EACA and TA have been demonstrated in multiple meta-analyses to reduce bleeding in cardiac surgery, when these agents are used prophylactically (i.e., initiated before CPB and maintained throughout CPB) rather than as rescue agents** [30]. *Dosing:* EACA 100 to 150 mg/kg bolus, 10 to 15 mg/kg/hr, *or* 4 to 10 g bolus, 1 g/hr. Reports suggest constant plasma activity may be best achieved with smaller initial boluses (approximately 50 mg/kg) followed by higher maintenance doses (20 to 25 mg/kg/hr). *Dosing range:* Low dose: TA 10 to 20 mg/kg bolus, 1 to 2 mg/kg/hr; Moderate dose: 30 to 50 mg/kg bolus, 15 to 30 mg/kg/hr; *or* High dose: 5-g bolus, repeat bolus to total 15 g. The latter dosing scheme probably is much higher than necessary and there is concern that high-dose TA may be associated with central nervous system adverse events.

b. Aprotinin, a high-molecular-weight proteinase inhibitor of bovine origin, inhibits plasmin, kallikrein, and other serine proteases. Aprotinin decreases activation of the hematologic system during CPB and subsequent fibrinolysis, resulting in a 30% to 40% decrease in chest tube drainage. It is the only agent found to be successful in reducing the rate of reoperation for bleeding in meta-analyses. However, an increased rate of mortality and renal morbidity has been reported with aprotinin that caused the drug to be removed from commercial use until the data were reevaluated [31–33]. Commercial availability of aprotinin going forward remains uncertain, and this may vary from country to country. Newer protease inhibitors are currently under investigation for use in cardiac surgery.

c. Investigational substances: Carbon monoxide releasing molecule-2 (CORM-2) significantly improved velocity of clot formation and clot strength in plasma in patients both before and following CPB. Pending further trials, CORM-2 may be of use in improving coagulation and decreasing fibrinolysis in patients with persistent bleeding after CPB [34].

3. Accurate heparin and protamine dosing. Attempts to individualize heparin and protamine doses in order to minimize bleeding rely on patient-specific doses of each drug based on patient sensitivity. **A number of different heparin and protamine management strategies have been reported to result in reduced perioperative bleeding.**

a. Higher heparin concentrations during CPB have been associated with increased mediastinal tube bleeding postoperatively. Higher doses might predispose to greater bleeding as a result of heparin rebound or platelet dysfunction. This leads to the practice of giving just enough heparin to maintain a "threshold" minimum acceptable ACT.

b. Some investigators postulate that higher heparin levels allow for reduced activation of the coagulation cascade and may blunt the consumptive coagulopathy that occurs with microvascular coagulation. This leads to the practice of maintaining heparin at a specific concentration in the blood, which leads to large doses of heparin and higher ACTs. Heparin management strategies are still highly variable and institution-specific.

c. Lower protamine doses have been used successfully to neutralize heparin after CPB and have been associated with reduced bleeding and transfusion requirements. This relationship between higher heparin and lower protamine doses has been suggested to result in less postoperative bleeding.

4. Inhibition of inflammation

a. Coated surfaces. Heparin-bonded CPB circuits make the extracorporeal circuit more biocompatible and thus effectively attenuate the inflammatory response to CPB. Despite this benefit, use of these circuits has not uniformly reduced morbidity. Use of a reduced heparin dose in conjunction with heparin-bonded circuits has shown reductions in postoperative chest tube drainage and transfusion requirements, but reduced heparin dosing in this scenario is not yet fully endorsed as the overall effect on safety for CPB is unclear.

b. Steroids. Methylprednisolone 500 to 1,000 mg has proved helpful in some studies but has not been universally adopted due to risks of hyperglycemia and immune suppression.

c. Aprotinin acts by kallikrein inhibition to reduce the inflammatory response, but this can only be achieved in the high-dose range (e.g., full Hammersmith protocol). As noted above, clinical availability of aprotinin in the future is uncertain (see Section C.2.b).

d. Modified ultrafiltration has a beneficial effect of reducing postoperative morbidity and improving organ function in pediatric patients.

e. Complement inhibitors are mostly experimental agents. They act to prevent activation of complement by kallikrein inhibition or direct complement antagonism. Reduction of the inflammatory response theoretically would reduce morbidity. Clinical trials are underway to evaluate different complement inhibitors but no one agent has been statistically proven to reduce adverse events.

V. Management of postbypass bleeding [1]

A. Evaluation of hemostasis

1. Achieve surgical hemostasis
2. Confirm adequate heparin neutralization
   a. Tests of heparin neutralization: heparinase ACT, protamine titration test, heparinase thromboelastography (TEG). *Note:* The standard ACT is not a specific test for complete heparin neutralization, that is, it is possible to have ACT return to normal while some residual heparin effect remains. **If the ACT has returned to baseline and residual heparin is either suspected or identified using a protamine titration technique, treat this by titrating in additional protamine. Most often protamine 25 to 50 mg completes the neutralization.**
3. Point-of-care testing to diagnose and treat bleeding. Point-of-care tests should be used appropriately in order to accurately and rapidly pinpoint the cause of a hemostasis defect. Etiologies of post-CPB bleeding should be prioritized by the clinician and should be tested in logical order. These tests should include heparin neutralization (see V.A.2.a), platelet function, platelet number, coagulation, and fibrinolysis (Table 19.6).
   a. Tests of platelet function: TEG maximal amplitude, Sonoclot, Platelet Works, Platelet Function Analyzer-100, VerifyNow, and whole blood aggregometry to name a few. **Treatment of platelet dysfunction may include administration of desmopressin acetate (DDAVP) 0.3 μg/kg slowly (over approximately 15 to 20 min, as vasodilation may occur). If platelet number is reduced or platelet dysfunction persists after DDAVP, a transfusion of platelet concentrates is recommended.**
   b. Coagulation tests: PT, aPTT, thrombin time, ACT, TEG-R, or TEG-K value. Treatment of this abnormality includes transfusion of FFP, or occasionally administration of recombinant factor VIIa (rVIIa) when the coagulopathy is unresponsive to FFP. Administration of rVIIa will also treat CPB or drug-induced platelet dysfunction by creating a thrombin burst; however, its safety has not been fully established.

TABLE 19.6 Point-of-care tests of platelet function

Test/monitor	Mechanism
Bleeding time	Collagen-activated in vivo adhesion
Thromboelastography/Sonoclot	Viscoelastic clot strength
Platelet Function Analyzer (PFA-100)	In vitro activated bleeding time
Platelet Works	Platelet count ratio
Standard aggregometry (PRP)	Optical density–light transmittance
Whole blood aggregometry	Electrical impedance
Ultegra/VerifyNow	Activated fibrinogen bead agglutination
Clot Signature Analyzer (research)	High shear and collagen activation
Hemodyne (PRP/whole blood) (research)	Platelet-mediated force transduction

Helena Cascade HMT
PRP, platelet-rich plasma.

c. Tests of fibrinolysis: Euglobulin lysis time, TEG lysis index, fibrin degradation products, D-dimers. Treatment of primary fibrinolysis includes administration of an antifibrinolytic agent. If an antifibrinolytic agent has already been administered and discontinued, this same agent should be re-started. Starting a different class of antifibrinolytic drug in the same patient is not recommended. Secondary fibrinolysis should be treated by replacement of consumed coagulation factors (FFP or cryoprecipitate).

d. ***Note*: Treatment of any abnormal laboratory value should not take place unless warranted by the clinical situation, that is, observation of clinical coagulopathy. Treat the patient, not the number!**

B. Treatment of postbypass hemostatic disorders

Follow the nine steps below in order. They reflect the causes of postoperative bleeding in decreasing frequency of occurrence. Remember to maintain intravascular volume to avoid generating or exacerbating a consumptive coagulopathy. These steps are designed to address the situation where urgency dictates that one must treat a presumed cause before obtaining laboratory results. Do not embrace any one presumed cause; rather, constantly re-evaluate and question your assumptions. **Instead of bedside empiricism, however, we encourage the development and use of transfusion algorithms using point-of-care testing** (see V.C).

14

1. Rule out a surgical cause. Copious chest tube drainage usually results from a vessel in need of suture. A generalized ooze suggests a non-surgical cause. Keep the blood pressure in the low normal range while the surgeons effect repair, and optimally for sometime thereafter to maximize the potential for clot formation.
2. Maintain normothermia. In the effort to restore intravascular volume rapidly, clinicians must infuse refrigerated blood products only with adequate warming, lest they cause or accentuate hypothermia, thereby decreasing platelet function and enzymatic activity of clotting proteins.
3. Determine the cause. While surgeons are checking anastomoses, assure complete heparin neutralization with an ACT and aPTT, the latter showing prolongation at smaller blood concentrations of heparin. Consider measuring fibrinogen concentration, D-dimer, and thrombin time, the last of which is prolonged only by residual heparin, inadequate amount or functionality of fibrinogen, and fibrin degradation products.
4. Give more protamine if the ACT exceeds its baseline (pre-heparin) value by >10 s (or the aPTT is more than 1.3 times its control value). A dose of 25 to 50 mg usually suffices. Do so upon learning the ACT results and while awaiting other laboratory results.
5. In the absence of hypovolemia, consider application of 5 cm of positive end-expiratory pressure (PEEP) to help tamponade open blood vessels in the chest. This maneuver may be most effective after the sternum is closed because of limitations in the ability of PEEP to effectively increase mediastinal end-expiratory pressure while the sternum remains open.
6. Platelet transfusion and/or DDAVP. If testing uncovers platelet dysfunction, or if it is highly suspected, give 1 unit of platelet concentrates per 10 kg body weight for an estimated effective platelet count below 100,000/μL. While awaiting platelet concentrates from the blood bank, consider administration of DDAVP 0.3 ug/kg especially if there is laboratory evidence of platelet dysfunction (e.g., decreased maximum amplitude [MA] on TEG). This may resolve the coagulopathy and avoid the need for platelet concentrates.
7. FFP. Give 15 mL/kg for a PT in excess of 1.5 times control, or an INR in excess of 2.0.
8. Give antifibrinolytic medication. Although these agents work best when administered prophylactically before and during CPB, about half of their benefit occurs if given (or continued) in the post-CPB period. An increased D-dimer value, or teardrop-shaped TEG tracing, suggests active fibrinolysis that would warrant antifibrinolytic agent administration or higher doses if antifibrinolytic agents are already being administered.
9. Give rVIIa or cryoprecipitate. rVIIa has been associated with "miracle cures" of post-CPB coagulopathy, but its use has been limited to rescue situations and very few prospective studies about its use have been published. In cardiac surgery, reductions in bleeding have clearly been documented; however, a dose of 80 ug/kg has been associated with some hypercoagulable complications [35]. The rVIIa probably makes the most sense when given

as a secondary intervention when two "rounds" of FFP 10 to 15 mL/kg and platelet concentrates 1 unit/10 kg have not resolved the coagulopathy. Overwhelming coagulopathy may at times call for earlier use of this potentially lifesaving agent, for which an initial dose of 30 to 40 ug/kg is recommended. Cryoprecipitate 1 unit/4 kg body weight (generally 15 to 20 units in adults) will correct fibrinogen deficiency (<100 mg/dL). Its use is best reserved for situations where hypofibrinogenemia has been documented.

C. **Transfusion medicine and the use of algorithms.** Allogeneic transfusions after CPB are common because of the wide range of hemostatic insults incurred. **The lack of adequate testing of hemostasis and the subjectivity of a diagnosis of microvascular bleeding lead to indiscriminate transfusion practices.**

1. Transfusion of red blood cells, platelets, and plasma is fraught with adverse effects, not least of which are infectious disease transmission, acute lung injury, and immunomodulation. The rational use of transfusion algorithms should create an approach to transfusion medicine that is stepwise, logical, and based on the hemostatic defects that are most common and easily treated. This usually starts with a specific test of heparin neutralization. After residual heparin is ruled out, other coagulation tests are measured.
2. **One of the most critical tests that should be measured "early" in a transfusion algorithm is an accurate point-of-care test of platelet function.** This will minimize the occurrence of indiscriminate transfusion practices because subjective assessment of microvascular bleeding often leads to empiric transfusion practices. Rapid and accurate diagnosis of a hemostasis abnormality after CPB is critical. TEG predicts abnormal bleeding after CPB and has been used successfully in a number of algorithms to reduce the incidence of transfusion [36,37]. Other point-of-care monitors (e.g., PT, aPTT, and platelet count) used in rational algorithms have proved effective in reducing transfusions in routine CPB patients and in patients who have been exposed to antithrombotic agents preoperatively [38].
3. Aside from confirming neutralization of heparin, the routine use of coagulation tests after CPB has not proven beneficial in the absence of a clinical coagulopathy.

REFERENCES

1. Horrow JC, Mueksch JN. Coagulation testing. In: Gravlee GP, Davis RF, Stammers AH, Ungerleider RM, eds. *Cardiopulmonary Bypass: Principles and Practice.* 3rd ed. Philadelphia, PA: Lippincott Williams & Wilkins; 2008:459–471.
2. Shore-Lesserson L, Gravlee GP. Anticoagulation for cardiopulmonary bypass. In: Gravlee GP, Davis RF, Stammers AH, Ungerleider RM, eds. *Cardiopulmonary Bypass: Principles and Practice.* 3rd ed. Philadelphia, PA: Lippincott Williams & Wilkins; 2008:472–501.
3. Merton RE, Curtis AD, Thomas DP. A comparison of heparin potency estimates obtained by activated partial thromboplastin time and British pharmacopoeial assays. *Thromb Haemost.* 1985;53:116–117.
4. Gravlee GP, Angert KC, Tucker WY, et al. Early anticoagulation peak and rapid distribution after intravenous heparin. *Anesthesiology.* 1988;68:126–129.
5. Heres EK, Speight K, Benckart D, et al. The clinical onset of heparin is rapid. *Anesth Analg.* 2001;92:1391–1395.
6. Olsson P, Lagergren H, Ek S. The elimination from plasma of intravenous heparin. An experimental study on dogs and humans. *Acta Med Scand.* 1963;173:619–630.
7. Bull BS, Korpman RA, Huse WM, et al. Heparin therapy during extracorporeal circulation. I. Problems inherent in existing heparin protocols. *J Thorac Cardiovasc Surg.* 1975;69:674–684.
8. Cohen EJ, Camerlengo LJ, Dearing JP. Activated clotting times and cardiopulmonary bypass I: The effect of hemodilution and hypothermia upon activated clotting time. *J Extracorp Technol.* 1980;12:139–141.
9. Gravlee GP, Case LD, Angert KC, et al. Variability of the activated coagulation time. *Anesth Analg.* 1988;67:469–472.
10. Despotis GJ, Summerfield AL, Joist JH. Comparison of activated coagulation time and whole blood heparin measurements with laboratory plasma anti-Xa heparin concentration in patients having cardiac operations. *J Thorac Cardiovasc Surg.* 1994;108:1076–1082.
11. Koster A, Despotis G, Gruendel M, et al. The plasma supplemented modified activated clotting time for monitoring of heparinization during cardiopulmonary bypass: A pilot investigation. *Anesth Analg.* 2002;95:26–30.
12. Chavez JJ, Foley DE, Snider CC, et al. A novel thrombelastograph tissue factor/kaolin assay of activated clotting times for monitoring heparin anticoagulation during cardiopulmonary bypass. *Anesth Analg.* 2004;99:1290–1294.
13. Hellstern P, Bach J, Simon M, et al. Heparin monitoring during cardiopulmonary bypass surgery using the one-step point-of-care whole blood anti-factor-Xa clotting assay heptest-POC-Hi. *J Extra Corpor Technol.* 2007;39:81–86.
14. Ganter MT, Monn A, Tavakoli R, et al. Kaolin-based activated coagulation time measured by sonoclot in patients undergoing cardiopulmonary bypass. *J Cardiothorac Vasc Anesth.* 2007;21:524–528.

15. Bennett-Guerrero E, Slaughter TF, White WD, et al. Preoperative anti-PF4/heparin antibody level predicts adverse outcome after cardiac surgery. *J Thorac Cardiovasc Surg.* 2005;130:1567–1572.
16. Warkentin TE, Kelton JG. Temporal aspects of heparin-induced thrombocytopenia. *N Engl J Med.* 2001;344:1286–1292.
17. Koster A, Meyer O, Hausmann H, et al. In vitro cross-reactivity of danaparoid sodium in patients with heparin-induced thrombocytopenia type II undergoing cardiovascular surgery. *J Clin Anesth.* 2000;12:324–327.
18. Greinacher A, Volpel H, Janssens U, et al. Recombinant hirudin (lepirudin) provides safe and effective anticoagulation in patients with heparin-induced thrombocytopenia. A prospective study. *Circulation.* 1999;99:73–80.
19. Koster A, Hansen R, Grauhan O, et al. Hirudin monitoring using the TAS ecarin clotting time in patients with heparin-induced thrombocytopenia type II. *J Cardiothorac Vasc Anesth.* 2000;14:249–252.
20. Metz S, Horrow JC. Pharmacologic manipulation of coagulation: protamine and other heparin antagonists. In: Lake CL, Moore RA, eds. *Blood: Hemostasis, Transfusion, and Alternatives in the Perioperative Period.* New York, NY: Raven Press; 1995:119–130.
21. Horrow JC. Protamine: A review of its toxicity. *Anesth Analg.* 1985;64:348–361.
22. Gale AJ, Elias DJ, Averell PM, et al. Engineered virus-like nanoparticles reverse heparin anticoagulation more consistently than protamine in plasma from heparin-treated patients. *Thromb Res.* 2011;128(suppl 4):e9–e13. Epub 2011 Apr 14.
23. Kamiński K, Szczubiałka K, Zazakowny K, et al. Chitosan derivatives as novel potential heparin reversal agents. *J Med Chem.* 2010;53:4141–4147.
24. Spiess BD, Horrow JC, Kaplan JA. Transfusion medicine and coagulation disorders. In: Kaplan JA, Reich DL, Savino JS, eds. *Kaplan's Cardiac Anesthesia: The Echo Era.* 6th ed. Philadelphia, PA: Elsevier Saunders; 2011:949–991.
25. Demeyere R, Gillardin S, Arnout J, et al. Comparison of fresh frozen plasma and prothrombin complex concentrate for the reversal of oral anticoagulants in patients undergoing cardiopulmonary bypass surgery: a randomized study. *Vox Sang.* 2010;99:251–260.
26. Brown DL, Fann CS, Chang CJ. Meta-analysis of effectiveness and safety of abciximab versus eptifibatide or tirofiban in percutaneous coronary intervention. *Am J Cardiol.* 2001;87:537–541.
27. Bertrand ME, Rupprecht HJ, Urban P, et al. Double-blind study of the safety of clopidogrel with and without a loading dose in combination with aspirin compared with ticlopidine in combination with aspirin after coronary stenting: the Clopidogrel Aspirin Stent International Cooperative Study (CLASSICS). *Circulation.* 2000;102:624–629.
28. Purkayastha S, Athanasiou T, Malinovski V, et al. Does clopidogrel affect outcome after coronary artery bypass grafting? A meta-analysis. *Heart.* 2006;92:531–532.
29. Levi M, Cromheecke ME, de Jonge E, et al. Pharmacologic strategies to decrease excessive blood loss in cardiac surgery: A meta-analysis of clinically relevant endpoints. *Lancet.* 1999;354:1940–1947.
30. Brown JR, Birkmeyer NJO, O'Connor JT. Meta-analysis comparing the effectiveness and adverse outcomes of antifibrinolytic agents in cardiac surgery. *Circulation.* 2007;115:2801–2813.
31. Mangano DT, Tudor IC, Dietzel C. The risk associated with aprotinin in cardiac surgery. *N Engl J Med.* 2006;354:353–365.
32. Fergusson DA, Hebert PC, Mazur CD, et al. A comparison of aprotinin and lysine analogues in high-risk cardiac surgery. *N Engl J Med.* 2008;358:2319–2331.
33. Henry D, Carless P, Fergusson D, et al. The safety of aprotinin and lysine-derived antifibrinolytic drugs in cardiac surgery: A meta-analysis. *CMAJ.* 2009;180(suppl 2):183–193.
34. Malayaman SN, Entwistle JW 3rd, Boateng P, et al. Carbon monoxide releasing molecule-2 improves coagulation in patient plasma in vitro following cardiopulmonary bypass. *Blood Coagul Fibrinolysis.* 2011;22:362–368.
35. Gill R, Herbertson M, Vuylsteke A, et al. Placebo-controlled trial in the setting of bleeding after cardiac surgery. Safety and efficacy of recombinant activated factor VII: a randomized placebo-controlled trial in the setting of bleeding after cardiac surgery. *Circulation.* 2009;120:21–27.
36. Shore-Lesserson L, Manspeizer HE, DePerio M, et al. Thromboelastography-guided transfusion algorithm reduces transfusions in complex cardiac surgery. *Anesth Analg.* 1999;88:312–319.
37. Nuttall GA, Oliver WC, Santrach PJ, et al. Efficacy of a simple intraoperative transfusion algorithm for nonerythrocyte component utilization after cardiopulmonary bypass. *Anesthesiology.* 2001;94:773–781.
38. Chen L, Bracey AW, Radovancevic R, et al. Clopidogrel and bleeding in patients undergoing elective coronary artery bypass grafting. *J Thorac Cardiovasc Surg.* 2004;128:425–431.

20 Anesthetic Considerations for Patients with Pericardial Disease

Matthew M. Townsley and Michael L. Shelton

KEY POINTS

1. Despite the many and varied etiologies, the manifestations of pericardial disease are primarily expressed as pericardial effusion, inflammation, and constriction. The common theme is impaired cardiac filling and diastolic dysfunction.
2. A relatively small amount of fluid (50 to 100 mL) that accumulates **acutely** within the closed pericardial space is sufficient to dramatically increase intrapericardial pressure and interfere with cardiac filling. Conversely, a **chronic** increase in pericardial fluid will produce tamponade only after a large volume of fluid accumulation, perhaps as great as a liter.
3. The primary abnormality in cardiac tamponade is impaired cardiac filling caused by increased intrapericardial pressure. The right heart is most vulnerable to compression due to its thin walls and lower chamber pressures.
4. Tamponade is often described as **Beck's Triad**: muffled heart sounds, jugular venous distension, and hypotension.
5. **Pulsus Paradoxus** (drop in systolic pressure during inspiration) occurs secondary to septal shift crowding the left ventricle during right ventricular filling. The opposite occurs during expiration. This phenomenon is described as enhanced ventricular interdependence.
6. **Electrical alternans** is due to the swinging motion of the heart in the pericardial sac.
7. Diastolic collapse lasting more than one-third of diastole demonstrated on echocardiography is fairly specific for tamponade.
8. Anesthetic induction in patients with tamponade can lead to cardiovascular collapse. If pericardiocentesis cannot be performed in a compromised patient and a surgical procedure is utilized instead, the patient should be prepped and draped prior to anesthetic induction so that surgery can proceed immediately after intubation. Volume loading prior to general anesthetic induction as well as inotropes may be required. Expect further deterioration after positive pressure ventilation is initiated.
9. Constrictive pericarditis (CP) is a diagnosis that encompasses a wide-spectrum of disease, from acute and subacute cases that may resolve spontaneously or with medical therapy to classic chronic progressive CP.
10. Although manifestations of hemodynamic instability are less with chronic pericarditis than with tamponade, induction and maintenance of anesthesia must encompass the same concerns.

I. Introduction. The clinical significance of pericardial disease encompasses a wide spectrum, ranging from asymptomatic subclinical disease to acute life-threatening emergencies. This spectrum is best appreciated with a thorough understanding of the physiologic derangements these disorders place upon the heart and its function. In addition, the perioperative care of these patients requires an appreciation of how this altered physiology is influenced by anesthetic techniques and pharmacology. Further complicating the management of these patients are the underlying conditions causing the pericardial dysfunction, which introduce additional management concerns of their own. Despite the many and varied etiologies, the manifestations of pericardial disease are primarily expressed
1 as pericardial effusion, inflammation, and constriction. Regardless, the common theme of most all pericardial pathology is **impaired cardiac filling** and **diastolic dysfunction**. This chapter reviews the normal structure and function of the pericardium, as well as the most common etiologies leading to pericardial disease. The two most clinically relevant pericardial disorders will be discussed in detail: **cardiac tamponade and constrictive pericarditis**.

II. Pericardial anatomy and physiology

A. The normal pericardium is a dual-enveloped sac surrounding the heart and great vessels. It comprises two layers: the parietal pericardium and the visceral pericardium. The **parietal pericardium** is a thick, fibrous outer layer composed primarily of collagen and elastin. It attaches to the adventitia of the great vessels, diaphragm, sternum, and the vertebral bodies. The inner **visceral pericardium** rests on the surface of the heart. It is composed of a single layer of mesothelial cells, which adhere to the pericardium. Normal pericardial thickness is 1 to 2 mm.

B. Two distinct sinuses are formed at points where the pericardium appears to fold onto itself. The **oblique sinus** forms posteriorly, between the left atrium and pulmonary veins, and is a common location for blood to collect after cardiac surgery. The **transverse sinus** also forms posteriorly behind the left atrium, situated behind the aorta and pulmonary artery (Fig. 20.1).

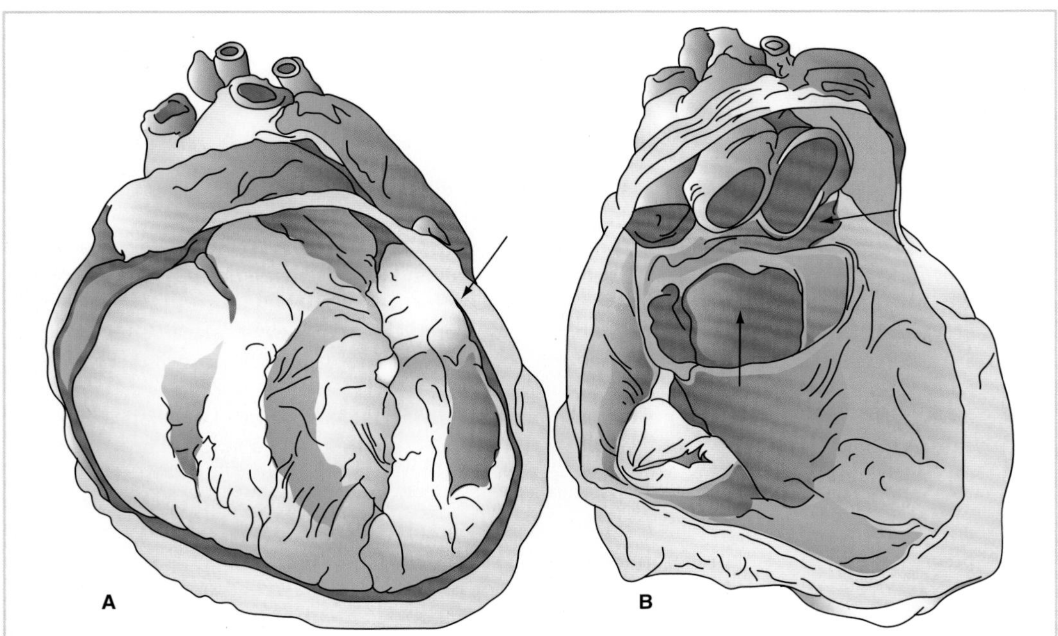

FIGURE 20.1 Anatomy of the pericardium and pericardial sinuses. The left image **(A)** demonstrates the heart in situ with a section of the parietal pericardium cut away. The left panel **(B)**, with the heart cut away, demonstrates the oblique sinus (*arrow at 6 o'clock*) and the transverse sinus (*arrow at 3 o'clock*). (Reused from Lachman N, Syed FF, Habib A, et al. Correlative anatomy for the electrophysiologist, part 1: The pericardial space, oblique sinus, transverse sinus. *J Cardiovasc Electrophysiol.* 2010;21(suppl 12):1421–1426).

C. Normal cardiac function can still occur in the absence of the pericardium, making it nonessential for survival. However, it does provide several useful physiologic functions. It aids in the reducing friction between the heart and surrounding structures, limits acute dilatation of cardiac chambers, provides a barrier to infection, optimizes coupling of left and right ventricular filling and function, and limits excessive motion of the heart within the chest cavity. The pericardium is also metabolically active, secreting prostaglandins that affect coronary artery tone and cardiac reflexes [1].

D. The pericardium is a highly innervated structure. Pericardial inflammation or manipulation may produce severe pain or vagally mediated reflexes.

III. Causes of pericardial disease. The etiologies of pericardial disease are numerous and can lead to pericardial inflammation, effusion, or both. Care of these patients must consider not only the pathological process of the pericardium, but the manifestations and complications of the underlying disease states. Pericardial disease can be caused by infection (e.g., viral, bacterial, fungal, tuberculosis), connective tissue disorders (e.g., systemic lupus erythematosus, sarcoidosis, rheumatoid arthritis), trauma, uremia, malignancy, post-myocardial infarction (Dressler's Syndrome), or following cardiac surgery and other invasive cardiac procedures.

IV. Pericardial tamponade

A. **Natural History**

1. **Etiology.** The visceral pericardium is responsible for the production of pericardial fluid, which is an ultrafiltrate of plasma. This fluid provides lubrication to decrease friction between the pericardial layers. The pericardial space normally contains **10 to 50 mL** of fluid, which is drained by the lymphatic system. As previously discussed, many conditions can cause fluid accumulation within the pericardial space, which may be serous, serosanguinous, purulent, or blood. However, the majority of cardiac effusions do not progress to tamponade. Tamponade occurs when the heart becomes extrinsically compressed by the contents of the pericardium, diminishing venous filling and, ultimately, cardiac output. In addition to effusion fluid, tamponade may also be caused by the accumulation of clot or air in the pericardial space. Acute, life-threatening tamponade most frequently results from bleeding into the pericardial space after cardiac surgery or other invasive cardiac procedures, following blunt chest trauma, or due to a ruptured ascending aortic aneurysm or aortic dissection [2]. Tamponade may occur in as many as 8.8% of patients presenting for cardiac surgery, although it is more commonly seen after valve surgery than coronary artery bypass grafting (CABG). The onset is often in the immediate postoperative period, but may occur as late as several days following surgery. Frequently there is localized clot or effusion, which causes nonuniform compression of the cardiac chambers and manifests without the classical clinical features of tamponade (Fig. 20.2). The diagnosis of post-cardiac surgery tamponade can therefore be challenging, especially when considering the many potential causes of hemodynamic instability during this time period. Unfortunately, morbidity and mortality increases significantly the longer the diagnosis is delayed [3].

2. **Symptomatology.** Symptoms of cardiac tamponade are usually rapid in onset, but depend upon the rate at which pericardial fluid accumulates. A relatively small amount of fluid (50 to 100 mL) that accumulates acutely within the closed pericardial space is sufficient to
2 dramatically increase intrapericardial pressure and interfere with cardiac filling. However, a chronic increase in pericardial fluid will produce tamponade only after a large volume is present (>1 L). A gradual accumulation of fluid stretches the parietal pericardium, allowing larger volumes to be tolerated before symptoms occur. Lack of this pericardial stretch explains the abrupt onset of symptoms and clinical deterioration in the setting of acute tamponade. The primary symptoms of cardiac tamponade include dyspnea, orthopnea, diaphoresis, and chest pain. Dyspnea is often the first and most sensitive symptom [4].

B. **Pathophysiology.** The primary abnormality in cardiac tamponade is impaired diastolic filling of the heart, caused by increased intrapericardial pressure that leads to compression of the
3 atria and ventricles. The right heart is most vulnerable to the compression due to its thinner walls and lower chamber pressures. Diastolic filling pressures (e.g., central venous pressure

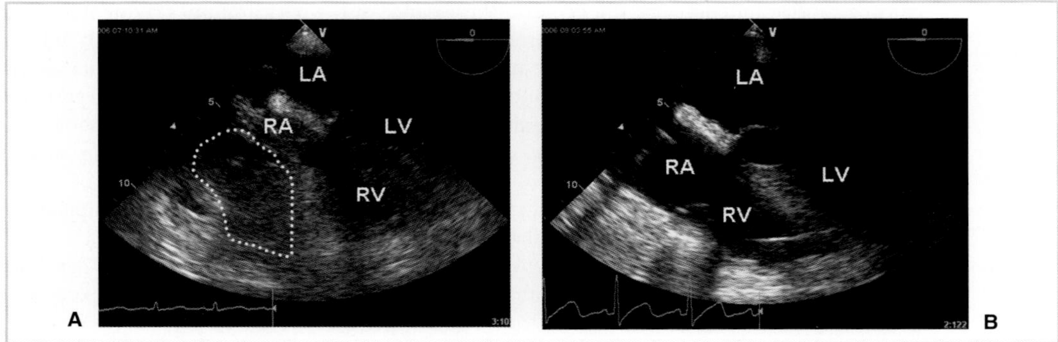

FIGURE 20.2 Regional tamponade following cardiac surgery. In this transesophageal (TEE) midesophageal four-chamber view, a localized clot is seen compressing both the right atrium and right ventricle **(A)**. Chamber compression is relieved following clot removal **(B)**. RA, right atrium; RV, right ventricle; LA, left atrium; LV, left ventricle. (Fontes ML, Skubas N, Osorio J. Cardiac tamponade. In: Yao FF, Fontes ML, Malhotra V, eds. *Yao & Artusio's Anesthesiology: Problem Oriented Patient Management.* 6th ed. Philadelphia, PA: Lippincott Williams & Wilkins; 2008:327.)

[CVP], left atrial pressure [LAP], pulmonary capillary wedge pressure [PCWP], left ventricular end-diastolic pressure [LVEDP] and right ventricular end-diastolic pressure [RVEDP]) become elevated and are nearly equal to each other, as well as the intrapericardial pressure, hence the terminology in tamponade of equalization of pressures. Physiologic manifestations of pericardial fluid, as previously discussed, are contingent upon the rate and amount of fluid accumulation, with a continuum ranging from clinically insignificant to severe hemodynamic collapse (Fig. 20.3). Ventricular preload and volume is critically reduced, which translates into

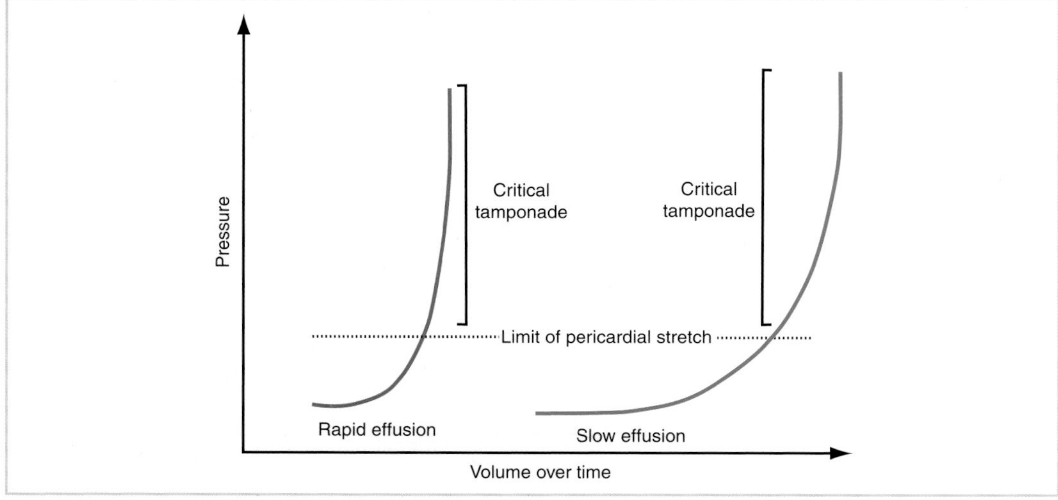

FIGURE 20.3 Pressure–volume relationship in acute versus chronic pericardial effusions. Intrapericardial pressure is contingent upon the change in intrapericardial volume. Pressure is relatively stable until a critical volume occurs. At this point, minimal increases in volume will lead to significant changes in intrapericardial pressure. With chronic effusions, pericardial stretch allows for a greater amount of volume to accumulate before critical increases in pressure occur. The lack of pericardial stretch explains the significant elevations in pressures seen with only small amounts of rapidly accumulating intrapericardial fluid. (Figure from Avery EG, Shernan SK. Echocardiographic evaluation of pericardial disease. In: Savage RM, Aronson SA, Shernan SK, eds. *Comprehensive Textbook of Perioperative Transesophageal Echocardiography.* 2nd ed. Philadelphia, PA: Lippincott Williams & Wilkins; 2011:726.)

decreased stroke volume, cardiac output, and systemic blood pressure. Compensatory sympathetic responses attempt to offset this reduction in stroke volume, with elevated levels of plasma catecholamines resulting in systemic vasoconstriction and tachycardia. This may temporarily maintain cardiac output and systemic perfusion; however, sudden hemodynamic collapse may rapidly occur with the depletion of catecholamines and/or continued elevation of intrapericardial pressure.

C. **Diagnostic evaluation and assessment**

1. **Clinical evaluation**

4 a. Acute tamponade is often described by **Beck's triad**: muffled heart sounds, jugular venous distention (JVD) due to increased venous pressure, and hypotension. Other common findings include tachypnea and tachycardia.

5 b. **Pulsus paradoxus** although not specific for tamponade, may be observed. This is defined as a decrease of more than 10 mm Hg in systolic arterial pressure occurring with inspiration. Tamponade physiology leads to respiratory variability in ventricular diastolic filling where the negative intrathoracic pressure accompanying inspiration leads to enhanced right-sided filling. Since total intrapericardial volume is fixed by the effusion, as the right ventricle (RV) fills, it will lead to a shift of the interventricular septum toward the left ventricle (LV). This crowding of the LV impedes its filling, decreasing LV stroke volume and explaining the exaggerated decline in systolic blood pressure seen with inspiration. The opposite is true during expiration, with diminished RV and enhanced LV filling. This phenomenon is described as enhanced ventricular interdependence, in which the diastolic filling characteristics of one ventricle can have pronounced influence on the filling of the other ventricle. Pulsus paradoxus is also seen in patients with chronic lung disease, right ventricular dysfunction, and CP.

c. Chest x-rays may show an enlarged, globular, bottle-shaped cardiac silhouette, with widening of the mediastinum. The right costophrenic angle is reduced to less than 90 degrees and the lung fields are clear. Pericardial fat lines in a lateral film are an uncommon, but highly specific, finding.

6 d. The ECG is nonspecific but may demonstrate sinus tachycardia, low-voltage QRS, nonspecific ST-T wave abnormalities, and electrical alternans. **Electrical alternans** (Fig. 20.4)

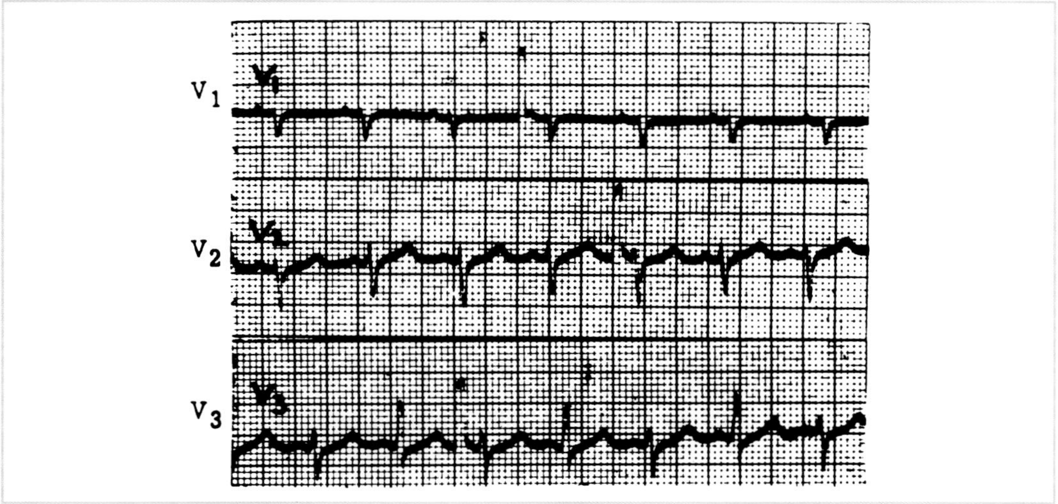

FIGURE 20.4 Electrical alternans with cardiac tamponade. Lead V_3 demonstrates the variation in the R-wave axis in alternate beats. Note that this phenomenon is not seen in all electrocardiographic leads. (Figure from Hensley FA, Martin DE, Gravlee GR. *A Practical Approach to Cardiac Anesthesia*. 3rd ed. Philadelphia, PA: Lippincott Williams & Wilkins; 2003:476.)

TABLE 20.1 Cardiac tamponade-clinical manifestations
Hypotension
Tachycardia
Widened mediastinum on chest x-ray
Elevation and near-equalization of filling pressures
Increasing inotrope requirements
Pulsus paradoxus
Electrical alternans
Initial high-output chest tube drainage that abruptly subsides

is due to a swinging motion of the heart in the pericardial sac, leading to beat-to-beat changes in the electrical axis.

e. Table 20.1 summarizes the classic clinical manifestations most commonly described in cardiac tamponade.

2. **Catheterization data.** Cardiac tamponade is a clinical diagnosis that cannot be made with catheterization data alone. However, common patterns of intracardiac pressures are usually seen. There is elevation and near equalization of the CVP, RVEDP, PCWP, LAP, and LVEDP. Increased central venous and right atrial pressures are seen with a prominent x-descent and a diminished or absent y-descent (Fig. 20.5).
3. **Echocardiography.** Echocardiography is the diagnostic modality of choice in evaluating cardiac tamponade. It is the most sensitive tool for making the diagnosis of pericardial effusion. Initial evaluation should focus on the presence, size, and extent (circumferential versus localized/loculated) of the pericardial effusion. This is seen as an echo-free space surrounding the heart. The effusion should be measured to estimate its severity (Table 20.2).

Although echocardiography alone cannot definitively diagnose tamponade, in the presence of a pericardial effusion, there are several echocardiographic features consistently associated with tamponade physiology. With tamponade, right atrial (RA) collapse is a sensitive sign, typically beginning in end-diastole and continuing through systole. Systolic RA collapse persisting for more than one-third of the cardiac cycle is specific for tamponade. Diastolic RV collapse is observed, and when lasting for more than one-third of diastole is thought to be even more specific than systolic RA collapse for the identification
7 of tamponade. End-diastolic dimensions of the RV will be reduced, reflective of diminished ventricular filling. Paradoxical motion of the interventricular septum is a frequent

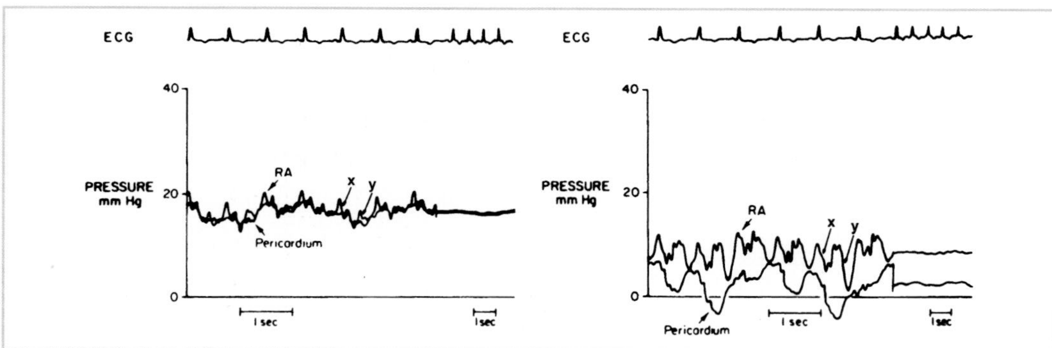

FIGURE 20.5 Right atrial (RA) and pericardial pressures in cardiac tamponade. **A:** Note equal RA and pericardial pressures and the diminished y-descent of the RA waveform. **B:** After removal of 100 mL of fluid, the pericardial pressure is lower than RA pressure, and the normal large descent has returned. (Figure from Hensley FA, Martin DE, Gravlee GR. *A Practical Approach to Cardiac Anesthesia.* 3rd ed. Philadelphia, PA: Lippincott Williams & Wilkins; 2003:475.)

TABLE 20.2 Estimation of effusion severity

	Size of Effusion
Minimal effusion (50–100 mL)	<5 mm
Small effusion (100–250 mL)	5–10 mm
Moderate effusion (250–500 mL)	11–20 mm
Large effusion (>500 mL)	>20 mm

finding, reflecting the reciprocal respiratory variability in diastolic filling. These changes are also reflected with Doppler transmitral and transtricuspid inflow velocity profiles (Figs. 20.6–20.9).

D. **Treatment.** Definitive treatment of cardiac tamponade is emergent drainage, which may be accomplished through either pericardiocentesis or surgical decompression.

1. **Pericardiocentesis.** Pericardiocentesis may be performed with or without imaging guidance (e.g., echocardiography, fluoroscopy). Imaging is often preferred to assist in safely guiding the needle tip through the pericardium to the most optimal location for drainage, as well as assessing the adequacy of fluid removal. Without imaging there is a significantly higher risk of complications, such as cardiac perforation, puncture of coronary or internal mammary arteries, and pneumothorax. In the setting of severe hemodynamic instability, however, it may be necessary to proceed without imaging due to the significant risk of rapid and profound clinical deterioration. A catheter is frequently left in the pericardial space to allow for continuous drainage (Fig. 20.10).

In addition to the previously discussed complications, several reports of post-pericardiocentesis pulmonary edema are reported in the literature. In some cases, severe pulmonary edema associated with life-threatening acute left ventricular dysfunction has been described. While the exact mechanism of this complication remains unclear, most agree that it is likely precipitated by the rapid removal of a large amount of fluid. Since systemic vascular resistance is usually elevated to compensate for tamponade physiology, rapid improvement in ventricular filling and volume following pericardiocentesis may

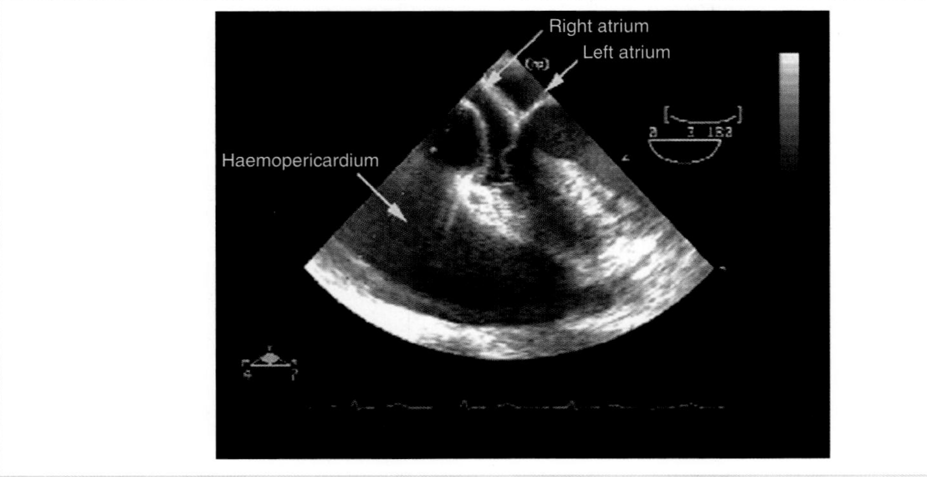

FIGURE 20.6 Pericardial tamponade. Compression of both the right atrium and right ventricle by a large pericardial fluid collection. (Reused from Lobato EB, Muehlschlegel JD. Transesophageal echocardiography in the intensive care unit. In: Perrino AC, Reeves ST, eds. *A Practical Approach to Transesophageal Echocardiography.* 2nd ed. Philadelphia, PA: Lippincott Williams & Wilkins; 2008:355.)

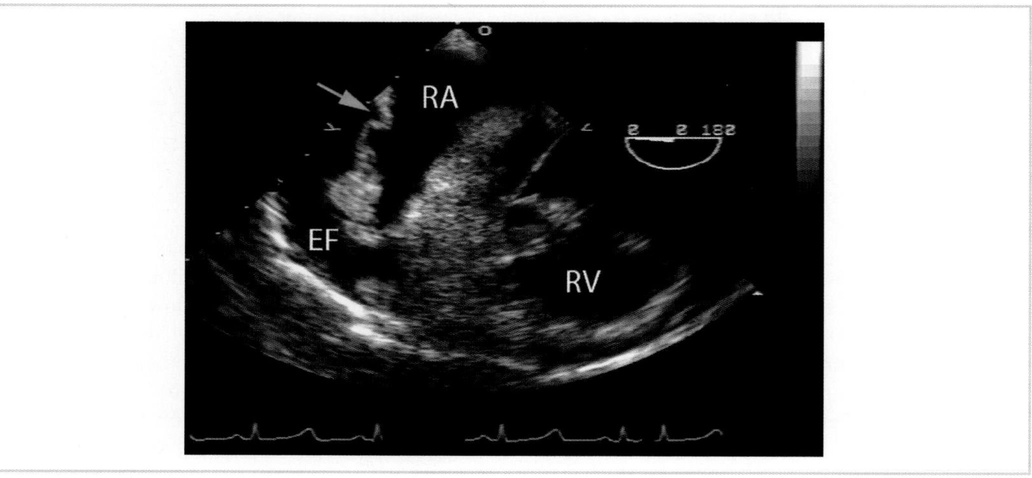

FIGURE 20.7 Pericardial effusion (EF) causing systolic right atrial (RA) collapse as seen in a TEE midesophageal four-chamber view. (From Avery EG, Shernan SK. Echocardiographic evaluation of pericardial disease. In: Savage RM, Aronson SA, Shernan SK, eds. *Comprehensive Textbook of Perioperative Transesophageal Echocardiography.* 2nd ed. Philadelphia, PA: Lippincott Williams & Wilkins; 2011:733.)

precipitate ventricular distension and a detrimental increase in LV wall stress, leading to diminished forward stroke volume and pulmonary edema. If LV dysfunction is observed, it usually transient, with ventricular function returning to baseline in most cases, leading many to believe that myocardial stunning is also a component of this phenomenon. Pulmonary edema may be observed following the drainage of both acute and chronic fluid collections, however, and the anesthesiologist must be especially

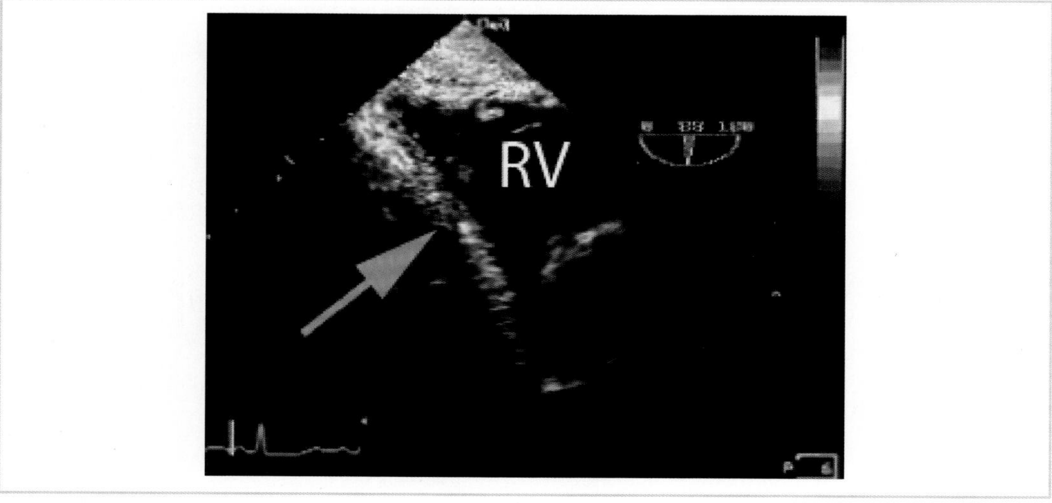

FIGURE 20.8 Diastolic right ventricular (RV) collapse in a patient with cardiac tamponade as seen in a TEE transgastric long-axis RV inflow view. RV collapse is indicated by the *orange arrow.* (From Avery EG, Shernan SK. Echocardiographic evaluation of pericardial disease. In: Savage RM, Aronson SA, Shernan SK, eds. *Comprehensive Textbook of Perioperative Transesophageal Echocardiography.* 2nd ed. Philadelphia, PA: Lippincott Williams & Wilkins; 2011:733.)

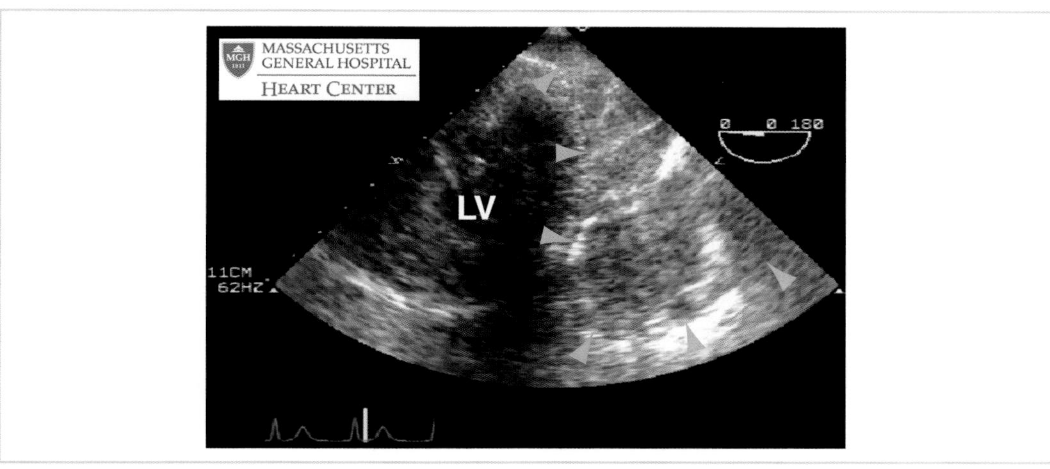

FIGURE 20.9 The pericardial space is occupied by a large amount of clot (marked by the *orange arrows*), seen adjacent to the lateral wall of the left ventricle (LV) in a transgastric short-axis midpapillary TEE view. (ECHO image from Avery EG, Shernan SK. Echocardiographic evaluation of pericardial disease. In: Savage RM, Aronson SA, Shernan SK, eds. *Comprehensive Textbook of Perioperative Transesophageal Echocardiography.* 2nd ed. Philadelphia, PA: Lippincott Williams & Wilkins; 2011:733.)

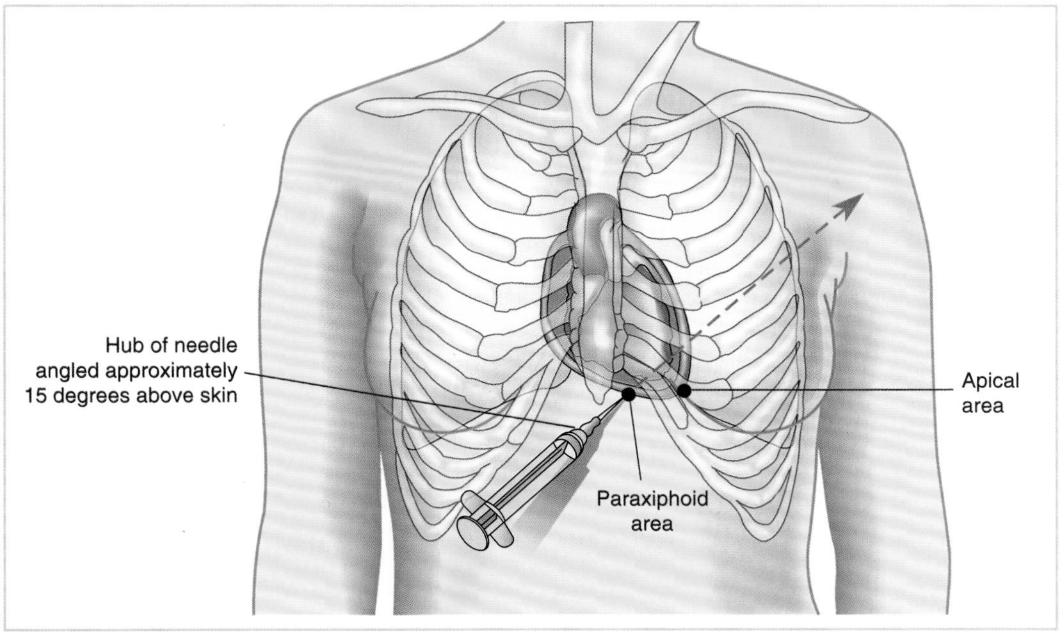

FIGURE 20.10 The most common needle insertion points for pericardiocentesis, including the paraxiphoid and apical approaches. When using the paraxiphoid approach, the needle tip should be directed toward the left shoulder. With the apical approach, the needle tip is aimed internally. (From Spodick DH. Acute cardiac tamponade. *N Engl J Med.* 2003;349:684–690.)

prepared for this complication whenever a large volume of fluid is rapidly removed in either circumstance [5].

2. **Surgical drainage.** Indications for surgical drainage include unsuccessful pericardiocentesis, localized/loculated effusions, removal of clot, and ongoing intrapericardial bleeding (e.g., acute aortic dissection, trauma, following cardiac surgery or percutaneous cardiac procedures). Surgical approach is primarily via subxiphoid pericardial window or a small anterior thoracotomy. The subxiphoid approach is easier to perform but offers a limited exposure, while a thoracotomy provides excellent exposure and is indicated if a larger surgical field is required. Both approaches allow for open exploration, facilitating the removal of clot and fibrinous debris. With hemorrhagic tamponade following cardiac surgery, full mediastinal exploration is needed to locate the source of bleeding and stabilize the patient. In the setting of malignant effusions, diagnostic pericardial biopsies can be obtained with a surgical approach to drainage [2]. Some patients may continue to experience recurrent pericardial effusions, requiring consideration of pericardiectomy. This is most commonly seen in patients with malignant effusions or uremia [6].

E. **Goals of perioperative management.** The hemodynamic state of the patient will dictate the
8 sequence of anesthesia and surgery. While general anesthesia is frequently used, it may contribute to clinical decompensation in severely compromised patients. Direct myocardial depression, systemic vasodilation, and diminished preload accompanying the induction of general anesthesia can lead to a profound decrease in cardiac output. Potentially life-threatening cardiac collapse can ensue. In this scenario, pericardiocentesis or subxiphoid pericardial window can be performed under local anesthesia. Frequently, hemodynamic instability is dramatically improved with the removal of only a small amount of fluid. This is due to the steep curve of the pressure-volume relationship of the pericardial contents [2]. Following this initial drainage, the patient may become stable enough to tolerate the institution of general anesthesia for the remainder of the procedure.

1. Premedication with anxiolytics or opioids is best avoided in patients with true cardiac tamponade. Even small doses of these medications can precipitate acute cardiac collapse.
2. To facilitate ventricular filling, preload must be optimized with intravenous fluids prior to induction. Any manipulations that decrease venous return should be avoided or minimized as much as possible.
3. In addition to standard noninvasive monitors, an arterial line should be considered prior to induction to allow for beat-to-beat monitoring of systemic blood pressure. Adequate intravenous access is needed for volume replacement and drug administration. Central venous access may be beneficial, but is not always essential. In a severely unstable patient, however, surgical intervention should not be delayed for the placement of lines or monitors.
4. Before proceeding with induction, the patient should be fully prepped and draped. The surgical team should be standing at the operating room table and ready to make an immediate incision in the event of hemodynamic collapse upon induction.
5. The perioperative anesthetic plan should have the following hemodynamic goals (Table 20.3):

   Heart rate should remain high and contractility optimized to preserve cardiac output, as these patients will have a fixed and reduced stroke volume. Adequate preload is essential to promote right ventricular filling. Decreases in systemic vascular resistance must be avoided, as this will reduce systemic perfusion pressure.

TABLE 20.3 Hemodynamic goals in cardiac tamponade

	Heart Rate	Contractility	Preload	Systemic Vascular Resistance
Tamponade	↑	↑	↑	↑

6. Positive-pressure ventilation can cause a dramatic decline in preload and cardiac output. It is suggested that patients with tamponade be allowed to breathe spontaneously until the pericardial sac is opened and drained. If spontaneous ventilation is not possible, ventilation with high respiratory rates and low tidal volumes should be considered to minimize mean airway pressure.
7. Careful consideration should be given to the selection of induction drugs, with particular attention aimed at minimizing myocardial depression and peripheral vasodilation. Etomidate is a reasonable induction agent, producing minimal decreases in contractility and systemic vascular resistance. Hypotension may still occur, however, as hypovolemia and tamponade physiology will magnify its typically minimal hemodynamic effects. Benzodiazepines are also a reasonable choice. Many advocate the use of ketamine in this setting, relying on the sympathetic stimulation it provides to minimize hemodynamic compromise. However, many patients have a diminished ability to increase their own sympathetic nervous system activity and these effects are not observed. In these patients, the myocardial depressant properties of ketamine will be unmasked and significant hypotension is likely to occur. Opioids should be given with caution, as vagally mediated bradycardia can lead to a decline in cardiac output.
8. Inotropes (e.g., epinephrine, norepinephrine) and vasoconstrictors (e.g., phenylephrine, vasopressin) may be needed to maintain cardiac output and peripheral perfusion, but serve only as a temporizing measure until tamponade can be definitively treated with drainage.
9. Tamponade physiology is rarely seen in patients presenting for surgical drainage of chronic, recurrent pericardial effusions. In this scenario, however, it is still essential to obtain as much information as possible regarding the clinical significance and severity of the effusion. This should include a review of the preoperative echocardiogram, a thorough discussion with the surgeon, and a detailed history and physical examination, focusing in particular on any vital sign abnormalities. Although tamponade physiology is rare, a high index of suspicion should be maintained for the potential of perioperative hemodynamic instability.

V. Constrictive pericarditis

A. Natural history

9

1. **Etiology.** CP is a diagnosis that encompasses a wide spectrum of disease, from acute or subacute cases that may resolve spontaneously or with medical therapy, to the classic chronic, progressive CP, which will be the focus of this section. Other entities noted in the literature include effusive-constrictive pericarditis, in which patients present with cardiac effusion or tamponade but retain characteristics of CP following drainage of the effusion; localized CP, involving only parts of the pericardium with variable hemodynamic sequelae; and occult CP, in which rapid infusion of intravenous fluids can provoke the signs and symptoms of the disease [7]. While many etiologies have been documented, the most common include idiopathic, viral, post-cardiac surgery, mediastinal radiation, and, in developing countries, tuberculosis.
2. **Symptomatology.** CP presents most commonly as chronic and progressive fatigue, orthopnea, dyspnea on exertion, peripheral edema, and abdominal distention. Given the nonspecific nature of these findings, care must be taken to differentiate this disease process from others such as hepatic failure, right ventricular failure, tricuspid valve disease, and, most importantly, restrictive cardiomyopathy. As the pathophysiology underlying these conditions is markedly different, the medical and surgical management will vary considerably as well.

B. Pathophysiology. The hallmark of CP is a thickened, often calcified, adherent pericardium, which effectively confines the heart inside a rigid shell. From a pathophysiologic perspective, this has three major consequences [8]:

1. *Impaired diastolic filling.* The noncompliant pericardium limits filling of all cardiac chambers, with elevation and near-equalization of end-diastolic pressures. Ventricular filling

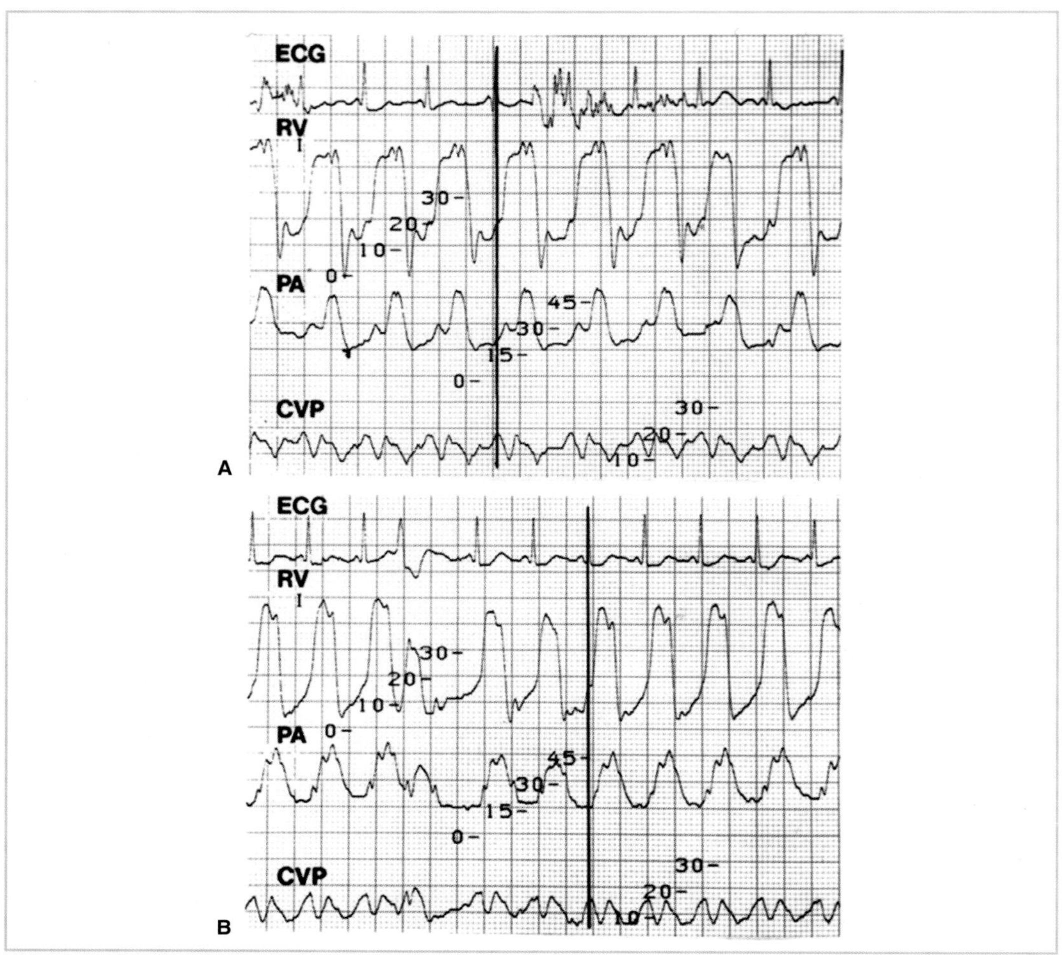

FIGURE 20.11 Waveform characteristics commonly seen during catheterization of patients with CP before **(A)** and after **(B)** pericardiectomy. Note the "square root sign" in the right ventricular (RV) pressure tracing, and the "M" waveform in the central venous pressure (CVP) tracing prior to pericardiectomy. ECG, electrocardiogram; PA, pulmonary artery. (Figure from Skubas NJ, Beardslee M, Barzilai B, et al. Constrictive pericarditis: intraoperative hemodynamic and echocardiographic evaluation of cardiac filling dynamics. *Anesth Analg.* 2001;92:1424–1426.)

occurs rapidly during early diastole but ceases abruptly as the volume, and thus pressure, in the ventricle reaches a critical point. This results in the characteristic "dip and plateau," or "square root sign," noted in ventricular pressure tracings (Fig. 20.11). Atrial systole does little to augment LV filling, and cardiac output is maintained by a compensatory increase in heart rate.

2. *Dissociation of intrathoracic pressures.* The rigid pericardium isolates the cardiac chambers from the negative pressure generated during inspiration, resulting in a decreased gradient between the pulmonary veins and the left atrium. Consequently, left heart filling, and thus cardiac output, are decreased.
3. *Ventricular interdependence.* As discussed previously, left and right heart filling are not independent events. Increases in right heart filling may cause a leftward shift in the interventricular septum at the expense of left heart filling. Expiration, as would be expected,

reverses this pattern. This phenomenon is known as ventricular interdependence, and is exaggerated in CP.

One of the most important consequences of pericardial constriction is significant respiratory variation in left and right ventricular filling patterns. This is an important consideration in the diagnosis of CP, and provides the foundation for the diagnostic workup to be discussed later. Of note, this respiratory variation is maintained, but reversed, in patients on mechanical ventilation [9].

C. Diagnostic evaluation and assessment

1. Clinical evaluation

a. The diagnosis of CP is difficult to make on history and physical examination alone, but must be considered in patients presenting with the signs and symptoms of venous congestion mentioned previously. On examination, JVD with Kussmaul's sign (an increase in JVD on inspiration) and Friedreich's sign (a rapid decrease in JVD during early diastole) may be present. Pulsus paradoxus, initially described by Kussmaul in patients with CP, may be present but is more common in patients with cardiac tamponade or in those with concurrent effusion with tamponade physiology [10]. On cardiac auscultation, a "***pericardial knock***" may be noted. This is a high-pitched sound in early diastole that is caused by the sudden cessation of ventricular filling, and is a highly specific but insensitive clue to the diagnosis. Pulmonary edema is often absent, and pulsatile hepatomegaly may be noted on abdominal examination.

b. Laboratory investigation may reveal organ dysfunction secondary to the disease process (e.g., kidney injury, elevated liver enzymes). Natriuretic peptide levels, which are released in response to myocardial stretch and are increased in many cases of heart failure, are usually normal or only slightly elevated. This is attributed to the rigid pericardium limiting the amount of chamber dilation possible.

c. ECG findings are nonspecific and may include sinus tachycardia, atrial fibrillation, conduction delays, p-mitrale, and ST-segment and T-wave changes.

d. While calcification of the pericardium is not universal, its presence on the lateral chest x-ray may suggest CP. A thickened pericardium (>2 mm) may be appreciated on CT or MRI, and other imaging techniques may demonstrate the pericardium adherent to the myocardium.

2. Catheterization data. As in tamponade, cardiac catheterization is not always necessary for the diagnosis of CP. However, it may be helpful in the diagnosis of effusive-constrictive pericarditis, with some suggesting its routine use during the drainage of pericardial effusions. Certain waveform characteristics may be seen during placement of invasive monitors in the operating room. Right atrial pressure tracings may show "***M***" or "***W***" waveforms with a prominent y-descent, the diagnostic equivalent of Friedreich's sign. Ventricular pressure tracings may show the characteristic "***dip and plateau,***" or "***square root sign,***" as previously described. The end-diastolic pressures in all chambers are elevated and nearly equal (≤5 mm Hg difference), and RV systolic pressures are usually <50 mm Hg with an RV end-diastolic to RV systolic ratio of >1:3.

3. Echocardiography. Echocardiography is essential to the diagnosis of CP, and more advanced techniques have become useful in its differentiation from other disease processes. Two-dimensional and M-mode examination may show a thickened, hyperechoic pericardium; diastolic flattening of the LV posterior wall, reflective of the abrupt cessation of ventricular filling; a ventricular septal "bounce," caused by the sudden changes in the transseptal pressure gradient; premature closure of the mitral valve and opening of the pulmonic valve, indicative of high chamber pressures; enlarged hepatic veins; and IVC plethora, where the vessel remains dilated and lacks the normal change in diameter during the respiratory cycle. Doppler evaluation of transmitral, transtricuspid, and pulmonary vein flow show characteristic tracings with profound respiratory variation (often >25%; Fig. 20.12), and newer techniques such as Doppler tissue imaging (DTI) of the mitral annulus and color Doppler M-mode of transmitral flow (propagation velocity; Fig. 20.13) allow further characterization and differentiation from restrictive cardiomyopathy [11] (Table 20.4).

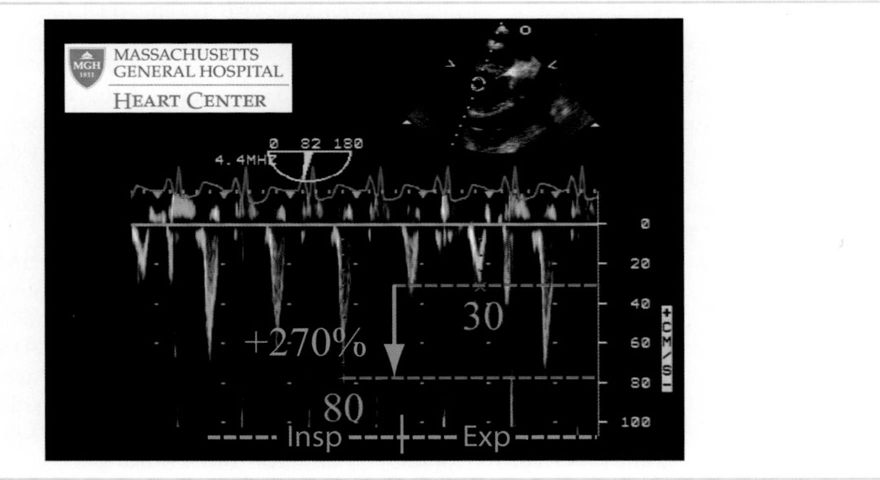

FIGURE 20.12 TEE pulsed wave transmitral Doppler profile in a patient with CP during positive pressure ventilation. Note the preserved, but reversed, respiratory variation as opposed to that which would be seen in a spontaneously ventilating patient. Insp, inspiration; Exp, expiration. (From Avery EG, Shernan SK. Echocardiographic evaluation of pericardial disease. In: Savage RM, Aronson SA, Shernan SK, eds. *Comprehensive Textbook of Perioperative Transesophageal Echocardiography.* 2nd ed. Philadelphia, PA: Lippincott Williams & Wilkins; 2011:737.)

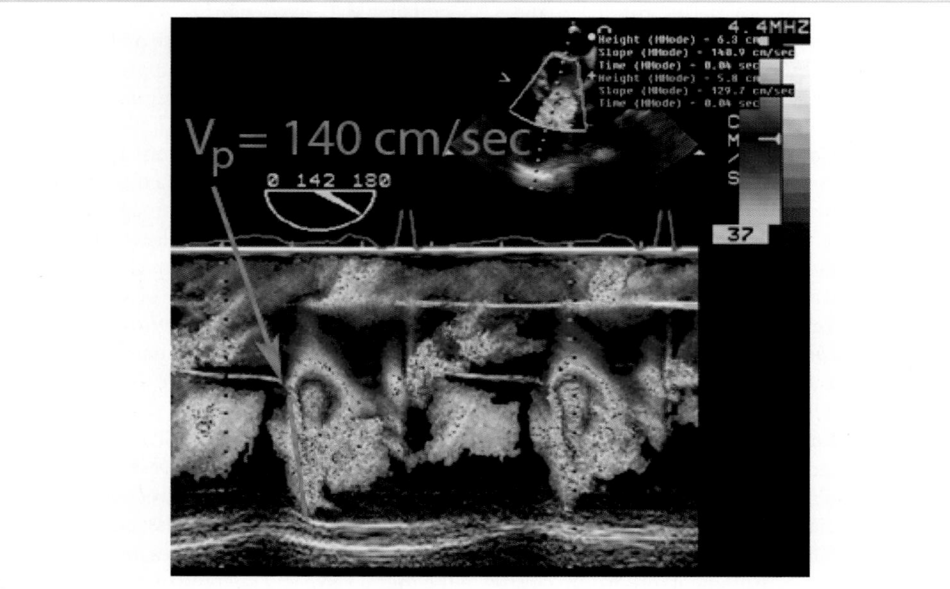

FIGURE 20.13 TEE image of the transmitral color M-mode (propagation velocity, V_p) profile of a patient with CP. The slope of the first aliasing velocity is used in this determination and is depicted by the pink line. (ECHO image from Avery EG, Shernan SK. Echocardiographic evaluation of pericardial disease. In: Savage RM, Aronson SA, Shernan SK, eds. *Comprehensive Textbook of Perioperative Transesophageal Echocardiography.* 2nd ed. Philadelphia, PA: Lippincott Williams & Wilkins; 2011:738.)

TABLE 20.4 Clues to the differentiation of constrictive pericarditis and restrictive cardiomyopathy

	Constrictive Pericarditis	**Restrictive Cardiomyopathy**
Pulsus Paradoxus	Variable	Absent
Kussmaul's sign	Common	Absent
Pericardial knock	Common	Absent
Chest x-ray	Pericardial calcification	No pericardial calcification
Computed tomography and Magnetic resonance imaging	Pericardial thickening (>2 mm)	Normal pericardium
B-type natriuretic peptide	Normal to mildly elevated	Significantly elevated
Catheterization data	LVEDP – RVEDP ≤5 mm Hg PASP < 40–50 mm Hg RVEDP : RVSP >1 : 3	LVEDP – RVEDP >5 mm Hg PASP > 40–50 mm Hg RVEDP : RVSP <1 : 3
Atrial size	Usually normal	Enlarged
Ventricular septal motion	Abnormal: septal "bounce"	Normal
Respiratory variation (Doppler flow patterns)	Exaggerated (often >25%)	Normal/minimal (<10%)
Color M-mode propagation velocity	>100 cm/s	<55 cm/s
Tissue Doppler imaging of mitral annulus	E′ >8 cm/s	E′ <8 cm/s

LVEDP, left ventricular end-diastolic pressure; RVEDP, right ventricular end-diastolic pressure; PASP, pulmonary artery systolic pressure; RVSP, right ventricular systolic pressure; E′, max E′ velocity on tissue Doppler imaging of the lateral mitral annulus.

D. **Treatment.** As mentioned, some cases of acute constriction may resolve spontaneously or with medical management. The definitive management of chronic CP, however, is usually surgical. Pericardiectomy, or pericardial decortication, is often performed via left thoracotomy or midline sternotomy, depending on the extent of resection necessary. The goal of treatment is total resection of both the visceral and parietal pericardium, and while this can often be performed without the use of cardiopulmonary bypass (CPB), its use may be indicated in more difficult dissections. Despite improvements in surgical technique, operative mortality remains as high as 10%, with poor predictors including prior cardiac surgery, radiation, malignancy, and advanced heart failure on presentation. As opposed to patients with tamponade, where surgical drainage may provide immediate improvement in hemodynamic and clinical status, an immediate improvement in symptoms is not generally observed.

E. **Goals of perioperative management.** The hemodynamic instability of patients with CP is generally less than those patients with acute tamponade, unless a concurrent effusion with tamponade physiology is present. However, many of the same principles can be applied to the
10 perioperative management of the patients.

1. Premedication with benzodiazepines and/or opioids must be titrated according to the patient's preoperative status.
2. In addition to standard noninvasive monitors, the intraoperative and postoperative management of patients with CP often requires invasive monitors. An arterial line is beneficial for blood gas analysis, especially with surgery via thoracotomy, as well as continuous blood pressure monitoring during cardiac manipulation and when CPB is utilized. The decision to place this preoperatively or after induction of anesthesia must take into account the patient's clinical status. Adequate intravenous access must be obtained given the possibility of marked and precipitous blood loss (cardiac chamber or coronary artery perforation, myocardial injury due to stripping of the pericardium, etc.), with central venous access allowing the rapid infusion of IV fluids, blood components, and vasoactive drugs, as well as the monitoring of CVP. Volume status and continuous cardiac output monitoring via a pulmonary artery catheter may be beneficial as well,

as low cardiac output syndrome may persist into the postoperative period [3]. While echocardiography plays a more important role in the preoperative diagnosis of CP, intraoperative TEE can provide useful information for both the surgeon and the anesthesiologist.

3. Pericardiectomy requires general anesthesia, and care must be taken to avoid hemodynamic deterioration during the induction and maintenance of anesthesia. Preload must be maintained, and often augmented, to ensure cardiac filling, and reductions in either preload or afterload may be poorly tolerated. Heart rate plays an important role in maintaining cardiac output, and bradycardia must be avoided. While the atrial "kick" does little to enhance ventricular filling in patients with CP, extreme tachycardia, such as atrial fibrillation with a rapid ventricular rate, may be poorly tolerated. Contractility should be maintained as well, as significant myocardial depression will adversely impact cardiac output and systemic flow.
4. Although the manifestations of hemodynamic instability are less than with tamponade, induction and maintenance of anesthesia must include the same considerations. Vasoactive medications must be readily available to offset any perturbations caused by the anesthetic agents or surgical manipulations, most notably decreased preload, afterload, contractility, and heart rate.

REFERENCES

1. Little WC, Freeman GL. Contemporary reviews in cardiovascular medicine: pericardial disease. *Circulation.* 2006;113: 1622–1632.
2. O'Connor CJ, Tuman KJ. The intraoperative management of patients with cardiac tamponade. *Anesthesiology Clin.* 2010;28: 87–96.
3. Oliver WC, Mauermann WJ, Nuttall GA. Uncommon cardiac diseases. In: Kaplan JA, Reich DL, Savino JS, eds. *Kaplan's Cardiac Anesthesia: The Echo Era.* 6th ed. St. Louis, MO: Elsevier Saunders; 2011:706–713.
4. Gandhi S, Schneider A, Mohiuddin S, et al. Has the clinical presentation and clinician's index of suspicion of cardiac tamponade changed over the past decade? *Echocardiography.* 2008;25:237–241.
5. Bernal JM, Pradhan J, Li T, et al. Acute pulmonary edema following pericardiocentesis for cardiac tamponade. *Can J Cardiol.* 2007;23(suppl 14):1155–1156.
6. Dinardo JA, Zvara DA. *Anesthesia for Cardiac Surgery.* 3rd ed. Malden, MA: Blackwell Publishing; 2008:289–303.
7. Sagrista-Salueda J. Pericardial constriction: Uncommon patterns. *Heart.* 2004;90:257–258.
8. Myers RB, Spodick DH. Constrictive pericarditis: Clinical and pathophysiologic characteristics. *Am Heart J.* 1999;138: 219–232.
9. Abdalla IA, Murray RD, Awad HE, et al. Reversal of the pattern of respiratory variation of Doppler inflow velocities in constrictive pericarditis during mechanical ventilation. *J Am Soc Echocardiogr.* 2000;13:827–831.
10. Bilchick KC, Wise RA. Paradoxical physical findings described by Kussmaul: Pulsus paradoxus and Kussmaul's sign. *Lancet.* 2002;359(suppl 9321):1940–1942.
11. Rajagopalan N, Garcia MJ, Rodriguez L, et al. Comparison of new Doppler echocardiographic methods to differentiate constrictive pericardial heart disease and restrictive cardiomyopathy. *Am J Cardiol.* 2001;87:86–94.

IV CIRCULATORY SUPPORT

21 Cardiopulmonary Bypass: Equipment, Circuits, and Pathophysiology

Eugene A. Hessel, II, Glenn S. Murphy, Robert C. Groom, and Joseph N. Ghansah

KEY POINTS

1. The goal of cardiopulmonary bypass is to provide adequate gas exchange, oxygen delivery, systemic blood flow with adequate perfusion pressure while minimizing the detrimental effects of bypass.
2. Roller pumps may cause more damage to blood elements and can result in massive air embolism if the venous reservoir becomes empty.
3. Membrane oxygenators function similarly to natural lungs, imposing a membrane between the ventilating gas and the flowing blood, thereby eliminating direct contact between blood and gas.
4. During bypass, excessive and rapid warming of blood with the bypass heat exchanger must be avoided to prevent gas coming out of solution risking embolism and to avoid excessive heating of the brain with subsequent potential neurologic damage.
5. Cardiotomy suction should be minimized or cell salvage techniques used to process the cardiotomy blood as it contains microaggregates of cells, fat, foreign debris, thrombogenic and fibrinolytic elements thought to be major sources of hemolysis, and microemboli during CPB.
6. More recent data have suggested that the lower limit of autoregulation of the brain is approximately a mean pressure of 70 mm Hg in awake, normotensive subjects. On the basis of this data some clinicians are now using higher (greater than 70 mm Hg) mean pressure on bypass.
7. Critical oxygen delivery is that point at which maximum oxygen extraction is reached and oxygen consumption starts to fall.

PART I: THE CARDIOPULMONARY BYPASS CIRCUIT

I. Introduction: It is critical that anesthesiologists who provide care for patients undergoing surgery using cardiopulmonary bypass (CPB) be intimately familiar with the function of the heart–lung (H–L) machine (also referred to as the extracorporeal circuit [ECC]). In this chapter, the components of the H–L machine, the physiologic principles and pathophysiologic consequences of CPB, and the important role the anesthesiologist should play in its optimal and safe conduct are described. In Chapter 8, the medical management of patients during CPB is described.

The primary goal and function of CPB is to divert blood away from the heart and lungs and return it to the systemic arterial system, thereby permitting surgery on the nonfunctioning heart. 1 In doing so, it must replace the function of both the heart and the lungs. **The goal is to provide adequate gas exchange, oxygen delivery, systemic blood flow, and arterial pressure, while minimizing the adverse effect of extracorporeal circulation.** This is accomplished by the two principal components of the H–L machine: The **artificial lung** (blood gas exchanging device or "oxygenator") and the **arterial pump**. The "oxygenator" removes carbon dioxide as well as adds oxygen to provide the desired P_aO_2 and P_aCO_2, while the arterial pump supplies the energy to maintain systemic blood for arterial pressure and organ perfusion. Because the proximal ascending aorta is often cross-clamped to arrest the heart to facilitate surgery, a **cardioplegia delivery system** is added to minimize myocardial ischemia. **Other components** of the ECC include cannulae that connect to the systemic venous and arterial systems, a venous reservoir, a heat exchanger to control body temperature, field or cardiotomy suction, and various safety and monitoring devices. These components will be described in this chapter. The interested reader may find further details on CPB components in the referenced texts [1–5].

II. Components of the circuit

A. Overview: The essential components of the H–L machine include the CBP console, oxygenator, venous reservoir, arterial pump, cardioplegia circuit, ventilating circuit, monitoring and safety systems, and various filters. These components can be assembled in a myriad of configurations depending on perfusionist/surgeon preference and patient need. Figure 21.1 shows a detailed schematic of a typical CPB circuit. Desaturated blood exits the patient's vena cava through a **right atrium (RA)/inferior vena cava (IVC) venous cannula** and is diverted to the **venous reservoir** by **gravity siphon drainage** through large-bore polyvinyl chloride (PVC) tubing. Blood is then drawn from the **venous reservoir** by the **systemic blood pump**, which can be either roller or kinetic, and pumped through a **heat exchanger** (integral to the membrane oxygenator [MO]). Blood then passes through the **oxygenator**, through an **arterial filter**, and back into the patient through the **arterial cannula** inserted into the ascending aorta. Additional parts of the circuit include a **recirculation line** from the arterial side of the oxygenator, which is used for priming the system and as a blood source for cardioplegia. A **purge line** is located on the housing of the arterial filter and is kept open during CPB to vent any air from the circuit back to the venous reservoir, or a second reservoir called **cardiotomy reservoir**.

Other roller pumps on the H–L machine are used for various functions including delivery of cardioplegic solution, return of shed blood via aspiration, venting of blood from intracardiac sources, or the removal of air from the venous reservoir when collapsible venous reservoir "bag" systems are used. Additional components of the CPB system include **microprocessors** for console control and electronic data recording, a **cooler/heater** which serves as an adjustable temperature water source used in conjunction with the **circuit heat exchangers**, an **anesthetic vaporizer** for the administration of volatile anesthetic agents, **cardioplegia delivery system**, various **sensors** for monitoring arterial and venous blood parameters as well as oxygen concentrations in the ventilating circuit, and various **safety devices**. Most of the components through which the blood passes are disposable and commercially custom-prepared to meet the specific requirements of individual cardiac teams.

B. Venous cannulation and drainage

1. **Overview:** Blood must be diverted into the H–L machine to keep it from passing through the heart and lungs and thereby permit access to the heart by the surgeon.
2. **Central venous cannulation (Fig. 21.2)**
   a. **Single simple cannula** in RA: Inserted through a purse-string suture in the RA free wall or atrial appendage. This type of cannulation tends to be unstable, does not reliably divert flow into the right ventricle (RV), and is rarely used in adult CPB.
   b. **Cavoatrial or "two-stage" single cannula:** A single-lumen cannula with a wide proximal portion with drainage slits situated in the RA, and a narrower distal end placed into the IVC. The tip in the IVC makes this cannula more stable. It is usually inserted through a purse-string suture in the atrial appendage. Insertion may be difficult in the presence of RA masses or hardware or a prominent Eustachian valve or Chiari network. Tears produced at the junction of the IVC with the RA are difficult to manage. This is the most common type of cannulation for coronary artery and aortic valve surgery. It may not reliably prevent blood from entering the RV, and may not provide optimal myocardial cooling (especially the RA and RV). Superior vena cava (SVC) drainage and hence venous return to the H–L machine can be compromised if the junction of the SVC to the RA is kinked (which occurs when the heart is lifted up for grafting of vessels in the inferior and posterior-lateral wall).
   c. **Bicaval cannulation:** Separate cannulae are placed into the SVC and IVC either directly or indirectly through the RA through purse-string sutures. **Bicaval cannulation is most effective at totally diverting blood away from the heart.** When the right heart must be opened, additional large ligatures or tapes are placed around the SVC and the IVC to prevent any caval blood from entering the atrium (and any air getting from the atrium into the venous drainage). When the caval tapes are tightened, this is termed "complete bypass." It is critical that when these tapes are tightened that the

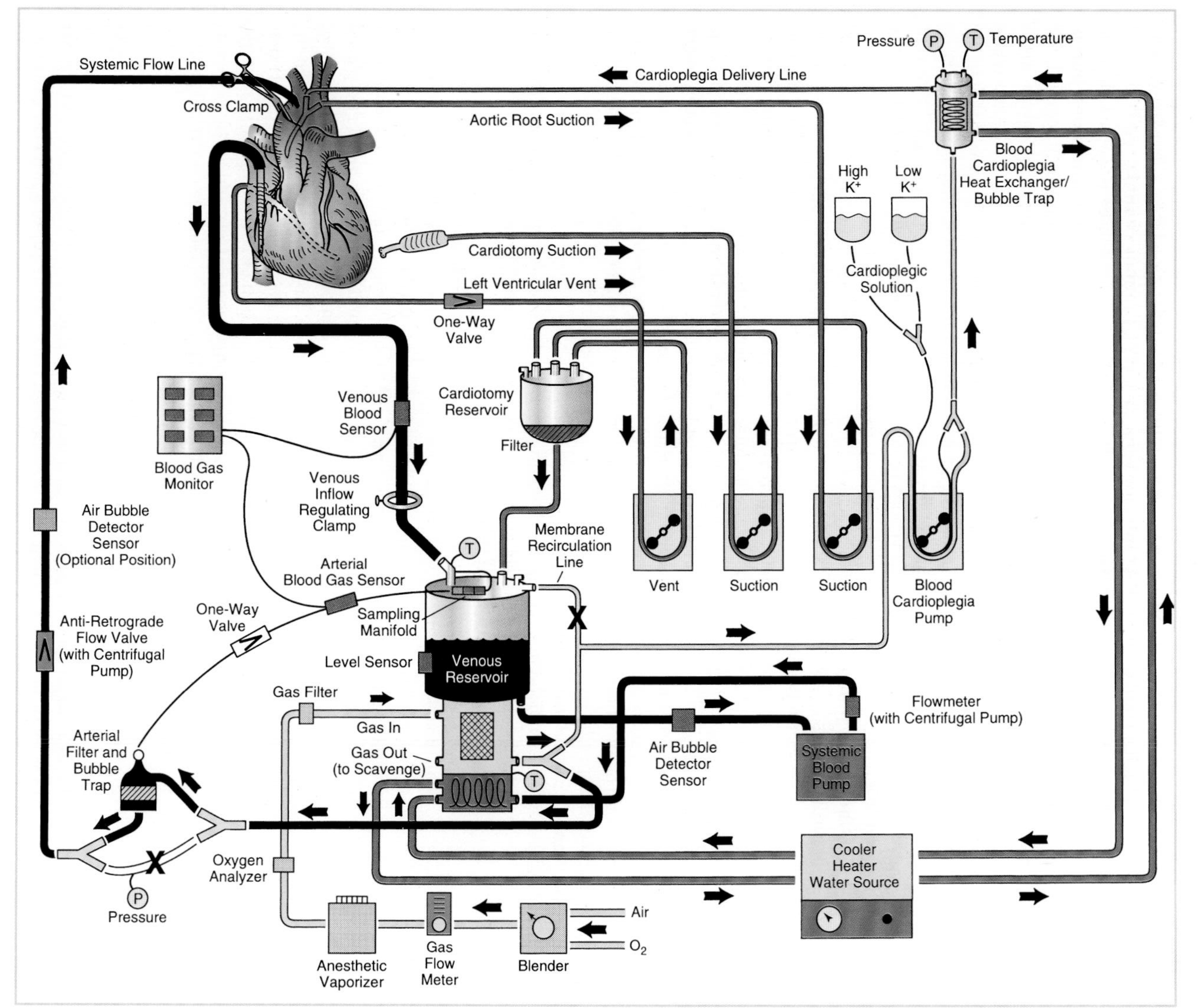

Pressure
Temperature
Systemic Flow Line
Cardioplegia Delivery Line
Cross Clamp
Aortic Root Suction
Blood Cardioplegia Heat Exchanger/ Bubble Trap
High K+
Low K+
Cardiotomy Suction
Left Ventricular Vent
Cardioplegic Solution
One-Way Valve
Cardiotomy Reservoir
Venous Blood Sensor
Blood Gas Monitor
Filter
Venous Inflow Regulating Clamp
Air Bubble Detector Sensor (Optional Position)
Membrane Recirculation Line
Arterial Blood Gas Sensor
Vent
Suction
Suction
Blood Cardioplegia Pump
Anti-Retrograde Flow Valve (with Centrifugal Pump)
One-Way Valve
Sampling Manifold
Level Sensor
Venous Reservoir
Gas Filter
Flowmeter (with Centrifugal Pump)
Gas In
Arterial Filter and Bubble Trap
Gas Out (to Scavenge)
Air Bubble Detector Sensor
Systemic Blood Pump
Cooler Heater Water Source
Oxygen Analyzer
Pressure
Air
O_2
Gas Flow Meter
Anesthetic Vaporizer
Blender

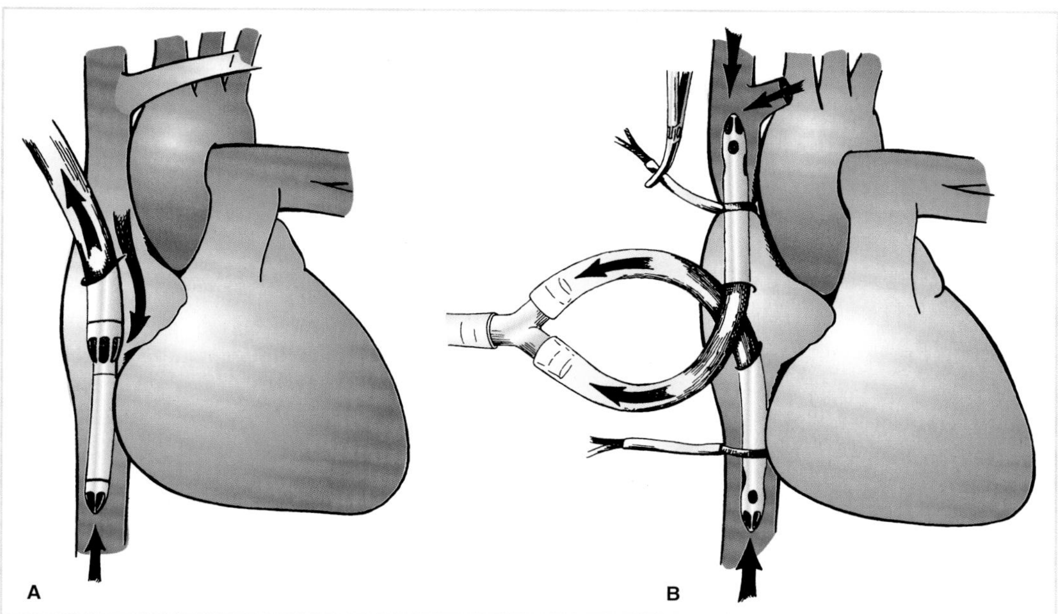

FIGURE 21.2 Venous cannulation (central, intra-thoracic). Methods of venous cannulation. **A:** Single cannulation of RA with a "two-stage" cavoatrial cannula. This is typically inserted through the RA appendage. Note that the narrower tip of the cannula is in the IVC, where it drains this vein. The wider portion, with additional drainage holes, resides in the RA, where blood is received from the coronary sinus and SVC. The SVC must drain via the RA when a cavoatrial cannula is used. **B:** Separate cannulation of the SVC and IVC. Note that there are loops placed around the cavae and venous cannulae and passed through tubing to act as tourniquets or snares. The tourniquet on the SVC has been tightened to divert all SVC flow into the SVC cannula and prevent communication with the RA. (From Hessel EA II. Circuitry and cannulation techniques. In: Gravlee GP, et al., eds. *Cardiopulmonary Bypass.* Philadelphia, PA: Lippincott Williams & Wilkins; 2008:67, with permission.)

cannulae or drainage do not become obstructed or venous hypertension (congestion) will occur. This is of particular concern in the SVC because of the potential adverse impact on cerebral perfusion; pressure in the SVC cephalad to the tip of the SVC cannula should be monitored. Bicaval cannulation is necessary whenever the surgeon plans to open the right heart (for surgery involving the tricuspid valve, RA masses, trans-atrial septal approaches to left heart, and for congenital heart surgery) and for mitral valve (MV)

FIGURE 21.1 Detailed schematic diagram of arrangement of a typical CPB circuit using an MO with integral hard-shell venous reservoir (lower center) and external cardiotomy reservoir. Venous cannulation is by a cavoatrial cannula and arterial cannulation is in the ascending aorta. Some circuits do not incorporate a membrane recirculation line; in these cases the cardioplegia blood source is a separate outlet connector built-in to the oxygenator near the arterial outlet. The systemic blood pump may be either a roller or centrifugal type. The cardioplegia delivery system (right) is a one-pass combination blood/crystalloid type. The cooler–heater water source may be operated to supply water to both the oxygenator heat exchanger and cardioplegia delivery system. The air bubble detector sensor may be placed on the line between the venous reservoir and systemic pump, between the pump and MO inlet or between the oxygenator outlet and arterial filter (neither shown) or on the line after the arterial filter (optional position on drawing). One-way valves prevent retrograde flow (some circuits with a centrifugal pump also incorporate a one-way valve after the pump and within the systemic flow line). Other safety devices include an oxygen analyzer placed between the anesthetic vaporizer (if used) and the oxygenator gas inlet and a reservoir-level sensor attached to the housing of the hard-shell venous reservoir (on the left). *Arrows,* directions of flow; *X,* placement of tubing clamps; *P and T,* pressure and temperature sensors, respectively. Hemoconcentrator (described in text) not shown. (From Hessel EA II. Circuitry and cannulation techniques. In: Gravlee GP, et al., eds. *Cardiopulmonary Bypass.* Philadelphia, PA: Lippincott Williams & Wilkins; 2008:64, with permission.)

surgery. The latter is because retraction of the RA to view the MV causes kinking of the junction of the cavae with the RA which interferes with venous drainage, or if the surgeon approaches the MV through the RA, or for Tricuspid Valve (TV) repair. Bicaval cannulation, by diverting blood away from the right heart, minimizes cardiac warming, especially of the RA and ventricle during cold cardioplegia.

d. **Impact of persistent left superior vena cava (LSVC)** on venous cannulation: About 0.3% of the general population (1% to 10% of patients with congenital heart disease) will have a persistent LSVC. This is a remnant of fetal development and drains blood from the junction of the left internal jugular (IJ) and left subclavian veins into the coronary sinus, and hence into the RA. Therefore, placing cannulae in the right SVC and IVC will not be effective in diverting all of the venous drainage away from the RA. One simple solution is for the surgeon to temporarily occlude (snare) the LSVC. However, in about two-thirds of these patients, the left innominate vein is absent or small, and this maneuver may result in venous hypertension and adverse cerebral consequences. In these cases, the surgeon may place a third venous cannula in the LSVC either retrograde via the coronary sinus, or directly into the LSVC through a purse-string suture.

3. **Peripheral venous cannulation:** Used for minimally invasive/"port-access" approaches, surgery via left thoracotomy, or for cannulation before entering the chest (electively or emergently when bleeding is anticipated or encountered). Most commonly, venous cannulae are placed via the femoral vein (and rarely the IJ vein). If the femoral vein is used, the cannula is positioned with the tip at the SVC–RA junction. Positioning of the cannula is often guided by transesophageal echocardiography (TEE). Bicaval cannulation is possible with a special IVC cannula designed for this purpose. If a separate IJ venous cannula is placed, it is often inserted by the anesthesiologists shortly after induction and requires special attention on their part in regards to sterile technique, heparinization, and clamping and unclamping of this line for CPB. As peripheral venous cannulae are smaller and longer than directly placed cannulae, resistance to drainage is greater and may require use of augmented venous drainage (see later).
4. **Venous cannulae** are plastic (Fig. 21.3). Some are wire-reinforced to minimize kinking. Others designed for direct caval cannulation have curved thin metal or plastic tips for a favorable internal diameter to external diameter (ID:OD) ratio.

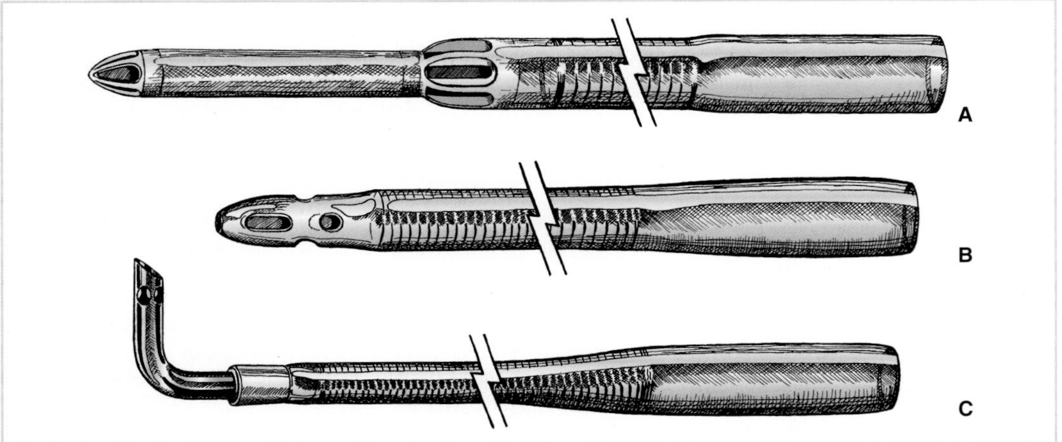

FIGURE 21.3 Venous cannulae. Drawings of commonly used venous cannulae. A: Tapered, "two-stage" RA–IVC cannula. **B:** Straight, wire-wound "lighthouse" tipped cannula for RA or separate cannulation of the SVC or IVC. **C:** Right-angled, metal-tipped cannula for cannulation of the SVC or IVC. (From Hessel EA II. Circuitry and cannulation techniques. In: Gravlee GP, et al., eds. *Cardiopulmonary Bypass.* Philadelphia, PA: Lippincott Williams & Wilkins; 2008:65, with permission.)

5. **Types of drainage**
   a. **Gravity:** Venous drainage is usually accomplished by gravity (siphon effect). This requires that the venous drainage tubing is full of fluid (blood). Drainage is based upon the pressure difference of the column of fluid between the level of the patient and that of the H–L machine (venous reservoir). Flow is influenced by central venous pressure (intravascular volume and venous tone), height differential between the patient and the H–L machine, and resistance in the venous cannula and tubing (length, internal diameter, mechanical obstruction, or malposition of cannulae). "Chattering" of the venous lines suggest excessive drainage or inadequate venous return. Since drainage depends on a siphon, this will be interrupted if the venous line becomes filled with air.
   b. **Augmented venous drainage:** Used when long or smaller cannulae or venous lines are employed and to permit elevation of the H–L machine to the level of the patients (all designed to decrease the prime volume or for peripheral or port-access cannulation). Two classes of systems are utilized: Vacuum-assisted and kinetic.
      (1) **Vacuum-assisted drainage** is accomplished by attaching the venous line to a closed "hard-shell" venous reservoir (see below) to which vacuum (usually negative 20 to 50 mm Hg) is applied. Whenever augmented venous drainage is employed there is increased risk of aspirating air from around the venous cannulae, and application of a second purse-string around this site is recommended. There is also additional risk of developing positive pressure in the closed reservoir which can lead to retrograde venous air embolism. This requires inclusion of a positive pressure release valve and heightened attention on the part of the perfusionist.
      (2) **Kinetic-assisted drainage** is accomplished by inserting a pump (usually centrifugal, but rarely a roller pump). The use of the former is easier to control and minimizes collapse of the cavae or atrium around the tip of the cannulae. This requires close attention by the perfusionist, and as with vacuum-assisted venous drainage increases the risk of air aspiration.
      (3) Studies have not found use of augmented venous return to increase destruction of blood elements nor to aggravate the inflammatory response to CPB.

C. **Arterial cannulation**
1. **Overview:** The blood from the H–L machine must be returned to the systemic arterial system through an arterial cannula. These cannulae are the narrowest part of the circuit and must carry the entire systemic blood flow ("cardiac output"). The size of cannula is based on the desired blood flow (mainly influenced by patient size) and is chosen to keep blood velocity less than 100 to 200 cm/s and pressure gradients less than 100 mm Hg. Higher flows and pressures (jets) may result in trauma to blood elements and the vessel wall ("sandblasting" and dissection) and potential for reduced flow into side branches. To maximize the ID/OD ratio, the tips of the cannulae are often constructed from metal or hard plastic and the narrowest part of the arterial line is kept as short as possible. Some special tips have been designed to minimize the exit velocities and jet effects (Fig. 21.4). Most commonly the arterial cannula is inserted in the distal ascending aorta, but other sites are also used.
2. **Cannulation site options (Table 21.1)**
   a. **Ascending aorta:** This is the most common approach. The cannula is inserted through one or two concentric purse-sting sutures in the distal ascending aorta and directed toward the transverse arch (NOT toward one of the arch vessels). Dislodgement of atheromatous material from the cannulation site is a primary concern. Palpation of the aorta may not be sensitive enough to detect atheroma, and many advocate imaging of the intended site for cannulation with epiaortic ultrasound. When placed in the ascending aorta, some groups use long cannulae directed into the proximal descending aorta to minimize jet effects in the arch, while others use very short cannulae inserted only 1 to 2 cm into the aorta. Dissection associated with ascending aortic cannulation occurs in less than 0.1% of patients. The ascending aorta may not be a suitable cannulation site for various reasons including presence of severe atherosclerotic disease,

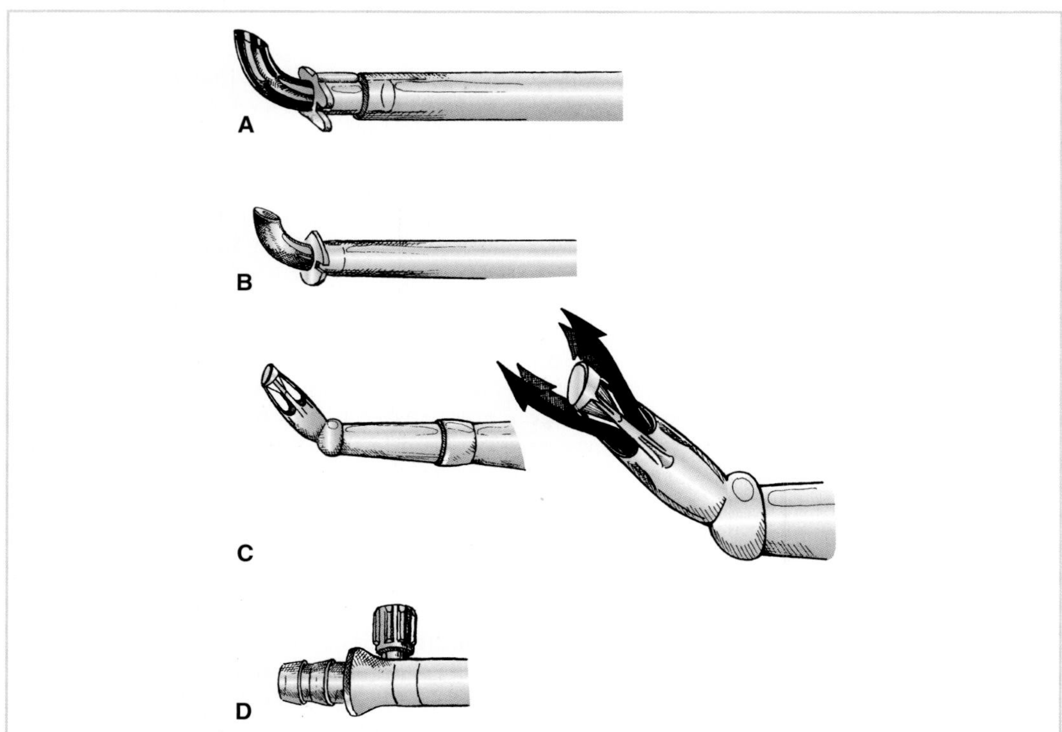

FIGURE 21.4 Arterial cannulae. Drawings of commonly used arterial cannulae. **A:** Tapered, bevel-tipped cannula with molded flange near tip. **B:** Angled, thin-walled, metal-tipped cannula with molded flange for securing cannula to aorta. **C:** Angled, diffusion-tipped cannula designed to direct systemic flow in four directions (right) to avoid a "jetting effect" that may occur with conventional single-lumen arterial cannulae. **D:** Integral cannula/tubing connector and luer port (for deairing) incorporated onto some newer arterial cannulae. (From Hessel EA II. Circuitry and cannulation techniques. In: Gravlee GP, et al., eds. *Cardiopulmonary Bypass.* Philadelphia, PA: Lippincott Williams & Wilkins; 2008:72, with permission.)

TABLE 21.1 Arterial cannulation sites

	Indications and advantages	**Limitations and hazards**
Ascending aorta	Convenient Lower risk of dissection (~0.1%)	Atheroembolism May not be available due to ascending aortic pathology (e.g., atherosclerotic, "porcelain aorta", aneurysm, dissection)
Femoral/Illiac	Ease For peripheral cannulation During re-entry, especially if developed bleeding Pre-incision if severe heart failure For minimal-access surgery	Retrograde dissection (~0.5–1.5%) Unavailable if peripheral vascular disease (PVD) Ischemia of cannulated extremity Compartment syndrome Post-release emboli Risk of malperfusion when used in patients with aortic dissection
Axillary/subclavian	Best for patients with aortic dissection Permits selective cerebral perfusion (SCP) Decrease risk of atheroemboli	More difficult and time consuming Not risk-free

aortic dissection, and for minimal access surgery, left thoracotomy surgery, and risk of or rescue from hemorrhage during repeat sternotomy.

b. **Femoral or external iliac artery:** This is the second most common approach and is used when ascending aortic cannulation is not desirable or feasible. However, this approach has a number of limitations including risk of dissection (0.5% to 1%), risk of atheroembolism (especially into brain and heart), malperfusion of the brain and other organs in the presence of extensive aortic dissection, and ischemia of the cannulated limb. The use of TEE surveillance of the descending aorta is recommended when CPB is initiated and periodically throughout CPB in order to detect the presence of a retrograde dissection. Prolonged femoral cannulation times may result in the release of emboli and acidotic products from the limb with reperfusion and for subsequent development of compartment syndrome in the limb. To minimize leg ischemia, some groups sew a graft onto the side of the femoral artery and insert the arterial cannula into this graft so that blood flows both retrograde and antegrade, while others insert a supplemental arterial cannula into the distal femoral artery.

c. **Axillary/subclavian artery cannulation** is often advocated in the presence of aortic dissection or severe atherosclerosis. These vessels are usually free of significant atherosclerosis, and malperfusion and iatrogenic dissection are probably less common than with femoral cannulation. The artery is approached through an infraclavicular incision, and the cannula can be placed either directly into the vessel, or via a graft sewn onto the side of the artery. The right artery is favored since it permits selective cerebral perfusion (SCP) if circulatory arrest is required (see later). If the vessel is cannulated directly (i.e., not through a side arm graft), then the artery in the contralateral upper extremity (radial or brachial) must be used for systemic arterial pressure monitoring during CPB.

d. **Innominate artery:** Rarely used approach. There is concern about adequacy of flow around the cannula (which is directed retrograde toward the ascending aorta) into the distal vessel and hence the brain.

D. **Venous reservoir**

1. **Overview:** The venous reservoir is designed to receive the venous drainage from the patient. The reservoir is placed immediately before the systemic arterial pump to serve as a "holding tank" and act as a buffer for fluctuation and imbalances between venous return and arterial flow. It also serves as a high-capacitance (i.e., low-pressure) receiving chamber for venous return and hence facilitates gravity drainage of venous blood. Additional venous blood may become available from the patient when CPB is initiated and systemic venous pressure is reduced to low levels. Thus, as much as 1 to 3 L of blood may need to be translocated from the patient to the ECC when full CPB begins. This reservoir may also serve as a gross bubble trap for air that enters the venous line, as the site where blood, fluids, or drugs may be added, and as a ready source of blood for transfusion into the patient. One of its most important functions, however, is to provide a source of blood if venous drainage is sharply reduced or stopped; this provides the perfusionist with **reaction time** in order to avoid "pumping the CPB system dry" and risking massive air embolism. These reservoirs usually include various filtering devices. There are two classes of reservoirs:

   a. **Rigid hard-shell plastic, "open" venous canisters:** Advantages include ability to handle venous air more effectively, simple to prime, larger capacity, and ability to apply suction for vacuum-assisted venous return. Most hard-shell venous reservoirs incorporate macro- and microfilters often coated with defoaming agents and can also serve as the cardiotomy reservoir (see later) by directly receiving suctioned and vented blood. Their ability to remove gaseous microemboli (GME) varies.

   b. **Soft-shell, collapsible plastic bag, "closed" venous reservoirs:** These reservoirs eliminate the gas–blood interface and reduce the risk of massive air embolism because they will collapse when emptied and do not permit air to enter the systemic pump. Closed collapsible reservoirs also make the aspiration of air by the venous cannulae more obvious to the perfusionist, but require a way of emptying the air out of the

TABLE 21.2 Comparison of roller versus centrifugal pumps

Centrifugal	Roller
Output inversely proportional to afterload (i.e., arterial pressure)	Output independent of afterload
Output not directly related to rpm Require flowmeter to determine output Will allow retrograde flow out of aorta when turned off if line not clamped	Output = rpm × volume per revolution
Will not blow out arterial line	Will blow out arterial line if line clamped
—	Must adjust occlusiveness
Would not pump massive air (but can pass amounts of air that can harm the patient)	Can pump massive air Wear (release particles of plastic ("spallation"); can rupture with prolonged use
Perhaps less blood trauma Perhaps safer Both require constant attention to adapt to available venous return.	

reservoir. When soft-shell reservoirs are used, a separate cardiotomy reservoir is required (see later). Because of reduction of the gas–blood interface, their use may be associated with less inflammatory activation. Data on comparative clinical outcome with use of the two types of venous reservoirs are conflicting and inconclusive [6].

E. **Systemic (arterial) pump:** There are currently two types of blood pumps used in the CPB circuit: Roller and kinetic (most commonly called centrifugal) (Table 21.2). In the United States, kinetic pumps are used in approximately 50% of all procedures.

1. **Roller pump (Fig. 21.5)**
   a. **Principles of operation:** Blood is moved through this pump by sequential compression of tubing by a roller against a horseshoe-shaped backing plate or raceway. A typical pump has two roller heads configured 180° apart to maintain continuous roller head contact with the tubing. The output is determined by the stroke volume of each revolution (the volume within the tubing which is dependent upon the tubing size [internal diameter] and the length of the compressed pathway times the revolutions per minute [rpm]). Flow from a systemic roller pump increases or decreases linearly with rpm. With larger ID tubing (e.g., 1/2-inch ID), lower rpm are required to achieve the same output compared to smaller ID tubing. The total pump output is displayed in milliliters or liters per minute on the pump control panel. Roller pumps are also used to deliver cardioplegia solution, remove blood and air from heart chambers or great vessels, and suction shed blood from the operative field (see later).

   b. **Adjustment of occlusion:** To minimize hemolysis, the occlusion must be properly set. Occlusion describes the degree to which the tubing is compressed between the rollers and the backing plate. An under-occlusive pump will allow retrograde movement of fluid when the pressure in the downstream location exceeds that generated by the pump, reducing forward flow. Conversely, an over-occlusive pump will create cellular damage (red blood cell [RBC] hemolysis, white blood cell [WBC] and platelet activation) and excessive wear on the tubing with release of microparticles ("spallation"). Occlusion is set by the perfusionist by adjusting the distance between the raceway and each of the roller heads. Typically, occlusion is adjusted to be barely nonocclusive.

   c. **Advantages and disadvantages:** Roller pumps have the advantages of being simple, effective, low-cost, having a low priming volume, and producing a reliable output which is afterload independent. A primary disadvantage is that since output is afterload independent, if the arterial line becomes occluded, high pressure will develop which may cause rupture of connections in the arterial line. If inflow is obstructed, roller pumps can generate high negative pressures creating microbubbles ("cavitation") and RBC damage.
2 **Roller pumps may cause more damage to blood components and can result in**

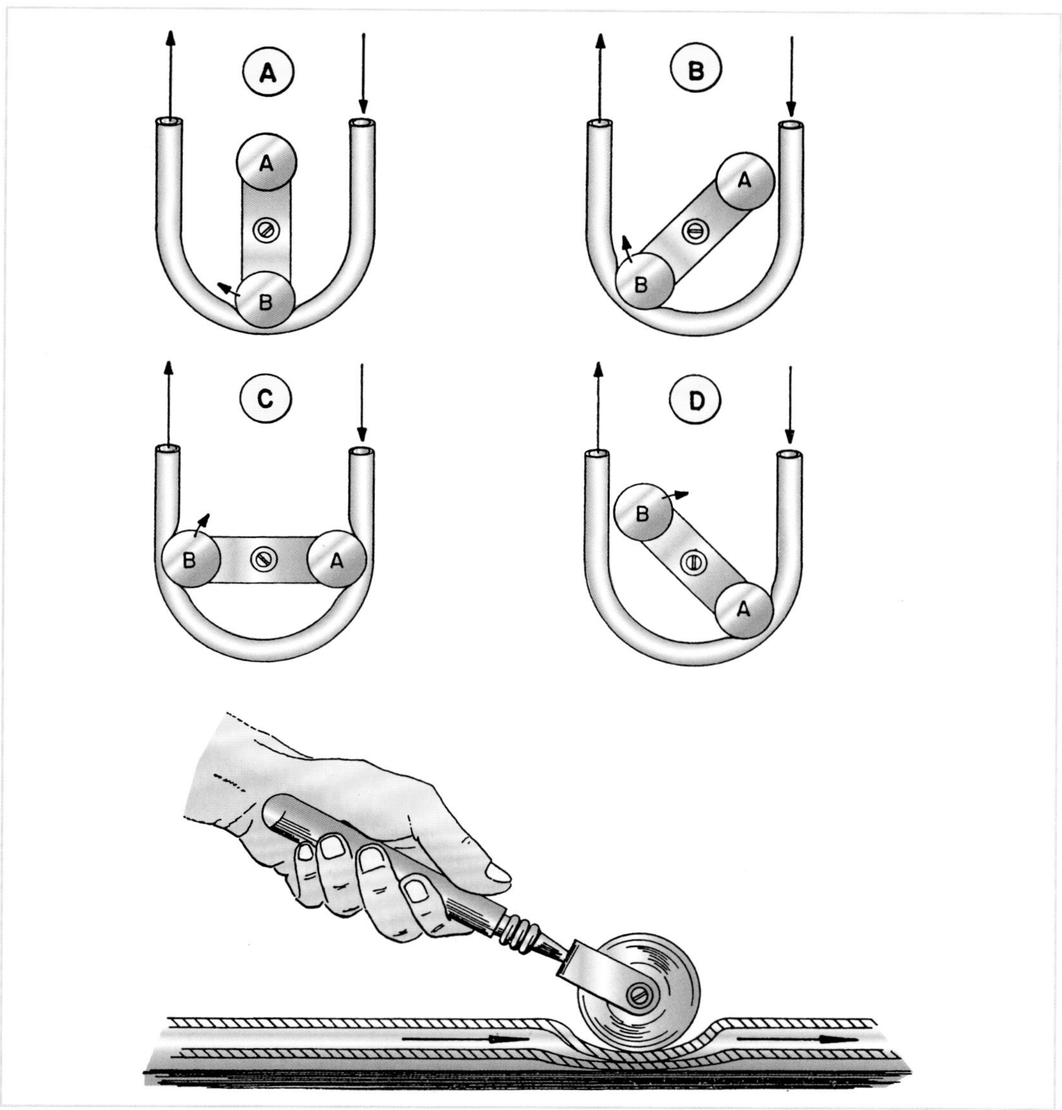

FIGURE 21.5 Roller pump. Drawing of a dual roller pump and tubing. The principle of the roller pump is demonstrated by the hand roller in the lower drawing moving along a section of tubing pushing fluid ahead of it and suctioning fluid behind it. The upper four drawings in sequence **(A–D)** show how roller pump B first moves fluid ahead of it and suctions fluid behind it **(A)**. As the pump rotates clockwise, the second roller A begins to engage the tubing **(B)**. As the rotation continues there is a very brief period with volume trapped between the two rollers **(C)** and no forward flow, which imparts some pulsatility. In position **D**, roller B leaves the tubing, while the second roller A continues to move fluid in the same direction. Not shown are the roller pump backing plate, tubing holders, and tube guides for maintaining the tubing within the raceway. Fluid flows in direction of the *arrows*. (From Stofer RC. *A Technic for Extracorporeal Circulation*. Springfield, IL: Charles C. Thomas; 1968:22, with permission.)

massive air embolism if the venous reservoir becomes empty. They do not adjust to changes in venous return and require more careful attention by the perfusionist.

2. **Centrifugal pumps (Fig. 21.6)**
   a. **Principles of operation:** Centrifugal pumps consist of a nest of smooth plastic cones or a vaned impeller located inside a plastic housing. When rotated rapidly (2,000 to

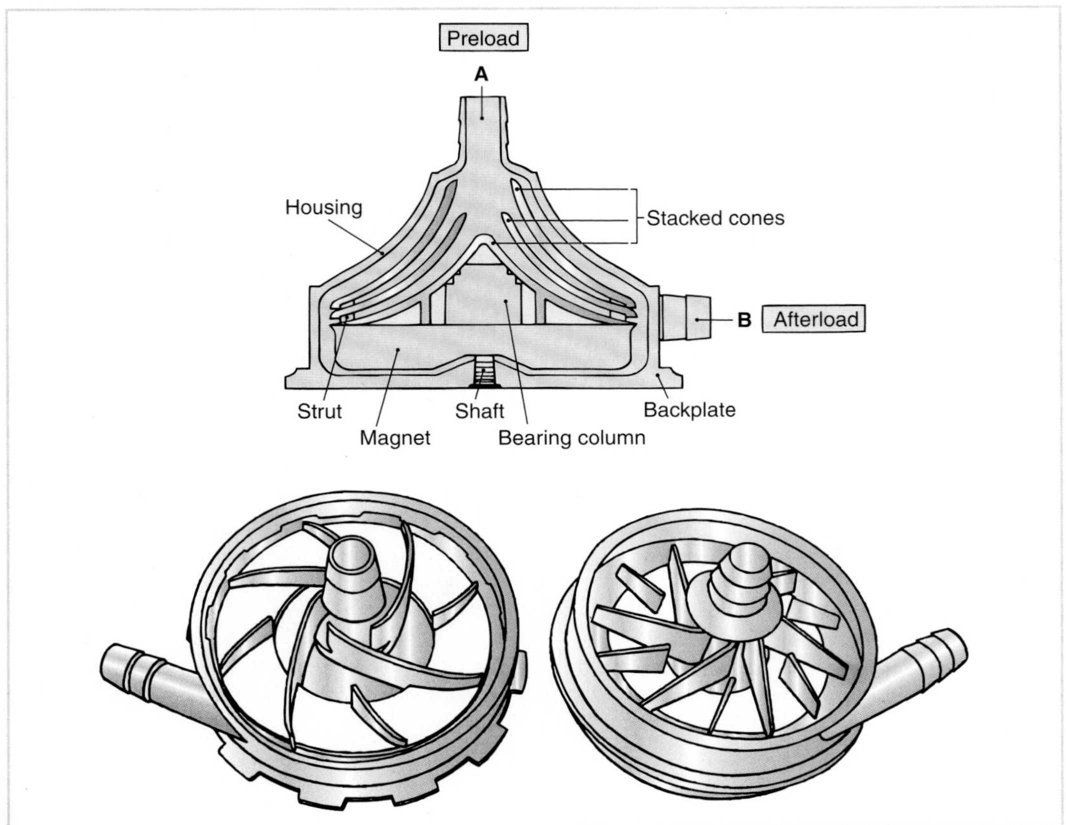

FIGURE 21.6 Centrifugal pumps. Drawings of centrifugal pump-heads. A cross-sectional view of a smooth, cone-type pump is shown on the top. Blood enters at A and is expelled on the right (B) due to kinetic forces created by the three rapidly spinning cones. Impeller-type pumps with vanes are shown in the bottom drawings. (Modified from Trocchio CR, Sketel JO. Mechanical pumps for extracorporeal circulation. In: Mora CT, ed. *Cardiopulmonary Bypass: Principles and Techniques of Extracorporeal Circulation.* New York, NY: Springer-Verlag; 1995:222, 223, with permission.)

3,000 rpm), these pumps generate a pressure differential that causes the movement of fluid. Smaller, vaned, impeller-type rotary (centrifugal) pumps are being used clinically in place of the traditional cone-type centrifugal pump These have smaller prime volumes and may cause less hemolysis.

b. Advantages and disadvantages: Unlike roller pumps, these devices are totally nonocclusive and afterload dependent (an increase in downstream resistance or pressure decreases forward flow). This has both favorable and unfavorable consequences. Flow is not determined by rotational rate alone, and therefore a **flowmeter** *must* be incorporated in the outflow line to quantify pump flow. Furthermore, when the pump is connected to the patient's arterial system but is not rotating, blood will flow backward through the pump and out of the patient unless the CPB systemic line is clamped or a one-way valve is incorporated into the arterial line. This can cause exsanguination of the patient or aspiration of air into the arterial line (from around the purse-string sutures). On the other hand, if the arterial line becomes occluded, these pumps will not generate excessive pressure and will not rupture the systemic flow line. Likewise, they will not generate as much negative pressure and hence as much cavitation and microembolus production as a roller pump if inflow becomes occluded.

A reputed advantage of centrifugal pumps over roller pumps is less risk of pumping massive air emboli into the arterial line; centrifugal pumps will become deprimed and stop pumping if more than approximately 50 mL of air is introduced into the circuit. **However, they will pass smaller but still potentially lethal quantities of smaller bubbles.** A number of studies have demonstrated that centrifugal pumps cause less trauma to blood elements, less activation of coagulation, produce fewer microemboli, and may be associated with better clinical outcomes than roller pumps [6].

3. **Pulsatile flow and pulsatile pumps**
   a. **Overview:** Most roller pumps produce only a low-amplitude, high-frequency pulsatile flow of little physiologic relevance, while centrifugal pumps produce a nonpulsatile flow. The importance of pulsatile flow has long been debated. (See later in this chapter and paper by Murphy et al. [6].)
   b. Many groups use roller pumps and centrifugal pumps that can be programmed to produce pulsatile flow.
   c. **A major problem** with efforts to produce physiologically effective pulsatile flow in the patient is the dampening effect of various components distal to the arterial pump including the MO, arterial filter, and the arterial cannula. It has been calculated that very little of the pulsatile energy generated is actually delivered into the patient's arterial system.

F. **The oxygenator (artificial lung or gas exchanging device)**

1. Although numerous **types of oxygenators** have been used in the past, currently only MOs are used in most parts of the world. These produce less blood trauma and microemboli, permit more precise control of arterial blood gases, and improve patient outcomes as compared with bubble oxygenators. Virtually all current MOs are positioned after the arterial pump because the resistance in the blood path requires blood to be pumped through them, and to minimize the risk of pulling air through the membrane and producing GME. Most oxygenators also include an integral heat exchanger (see later).

   MOs function similarly to natural lungs, **imposing a membrane between the ventilating gas and the flowing blood and eliminating direct contact between the blood and the gas**. At least three types of membranes are used:
   a. **True membranes:** These usually consist of thin sheets of silicone rubber wrapped circumferentially over a spool.
   b. **Microporous polypropylene (PPL) membranes:** Usually configured in longitudinal bundles of narrow hollow fibers, but occasionally as folded sheets of membrane. The pores fill with autologous plasma which serves as the "membrane" through which gas exchange occurs. With excessive pressure in the blood path or over prolonged time, plasma may leak through the membrane (which degrades gas transfer), while excessive negative pressure can lead to entrainment of air emboli. In hollow fiber MOs, the blood typically flows outside the hollow fibers, while ventilating gases flow through the hollow fibers (in a counter-current direction).
   c. **Poly-methyl pentene (PMP) diffusion membranes:** Hollow fiber MOs made of a new non porous plastic, PMP, are true membranes. This has the advantage of minimizing the risk of plasma leak and microair aspiration and permits prolonged oxygenation(days). Gas exchange occurs by diffusion across this true membrane. An important limitation is that it does not appear to allow transfer of volatile anesthetics and therefore intravenous anesthetics must be employed during CPB. Because of this limitation and because they are more expensive, PMP "diffusion" MOs are not commonly used for conventional CPB, at least in the United States, but because of their reduced risk of plasma leak ("oxygenator pulmonary edema") are commonly used for long term extracorporeal support (e.g., extracorporeal membrane oxygenation [ECMO]).

2. MOs were thought to serve as bubble filters and to prevent venous GME from passing into the arterial system, but it is now recognized that the majority of venous gas emboli transit through MOs. The effectiveness of GME removal varies among MOs [6]. This limitation is

why teams must make every effort to minimize the entrainment and administration of air into the venous drainage system.

3. **Control of gas exchange and gas supply to the MO:** Gas exchange by MO is controlled similarly to normal lungs. Arterial carbon dioxide levels are controlled by flow of fresh gas (commonly called "sweep gas flow") through the oxygenator (comparable to alveolar ventilation), and arterial PO_2 is controlled by varying fractional inspired oxygen (F_IO_2). Oxygenators require a **gas supply system**. This typically includes a source of oxygen and air (and occasionally carbon dioxide), which passes through a **blender**. An **oxygen analyzer** should be incorporated in the gas supply line after the blender. An **anesthetic vaporizer** is also placed in the gas supply line near the oxygenator. Volatile anesthetic liquids may be destructive to the plastic components of ECCs; therefore, care must be taken when filling them with volatile agents. A method of **scavenging** waste gas from the oxygenator outlet should be provided.

G. Heat exchanger

1. **Overview:** The passage of blood through the ECC results in heat loss and patient cooling. To maintain normothermia, heat must be added to the circuit. This is accomplished with a **heat exchanger**, which may also be used to intentionally cool and rewarm the patient. Heat exchangers consist of heat-exchanging tubes (often metal) through which the blood flows. These tubes are surrounded by water of varying temperatures. As mentioned earlier, heat exchangers are often incorporated in the oxygenator.
2. **Heater–cooler.** To control the temperature of the water flowing through the heat exchanger, a heater–cooler device adjusts the water temperature and pumps it through the heat exchanger (counter-current with the blood flow).
3. Excessive gradients between the blood and water temperature should be avoided. Most groups avoid gradients greater than 10°C. Proper conduct of heating and cooling requires monitoring of the temperature of the water going to the heat exchanger, and of the venous and arterial blood entering and leaving the H–L machine. **Excessive warming can lead to gases coming out of solution and causing GME and could cause excessive heating of the**
4 **brain. Currently, most groups limit the inflow temperature of the arterial blood to 37°C** and limit the inflow temperature of the water entering the heat exhanger to 40°C. However, acceptable or optimal temperature gradients have not been conclusively determined.
4. Separate heat exchangers are also used in the cardioplegia circuits (see below).

H. Cardioplegia delivery system or circuit

1. **Overview:** When the aorta is cross-clamped (distal to the aortic valve but proximal to the arterial inflow cannula) to provide a quiet operative field or access to the aortic valve, the heart is deprived of coronary perfusion and becomes ischemic. This is usually managed by perfusing the heart with cardioplegia solutions. (See also Chapter 23 for further discussion on myocardial protection.)
2. **Route of delivery of cardioplegia solutions**
    a. **Aortic root:** A cannula is inserted in the aortic root (proximal to the cross-clamp). Typically this has a "Y" connector: One limb is connected to the cardioplegia delivery system and the other to suction (to vent the left ventricle [LV] or aspirate air). The cardioplegia solution is delivered into the aortic root and thence into the coronary arteries. **This is not effective in the presence of severe aortic regurgitation or when the aortic root is open;** it is also less effective in the presence of severe proximal coronary artery stenosis. Ideally, pressure in the aortic root should be measured during administration of the cardioplegia to assure adequate coronary flow.

    b. **Directly into the coronary ostia:** Special hand-held cannulae are placed directly into the right and left main coronary arteries for delivery of the cardioplegia solutions. This is commonly done in the presence of aortic regurgitation or when the aortic root is open.

    c. **Retrograde into the coronary sinus:** Balloon-tipped cannulae are inserted blindly (or under direct vision if the RA is opened) into the coronary sinus through a purse-string suture in the low lateral wall of the RA. TEE may be helpful in guiding and assessing placement. Many of these cannulae have a pressure port near the tip so that the pressure in the coronary sinus can be monitored during perfusion (ideally maintained between 30 and 50 mm Hg). Retrograde administration of cardioplegia may be advantageous in the presence of severe coronary artery stenosis or aortic regurgitation and during aortic valve surgery. **However, it may provide inferior protection of the RV.**

3. **Delivery systems.** These vary in their complexity. If blood cardioplegia is being used, blood is taken out of the arterial perfusion line following oxygenation and mixed with the crystalloid cardioplegia solution (usually at a blood:crystalloid ratio of 4 to 6:1). This may be accomplished by using two separate roller pumps, or with a single roller pump which drives two sets of tubing of different sizes (to produce the proper flow ratio). The mixture is then passed through a dedicated heat exchanger. Microfiltration may be added and pressures and temperatures are monitored. More complex delivery systems are in use which permit rapid change of the concentration of various components in the cardioplegia solution.

I. **Cardiotomy, field suction, cell salvage processors, and savers**

1. **Overview:** During CPB there is often considerable bleeding into the surgical field due to systemic heparinization and persistent pulmonary and coronary venous drainage. It is usually not feasible to discard this large volume of blood via conventional discard suction. Traditionally, this blood is removed from the field by roller pumps on the H–L machine **("cardiotomy suckers")** and returned to the H–L machine via the **cardiotomy reservoir** (which includes filters and, as noted above, is commonly incorporated into the hard-shell venous reservoir, but must be added separately when a soft-shell reservoir is used). The cardiotomy suction should not be used until the patient is adequately anticoagulated and should be discontinued as soon as reversal with protamine is commenced (to avoid clotting of blood in the H–L machine).

5 2. **Hazards of cardiotomy blood:** Cardiotomy blood contains microaggregates of cells, fat, foreign debris, and thrombogenic and fibrinolytic factors, and is thought to be a major source of microemboli and hemolysis during CPB. **For these reasons cardiotomy suction should be used sparingly.**

3. **An alternative strategy** is to suction the field blood into a **cell salvage washer/processor/saver system** (or to process the blood that has been suctioned into a stand-alone cardiotomy reservoir with this cell salvage system before returning it to the H–L machine). These devices wash the blood with saline, and separate the red cells from the plasma and saline by centrifugation with the intent of reducing the microemboli, fat, etc. It also removes plasma proteins, platelets, heparin, and some of the WBCs, retaining concentrated RBCs (hematocrit about 70%). Not all processors are equally effective at removing fat, and the salvaged blood may have to be specially filtered before administration. Some of the problems associated with the use of cell processors include delayed availability and turnover time (not adequate in the face of rapid hemorrhage) and loss of platelets and coagulation factors (resulting in a consumptive coagulopathy if >6 bowls or 1,500 mL of blood is processed). Comparative studies of cardiotomy suction versus cell processors have produced conflicting results [6].

J. **Venting**

1. **Overview:** It is important that both the RV and LV are decompressed during CPB to improve surgical exposure, reduce oxygen demands of the myocardium, and attenuate damage to the heart from overdistention.
2. The RV is readily visible to the surgeon, and decompression depends on adequacy of venous drainage. The LV is more difficult to observe, has more adverse consequences if distended, and requires various strategies for venting.
3. **Consequences of distention of the left heart:**
   a. Stretches myocardium causing ventricular dysfunction
   b. Myocardial ischemia: Impairs subendocardial perfusion and increases myocardial oxygen needs
   c. Increases left atrial pressure, leading to pulmonary edema and hemorrhage
   d. Interferes with surgical exposure
4. **Distention of the left heart is likely to occur** when the LV is unable to empty (e.g., on initiation of CPB, in the presence of aortic regurgitation, during cardiac arrest, aortic cross-clamping, and administration of antegrade cardioplegia, during ventricular fibrillation, and following aortic cross-clamp release).

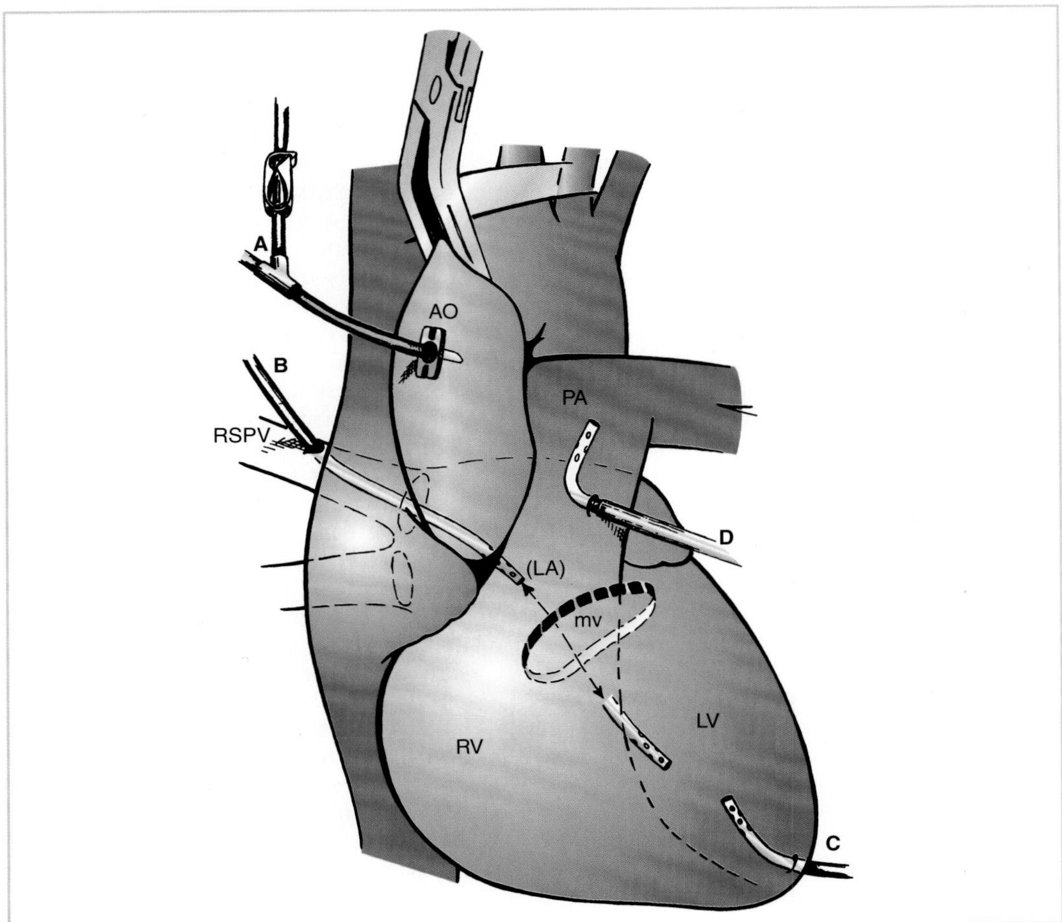

FIGURE 21.7 Sites for venting the left heart. A: Aortic root cannula; one limb of the "Y" is connected to the cardioplegia delivery system and the other limb to suction (siphon or roller pump) for venting the aortic root and hence the LV. **B:** Cannula inserted at the junction of the right superior pulmonary vein with the left atrium and then threaded through the left atrium and MV and into the LV. **C:** Cannula inserted directly into the apex of the LV. **D:** Cannula is inserted into the pulmonary artery. AO, aorta; PA pulmonary artery; LA, left atrium. (From Hessel EA II. Circuitry and cannulation techniques. In: Gravlee GP, et al., eds. *Cardiopulmonary Bypass*. Philadelphia, PA: Lippincott Williams & Wilkins; 2008:90, with permission.)

5. **Sources of blood coming into the left heart during CPB:**
   a. Bronchial venous drainage (normal ~100 mL/min)
   b. Systemic venous blood that bypasses venous cannulae and passes through right heart and lungs
   c. Aortic regurgitation
   d. Patent ductus arteriosus (PDA) (~1/3,500 adults)
   e. Atrial septal defect (ASD), Ventricular septal defect (VSD)
6. **Assessment of adequacy of decompression of the left heart** by inspection or palpation is difficult because of its position and thick walls of the LV. The best method of evaluating the adequacy of LV decompression is TEE.
7. **Methods of venting or decompressing the left heart** (see Fig. 21.7 and Table 21.3): Cannulae are inserted in various locations and attached to tubing connected to roller pumps which transfers the blood to the venous or cardiotomy reservoirs. The tubing should first be placed under a level of fluid to assure that it is sucking and not emitting air,

TABLE 21.3 Methods of venting the left heart

Method	Advantages	Disadvantages
Ascending aortic (cardioplegia cannula)	Simple; no additional cannula	Only works when aorta is cross-clamped
	Also vents air when unclamp aorta and when LV starts to eject	Does not work during administration of antegrade cardioplegia
	Can be used to monitor aortic root infusion pressure	Can cause air to be aspirated into the aortic root
Indirect LV (via stab wound in RSPV, through LA and MV)	Handles all sources of blood causing LV distension	Somewhat difficult exposure of insertion site
	Best for aortic regurgitation	May be difficult to thread cannula into LV and position correctly
	Provides optimal decompression of LV	Risk of bleeding and tears at insertion site in RSPV
	Avoids problems of direct LV vent	Potential for air entry into left heart
		Potential problem if mechanical prosthesis in MV
		Potential embolism if tumor or clots in LA or LV
Direct LV (through stab wound in apex)	Direct and simple	Positioning may be a problem—tip becomes easily obstructed by LV wall or MV apparatus
	Avoids going across prosthetic MV	Risk of damage to LV and injury to coronary arteries and collaterals (myocardial ischemia)
	Handles all sources of blood causing LV distension	May be difficult to control bleeding from stab wound
		Late LV aneurysm
		Potential embolism if clots in LV
		Potential for air entry into the left heart
Direct LV (via LA appendage, roof of LA, or RSPV)	Relatively simple	Does not handle AR
	Avoids going across the MV	Potential embolism if clots in LA
		Potential for air entry into the left heart
Pulmonary artery	Simple, easy access	Does not handle AR
	Reduces risk of admitting air into the left heart (but still can occur)	Renders use of PA pressure as a monitor of LV distention invalid
		Risk of damage and bleeding from pulmonary artery

LA, left atrium; PA, pulmonary artery; RSPV, right superior pulmonary vein; AR, aortic regurgitation.
Modified from Table 5 in Chapter 5 in Gravlee GP, et al. *Cardiopulmonary Bypass.* 3rd ed. Philadelphia, PA: Wolters Kluwer/Lippincott Williams & Wilkins; 2008.

and the rate of suction must be constantly adjusted to avoid excessive (risk of damage to heart or aspirating air) or inadequate (overdistention) venting.

a. **Aortic root vent** (one limb of the antegrade cardioplegia cannula): This is the most common technique used during coronary artery bypass graft (CABG) surgery. Suction is applied to the antegrade cardioplegia cannula (directly or via a side branch). Aortic root venting of the LV is only effective when the aorta is cross-clamped, when antegrade cardioplegia is not being administered, and when the aortic root is not opened.
b. **LV vent placed via the right superior pulmonary vein:** A cannula is inserted at the junction of the right superior pulmonary vein with the left atrium and then threaded through the left atrium and MV into the LV. This method is used during aortic and MV surgery (especially in the presence of aortic regurgitation) and for patients with poor LV function.

c. **LV vent placed directly through the LV apex:** This is rarely used today because of difficulty in positioning and bleeding after removal.

d. **Vent placed through the left atrial appendage or the top of the left atrium** (into either the left atrium or LV). Rarely used.

e. **Vent placed in the main pulmonary artery:** This method minimizes the risk of air entry into the left heart (although it can still occur). It does **not** provide reliable decompression of the LV in the presence of aortic regurgitation, and closure of the incision in the pulmonary artery can be problematic in patients with pulmonary hypertension.

8. **Complications of venting the left heart** include systemic air embolism, bleeding, damage to cardiac structures, dislodgement of thrombi, calcium, tumor, etc., and MV incompetence. A critical complication is inadvertent pumping of air into the heart via these vent lines. This occurs if tubing is misaligned in the roller pump-head or if the pump is in reverse mode. Air can also enter the left heart when these lines are inserted or removed; therefore, the volume and pressure in the left heart should be high at these times and ventilation interrupted.

9. Any time the heart is opened, even by simply placing a catheter in a chamber, air may collect in the heart. If not removed, this air will embolize with resumption of cardiac contractions. Even right-heart air has the potential to pass into the left heart via septal defects or through the lungs. In addition to vigorous attempts at removal of all air before closing the left heart, **the use of venting at the highest point of the aorta is considered the final safety maneuver against systemic air embolism.** This is most commonly accomplished using the **antegrade cardioplegia cannula** (see above) which is placed on suction. TEE is particularly useful in assessing the adequacy of deairing. Some surgical teams often flood the surgical field with carbon dioxide during open cardiac procedures. Because of carbon dioxide's increased solubility there is a potential for reduction of microemboli.

K. **Ultrafiltration/hemoconcentrators.** A hemofiltration device (also referred to as ultrafiltration) consists of a semipermeable membrane which separates blood flowing on one side (under pressure) and air (sometimes under vacuum) on the other side. **Water and small molecules (sodium, potassium, water-soluble non–protein-bound anesthetic agents) can pass through it and be removed from the blood, but not protein or cellular components of the blood.** Hemoconcentrators are used to eliminate excess crystalloid and potassium, and to raise hematocrit (hemoconcentrate). They may also remove inflammatory mediators and hence reduce the systemic inflammatory response syndrome (SIRS). The device is usually placed distal or after the arterial pump with drainage into the venous limb or reservoir. It can be placed in the venous limb of the circuit but would require a separate pump. Five hundred to 2,000 mL or more of fluid may be removed during an adult case. When using post-bypass (but before reversing heparin) it is referred to as **"modified ultrafiltration" or "MUF."** MUF is commonly used in pediatric cases but rarely in adult cases [4,7].

L. **Filters and bubble traps**

1. **Overview:** CPB generates macro- and microemboli of gas, lipids, and other microparticles (WBCs, platelets, foreign debris) which must be filtered out.
2. **Types and location:** Many different types of filters (screen and packed fibers ["in-depth"], made of various materials) with various pore sizes are employed in multiple locations in the ECC. These sites include the venous and cardiotomy reservoirs, as part of the oxygenator, in the arterial and cardioplegia lines, and blood administration sets (including the cell processor), and the gas going to the oxygenator. The "in-depth filters" mainly work by adsorption. The clinical importance of the various types of filters remains controversial [6].
3. **Arterial line filter/bubble trap:** Most groups employ a microfilter/bubble trap on the arterial line, especially to reduce air embolization [6]. If used, often a clamped bypass line is placed around the filter in case the filter becomes obstructed and a vent line with a one-way valve runs from the filter/bubble trap to the venous reservoir to vent any trapped air.
4. The employment of **leukocyte-depleting filters** in various locations in the circuit is advocated by some, but their benefit remains to be proven.

TABLE 21.4 Monitors and safety devices

Monitors	Safety devices
Pressure in arterial line	High arterial line pressure alarm ± servo control or turn-off of arterial pump
Level sensor in venous reservoir	Low level in venous reservoir alarm ± servo control or turn off of arterial pump
Bubble/air detector	Air/bubble detector alarm ± servo control or turn off of arterial pump
Microprocessor/console monitor and control	One-way check valves in arterial line, cardiac vents, and arterial line filter/bubble-trap purge line
Inline venous and/or arterial oxygen saturation or PO_2 monitor ± of other gases, electrolytes, glucose, lactates, and hematocrit/hemoglobin	Arterial line filter
Arterial line flowmeter	Bypass line around arterial line filter/bubble trap
Temperature of systemic blood coming out of and going into the patient, and of water going into the heat exchangers, and of the cardioplegia solution	Purge line off of the arterial line filter/bubble trap
Oxygen analyzer of gas going into the oxygenator	

M. Safety devices and monitors on the H–L machine

1. **Monitors (see Table 21.4)**
   - **a.** Microprocessor/console monitor and control. Many of the current commercial H–L machines include a microprocessor-driven monitor that displays and controls various functions of the machine and hemodynamic data from the patient.
   - **b.** Inline venous and arterial oxygen saturation, ± other blood gases, electrolytes, glucose, and hematocrit.
   - **c.** Pressure in arterial line: This should be measured proximal to the arterial line filter/ bubble trap and distal to the oxygenator. Prior to initiation of CPB, the pressure should reflect a pulsatile wave that correlates with patient's arterial pressure (to confirm proper intra-arterial placement of the arterial cannula). Excessively high arterial infusion line pressure during CPB (relative to patient's arterial pressure) indicates a problem in the arterial flow delivery system or at the cannula tip, bearing in mind that there should always be a considerable (50 to 150 mm Hg) pressure gradient across the aortic cannula. Pressures in the line post-CPB can give clues to true systemic pressures. Some also advocate monitoring the pressure proximal to the MO; high gradients (>100 mm Hg) suggest oxygenator dysfunction.
   - **d.** Level sensor in venous reservoir
   - **e.** Bubble/air detector
   - **f.** Arterial line flowmeter: This is required when using a centrifugal systemic arterial pump, and desirable even when using a roller pump.
   - **g.** Temperature: Water-to-heat exchanger and of blood being delivered to the patient
   - **h.** Oxygen analyzer of gas delivered to oxygenator
2. **Safety devices (see Table 21.4)**
   - **a.** Low-level alarm ± servo control/turn-off of arterial pump
   - **b.** High arterial line pressure alarm ± servo control/turn-off of arterial pump
   - **c.** Air/bubble detector and alarm ± servo control/turn-off of arterial pump
   - **d.** One-way check valves in the arterial lines, cardiac vents, and arterial filter/bubble-trap purge lines
   - **e.** Arterial line filter
   - **f.** Bypass line around arterial line filter/bubble trap
   - **g.** Purge line off of arterial line filter/bubble trap

3. **Emergency personnel, supplies, and equipment**
   a. Second perfusionist
   b. Battery backup for H–L machine including the pumps and monitors
   c. Portable lighting and flashlights
   d. Backup-oxygen supply (cylinders with regulators)
   e. Hand cranks to drive arterial and other pumps
   f. Spare oxygenator

III. Special topics

A. **Surface coating.** Many commercial circuits coat all of the surfaces which come in contact with blood (tubing, reservoirs, oxygenators) with various substances (proprietary) designed to minimize the activation of blood components. Many of these coatings include heparin (which should be avoided in patients with heparin-induced thrombocytopenia [HIT]). The clinical benefits of any or of one type of coating over another remains controversial [6].

B. **Miniaturized or minimized circuits:** By reducing the surface area and prime volume, miniaturized circuits reduce the amount of hemodilution (resulting in less transfusions) and are purported to reduce the inflammatory response to CPB (producing improved clinical outcomes) [8]. They often feature a closed (veno-arterial loop) circuit (i.e., no venous reservoir or cardiotomy suction) and kinetic-assisted venous drainage. A sophisticated air detection and elimination system is required, as well as stringent avoidance of air entrance in the venous line. Concerns about safety (especially air embolization), inability to handle fluctuations in venous return (especially if the patient has a large blood volume or experiences exsanguination), and lack of cardiotomy and field suction require careful consideration. These systems require close communication amongst all team members. Miniaturized circuits are rarely used in the United States, but may be used more commonly in Europe. Their use is usually limited to uncomplicated CABG and aortic valve surgery, cases associated with minimal intravascular volume shifts and limited need to scavenge much blood from the surgical field.

C. **Pediatric circuits.** The major challenges with pediatric CPB are related to the small blood volume of the patient compared with the prime volume of the ECC, and the small venous and arterial cannulae required by the small-sized vessels. Pediatric cardiac surgery groups and industry have made great strides in miniaturization and reduction of priming volumes (some a little at 100 to 200 mL) by including augmented venous return and elevating and the H–L machine closer to the patient (allowing the use of shorter and narrower tubing). Most pediatric surgery centers in North America include albumen in the prime; packed red blood cell or whole blood and fresh frozen plasma are often used for infants [7]. Some groups exclude arterial microfilters and others use an oxygenator which has an integrated "arterial" microfilter. In distinction to adult CPB, inline arterial blood gas monitoring is employed by the vast majority of North American pediatric centers. (See additional discussion in Chapter 14.)

D. **Cerebral perfusion during circulatory arrest**
   1. **Overview:** Circulatory arrest is often required for conduct of surgery involving the aortic arch, and in congenital heart surgery. Deep hypothermia (<18°C) is used to minimize cerebral injury. For periods of circulatory arrest exceeding 25 to 30 min, two strategies for cerebral perfusion are utilized. The benefits and preference of one over the other remain controversial. (See additional discussion in Chapters 24 and 25.)
   2. **Retrograde cerebral perfusion (RCP):** The arterial line from the H–L machine is connected to the SVC cannula (in the case of bicaval cannulation), or to a cannula inserted through a purse-string in the SVC. The SVC is occluded between the entrance of the catheter and the junction with the RA. Cold blood (15 to 18°C) is then pumped at flow rates of 250 to 500 mL/min and pressures maintained between 20 and 40 mm Hg. It may be desirable to measure the pressure via a catheter placed directly into the right internal jugular (IJ) vein, since valves may reduce the amount of flow and pressure being delivered into this vein. If pressure is measured in this location, it is probably prudent to keep the pressure <25 mm Hg to minimize cerebral edema. An additional benefit of RCP is that atheroemboli and air in the carotid vessels may be "washed out."

3. **Antegrade cerebral perfusion or selective cerebral perfusion (SCP):** Catheter(s) (sometimes with balloon cuffs) connected to the arterial line are inserted into the right innominate or carotid artery or the left carotid and subclavian artery. Cold blood is then infused at a rate of about 10 mL/kg/min and a pressure of about 30 to 70 mm Hg. This technique provides more cerebral blood flow than RCP but adds a risk of arterial trauma and embolization. If the systemic arterial cannula had been inserted into the right subclavian artery (see above), then selective perfusion of the right carotid artery can be accomplished by occluding the proximal innominate artery. If the arterial cannula in the subclavian has been placed via a graft sewn onto the side of the artery, the pressure in the right radial or brachial line provides monitoring of the cerebral perfusion pressure. Obviously this provides only unilateral perfusion and relies on an adequate Circle of Willis to perfuse the left side of the brain.

E. **Less common cannulation**

1. **Minimally invasive or port access CPB** involves use of smaller incision and often smaller or specially designed venous and arterial cannulae for transthoracic placement, or peripheral cannulation. This may require use of augmented venous drainage and increase the risk of aortic dissection associated with femoral artery inflow. Peripherally placed retrograde coronary sinus catheters (via the right IJ vein by the anesthesiologist), and aortic balloon occlusion catheters and antegrade cardioplegia cannulae (passed via the femoral artery) are used. These require TEE and fluoroscopic guidance for proper placement.
2. **Right thoracotomy.** This approach gives excellent views of the MV and RA, but aortic cannulation, occlusion of the ascending aorta, administration of antegrade cardioplegia, and deairing of the LV are problematic. Often some of the minimally invasive cannulation techniques mentioned above are employed.
3. **Left thoracotomy.** This approach is used for surgery on the descending thoracic aorta and occasionally for redo MV surgery and CABG surgery for revascularization of the lateral or posterior heart. Venous cannulation is problematic. Peripheral cannulation of the RA via the femoral vein is a commonly employed option (see above). For descending thoracic aortic surgery, isolated partial left heart bypass (LHB) can be accomplished cannulating the left atrium or ventricle directly or via a purse-string in the left superior pulmonary vein or left atrial appendage for venous outflow and the distal aorta or femoral artery for arterial return. The ECC for partial LHB does not require an oxygenator or reservoir and may not include a heat exchanger, typically employs a centrifugal pump and is heparin coated and permits minimal systemic heparinization, but it only supplies oxygenated blood to the lower half of the body. Flows are typically about 1 to 1.5 L/min/M^2 and adjusted to adequately decompress the left heart and maintain adequate pressures in the lower and upper part of the body. Perfusion of the upper half of the body (especially to the heart and brain) is provided by the LV and oxygenation to both parts must be provided by the patient's own lung. Management of partial LHB is quite challenging and requires excellent communication between the anesthesiologist and perfusionist. TEE assessment of LV filling is extremely valuable [9]. See also Chapter 25.

IV. Priming

A. **Overview:** The ECC (including venous and arterial lines) must be filled with fluid ("primed") before use and all air in the circuit eliminated. Circuits are usually primed with asanguineous fluids. To minimize hemodilution much effort has recently been directed at reducing the priming volume of ECC (as low as 1,000 to 1,250 mL for adults).

B. **Consequence of asanguineous primes:** Priming results in hemodilution with reduction of hematocrit, plasma proteins (decreased oncotic pressure), and coagulation factors. Controversy surrounds the acceptable lower level of hematocrit [6]. However, prior to initiation of CPB, the predicted hematocrit should be estimated to determine if the team wishes to add RBCs to the prime.

Predicted hematocrit = (Baseline hematocrit × Estimated blood volume [EBV])/ (EBV + prime volume + first dose of crystaloid in the cardioplegia solution).

Baseline hematocrit used for this calculation should be obtained immediately prior to CPB to account for any crystalloids administered prior to CPB.

C. **Retrograde autologous priming (RAP)** is a method of reducing hemodilution. Before commencing CPB, arterial blood is drained retrograde to displace asanguineous prime in the arterial line (which is sequestered in a collection bag). Immediately before going on CPB, venous blood is also allowed to drain out of the patient through the venous line into the collection bag **("antegrade autologous priming")**. With this method 500 to 1,000 mL of asanguineous prime may be eliminated. However, it is associated with a reduction of the patient's blood volume and may result in hypotension. Placing the patient in Trendelenburg position and administration of a vasopressor is usually required. The majority of randomized trials have demonstrated that RAP reduces perioperative packed RBC transfusions and is usually safe. However, this technique can be very dangerous in certain high-risk patients, leading to hypotension and requiring initiation of immediate bypass to rescue the patient. Further studies are needed to determine the effect of retrograde priming on major morbidity and mortality.

D. **Composition of the prime:** Many formulations are in use. Most use a balanced electrolyte solution without glucose. Much controversy surrounds the need to add colloid, and use of both albumen and hydroxyethyl starches (HES) have been advocated (although use of high-molecular-weight HES [Hetastarch™] is not recommended by the FDA in the United States). Many add mannitol to the prime and most include heparin (about 2,500 units/L).

E. **Priming of the circuit.** The perfusionist fills the circuit with the priming fluid and circulates it employing various maneuvers to remove all air. Often before introducing the prime the circuit is flushed with carbon dioxide which is more easily removed from the prime than air bubbles. Usually, a **prebypass microfilter** is temporarily included in the circuit during this recirculation process to remove any foreign particles.

F. **Final disposition of prime at the end of CPB:** Usually, as much of this volume as possible is returned to the patient before removing the arterial line. That which is left may either be pumped directly (sometimes through a hemoconcentrator) into an IV line in the patient, or placed in an IV bag for administration by the anesthesiologist (preserving platelets and protein but also containing heparin which will require neutralization), or first processed by a cell-washing device and hemoconcentrated (does not contain heparin).

V. Complications, safety, and risk containment

A. **Incidence of adverse events:** Three surveys covering practice between 1994 and 2005 have reported rates of adverse events associated with CPB of 1/35, 1/135, and 1/198 (average 1.3%), with a severe injury or death rates of 1/1,286, 1/1,453, and 1/3,220 (average 0.04%) [10–12].

B. **Specific complications**

1. **Aortic dissection** occurs in about 0.06% of cases (about 0.05% following cannulation of ascending aorta, 1% with femoral artery cannulation, and 0.8% with axillary/subclavian cannulation); adverse outcome occurs in about 20% of these cases. It is usually associated with arterial cannulation but can also be related to cross-clamping, aortic vents, and aorto-coronary anastomoses. Dissection often presents as low arterial pressure, high arterial line pressure, loss of venous return (hidden blood loss), bluish discoloration of ascending aorta, and signs of ischemia in various organs. It is best diagnosed with ultrasound imaging (TEE or epiaortic ultrasound). Although dissection usually presents early it can occur at any time during CPB. Repair of the dissection is usually required (after moving the arterial cannula to an alternate site, and induction of deep hypothermic circulatory arrest). If recognized early in the course of CPB, especially when associated with femoral cannulation, the situation may resolve by simply coming off CPB.
2. **Massive air embolism** occurs in about 0.01% of cases with an adverse outcome in 35% of events. It is almost always preventable with vigilance and employment of various safety devices and techniques. The most common cause is pumping air out of an empty venous reservoir; other causes are related to LV vents, pressurization of cardiotomy or venous reservoirs, and premature ejection by the LV before adequate deairing. Prevention is key. Successful management, when it occurs, requires the collaborative efforts of **all members**

of the team. Establishment of protocols and team practice during simulation are essential. Further discussion can be found in Chapter 8 and management is detailed in Table 8.3.

3. **Oxygenator failure** occurs in about 0.05% of cases with adverse outcomes in 10% of cases. This is usually manifested by hypoxemia, but can also present with hypercapnia. Excessive oxygen consumption (reflected by a low venous saturation) or excessive carbon dioxide production (often related to uptake from the field suction if the field is being flooded with carbon dioxide) should be ruled out. Failure of an oxygenator is often preceded by increased pressure gradients through the oxygenator. Systematic examination of entire oxygen supply system to the oxygenator should be conducted. Disconnections, especially at the anesthesia vaporizer, are common causes, as is malfunction of the blender. An alternate source of oxygen should be explored. If the cause is thought to be the MO and the heart is still functioning, separation from bypass should be considered. If the heart is arrested, then the oxygenator must be replaced. To accomplish this, circulation must be interrupted. If time permits, cooling the patient as rapidly as possible is prudent. With proper training, supplies, and practice, perfusionists should be able to do this in less than 3 min [13].
4. **Arterial pump malfunction:** Malfunction of the arterial pump occurs in about 0.06% of cases. This can be due to electrical or mechanical failure and can result in either excessive flow ("run-away") or cessation of function. Hand cranks must be available.
5. **Inadequate anticoagulation and clotting of the circuit** has been encountered in about 0.03% of cases. It is usually related to inadequate heparinization. Periodic monitoring of anticoagulation is required (see also Chapter 19). While on CPB the ACT can overestimate heparin levels, therefore most groups advocate adding heparin (~100 units/kg) hourly even if the ACT is satisfactory. Monitoring heparin levels (e.g., by protamine titration) may alleviate this discrepancy. A catastrophic accident is inadvertent administration of protamine during CPB (often due to miscommunication). Another potential problem is clotting of the ECC after CPB due to continued use of the cardiotomy suction after administration of protamine. If this occurs, it is impossible to resume bypass if required urgently to rescue a patient [11]. It is therefore prudent to discontinue the use of cardiotomy suction as soon as protamine administration is initiated.
6. **Dislodgment of cannulae** is encountered in about 0.06% of cases and tubing rupture in about 0.03%. Vigilant care of these cannulae must be maintained. If a venous line dislodges, an "air-lock" occurs (see below), and arterial flow will have to be stopped to avoid pumping air out of a depleted venous reservoir. Dislodged arterial cannulae also require that the arterial pump be stopped until the cannula is placed back into the arterial system (after excluding all air). Tubing rupture (usually in the high-pressure part of the circuit) again requires cessation of CPB while the defect is repaired.
7. **Obstructed venous return and air-lock.** This complication poses two problems: elevation of venous pressure (with possible decreased cerebral perfusion, distention of the right heart, and decreased venous return to the H–L machine) and risk of pumping air if the reservoir becomes empty. Vigilant monitoring of the pressure in the SVC and of the level in the venous reservoir is essential. The entire venous drainage circuit must be examined. Sites of obstruction include clamps, kinks, malposition of cannulae, and an air-lock. An air-lock occurs when a bolus of air fills the venous drainage line and interrupts the siphon. The source of the air leak must be corrected and then the air emptied into the venous reservoir by sequential elevation and lowering of the venous line.
8. **Erroneous systemic blood flow:** Due to miscalibration or malfunction of the arterial pump or the flowmeter; may lead to excessive or inadequate blood flow.
9. **Vasoplegia.** Vasodilation during and following CPB is a frequently encountered problem which if persists is associated with adverse outcome. It is defined as low arterial pressure despite a normal or elevated systemic blood flow (cardiac output). Evaluation begins with the differential diagnosis of low arterial pressure (e.g., artifactual measurement, low blood flow [malfunctioning or miss calibrated arterial pump, open arteriovenous shunts], reduced viscosity [severe anemia], allergic reaction, infusion of vasodilating drugs, aortic dissection and sepsis). Purported risk factors for the vasoplegic syndrome include

preoperative Angiotensin conversion enzyme-1 (ACE-I), angiotensin receptor blockers (ARBs) and calcium-channel blockers, and Ventricular assist device (VAD) placement. The next decision is whether or not to treat the low pressure (see discussion in subsequent section on pathophysiology). This is based upon the severity of the hypotension, patient factors [e.g., age, coexisting disease (vascular, renal, diabetes, central nervous system [CNS])] and whether there is evidence of inadequate tissue perfusion (venous saturation, acid–base status and lactates, cerebral oximetry, urine output). Therapeutic options include raising blood flow, raising hematocrit, and adding a vasoconstrictor. Phenylephrine and norepinephrine are most commonly used initially, with vasopressin (2 to 4 units/hr) and methylene blue (1.5 mg/kg bolus ± 1 mg/kg/hr) often used as second-line agents.

10. **Heater–cooler dysfunction** occurs in about 0.16% cases and can lead to excessive heating or cooling. Close monitoring of water inflow temperature and temperature of arterial blood leaving the oxygenator (which contains the heat exchanger) is essential to detect these problems. If malfunction is detected, the heater–cooler must be inactivated and other means of temperature control initiated.
11. **Electrical failure** (H–L machine only or entire room) has been reported in 0.08% of cases. All modern H–L machines should have battery backup which should be tested before each case. If battery backup fails, hand cranking of the arterial pump must be initiated immediately. Often overlooked is the loss of field suction and left heart vents, which could impair surgical exposure and lead to loss of venous return; thus, the pumps driving these systems must also be hand cranked. Electrical failure may also cause loss of critical monitoring and lighting.
12. **Gas (oxygen) supply failure** is encountered in about 0.03% of cases. Since most teams do not monitor flow into the oxygenator, this complication may present as a cause of oxygenator failure (see above). A standby oxygen supply (cylinder) must be available.
13. **High arterial line pressure** demands immediate attention. It may be a sign of systemic arterial hypertension, malposition of the arterial cannula, arterial dissection, kinks or clamps in the arterial cannula or line, inadequate cannula size, excessive flow, or an obstructed arterial line filter. Arterial flow must be reduced until the problem is identified and rectified.
14. **Distension of right and/or left heart** (see section on venting above)

C. **Risk containment.** This requires the active and continuing participation of all members of the team (surgeons, perfusionists, anesthesiologists, and nurses).

1. Vigilance on the part of all members of the team
2. **Special monitoring** of the adequacy of perfusion is discussed in Part II of this chapter and in Chapter 8 and by Murphy et al. [6]. Two issues deserve special attention:
   a. **The CNS.** Many advocate the use of cerebral near-infrared spectroscopy (NIRS) (i.e., cerebral oximetry) or other monitors of cerebral perfusion/function (e.g., transcranial Doppler, processed electroencephalography) to detect problems with venous drainage and arterial cannulation and malperfusion (e.g. with dissection) [14]. This is discussed further in Chapter 24.
   b. **TEE.** TEE is useful not only to diagnose cardiac abnormalities pre-CPB and evaluate surgical repairs but to assist with the conduct of CPB. Some of these applications include the following:
      (1) Evaluating atherosclerosis in the aorta (often adding epiaortic scanning) as it relates to cannulation and placement of clamps
      (2) Evaluating placement of cannulae, especially retrograde coronary sinus cannula, LV vents, and transfemorally placed IVC cannulae, and intra-aortic balloon pump (IABP)
      (3) Detect devices, masses (thrombi and tumors), and anatomic abnormalities that could affect cannulation
      (4) Assess adequacy of decompression of the LV
      (5) Detect and evaluate deairing of left heart
      (6) Detect aortic dissection and malperfusion of arch vessels
3. Education, practice, experience, retraining, certification, and recertification
4. Communication between surgeon, perfusionist, and anesthesiologist. Each must warn team members of actions that could impact all the others, and of any variance with normal

course of CPB or deviations in expected parameters. Commands must be positively and verbally acknowledged.

5. **The "two-minute drill":** Although serious complications occur in only about 0.25% to 0.1% of the time, it is prudent to wait about 2 min after going on "full bypass" and arresting the heart, to assure that all is going well and to rule out serious complications which can be most easily managed by discontinuing CPB before the heart is arrested, and resuming normal circulation. One should confirm the following endpoints:
   a. Able to achieve targeted flow
   b. Adequate venous return and not losing volume
   c. Adequate oxygenation from the oxygenator
   d. Acceptable arterial pressure and have excluded arterial dissection as the cause of hypotension
   e. RV and LV are decompressed
   f. Acceptable systemic venous pressure
   g. Acceptable arterial line pressure
   h. Acceptable venous oxygen saturation
6. Planning, development of, and adherence to **protocols** for routine as well as unusual types of CPB and of complications
7. Use of prebypass **check-lists** and for other key times during CPB and for adverse events
8. Use of safety equipment and alarms
9. Appropriate preventive maintenance program, replacement of old equipment, and familiarity and testing of new equipment
10. Team practice at diagnosing and management of major complications
11. Periodic audit, team meetings, quality assurance (QA) and quality improvement (QI). Use of a registry to measure variation and benchmarking
12. Automated control and regulation of the H–L machine

D. **Key role of the anesthesiologist in the conduct of CPB.** Anesthesiologists are in a unique position to assist with the conduct and management of CPB. They are able to observe both the surgical field and the H–L machine, and can facilitate communication between the perfusionist and surgeon. Their detailed knowledge about the patient's medical history and the patient's course prior to arrival in the operation room and prior to CPB gives them a unique perspective.

Anesthesiologists should oversee the anesthetic and vasoactive drug management and patient monitoring during CPB and make recommendations concerning the safe and appropriate conduct of the CPB. They should be vigilant for any adverse events and assist with the management of the complications mentioned above. Finally, anesthesiologists should be involved in collaboration with the surgeons and perfusionists in the development of protocols for the conduct of safe CPB, participate in practice sessions for handling emergency situations and complications, and be involved in education, and QA/QI activities related to perfusion.

PART II: PATHOPHYSIOLOGY OF CARDIOPULMONARY BYPASS

I. Introduction

Improvements in the design of the CPB circuit and greater understanding of the physiologic insult of CPB have contributed to the relative safety of modern cardiac surgery. Despite advancements in technology and knowledge during the past several decades, a variety of minor and major complications are observed following CPB.

Major physiologic trespasses introduced by CPB include: (i) Alterations of pulsatility, blood flow patterns, and pressure; (ii) exposure of blood to nonphysiologic surfaces and shear stresses; (iii) hemodilution; (iv) systemic stress response; and (v) varying degrees of hypothermia (or hyperthermia during rewarming). Improving the safety of CPB will depend on greater understanding of these aberrations [15].

II. CPB as a perfusion system

A. **Circulatory control during CPB.** "Cardiac output" on CPB is the pump flow rate, which can be set at any level desired, but is limited by the amount of venous return. Systemic and venous blood pressures are partially dependent on the patient's autonomic tone, but can be manipulated by increasing or decreasing venous drainage and by administering vasopressors or vasodilators. Thus, the circulation during CPB is controlled in large part by the perfusionist and the anesthesiologist.

1. **Systemic blood flow.** Systemic blood flow is determined by pump flow of the H–L machine, which is set by the perfusionist. This should be guided by the patient's age, temperature, depth of anesthesia, and hematocrit.
   a. Pump flow rates are usually expressed as L/min/M^2. In awake patients, it is generally accepted that a cardiac index less than 2.0 to 2.2 L/min/M^2 is not sufficient to provide tissues with an adequate oxygen supply. **This also appears to be the lower limit of sufficient cardiac output during normothermic CPB.**
   b. At moderate hypothermia (about 30°C) and with a hematocrit of about 24% in an adult, flow is often set at about 2.4 L/min/M^2, which meets the oxygen needs of an anesthetized patient. Whether this remains true at higher temperatures (e.g., 35°C) remains to be determined.
   c. With increasing degrees of hypothermia, the patient's oxygen demand decreases, and consequently pump flow rates may be reduced significantly. Kirklin and Barratt-Boyes [16] calculated curves relating oxygen consumption to pump flow rates at different temperatures and describe "best-fit" lines for measured oxygen consumption (VO_2) at varying nonpulsatile flow rates (*Q*) from several animal studies (Fig. 21.8). The small *x*s on each curve represent flow rates at each temperature used clinically during CPB at the University of Alabama at that time.
   d. Maximal flow rate during CPB is limited by venous return from the patient, which is influenced by the height of the operating table above the H–L machine, placement, resistance, and size of venous cannulae and lines, blood volume, and venous tone. Maximal flow is also limited by the capacity of the H–L machine and size of the arterial cannula. High flows through the arterial cannula produce high pressure gradients and turbulence, which damage the blood and produce adverse jet effects (e.g., dislodgment of atheroemboli).

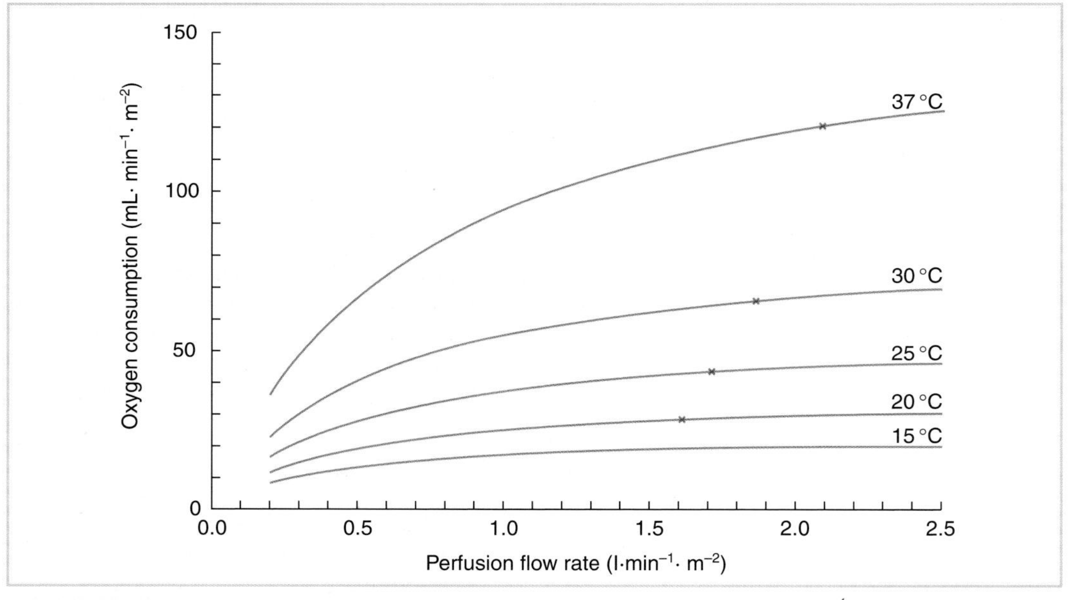

FIGURE 21.8 Nomogram relating oxygen consumption (VO_2) to perfusion flow rate (*Q*) and temperature. (From Kirklin JW, Barratt-Boyes BG. Hypothermia, circulatory arrest, and cardiopulmonary bypass. In: Kirklin JW, Barratt-Boyes BG, eds. *Cardiac Surgery.* 2nd ed. New York, NY: Churchill-Livingstone; 1993:91, with permission.)

   e. At the present time, there are no data defining a minimal (or maximal) safe flow rate during hypothermic or normothermic CPB, nor has the optimal flow rate which results in the most favorable organ perfusion (and best clinical outcomes) been determined.

2. **Arterial pressure.** As in the normal state, arterial pressure is the product of cardiac output (i.e., pump flow during CPB) and systemic vascular resistance (SVR). The latter is determined by blood viscosity and by smooth muscle tone in the arterioles. Viscosity is principally influenced by hematocrit and temperature, both of which often change considerably during CPB.
   a. At normothermia, if hematocrit falls from 40% to 20%, viscosity (and hence SVR) will fall about 50% and at a constant pump flow (cardiac output) the mean arterial pressure (MAP) will fall about 50%.
   b. SVR is also determined by vascular tone, which is influenced by pulsatility (SVR lower with pulsatile flow), sympathetic nervous system activity, depth of anesthesia, catecholamines, angiotensin and arginine vasopressin (AVP) and other local vasoactive substances (e.g., nitric oxide and endothelin), acid–base and electrolyte status, various mediators of the systemic inflammation reaction (SIR), and administration of vasoactive drugs.
   c. The optimal range of arterial pressures during CPB remains controversial. If pressure is too low, perfusion of critical vascular beds may be compromised, especially if vascular disease is present. Conversely, excessive arterial pressure increases noncoronary collateral flow to the heart during aortic cross-clamping (hence "washing out" myocardial protection with cardioplegia) and bronchial flow to the lungs (which increases blood return to left heart) and places strain on arterial clamps and suture lines.
   d. Many clinicians maintain MAP of 50 to 60 mm Hg during adult CPB. This value is based on data suggesting a lower limit of autoregulation of the brain of 50 mm Hg in awake subjects. However, the lower limit of cerebral autoregulation may be as low as 20 to 30 mm Hg during hypothermic bypass with moderate hemodilution [17]. This explains why short periods of hypotension (MAP of 30 mm Hg or less) are well tolerated for brief periods of time.

6

   e. More recent data have suggested that **the lower limit of autoregulation of the brain is approximately 70 mm Hg in awake, normotensive subjects, while during CPB in adults it has been found to average 66 mm Hg (but with a 95% prediction interval of between 43 and 90 mm Hg) and to NOT be related to preoperative blood pressure or hypertension, age, gender, diabetes or a history of prior cerebrovascular accident** [6,18]. On the basis of these data, some clinicians use higher MAP (≥70 mm Hg) on CPB. Higher perfusion pressures may improve tissue perfusion in high-risk patients (older, hypertensive, peripheral vascular disease) and enhance collateral blood flow when emboli obstruct blood vessels.
   f. Observational studies examining the association between hypotension on CPB (usually defined as an MAP <50 mm Hg) and adverse outcomes have yielded conflicting results (outcomes either unchanged or worsened) [6]. In a randomized trial of low (targeted pressures of 50 to 60 mm Hg) or high (targeted pressures of 80 to 100 mm Hg) pressure on CPB, the combined incidence of adverse cardiac and neurologic outcomes was lower in the high-pressure group [19].
   g. There is insufficient evidence to recommend an optimal arterial pressure during CPB. In addition, the best method of increasing arterial pressure which may beneficially impact clinical outcomes is undetermined (increasing flow, increasing hematocrit, use of vasoactive medications). The decisions relating to arterial pressure on CPB should be based on an assessment of the benefits and risks of higher or lower perfusion pressures for each patient. In the near future it may be possible to individualize MAP during CPB utilizing real-time monitoring of cerebral autoregulation [18].

3. **Venous pressure.** Venous pressure is determined by blood volume, venous tone (sympathetic nervous system, depth of anesthesia, vasoactive drugs), resistance to flow out of the venous cannula (placement, size, kinks, distortion of heart), height of operating table, and total systemic flow.

Venous return is normally by gravity (siphon), but sometimes is augmented by applying vacuum or suction to the venous lines. Elevated venous pressure can seriously compromise organ perfusion and can lead to peripheral edema.

4. **Distribution of blood flow.** In addition to total blood flow, one must be concerned about flow in each organ [20]. Recent studies have noted a **hierarchy** of distribution of blood flow during normothermia and hypothermia as total flow is reduced [21]. Even at "normal flow" (i.e., 2.4 L/min/M^2), muscle flow is significantly reduced during CPB. **As flow is progressively reduced, first splanchnic, then renal, and eventually (only at extremely low flows) cerebral flows are reduced.**

B. Circulatory changes during CPB

1. **Changes at onset of CPB.** At commencement of CPB, there is usually a fall in systemic blood pressure due to a decrease in SVR. This phenomenon results from the following:
   - **a.** Decreased blood viscosity secondary to hemodilution by the pump-priming fluid
   - **b.** Decreased vascular tone secondary to the following:
     - **(1)** Dilution of circulating catecholamines
     - **(2)** Temporary hypoxemia. Hypoxemia from initial circulation of pump asanguineous priming fluid may lead to decreased vascular tone.
     - **(3)** Low pH and low calcium and magnesium levels in the priming fluid
2. **Circulatory changes during hypothermic CPB**
   - **a. Increased SVR.** There may be considerable patient-to-patient variations in SVR during CPB. However, as CPB progresses, there will generally be a steady increase in systemic pressure due to increasing SVR if flow rates are kept constant. The observed increase in SVR during the course of CPB is due to several factors:
     - **(1)** Decreased vascular cross-sectional area from closure of portions of the microvasculature
     - **(2)** Vasoconstriction brought on by the following factors:
       - **(a)** Hypothermia
       - **(b)** Increasing levels of circulating catecholamines, AVP, endothelin, and angiotensin II
     - **(3)** Increase in blood viscosity secondary to hypothermia and rising hematocrit (due to urine output or translocation of fluid into the interstitial compartment)
   - **b. Decreased SVR.** Transient decreases in SVR and systemic pressure may be observed shortly after infusion of cardioplegic solutions, especially if the solutions contain nitroglycerin.
3. **Circulatory changes during the rewarming phase of CPB**
   - **a.** As the perfusate temperature is increased to rewarm the patient, variable circulatory responses are observed depending on the anesthetics used, patient hematocrit, underlying disease, and other factors. SVR and MAP increase frequently during initial rewarming from 25 to 32°C, but then usually decrease as temperature increases above 32°C.
   - **b.** A more consistent decrease in SVR and MAP usually occurs with release of the aortic cross-clamp and reperfusion of the heart. Despite cardioplegia and hypothermia, there is some degree of ongoing metabolic activity and utilization of myocardial energy stores during the ischemic period. This results in coronary vasodilation and a marked increase in coronary blood flow and a decrease in arterial pressure. In addition, when the heart is reperfused, accumulated metabolites are washed out of the heart into the general circulation. Some of these metabolites, most notably **adenosine**, are potent vasodilators which aggravate the decrease in SVR.
4. **Changes in the microcirculation and adequacy of tissue perfusion during CPB**
   - **a.** During CPB, cardiac output and arterial pressure can be easily maintained at "normal" values. However, several observations suggest that tissue perfusion and oxygen delivery can be impaired to varying degrees during CPB, including the following:
     - **(1)** Postoperative organ dysfunction, both temporary and permanent
     - **(2)** Variable decreases in oxygen consumption during normothermic CPB at flows and pressures that are comparable to pre-CPB values
     - **(3)** Increases in serum lactate levels

b. The microcirculation lies between the precapillary arterioles and the postcapillary venules and includes the capillary bed, interstitial fluid space, and microcirculatory lymphatics. Normal microcirculatory physiology is poorly understood and requires further clarification. However, it is clear that microcirculatory function during CPB may be impaired by the following:

(1) Constriction of precapillary arteriolar sphincters caused by catecholamines, angiotensin, vasopressin, thromboxane, endothelin, and decreased release of nitric oxide (NO)

(2) Increased interstitial fluid volume (edema)

(3) Decreased lymphatic drainage

(4) Loss of pulsatile flow

(5) "Sludging" in the capillaries due to hypothermia

(6) Altered deformability of RBCs

(7) Microaggregation and adhesion of white cells, platelets, and fibrin onto the endothelium related to the SIR

(8) Microemboli (gas, lipids, cellular aggregates), primarily from the cardiotomy suction

c. Attempts to optimize microcirculatory function during CPB may include use of vasodilators to inhibit arteriolar constriction, addition of mannitol and colloid (e.g., albumin) to the pump-priming fluid to inhibit interstitial fluid accumulation, use of pulsatile perfusion techniques, hemodilution to a hematocrit between 20% and 30% to optimize capillary flow, use of microfiltration, minimizing return of unprocessed cardiotomy suction blood directly into the H–L machine, and anti-inflammatory strategies.

5. Pulsatile versus nonpulsatile flow during CPB. One of the major physiologic derangements introduced by CPB is loss of pulsatility of flow. Intuitively, it seems desirable to reproduce normal flow patterns as closely as possible during CPB. However, there is considerable controversy about the merits of and need for pulsatile perfusion compared with conventional nonpulsatile perfusion [6].

a. How to produce pulsatile flow. Several methods are commonly used to achieve arterial pulsations during CPB:

(1) If partial CPB is being used, venous drainage can be reduced to permit some cardiac ejection.

(2) If an intra-aortic balloon is in place, it can be used to impart pulsatility to the flow.

(3) Pulsations can be produced by roller pumps, and to a lesser degree by centrifugal pumps, designed to rotate at varying speeds.

b. Damping effects of the aortic cannula. The first two methods of producing pulsations are more effective because they generate the pulse in the aorta itself. Although many pumps can generate a pulsatile outflow, the amount of pulsatile energy transmitted into the aorta is limited by the damping effects caused by the narrow aortic cannula, MOs, and arterial microfilters. This makes it unlikely that much pulsatile power can be transferred into the patient by roller pumps [22].

c. Putative benefits of pulsatile flow

(1) Transmission of more energy to the microcirculation, which improves tissue perfusion, lymphatic flow, and cellular metabolism

(2) Reduction of adverse neuroendocrine responses (mainly vasoconstrictive) to nonpulsatile flow that emanate from baroreceptors, the kidneys, and the endothelium

d. Liabilities of attempting to generate pulsatile flow

(1) Increased cost and complexities

(2) Requires use of larger arterial cannulae

(3) Is associated with higher nozzle velocities out of the arterial cannula (risking vascular injury and thromboembolism)

e. Clinical outcome. Clinical outcome data have been conflicting. A recent evidence-based review concluded that existing data were insufficient to support recommendations for or against pulsatile perfusion to reduce the incidence of complications following CPB [6].

III. Adequacy of perfusion

A. How to define. There is no generally accepted definition of optimal perfusion during CPB. Perfusion can be considered acceptable if the patient survives without evidence of organ dysfunction. However, the primary objective of optimal perfusion is to produce a healthy, productive long-term survivor of cardiac surgery. Therefore, perfusion during CPB should accomplish the following goals:

1. **Maintain adequate oxygen delivery to all organs (arterial oxygen content and delivery)**
2. **Avoid activation of undesirable reactions, e.g., neuroendocrine stress response and inflammation**
3. **Minimize microembolization and disturbance of the coagulation system**
4. **Maintain adequate systemic blood flow and arterial pressure**

B. Monitoring. Detailed monitoring of organ perfusion and function during CPB is not usually employed during clinical CPB; however, research studies of this nature have provided much useful information to guide improvements in conducting CPB.

1. **Global perfusion**

   a. **Oxygen consumption (VO_2)** measurement, although not commonly used clinically, has provided much insight into the proper conduct of CPB. It can be easily calculated from simultaneously measured arterial and venous oxygen contents and pump flow rate:

   $$Vo_2 = \text{Pump flow} \times (C_ao_2 - C_vo_2)$$

   Kirklin and Barratt-Boyes [16] suggested that maintaining VO_2 at 85% of the predicted maximum for a given temperature will provide adequate oxygen delivery (Fig. 21.8).

   Normal oxygen consumption in an awake normothermic resting person is about 120 to 140 mL/min/M^2 and during deep general anesthesia may be about 90 to 110 mL/min/M^2 [23], and falls about 5% per degree centigrade of hypothermia (i.e., below 37°C).

   A fall in oxygen consumption during CPB while the other determinants of oxygen consumption (e.g., depth of anesthesia, muscle relaxation, temperature) remain stable suggests impaired oxygen delivery (even if mixed venous oxygen saturation remains stable).

   b. **Oxygen delivery ($DO_2 = C_aO_2 \times$ pump flow)** may be one of the most important determinants of adequacy of perfusion. The DO_2 calculation incorporates two critical variables that determine tissue oxygenation (arterial oxygen content and pump flow rate) into a single measure. During CPB, DO_2 can be improved by raising hematocrit values (transfusion or hemoconcentration), increasing inspired oxygen concentrations, or increasing pump flow rates (e.g., significant hemodilution on CPB can be compensated for by increasing flow rates). Normal oxygen delivery in awake subjects is about 700 mL/min/M^2 and the lower limit of normal is about 350 mL/min/M^2. This value is lower in the hemodiluted patient under CPB (typically 200 to 300 mL/min/M^2). Therefore, the safe margin between oxygen supply and demand may be reduced on bypass.

7 ***Critical oxygen delivery*** **is that point at which maximum oxygen extraction is reached and oxygen consumption starts to fall (i.e., become flow dependent).** Tissue hypoxemia and systemic acidosis (lactic) begin to occur at this point. The existence of a critical level of oxygen delivery during CPB has been the subject of active debate. Some studies have found this threshold to be 330 mL/min/M^2 at 35°C, 272 mL/min/M^2 at 32 to 34°C, and 243 mL/min/M^2 at 32°C in humans prior to or during CPB [23,24]. However, other investigators have observed a direct linear relationship between DO_2 and VO_2, and have been unable to define a critical DO_2 level.

   c. **Mixed venous oxygen saturation (SvO_2),** content **(C_vo_2),** partial pressure **(PvO_2),** or oxygen extraction ratio **(OER)** provide clues to the adequacy of the balance of oxygen delivery (DO_2) to oxygen demand (VO_2). OER is the ratio of VO_2/DO_2. Normally, SvO_2 is about 75% and OER about 25%. When these two values approach 50%, critically compromised oxygen delivery is suggested. Inline monitoring of mixed venous saturation or partial pressure is advocated during CPB, and clinicians should strive to maintain the SvO_2 at ≥80%. Unfortunately, global venous oxygen saturation values can fail to detect regional ischemia if the vascular bed is small or if there is too little desaturated blood returning from a poorly perfused bed [25]. Furthermore, SvO_2 has been found not to be sensitive to critical oxygen delivery nor to the development of hyperlactatemia during CPB [26]. **Thus, although a low venous oxygen saturation should always be remedied, a normal or high venous saturation does not assure adequate perfusion to all organs.**

d. **Metabolic and lactic acidosis**

e. **Cerebral oximetry** (e.g., NIRS). In addition to its role as a monitor of the adequacy of cerebral oxygen delivery, recent studies have suggested that it may be a useful surrogate to assess adequacy to total body oxygen delivery [27]. As flow is maintained to the brain at the expense of other organs, decreases in cerebral oxygenation suggest that flow to all other tissues is impaired. A critical issue with this technology is categorizing thresholds which identify pathologic brain perfusion. At the present time, clinical studies suggest that reductions in cerebral oxygenation of ≥20% to 25% relative to baseline are associated with organ dysfunction and adverse outcomes [27].

2. **Organ-specific perfusion**

a. **Brain.** Electroencephalography (raw and processed, e.g., bispectral index) and transcranial Doppler are used to monitor cerebral perfusion, but their value is debated. **Cerebral oximetry** can be used as an indirect monitor of cerebral blood flow; **however, only limited data support a beneficial effect of this monitoring on clinical outcomes** [28]. Although some have suggested that such monitoring should be a standard of care, this is an unresolved controversy [14,29,30]. Jugular venous saturation, pressure, and temperature may give additional insight into how well the brain is being supported. In the research setting, release of cerebral enzymes (e.g., S-100, enolase) into cerebrospinal fluid or systemic blood is used as sensitive indicators of CNS injury.

b. **Heart.** Monitoring the electrocardiography (ECG), TEE, myocardial temperature, myocardial tissue pH, Pco_2, PO_2, coronary sinus lactates, and cardiac enzymes have been advocated to assure adequate support of the heart.

c. **Kidney.** Urine output is the simplest measure of renal function. However, different blood flow patterns, varying perfusion pressures, hypothermia, and the presence or absence of diuretics in the pump-priming fluid may affect urine output and render it an inaccurate indicator of overall tissue perfusion. Measurement of kidney-specific tubular proteins (e.g., cystatin C, KIM, NGAL, GST, NAG, α1-MG, NEP, and RBP) in the urine may represent more sensitive indicators of renal injury than changes in postoperative creatinine and creatinine clearance/glomerular filtration rate [31].

d. **Splanchnic bed.** No monitoring is usually employed clinically at this time, but use of gastric tonometry (saline or air, pH, or Pco_2), Doppler assessments of mucosal blood flow, hepatic blood flow measurement, and hepatic venous oxygen saturation monitoring have been used in clinical investigations.

IV. Hypothermia and CPB

A. **Effects of hypothermia on biochemical reactions.** The Q_{10} for **chemical reactions** is a measure of **changes in rate of reaction** for each 10°C change in temperature. **For human tissues, Q_{10} is approximately 2.** That is, for each 10°C decrease in body temperature, the rate of reaction (i.e., metabolic rate or oxygen consumption) is roughly halved.

B. **Effects of hypothermia on blood viscosity.** Hypothermia increases blood viscosity. In the early history of CPB, hemodilution was not performed. In contemporary cardiac surgical practices, patients are typically hemodiluted to hematocrits of 20% to 30% during CPB (due to the inevitable hemodilution of the patient's red cell mass with the asanguineous pump-priming solution). Although oxygen-carrying capacity is decreased from hemodilution, oxygen delivery may be improved due to decreased viscosity and enhanced microcirculatory flow. Data suggest that viscosity remains stable if hematocrit (%) matches temperature (in °C) during hypothermia. The optimal degree of hemodilution during hypothermic CPB has not been determined. Recent studies have demonstrated an association between severity of hemodilution on CPB (hematocrits below 22% to 23%) and morbidity and mortality [32]. Clinicians should avoid both excessively high hematocrits (increased blood viscosity and decreased microcirculatory flow) and low hematocrits (inadequate oxygen content) during hypothermic CPB.

C. Changes in blood gases associated with hypothermia

1. **Changes in oxygen–hemoglobin dissociation curve.** As the temperature decreases, the affinity of oxygen for hemoglobin increases (i.e., the oxygen–hemoglobin dissociation curve is shifted to the left). A lower partial pressure of oxygen in the tissues is required to remove the same amount of oxygen from the hemoglobin molecule.
2. **Changes in solubility of O_2 and CO_2.** As temperature decreases, gases become more soluble in liquid. For a given partial pressure more gas will be dissolved in the plasma. This is more significant for CO_2 due to a higher solubility in plasma at any given temperature.
3. **Neutrality of water.** Neutral water is water in which the [H+] is equal to the [OH−]. At 37°C, the pH of neutral water is 6.8. At 25°C the pH of neutral water is 7. As temperature decreases, the pH at which water is "neutral" changes in a linear fashion. The neutral pH increases 0.017 units for each degree Celsius decrease in temperature (Fig. 21.9).
4. **Differing strategies for measuring and managing blood gases during CPB.** Blood gases are measured at 37°C in blood gas analyzing machines. If the patient's body temperature is lower than 37°C, pH and P_aCO_2 can be corrected to determine their actual values at the patient's temperature. If the patient's temperature is 27°C and the pH and PCO_2 as measured at 37°C are 7.4 and 40, respectively, then the pH and P_aCO_2 corrected to a body temperature of 27°C would be about 7.55 and 25. Conversely, if the pH and P_aCO_2 as measured at 37°C are 7.25 and 55, then the corrected values at 27°C would be about 7.4 and 40.

   At issue are the appropriate temperature-corrected pH and P_aCO_2 values during hypothermia. One method (*pH-stat*) attempts to keep the temperature-corrected pH and P_aCO_2 at 7.4 and 40, respectively. The other method (*α-stat*) attempts to keep the ratio of OH−/H+ ions constant so that enzyme systems function appropriately. This will be accomplished if the uncorrected pH and P_aCO_2 as measured at 37°C are 7.4 and 40 mm Hg, respectively. The rationale for these two regimens is discussed in further detail in Chapters 8, 14, and 24.

V. Normothermia and CPB

A. Potential advantages of normothermic CPB. By the late 1960s, hypothermia became a near-ubiquitous practice for patients undergoing CPB. Recently, there has been a trend to conduct CPB at near-normothermic levels [33]. The putative advantages include avoiding adverse effects of hypothermia (increased viscosity, reduced microcirculatory flow, leftward shift of the oxygen–hemoglobin dissociation curve), decreased duration of bypass (time spent cooling and rewarming not required), and avoiding the hazards of overheating (especially of the brain).

B. Potential disadvantages of normothermic CPB. Normothermic bypass narrows the ratio of oxygen demand (VO_2) to oxygen delivery (DO_2). This suggests the need to maintain hematocrit

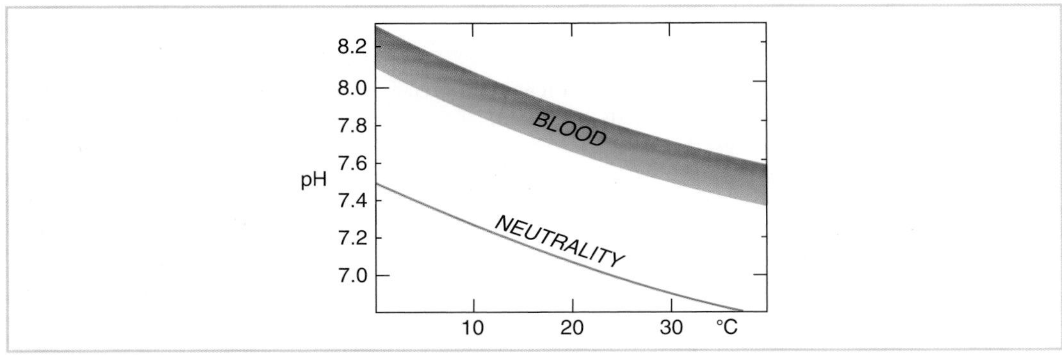

FIGURE 21.9 Blood pH of exotherms and homeotherms, and pH of neutral water as a function of body temperature. (From Ream AF, Reitz BA, Silverberg G. Temperature correction of Pco2 and pH in estimating acid-base status: An example of the Emperor's new clothes? *Anesthesiology.* 1992;56:42, with permission.)

and pump flow rates higher than accepted during hypothermic CPB. However, minimal safe pump flow rates and hematocrit values during normothermic CPB have not been determined. SVR and MAP also tend to be lower; more fluids and vasoconstrictors and higher pump flow rates are typically used at higher CPB temperatures.

C. **Clinical outcomes following normothermic CPB.** Neurologic injury is a primary concern of conducting bypass at normothermia. The two largest randomized studies examining the effect of temperature management on neurologic outcomes reached conflicting conclusions; in patients undergoing warm CPB, the incidence of stroke was reported to be increased or not different compared to patients undergoing hypothermic bypass [34,35]. Normothermic CPB was introduced primarily to improve myocardial protection, and some evidence suggests that myocardial injury is reduced and myocardial function is improved following bypass at warmer temperatures [6]. Renal or hematologic function does not appear to be improved by normothermic CPB [6]. At the present time, many cardiac centers are using mild degrees of hypothermia (about 35°C), the so-called "tepid" bypass, which may offer substantial cerebral protection without the disadvantages of deeper levels of hypothermia. Current evidence does not clearly support one temperature management strategy over another, and it is likely that the ideal temperature for CPB varies with the physiologic requirements of the patient and surgery.

VI. Systemic effects of the CPB

CPB is a highly unphysiologic experience that triggers an "explosion" of adverse events (Fig. 21.10).

A. **Causes and contributors of adverse systemic effects of CPB:**

1. Microemboli (gas and particulate matter)
2. Activation of the inflammatory and coagulation systems
3. Altered temperature, cooling and warming
4. Exposure of blood to foreign surfaces
5. Reinfusion of shed blood and transfusion of blood products
6. Hemodynamic alterations (abnormal flow rate and pattern, abnormal arterial and venous pressures)
7. Ischemia and reperfusion (especially of heart, lungs, and gut)
8. Hyperoxia
9. Hemodilution (with anemia and reduced oncotic pressure)

B. **Blood**

1. **Coagulation and fibrinolytic systems and tissue factor (TF).** Changes in the coagulation cascade, platelets, and the fibrinolytic cascade are discussed in Chapter 19.
2. Changes in formed elements
   a. **RBCs**
      (1) RBCs become stiffer and less deformable during CPB, which may interfere with microcirculatory blood flow and increase susceptibility to hemolysis.
      (2) During CPB, RBCs are exposed to nonphysiologic surfaces and shear stresses which may cause their destruction. The degree of hemolysis is increased by both higher flow rates and the accompanying increase in rate of shear, and by gas–fluid interfaces in the ECC. As red cells are lysed, the free hemoglobin produced is bound to haptoglobin. When the amount of free hemoglobin generated exceeds the binding capacity of haptoglobin, serum hemoglobin concentrations increase and hemoglobin is filtered by the kidney, resulting in hemoglobinuria. Cardiotomy suction is a major contributor to hemolysis during CPB.

   b. **Leukocytes.** CPB affects primarily neutrophils (polymorphonuclear leukocytes [PMNs]) and, to a lesser degree, monocytes. Shortly after the onset of CPB there is a marked decrease in circulating PMNs. This is due to sequestration in the pulmonary circulation and intravascular and extravascular accumulation in the microcirculation of heart and skeletal muscle. Blockage of vessels by PMNs or microcirculatory derangements induced by substances released from PMNs may contribute to organ dysfunction after CPB. Circulating PMN levels increase dramatically with rewarming. Neutrophils released from the pulmonary circulation and younger cells released from the bone marrow contribute to the observed neutrophilia.

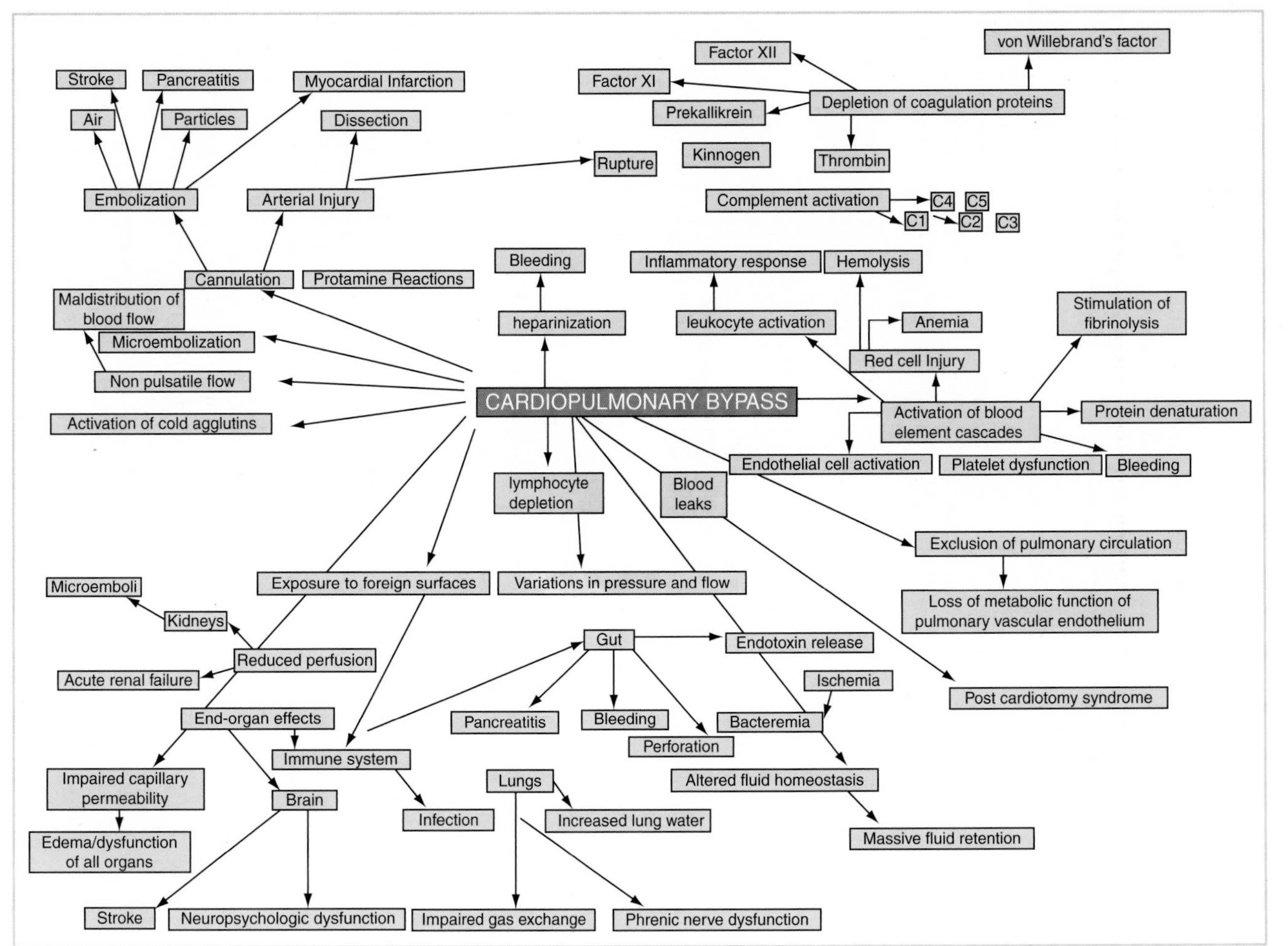

FIGURE 21.10 The "explosion" of adverse events triggered by cardiopulmonary bypass. (From Eleferiades JA. Mini-CABG. A step forward or backward? The "pro" point of view. *J Cardiothorac Vasc Anesth.* 1997;11:661, with permission.)

Effects of CPB on host defense functions of PMNs are controversial. Studies demonstrating decreased responsiveness of PMNs to chemotactic and aggregating stimuli indicate impaired defense mechanisms. However, other studies show that the bacteriocidal activity of PMNs is increased for up to 3 days after CPB.

3. **Changes in plasma proteins**
   a. **Denaturation.** Proteins are molecules with highly specific structures. When proteins approach a gas–liquid interface, strong electrostatic forces at that interface produce varying degrees of molecular unfolding by disrupting internal bonds (i.e., denaturation). Some of the consequences of this protein denaturation include the following:
      (1) **Altered enzymatic function.** Denatured proteins lose some or all of their function. This may be one mechanism by which coagulation becomes impaired during and after CPB.
      (2) **Aggregation of proteins.** Denatured proteins have a tendency to aggregate and produce precipitates.
      (3) **Altered solubility characteristics.** Denatured proteins are less soluble in plasma and cause increased blood viscosity.
      (4) **Release of lipids.** Denaturation of lipoproteins and the protein fractions of chylomicrons may result in aggregates which occlude small vessels.
      (5) **Absorption of denatured proteins** onto RBC membranes may cause them to become "sticky." The resulting RBC aggregates promote capillary sludging and microcirculatory dysfunction.
   b. **Reduced colloid osmotic (oncotic) pressure (COP).** Because of the hemodilution associated with use of asanguineous priming solutions, plasma protein concentration and hence COP fall with onset of CPB if no colloids are added to the CPB circuit. There is controversy about the need and benefits of avoiding the fall in COP by use of albumin or artificial colloids (e.g., dextrans, starches) in the prime.
4. **Activation of humoral cascade systems—see later.**

C. **Fluid balance and interstitial fluid accumulation during CPB.** The following equation, based upon Starling's hypothesis, is thought to describe the fluid fluxes at the microcirculatory level:

$$\text{Tissue fluid accumulation} = K[(P_c - P_{is}) - \delta(\pi_c - \pi_{is})] - Q_{lymph}$$

where K is the filtration coefficient ("permeability") of capillary membrane, P_c the mean intracapillary hydrostatic pressure, P_{is} the mean interstitial hydrostatic pressure, δ the reflection coefficient to macromolecules, π_c the intracapillary oncotic pressure, π_{is} the interstitial oncotic pressure, and Q_{lymph} the lymph flow out of interstitium.

CPB shifts this balance toward accumulation of interstitial fluid by affecting several of these variables. Membrane permeability is increased by activation of the SIR and intermittent ischemia/reperfusion. Plasma oncotic pressure falls due to the use of asanguineous priming fluids. Inadequate venous drainage may increase mean capillary hydrostatic pressure, whereas immobility, lack of pulsatile flow, and loss of negative intrathoracic pressure impede lymphatic flow.

D. **Heart.** Some degree of myocardial injury and cell necrosis occurs during CPB which may result in myocardial stunning and dysfunction. However, frank myocardial infarction is relatively uncommon (although the ECG and cardiac enzyme changes which identify myocardial infarction have not been precisely defined).

Factors that contribute to myocardial injury include those that affect microcapillary perfusion in general, but also ventricular distention, prolonged ventricular fibrillation, coronary air embolization, hypotension, catecholamines, endotoxemia, and ischemia/reperfusion associated with aortic cross-clamping. **It is thought that higher perfusion pressures are desirable to maintain adequate myocardial perfusion in patients with cardiac hypertrophy or severe coronary artery disease during those periods of CPB when the ascending aorta is unclamped.** Potent volatile anesthetics appear to be protective of the heart. (See also Chapter 23.)

E. **CNS.** Cerebral dysfunction (ranging from subtle neurocognitive dysfunction to frank stroke or coma) is not infrequent following CPB. Its etiology is multifactorial and includes hypoperfusion, macroemboli, microemboli, and the inflammatory response to CPB. The causes of cerebral dysfunction and strategies to minimize adverse cerebral outcomes are discussed further in Chapter 24.

F. **Kidneys.** Renal dysfunction after CPB, which ranges from a rise in creatinine and release of renal tubular proteins to frank renal failure requiring renal replacement therapy (e.g., hemodialysis), is a persistent cause of morbidity and mortality in cardiac surgical patients.

1. **Significance of urine output during CPB.** Urine output is a crude indicator of renal function, but there is no correlation between the amount of urine output during CPB and the incidence of postoperative renal failure. Urine output is greater when MAP is higher, when pulsatile perfusion is used, and when mannitol is added to pump-priming fluids.
2. **Decreased glomerular and tubular function.** Evidence of temporary glomerular and tubular dysfunction is present in many patients early post-CPB [36]. Tubular function is depressed by hypothermia and by reductions in renal blood flow.
3. **Renal blood flow.** Global renal blood flow usually decreases during CPB as a result of diminished flow rates and pressures or loss of pulsatility. As in other low-flow states, there is a redistribution of renal blood flow from the cortex to the outer medulla. This redistribution of blood flow appears to be less severe during pulsatile perfusion.
4. **Hemoglobinuria.** Intravascular hemolysis and hemoglobinuria can cause acute tubular necrosis. The mechanism is precipitation of pigment in the renal tubules with subsequent blockage of tubular flow or glomerular–tubular injuries caused by red cell stroma and other substances liberated from lysed RBCs.
5. **Renal failure.** The reported incidence of acute renal failure requiring renal replacement therapy ranges from 1% to 3%. **Development of renal failure appears to depend more on the preoperative renal function and postoperative hemodynamic status than on various manipulations used to maintain urine output during CPB** [36]. However, Ranucci et al. [24] observed that a critically low oxygen delivery during CPB was an important predictor of acute renal failure after coronary artery surgery.

G. **Splanchnic, visceral, and hepatic effects.** The incidence of major gastrointestinal (GI) complications (e.g., bleeding, ulcers, mesenteric ischemia or infarction, cholecystitis, pancreatitis), postoperatively, is low (1% to 2%), but is associated with high mortality rates (36% to 65%). Risk factors include advanced age, open ventricle operations, emergency procedures, prolonged bypass times, use of vasopressors, and postbypass low cardiac output syndrome [37].

Although global splanchnic blood flow (and hepatic venous oxygen saturation) appears to be preserved during CPB, the hierarchy of regional blood flow suggests that splanchnic flow will be compromised early whenever systemic flow is reduced during CPB [20,21] (and is likely reduced further with administration of vasoconstrictors, such as phenylephrine, norepinephrine, and AVP). Furthermore, many subjects exhibit increased intestinal permeability, decreased gastric or intestinal mucosal pH and increased mucosal Pco_2 (by tonometry), decreased mucosal blood flow (by Doppler flowmetry), and endotoxemia, all of which suggest that mucosal ischemia occurs frequently during CPB. GI ischemia may play a primary role in the development of SIR syndrome and other GI complications.

As with renal failure, hepatic dysfunction is more dependent on hemodynamic status before and after CPB than on any direct effect of CPB. Jaundice may occur in up to 23% of patients after cardiac surgery, but severe jaundice (bilirubin levels at least 6 mg/dL) occurs in only 6% of patients. The risk of postoperative jaundice is increased in the setting of high RA pressures, persistent hypotension after CPB, or significant transfusion.

H. **Lungs.** Pulmonary dysfunction after CPB may range from mild decreases in P_ao_2, related to the nearly ubiquitous postoperative atelectasis, to full-blown respiratory failure resembling the adult respiratory distress syndrome (ARDS).

1. **Pulmonary dead space and ventilation–perfusion mismatching after CPB.** Extravascular lung water increases during CPB. Development of intrapulmonary shunts and increased dead space ventilation result in less efficient matching of ventilation to perfusion. Increased dead space is reflected in greater end-tidal–arterial CO_2 gradients

after CPB in the majority of patients. Ventilation–perfusion (*V/Q*) mismatching results in increased alveolar-arterial O_2 gradients and decreased P_aO_2. These are the most consistent abnormalities noted after CPB.

2. **Pulmonary sequestration of neutrophils and release of vasoactive compounds.** PMNs sequestered in the lung during CPB may undergo release reactions causing localized, intense vasoconstriction or membrane damage with subsequent edema formation, resulting in increased dead space ventilation and *V/Q* mismatching.
3. **Changes in pulmonary vascular resistance (PVR) and hypoxic pulmonary vasoconstriction**
   a. **PVR.** Numerous factors influence pulmonary vascular tone after CPB. Many congenital cardiac lesions are associated with increased PVR. Catecholamine and endothelin levels rise during and after CPB, which may also contribute to increases in PVR. Efforts to limit increases in PVR include hyperventilation and administration of sodium bicarbonate to maintain an alkaline pH, maintenance of high inspired oxygen concentrations, and avoidance of catecholamine infusions that can induce pulmonary vasoconstriction.
   b. **Hypoxic pulmonary vasoconstriction.** Direct effects of CPB and hypothermia on hypoxic pulmonary vasoconstriction are poorly understood. However, use of volatile anesthetics and vasodilators after CPB may interfere with hypoxic pulmonary vasoconstriction, leading to *V/Q* mismatching and decreasing P_aO_2.
4. **Postpump pulmonary dysfunction.** Most patients exhibit some immediate decrease in P_aO_2 postoperatively, and it is difficult to predict which patients will go on to develop more serious pulmonary insufficiency. Although full-blown respiratory failure after CPB is now relatively rare, its incidence is directly related to preoperative pulmonary dysfunction, duration of CPB, and postoperative hemodynamic status. Events during CPB that may contribute to development of pulmonary dysfunction include the following:
   a. **Decreased pulmonary blood flow** resulting from the following:
      (1) Emboli of various compositions leading to localized areas of ventilation/perfusion (*V/Q*) mismatching
      (2) Localized vasoconstriction due to elevated endogenous and exogenous catecholamines, endothelin, or substances released from PMNs trapped in the pulmonary capillaries
   b. **Membrane damage resulting in increased capillary permeability and edema formation** from the following:
      (1) Complement activation
      (2) Vasoactive compounds released from PMNs
      (3) Oxygen-free radicals
   c. **Edema formation from increased pulmonary hydrostatic pressure** caused by inadequate LV venting and increased bronchial blood flow
   d. **Ischemia/reperfusion** of the lungs and remote organs
   e. **Atelectasis from lung deflation during CPB**, which occurs in up to 60% of patients
   f. **SIR**
5. **Methods to reduce lung injury associated with CPB**
   a. **Optimal lung management during CPB.** Most data suggest that ventilation with 100% oxygen during CPB is detrimental to the lungs. The majority of studies suggest that application of 5 cm of water PEEP and/or continuous ventilation utilizing low tidal volumes during CPB does not improve pulmonary function or gas exchange following CPB. In contrast, the use of recruitment maneuvers at the end of CPB before resuming ventilation does appear to improve post-CPB oxygenation, particularly if PEEP is used after the recruitment maneuver.
   b. Prophylactic administration of anti-inflammatory drugs such as aprotinin and corticosteroids to help preserve lung function during CPB has been advocated by some investigators. Although both drugs reduce the SIR to CPB, the effect of these agents on postoperative gas exchange and pulmonary complications remains controversial.

I. **Inflammation.** All patients undergoing cardiac surgery will experience a systemic proinflammatory response to the procedure. Although the trauma of surgery itself leads to a degree of inflammation, the CPB circuit seems to accentuate this inflammatory response.

This syndrome represents an unphysiologic activation of the innate immune system resulting in a whole-body SIR resembling that associated with sepsis and trauma [38]. It presents as a spectrum of responses ranging from near-universal evidence of mild inflammation (fever, leukocytosis), to more significant clinical signs (tachycardia, increased cardiac output, decreased SVR, increased oxygen consumption, increased capillary permeability) to frank organ dysfunction (cardiac, renal, pulmonary, GI, hepatic, CNS) and finally to the multiple organ dysfunction syndrome (MODS) and death. There are several possible variables that may explain why the SIR differs significantly between patients. These factors include pre-existing medical conditions, extremes of age, the extent and duration of the surgery, and genomic makeup of the patient.

Normal inflammation is a localized protective response that is composed of cellular as well as humeral components. When the localized inflammatory response is excessive, it may spill over to the rest of the body; the same appears to be true when the injurious agent is systemic (e.g., CPB), and thus the inflammatory response becomes generalized leading to diffuse and remote end-organ damage [39–42].

1. **Activation.** Nonspecific activators of the inflammatory response include surgical trauma, blood loss or transfusion, and hypothermia. CPB may also activate the inflammatory response by three distinct mechanisms, which include the following:
   a. **Contact activation.** When blood comes into contact with the CPB circuit, plasma proteins are adsorbed to the surface of the circuit. Platelets then adhere to the surface of this protein layer. Contact activation results in the activation of the complement, coagulation, and fibrinolytic systems and the kallikrein–bradykinin cascades.

      Another cause of contact activation is the use of cardiotomy suction. Blood aspirated with the cardiotomy suction is contaminated with TF, tissue and fat fragments, free plasma hemoglobin, thrombin, TF activator, and fibrin degradation products. These contaminants as well as a blood–air interface and turbulent flow lead to activation of complement and coagulation systems.

   b. **Ischemia–reperfusion.** Reperfusion injury refers to damage to tissue caused when blood supply returns to the tissue after a period of ischemia. The absence of oxygen and nutrients from blood creates a condition in which the restoration of circulation results in inflammation and oxidative damage from the oxygen rather than re-establishment of normal function. The reintroduction of oxygen with restored blood flow results in formation of oxygen-free radicals that damage cellular proteins, DNA, and plasma membranes. WBCs carried to the area release a host of inflammatory substances such as interleukins. In addition, leukocytes may also build up in small capillaries leading to obstruction and more ischemia.
   c. **Endotoxemia.** Endotoxin is a lipopolysaccharide from the cell wall of gram-negative bacteria. Endotoxin binds with lipopolysaccharide-binding protein and this complex stimulates the release of tumor necrosis factor (TNF) by macrophages, potentially triggering the development of SIRS. During CPB there is transient endotoxemia. This phenomenon is thought to result from splanchnic hypoperfusion, which causes damage to the GI mucosa and translocation of endotoxin.
2. **Propagation.** Once the inflammatory response is triggered, components of the immune and coagulation systems are activated (as well as the endothelium), which propagate the SIR. These components include the following:
   a. **Complement.** The complement system is a cytotoxic host immune defense system composed of a cascade of 30 or so proteins that interact to recognize and kill pathogens. Activation is triggered by one of three pathways—classical, alternative, and lectin. Mechanisms of activation and propagation include the following:
      (1) Exposure of blood to the foreign surface and the blood–gas interface of the CPB circuit activates the alternative pathway.

(2) Endotoxin from the GI tract during CPB activates both the alternative and classical pathways.

(3) Heparin–protamine complexes in the post-CPB period activate the classical pathway.

The result of complement activation is the release of several active substances including the following:

(a) The anaphylatoxins C3a and C5a, which stimulate leukocyte activation and chemotaxis, increase production of proinflammatory cytokines, oxygen-derived free radicals, proteolytic enzymes, and leukotrienes, and increase capillary permeability.

(b) iC3b, which binds to the CPB circuit and the vascular endothelium and acts as a ligand for leukocyte adhesion

(c) C5b-9, which causes cell lysis, increases leukocyte adhesion molecule expression, and stimulates proinflammatory cytokine production

The degree of complement activation in patients undergoing CPB appears to correlate with the extent of postoperative complications.

b. The release of other mediators

(1) Cytokines

Cytokines are small proteins and polypeptides that mediate and regulate immunity, inflammation, and hematopoiesis. They are released by activated monocytes, tissue macrophages, lymphocytes, and endothelial cells. In addition, blood products and reinfused shed blood contain significant concentrations of cytokines.

Cytokines may exert proinflammatory or anti-inflammatory effects. **Proinflammatory cytokines** are produced predominantly by activated macrophages and are involved in the upregulation of inflammatory reactions. These include TNF-α, interleukin (IL)-1, IL-2, IL-6, IL-8, and interferon γ. Elevations of proinflammatory cytokine levels post-CPB have been associated with adverse outcome following cardiac surgery.

Anti-inflammatory cytokines belong to the T-cell–derived cytokines and are involved in the downregulation of inflammatory reactions. Those released during CPB include IL-10, IL-1 receptor antagonist (IL-1ra), and transforming growth factor-β (TGF-β) [41].

(2) **Nitric oxide.** NO is produced by the vascular endothelium by the conversion of L-arginine to L-citrulline by constitutive NO synthase (cNOS). The effects of NO include regulation of vasomotor tone, inhibition of platelet and neutrophil aggregation, and immunomodulation. CPB leads to the upregulation and release of inducible NO synthase (iNOS), potentially resulting in post-CPB vasodilation, vascular permeability, and end-organ dysfunction [38].

(3) **Leukotrienes.** Leukotrienes are released during CPB and act as chemokines and potent vasoconstrictors of smooth muscle. They may also play a role in neutrophil-related injury, ARDS, and MOF.

(4) **Platelet-activating factor (PAF).** PAF is an endogenous phospholipid intracellular signaling messenger as well as an inflammatory and neurotoxic agent. Its neurotoxic actions include increasing intracellular calcium concentrations, disrupting the blood–brain barrier, and reducing cerebral blood flow.

(5) **Tissue factor.** During CPB, TF is expressed by many cells including the endothelium and blood monocytes. TF-initiated blood coagulation through the extrinsic pathway leads to the release of a myriad of proinflammatory cytokines.

(6) **Kallikrein–bradykinin.** Kallikrein plays a seminal role in activation and amplification of the inflammatory response. Bradykinin increases vascular permeability and release of tissue plasminogen activator.

(7) **Collagenases, gelatinases, and metalloproteases**

(8) **Endothelins.** These are a family of peptides, the most important of which is endothelin-1, which are produced by endothelial cells (as well as smooth

muscle and cardiac myocytes). Endothelin-1 is a potent vasoconstrictor that has been associated with pulmonary and systemic hypertension and myocardial dysfunction.

c. **The endothelium.** The endothelium is an active participant in a variety of physiologic and pathologic processes. It plays a major role in regulating vascular tone, membrane permeability, coagulation and thrombosis, fibrinolysis, and inflammation. It attracts and directs the passage of leukocytes into areas of inflammation through the expression of adhesion molecules [42].

CPB causes extensive activation and dysfunction of the endothelium due to ischemia/reperfusion, exposure to inflammatory mediators, surgical manipulation, and hemodynamic shear stresses. Expression of adhesion molecules mediates the binding of neutrophils to the endothelium and translocation into the interstitium. Resultant neutrophil degranulation worsens the state of the endothelium further, leading to capillary leak and edema. Proinflammatory cytokines inhibit the production of NO, shifting the balance from vasodilation to vasoconstriction. Endothelial cell activation also shifts the endothelial anticoagulant phenotype to a procoagulant phenotype.

d. **Coagulation and fibrinolysis.** The coagulation–fibrinolysis cascade is closely intertwined with the inflammatory response. The activation of one system plays a key role in the other.

e. **The cellular immune response.** Leukocytes are made up of granulocytes, monocytes, and lymphocytes. Granulocytes include neutrophils, eosinophils, and basophils. Monocytes become tissue macrophages after they migrate into tissue. Lymphocytes are made up of B- and T-cells and natural killer cells.

CPB results in the activation of leukocytes, leukocyte-endothelial cell adhesion, and transmigration. The activation may be mediated by contact activation through the CPB circuit and via a variety of inflammatory mediators.

(1) **Neutrophils.** Interaction of neutrophils with the endothelium takes place in distinct steps:

(a) **Neutrophil "rolling"** on the endothelium. This process is thought to be mediated by P-selectin, an adhesion molecule, which is expressed on both endothelial cells and neutrophils during CPB.

(b) **Interaction of more adhesion molecules** on the neutrophils and endothelium causes a firm neutrophil adherence: $\beta 2$ integrins (e.g., CD11a/CD18, CD11b/CD18, ICAM-1).

(c) **Migration** of the neutrophils into the interstitial space

Activated neutrophils can cause tissue damage and end-organ dysfunction via microvascular occlusion or release toxic metabolites and enzymes.

(2) **Monocytes and macrophages.** Monocytes phagocytize microorganisms and cell fragments, produce and secrete chemical mediators, and produce cytotoxins. The cytokine monocytes release play an important role in directing neutrophils and monocytes to sites of inflammation.

(3) **Lymphocytes.** B and T lymphocytes decrease in number and function following CPB, which may render the patient immunosuppressed and at risk for infections.

(4) **Platelets.** Through the production and release of leukotrienes, serotonin, chemokines, PF4, and other substances, platelets contribute to the inflammatory response.

(5) **Endothelium.** See above.

3. **Consequences of the inflammatory response to CPB.** In most patients, the early SIR resolves without significant injury as a result of discontinuation of the stimulus, dissipation of mediators, or the action of naturally occurring antagonists (e.g., IL-10). The variability in the expression, consequences, and outcome of the inflammatory response to CPB is the subject of much speculation. Some factors which influence this include the preoperative condition of the patient, type and complexity of the surgery, and, perhaps most importantly, underlying genetic polymorphism.

4. **Strategies to minimize the inflammatory response to CPB.** Various strategies have been promoted to minimize the SIR syndrome, including surface modification of the ECC (e.g., heparin-coated circuits), use of centrifugal pumps, pulsatile flow, and MOs, priming with colloids, ultrafiltration, leukodepletion or leukofiltration, use of minimized circuits (reduced surface area and elimination of the venous reservoir), improved management of shed blood (e.g., elimination of or minimizing use of cardiotomy suction, use of RBC-washer/salvage devices), off-pump techniques, administration of corticosteroids or aprotinin, complement inhibitors, protease inhibitors (e.g., aprotinin), anticytokine therapy, antiendotoxin therapy, digestive decontamination, and administration of antibodies to block adhesion molecules or their activation [38,41,43]. **Although many of these strategies have been effective in attenuating the inflammatory response to CPB, few have been proven to reduce major complications in the postoperative period.**

J. **"Stress response" to CPB—Endocrine, metabolic, and electrolyte effects.** CPB is associated with a marked exaggeration of the **stress response** associated with all types of surgery. This is manifested by large increases in epinephrine, norepinephrine, AVP (or antidiuretic hormone), adrenocorticotropic hormone, cortisol (mainly after bypass), growth hormone, and glucagon. Elevated catecholamines may have adverse effects on regional and organ blood flow patterns. Catecholamines also increase myocardial oxygen consumption, which may adversely affect the balance of myocardial oxygen supply and demand at the time of reperfusion. Other stress hormones also increase catabolic reactions, leading to increased energy consumption, tissue breakdown, and possible impairment of wound healing.

Hyperglycemia is invariably encountered during CPB, especially in patients with diabetes mellitus. Contributors to hyperglycemia include decreased insulin production, insulin resistance (possibly related to stress hormones), decreased consumption (related to insulin resistance and hypothermia), increased glycogenolysis and gluconeogenesis (related to stress hormones), and increased reabsorption of glucose by the kidney. Observational studies have demonstrated an association between post-CPB hyperglycemia and increased morbidity and mortality. Although control of blood glucose values during and following CPB is currently strongly advocated, the optimal "target range" for serum glucose concentrations has not been determined.

Renin, angiotensin II, and aldosterone levels all tend to rise during CPB. Many patients display the so-called **sick euthyroid syndrome** with reduced tri-iodothyronine (T3), thyroxine (T4), and free thyroxin levels but normal thyroid-stimulating hormone levels. The etiology of this phenomenon is unclear, but it provides the rationale for administration of thyroid hormone in some patients with low cardiac output syndrome.

Calcium and magnesium. Both ionized calcium and total and unfiltratable fractions of magnesium commonly fall, whereas potassium levels may fluctuate widely during CPB. The latter may be related to diuretics, catecholamines, preoperative spironolactone (aldactone) and β-blockers, potassium-containing cardioplegia, and renal dysfunction. The importance of maintaining normal levels of these ions to preserve normal muscle and cardiac function and prevent dysrhythmias is apparent.

VII. Summary

CPB is performed safely and effectively throughout the world. This is a result of a combination of sophisticated equipment used for extracorporeal circulation and well-trained and educated perfusionists. The responsibility for safe CPB is shared by surgeons, anesthesiologists, and perfusionists in order to manage cardiovascular surgery with the lowest possible patient risk. Despite technologic advances in circuit design that have occurred over the past several decades, aberrations of normal physiology are imposed by CPB, which may result in postoperative organ dysfunction. Post-CPB organ dysfunction constitutes a spectrum ranging from mild dysfunction in one or more organ systems to death resulting from multiorgan failure. **It should be emphasized that placing a patient on CPB is a physiologic trespass against that patient.** Absence of significant damage caused by CPB depends primarily on a particular patient's ability to compensate for the derangements introduced by that trespass.

REFERENCES

1. Ghosh S, Falter F, Cook DJ. *Cardiopulmonary Bypass.* Cambridge, MA: Cambridge University Press; 2009.
2. Hessel EA. Cardiopulmonary bypass equipment. In: Estafanous FG, et al., eds. *Cardiac Anesthesia.* 2nd ed. Philadelphia, PA: Lippincott Williams & Wilkins; 2001.
3. Schell RM, Hessel, EA II, Reves JG. Cardiopulmonary bypass. Chapter 10. In: Reves JG, Reeves S, Abernathy JH III, eds. *Atlas of Cardiothoracic Anesthesia.* 2nd ed. New York, NY: Springer; 2009.
4. Groom RC, Stammers AH. Extracorporeal devices and related technologies. In: Kaplan JA, et al., eds. *Kaplan's Cardiac Anesthesia.* 6th ed. St. Louis, MO: Elsevier/Saunders; 2011.
5. Hessel EA II. Circuitry and cannulation techniques. In: Gravlee GP, Davis RF, Stammers AH, et al., eds. *Cardiopulmonary Bypass: Principles and Practice.* 3rd ed. Philadelphia, PA: Lippincott Williams & Wilkins; 2008.
6. Murphy GS, Hessel EA, Groom RC. Optimal perfusion during cardiopulmonary bypass: An evidence-based approach. *Anesth Analg.* 2009;108:1394–1417.
7. Groom RC, Froebe S, Martin J, et al. Update on pediatric perfusion practice in North America: 2005 survey. *J Extra Corpor Technol.* 2005;37:343–350.
8. Zangrillo A, Garozzo FA, Biondi-Zoccai G, et al. Miniaturized cardiopulmonary bypass improves short-term outcome in cardiac surgery: A meta-analysis of randomized controlled studies. *J Thorac Cardiovasc Surg.* 2010;139:1162–1169.
9. Hessel EA. Bypass techniques for descending thoracic aortic surgery. *Semin Cardiothoracic Vasc Anesth.* 2001;5:293–320.
10. Charrière JM, Pélissié J, Verd C, et al. Survey: Retrospective survey of monitoring/safety devices and incidents of cardiopulmonary bypass for cardiac surgery in France. *J Extra Corpor Technol.* 2007;39:142–157.
11. Jenkins OF, Morris R, Simpson JM. Australasian perfusion incident survey. *Perfusion.* 1997;12:279–288.
12. Mejak BL, Stammers A, Rauch E, et al. A retrospective study on perfusion incidents and safety devices. *Perfusion.* 2000;15: 51–61.
13. Groom RC, Forest RJ, Cormack JE, et al. Parallel replacement of the oxygenator that is not transferring oxygen: The PRONTO procedure. *Perfusion.* 2002;17:447–450.
14. Edmonds HL Jr. 2010 Standard of care for central nervous system monitoring during cardiac surgery. *J Cardiothorac Vasc Anesth.* 2010;24:541–543.
15. Gravlee GP, Davis RF, Kurusz M, eds. *Cardiopulmonary Bypass: Principles and Practice.* 3rd ed. Philadelphia, PA: Lippincott Williams & Wilkins; 2007.
16. Kirklin JW, Barratt-Boyes BG. Hypothermia, circulatory arrest, and cardiopulmonary bypass. In: Kirklin JW, Barratt-Boyes BG, eds. *Cardiac Surgery.* 2nd ed. New York, NY: Churchill Livingstone; 1993:61–127.
17. Grovier AV, Reves JG, McKay RD, et al. Factors and their influence on regional cerebral blood flow during nonpulsatile cardiopulmonary bypass. *Ann Thorac Surg.* 1984;38:592–600.
18. Joshi B, Ono M, Brown C, et al. Predicting the limits of cerebral autoregulation during cardiopulmonary bypass. *Anesth Analg.* 2012;114(3):503–510.
19. Gold JP, Charlson ME, Williams-Russo P, et al. Improvement of outcomes after coronary artery bypass. A randomized trial comparing intraoperative high versus low mean arterial pressure. *J Thorac Cardiovasc Surg.* 1995;110:1302–1311.
20. Rudy LW, Heymann MA, Edmunds LH. Distribution of systemic blood flow during cardiopulmonary bypass. *J Appl Physiol.* 1973;34:194–200.
21. Slater JM, Orszulak TA, Cook DJ. Distribution and hierarchy of regional blood flow during hypothermic cardiopulmonary bypass. *Ann Thorac Surg.* 2001;72:542–547.
22. Wright G. Mechanical simulation of cardiac function by means of pulsatile blood pumps. *J Cardiothorac Vasc Anesth.* 1997;11:299–309.
23. Cavaliere F, Gennari A, Martinelli L, et al. The relationship between systemic oxygen uptake and delivery during moderate hypothermic cardiopulmonary bypass: Critical values and effects of vasodilation by hydralazine. *Perfusion.* 1995;10:315–321.
24. Ranucci M, Romitti F, Isgro G, et al. Oxygen delivery during cardiopulmonary bypass and acute renal failure after coronary operations. *Ann Thorac Surg.* 2005;80:2213–2220.
25. Schmidt FX, Philipp A, Foltan M, et al. Adequacy of perfusion during hypothermia: Regional distribution of cardiopulmonary bypass flow, mixed venous and regional venous oxygen saturation. *Thorac Cardiovasc Surg.* 2003;51:306–311.
26. Ranucci M, Isgro G, Romitti F, et al. Anaerobic metabolism during cardiopulmonary bypass: Predictive value of carbon dioxide derived parameters. *Ann Thorac Surg.* 2006;81:2189–2195.
27. Murkin JM, Adams SJ, Novick RJ, et al. Monitoring brain oxygen saturation during coronary bypass surgery: A randomized, prospective study. *Anesth Analg.* 2007;104(1):51–58.
28. Taillefer M-C, Denault AY. Cerebral near-infrared spectroscopy in adult heart surgery: Systematic review of its clinical efficacy. *Can J Anaesth.* 2005;52:79–87.
29. Hessel EA. CNS monitoring: The current weak state of the evidence. *J Cardiothorac Vasc Anesth.* 2011;25(4):e15 [Online only article].
30. Edmunds HL, Jr. Reply to Dr. Hessel. *J Cardiothorac Vasc Anesth.* 2011;25(4):e16.
31. Wagener G, Jan M, Kim M, et al. Association between increases in urinary neutrophil gelatinase-associated lipocalin and acute renal dysfunction after adult cardiac surgery. *Anesthesiology.* 2006;103:485–491.
32. Habib RH, Zacharias A, Schwann TA, et al. Adverse effects of low hematocrit during cardiopulmonary bypass in the adult: Should current practice be changed? *J Thorac Cardiovasc Surg.* 2003;125:1438–1450.
33. Cook DJ. Changing temperature management for cardiopulmonary bypass. *Anesth Analg.* 1999;88:1254–1271.
34. The Warm Heart Investigators. Randomized trial of normothermic versus hypothermic coronary bypass surgery. *Lancet.* 1994;343:559–563.

35. Martin TD, Craver JM, Gott JP, et al. Prospective, randomized trial of retrograde warm blood cardioplegia: Myocardial benefit and neurological threat. *Ann Thorac Surg.* 1994;57:298–304.
36. Aronson S, Blumenthal R. Perioperative renal dysfunction and cardiovascular anesthesia: Concerns and controversies. *J Cardiothorac Vasc Anesth.* 1998;12:567–586.
37. Hessel EA II. Abdominal organ injury after cardiac surgery. *Semin Cardiothorac Vasc Anesth.* 2004;8:243–263.
38. Laffey JG, Boylan JF, Cheng DCH. The systemic inflammatory response to cardiac surgery. Implications for the anesthesiologist. *Anesthesiology.* 2002;97:215–252.
39. Pintar T, Collard CD. The systemic inflammatory response to cardiopulmonary bypass. *Anesthesiol Clin North America.* 2003;21:453–464.
40. Menasche P, Edmunds LH Jr. The inflammatory response. In: Cohn LH, Edmunds LH, eds. *Cardiac Surgery in the Adult Patient.* New York, NY: McGraw-Hill Professional; 2003:349–360.
41. Bennett-Guerrero E. Systemic inflammation. In: Kaplan JA, Reich DL, Savino JS, eds. *Kaplan's Cardiac Anesthesia.* 6th ed. Philadelphia, PA: Elsevier/Saunders; 2011:178–192.
42. O'Brien ERM, Nathan HJ. Coronary physiology and atherosclerosis. In: Kaplan JA, Reich DL, Lake CL, et al., eds. *Kaplan's Cardiac Anesthesia.* 5th ed. Philadelphia, PA: Elsevier/Saunders; 2006:94–96.
43. Asimakopoulos G, Gourlay T. A review of anti-inflammatory strategies in cardiac surgery. *Perfusion.* 2003;18:7–12.

22 Devices for Cardiac Support and Replacement

Joseph C. Cleveland, Jr., Benjamin C. Sun, Ronald L. Harter, and Glenn P. Gravlee

KEY POINTS

1. Mechanical circulatory support devices most often are ventricular assist devices, which are indicated for bridging to myocardial recovery or cardiac transplantation or as a permanent assist device (destination therapy).
2. The principal growth area for ventricular assist devices in recent years has been destination therapy. The predominant device used for this purpose has changed from the pulsatile, bulky Heartmate XVE to the compact nonpulsatile (continuous flow) Heartmate II device.
3. In New York Heart Association Class IV Heart Failure (minimal activity induces symptoms), both the Heartmate XVE and Heartmate II provide better survival and quality of life than medical therapy, but Heartmate II outcomes are superior to those for Heartmate XVE.
4. A variety of nonpulsatile right ventricular assist devices (RVAD) and a pulsatile total artificial heart are Food and Drug Administration-approved for bridging to recovery or to transplantation. RVADs are sometimes needed as a bridge to RV recovery for patients undergoing destination LVAD placement.
5. Newer short-term bridging VADs include the CentriMag, Tandem Heart, and Impella pumps, all of which are continuous-flow pumps that implant and operate in separate and distinct ways.
6. Placement of a destination LVAD most often requires a median sternotomy and cardiopulmonary bypass. Anesthetic management is similar to that for orthotopic cardiac transplantation in that it requires recognition that preoperative LV systolic function is abysmal.

7. Separation from CPB after LVAD placement is often complicated by either primary or secondary RV failure, which may require various combinations of pulmonary arterial vasodilators (e.g., milrinone, nitric oxide), inotropes (e.g., dobutamine, epinephrine), and systemic arterial vasoconstrictors (e.g., vasopressin).
8. Transesophageal echocardiography is essential to VAD placement for its assessment of biventricular preload, valve function, RV function, presence or absence of a patent foramen ovale, and VAD inflow and outflow. Aortic valve insufficiency is particularly troublesome for LVAD patients.
9. Early postoperative problems include bleeding and thromboembolism. Late postoperative problems include device malfunction and infection, especially for pulsatile VADs.
10. Continuous-flow VAD patients presenting for noncardiac surgery pose a variety of clinical problems, which may include obtaining accurate measurements of blood pressure, VAD blood flow, and pulse oximetry as well as acquired von Willebrand's syndrome and aortic valve insufficiency.
11. Intra-aortic balloon pumps (IABPs) are most often used to provide temporary LV support to patients undergoing interventional cardiology or cardiac surgical procedures. IABPs augment diastolic blood flow to reduce LV afterload, while simultaneously potentially increasing coronary artery blood flow.
12. IABP inflation and deflation must be synchronized to the cardiac cycle, which can be done using either electrocardiography or an intra-arterial waveform. Inflation should commence just after systole ends, and deflation should end just before systole begins.
13. The most common serious IABP complication is lower limb ischemia.

I. Introduction

Aside from the intra-aortic balloon pump (IABP), the use of a **mechanical circulatory support device (MCSD)** has historically been relegated to "salvage" therapy. Although a selective role continues for this type of intervention, MCSDs are taking their place as part of a therapeutic continuum that can be successfully used to treat a multitude of cardiovascular problems. Indeed, many therapeutic interventions using MCSDs are performed on an elective or urgent basis rather than as a life-saving emergency. Most current devices and devices in development are designed for long-term outpatient therapy with excellent quality of life.

Devices are getting smaller, easier to implant, and more durable. The potential growth for this emerging therapy is quite substantial. This chapter will discuss the current state of MCSDs, future directions, and also will review the most common circulatory assist device, the IABP.

II. History

Dr. Michael DeBakey performed the first successful clinical implant of a ventricular assist device (VAD) for postcardiotomy cardiac failure in 1966 [1]. The patient was mechanically supported for 4 days. The first successful use of MCSD for a "bridge" to transplantation occurred in 1978 at the Texas Heart Institute. That patient was supported for 5 days by a pneumatically actuated paracorporeal device. The first implant of a total artificial heart (TAH) was performed on Dr. Barney Clarke, a retired dentist, by Dr. William DeVries in 1982 at the University of Utah. The pump was a Jarvik TAH designed by Dr. Robert Jarvik. Dr. Clarke lived for 112 days; unfortunately, the world watched him slowly and courageously die over the ensuing months from sepsis and embolic events. As with the pioneering experience with cardiac transplantation in the 1960s, there was public criticism of TAH as an "advancement" that was not worthwhile. Nevertheless, development of more sophisticated devices for short-term and long-term use quietly persisted. Successful recovery of patients in acute cardiogenic shock using short-term VADs occurred and the data improved. The first pump to receive Food and Drug Administration (FDA) approval in the United States was the Abiomed BVS 5000 (Abiomed, Danvers, MA, USA) in November, 1992. Two implantable pumps were then approved for inpatient long-term use, the Heartmate IP system (Thoratec Corp., Pleasanton, CA, USA) and the Novacor system (Worldheart, Ontario, Canada). In 1995, both the Heartmate Vented Electric (VE) system and the Novacor system were subsequently approved for outpatient use. This was followed by the Thoratec VAD system (Thoratec Corp., Pleasanton, CA, USA), which was approved as a long-term support system in 1996. The TAH also quietly evolved during this time. There were three different systems that developed with the support of the National Institutes of Health (NIH): (a) The Penn State TAH (Hershey, PA, USA; Minnesota Mining and Manufacturing, Minneapolis, MN, USA); (b) the Abiomed AbioCor TAH (Abiomed, Danvers, MA, USA); (c) the Cardiowest TAH (Syncardia, Tucson, AZ, USA). The Penn State TAH was purchased by Abiomed and is being developed as the AbioCor II. AbioCor I (the original AbioCor) was implanted in 14 patients as a Phase I clinical trial for destination (i.e., permanent) therapy. It was approved for clinical use by the FDA in September, 2006. The Cardiowest TAH represented the evolution of the Jarvik TAH and has had over 1,000 implants worldwide. It received FDA approval as a bridge to transplantation in 2005.

The period of 2007 to 2012 has marked an exciting and exponential rise in the use of newer, smaller rotary and centrifugal left ventricular assist devices (LVADs). The Heartmate II (HM II) LVAD (Thoratec Corp., Pleasanton, CA, USA) received FDA approval for bridge to transplantation in 2007 and destination therapy in 2009. The Jarvik rotary LVAD (Jarvik Heart, Inc., New York, NY, USA) remains in clinical trials, but offers implantation through a left thoracotomy, which may be advantageous in certain circumstances. The Heartware HVAD (HeartWare International, Framingham, MA, USA) is a centrifugal pump which has the advantage of implantation directly into the LV apex without requiring an additional extrapericardial pocket. Since an additional pump pocket is not required, there will likely be fewer infectious complications and faster implant times for this pump when compared with contemporary rotary pumps. In addition, the HVAD is the first long-term centrifugal pump to be tested in clinical trials.

III. Indications

There are three commonly described indications for the use of MCSDs: Bridge to myocardial or hemodynamic recovery, bridge to cardiac transplantation, and alternative to cardiac transplant or "destination therapy."

A. Bridge to recovery. The use of an MCSD as a recovery system has focused on short-term use. **Traditionally, this has been thought of as support for days to weeks.** Clinical indications for this use include cardiogenic shock in the following settings:

1. Postcardiotomy
2. Acute myocardial infarction (MI)
3. Viral cardiomyopathies
4. 1 Inadequate preservation of donor heart after cardiac transplantation
5. Other causes

The postcardiotomy use of these pumps has declined over the past several years [2]. This likely derives from improved perfusion and preservation techniques. Nevertheless, in this patient population the anticipated recovery time was 3 to 5 days. Animal data for support to recovery supported this timeline, as recovery was seen quite early [3]. **We now recognize that there may be substantial variability in the time it may take for patients' hearts to recover while on support. This is likely to be diagnosis specific.** Data from the Abiomed voluntary registry showed that mean support time to successful recovery may exceed 30 days [2]. Several devices are now employed as short-term bridge-to-recovery devices: The Abiomed system, the Centrimag (centrifugal system, Thoratec Corp., Pleasanton, CA, USA), the Impella 2.5 or 5.0 and the Tandem Heart (CardiacAssist Inc., Pittsburgh, PA, USA), and lastly conventional veno-arterial extracorporeal membrane oxygenation (ECMO). The goal of short-term bridge-to-recovery device is to provide end-organ perfusion while the heart is recovering. These short-term devices are especially useful in catastrophic, sudden presentations of cardiogenic shock (e.g., prolonged cardiac arrest during high-risk percutaneous coronary interventions) situations in which the likelihood of intact neurologic recovery remains unknown. These devices allow time to determine whether an irreversible neurologic injury would preclude a successful recovery or transplantation.

B. Bridge to transplantation. The use of MCSDs as a bridge to cardiac transplantation constituted the early human laboratory to understand the long-term effects of support on many physiologic parameters as well as on quality-of-life measures. The therapy was instituted in

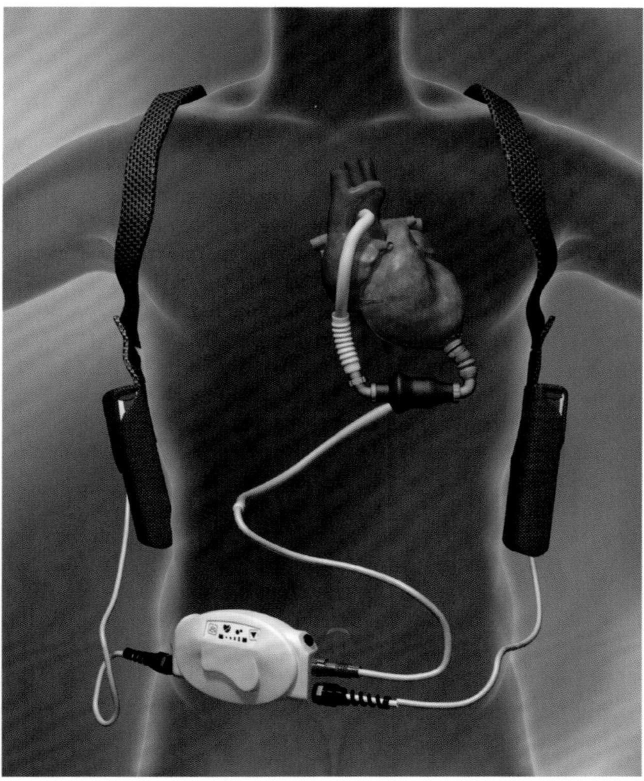

FIGURE 22.1 Diagram of a patient with an implanted HM II continuous-flow LVAD including driveline and portable power source. (Reproduced with permission from Thoratec, Inc., Pleasanton, CA, USA.)

individuals who were listed for cardiac transplantation, but failing conventional or inotropic therapy. **The MCSD would be employed to support the patient and improve the physiologic condition until a donor heart became available.** The MCSD would then be explanted at the time of cardiac transplantation.

Many of the VADs (Thoratec IVAD [implantable VAD]/PVAD [paracorporeal VAD], Heartmate XVE, Novacor) or the Cardiowest TAH are approved for this indication. The Thoratec HM II pump (Fig. 22.1) has become the mainstay of pumps implanted for a bridge-to-transplantation indication. However, a randomized clinical trial comparing the HM II LVAD to the Heartware HVAD has recently been completed and the data submitted to the FDA seeking a bridge-to-transplantation indication for the Heartware HVAD [4,5].

2 C. **Destination therapy.** As experience with long-term use of MCSD led to successful outpatient use of this therapy, the concept of using MCSD as another option for patients with end-stage heart failure who were not transplant candidates emerged.

A landmark study called Randomized Evaluation of Mechanical Assistance in the Treatment of Congestive Heart failure (REMATCH) concluded that **end-stage heart-failure patients who received a Thoratec Heartmate VE LVAD experienced improved survival and quality of life when compared to optimal medical therapy.** The use of MCSD as permanent support for end-stage heart failure is now an accepted and viable therapy that is also supported by the Center for Medicare Services (CMS). The Heartmate XVE was the first LVAD approved for this indication. Although the Heartmate XVE provided superior outcomes to medical therapy, this device was found to only support patients for approximately 2 yrs before

the device failed. In a subsequent randomized trial comparing the Heartmate XVE with the
3 HM II LVAD (continuous-flow pump), the HM II LVAD proved superior to the Heartmate XVE, with 2-yr survival in the HM II cohort of 58% versus 25% in the XVE group. The HM II received FDA approval for destination therapy in 2009 and the most recent Interagency Registry for Mechanically Assisted Circulatory Support (INTERMACS) database documented that more than 99% of destination therapy implants in 2010 were continuous-flow pumps [6].

IV. Classification and attachment sites of VADs

VADs can be used as an isolated LVAD, an isolated right ventricular assist device (RVAD), or as a biventricular assist device (BIVAD). These devices are attached to the heart through cannulae that allow the blood to enter the pumping chamber from which it is ejected into the systemic or pulmonary circulation. TAHs differ from VADs in that a TAH removes all of the native ventricles and part of the atria. In contrast, if a BIVAD is implanted, the LV and RV remain in place, but the majority of the cardiac output emanates from the BIVAD.

A. **LVAD.** For left-sided circulatory support, all of the devices can be attached to the left ventricular (LV) apex as the inflow connection to the pumping chamber. **The LV apex is the preferred site of LVAD attachment for most of the devices and is the only option for some devices (HM II LVAD and Heartware HVAD).** Some devices can function through cannulation of the left atrium either directly or percutaneously through the interatrial septum. The left atrium is not the ideal cannulation site for long-term support as the left ventricle may then form large thrombi as a result of blood stasis [7]. In addition, flows through the LVAD are generally higher with LV versus LA cannulation for VAD inflow. For cardiogenic shock where short-term LVAD support is anticipated, left atrial cannulation is a reasonable option. **The LVAD outflow graft is routinely anastomosed to the aorta,** usually the ascending aorta (Fig. 22.2).

B. **RVAD.** For right-sided support, either **right atrial or right ventricular (RV) cannulation can be used successfully.** Substantial thrombus formation in the RV does not appear to result
4 from right atrial cannulation even in long-term support. **The RVAD outflow graft is anastomosed to the pulmonary artery.** VADs can be implanted without the support of cardiopulmonary bypass (CPB), but CPB is generally used to maintain patient stability [8].

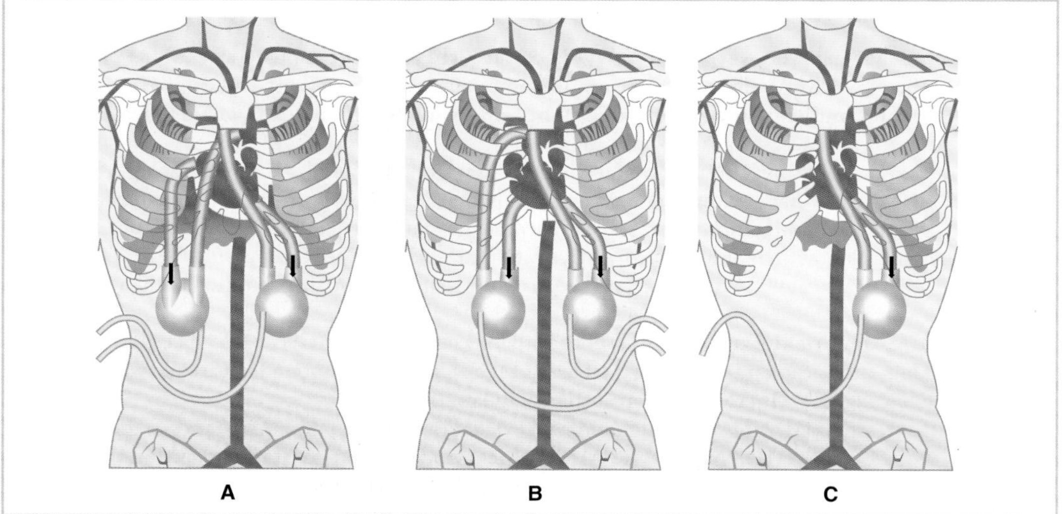

FIGURE 22.2 Cannulation configurations for the Thoratec VAD either as a BIVAD on the left and right sides (as shown in **A** and **B**) or left side (LVAD) only (shown in **C**). **A** shows right-atrial inflow to pulmonary artery outflow configuration for the **RVAD. B** shows an RV inflow to pulmonary artery outflow for the RVAD. **A, B,** and **C** all show the traditional LV inflow to aortic outflow configuration for the LVAD. (Reprinted with permission from Thoratec Corporation.)

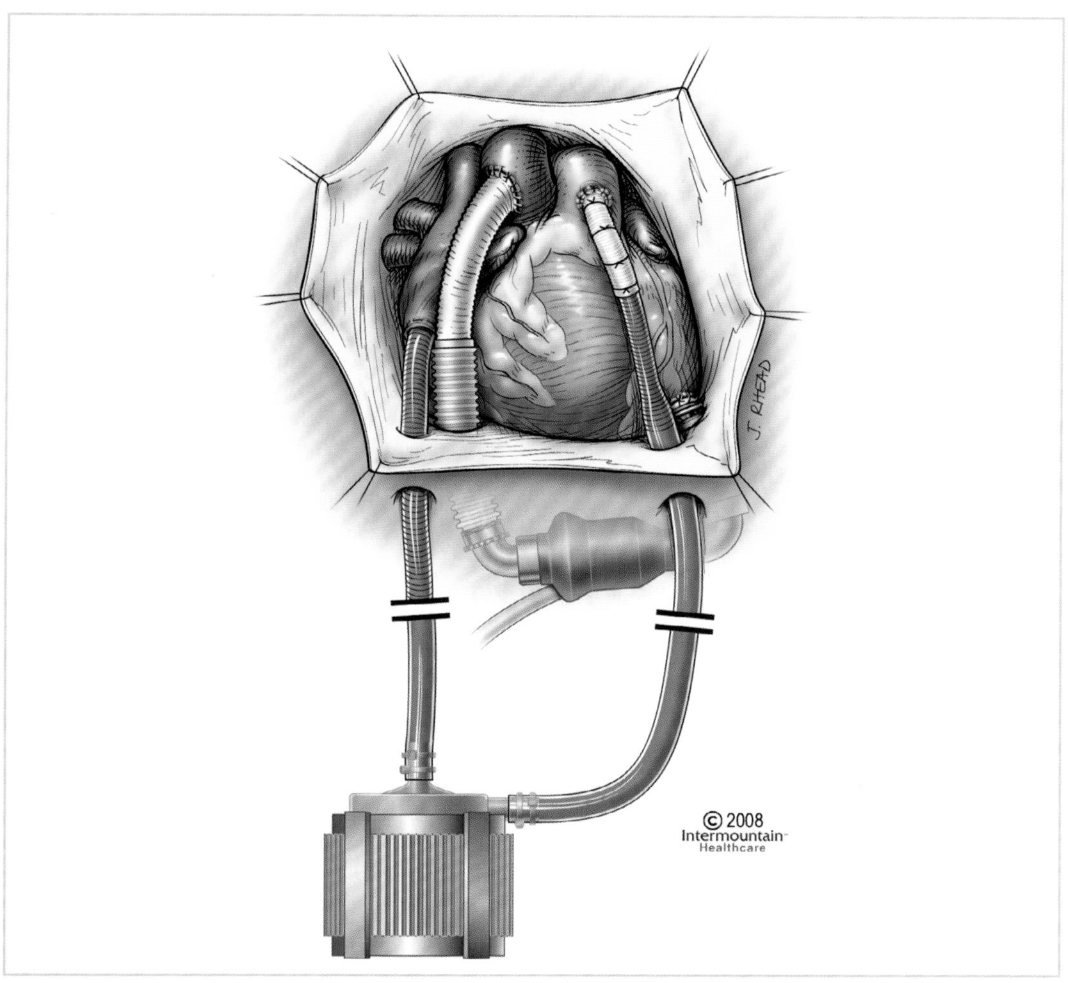

FIGURE 22.3 Illustration of the Centrimag continuous-flow VAD positioned as an RVAD with inflow from the right atrium and outflow into the pulmonary artery. Also pictured is an HM II LVAD with inflow from the LV apex and outflow into the ascending aorta. (Reproduced with permission from Thoratec, Inc., Pleasanton, CA, USA.)

C. **BIVAD.** A BIVAD (Fig. 22.3) consists of the simultaneous use of RVAD and LVAD with connections as noted earlier for the individual assist devices.

D. **TAH.** Placement of a TAH requires excision of the native heart. The current systems require removal of the ventricles, preserving the atria for securing the device. Sewing cuffs connect the TAH pumping chambers to the atria. Both of the current clinical systems have valves in both inlet (atrioventricular) and outlet (aortic or pulmonary) positions. Separate graft conduits connect the two pumping chambers to the aorta and main pulmonary artery. Once these grafts and cuffs are sewn, pressurized saline is used to test for leaks.

V. Mechanical assistance systems

A variety of mechanical support systems are used to treat patients with end-stage heart failure. However, there are only two distinct methods of blood flow delivery by these assist devices, which are essentially pumps. One method provides a constant flow to the patient's circulatory system through a high-speed rotor pump. The other method provides pulsatile flow generated by a volume displacement pump (unsynchronized with the patient's native heartbeat). Although the implantation of these devices is identical, there are differences in how the two systems fill and empty the heart and in the afterload the heart will experience. These differences may influence the right side of the heart (in the case of isolated LVADs) as well as end-organ function (e.g., brain, kidneys, liver). Both types of pumping systems may be used for short-term or long-term support.

A. **Pulsatile. Pulsatile pumps are generally volume displacement pumps that work like the native heart.** These are often called first-generation pumps. A chamber fills until a set volume is achieved, and this volume of blood is ejected into the aorta. Pulsatile pumps all have inflow and outflow valves mimicking the native mitral and aortic valves. The method of energy delivery used to eject the blood from the chamber may be air (pneumatic), fluid (hydraulic), or a mechanical pusher plate.

1. **Short-term support. The Abiomed BVS 5000/AB ventricle system serves as an example of a pulsatile pump used for short-term support.** These pumps can be used for single ventricle support of either the right or left side as well as for biventricular support (using two pumps). They are easily implanted and require minimal setup to initiate support. This "plug and play" implantability as well as relatively low cost has kept them in most institutions as the emergency support system. Recently, there has been a shift to using the Levitronix Centrimag system. This system is also an extracorporeal VAD; however, in contradistinction to the ABIOMED system, the Centrimag provides nonpulsatile continuous flow. The Thoratec PVAD has also been FDA-approved for potential short-term recovery, but it is more expensive and more complex to initiate. Its advantages are an excellent safety profile and durability. It is also approved for long-term outpatient use, should the patient require bridge to transplantation.
2. **Long-term support.** Five systems are currently FDA-approved for bridge to transplantation: Thoratec PVAD/IVAD, Thoratec Heartmate XVE, Thoratec HM II LVAD, Worldheart Novacor System, and Syncardia Cardiowest TAH. **The Heartmate XVE and HM II LVAD are also the only devices that are currently FDA-approved for destination therapy,** although other devices, notably the Heartware HVAD, are undergoing clinical trials for this indication.

B. **Continuous flow.** Continuous-flow devices come in different variations: Axial flow or centrifugal flow, and with different bearings: Mechanical (ball bearing, ruby bearing, fluid bearing) or magnetic (mag-lev or bearingless). **Continuous-flow devices with bearings are considered "second-generation" devices, whereas the mag-lev pumps are considered "third-generation" devices.**

1. **Short-term support.** Three continuous-flow pumps are currently being utilized in the United States as short-term support devices: CentriMag (Levitronix, Waltham, MA, USA), the Tandem Heart (CardiacAssist, Inc., Pittsburgh, PA, USA), and Impella (Abiomed, Danvers, MA, USA). The Centrimag pump (Fig. 22.3) is most commonly utilized with an open chest implantation with left atrial or LV inflow cannulation for the LVAD, and ascending aortic cannulation for outflow. The right atrium or right ventricle can be cannulated for inflow for an RVAD and the pulmonary artery as outflow for an RVAD. The Tandem Heart pump is attractive as a percutaneous LVAD. The inflow is placed via the right common femoral vein, across the intra-atrial septum into the left atrium. The outflow is in the descending thoracic aorta via a cannula placed in the femoral artery. The Impella pump is placed percutaneously via the common femoral artery retrograde across the aortic valve into the left ventricle. Inflow is through the left ventricle and outflow is into the ascending aorta—the VAD is placed across the aortic valve.
2. **Long-term support.** The Thoratec HM II LVAD was FDA-approved for bridge to transplantation in 2008. The HM II received FDA approval in January 2010 for use as destination therapy. The ENDURANCE trial is currently in progress and is a randomized clinical trial comparing Heartware HVAD to the HM II LVAD for destination therapy.
3. **Advantages and disadvantages. Continuous-flow devices offer the advantage of being much smaller than their pulsatile counterparts, as no "blood chamber" is needed.** Their smaller size often leads to easier implantation with less intraoperative dissection. This can reduce blood loss, shorten operative times, reduce infection rates, and provide the potential for more rapid recovery. The data generated from the outcomes with

utilization of continuous-flow devices as a bridge-to-transplant indication show excellent 1-yr survival, approaching 90%. The 2-yr survival for the cohort that received the HM II for destination therapy was 58%. This was double the survival in the cohort that received the XVE.

Continuous-flow devices pose inherent challenges. These devices do not have valves and need to flow a minimum rate to prevent "device insufficiency." This regurgitant flow can be catastrophic if power to the device is suddenly turned off. In addition, as patients are managed with longer-term nonpulsatile devices, certain complications that are device related have emerged, The HM II LVAD universally cleaves von-Willebrand's factor (VWF). Nearly all patients with a HM II LVAD acquire a deficiency in VWF and are prone to mucosal bleeding events—particularly in the gastrointestinal tract [9]. Ongoing research into this phenomenon will hopefully gain more insight into who is at risk and how to optimally manage patients with bleeding. For the present, it appears likely that these patients would respond favorably to a desmopressin bolus (30 mcg/kg). Additionally, **many patients have minimal arterial pulsatility when on full support.** This is not generally problematic when arterial pressure is monitored with an indwelling arterial catheter, but may become so when the patient leaves the intensive care unit (ICU) or leaves the hospital for home or an extended care facility. In those settings, if a patient with a continuous-flow LVAD were found unresponsive, it would be challenging for the first responder to determine whether "circulation" is present or not.

VI. Intraoperative considerations

A. Anesthetic considerations

1. **Monitoring and vascular access. Large-bore vascular access is required** because blood loss and coagulopathy can be substantial. This can be achieved with one large-bore (16 gauge or larger) peripheral intravenous catheter and a large-lumen (e.g., 9 Fr) central-access introducer or with its equivalent via central venous access (e.g., a pulmonary artery catheter introducer with additional double-lumen large-bore integral ports). Standard American Society of Anesthesiologists monitors (electrocardiography [ECG], pulse oximetry, temperature) are used with the possible exception of a noninvasive blood pressure (BP) cuff. As noted earlier, an arterial catheter is essential and consideration might be given to its placement in a larger central artery such as the femoral artery, in order to minimize the potential problem of central-to-peripheral BP discrepancies at separation from CPB or thereafter. Pulmonary artery catheters can be very helpful for the assessment of RV function and pulmonary vascular resistance, but they may be mechanically infeasible after initiation of therapy with RVAD, BIVAD, or TAH. **Intraoperative transesophageal echocardiography is essential** for the assessment of aortic valve competency, patent foramen ovale (PFO), LV thrombus, adequacy of VAD inflow and outflow, cardiac preload assessment, and RV function (for isolated LVADs).

6

2. **Anesthetic techniques. General endotracheal anesthesia is used, and most practitioners probably place emphasis on intravenous techniques that minimize hemodynamic impact.** For example, a total intravenous technique using an opioid (e.g., fentanyl or sufentanil), a benzodiazepine such as midazolam, and a muscle relaxant, such as vecuronium or rocuronium may be selected. If renal or hepatic function is markedly impaired, cisatracurium can be a wise choice. In most centers, there is no advantage to attempting a "fast-track" approach, because these patients will generally remain intubated overnight or longer regardless of the type of device implanted. This may change as experience grows and as the devices become less and less cumbersome to implant. Consequently, these cases present a good opportunity for medium- (e.g., fentanyl 20 to 40 μg/kg total dose) to high-dose opioids (e.g., fentanyl 50 to 75 μg/kg total dose) as a means to ensure hemodynamic stability without concern for early extubation. If hepatic function is compromised, medium or lower doses may be more appropriate. Volatile anesthetic agents such as desflurane, sevoflurane, and isoflurane can be used as hemodynamically tolerated. Nitrous oxide probably should be avoided because of its potential to increase pulmonary vascular resistance (PVR) and because of the high risk of intravascular air.

B. Surgical techniques

1. Cannulation techniques

a. VADs. Atrial cannulation is the most common approach to gain inflow for short-term support when using either a right- or left-sided VAD system. The atria are easily accessed and the low pressures in these chambers facilitate hemostasis upon decannulation when the heart has recovered. The right atrial appendage is used for right-sided support. For left-sided support, the interatrial groove at the junction of the right superior pulmonary vein is the most common site for cannulation. Other cannulation options for left-sided support include the dome of the left atrium (between the aorta and superior vena cava), the left atrial appendage, or through the apex of the LV. Cannulation of the LV apex for inflow minimizes blood stasis and provides the best decompression of the heart. However, decannulation and repair of this high-pressure chamber can be difficult and often requires placement back onto CPB. LV apex cannulation is highly recommended when a prosthetic mitral valve is present to maintain blood flow through the valve and prevent thrombus formation. **The LV apex is the sole acceptable inflow cannulation site for most long-term LVADs** (Heartmate XVE, HM II, Heartware HVAD, Micromed, Novacor). The ventricular chamber empties into a long tube attached to a coated Dacron vascular outflow graft that is sewn to the ascending aorta or the pulmonary artery.

b. TAH. For implantation of a TAH, excision of the native heart must be performed while preserving the atria. First, the surgeon attaches sewing cuffs that will connect the atria to the TAH pumping chambers, after which the surgeon sews grafts to both the aorta and the main pulmonary artery. After these grafts and cuffs are sewn, leak testing with pressurized saline (tinged with methylene blue) is used. Leak testing is imperative as the suture lines are often inaccessible if bleeding occurs once the TAH is in place. The TAH is then attached to the atrial cuffs followed by the arterial grafts.

C. Initiation of support for LVAD

1. Initial considerations. Techniques for the initiation of support are similar in all of the pulsatile systems. Ventilation is re-established and the heart is gradually filled. The assist device is manually actuated until adequate preload and afterload are established. **If the**
7 **ventricle(s) are not decompressed with the initiation of support, inflow obstruction (into the VAD) must be considered.** A distended ventricle will not be unloaded and will not recover. Pulmonary edema may also develop as the blood backs up into the pulmonary vasculature. If appropriate inflow and outflow cannula placement and decompression of the LV are achieved, TEE should identify interventricular septal displacement toward the LV. This often compromises right heart function by impairing the septal component of RV contraction, and the physical distortion may also induce tricuspid regurgitation. **Right-sided function may be further compromised by increased** PVR caused by thromboxane A2 [10] and transfusion-induced cytokine activation [11] as a result of CPB.

2. Role of TEE. Use of TEE to separate from CPB is essential. TEE is used to assess the presence of air in the ventricle or ejecting from the LVAD into the ascending aorta. The
8 chamber that has been cannulated for the inflow of the MCSD should be decompressed. **If the chamber is full, and there is poor device flow, there is a technical issue that needs to be identified and corrected.** In the case of an LVAD, the LV should be decompressed; if it is full, there is a technical impingement of flow into the pump (typically faulty inflow or outflow). If the LV is empty and there is poor flow through the VAD, then there is either inadequate RV preload or right heart failure (which may be primary or secondary to high PVR). As the LV is decompressed and global cardiac output increases, there may be some tolerable physiologic right heart dilation, which may at times be difficult to distinguish from right heart failure. The apical interventricular septum can occasionally deflect leftward and obstruct inflow into the LVAD. When this occurs, it is easily identified by TEE. TEE is also used to identify aortic insufficiency and the presence of intracardiac shunts, either of which may arise at the time of VAD support even if absent before that time.

3. **Aortic insufficiency. Aortic valve insufficiency (AI) can be catastrophic, and TEE is essential to identify its presence or absence and severity.** Even mild preoperative AI can be problematic since patients in cardiogenic shock will have a low mean arterial pressure (MAP) and a high LV end-diastolic pressure (LVEDP) to produce a relatively low aortic transvalvular diastolic gradient. With implementation of LVAD support, the LVEDP will become very low and the MAP will be higher, so the aortic transvalvular gradient (MAP–LVEDP) will be much greater. Mild preoperative AI, therefore, can become severe AI with LVAD support. This induces high LVAD flows as the insufficient valve fills the LV and subsequently the VAD. The resulting high LVAD flow rates are deceptive, because much of the flow is "circular" from LV to LVAD to ascending aorta and back via the incompetent aortic valve to the LV, so the net forward "perfusion" flow will be low. The aortic valve incompetence must be eliminated in this situation, but the approach is controversial depending on the indications for device implant and expected duration of support (valve replacement versus permanent valve closure) [12–14].
4. **Intracardiac shunts: Quiescent intracardiac shunts may become clinically apparent and significant as a result of changes in chamber pressures when VAD support is initiated.** A PFO is present in up to 20% of the population, but is clinically quiescent in the vast majority of these patients. Upon unloading the LV and left atrium with LVAD support, right atrial pressure will become higher than left atrial pressure. Under these circumstances, even a small PFO can produce a large right-to-left shunt manifested by arterial desaturation and potential paradoxical air embolism. These shunts should be closed when identified and should be assessed by TEE both before and after initiation of VAD support. If identified preoperatively, cannulation techniques for CPB may be altered to facilitate repair.
5. **Pharmacologic support. Inotropic agents (e.g., dobutamine or epinephrine) are important to support the right heart when only left-sided support is used. Inhaled nitric oxide (20 to 40 ppm) may be invaluable in the early management of these patients because of its capacity to vasodilate the pulmonary vasculature without the systemic hypotensive effects seen with other pulmonary artery vasodilators.** Alternative approaches include the use of a phosphodiesterase inhibitor (e.g., milrinone, which decreases pulmonary and systemic vascular resistances) or nesiritide usually in combination with a systemic vasoconstrictor such as vasopressin. **Vasopressin offers an advantage over α-adrenergic agonists because it possesses minimal vasoconstrictive effects on the pulmonary arterial vasculature.**

   For a variety of reasons, systemic arterial vasodilation commonly occurs after initiation of LVAD support, so a need for a systemic vasoconstrictor is common. Experimental approaches to pulmonary vasodilation include inhaled nitroglycerin, inhaled prostacyclin, and sildenafil. Antiarrhythmics are often initiated before weaning from bypass onto device support as well.

D. Initiation of support for BIVAD

1. **Initial considerations.** When initiating biventricular support, **the left system should be actuated first.** Alternatively, both right and left systems may be actuated together. This prevents LV overdistention as well as pulmonary edema. Inotropic support can often be totally discontinued as the heart need not work. Biventricular support allows more complete resting of the heart and usually allows total decompression of the venous system as well. This minimizes hepatic and other end-organ congestion. The PA catheter should not be withdrawn as it will be difficult to reinsert it. Thermodilution cardiac outputs are not calculable when an RVAD is functioning.
2. **Flow rates.** The RVAD and LVAD should both have similar flow rates. The LVAD often has higher flow rates due to physiologic shunts (bronchial arterial return). RVAD flow that exceeds LVAD flow early after initiating BIVAD support is worrisome. This can occur with two common scenarios:
   a. One or both left-sided cannulae are malpositioned to impede inflow to or from the device. If the obstruction is not corrected, the lungs can become flooded with the increased blood flow from the RVAD.

b. The LV is beginning to recover and is ejecting some blood over and above the LVAD flow. This can be identified by the appearance of an arterial pressure waveform corresponding to the QRS complex of the ECG (see weaning from device support). Remember that pulsatile LVADs are not synchronized with the ECG. Initiating TAH differs in that both ventricles will beat immediately, so one can rapidly wean off of bypass onto TAH support.

E. Initiation of support for RVAD

1. **Initial considerations.** Isolated RVAD support is less common than LVAD or BIVAD support, but when used, the essential considerations are similar to LVAD (air elimination, adequate RV decompression) in some ways, and different in others.
2. **Pulmonary circulation.** If the RVAD is a pulsatile pump and RV preload is adequate, the pump will function adequately even if the PVR is very high. Even if flow is normal, excessive PA pressures may lead to pulmonary edema, so monitoring and control of PA pressures may be helpful. If the RVAD is a continuous-flow pump, however, excessively high PVR may limit flow.
3. **Pharmacologic support.** In most instances, some inotropic support of the LV will be necessary.

VII. Postoperative management and complications

A. Right-sided circulatory failure. Right-sided circulatory management is the key to perioperative care for MCSD patients. This is less important for a patient on a TAH or a BIVAD. However, as isolated LVAD is the most common use of this therapy, attention to right heart management and PVR is critical. Strategies include pacing (chronotropy), inotropes, and pulmonary vasodilators to increase flow through the pulmonary vascular bed. For additional considerations, see LVAD initiation.

B. Hemorrhage. Postoperative hemorrhage is common in this patient population. Cardiogenic shock often leads to hepatic congestion and renal insufficiency. Both of these processes lead to imbalances in platelet function and the coagulation cascade. The addition of CPB and the consumptive coagulopathy that can be initiated can exacerbate postoperative bleeding. In addition, exposing the blood to the foreign surfaces of the extracorporeal circuit and of the conduit cannulae can also lead to a consumptive coagulopathy. It should not be a surprise that postoperative hemorrhage and re-exploration for bleeding is a common occurrence. Warming the patient and replenishing platelets and factors of the coagulation cascade is often best accomplished in the ICU with the chest closed. Re-exploration for bleeding/tamponade can then be performed when the patient is adequately resuscitated. Use of a thromboelastogram (TEG) to help target the deficiency in the clotting process is gaining popularity. Transfused platelets and
9 red blood cells (packed cells or whole blood) in transplant candidates should ideally be leukoreduced, because exogenous leukocytes induce alloimmunization that can develop antibodies against future potential donated organs. High levels of these preformed antibodies reduce the pool of otherwise-suitable donor organs for these patients. Fresh frozen plasma and cryoprecipitate do not have high leukocyte content and do not need filtration.

C. Thromboembolism. Thromboembolism is associated with all current assist systems. The unique design characteristics of each system as well as the patient's underlying pathology establish the overall risk. Anticoagulation with warfarin is required with all assist devices except the Heartmate IP/XVE, which appears to have the lowest overall thromboembolic rate [15,16].

D. Infection. Device-related infection is the most common cause of morbidity in the chronically supported patient. Driveline and device "pocket" infections occur in up to 40% of these patients. The vast majority of these infections may be managed with chronic antibiotic therapy until transplantation. Infection of the blood-contacting surfaces of the device (valves or diaphragm) necessitates device change.

E. Device malfunction. Catastrophic device malfunctions occur infrequently but can be life-threatening. These include mechanical device failure, device separation or fracture, graft or valve rupture, and console failure. Minor device malfunctions occur more frequently and are usually addressed at the bedside. These include driveline cover tears and controller malfunctions. All of these malfunctions are becoming increasingly rare as yearly device modifications and software upgrades are introduced.

VIII. Weaning from VAD support

All the support systems (except the IABP) function independent of the cardiac cycle, and the arterial waveforms will not correspond to the patient's QRS complex. For patients in whom the heart recovers, the heart will be able to eject and the arterial waveform will begin to display pulses corresponding to the QRS complex. When the device flows are weaned downward and cardiac preload conditions move toward normal, these ejections will become more prominent. **If the device can be weaned to 1 L/min flow and the patient can maintain adequate perfusion with reasonable inotropic support, explantation can be considered.** This evaluation can be performed in the ICU. TEE can once again be very helpful in assessing cardiac function as the heart is loaded. **Final weaning from the device should be accomplished only in the operating room, as CPB is usually needed for device explantation.**

IX. Management of the VAD patient for noncardiac surgery

These patients can be very ill if surgery is contemplated early after MCSD implantation. However, patients will often recover physiologically over the ensuing weeks and months. Patients who are weeks to months on support may safely undergo noncardiac surgical procedures more routinely
10 [17]. The optimal approach involves asking some basic questions:

A. What chamber(s) are being assisted (LVAD, RVAD, BIVAD, or TAH)?

B. What type of pump is being used? Is it a pulsatile pump (generally afterload insensitive) or a continuous-flow pump (afterload sensitive)?

C. Is technical support personnel available to help troubleshoot the pump? This is critical for transport as well as intraoperative management.

D. **How does one determine flow through the pump?** This can be quantitative or qualitative, depending upon the pump, but knowledge of pump flow clearly assists in determining systemic vascular resistance and PVR, which in turn guide anesthetic drug selection, pharmacologic support, and volume management.

E. Will TEE be helpful? If major volume shifts are anticipated, use of TEE can be very helpful in assessing preload, valvular function, and intracardiac shunts.

F. What is the patient's clotting status? For most pumps, multidrug anticoagulation may be required, whereas the Heartmate XVE systems do not require any anticoagulation or anti-platelet agents. This has major implications for reversal of anticoagulation (if safely possible) and blood component use. Reversal of warfarin and conversion to intravenous heparin may be indicated. In general, be prepared for transfusion of RBCs and other components.

G. What is the patient's intravenous access? The more and the larger the intravenous cannulae, the better. Central venous access is desirable in most situations.

H. What pharmacologic support is the patient receiving? This will vary from no support to multiple inotropes, antiarrhythmics, vasoconstrictors, and pulmonary vasodilators. If nitric oxide is in use, this will require planning for transport and operating room use.

I. **Will electrocautery affect the assist device?** For most devices, this will not be a problem, but excessive electrocautery can intermittently interfere with the function of some pumps. If electrocautery poses a problem, either short (1 s) bursts may suffice or the use of an ultrasonic scalpel can be considered.

J. If defibrillation or electrical cardioversion is needed, how will it be most safely applied? In some cases, the pump may need to be separated from the driveline and operated manually during cardioversion, though most will tolerate DC cardioversion.

X. Future considerations

A. **Totally implantable LVAD.** The totally implantable LVAD will need to employ a replenishable source of power with an internal battery reserve. A transcutaneous energy transfer system (TETS) system has been employed in the AbioCor as well as the discontinued LionHeart (Arrow International, Inc., Reading, PA, USA). This has the potential advantage of improved infection risk, as it obviates the percutaneous driveline. Many of the current systems could adopt this technology.

B. **TAH.** Use of a TAH is gaining traction in the field of MCSD. There has historically been a psychosocial reluctance to pursue this technology as well as a perceived lack of need for this type of MCSD. The highly publicized struggle of the first TAH implant patient, Dr Barney

Clarke, accounts for some of the psychological impact, as does the thought of excising one's heart (often perceived as one's soul) to replace it with a manmade pump. In addition, many physicians believe that the use of BIVADs provides a good alternative to TAH. Nevertheless, the higher flow rates that can be achieved with a TAH offer an advantage over BIVADs in large patients or in those with multisystem organ dysfunction.

C. **"Platform" therapy. Many patients with end-stage congestive heart failure who are chronically supported by VADs will demonstrate some level of functional myocardial recovery. On rare occasions, recovery may be robust enough for removal of the device** [18–20]. This phenomenon is currently being studied, as it remains unclear in whom this phenomenon will occur. The use of long-term mechanical support as a therapy for de novo myocardial recovery is a very promising area of investigation. Therapies could be instituted to enhance myocardial recovery such as clenbuterol [21,22], cellular transplantation [23], myocardial exercise, or vascular regeneration.

XI. IABP circulatory assistance

A. **Indications for placement.** Thought by some to be reserved for placement after one or more failed attempts at separation from CPB, the number of IABPs placed in the cardiac catheterization laboratory approaches or exceeds the number placed intraoperatively. Interventional cardiologists often place IABPs when high-grade lesions of proximal coronary vessels
11 supplying large regions of myocardium are diagnosed, or when myocardial ischemia persists or MI occurs after an intervention such as coronary stent placement. Retrospective outcome studies for preoperative versus intraoperative placement of IABP for coronary artery bypass graft (CABG) patients suggest that preoperative IABP placement improves outcome and shortens hospital stay, especially for patients with low ejection fractions or those undergoing urgent or emergent CABG [24]. Indications for intraoperative IABP placement vary widely among centers and even among or within surgical teams. LV failure despite moderate-to-high-dose inotropic support and/or evidence of ongoing regional myocardial ischemia that is not amenable to surgical revascularization constitute the primary intraoperative indications. Moderately severe LV failure despite reasonable inotropic support that is thought to derive from an injury that will resolve (or greatly improve) within 24 to 48 hrs (e.g., LV stunning) constitutes the most common intraoperative indication. The definitions of "LV failure," "maximal inotropic support," and "ongoing regional myocardial ischemia" may vary widely among surgeons and anesthesiologists. Independent predictors of death among patients with intraoperative IABP insertion include New York Heart Association Class III or IV symptom level, mitral valve replacement or repair, prolonged CPB, urgent or emergent operation, emergent reinstitution of CPB, preoperative renal dysfunction, diabetes mellitus, RV failure, complex ventricular ectopy, pacer dependence, and IABP placement via the ascending aorta [24]. IABP assistance can be used during high-risk off-pump CABG as well, where the support of coronary perfusion pressure may be especially helpful while the heart is placed in positions that compromise cardiac filling or emptying. Rarely, prophylactic IABP placement may be appropriate for high-risk urgent noncardiac surgery. As an example, suppose a patient who has unstable angina pectoris and compromised LV function requires an urgent radical nephrectomy for cancer.

B. **Contraindications to placement**

1. **Aortic insufficiency.** Use of the IABP is relatively contraindicated in patients with AI. As the IABP inflates in the descending aorta during diastole to promote retrograde flow into the ascending aorta, this potentially increases aortic valvular regurgitation, further distending the LV at the expense of coronary perfusion.
2. **Sepsis.** As with any prosthetic intravascular device, bacteremic infections are difficult to treat if the prosthetic surfaces become seeded with bacteria.
3. **Severe vascular disease.** Placement of an IABP may be technically difficult in patients with atherosclerosis or other vascular pathologies. Such patients are more prone to arterial thrombosis during use of an IABP. Patients with abdominal aortic aneurysms are at increased risk for aortic rupture, although balloons have been successfully passed and used in such patients. For patients with severe aortoiliac or femoral arterial disease, another option is to place the balloon directly into the descending thoracic aorta. Alternatively,

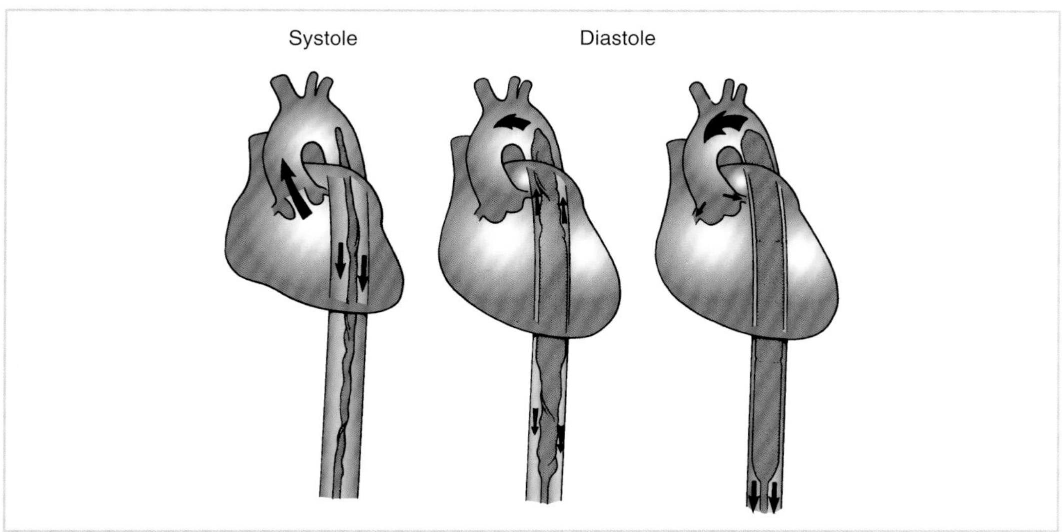

FIGURE 22.4 Placement of the IABP in the aorta. The IABP is shown in the descending aorta, with the tip at the distal aortic arch. During systole the balloon is deflated to enhance ventricular ejection. During diastole the balloon inflates, forcing blood from the proximal aorta into the coronary and peripheral vessels.

placement may be performed through a small vascular graft sewn to the subclavian artery. These options require a subsequent trip to the operating room to remove the device when such support becomes unnecessary.

C. **Functional design.** The IABP consists of an inflatable balloon at the end of a catheter that is typically advanced into the descending thoracic aorta percutaneously from the groin (Fig. 22.4). The balloon inflates during diastole, displacing blood from the thoracic aorta and increasing aortic diastolic pressure. Balloon inflation improves coronary perfusion pressure, increasing coronary blood flow to both the LV and the RV. During early systole, rapid balloon deflation reduces LV afterload and wall tension. IABP can improve myocardial energy balance at most by 15%. The IABP drive console consists of a pressurized gas reservoir that is connected to the balloon supply line through an electronically controlled solenoid valve. The gas used to inflate the balloon is either CO_2 or helium. The advantage of CO_2 is its high blood solubility, which reduces the consequences of balloon rupture with potential gas embolization. The advantage of helium is its low density, which thereby decreases the Reynolds number and allows the same flow through a smaller driveline. A tube with a smaller diameter decreases the potential for injury to the artery.

D. **IABP placement**

1. Insertion of the IABP is usually accomplished either percutaneously or by surgical cutdown into the femoral artery using the Seldinger technique for placement of a large-diameter introducer. Accurate placement of the Seldinger wire is often confirmed intraoperatively using TEE.
2. The balloon is passed through the introducer.
3. The balloon is ideally positioned so that its tip is at the junction of the descending aorta and the aortic arch, just distal to the origin of the subclavian artery, as shown in Figure 22.4. This positioning minimizes the risk of subclavian or renal artery injury or occlusion. Radiographically, the tip should lie between the anterior portion of the second intercostal space and the first lumbar vertebra.
4. When the IABP is placed intraoperatively, transesophageal echocardiography can confirm proper tip location before initiation of balloon assistance. Fluoroscopy, if available, can also facilitate positioning.

E. **IABP control.** Several parameters are important during the setup and operation of an IABP.

1. **Synchronization of the IABP.** Synchronization of the IABP with the cardiac rhythm is accomplished by using either the electrocardiographic QRS complex or the arterial 12 pressure waveform. If there is a natural pulse pressure greater than 40 mm Hg, use of the arterial waveform for synchronization is often preferred in the operating room because the electrical artifact produced by electrocautery inhibits ECG-triggered IABP control units. Recent monitoring systems have advanced suppression circuitry designed to reduce electrical noise from electrocautery. Most current consoles can differentiate pacer spikes from a QRS complex, allowing proper timing of IABP inflation even when atrial or atrioventricular pacing is in use, but pacer interference should be considered in the differential diagnosis of faulty IABP timing.
2. **Timing of balloon inflation and deflation.** When setting the timing of IABP inflation (Fig. 22.5), it is important to time the onset of the pressure rise caused by balloon inflation with the dicrotic notch of the arterial waveform, which signifies aortic valve closure and the start of diastole. If inflation begins sooner, the IABP will impede ventricular ejection. If it begins later, the effectiveness of the balloon in augmenting coronary perfusion and reducing afterload will be limited. Deflation should be timed so that the arterial pressure just reaches its minimum level at the onset of the next ventricular pulse. If it deflates too soon, the aorta will not be maximally evacuated before ventricular contraction, and coronary perfusion will not be optimized. If the balloon deflates too late, it will impede LV ejection. Most modern balloon devices use an intra-aortic arterial waveform obtained from the tip of the balloon catheter. If this mechanism should fail and synchronization should be monitored from another site, subtle differences in optimal timing may occur (e.g., balloon inflation and deflation as judged by a femoral arterial waveform are delayed in comparison to an intra-aortic or radial arterial waveform).
3. **Ratio of native ventricle pulsations to IABP pulsation.** Pumping is frequently initiated at a ratio of 1:2 (one IABP beat for every two cardiac beats), so the natural ventricular beats and augmented beats can be compared to determine IABP timing and efficacy. Depending on the patient's condition, the ratio will often be increased to 1:1 to obtain maximal benefit.
4. **Stroke volume of the balloon.** The volume of gas used to inflate the balloon is determined by the balloon used and the patient's size. Exceeding the volume for which the balloon was designed risks rupture with arterial gas embolization. Typically, balloon volume is set to 50% to 60% of the patient's ideal stroke volume [25].
5. **Balloon filling.** The time required for the balloon to fill and empty is determined by the density of the gas used, gas pressure, the length and diameter of the gas line, and balloon volume. These values are usually constant for any particular balloon. At high heart rates, the time required for balloon filling may limit balloon stroke volume.

F. **IABP weaning.** Weaning the patient from IABP circulatory assistance should be considered when inotropic support has been reduced substantially, allowing "room" to increase inotropic support as IABP support is reduced. Weaning is done primarily by gradually (over 6 to 12 hrs) decreasing the ratio of augmented to native heartbeats (from 1:1 to 1:2 to 1:4 or less) and/or decreasing balloon inflation volume while maintaining acceptable hemodynamics, which often necessitates a concomitant increase in inotropic support. The balloon is never turned off while it remains in the aorta except when the patient is anticoagulated, as during CPB, because of the risk of thrombus formation on the balloon or balloon catheter. Comparison of intra-arterial pressure tracings of augmented ventricular pulsations to native pulsations can serve as an indicator of ventricular performance. As ventricular performance improves, the amplitude of the native pressure tracing will increase relative to the augmented pressure tracing. By comparing the magnitude of these two pulses over time, one can obtain a qualitative assessment of ventricular performance. Once the IABP is removed, it is important to continue close examination of the distal ipsilateral leg because partial or total femoral arterial occlusion may occur.

G. **Management of anticoagulation during IABP assistance.** During extended IABP use, anticoagulation is generally indicated. In the immediate post-CPB period, anticoagulants may not be required for the first few hours or until drainage from the chest tubes is acceptable (less than

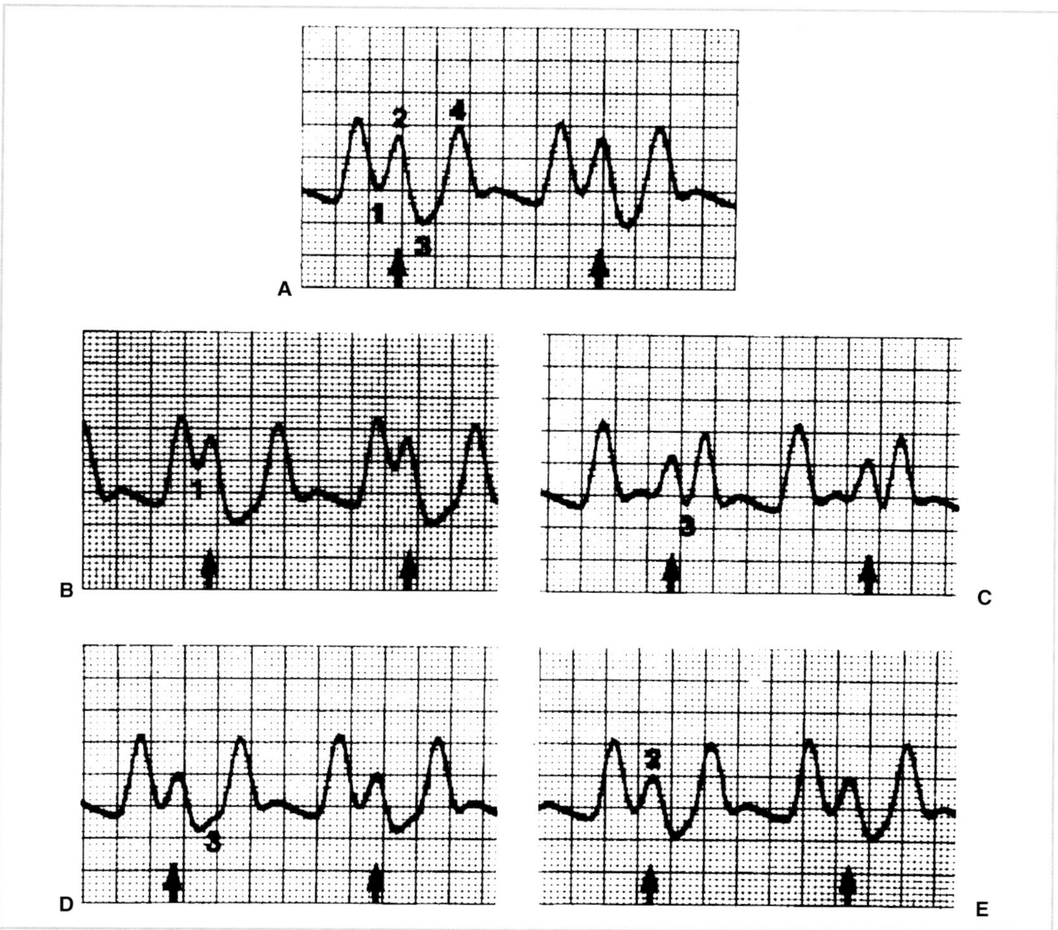

FIGURE 22.5 Manipulation of the timing of inflation and deflation of IABP. Tracings illustrate 1:2 support for the sake of clarity. **A:** Normal tracing. Augmentation commences after the dicrotic notch (*1*) augments diastolic pressure (*2*) and reaches its nadir just before the next contraction (*3*). Peak systolic pressure in the next (nonaugmented) beat is decreased (*4*). **B:** Early inflation. Augmentation commences before aortic valve closure (*1*), thereby increasing afterload and possibly inducing aortic regurgitation. **C:** Late inflation. Diastolic augmentation is inadequate, and end-diastolic pressure is not different from that in the unassisted cycle (*3*). **D:** Early deflation. Diastolic augmentation and afterload reduction are impaired. **E:** Inadequate filling time. Timing is satisfactory, but diastolic augmentation is impaired. (From Sladen RN. Management of the adult cardiac patient in the intensive care unit. In: Ream AK, Fogdall RP, eds. *Acute Cardiovascular Management in Anesthesia and Intensive Care.* Philadelphia, PA: Lippincott; 1982:509.)

100 to 150 mL/hr). Low-molecular-weight dextran is sometimes chosen to prevent thrombosis in patients with IABP because its antithrombotic effects are fairly mild, although no reversal agent exists. Heparin can prevent IABP-related thrombosis and its ready reversibility offers appeal, but many surgeons are understandably reluctant to initiate heparin therapy within the first 6 hrs after CPB. If heparin is used, adequate anticoagulation should be confirmed every 4 to 6 hrs with activated clotting time (ACT) or activated partial thromboplastin time (aPTT) maintained at 1.5 to 2 times normal values.

13

H. **Complications.** The incidence of IABP complications has decreased significantly from its early use, but significant morbidities persist. The most frequent complications are vascular in nature, with a reported incidence of 6% to 33% [24]. These complications include events such as limb ischemia, compartment syndrome, mesenteric infarction, aortic perforation, and aortic dissection. Risk factors for these complications include a history of peripheral vascular disease, female gender, tobacco smoking, diabetes mellitus, and postoperative IABP placement. Because of small femoral artery size and the likelihood of concurrent peripheral vascular disease, a common expression among cardiac surgeons is "Little old ladies and balloon pumps don't mix." Other complications include infection, primarily at the groin site of a transcutaneous introducer, and coagulopathies (especially thrombocytopenia). Neurologic complications include paresthesia, ischemic neuritis, neuralgia, footdrop, and rarely paraplegia [26]. Balloon rupture with gas embolus can occur presumably as a result of severe aortic atherosclerotic calcifications. When this occurs, blood is usually seen in the gas driveline and the arterial pressure deflection caused by the IABP is lost. Most pumps have an alarm that indicates low balloon pressure. Air embolism from the pressure monitoring line to the brain is a larger risk from the IABP than from a radial artery catheter, because the monitoring port is located at the tip of the balloon catheter, which is close to the origin of the carotid arteries. Arterial blood gases should be drawn through the IABP pressure monitoring line only if no other locations are available, paying meticulous attention to ensure that no air bubbles or other debris are flushed through the tubing.

I. **Limitations.** The ability of the IABP to augment cardiac output and unload the LV is limited, because the IABP does not directly affect LV function. With severe LV failure, an IABP will not provide sufficient flow to sustain the circulation. When the LV cannot eject blood into the aorta, the IABP will simply cause pulsations in the arterial waveform without increasing blood flow. In this situation, a VAD must be considered, although readily correctable technical problems with the IABP, such as malpositioning, kinking of the gas line, or improper inflation–deflation timing, should be considered. Early IABPs were not effective during rapid cardiac rhythms. Improvements in the pneumatic circuitry and compressor response time now permit some IABP models to provide hemodynamic improvement at rates up to 190 beats/min. Irregular heart rhythms persist as a limitation to IABP efficacy, because optimal timing of inflation and deflation cannot be achieved with large variations in the R–R interval.

REFERENCES

1. Ross JN Jr, Akers WW, O'Bannon W, et al. Problems encountered during the development and implantation of the Baylor-Rice orthotopic cardiac prosthesis. *Trans Am Soc Artif Intern Organs.* 1972;18:168–175.
2. ABIOMED Voluntary Data Registry for AB5000 as of April 2005.
3. Konstantinov BA, Dzemeshkevich SL, Rogov KA, et al. Extracorporeal mechanical pulsatile pump and its significance for myocardial function recovery and circulatory support. *Artif Organs.* 1991;15:363–368.
4. Miller LW, Pagani FD, Russell SD, et al. Use of a continuous flow device in patients awaiting heart transplantation. *N Engl J Med.* 2007;357:885–896.
5. Slaughter MS, Rogers JG, Milano CA, et al. Advanced heart failure treated with continuous flow left ventricular assist device. *N Engl J Med.* 2009;361:2241–2251.
6. Kirklin JK, Naftel DC, Kormos RL, et al. Second INTERMACS annual report: More than 1,000 primary left ventricular assist device implants. *J Heart Lung Transplant.* 2010;29:1–10.
7. Farrar D. Atrial versus ventricular cannulation for bridge to transplantation with the Thoratec VAD system. Presentation at Cardiovascular Technology and Science Meeting, Bethesda, MD. December 12, 1992.
8. Piacentino V III, Jones J, Fisher CA, et al. Off-pump technique for insertion of a HeartMate vented electric left ventricular assist device. *J Thorac Cardiovasc Surg.* 2004;127:262–264.
9. Crow S, Chen D, Milano CA, et al. Acquired von Willebrand syndrome in continuous flow ventricular assist device recipients. *Ann Thorac Surg.* 2010;90:1263–1269.
10. Cave AC, Manche A, Derias NW, et al. Thromboxane A2 mediates pulmonary hypertension after cardiopulmonary bypass in the rabbit. *J Thorac Cardiovasc Surg.* 1993;106:959–967.
11. Shenkar R, Coulson WF, Abraham E. Hemorrhage and resuscitation induce alterations in cytokine expression and the development of acute lung injury. *Am J Respir Cell Mol Biol.* 1994;10:290–297.
12. Bryant AS, Holman WL, Nanda NC, et al. Native aortic valve insufficiency in patients with left ventricular assist devices. *Ann Thorac Surg.* 2006;81:E6–E8.
13. Samuels LE, Thomas MP, Holmes EC, et al. Insufficiency of the native aortic valve and left ventricular assist system inflow valve after support with an implantable left ventricular assist system: Signs, symptoms, and concerns. *J Thorac Cardiovasc Surg.* 2001;122:380–381.
14. Savage EB, d'Amato TA, Magovern JA. Aortic valve patch closure: An alternative to replacement with HeartMate LVAS insertion. *Eur J Cardiothorac Surg.* 1999;16:359–361.
15. Slater JP, Rose EA, Levin HR, et al. Low thromboembolic risk without anticoagulation using advanced-design left ventricular assist devices. *Ann Thorac Surg.* 1996;62:1321–1327.

16. Schmid C, Weyand M, Nabavi DG, et al. Cerebral and systemic embolization during left ventricular support with the Novacor N100 device. *Ann Thorac Surg.* 1998;65:1703–1710.
17. Goldstein DJ, Mullis SL, Delphin ES, et al. Noncardiac surgery in long-term implantable left ventricular assist-device recipients. *Ann Surg.* 1995;222:203–207.
18. Mancini DM, Beniaminovitz A, Levin H, et al. Low incidence of myocardial recovery after left ventricular assist device implantation in patients with chronic heart failure. *Circulation.* 1998;98:2383–2389.
19. Helman DN, Maybaum SW, Morales DL, et al. Recurrent remodeling after ventricular assistance: Is long-term myocardial recovery attainable? *Ann Thorac Surg.* 2000;70:1255–1258.
20. Dandel M, Weng Y, Siniawski H, et al. Long-term results in patients with idiopathic dilated cardiomyopathy after weaning from left ventricular assist devices. *Circulation.* 2005;112:I37–I45.
21. George I, Xydas S, Mancini DM, et al. Effect of clenbuterol on cardiac and skeletal muscle function during left ventricular assist device support. *J Heart Lung Transplant.* 2006;25:1084–1090.
22. Birks EJ, Tansley PD, Hardy J, et al. Left ventricular assist device and drug therapy for the reversal of heart failure. *N Engl J Med.* 2006;355:1873–1884.
23. Dib N, Michler RE, Pagani FD, et al. Safety and feasibility of autologous myoblast transplantation in patients with ischemic cardiomyopathy: Four-year follow-up. *Circulation.* 2005;112:1748–1755.
24. Melhorn U, Kroner A, deVivie ER. 30 years of clinical intra-aortic balloon pumping: Facts and figures. *Thorac Cardiovasc Surg.* 1999;47:298–303.
25. Booker PD. Intra-aortic balloon pumping in young children. *Paediatr Anaesth.* 1997;7:501–507.
26. Hurle A, Llamas P, Meseguer J, et al. Paraplegia complicating intra-aortic balloon pumping. *Ann Thorac Surg.* 1997;63:1217–1218.

23 Intraoperative Myocardial Protection

John W.C. Entwistle, III, Percy Boateng, and Andrew S. Wechsler

KEY POINTS

1. Mechanisms of myocardial ischemic injury are multifactorial and include some of the following: Depletion of high-energy phosphates, intracellular acidosis, alterations in intracellular calcium homeostasis, complement activation, generation of oxygen-free radicals upon reperfusion, and myocardial edema.
2. **Myocardial stunning** represents viable myocardium that has systolic and/or diastolic dysfunction in the presence of normal myocardial perfusion.
3. **Hibernating myocardium** is viable myocardium that is chronically underperfused and subsequently has downregulated its contractile elements.
4. The ultimate measure of improved myocardial protection is improved survival or lessening of low-output syndrome (LOS). While LOS has declined in frequency over the decades, its prognosis has worsened with a high mortality associated with LOS.
5. The purpose of cardioplegia in addition to preservation of cardiac function is to provide cardiac quiescence and a bloodless operative field.
6. Diastolic arrest with potassium-rich solution and hypothermia are the mainstays of cardioplegic protection.

7. Although benefits to blood cardioplegia may include improved systolic functional recovery, decreased ischemic injury, and decreased myocardial anaerobic metabolism, it appears that there is no difference in operative mortality or long-term ventricular function when compared to crystalloid cardioplegia. However, most operative centers in the United States use blood cardioplegia.
8. Cardioplegia can be delivered anterograde through the aorta or coronary ostia or retrograde through the coronary sinus. There are advantages and disadvantages to each and both are often combined in the same procedure.

I. Introduction

Cardiac surgery is performed to preserve or restore cardiac function in a diseased heart. However, the performance of the procedure is, by necessity, accompanied by myocardial injury. This injury occurs when there is a significant imbalance between myocardial oxygen delivery and energy requirements. In the vast majority of cases, perioperative myocardial injury is minimal and is well tolerated. However, severe perioperative myocardial dysfunction is often lethal. Unlike the situation of a myocardial infarction, ischemia during cardiac surgery is usually planned, global in nature, and starts with the application of the aortic cross-clamp or some other intentional maneuver. The ischemic period may be continuous or intermittent, depending on the conduct of the operation.

Adequate myocardial protection can minimize the detrimental effects of the operation on the heart and can allow the heart to tolerate the prolonged periods of planned ischemia that are often necessary to conduct the operation. A proper strategy of myocardial protection encompasses events before, during, and after the initiation of planned myocardial ischemia, including treatment of the patient both preoperatively and postoperatively. As such, all medical personnel involved in the perioperative care of the cardiac patient should be cognizant of the implications of their actions toward myocardial preservation. A strategy of myocardial protection may be made infinitely complex, but most patients will be adequately served through the use of a limited number of techniques and agents designed to minimize the difference between oxygen delivery and utilization during ischemia. Beating heart surgery requires different strategies for myocardial protection, but they remain based on the balance between the supply and demand of oxygen. In addition, the use of minimally invasive techniques, such as port access, has increased the role of the anesthesiologist in the perioperative aspects of myocardial protection.

II. History of myocardial protection

A. Before the introduction of the cardiopulmonary bypass machine, the earliest cardiac procedures were performed without myocardial protection. Topical cooling and **systemic hypothermia** were used to facilitate the conduct of the operation with relatively little regard to the metabolic needs of the heart.

B. In 1955, Melrose advocated the use of hyperkalemic cardioplegia to provide cardiac quiescence during the operation. This approach was later abandoned because of the permanent myocardial injury (**"stone heart"**) produced by the high potassium concentrations used.

C. In 1956, Lillehei introduced the technique of administration of cardioplegia through the right atrium or coronary sinus (**"retrograde cardioplegia"**) for use in operations on the aortic valve.

D. Procedures used to provide myocardial standstill, such as intermittent aortic cross-clamping, were primarily performed to facilitate the conduct of the operation, with less regard to the ischemic consequences to the myocardium. Interest and research in chemical cardioplegia persisted but was not used clinically.

E. **Topical myocardial cooling** with iced saline or slush was used as an early form of myocardial protection once it was possible to support the circulation with cardiopulmonary bypass.

F. A correlation was made between poor myocardial protection and the development of **myocardial necrosis** in patients who succumbed to postoperative cardiogenic shock. Clinical confirmation was obtained when a high rate of perioperative myocardial infarction was demonstrated in patients undergoing either coronary artery bypass grafting (CABG) or valvular procedures.

G. In 1973, Gay and Ebert reintroduced **hyperkalemic cardiac arrest** but with potassium concentrations less than 20 mmol, thus preventing the occurrence of stone heart syndrome seen with the earlier use of potassium cardioplegia. This marked the beginning of the use of a technique that provided a combination of effective myocardial protection and cardiac quiescence.

H. In the late 1970s, Follette et al. [1] and Buckberg popularized the use of **blood cardioplegia**, citing the advantages gained by using the intrinsic characteristics of potassium-enriched blood, such as its natural buffers and oxygen delivery capabilities.

III. Cardiac physiology

A. The myocardium has a high rate of energy consumption under normal circumstances. This requires a constant supply of oxygen to the myocardium. **Myocardial ischemia** occurs when the supply of oxygen is exceeded by the demand, and infarction occurs when this occurs for a prolonged period of time.

B. **Oxygen delivery** to the myocardium is dependent upon the concentration of hemoglobin in the blood, the arterial oxygen saturation, and the flow of oxygenated blood to the myocardium. Under normal conditions, the blood flow to the myocardium is controlled by **autoregulation,** in which blood flow is matched to myocardial requirements. Autoregulation is not active when the blood pressure is above or below the autoregulatory range (roughly 60 to 180 mm Hg).

C. The **subendocardium** receives its nutritive flow primarily during diastole and is vulnerable to variations in blood flow.

1. Flow is dependent upon the transmural gradient, which is the difference between the aortic diastolic pressure and the intraventricular end-diastolic pressure.
2. Oxygen delivery may be insufficient because of either a decrease in perfusion pressure (systemic hypotension or coronary artery disease) or an increase in ventricular end-diastolic pressure (aortic stenosis, ventricular fibrillation, or ventricular distension).
3. The right ventricle may be less susceptible to injury since its subendocardium receives nutritive flow throughout the cardiac cycle as a consequence of RV systolic pressures well below systemic levels, with the exception of instances of severe pulmonary hypertension.

D. The heart depends upon a continuous supply of oxygen to maintain full function.

1. Adenosine triphosphate (ATP) is generated at a rate of 36 moles per mole of glucose in the presence of oxygen.
2. Under anaerobic conditions, ATP production falls to 2 moles of ATP per mole of glucose. Lactate and hydrogen accumulate in the tissues, which further inhibit glycolysis and other cellular functions.

E. Myocardial **oxygen consumption** is dependent upon the work performed by the heart (Fig. 23.1) [2,3].

1. Normal working ventricular myocardium consumes 8 mL of O_2 per 100 g of myocardium per minute.

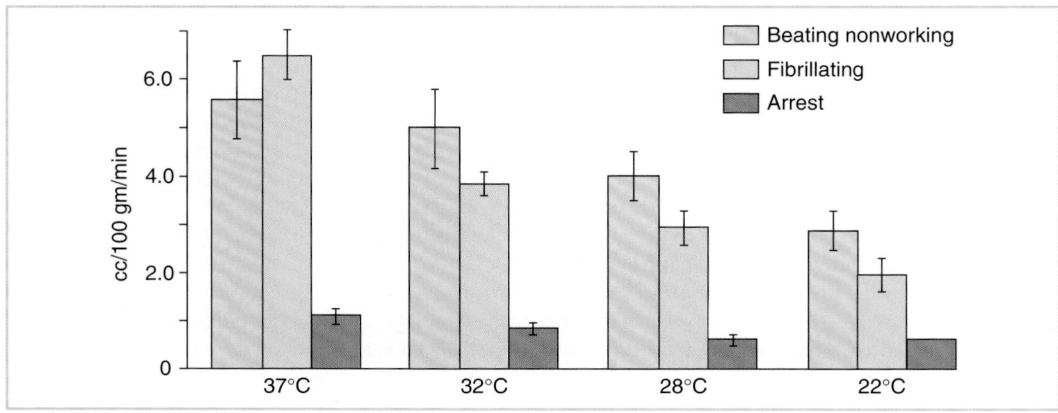

FIGURE 23.1 LV myocardial oxygen uptake of the beating empty, fibrillating, and arrested perfused hearts at varying myocardial temperatures. The greatest decrease in myocardial oxygen uptake at a given temperature occurs with mechanical arrest. The addition of hypothermia decreases the oxygen consumption to a lesser degree. (From Buckberg GD, Brazier JR, Nelson RL, et al. Studies of the effects of hypothermia on regional myocardial blood flow and metabolism during cardiopulmonary bypass. I. The adequately perfused beating, fibrillating, and arrested heart. *J Thorac Cardiovasc Surg.* 1977;73:87–94, with permission.)

2. This decreases to 5.6 mL of O_2 per 100 g of myocardium in the empty beating heart and to 1.1 mL of O_2 per 100 g of myocardium per minute in the potassium-arrested heart.
3. Myocardial cooling provides an additional decrease to 0.3 mL of O_2 per 100 g of myocardium.

IV. Mechanisms of myocardial ischemic injury. The mechanisms by which ischemia and reperfusion
1 injure the heart are complex, and the contributions of the individual components to this process are hotly debated. It is possible that the process of reperfusion may be equally as harmful to the myocardium as the ischemic insult itself. Thus, in the field of myocardial protection, it is important to have an understanding of the components thought to contribute to the damage. Strategies to ameliorate these factors may lessen the injury, whereas ignoring important aspects of ischemia–reperfusion injury may make all other protective interventions ineffective.

A. **Depletion of high-energy phosphates** occurs during ischemia. Breakdown products may be washed away with reperfusion, prohibiting the rapid conversion back to ATP once perfusion is restored.

B. **Intracellular acidosis** develops during anaerobic metabolism, and the accumulation of hydrogen ions interferes with the function of many intracellular enzymes.

C. Calcium is important in numerous cellular functions. The intracellular fluxes in calcium concentration are responsible, in part, for contraction and relaxation of the myocardium. Alterations in intracellular **calcium homeostasis** have been documented after ischemia and reperfusion. Changes in the rate of calcium uptake or release within the cell can have profound functional consequence and injured ischemic myocardium rapidly becomes calcium overloaded.

D. **Direct myocellular injury** from ischemia may cause myocardial dysfunction.

E. In addition to the alterations in calcium homeostasis that have been documented, intracellular **calcium overload** can occur at the time of reperfusion as calcium is released from the sarcoplasmic reticulum or enters the cell through calcium channels, such as the sodium–calcium exchanger or the L-type calcium channel. Alterations in intracellular calcium levels may activate enzymes, trigger second messenger cascades, or alter excitation–contraction coupling. Calcium concentrations may be so high that contracture develops. In the presence of ischemia, ATP necessary for extrusion of sodium is absent and cells become sodium loaded which leads to intracellular calcium loading through the sodium–calcium exchanger.

F. Generation of **oxygen-derived free radicals** occurs upon reperfusion. These are highly unstable compounds that are capable of damaging proteins, nucleic acids, phospholipids, and other cellular components. Natural free-radical scavengers prevent damage under normal circumstances, but these endogenous systems are depleted during a significant period of ischemia and are quickly overwhelmed.

G. **Complement activation** may occur as part of the generalized inflammatory process that occurs with injury.

H. Adverse **endothelial cell–leukocyte interactions** occur after ischemia and reperfusion. Under normal conditions, the endothelium and neutrophils are the producers of, and responsive to, numerous signaling compounds. There is a delicate balance between vasoconstriction and vasodilation, as well as between the promotion and prevention of thrombosis. Adenosine, nitric oxide, endothelin, and thromboxane are a few of the potent substances whose production and effects are altered after ischemia and reperfusion. This may produce a state of altered endothelial cell–leukocyte interaction, leading to areas of myocardial malperfusion and damage from increased endothelial adherence [4].

I. Myocellular **edema** may result from ischemia–reperfusion injury. Edema may occur in response to numerous injurious events and can alter the function of all of the cells within the myocardium. Edema has been implicated in contractile dysfunction, decreased ventricular compliance, and capillary plugging that inhibits reperfusion of the coronary microcirculation.

J. Damage to **non-myocyte components** of the heart may cause systolic and diastolic dysfunction. This includes injury to the endothelium of the coronary circulation, as well as to fibroblasts and other structural components of the heart.

V. Consequences of ischemia–reperfusion injury. The severity of myocardial injury after a period of ischemia and reperfusion depends on numerous factors, including the length of ischemia

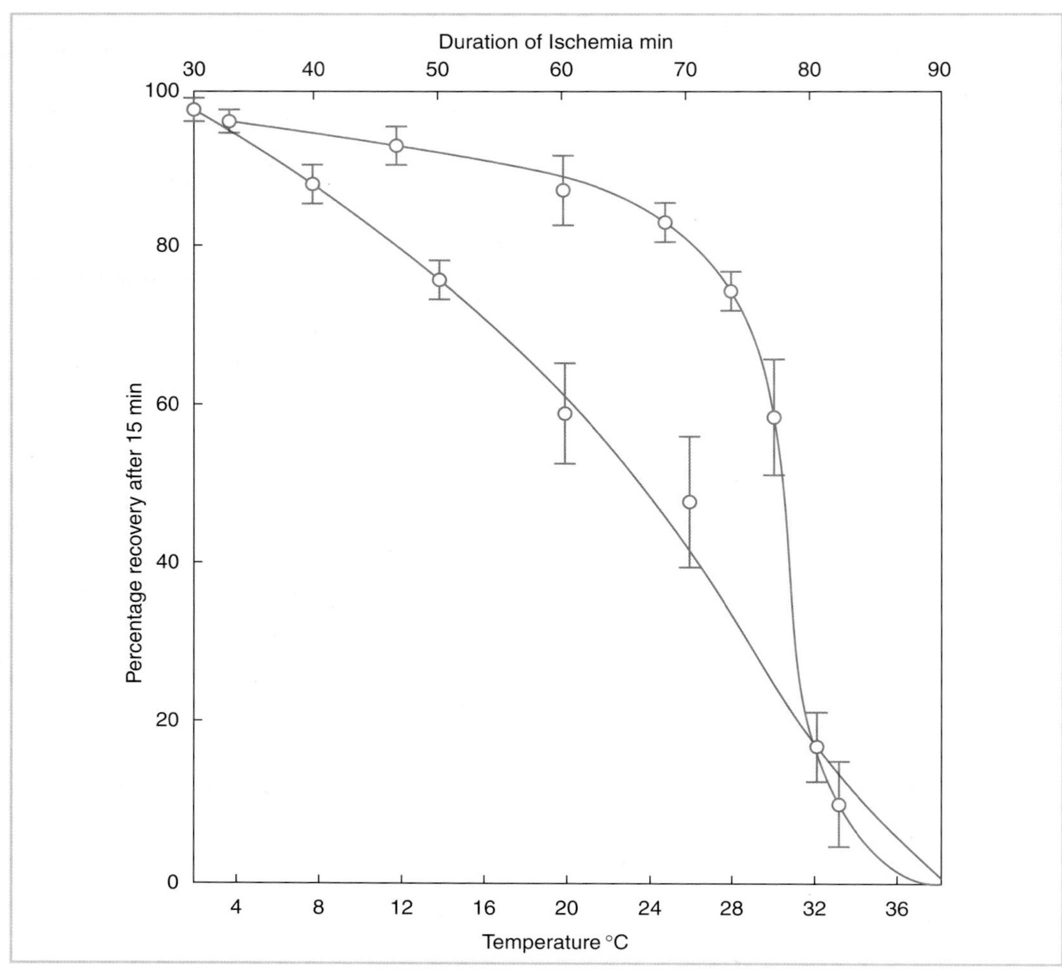

FIGURE 23.2 Relationship among myocardial temperature, duration of ischemia, and recovery of aortic blood flow. Two sets of experiments are shown. In the duration of ischemia studies (*top horizontal axis, blue line*), the heart was made ischemic for varying times at 30°C and then reperfused. The percentage myocardial recovery is shown on the *vertical axis,* and it declines steadily with time. In the temperature studies (*lower horizontal axis, red line*), hearts were subjected to 60 min of ischemia at varying myocardial temperatures and then reperfused. As the temperature of the myocardium is decreased below 28°C, myocardial recovery increases. (From Hearse DJ, Stewart DA, Braimbridge MV. Cellular protection during myocardial ischemia. The development and characterization of a procedure for the induction of reversible ischemic arrest. *Circulation.* 1976;54:193–202, with permission from Lippincott Williams & Wilkins.)

(Fig. 23.2) [5], the temperature of the myocardium, the conditions of the myocardium before, during, and after the ischemia, and the method in which the myocardium is reperfused. The resulting myocardial injury can be described according to the established criteria.

A. Brief periods of ischemia may produce no readily identifiable functional deficit.

2 B. **Myocardial stunning** represents ischemia–reperfusion injury in its mildest form. Although stunning may be severe, it represents **viable myocardium that has systolic and/or diastolic dysfunction in the presence of normal myocardial perfusion.** The etiology of the functional changes seen in stunning is multifactorial and likely includes altered calcium handling, cellular edema, and other factors. By definition, there is no necrosis in stunned myocardium. Given sufficient time, stunned myocardium will manifest complete functional recovery in the absence
3 of additional injury. Stunned myocardium is distinct from **hibernating myocardium, which**

is viable myocardium that is chronically underperfused and subsequently has down-regulated its contractile elements. Upon revascularization, hibernating myocardium begins to return to its normal phenotype and subsequently returns to normal function.

C. **Myocardial necrosis** occurs when myocytes are irreversibly injured. Necrosis may not be readily identifiable by functional or histologic means early after injury and thus may not be distinguishable from stunned myocardium at this early time point. However, these cells eventually die despite reperfusion and are replaced by a noncontractile scar.

VI. **Measuring success.** Myocardial protection in cardiac surgery has advanced a long way since the first cardiac operations were performed, and morbidity and mortality rates have dropped
4 significantly. The ultimate measure of improved myocardial protection is improved survival or a lessening in the occurrence of "low-output syndrome" (LOS). While the occurrence of LOS has declined in frequency over the decades, its prognosis has worsened with a higher mortality rate associated with LOS [6]. Since mortality and LOS are rather uncommon in elective cardiac cases today and the incremental benefit of a new protection strategy is likely to be small, randomized trials to demonstrate a benefit in terms of survival or LOS will have to be large. Due to this impracticality, many current trials use surrogate endpoints such as lowered levels of cardiac enzymes or shorter ICU stays. However, the clinical significance of these endpoints is less well defined. Importantly, many agents touted to improve myocardial protection have shown remarkable results in animal studies only to fail to achieve significance in humans. Thus, it is important to determine if a protective strategy has a clinically meaningful endpoint in humans, and to ensure that not too much weight is given to results from animal studies, regardless of the degree of benefit seen.

VII. **Purpose of cardioplegia.** Historically, most cardiac operations performed over the past few
5 decades have been done under conditions of cardiac arrest. Despite the availability of beating heart surgery techniques, cardiac arrest is still predominantly used during valve repair/replacement, cardiac transplantation, procedures on the aortic root, and most cases of cardiac revascularization. Cardioplegia serves separate, but often interrelated, purposes.

A. **Cardiac quiescence** facilitates most cardiac procedures as they are more easily performed on the flaccid, noncontracting heart than on the beating heart. Additionally, this lessens the possibility of air embolism occurring during open procedures performed on the left-sided chambers of the heart. Although cardiac standstill was originally produced via cooling of the heart, potassium-based cardioplegia can provide rapid and reversible arrest.

B. Interruption of myocardial blood flow facilitates the operation by providing a **bloodless field**, enhancing visibility. During most cardiac procedures, a cross-clamp is applied across the ascending aorta, which eliminates continuous coronary blood flow. Through the use of cardioplegia, the energy requirements of the myocardium can be significantly reduced, thus increasing the safety and allowable duration of this interruption of blood flow.

C. Through the reduction in myocardial energy consumption produced by electromechanical arrest, there is preservation of myocardial function, despite significant periods of myocardial ischemia.

D. Current methods of cardioplegic myocardial arrest allow for the rapid resumption of contractile activity at the end of the procedure. The period of contractile arrest can be lengthened by the administration of additional doses of cardioplegia, and it can be shortened by the restoration of myocardial blood flow with washout of the cardioplegia. This control allows the surgeon to minimize the time of cardiopulmonary bypass awaiting the return of cardiac function while providing maximal myocardial protection during the performance of the procedure.

VIII. **Interventions before the onset of ischemia (aortic cross-clamping).** Optimal myocardial protection requires a complete, well-conceived strategy that takes into consideration the unique characteristics of the individual patient. While it may be possible to treat every patient the same, a tailored approach is more likely to minimize cardiac damage and thus mortality. Aortic insufficiency, ventricular hypertrophy, and severe obstructive coronary disease are a few of the factors that may alter the intraoperative management in order to obtain maximal cardiac protection. As a part of planning ahead, there are several interventions before the onset of global cardiac ischemia (aortic cross-clamping) that influence the effectiveness of myocardial protection. Almost all aspects of myocardial protection involve maintaining balance between myocardial oxygen supply and demand.

A. **Minimization of ongoing ischemia** may require the use of nitrates, anticoagulants, antiplatelet agents, or insertion of an intra-aortic balloon pump in the preoperative period. Since there may be asymptomatic cardiac ischemia at baseline, hypertension, tachycardia, and patient anxiety should be controlled. Supplemental oxygen should be used liberally.

B. **Perioperative *β*-blockade** has been shown to decrease cardiac-related mortality in most patients undergoing surgical revascularization, although there may be a slight increase in mortality in those patients with an ejection fraction less than 30% who are treated with preoperative *β*-blockers. Unless contraindicated, preoperative *β*-blockers should be given in patients undergoing CABG surgery in the absence of severe depression of left ventricular (LV) function.

C. **Rapid revascularization.** Any sign of ischemia should warrant aggressive diagnosis and management. If ischemia cannot be readily controlled and infarction is imminent, then emergent operation to alleviate ischemia is required unless otherwise contraindicated. This requires the active involvement of all members of the surgical team so that the operation can proceed without delay. In this setting, rapid reversal of ischemia may require the use of saphenous vein grafts as opposed to arterial conduits if the harvesting of the internal mammary artery would unduly delay resolution of the ischemia. Similarly, the choice between on-pump and beating heart revascularization may depend upon the urgency of the operation and stability of the patient.

D. **Nutritional repletion** may be possible in the setting of elective cardiac surgery. The depleted heart has little reserve and may not tolerate ischemia well. Depressed glycogen levels have been correlated with poor postoperative outcomes, and repletion with the preoperative administration of **GIK solution** (glucose, insulin, potassium) [7] has been demonstrated to reduce complications and improve early postoperative cardiac function.

E. **Avoidance of ischemia.** Although some regional myocardial ischemia is required during any bypass operation, the intraoperative global cardiac ischemia that accompanies aortic cross-clamping may be avoided through one of several mechanisms.

1. CABG may be performed using beating heart techniques. This strategy allows continuous perfusion of the coronary vasculature, with the exception of the territory being bypassed while the anastomosis is being performed. With the use of an **intraluminal flow-through device (shunt)**, some blood flow can be maintained to the distal vessel during the creation of the anastomosis, except for brief periods of time. However, perfusion pressure must be maintained within the physiologic range to avoid cardiac and peripheral ischemia. Insertion of an intra-aortic balloon pump may be useful in this setting if hemodynamic instability results from cardiac manipulation.
2. Bypass grafting may be performed with minimal cardiac ischemia through the use of cardiopulmonary bypass without aortic cross-clamping. In the setting of the empty beating heart, perfusion to both the body and coronary arteries is supported by the bypass machine, eliminating the hemodynamic instability and subsequent hypoperfusion that may be associated with cardiac manipulation in some off-pump patients. Although this technique does not avoid the systemic effects of extracorporeal perfusion, it eliminates the effects of systemic hypothermia and avoids the myocardial effects of cardioplegia. By eliminating the work performed by the heart, myocardial energy requirements may drop by 20% to 30% of those in the working heart.
3. Intracardiac procedures may be performed without significant cardiac ischemia with the patient on bypass, without aortic cross-clamping. Although visibility may be limited, procedures such as tricuspid or mitral valve repair or replacement, or atrial or ventricular septal defect repair may be performed with continuous coronary perfusion. On procedures of the left heart, the heart is often briefly fibrillated while the chambers are opened. The LV must remain decompressed to avoid the ejection of air through the aortic valve and subsequent air embolization.

F. **Fibrillatory arrest** creates a nearly motionless heart to allow the performance of many cardiac procedures. It may be produced through either electrical stimulation or myocardial cooling.

1. **Normothermic fibrillatory arrest** is produced by placing an alternating current generator in contact with the ventricular myocardium. As long as contact is maintained, the ventricle will remain in fibrillation, allowing procedures to be performed upon the heart with little

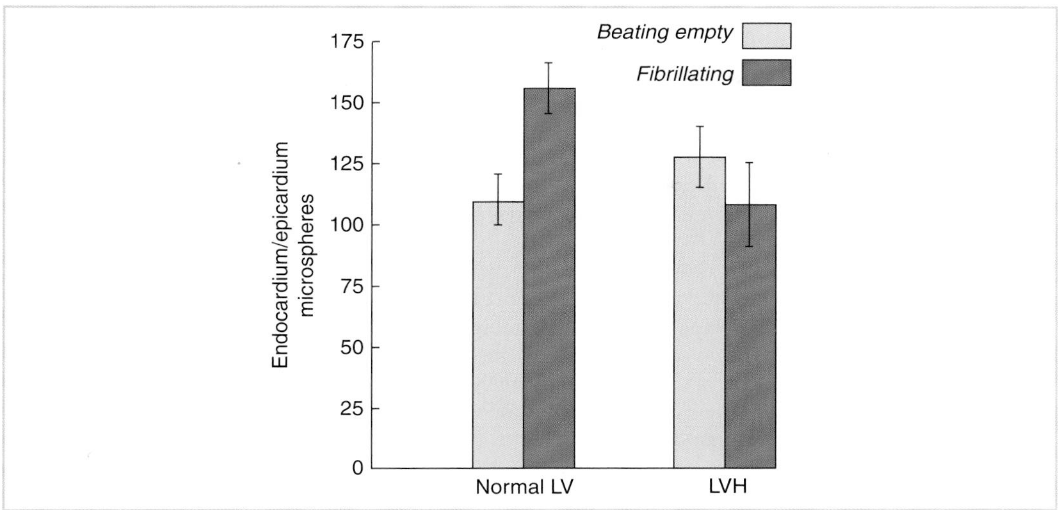

FIGURE 23.3 LV myocardial flow distribution in the normal and hypertrophied heart. In LV hypertrophy, endocardial blood flow is compromised during fibrillation, as the ratio of endocardial to epicardial flow decreases. This does not occur in the normal ventricle. (From Hottenrott CE, Towers B, Kurkji HJ, et al. The hazard of ventricular fibrillation in hypertrophied ventricles during cardiopulmonary bypass. *J Thorac Cardiovasc Surg.* 1973;66:742–753, with permission.)

ventricular motion. In this state, the left side of the heart can be opened to allow procedures such as closure of an atrial septal defect, without the fear of ejecting air into the arterial circulation.

   a. Since the myocardium remains warm and the heart is essentially in a continuous state of contraction, energy consumption remains high.

   b. The fibrillating myocardium has increased wall tension since it is in a state of continuous systole.

   c. Since perfusion to the endocardium occurs primarily during diastole, endocardial perfusion is compromised, thus allowing possible subendocardial infarction.

   d. Thus, it is impossible to produce a balance between oxygen supply and demand. Since myocardial ischemia is the inevitable result, this technique is not recommended.

2. **Hypothermic fibrillatory arrest** [8] occurs as the myocardial temperature falls when the body is cooled. Energy consumption of the myocardium is less than during warm ventricular fibrillation, but not as low as during complete arrest. Procedures such as CABG or mitral valve replacement may be performed without interruption of myocardial perfusion in the cold fibrillating heart. Fibrillation should be avoided in the setting of ventricular hypertrophy (Fig. 23.3) [9] or significant aortic insufficiency (see "Prevention of ventricular distention").

3. **Intermittent aortic cross-clamping** may be combined with hypothermic myocardial ventricular fibrillation (or brief periods of ischemic arrest) during performance of the distal anastomoses of a bypass operation to improve visibility while minimizing the time of myocardial ischemia. The aorta is unclamped between each distal anastomosis to reperfuse the myocardium intermittently.

G. Prevention of ventricular distention is important because increases in wall tension dramatically increase oxygen consumption while at the same time decreasing oxygen delivery to the subendocardium. Ventricular distention is more likely to occur in the setting of aortic valve insufficiency. This can be due to either native aortic valve disease or distortion of the valve during manipulation of the heart. This is particularly dangerous in the setting of ventricular hypertrophy or fibrillation where subendocardial perfusion is already jeopardized. Since the LV is out of sight during many portions of a cardiac procedure, distention can go unrecognized.

Intermittent palpation of the LV or monitoring of the pulmonary artery pressure for increases may alert the surgeon to a potential problem.

1. After the patient is on bypass and the heart is no longer ejecting blood into the aorta, a vent is inserted into the LV. This is usually performed through the right superior pulmonary vein.
2. The vent is actively drained into the cardiotomy reservoir of the cardiopulmonary bypass machine at a rate of 100 to 300 mL/min to keep the LV decompressed.

H. **Myocardial preconditioning** refers to the concept that myocardium that has undergone a brief limited period of ischemia may be better able to tolerate a subsequent, longer period of ischemia [10].

1. Experimentally, hearts exposed to a brief ischemic stimulus sustain a smaller area of necrosis following a second longer period of ischemia. Numerous stimuli may induce the preconditioning response, including ischemia, hyperthermia, or the use of drugs (bradykinin, nitric oxide, phenylephrine, endotoxin, and adenosine). Some experimental data have also implicated the role of inhalational anesthetic agents (sevoflurane, desflurane, and isoflurane) in myocardial protection through a preconditioning process, with potential improvements in mortality as well as troponin release [11]. Remote preconditioning is the process where brief ischemia to a remote area of the body (arm or leg through the use of a blood pressure cuff) may lead to cardiac protection [12].
2. Clinically, the effect of preconditioning is controversial. Adenosine has been demonstrated in one randomized trial to provide improved cardiac function in patients undergoing elective revascularization. However, it is more likely to be relevant in the absence of myocardial protection, making it potentially more applicable in the setting of beating heart surgery or when myocardial protection is suboptimal, as with severe ventricular hypertrophy or occlusive coronary artery disease.

I. The use of warm, oxygenated cardioplegic solution to induce myocardial arrest (**warm induction**) minimizes energy consumption by arresting the ventricle while it provides oxygen and substrates to the myocardium. Distribution of the cardioplegia to the subendocardium is maximized because the heart is arrested in diastole. This preischemic administration of cardioplegia has been shown to be beneficial in myocardial protection [13].

6 J. **Diastolic arrest** is the most common method of myocardial protection when aortic cross-clamping is used. Potassium-rich solutions are used to produce and maintain arrest until reperfusion. The electrical potential across the cellular membrane is determined by the concentrations of the ions on either side of the membrane at any given time. The resting potential across the cellular membrane is about −90 mV. During activation, the membrane depolarizes (becomes less negative), which allows the influx of sodium through voltage- and time-dependent sodium channels. Intracellular calcium concentrations rise, producing contraction. Relaxation occurs when calcium is sequestered into its intracellular sites. When cardioplegia is administered, with a potassium concentration of 8 to 10 mEq/L, depolarization occurs. Sodium influx occurs, and the channels close in a time-dependent manner. However, because the concentration of potassium remains elevated in the extracellular space, the membrane remains depolarized, and the sodium channels remain closed and inactivated. Thus, the cell is unexcitable in a state of diastolic arrest. As the cardioplegia washes out of the extracellular space, the cell will repolarize and become excitable again. This is one reason why cardioplegia may require multiple doses over the course of the procedure.

IX. Interventions during ischemia.

IX. Interventions during ischemia. The period of myocardial ischemia is when the myocardium is most vulnerable to injury. Numerous interventions are possible in order to minimize the injury, but not all are required in every circumstance. The overall strategy of myocardial protection must be individualized to the situation at hand.

A. Determination of the desired **myocardial temperature** is central to planning the protective strategy [14–16]. Although procedures can be performed on either the warm or hypothermic heart, the other components of the protective strategy must be chosen with the myocardial temperature in mind.

1. **Hypothermia** is useful because the myocardial oxygen consumption decreases by 50% for every 10°C decrease in myocardial temperature (**Q_{10} effect**). Thus, the greatest absolute decrease in myocardial energy consumption occurs as the myocardial temperature decreases

to 25°C, with relatively lesser gains with a progression to profound hypothermia. The major advantage of hypothermia is that it allows the interruption of myocardial blood flow for short periods of time, enabling the conduct of the operation to occur with minimal myocardial ischemic damage [2]. However, hypothermia itself is associated with injury to the myocardium, including alterations in cellular fluidity and transmembrane gradients, with the production of myocardial edema and a resultant decrease in ventricular performance. Intracellular pumps normally critical for ionic homeostasis are inhibited during hypothermia, thus favoring sodium and calcium loading of cells, which can have detrimental effects upon the myocardium. When desired, myocardial cooling can be produced through several mechanisms:

a. Myocardial cooling is most frequently produced through the **administration of cold cardioplegia**. Cardioplegia is usually given at a temperature of 4 to 10°C and will produce myocardial cooling to 15 to 16°C. Cardioplegia may be administered through either the antegrade route via the native coronary arteries or the retrograde route through a special cannula placed in the coronary sinus.

b. Profound systemic hypothermia as a method of routine myocardial protection is impractical, because it takes a long time to cool and rewarm the patient. However, myocardial cooling in the absence of systemic hypothermia can allow the unintentional rewarming of the myocardium through contact of the heart with the body and the return of warm blood to the heart through the cavae and noncoronary collaterals.

c. **Topical cooling** of the myocardium can be achieved through the use of chilled saline or slush, or through the use of a cooling jacket. Ice may produce uneven myocardial cooling. Slush may produce injury to the phrenic nerve through prolonged contact and increase atelectasis and pleural effusions. In addition, topical methods of cooling do not provide cooling to the deep myocardium and thus are better suited for cooling the less muscular and relatively thin RV than the LV. In the setting of LV hypertrophy, topical methods are clearly inadequate. Although data to support the use of topical cooling are sparse, it is still occasionally used as an adjunct to cooling with cardioplegia, especially with retrograde cardioplegia to improve cooling of the RV.

2. Warm cardioplegia may be used before the initiation of ischemia as warm induction (discussed previously). However, the entire operation may be conducted with **warm cardioplegia**. Since the myocardium is maintained at a warm temperature, metabolic activity continues, albeit at a lesser degree because mechanical activity of the heart is abolished. This constant oxygen requirement prohibits the use of significant periods of ischemia during the conduct of the operation [17,18].

a. Warm cardioplegia must be supplied continuously to avoid ischemic injury.

b. Its use is associated with less postoperative myocardial infarction and a lower incidence of low-output state.

c. It requires the use of blood cardioplegia because crystalloid-based cardioplegia cannot carry enough oxygen to meet the demands of warm myocardium.

d. Warm cardioplegia may not provide adequate protection in the presence of severe coronary artery disease, where uneven distribution may lead to poor protection.

3. **Tepid cardioplegia**, administered at 29°C, may provide some of the benefits of warm cardioplegia while minimizing the effects of hypothermia upon the myocardium.

B. The ideal **composition of cardioplegia** is hotly debated. Cardioplegia comes in two basic varieties, namely, crystalloid and blood. Blood cardioplegia is the most commonly used solution in adult cardiac surgery today, although the "recipe" varies significantly between surgeons. Cardioplegia can be made infinitely complex in nature by the use of additives and variations in administration. Most of these additives are chosen to combat the presumed causes of ischemia–reperfusion outlined in Section IV. The available evidence is controversial concerning the superiority of one cardioplegic regimen over the other, and any differences that exist
7 are likely to be small [19,20]. Although benefits to blood cardioplegia may include improved systolic functional recovery, decreased ischemic injury, and decreased myocardial anaerobic metabolism, it appears that there is no difference in operative mortality or long-term ventricular function when compared to crystalloid cardioplegia.

1. **Crystalloid cardioplegia** is uncommonly used in adult patients in the United States. A notable exception is in the preservation of the donor heart during cardiac transplantation.
   a. Crystalloid solutions do not contain hemoglobin and thus deliver dissolved oxygen only. This small amount of oxygen is adequate to sustain the myocardium at cold temperatures, but is insufficient in warm myocardium. Therefore, crystalloid cardioplegia can be used only with a strategy of myocardial hypothermia.
   b. All components may be rigorously controlled. However, each additive increases the complexity of the cardioplegia. In addition, most additives serve to replace substances already present in blood cardioplegia.
2. **Blood cardioplegia** is produced by mixing blood to crystalloid in a defined ratio (often 4 to 1), with a final hematocrit usually of 16 to 20 vol%.
   a. Blood contains hemoglobin and thus has a high oxygen-carrying capacity. However, at low temperatures, the oxygen–hemoglobin dissociation curve is shifted to the left, diminishing the amount of oxygen available to the myocardium. Due to the hemoglobin and the resultant increase in oxygen-carrying capacity compared to crystalloid solutions, blood cardioplegia may be administered either warm or cold. The frequency of administration varies with the temperature.
   b. Blood contains buffers, free-radical scavengers, colloids, and numerous other substances that may have important benefits in myocardial protection. Because of these components, fewer additives may be required with blood cardioplegia.
   c. Blood has increased viscosity compared to crystalloid, and this is compounded with the addition of hypothermia. However, blood cardioplegia produces good myocardial protection, suggesting that the concerns over viscosity and capillary sludging are overstated.
   d. The ideal hematocrit for blood cardioplegia is unknown, but it may depend on the temperature of the myocardium and the frequency of administration. **Microplegia** refers to the use of blood that is minimally diluted with crystalloid containing only the elements necessary for achieving cardiac arrest. Theoretically, the avoidance of hemodilution lessens myocardial edema and thus improves postoperative LV function. Clinical studies using microplegia have been small, and have shown a possible advantage over standard 4:1 diluted blood cardioplegia [21].

C. **Route of cardioplegia delivery.** Cardioplegia may be administered in either an antegrade or a retrograde direction.
1. **Antegrade cardioplegia** is delivered to the myocardium through the coronary arteries.
   a. Usually, it is delivered through a cannula placed into the aortic root, after the aortic cross-clamp is applied. Flow is often started at a rate of 150 mL/(min · m^2) and adjusted to maintain an optimal aortic root pressure. Rapid infusion leads to uneven distribution and poor protection. A typical initial dose is 10 to 15 mL/kg, up to 1,000 mL. A low perfusion pressure results in uneven distribution of cardioplegia, and high perfusion pressure may cause damage to the endothelium. **Perfusion pressure is typically between 70 and 100 mm Hg.**
   b. Antegrade cardioplegia through the aortic root cannot be used in the presence of significant aortic valve insufficiency. First, it is difficult to obtain adequate aortic root pressure when the aortic valve is incompetent. Second, cardioplegia enters the LV, causing increased intraventricular pressure and wall tension and impeding delivery of the cardioplegia to the subendocardium. Finally, a significant portion of the cardioplegia fails to perfuse the coronary arteries, further leading to inadequate protection. In this setting, antegrade cardioplegia may be administered directly down the left and right coronary arteries by using special cannulae that are placed into the coronary ostia after the aortic root is opened.
   c. In the presence of severe occlusive coronary artery disease, especially in the absence of collateral vessels, uneven distribution of cardioplegia may occur through the antegrade route. Topical cooling with iced saline or slush may improve cooling in this setting. Supplemental cardioplegia administered retrograde may also augment the myocardial protection in this setting (see "Retrograde delivery").

   d. During CABG, additional doses of cardioplegia can be given down each graft as it is completed. Not only does this allow the surgeon to check the flow of the graft, but it allows cardioplegia to be given distal to a flow-limiting lesion where the initial dose of cardioplegia may not have been adequate.

2. **Retrograde delivery** of cardioplegia may be used as either an adjunct to antegrade delivery or as the primary route of myocardial protection [22]. Cardioplegia is administered to the myocardium through the coronary veins by way of the coronary sinus.
   a. A special cannula is directed into the coronary sinus through a small hole in the right atrium. **Cardioplegia is delivered at a pressure of less than 40 mm Hg.** Higher pressures may cause damage.
   b. Improper placement of the catheter can cause injury to the coronary sinus.
   c. Since the coronary veins draining the RV enter the coronary sinus near the right atrium, or enter the right atrium directly, retrograde cardioplegia may not adequately protect the RV because the tip of the cardioplegia catheter is positioned further into the coronary sinus.
   d. Retrograde delivery has been associated with a larger leak of cardiac enzymes in the postoperative period, but there have not been associated clinical consequences of this leak.
   e. The primary advantage of retrograde cardioplegia is in the performance of valvular procedures. In aortic valve replacement, multiple doses of cardioplegia can be administered without stopping the procedure and cannulating the coronary ostia individually. In mitral procedures, retraction on the heart limits the effective distribution of antegrade cardioplegia, so repeat doses require release of the retractors. However, in retrograde cardioplegia, multiple doses can be given without changing the retractors, thus simplifying the procedure.
   f. During all arterial grafting with in situ (internal mammary and gastroepiploic) arteries, additional doses of cardioplegia can be administered through the retrograde route to achieve protection in areas supplied by diseased coronaries because cardioplegia cannot be given down the completed grafts.
   g. During acute coronary artery occlusion, where collateral vessels have not developed, retrograde cardioplegia may provide some protection to the ischemic myocardium before the bypass can be completed.

3. **Antegrade and retrograde cardioplegia are often used together**, in a variety of different combinations. Studies have demonstrated that the combined use provides better myocardial protection than with either method alone (Fig. 23.4) [23], particularly in the presence of left main coronary artery disease.
   a. Antegrade cardioplegia can be used to arrest the myocardium, with additional doses given retrograde with venting of the aortic root. This maximizes the distribution of cardioplegia.
   b. Antegrade and retrograde cardioplegia can be administered throughout the procedure in either an alternating or a simultaneous manner [24]. With the alternating technique, retrograde cardioplegia is administered frequently and interrupted for antegrade cardioplegia down each completed graft or through the aortic root. With the simultaneous method, retrograde cardioplegia is continued while antegrade cardioplegia is given down each graft, minimizing the time spent administering cardioplegia. Venovenous collaterals prevent venous hypertension in the coronary sinus. Clinical outcomes are similar between the two methods.

4. The **frequency of cardioplegia administration** is determined by several factors, most importantly the temperature of the myocardium.
   a. Warm myocardium requires a constant supply of oxygen and thus constant administration of cardioplegia. The cardioplegia may be interrupted for brief periods to allow improved visualization. Significant hemodilution is possible when cardioplegia with a high crystalloid content is used continuously because of the high volume of cardioplegia required. In addition, large doses of potassium are required to maintain electromechanical quiescence in the warm perfused myocardium.

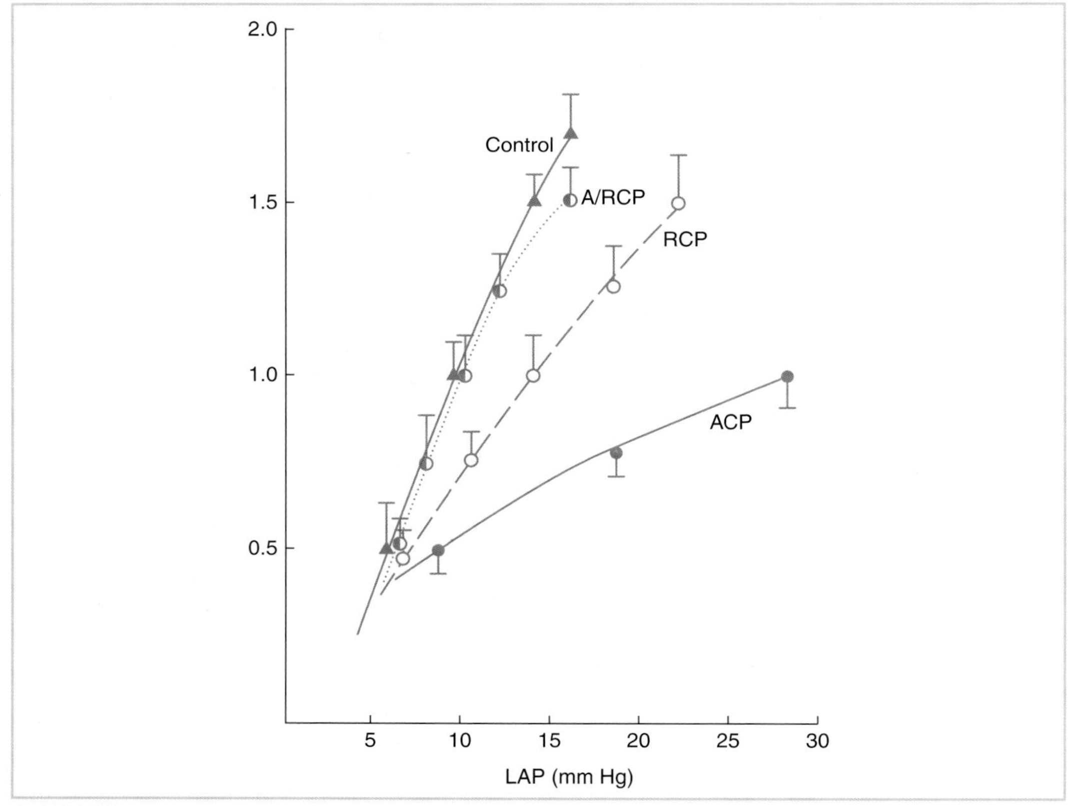

FIGURE 23.4 Global recovery of left ventricular stroke work index (LVSWI) 30 min after discontinuation of extracorporeal circulation. As left atrial pressure (LAP) increases, LVSWI increases in control hearts. Hearts protected with antegrade perfusion only (ACP, ●) recover less function compared to hearts protected with retrograde perfusion (RCP, ○). Hearts with combined antegrade and retrograde perfusion (A/RCP,◐) exhibit recovery of LVSWI similar to control values (▲) in this model. (From Partington MT, Acar C, Buckberg GD, et al. Studies of retrograde cardioplegia. II. Advantages of antegrade/retrograde cardioplegia to optimize distribution in jeopardized myocardium. *J Thorac Cardiovasc Surg.* 1989;97:613–622, with permission.)

b. With cold myocardium, visualization can be maximized with intermittent administration of cardioplegia. Each administration is essentially a period of reperfusion, so the initial pressure of cardioplegia should be controlled as it is during reperfusion.

c. Single-dose cardioplegia can be used with cold myocardium if the duration of the operation will be limited and if there is no significant coronary artery disease to limit the distribution of cardioplegia.

d. Multidose regimens are preferable in most circumstances. The initial dose produces cardiac arrest. Subsequent doses, through the aortic root, down a completed graft, or retrograde, serve to wash out metabolic byproducts and replenish substrates. These advantages may not hold in the immature myocardium. In addition, multidose regimens will help to maintain myocardial hypothermia, especially when the operation is being performed with mild or no systemic hypothermia. Some surgeons monitor the myocardial temperature with a probe and re-dose the cardioplegia with a rise in temperature, but more commonly cardioplegia is re-dosed at time intervals or with the return of electrical or mechanical myocardial activity.

D. The list of **potential additives to cardioplegia** is tremendous, and a comprehensive listing and discussion would be overwhelming. Table 23.1 gives a partial list of common additives. The vast majority of additives available serve to combat one or more of the putative causes of ischemia–

TABLE 23.1 Common additives to cardioplegia

Component	Purpose
KCl	Produce/maintain diastolic arrest
THAM/histidine	Buffer
Mannitol	Osmolarity, free-radical scavenger
Aspartate/glutamate	Metabolic substrate
$MgCl_2$	Mitigates against effects of calcium
CPD	Lowers free calcium concentration
Glucose	Metabolic substrate
Blood	Oxygen-carrying capacity

CPD, citrate–phosphate–dextrose; THAM, tromethamine.

reperfusion injury. In addition, most additives have functions similar to substances already found in the blood. The cardioplegic solution must balance the goals of simplicity, cost, and effectiveness.

1. The **electrolyte composition** of cardioplegia is important for producing and maintaining rapid myocardial arrest and limiting myocardial edema.
   a. **"Intracellular" cardioplegia** has an electrolyte composition that mimics that of the intracellular space. **It produces myocardial arrest by eliminating the sodium gradient across the cellular membrane and thereby eliminating phase 0 of the action potential**.
      (1) Intracellular solutions are crystalloid. Bretschneider solution is a popular example.
      (2) The osmolar gap produced by the low sodium concentration allows the use of several additives without producing a hyperosmolar solution.
      (3) In North America, these solutions are primarily used today for organ preservation in cardiac transplantation. However, intracellular solutions are more popular for use routinely in Europe than in the North America.
   b. **"Extracellular" solutions** have an electrolyte concentration similar to serum with a higher level of potassium. **Diastolic arrest is produced by depolarization of the cellular membrane by high potassium concentrations.**
      (1) Potassium concentrations of 8 to 30 mM are used to produce arrest. Cardioplegia administration must continue until there is electrical silence, because persistent electrical activity utilizes ATP stores. Especially when hypothermia is used, subsequent doses of cardioplegia can use lower concentrations of potassium as long as electrical arrest persists.
      (2) Other methods of producing cardiac arrest include the use of magnesium or local anesthetics. However, due to the simplicity of potassium-induced arrest, these methods are not commonly used.
   c. **Calcium** is critical to cardiac function. However, high calcium concentrations are detrimental to the myocardium. Limiting the calcium in the cardioplegia helps to maintain arrest.
      (1) Calcium-free cardioplegia produces arrest due to lack of calcium influx across the plasma membrane. However, this may lead to the **"calcium paradox"** in which calcium is depleted from the cell. Upon reperfusion, calcium re-enters the cell and can cause severe damage. Therefore, solutions devoid of calcium are not used.
      (2) Instead of limiting calcium concentration, the effects of calcium can be limited with nifedipine or diltiazem, which are calcium-channel blockers. These drugs may improve myocardial metabolism, but the negative inotropic properties limit their clinical use.
   d. The addition of **magnesium** to cardioplegia may counter the effects of calcium by competing with calcium for entry via calcium channels, eliminating the need to reduce calcium levels in blood cardioplegia [25]. The benefits of magnesium addition depend on the relative concentrations of the two ions, and there is no benefit to the addition of magnesium to calcium-free cardioplegia.

2. The **pH** of the myocardium is critical to the function of the heart. During ischemia, there is a fall in intracellular pH as lactate accumulates within the cell. Buffers in the cardioplegia are important to limit the change in pH associated with the period of ischemia.
   a. Blood contains many naturally occurring buffers, including the **histidine** and **imidazole groups** on proteins.
   b. Buffers commonly added to cardioplegia include tromethamine (THAM), Tris, and histidine. These can buffer large amounts of hydrogen ion and have a pK_a in the vicinity of 7.4, which makes them good choices. The addition of buffers is probably more important when using crystalloid cardioplegia than with blood.
   c. The method used to monitor pH during hypothermia is important because of the normal rise in pH associated with a fall in temperature.
      (1) With the **α-stat protocol**, the pH of the blood sample is corrected to 37°C to provide a pH value that is independent of patient temperature.
      (2) Under the **pH-stat** protocol, the pH value is measured at the temperature of the patient and is corrected to 7.4 by the addition of CO_2 into the perfusion circuit. Although this protocol may lead to improved cerebral protection, it results in impaired ventricular function compared to the other method.
3. The **osmolality** of cardioplegia is important in limiting the myocardial edema, which may be detrimental to ventricular recovery. Since blood is iso-osmolar, additives serve to make it hyperosmolar with respect to unmodified blood, unless the blood is diluted with hypotonic crystalloid. With crystalloid cardioplegia, on the other hand, the final solution may range from hypotonic to hypertonic, depending on the type and amount of additives used. Mannitol, glucose, and albumin are commonly used to increase the osmolality of the cardioplegia. Mannitol has been shown to lessen myocellular edema and improve postoperative ventricular function when used to produce a mildly hypertonic solution.
4. **Glutamate and aspartate** are intermediates in the Krebs cycle and serve to restore high-energy phosphate levels. The addition of these amino acids has been demonstrated to be beneficial in preserving myocardial function, both experimentally and clinically, although the benefit may be limited to substrate-depleted myocardium [26].
5. The addition of insulin to warm blood cardioplegia has been shown to provide superior protection in patients undergoing revascularization for unstable angina or with ventricular hypertrophy, although such a benefit was not demonstrated in the general population. This effect may be separate from the improved results seen in cardiac surgery patients who have serum glucose tightly controlled.

E. **Intermittent aortic cross-clamping** is used by some surgeons during revascularization procedures with good results [27]. In this technique, a cross-clamp is applied and the heart fibrillates or arrests during the performance of a distal anastomosis. The clamp is removed to restore perfusion, and is reapplied for each distal anastomosis. To be successful, each ischemic interval needs to be short to minimize irreversible damage. Potential problems associated with this technique include the necessity to perform each anastomosis quickly to minimize the length of each ischemic interval, and the risk of embolism of aortic debris with each application and removal of the cross-clamp.

X. Interventions during reperfusion

The period of reperfusion is critical to preserving myocardial function. Several potential mechanisms of ischemia–reperfusion injury are active in the reperfusion period, and any chance of minimizing these sources of injury requires action at, or slightly before, the time of reperfusion. If the conditions of reperfusion are not optimized, then potentially viable myocardium may be irreversibly injured. There are many components of the reperfusion period that are important in determining the amount of myocardium that is salvaged.

A. **Substrate washout and terminal warm blood cardioplegia.** The final dose of cardioplegia can be used to improve cardiac function after reperfusion through one of two mechanisms:
   1. **Substrate washout:** In cold myocardium, continued arrest can often be maintained even with removal of potassium from the cardioplegia, allowing washout of metabolic byproducts without continued exposure of the myocardium to a high potassium solution. Since the

heart is cold, there is no efficient replenishment of substrates within the myocardium. As the heart rewarms, function returns slowly. If the heart fibrillates, prompt electrical cardioversion minimizes the period of increased wall tension.

2. **Terminal warm blood cardioplegia:** Warm hyperkalemic blood cardioplegia administered at the end of the procedure is termed a **"hot shot"** or terminal warm blood cardioplegia [28,29]. This allows the maintenance of electromechanical arrest with replenishment of metabolic substrates. It has been shown to preserve intracellular ATP and amino acid levels and to produce improved metabolic recovery.

B. **Controlled reperfusion.** The pressure of reperfusion is important in limiting the damage to the myocardium [30]. The endothelium is injured during ischemia, and its vasoregulatory properties are limited. This damage can be worsened through unregulated reperfusion.
   1. **After cross-clamp removal, the perfusion pressure should be limited to 40 mm Hg for the first 1 to 2 min of reperfusion by decreasing pump flows. The pressure during this period should not be increased abruptly with phenylephrine, or other agents, until after 1 or 2 min.**
   2. Pump flows are increased to maintain a mean pressure of 70 mm Hg subsequently. Pressors may be required to achieve this. Hypertension should be avoided.

C. **Postconditioning.** Brief periods of reperfusion interrupted by brief periods of reocclusion reduce many of the consequences of ischemic injury such as infarct size through a process termed postconditioning, although there is no convincing evidence that this is useful in clinical cardiac operations.

D. **Avoiding ventricular distention.** The contractile state of the ventricle is critical to recovery, particularly in the early postischemic period. Ventricular distention is detrimental to the myocardium, especially during this period.
   1. The ventricle should remain empty during the early period of reperfusion, while contractile function is recovering. This can occur by maintaining full bypass with right heart decompression or rapidly introducing a vent into the left ventricle if this is not sufficient.
   2. In the presence of aortic insufficiency, not severe enough to require valve replacement, venting of the LV through a vent placed via the superior pulmonary vein can maintain decompression.
   3. Ventricular fibrillation is likewise harmful in the warm myocardium, especially as the ventricle begins to fill with blood. Rapid electrical **cardioversion** is required to prevent the rapid depletion of substrates. Prophylactic lidocaine is given near the completion of bypass to lessen the frequency of arrhythmia.

E. **Deairing of the heart** is important to prevent the embolization of air, either down the coronary arteries or into the cerebral or peripheral vessels. The right coronary artery is particularly vulnerable due to its anterior location on the aortic root. Air down this coronary can lead to malperfusion in its distribution and subsequent RV dysfunction in the early postoperative period. Techniques for removal can include the following:
   1. Placement of a vent through the right superior pulmonary vein into the LV, particularly in the case of mitral valve procedures
   2. Venting of the aortic root with a small cannula placed to suction controlled by the perfusionist
   3. Aspiration of the LV by piercing the apex of the heart with an intravenous catheter
   4. Restoring some blood flow through the heart. The perfusionist fills the right atrium with blood by temporarily impeding venous return, then the anesthesiologist fills the lungs with air. This produces increased blood flow through the pulmonary vasculature and into the left side of the heart to displace air that can then be removed with a vent.

      Adequacy of air removal from the left cardiac chambers can be assessed with the use of intraoperative transesophageal echocardiography. It is important that air removal from the left chambers precede the onset of LV ejection, to minimize the incidence of air embolization.
   5. The deleterious consequences of air embolism may be mitigated by flooding the operative field with carbon dioxide during open heart portions of the procedure, thereby displacing nitrogen-rich gas with highly soluble CO_2 which dissolves rapidly in the event of an embolic occurrence.

F. **Oxygen-derived free radicals** are normally produced in living cells, but the rate of production increases significantly at the moment of reperfusion. At the same time, the natural defense mechanisms are weakened.

1. To be effective, scavengers must be present and active at the initial moment of reperfusion.
2. Since each dose of cardioplegia in a multidose protocol is a period of reperfusion, scavengers may be important in the cardioplegia.
3. Free-radical injury involves a cascade of radicals. Different scavengers are active at different points along the cascade. The physical properties of scavengers dictate their distribution within the myocardium, potentially limiting access to areas of free-radical production. Therefore, the optimal use of free-radical scavengers likely involves the use of several agents with activity at different points along the cascade.
4. Blood cardioplegia contains many natural free-radical scavengers. Addition of extra scavengers may not be critical [31].

G. **Calcium management.** Intracellular hypercalcemia at the time of reperfusion can have detrimental effects. Although calcium is necessary at the time of reperfusion, the calcium concentration in the initial reperfusate may be effectively decreased with citrate or calcium-channel blockers (diltiazem).

XI. Special circumstances

A. **Beating heart surgery.** The popularity of beating heart surgery appears to have plateaued, with approximately 20% of surgical revascularization procedures performed in the United States using these techniques. However, the rate of beating heart revascularization varies among surgeons between 0% and nearly 100%. The anesthetic management in beating heart surgery is discussed elsewhere in this text. There are a few caveats of myocardial protection that deserve mention.

1. Coronary perfusion pressure must remain adequate, especially because there are already flow-limiting lesions in the vessels. Similarly, hypertension increases the afterload and ventricular wall tension, decreasing subendocardial perfusion. Options to maintain perfusion pressure include volume loading, altering the position of the table to increase venous return, the judicious use of pressors, the use of an intra-aortic balloon pump, and appropriate positioning of the heart to provide a balance between visualization of the target vessels and cardiac function.
2. The order in which bypasses are performed is often critical. If required, the internal mammary artery to the left anterior descending artery is often a good choice for the first bypass, because an open graft can provide perfusion and stability to the myocardium during manipulation of the heart for subsequent bypasses.
3. Proximal anastomoses may be performed early, such that flow may be delivered down each graft after the distal is completed.
4. The use of flow-through shunts may permit adequate perfusion of the distal vessel while the anastomosis is completed. However, a shunt does not guarantee adequate myocardial perfusion, and injury or instability may still occur.
5. Bypasses to totally occluded vessels are often well tolerated by the heart because occlusion during the anastomosis does not usually cause additional significant ischemia. This is especially true when collateral vessels are well established.
6. Off-pump surgery probably represents a hypercoagulable state compared to its on-pump counterpart. The coagulopathy from extracorporeal circulation and the establishment of hypothermia are avoided. Many surgeons do not fully reverse the heparinization with protamine, instead aiming for an activated clotting time (ACT) of approximately 180 s at the conclusion of the procedure. In addition, many surgeons use antiplatelet agents, such as clopidogrel (Plavix), to inhibit graft thrombosis in the early postoperative period, although data regarding this are lacking.

B. **Redo operations** often present unique challenges to myocardial preservation.

1. Patent bypass grafts are a potential source of atheroemboli and subsequent myocardial infarction. The rate of postoperative infarction is higher in redo operations than for primary grafting procedures. Avoidance of graft manipulation can minimize the embolization of loose debris.

2. Dense adhesions from the prior operation may limit the safe dissection required to perform the standard maneuvers required for myocardial protection. Therefore, the risk of obtaining exposure to permit topical cooling of the RV, placement of an LV vent, or temporary occlusion of a patent internal mammary graft may outweigh the potential benefits of these maneuvers. Therefore, the surgeon must be well versed in alternative exposures or methods of myocardial protection.
   a. For a patent internal mammary artery that cannot be safely occluded, hypothermic fibrillatory arrest may represent the best alternative.
   b. A right thoracotomy approach to the mitral valve provides excellent exposure, especially in a reoperation. Dissection of the aorta through the right chest is possible for placement of a cross-clamp, but many procedures can be done with femoral cannulation and a beating or fibrillating heart on bypass.

C. **Port-access surgery.** Popularized by Heartport, Inc. (now a Johnson and Johnson subsidiary), port-access surgery allows common cardiac procedures to be performed through smaller incisions. The operative procedure should be similar to that for standard cardiac surgery, but the limited exposure requires alternative methods of cardioplegia administration, ventricular venting, and aortic occlusion. The technology provides the surgeon with the ability to use the limited exposure, but the entire operative team must embrace the technology for it to be successful. Transesophageal echocardiography is important for the preparation and conduct of the operation. Myocardial protection requires vigilance of the surgeon, anesthesiologist, and perfusionist. Since very little of the heart is exposed, the monitors play an increased role in the assessment of the electromechanical state of the heart and provide vital information with regard to the pressures within the unseen cardiac chambers.

D. **Acutely ischemic myocardium** requires that energy demands on the myocardium be diminished as soon as possible and that delivery of oxygen to the ischemic territory is prompt.
   1. The patient should be prepared for surgery promptly. Delays should be minimized to those necessary for patient safety. The patient should be well oxygenated, and perfusion pressure is critical. A preoperative intra-aortic balloon pump may be useful.
   2. Once on bypass, normothermic induction of cardioplegia can provide substrate to the stressed myocardium that is still perfused.
   3. Retrograde cardioplegia is often used in this situation to provide cardioplegia to the territory that is served by the occluded vessel.
   4. The acutely ischemic area should be revascularized first, with cardioplegia administered down the graft to the occluded vessel. There may be advantages to warm reperfusion to this segment of myocardium, and perfusion can be continued at a controlled pressure while other grafts are placed.
   5. Special attention is directed to the period of time at which cardiopulmonary bypass is terminated, as the ischemic myocardium is likely to exhibit contractile dysfunction. It may be necessary to place the patient back on bypass temporarily to adjust inotropes or volume status and to give the myocardium additional time to recover contractile function before permanent separation from bypass is possible. Improper weaning may result in myocardial infarction in regions that are potentially recoverable.

E. **Pediatric heart.** The pediatric heart is unique in its physiology and thus requires special attention. Some of the differences are due to the disease states seen in the pediatric population, whereas others are inherent differences in the immature myocardium. Many of these are due to differences in myocardial gene expression seen in the fetal and neonatal heart, and result in differences in myocardial metabolism and energy consumption compared to the adult heart. For a complete discussion of the management of the pediatric myocardium, see the review by Allen et al. [32].
   1. The normal immature myocardium is more resistant to ischemic injury than adult myocardium. However, cyanosis, pressure overload, or volume overload, which are all common in hearts with congenital defects, make these hearts more susceptible to ischemic injury.
   2. In contrast to the cardiac surgery in the adult heart, crystalloid cardioplegia is frequently used in pediatric cardiac surgery. Although most studies have not demonstrated a

difference in outcome, blood cardioplegia may be beneficial in the neonatal heart that has been subjected to hypoxic stress.

3. The immature myocardium is more susceptible to damage from high calcium concentrations due to its diminished capacity for calcium sequestration. Calcium levels may be reduced with citrate. In addition, magnesium supplementation of the cardioplegia provides increased protection from transient increases in intracellular calcium concentration.
4. The hypoxic immature heart is sensitive to the delivery pressure of cardioplegia. This must be controlled to both provide adequate distribution yet prevent myocardial edema and damage from high-pressure delivery.

XII. Conclusion

This chapter has covered many of the facets of contemporary myocardial preservation during heart operations. However, effective myocardial preservation should not be thought of as a "technique" but rather a **strategy** that utilizes an array of techniques best suited for an individual patient. Moreover, the operating team must be ready at any moment to pursue alternate strategies and tactics when previously unanticipated intraoperative events occur. It is important to remember that myocardial protection begins **before** the patient enters the operating room, and does not end until after the operation is over.

REFERENCES

1. Follette DM, Mulder DG, Maloney JV, et al. Advantages of blood cardioplegia over continuous coronary perfusion or intermittent ischemia. Experimental and clinical study. *J Thorac Cardiovasc Surg.* 1978;76:604–619.
2. Buckberg GD, Brazier JR, Nelson RL, et al. Studies of the effects of hypothermia on regional myocardial blood flow and metabolism during cardiopulmonary bypass. I. The adequately perfused beating, fibrillating, and arrested heart. *J Thorac Cardiovasc Surg.* 1977;73:87–94.
3. Sink JD, Hill RC, Attarian DE, et al. Myocardial blood flow and oxygen consumption in the empty-beating, fibrillating, and potassium-arrested hypertrophied canine heart. *Ann Thorac Surg.* 1983;35:372–379.
4. Nakanishi K, Zhao Z-Q, Vinten-Johansen J, et al. Coronary artery endothelial dysfunction after ischemia, blood cardioplegia, and reperfusion. *Ann Thorac Surg.* 1994;58:191–199.
5. Hearse DJ, Stewart DA, Braimbridge MV. Cellular protection during myocardial ischemia. The development and characterization of a procedure for the induction of reversible ischemic arrest. *Circulation.* 1976;54:193–202.
6. Algarni KD, Maganti M, Yau TM. Predictors of low cardiac output syndrome after isolated coronary artery bypass surgery: Trends over 20 years. *Ann Thorac Surg.* 2011; 92(5):1678–1684. doi:10.1016/j.athoracsur.2011.06.017
7. Quinn DW, Pagano D, Bonser RS, et al. Improved myocardial protection during coronary artery surgery with glucose-insulin-potassium: A randomized controlled trial. *J Thorac Cardiovasc Surg.* 2006;131:34–42.
8. Akins CW, Carroll DL. Event-free survival following nonemergency myocardial revascularization during hypothermic fibrillatory arrest. *Ann Thorac Surg.* 1987;43:628–633.
9. Hottenrott CE, Towers B, Kurkji HJ, et al. The hazard of ventricular fibrillation in hypertrophied ventricles during cardiopulmonary bypass. *J Thorac Cardiovasc Surg.* 1973;66:742–753.
10. Perrault LP, Menasche P. Preconditioning: Can nature's shield be raised against surgical ischemic-reperfusion injury? *Ann Thorac Surg.* 1999;68:1988–1994.
11. Landoni G, Bignami E, Oliviero F, et al. Halogenated anaesthetics and cardiac protection in cardiac and non-cardiac anaesthesia. *Ann Card Anaesth.* 2009;12:4–9.
12. Yong SC, Shim JK, Kim JC, et al. Effect of remote ischemic preconditioning on renal dysfunction after complex valvular heart surgery: A randomized controlled trial. *J Thorac Cardiovasc Surg.* 2011;142:148–154.
13. Rosenkranz ER, Vinten-Johansen J, Buckberg GD, et al. Benefits of normothermic induction of blood cardioplegia in energy-depleted hearts with maintenance of arrest by multidose cold blood cardioplegic infusions. *J Thorac Cardiovasc Surg.* 1982; 84:667–677.
14. Bufkin BL, Mellitt RJ, Gott JP, et al. Aerobic blood cardioplegia for revascularization of acute infarct: Effects of delivery temperature. *Ann Thorac Surg.* 1994;58:953–960.
15. Hayashida N, Ikonomidis JS, Weisel RD, et al. The optimal cardioplegic temperature. *Ann Thorac Surg.* 1994;58:961–971.
16. Yau TM, Weisel RD, Mickle DAG, et al. Optimal delivery of blood cardioplegia. *Circulation.* 1991;84(suppl III):III-380–III-388.
17. Naylor CD, Lichtenstein SV, Fremes SE, et al. Randomised trial of normothermic versus hypothermic coronary bypass surgery. *Lancet.* 1994;343:559–563.
18. Yau TM, Ikonomidis JS, Weisel RD, et al. Ventricular function after normothermic versus hypothermic cardioplegia. *J Thorac Cardiovasc Surg.* 1993;105:833–843.
19. Fremes SE, Christakis GT, Weisel RD, et al. A clinical trial of blood and crystalloid cardioplegia. *J Thorac Cardiovasc Surg.* 1984;88:726–741.
20. Jacob S, Kallikourdis A, Sellke F, et al. Is blood cardioplegia superior to crystalloid cardioplegia? *Interact Cardiovasc Thorac Surg.* 2008;7:491–498.
21. Hayashi Y, Ohtani M, Sawa Y, et al. Minimally-diluted blood cardioplegia supplemented with potassium and magnesium for combination of 'initial, continuous and intermittent bolus' administration. *Circ J.* 2004;68:467–472.

22. Schaper J, Walter P, Scheld H, et al. The effects of retrograde perfusion of cardioplegic solution in cardiac operations. *J Thorac Cardiovasc Surg.* 1985;90:882–887.
23. Partington MT, Acar C, Buckberg GD, et al. Studies of retrograde cardioplegia. II. Advantages of antegrade/retrograde cardioplegia to optimize distribution in jeopardized myocardium. *J Thorac Cardiovasc Surg.* 1989;97:613–622.
24. Shirai T, Rao V, Weisel RD, et al. Antegrade and retrograde cardioplegia: Alternate or simultaneous? *J Thorac Cardiovasc Surg.* 1996;112:787–796.
25. Hearse DJ, Stewart DA, Braimbridge MV. Myocardial protection during ischemic cardiac arrest. The importance of magnesium in cardioplegic infusates. *J Thorac Cardiovasc Surg.* 1978;75:877–885.
26. Rosenkranz ER, Okamoto F, Buckberg GD, et al. Safety of prolonged aortic clamping with blood cardioplegia. III. Aspartate enrichment of glutamate-blood cardioplegia in energy-depleted hearts after ischemic and reperfusion injury. *J Thorac Cardiovasc Surg.* 1986;91:428–435.
27. Korbmacher B, Simic O, Schulte HD, et al. Intermittent aortic cross-clamping for coronary artery bypass grafting: A review of a safe, fast, simple, and successful technique. *J Cardiovasc Surg (Torino).* 2004;45:535–543.
28. Caputo M, Dihmis WC, Bryan AJ, et al. Warm blood hyperkalemic reperfusion ("hot shot") prevents myocardial substrate derangement in patients undergoing coronary artery bypass surgery. *Eur J Cardiothorac Surg.* 1998;13:559–564.
29. Teoh KH, Christakis GT, Weisel RD, et al. Accelerated myocardial metabolic recovery with terminal warm cardioplegia. *J Thorac Cardiovasc Surg.* 1986;91:888–895.
30. Okamoto F, Allen BS, Buckberg GD, et al. Studies of controlled reperfusion after ischemia. XIV. Reperfusion conditions: Importance of ensuring gentle versus sudden reperfusion during relief of coronary occlusion. *J Thorac Cardiovasc Surg.* 1986; 92:613–620.
31. Julia PL, Buckberg GD, Acar C, et al. Studies of controlled reperfusion after ischemia. XXI. Reperfusate composition: Superiority of blood cardioplegia over crystalloid cardioplegia in limiting reperfusion damage—Importance of endogenous oxygen free radical scavengers in red blood cells. *J Thorac Cardiovasc Surg.* 1991;101:303–313.
32. Allen BS, Barth MJ, Ilbawi MN. Pediatric myocardial protection: An overview. *Semin Thorac Cardiovasc Surg.* 2001;13:56–72.

24 Protection of the Brain during Cardiac Surgery

John M. Murkin

KEY POINTS

1. The incidence of overt stroke is 2% to 6% for closed-chamber cardiac procedures. For open-chamber procedures, the incidence of stroke is increased to 4.2% to 13%.
2. Risk factors for early stroke have been found to be advanced age, duration of cardiopulmonary bypass (CPB), high postoperative creatinine, and extensive aortic atherosclerosis, while delayed stroke was associated with female gender, postoperative atrial fibrillation, cerebrovascular disease and requirement for inotropic support.
3. Within the first postoperative week, up to 83% of all patients undergoing bypass surgery using CPB demonstrate a degree of cognitive dysfunction. Efforts to mitigate against early postoperative cognitive dysfunction are warranted since early postoperative cognitive issues are in part reflective of subclinical brain injury.

4. Watershed lesions are commonly due to profound hypotensive episodes but may also be the result of cerebral embolism. Embolization and hypotension acting together may magnify CNS injury.
5. The etiology of CNS damage associated with embolization is from multiple sources that are patient related, procedure related, and equipment related.
6. Leukocytosis is associated with a higher risk for ischemic stroke. The results strongly implicate inflammation and white cell activation as etiologic factors in both the extent and severity of perioperative cerebral events.
7. α-Stat blood gas management, which maintains a normal transmembrane pH gradient and maintains cerebral autoregulation of blood flow, should be used in adult patients undergoing bypass. This modality may help prevent cerebral embolization. See Table 24.7 for additional evidence-based practice guidelines.
8. A wide variety of autoregulation thresholds occurs even with α-stat blood gas management and is likely a consequence of increased age and cerebrovascular disease. There is an emerging consensus during normothermic and tepid bypass to maintain MAP greater than 70 mm Hg. See Table 24.8 for other management strategies to decrease CNS brain injury.

I. Central nervous system (CNS) dysfunction associated with cardiac surgery

A. Overview. Despite the continuing improvements in surgical and cardiopulmonary bypass (CPB) techniques during cardiac surgery, stroke remains a devastating postoperative complication for patients and their families. In a recent study in which 1,800 patients with three-vessel or left mainstem coronary artery disease were randomized to percutaneous intervention (PCI) or conventional coronary artery bypass (CAB) surgery, there was no difference in mortality at 1 yr but a significantly lower incidence of primary composite endpoint of major adverse cardiac or cerebrovascular event in CAB (12.4%) versus PCI (17.8%) patients [1]. However, while the overall outcome should argue strongly in favor of CAB surgery, the stroke rate was significantly higher in CAB (2.2%) than PCI (0.6%) patients. Given the relatively equivalent risk factors between PCI and CAB patients in this study, the mechanism of perioperative stroke must be better understood if we are to further reduce the risk of CNS morbidity related to cardiac surgery. This chapter will review the current incidence and risk factors for brain damage in cardiac surgery and will outline strategies aimed at protection of the brain during cardiac surgical procedures.

B. Stroke incidence. In most series reported to date, the incidence of clinically apparent neurologic
1 injury or overt stroke is 2% to 6% for closed-chamber cardiac procedures (e.g., CAB surgery). Up to 25% to 65% of strokes after CAB surgeries are bilateral or multiple, suggestive of an embolic etiology [2]. For open-chamber procedures (e.g., valve surgery), the reported incidence varies from 4.2% to 13%, which could be related to increased risk of embolization, increased hemodynamic instability, or prolonged CPB time. However, more subtle neurologic changes, such as development of primitive reflexes (e.g., snouting, palmomental reflex), visual field defects, and subtle motor-sensory abnormalities, can be demonstrated in the early postoperative period in up to 61% of all patients undergoing CPB. By 2 mos postoperatively, the prevalence of such new subtle neurologic dysfunction decreases to about 20% and persists for at least 1 yr [3].

C. Early versus delayed stroke. In considering the incidence of perioperative stroke, it is apparent that distinguishing stroke as early (i.e., neurologic deficit apparent on emergence from anesthesia) or delayed (i.e., neurologic deficit developing after awakening from anesthesia) is important to better discriminate etiology and assess potential risk-reduction strategies, as it is apparent that only approximately 50% of perioperative strokes present during the first 24 hrs postsurgery [3], and tend to be more severe with a higher permanent deficit and a higher impact on mortality [3–5]. The higher mortality could be related to sicker patients, or that stroke is just one manifestation of other concomitant embolic/hypoperfusion-mediated complications. Stroke can also have a long-term effect on mortality (Fig. 24.1). In a prospective study on CAB patients, the adjusted survival rates at 1, 5, and 10 yrs were 94.1%, 83.3%, and 61.9% among patients free from stroke versus 83%, 58.7%, and 26.9% for those suffering perioperative stroke [6]. Risk factors for
2 early stroke have been found to be advanced age, duration of CPB, high preoperative creatinine,

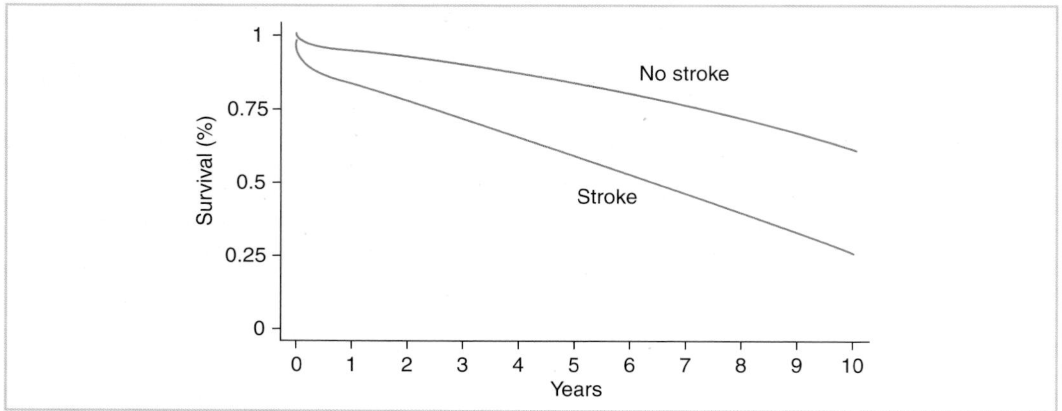

FIGURE 24.1 Effect of stroke on 10-yr survival after CAB graft. The crude annual incidence of death was 18.1/100 person-years among patients with strokes and 3.7/100 person-years among patients without strokes (p <0.001). (From Dacey LJ, Likosky DS, Leavitt BJ, et al. Perioperative stroke and long-term survival after coronary bypass graft surgery. *Ann Thorac Surg.* 2005;79:532–536, with permission.)

and extensive aortic atherosclerosis, while delayed stroke was associated with female gender, postoperative atrial fibrillation, cerebrovascular disease, and requirements for inotropic support [5]. **Delayed but not early stroke was associated with long-term mortality.**

D. Cognitive dysfunction. It has been demonstrated that within the first postoperative week, up to 83% of all patients undergoing CAB surgery using CPB demonstrate a degree of cognitive dysfunction. Of these patients, 38% have symptoms of intellectual impairment and 10% are considered to be overtly disabled. Concentration, retention, and processing of new information and visuospatial organization are the most frequently affected domains. At 5-yr follow-up, more than 35% of CAB patients exhibit some degree of neuropsychologic dysfunction [7]. Variable definitions, different measurement techniques, and different intervals of post-operative cognitive testing confound this issue, however, giving rise to reported incidences of perioperative cognitive decline that vary from 4% to 90%. Additional confounders include the variability in performance to repeated neuropsychometric testing even in healthy subjects, and an innate decline in cognitive function associated with both aging and the various comorbidities found in cardiac surgical patients. The challenge lies in discerning whether a specific event, for example, cardiac surgery, is causal or coincidental to deterioration in cognitive function. On the basis of more recent studies, the consensus is that longer-term cognitive dysfunction has a similar incidence whether patients undergo cardiac surgery with or without use of CPB, or instead undergo PCI or are managed medically, with the implication that aging and progression of underlying atherosclerosis and related comorbidities are of most significance [8].

E. Comparison groups. The incidence of new postoperative CNS dysfunction in CAB patients has been compared with that of patients undergoing major abdominal vascular or thoracic surgical procedures. Most of these patients usually have concomitant disease including hypertension, diabetes mellitus, diffuse atherosclerosis, and chronic lung disease. After adjusting for identified risk factors, patients undergoing any surgical procedure have been found more likely to suffer a cerebrovascular accident (CVA) than nonoperated controls with an odds ratio of 3.9. Even after excluding high-risk surgery (cardiac, vascular, and neurologic), the odds ratio is 2.9, which suggests the perioperative period itself predisposes patients to stroke. This observation is of particular relevance in considering the role of inflammatory processes and the salutary effect of statins as discussed below.

Studies on patients undergoing CAB surgery have demonstrated minimal difference in long-term cognitive function between patients undergoing on-pump versus off-pump procedures [9]. However, in general, it does appear that compared with other noncardiac surgical groups, the incidence of **early postoperative cognitive dysfunction is higher in CAB**

TABLE 24.1 Risk factors for neurologic complications in cardiac surgery

Common risk factors for both stroke and cognitive decline	
Advanced age (>75 yrs)	
Hypertension	
Severe carotid stenosis	
Diabetes mellitus	
Prior cerebrovascular disease	
Aortic atheromatosis	
Postbypass hypotension	
Postoperative arrhythmias	
Hemodynamic unstability during CPB	
Risk factors for stroke	**Risk factors for cognitive decline**
Type of surgery (complex procedures)	Cerebral oxygen desaturation during CPB
Emergency surgery	Cerebral hypoperfusion during CPB
	Brain hyperthermia during rewarming from CPB
Vascular disease	
CPB longer than 2 hr	
Elevated preoperative creatinine	
Postoperative atrial fibrillation	

patients, and since new ischemic lesions on magnetic resonance imaging (MRI) studies in valve surgery patients have been correlated with early postoperative cognitive dysfunction [10], as has intraoperative cerebral oxygen desaturation and early postoperative cognitive dysfunction in CAB patients, it does appear as though **efforts to mitigate against early postoperative cognitive dysfunction are warranted since early postoperative cognitive dysfunction is in part reflective of subclinical brain injury**.

F. **Risk factors.** Table 24.1 shows risk factors for both stroke and cognitive dysfunction. Risk factors have been pooled into various risk prediction models, which, while useful to compare patient groups, are still not predictive of a particular individual's outcome, although the presence of key risk factors may help in deciding the best procedure for a particular high-risk patient (i.e., surgery vs. angioplasty or valvuloplasty). Specific risk factors (i.e., aortic atherosclerosis, recent stroke) should prompt further preoperative investigations (e.g., carotid scanning, modification of intraoperative management) and may even suggest a change in surgical approach (i.e., off-pump CAB [OPCAB] with no instrumentation of the aorta) to minimize the potential for neurologic complications.

II. Cerebral physiology

A. **Cerebral autoregulation.** In normal subjects, cerebral blood flow (CBF) remains constant at 50 mL/(100 g·min) over a wide range of mean arterial pressure (MAP) from 50 to 150 mm Hg. This **autoregulatory plateau** reflects the tight matching between cerebral metabolic rate for O_2 ($CMRo_2$) and CBF, mediated in part by endothelium-derived relaxing factor (EDRF-nitric oxide [NO]). With decreased metabolic activity resulting from certain anesthetics or hypothermia, lowered $CMRO_2$ produces a resultant reduction in CBF and establishment of a lower autoregulatory plateau. It is apparent and should be considered that rather than a single cerebral autoregulatory curve, there are instead a series of autoregulatory curves. Each autoregulatory curve represents a differing set of metabolic conditions of the brain (e.g., normal metabolic activity) at 37°C versus lowered metabolic activity at 28°C. The autoregulatory plateau is a manifestation of intact cerebral flow and metabolism coupling, and it varies with metabolic rate.

With intact autoregulation, adequate substrate (blood flow) can be delivered at a lower perfusion pressure during conditions of lowered metabolic rate (e.g., anesthesia, hypothermia) in the absence of cerebral vasodilators (Fig. 24.2). Cerebral autoregulation is lacking in patients with diabetes mellitus and appears to be lost during deep hypothermia (e.g., less than 20°C) and for several hours after deep hypothermic circulatory arrest (DHCA). This results in pressure-passive CBF; in these instances, hypotension may entail increased risk for cerebral

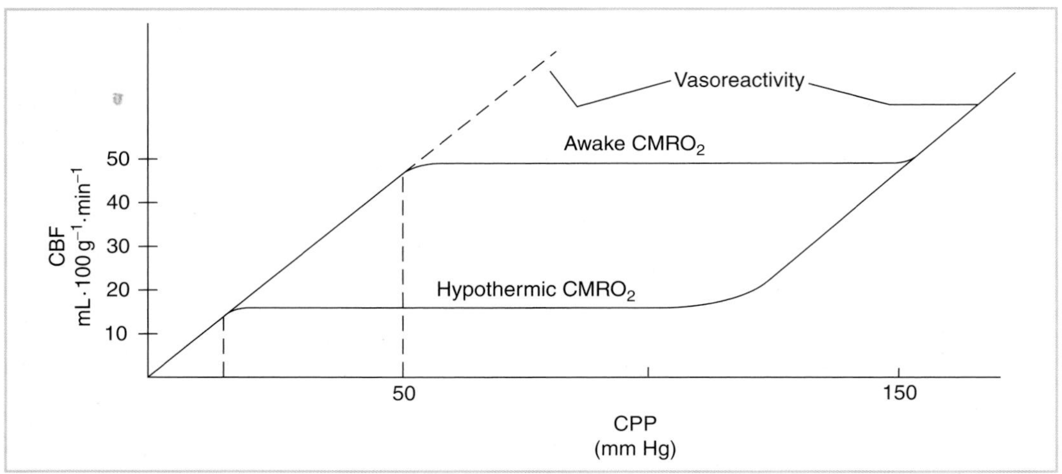

FIGURE 24.2 Cerebral autoregulatory curves during normothermia and hypothermia. The *upper curve* demonstrates a higher CBF autoregulatory plateau that is appropriate for the higher $CMRO_2$ in the awake state, versus a lower CBF plateau during hypothermia. With maximal cerebral vasodilation, lower CPP results in lower CBF that is appropriate at a lower $CMRO_2$ (hypothermia), but not at higher $CMRO_2$. (From Murkin JM. The pathophysiology of cardiopulmonary bypass. *Can J Anesth.* 1989;36:S41–S44, with permission.)

hypoperfusion. Similarly, in patients with chronic hypertension, cerebral autoregulation has been reset and higher perfusion pressures might be needed during CPB. In these circumstances, an uncoupling of CBF and cerebral metabolism could be related to neurocognitive decline [11].

It is notable that most of the initial studies on CBF and $CMRo_2$ specifically excluded patients with overt cerebrovascular disease while more recent studies which included elderly patients and those with previous CVA have indicated a striking variability in the autoregulatory threshold [12]. Using transcranial Doppler (TCD) or cerebral near-infrared spectroscopy (cNIRS), lower limits of cerebral autoregulation ranging from 45 to 80 mm Hg have been demonstrated, and in a study of 127 adult patients during CPB, a correlation has been made between loss of cerebral autoregulation during rewarming and postoperative neurologic events [13,14].

B. pH management. There is an inverse relationship between solubility of respiratory gases and blood temperature. With cooling of blood, CO_2 partial pressure ($PaCO_2$) decreases and arterial pH (pH_a) increases, producing an apparent respiratory alkalosis in vivo. To compensate for this condition during hypothermic CPB, total CO_2 must be increased by addition of exogenous CO_2 to the oxygenator, known as **pH-stat pH management**.

1. **α-Stat maintains pH_a 7.4 and $PaCO_2$ 40 mm Hg at 37°C without addition of exogenous CO_2.** Intracellular pH is primarily determined by the neutral pH (pH_N) of water. Since pH_N becomes progressively more alkaline with decreasing temperature, intracellular pH becomes correspondingly more alkaline during hypothermia. Since this intracellular alkalosis occurs in parallel with the hypothermia-induced increased solubility of CO_2 and increased blood pH, the normal transmembrane pH gradient of approximately 0.6 units remains unchanged, thus preserving optimal function of various intracellular enzyme systems. **This preservation of normal transmembrane pH gradient is the crux of α-stat pH theory**, and, in fact, we function in vivo according to α-stat principles. Since different tissues have differing temperatures (e.g., exercising muscle at 41°C vs. skin at 25°C), they also will have correspondingly different pH_a values (e.g., 7.34 vs. 7.6, respectively), although the net pH_a at 37°C will be 7.4. **α-Stat management acknowledges the temperature dependence of normal pH_a** and strives to maintain a constant transmembrane pH

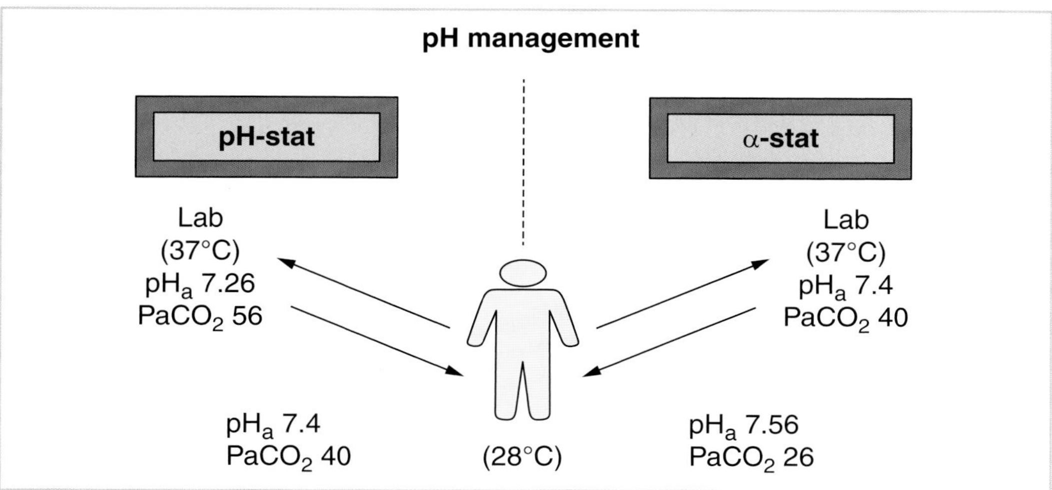

FIGURE 24.3 Contrasting arterial blood gas values as seen in vitro at 37°C or in vivo at 28°C when using α-stat or pH-stat management. Using pH-stat, laboratory values in vitro would be pH_a 7.26 and $PaCO_2$ 56 mm Hg, whereas temperature-corrected values in vivo would be pH_a 7.4 and $PaCO_2$ 40 mm Hg. If α-stat were used, laboratory values in vitro would be pH_a 7.4 and $PaCO_2$ 40 mm Hg, whereas temperature-corrected values in vivo would be pH_a 7.56 and $PaCO_2$ 26 mm Hg.

gradient by maintaining $PaCO_2$ at **40 mm Hg** and pH_a at 7.4 as measured in vitro at 37°C. For this strategy during CPB, total CO_2 is kept constant by not adding exogenous CO_2 and thus not compensating for increased solubility of CO_2. Blood samples measured at 37°C will show pH_a 7.4 and $PaCO_2$ 40 mm Hg, but those same samples measured at 28°C would have pH_a 7.56 and $PaCO_2$ 26 mm Hg (Fig. 24.3).

2. **pH-stat management involves addition of exogenous CO_2 to maintain $PaCO_2$ 40 mm Hg and pH_a 7.4 when corrected for the patient's body temperature in vivo.** Until the mid-1980s, pH-stat management was generally the most common mode of pH management during moderate hypothermic CPB. Since it is a potent cerebral vasodilator, such increases in total $PaCO_2$ associated with pH-stat have been shown to produce cerebral vasodilation, impairing cerebral flow and metabolism coupling and producing loss of cerebral autoregulation (Fig. 24.4). There is evidence that pH-stat management can increase the incidence of postoperative cognitive dysfunction when CPB duration exceeds 90 min [15]. This likely reflects both increased delivery of microemboli into the brain resulting from CO_2-induced vasodilation, and impairment of regional cerebral autoregulation. **It is notable that in recent studies even with use of α-stat, a wide variability of autoregulatory threshold has been found likely as a consequence of the increased age and presence of overt cerebrovascular disease in current surgical populations [12,14].**

III. Etiology of CNS damage

A. **Embolization.** In the context of CPB, focal ischemia is most often a consequence of isolated cerebral arteriolar obstruction by a particulate or gaseous embolus. Emboli vary in size, nature (particulate vs. gaseous), and origin (patient vs. equipment). Embolus factors influencing potential for damage include size, solubility, viscosity, and buoyancy relative to blood. Vessel diameter, anatomical location, and inflammatory responsivity influence tissue vulnerability. Open-chamber procedures generally entail greater risk of embolization than closed-chamber procedures. Calcific or atheromatous macroembolic debris from the ascending aorta or aortic arch appears to be a prime factor in the production of clinical stroke syndromes. It was formerly thought that microembolic elements, either gaseous or particulate, produced cognitive dysfunction. Studies from beating-heart surgery in which CPB is avoided, despite a much

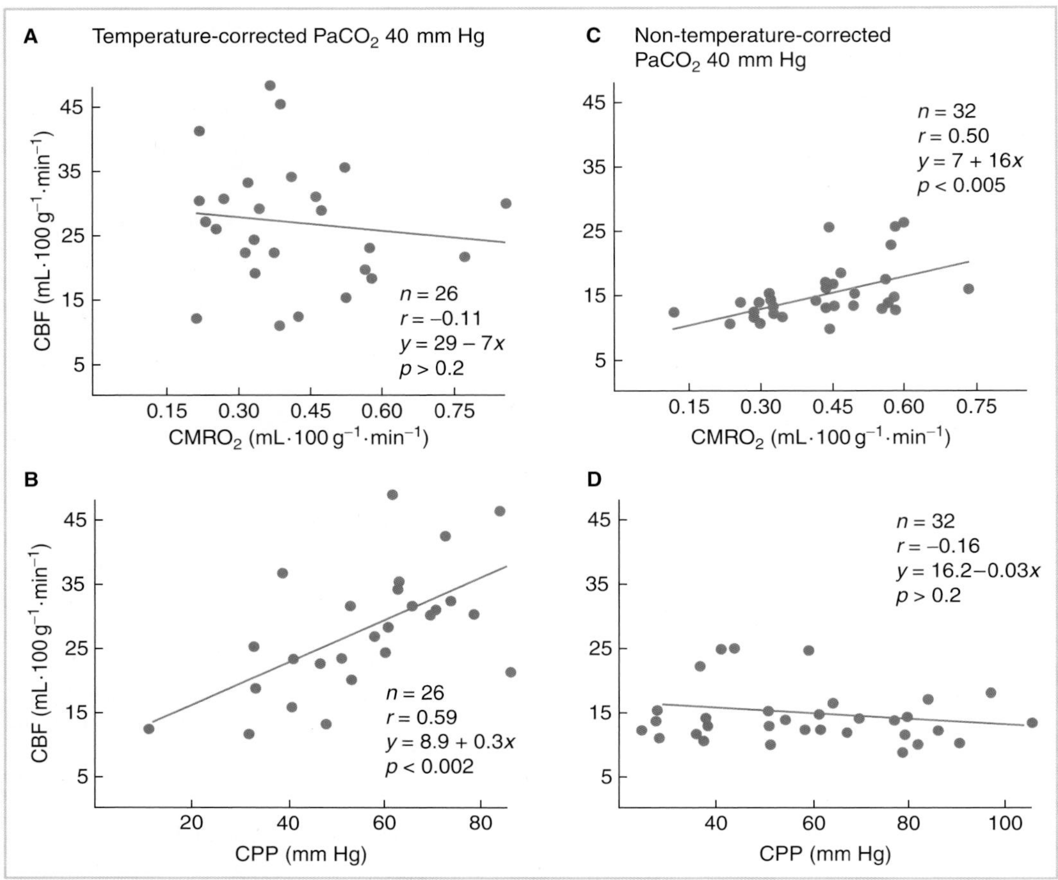

FIGURE 24.4 Linear regression analysis of CBF and $CMRO_2$, or CPP, for patients managed using α-stat (non-temperature-corrected) or pH-stat (temperature-corrected) management during moderate hypothermia (28°C). With pH-stat **(A)**, there is no correlation between CBF and $CMRO_2$, demonstrating loss of cerebral flow and metabolism coupling, whereas with α-stat **(C)** there is a highly significant (p <0.005) correlation. CBF significantly (p <0.002) correlates with CPP using pH-stat **(B)**, reflecting pressure-passive CBF and loss of autoregulation, whereas with α-stat **(D)**, CBF is independent of CPP. (From Murkin JM, Farrar JK, Tweed WA, et al. Cerebral autoregulation and flow/metabolism coupling during cardiopulmonary bypass: The influence of $PaCO_2$. *Anesth Analg.* 1987;66:825–832, with permission.)

lower incidence of embolic events, appear to have a relatively similar incidence of long-term cognitive dysfunction when compared to CAB using conventional CPB. Microgaseous emboli, the numbers of which are greatly reduced by avoidance of CPB, paradoxically appear to be relatively less injurious than otherwise predicted. The use of heparin anticoagulation in cardiac surgical patients has been demonstrated to ameliorate some of the overt effects of cerebral gas emboli [16].

Areas of brain localized at the boundary limits of major cerebral arteries (e.g., anterior and middle, or middle and posterior cerebral arteries, or superior and posterioinferior cerebellar arteries) are known as **arterial boundary zones or watershed zones** (Fig. 24.5), and these can manifest as isolated lesions as a consequence of transient global ischemia (see following sections). **Although they are commonly due to profoundly hypotensive episodes, watershed lesions are not pathognomonic of a hypotensive episode and may be the result of cerebral emboli. Embolization and hypoperfusion acting together can play a synergistic**
4 **role and either cause or magnify CNS injury in cardiac surgical patients.**

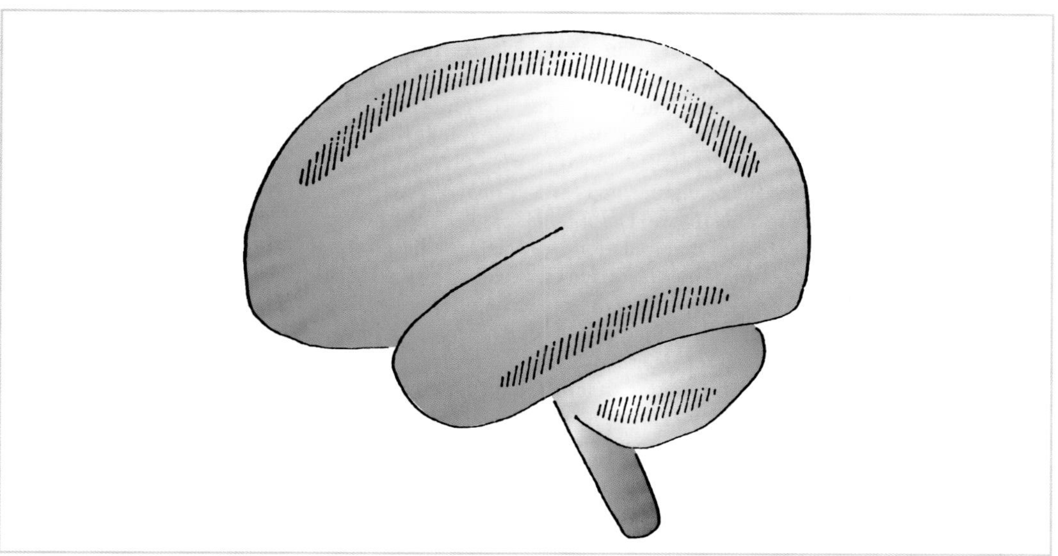

FIGURE 24.5 *Hatched areas* showing the most frequent locations of boundary area, or watershed zone infarcts in the brain, situated between the territories of major cerebral or cerebellar arteries. (From Torvik A. The pathogenesis of watershed infarcts in the brain. *Stroke.* 1984;2:221–223, with permission.)

1. **Detection of emboli**
   a. **Brain histology.** Isolated areas of perivascular and focal subarachnoid hemorrhage, neuronal swelling, and axonal degeneration are seen with higher frequency in the brains of patients dying after cardiac surgery than after non-CPB major vascular surgery. After surgery using unfiltered CPB circuits, fibrin and platelet emboli and calcific and atheromatous debris were seen frequently in small arterioles and capillary beds. **Small cerebral capillary and arterial dilatations (SCADS)** have been demonstrated histologically, occurring in nonsurvivors after proximal aortic instrumentation after either CPB or coronary angiography. **These SCADS are increasingly believed to be due in part to lipid microemboli from usage of unprocessed cardiotomy suction blood.**
   b. **Intraoperative emboli detection.** Intraoperative fluorescein retinal angiography has demonstrated that extensive retinal microvascular embolization occurs during CPB. The incidence and extent of retinal obstruction are much greater with bubble than with membrane oxygenators, despite use of 40 μm arterial line filters. Use of TCD insonation enables assessment of blood flow perfusion characteristics through the middle cerebral artery (MCA). TCD insonation permits measurement of blood flow velocity and detection and quantification of emboli, though discrimination of gaseous from particulate emboli remains unreliable. **Proximal aortic instrumentation and initiation of CPB have been identified as particularly embologenic events.** After open-chamber surgery, cerebral emboli are detected as the heart fills and begins to eject, underscoring the importance of meticulous deairing techniques (see the following sections).

5 2. **Sources of emboli**
   a. **Patient-related sources**
      (1) **Aortic atheroma.** Atheromatous debris can be embolized during aortic clamping or cannulation. Intraoperative aortic ultrasonography using either transesophageal echocardiography (TEE; high sensitivity, low specificity) or epiaortic scanning (EAS) (high sensitivity, high specificity) enables visualization of aortic wall and can be used to guide cannulation sites. Ultrasonography has demonstrated that plaque may fracture or shear off and embolize during CPB as a consequence of trauma

from aortic clamping and cannulation or from blood "jetting" from the aortic cannula or may result in intimal flap formation with potential for delayed postoperative embolization [17]. Using EAS, Ura et al. compared images before and after CPB in 472 patients undergoing cardiac surgery, and noted new lesions in the ascending aortic intima in 16 patients (3.4%) following decannulation [17]. In 10 patients, 3 of whom suffered postoperative CVA, the new lesions were severe with mobile lesions or disruption of the intima, of which 6 were related to aortic clamping and the other 4 to aortic cannulation. Only the maximal thickness of the atheroma near the aorta manipulation site was a predictor of new lesions. If the atheroma was 3 to 4 mm, the incidence of new lesions was 11.8% and was as high as 33.3% if the atheroma was >4 mm. As such, embolization of plaque or thrombus from such intimal fractures may explain one mechanism of delayed stroke cited above. Proximal aortic atherosclerosis is thus a significant risk factor for neurologic injury.

(2) **Intraventricular thrombi.** During closed-chamber procedures in patients with recent mural thrombi, manipulation of the heart can dislodge thrombi that embolize once the heart begins to fill and eject.

(3) **Valvular calcifications.** Valve surgery, particularly valve replacement surgery, is associated with increased risk of CVA resulting from embolization of intracavitary valve debris.

(4) **Postoperative atrial fibrillation.** Early-onset atrial fibrillation is associated with a variety of adverse outcomes and has been strongly linked to increased perioperative stroke risk, and is particularly associated with increased risk of delayed-onset postoperative stroke [5]. Even transient new-onset atrial fibrillation is associated with increased risk of 30-day and 1-yr cardiovascular events composed of stroke, cardiac death, and myocardial infarction (MI). In cardiac surgical patients a decreased incidence of atrial fibrillation has been associated with perioperative statin therapy as discussed below. **Increased efforts should thus be aimed in part at reducing even transient new-onset postoperative atrial fibrillation.**

b. Procedure-related sources

(1) While open-chamber procedures (e.g., septal repair, ventricular aneurysmectomy, valve surgery) expose the arterial circulation to air or particulate debris, closed-chamber procedures also can be associated with ventricular air. Use of a ventricular vent, particularly if active suction is applied and the heart is empty, produces localized subatmospheric pressure at the vent tip within the left ventricle (LV) and cause air to be entrained retrograde from the vent insertion site (usually through the superior pulmonary vein) into the LV. Use of TEE can assist in visualization and guide the removal of residual intracavitary air (see following discussion). Inadvertent opening of the left atrium (LA) or LV while the heart is beating also caused rapid air entrainment and increased potential for cerebral emboli.

(2) Aortic cannulation and clamping are associated with cerebral embolization, particularly in the presence of extensive aortic atherosclerosis.

(3) **Duration of CPB is an independent risk for postoperative brain dysfunction.** After 90 min of CPB, the incidence of cognitive dysfunction is increased compared to CPB of shorter duration. It is important to note that duration of CPB may be increased by factors (e.g., extensive atherosclerotic disease), which may independently contribute to neurologic injury [3,4].

c. Equipment-related sources

(1) Incorporation of a 25 μm filter into the aortic inflow line effectively reduces cerebral embolic load and has been shown to decrease the incidence of postoperative cognitive dysfunction.

(2) Membrane oxygenators give rise to markedly fewer gaseous microemboli than bubble oxygenators, but this does not entirely eliminate the risk of air emboli. Similarly, air entrained into the venous side of a membrane oxygenator, or gaseous emboli resulting from drug administration via injection directly into CPB circuitry

can transit the membrane and appear in the arterial inflow line, despite use of arterial line filters.

(3) Use of 20 to 40 μm filters in the cardiotomy return line prevents particulate debris from the operative site from entering the CPB circuit. Use of cardiotomy blood washing techniques (cell saver) is associated with reduced amounts of cerebral lipid microemboli but has also been shown to result in greater transfusion requirements and has not been shown to consistently improve CNS outcomes.

(4) Use of nitrous oxide (N_2O) before commencement of CPB has been associated with increased evidence of ischemic damage, likely because residual N_2O increases the size of any microgaseous emboli in the cerebral circulation. This is especially true for several hours after CPB when high fractional inspired oxygen (FIO_2) should be used to minimize the size of residual gaseous microemboli.

B. Hypoperfusion

1. **Watershed areas.** Collateral perfusion of the brain can occur via extracerebral anastomoses (primarily through the circle of Willis) or by way of intracerebral anastomoses between major cerebral arteries, known as **arterial boundary zones** (watershed zones; Fig. 24.5). Rapid severe hypoperfusion can produce ischemic lesions within these boundary zones found at the territorial limits of the major cerebral arteries. The most frequently affected area is the parieto-occipital sulci located at the limits of the anterior, middle, and posterior cerebral arteries. Despite a global ischemic stress, these watershed lesions may be focal and asymmetrical. Placement of electroencephalogram (EEG) electrodes using a parasagittal montage (see following) may allow increased sensitivity for border zone ischemia detection.
2. **Cerebral perfusion pressure (CPP).** During moderate hypothermia (28 to 30°C) using α-stat pH management, autoregulation is preserved in patients without overt cerebrovascular disease over the CPP range from 20 to 100 mm Hg. However, studies in elderly cardiac surgical patients and those with cerebrovascular disease indicate a wide variability of lower limit of autoregulation between 45 and 80 mm Hg [12]. Additionally, there are several conditions in which autoregulation may be lost (Table 24.2). With profound hypothermia (15 to 20°C), there appears to be loss of autoregulation as a result of hypothermia-induced vasoparesis, while diabetic patients have been shown to have impaired cerebral autoregulation even at moderate hypothermia.

   During CPB, there may be dissociation between MAP and CPP as a result of unrecognized cerebral venous hypertension. Particularly with use of a single two-stage venous cannula, cerebral venous drainage may be impaired specially during performance of posterior distal anastomoses (Fig. 24.6). Consequently, jugular venous pressure should be measured proximally within the superior vena cava (SVC; e.g., via introducer port of pulmonary artery or central venous catheter). CPP can also be compromised during performance of off-pump coronary surgery especially while performing multiple-graft procedures. During these operations the patient is often placed head-down and the heart is lifted to expose the distal targets, two factors which can increase central venous pressure and thus decrease CPP. Concurrent systemic arterial hypotension and low cardiac output often occur concomitantly with resultant cerebral hypoperfusion.
3. **Circulatory arrest.** During circulatory arrest for surgical procedures, profound hypothermia (16 to 18°C) is used to minimize $CMRO_2$ and increase tolerance for ischemia (see following). During circulatory arrest under normothermic conditions, O_2 levels are depleted within a

TABLE 24.2 Factors associated with loss of cerebral autoregulation

- pH-stat management (Fig. 24.4)
- Diabetes mellitus
- Profound hypothermia (<20°C)
- Deep hypothermic circulatory arrest
- Previous cerebrovascular accident
- Advanced age

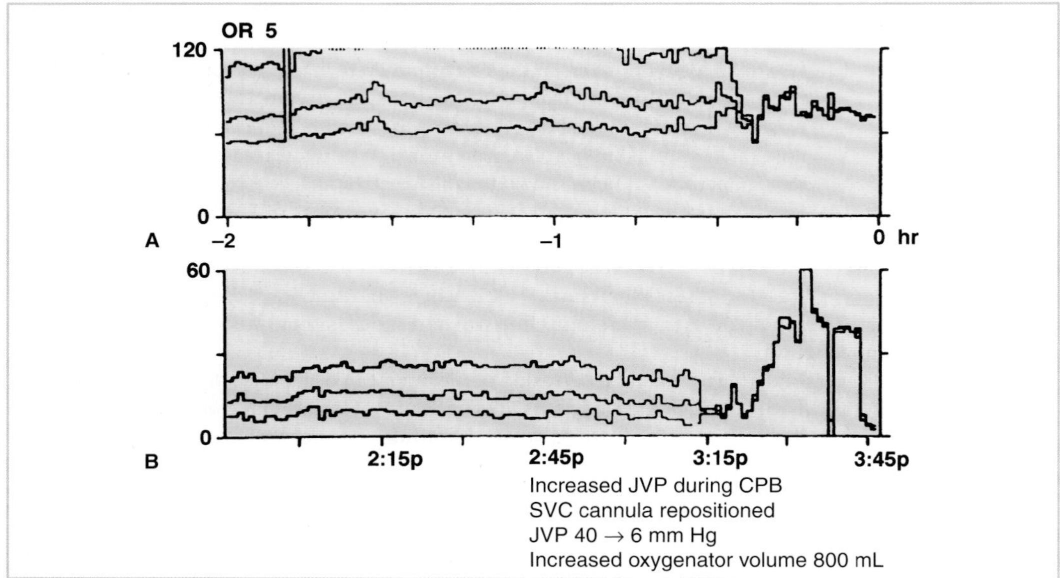

FIGURE 24.6 **A:** Systolic, mean, and diastolic arterial blood pressures, with commencement of CPB indicated at 3:15 p.m., after which MAP is shown. **B:** Pulmonary artery systolic, mean, and diastolic pressures with proximal jugular venous pressure (JVP) recorded at 3:15 p.m., with commencement of CPB. A single two-stage venous cannula was used for CPB. With rotation of the heart, venous return to the oxygenator decreased and JVP approached MAP values. (Modified from Murkin JM. Intraoperative management. In: Estaphanous FG, Barash PG, Reves JG, eds. *Cardiac Anesthesia: Principles and Clinical Practice.* Philadelphia, PA: J.B. Lippincott Company; 1994:326, with permission.)

few seconds of onset of ischemia, EEG activity is lost (isoelectric EEG) within 30 s, high-energy phosphates are exhausted within 1 min, and ischemic neuronal damage is found after periods of anoxia as brief as 5 min.

For certain cardiac electrophysiologic procedures (e.g., diagnosis and treatment of certain refractory arrhythmias), transient ventricular fibrillation (VF) is often induced at normothermia and without circulatory support. Duration of VF must be limited to less than 1 min, and prompt hemodynamic resuscitation with at least 4 min of reperfusion should be maintained between episodes of VF [18]. Monitoring and management of these patients should follow the principles outlined herein.

4. **Intracerebral and extracerebral atherosclerosis.** Patient-related factors including intracerebral and extracerebral atherosclerosis also modify the impact of perioperative hypotension. Neurologic injury after cardiac surgery is higher in patients with previous stroke, hypertension, advanced age, diabetes, and carotid bruit [2–5], which are all factors related to more extensive cerebrovascular disease. In one series of 206 perioperative CABG patients, over 50% exhibited concomitant cerebrovascular disease [19]. Such patients are more prone to cerebral ischemia secondary to perioperative hemodynamic instability.

IV. Pathophysiology of neuronal ischemia

Ischemia is defined as diminution of blood flow below a critical level that propagates tissue damage. Whether from embolization or hypoperfusion, neuronal ischemia is the final common pathway leading to cerebral damage. The extent of ischemic changes will depend on the duration of the ischemic insult, the affected vascular territory, the presence of collateral circulation, and factors that either ameliorate (e.g., hypothermia) or increase (e.g., hyperglycemia) the impact of ischemia on neuronal tissue [20].

A. **Lactic acidosis.** Glucose is essentially the sole substrate for energy production by the brain, being metabolized to produce 36 moles of adenosine triphosphate (ATP) per mole glucose. Oxygen is essential for oxidative phosphorylation, and in the presence of ischemia, anaerobic glucose metabolism yields only 2 moles of ATP and results in lactate production with accumulation of hydrogen ion (H^+). Anaerobic glycolysis is the primary cause of acidosis during ischemia, and the severity of lactic acidosis is directly related to preischemia glucose concentrations. Hyperglycemia is associated with worsening of neurologic injury after cerebral ischemia, and should be avoided in the perioperative interval.

B. **Apoptosis, necrosis, and inflammation.** Two distinct phases of cellular death have been described after cerebral ischemia: apoptosis and necrosis. These are related to the intensity and duration of ischemic insult. Apoptosis is programmed cerebral cell death. Its main features include cell shrinkage with preservation of cell membrane and mitochondrial integrity and lack of inflammation and injury to surrounding tissue. There is some evidence that CPB may exacerbate apoptotic processes accelerating neuronal loss manifest as delayed postoperative CNS injury. Necrosis is a nonprogrammed event leading to cellular swelling, disruption of cell membrane and mitochondrial damage with inflammatory reaction, vascular damage, and edema formation [20]. The core of the ischemic tissue will show predominantly necrosis, and apoptosis will be found mostly in the periphery of the ischemic area. The sensitivity of neurons to ischemic insult varies by region with hippocampal areas exhibiting marked vulnerability.

C. **Ion gradients and role of calcium.** Neuronal function and structural integrity are dependent on ionic gradients, such that up to 75% of ATP produced by resting neurons is utilized by sodium–potassium ATPase and for extrusion of calcium by calcium-dependent ATPase. With ischemia, decreased ATP production and evolving lactic acidosis impair transmembrane ionic pumps and consequently diminish cellular electrochemical gradients leading to cell depolarization. Extraneuronal leakage of K^+ depolarizes adjacent neurons, thereby decreasing synaptic transmission and, along with calcium, promoting vasospasm in adjacent vasculature.

D. **Calcium.** With ischemia, ATP depletion causes loss of ionic gradients, resulting in cell membrane depolarization and influx of calcium ion (Ca^{2+}) through voltage-sensitive channels. Intracellular accumulation of Ca^{2+} is likely the final common pathway leading to neuronal death through enhanced protein and lipid catabolism. Elevated intracellular calcium will activate both phospholipases, which leads to membrane cell breakdown and arachidonic acid and free radical formation, and endonucleases, which induces fragmentation of genomic DNA, mitochondrial dysfunction, and energy failure. The intensity of intracellular calcium overload is the key element leading to irreversible cellular damage. Influx of Ca^{2+} can be minimized by calcium antagonists. Nimodipine has shown clinical benefit in decreasing vasospasm after subarachnoid hemorrhage, but has been associated with increased bleeding and mortality in cardiac surgical patients.

E. **Free fatty acids.** Some of the earliest cell membrane changes with ischemia involve production of free fatty acids (FFAs) from membrane phospholipids. Intracellular Ca^{2+} activates calcium-dependent phospholipases C and A2, transforming membrane phospholipids into FFAs, which themselves are neurotoxic. FFAs are powerful uncouplers of oxidative phosphorylation and can undergo further oxidation from arachidonic acid, with resultant free radical formation. During cerebral ischemia, FFA production is decreased by administration of calcium antagonists and 21-aminosteroids (**lazaroids**), potent inhibitors of lipid peroxidation. Despite laboratory promise, clinical trials have so far been disappointing.

F. **Excitotoxicity.** Glutamate is the most abundant excitatory amino acid (EAA) in the brain. It serves metabolic, neurotransmitter, and neurotropic functions and is normally compartmentalized in the neuron. Under normal conditions the brain has the ability to quickly uptake extracellular glutamate. Glutamate stimulates two kinds of receptors: Ionophore-linked receptors and metabotropic receptors; the last ones act only as modifiers of the excitotoxic injury. The main excitotoxic role lies in the ionophore-linked receptors, and these include NMDA (N-methyl-D-aspartate), AMPA (alpha-amino-methylisoxazole-propionic acid), and kainate, responsible for mediating transmembrane Ca^{2+} and Na^+K^+ passage. Ischemia produces enhanced presynaptic EAA release and decreased reuptake, which causes activation of postsynaptic NMDA and AMPA receptors and produces massive efflux of K^+ and influx of Na^+ and Ca^+ and resultant osmolysis and calcium-related damage. EAAs also are increasingly implicated in free radical formation. Administration of ketamine, an NMDA receptor antagonist, has shown variable efficacy to decrease neuronal ischemic injury (see later).

G. **Nitric oxide.** NO is a free-radical gas synthesized from L-arginine by NO synthase (NOS). NO functions as a neurotransmitter and has a role in regulating CBF and inflammation. In brain ischemia, the elevation of intracellular calcium markedly increases the activity of NOS. Increased NO combined with superoxide anion leads to formation of other reactive oxygen species, hydroxyl free radicals, and nitrogen dioxide producing proteolysis and cell damage. NO also mediates activation of ADP-polymerase leading to ATP and nicotinamide consumption and cell death [20]. Experimentally, lazaroids ameliorate neuronal ischemic damage when administered for ischemic stress, but results of clinical trials have not been positive.

H. **Leukocytosis.** In a subanalysis of a trial randomizing 18,558 patients with symptomatic vascular disease to aspirin or clopidogrel, it was observed that in the week prior to a second vascular event, **the quartile with highest leukocyte counts had higher risks for ischemic stroke**, myocardial infarction, and vascular death after adjustment for other risk factors [21]. In the week before a recurrent event, but not at earlier time points, the leukocyte count was significantly increased over baseline levels, suggesting that leukocyte counts and mainly neutrophil counts are independently associated with ischemic events in these high-risk populations. Consistent with this, in a prospective study of 7,483 patients who underwent CAB or valvular surgery or both, leukocyte count was compared with the occurrence of postoperative stroke [22]. There were a total of 125 postoperative strokes and it was demonstrated that leukocyte count was significantly higher preoperatively and directly postoperatively in patients with stroke and that the magnitude of elevation of leukocyte count was correlated with magnitude
6 and extent of stroke. **These results strongly implicate inflammation and white cell activation as etiologic in both the extent and severity of perioperative cerebrovascular events.**

V. Intraoperative cerebral monitoring

As shown in Table 24.3, there are various confounds for EEG monitoring, which along with the complex etiology of perioperative neurologic morbidity, suggest multimodal neuromonitoring as the best approach for systematic detection and avoidance of perioperative cerebral complications.

A. **Brain temperature.** Accurate monitoring of brain temperature is essential because temperature profoundly influences CMR and thus tolerance for ischemia. Mild hypothermia (less than 35°C) is disproportionately effective in decreasing ischemia-related injury due to inhibition of EAA release (see previous sections). During CPB, thermal gradients exist between various tissues; thus, brain temperature must be measured independent of other sites. Because of the small risk of trauma associated with placement of a tympanic thermistor, nasopharyngeal temperature (NPT) is the preferred site for clinical monitoring of brain temperature. Thermistor insertion should be through the nares to the level of the midpoint of the zygoma, a depth of 7 to 10 cm in an adult. Insertion of the thermistor before heparinization, using lubrication and exerting gentle pressure parallel to the floor of the nose, will prevent epistaxis and trauma to mucosa and turbinates. Esophageal temperature is a poor substitute for NPT because it variously reflects aortic inflow temperature, temperature of surrounding tissue, and the influence of residual ice or cooled fluid within the pericardial sac. For DHCA and high-risk patients, a thermistor/oximetric catheter can be placed retrograde into the jugular bulb, thus providing the most sensitive clinical measure of global brain temperature and oxygenation.

TABLE 24.3 Electroencephalogram confounds
• Anesthetic agents (e.g., propofol, sevoflurane, desflurane, thiopental, etomidate) producing EEG burst suppression (Fig. 24.10)
• High-dose enflurane (EEG pattern indistinguishable from electrocortical seizure activity)
• High-dose narcotics or cerebral ischemia (similar EEG δ-wave activity)
• Biopotentials (e.g., cardiac depolarization [electrocardiogram], skeletal muscle [shivering], eye movement myopotentials, blood flow through aortic cannula)
• 60-Hz activity from electrical equipment (e.g., cardiopulmonary bypass pump motor, electrocautery, EEG).

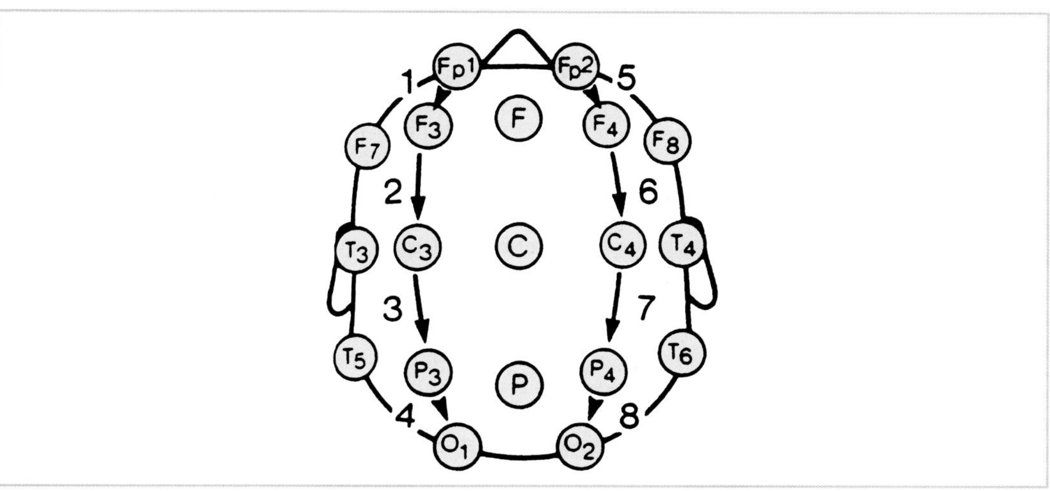

FIGURE 24.7 Standard bipolar parasagittal montage based on the international 10–20 system. F_{P1} and F_{P2} refers to frontal pole; F_3, F_4, F_7, and F_8 refer to frontal; C_3 and C_4 refer to central; P_3 and P_4 refer to parietal; O_1 and O_2 refer to occipital; and T_3, T_4, T_5, and T_6 refer to temporal positions. (From Murkin JM, Moldenhauer CC, Hug CC Jr, et al. Absence of seizures during induction of anesthesia with high-dose fentanyl. *Anesth Analg.* 1984;63:489–494.)

B. **EEG.** EEG represents the amplified, summated, spontaneous electrical activity of the superficial cerebral cortex. Each electrode reflects microcurrent (10 to 200 μV) generated by electrical gradients across layers of neurons aligned at right angles to the monitored cortical surface in a 2 to 3 cm radius. Electrode placement should be based on the standard 10- to 20-electrode system and modified according to the number of channels being monitored (Fig. 24.7). EEG activity is commonly divided into four bands according to frequency: δ less than 4 Hz; θ 4 to 8 Hz; α 9 to 12 Hz; and β greater than 13 Hz. In general, slower frequencies indicate a deeper level of anesthesia. Several factors can confound interpretation of intraoperative EEG (Table 24.3) which, along with its technical complexity, have limited its clinical use to monitoring cooling during DHCA. Recordings are potentially made in the presence of various anesthetic agents, during profound changes in body temperature, and in the electrically hostile environment found in an operating room. Although subtle EEG changes may be difficult to interpret, development of asymmetric EEG activity should be considered to represent hemispheric compromise (Table 24.4).

1. **Processed EEG.** After initial electronic filtering, analog EEG voltages are rapidly digitized (150/s) and analyzed over "epochs" (generally 2 to 4 s in duration) using analyses based on either frequency-domain or time-domain processing.
   a. **Compressed spectral array (CSA) and density-modulated display of power spectrum analysis (DSA).** For frequency-domain processing, many EEG applications use power spectral analysis. In this application, each EEG epoch is converted into a series

TABLE 24.4 Causes of electroencephalographic asymmetry
• Unilateral carotid perfusion from aortic miscannulation
• Cerebral venous hypertension from kinking of atrial cannulas
• Cerebral hypoperfusion from low pump flow or systemic arterial hypotension unmasking unilateral cerebrovascular disease
• Cerebral ischemia from embolus
• Unmasking of previous cerebrovascular accident
• Artifact from proximity of arterial inflow cannula blood flow to ground electroencephalographic electrode

of sine-wave components using Fourier transformation that treats the digitized EEG as a sum of sine waves of variable frequency and power. The amplitude (power) of each of the sine-wave components is indicated as a function of its frequency, and in the CSA each EEG epoch is shown over time in a three-dimensional representation (frequency vs. power vs. time) with the most current epoch in the foreground. The vertical displacement, representing both power and time, hinders recognition of low-amplitude activity followed by high-amplitude activity in the same frequency band. DSA is a representation in which each epoch is displayed using gray-scale intensity or dot size proportional to the power of the individual frequency band plotted. Consequently, it can be difficult to recognize small changes in frequency using this display.

   b. **Spectral edge frequency (aperiodic analysis).** Aperiodic analysis is time-domain–based processing and does not use Fourier transformation. Instead it is based on assessing voltage versus time of the raw EEG. For each component EEG wave in an epoch, the frequency is determined as the reciprocal of the time interval measured between zero axis voltage crossings, the zero-crossing frequency (ZXF), while the amplitude is the square root of the sum of squares of the voltages of the wavelets. Fast- and slow-wave components are analyzed separately, then combined for display. This model of analysis is also used to calculate the burst-suppression ratio, which can be an indicator of anesthetic depth and cerebral metabolism depression. Epileptiform activity and artifact have been reported to be most readily identified by time-domain processing. EEG frequency carrying the median power (median frequency power) correlates with plasma levels of several narcotics. The spectral edge frequency (frequency below which 95% of summated EEG power is contained) correlates with clinical assessment of anesthetic depth achieved with barbiturates or volatile anesthetics.

2. **Bispectral (BIS) index.** Most frequency-domain processing (CSA, DSA) treats those component waveforms resulting from Fourier transformation as independent. Bispectral (BIS) analysis measures potential interactions between the waves to determine the presence of interactive components (harmonics) indicative of phase coupling (biocoherence), information that is not present in power spectral analysis. It has been recognized that EEG slowing and synchrony often occur in relation to increasing depth of anesthesia. The BIS measurement is the first device specifically for the measurement of the hypnotic effects of drugs approved by the US Food and Drug Administration (FDA).

3. **Evoked potentials.** Metabolic and hemodynamic homeostasis determines the state of cerebral functional integrity. The latter can be inferred from EEG changes in response to repeated stimulation of intact afferent pathways. Separated from raw EEG and averaged, these evoked potentials (EPs) are described in terms of latency (time between the stimulus and respective EEG change) and amplitude (cortical microcurrent 1 to 5 μV). Reduction in CBF below 18 mL/(100 g·min) causes progressive decrease of the latter, which disappears at CBF below 15 mL/(100 g·min). In clinical practice, only the response of sensory neurons of gray matter can be tested in this way. More commonly, EPs serve to monitor the function of sensory tracts. Certain anesthetic agents complicate the recognition of specific effects of changing metabolic environment on EPs (e.g., isoflurane increases latency and decreases amplitude of somatosensory EPs) and have opposite effects on different EPs (visual somatosensory). As temperature changes also affect the latency and amplitude of EPs, the net result is potential intraoperative variability in EP during cardiac surgery potentially limiting its clinical applicability.

C. **TCD.** Insonation of blood moving within a vessel produces a characteristic shift in signal frequency (Doppler shift) that is proportional to the flow velocity. Use of low-frequency sound waves (2 to 4 MHz) from depth-gated, direction-sensitive probes allows transmission through thin areas of skull (e.g., **temporal window located above zygomatic arch between ear and orbit**). This transmission enables continuous assessment of blood flow velocity within major intracerebral arteries (e.g., proximal MCA). Cerebral perfusion characteristics also can be assessed using TCD insonation for demonstration of laminar versus pulsatile flow or for detection of emboli. Because dissimilar acoustic echoes reflect inhomogeneities in the insonated

TABLE 24.5 Transcranial Doppler characteristics of emboli versus noise

	Emboli	Noise
Duration(s)	<0.1	0.5
Directionality	Unidirectional	Bidirectional
Frequency range (db)	3–60	1–20
Sound	Chirpy	Noisy
Time delay (ms; bigate 10-mm distance)	11	0.08

substrate, microaggregate or microgaseous emboli can be detected within the bloodstream. Because TCD essentially functions as a microphone, artifactual noise transients can register as emboli. However, certain criteria have been employed to distinguish embolic signals from noise artifact (Table 24.5). Much greater acoustic resonance of gas emboli relative to formed elements creates limits of TCD detection for formed elements greater than 100 μm. In addition, the amplitude of signal is proportional to the size of the embolus, whereas for bubble emboli, limits of resolution are 50 μm and the amplitude of the reflected signal is unrelated to size of the bubble.

Because of the ability to focus a pulsed U/S beam, however, by using a dual gating technique in which the vessel is insonated at two discrete sites, emboli can be discriminated from artifacts. This reflects the fact that emboli propagate with blood motion and artifact does not and thus emboli but not artifact will be detected sequentially at different depths along the insonated cerebral artery.

One of the major goals in intraoperative TCD monitoring is discriminating solid versus gaseous cerebral emboli. Solid and gaseous microemboli may be differentiated with a new generation of multifrequency transducers, using both 2- and 2.5-MHz crystals, based on the principle that solid microemboli reflect more ultrasound at the higher than at the lower frequency, whereas the opposite is the case for gaseous microemboli. How robust this will prove in clinical practice remains to be seen and the results to date remain unconvincing.

D. **Jugular oximetry.** The characteristic attenuation of 650 to 1,100 nm infrared light by a few specific light-absorbing chromophores (primarily oxyhemoglobin, deoxyhemoglobin, and oxidized cytochrome c oxydase) imparts wavelength (color) shift on the incident light. This spectral shift is proportionate to the degree of oxygenation enabling quantification of tissue oxygenation using optical spectroscopic devices. Placement of a fiberoptic oximetric catheter into the jugular bulb provides continuous monitoring of the hemoglobin saturation of effluent cerebral venous blood and reflects global cerebral O_2 supply and demand balance. **Jugular oximetry may provide an appropriate endpoint for termination of cooling before DHCA (see below).** After jugular saturation has increased maximally and stabilized, $CMRO_2$ is at its lowest. Such monitoring has identified an association between rewarming after hypothermic CPB and significant cerebral venous blood desaturation. This indicates mismatching between cerebral O_2 supply and metabolic rate, and increasing either hemoglobin concentration or depth of anesthesia (greater metabolic suppression) may be appropriate.

E. **NIRS.** Similar principles of light absorbance are used during noninvasive cerebral optical spectroscopy using scalp-attached probes. Most of the currently available commercial devices employ two-channel monitoring using adhesive pads with one or more transmitting and two or more separately spaced receiving optodes. Differential spacing of the receiving optodes enables correction for extracerebral tissues to be made, allowing an assessment of regional oxygen saturation (rSO_2) of cerebral cortex (Fig. 24.8). Current studies estimate that there is between 5% and 15% influence of extracerebral tissue on cerebral oximetry values as measured. Advantages and limitations of NIRS cerebral oximetry monitoring are shown in Table 24.6. This device enables indices of cerebral oxygenation to be determined in a continuous manner in a variety of clinical circumstances. There is no requirement for pulsatile blood flow enabling continuous monitoring during CPB, and there are no temperature-related artifacts. A potential limitation is the fact that the cerebral sample volumes are on the order of 1 mL of frontal cortical

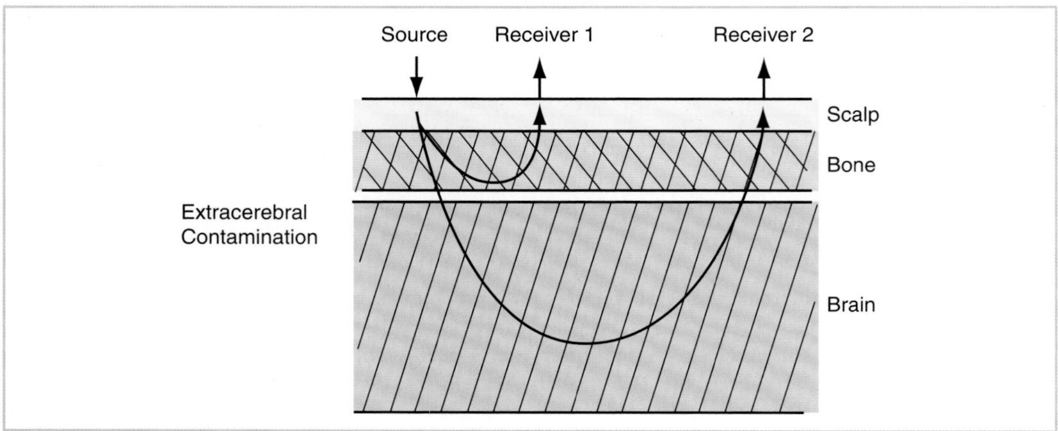

FIGURE 24.8 Schematic representation of tissue layers through which light must propagate to reach the brain. Light propagating from source to receiver 1 has a mean tissue path length such that it predominantly samples superficial tissue (scalp and skull), whereas light propagating to receiver 2 has a deeper mean path length into brain. The signal from receiver 1 is used to correct the signal from receiver 2 for superficial tissue contamination. (From McCormick PW, Stewart M, Goetting MG, et al. Noninvasive optical spectroscopy for monitoring cerebral oxygen delivery and hemodynamics. *Crit Care Med.* 1991;19:89–97, with permission.)

tissue, thus rendering them highly localized in nature. It is also apparent that since NIRS measures total tissue oxygenation, various factors including patient age, hemoglobin concentration at the measurement site, and sensor location can affect rSO_2 values. A prospective study demonstrated that avoidance of low intraoperative cerebral oximetry values decreases major organ morbidity and death in patients undergoing CABG surgery [23], and a strong correlation has also been made between low preoperative baseline cerebral oximetry values and short- and long-term morbidity and mortality in cardiac surgical patients [13]. While there is increasing clinical consensus that cerebral oximetry is beneficial in patients undergoing hypothermic circulatory arrest with direct cerebral perfusion [24], other studies report skeptical results about cerebral oximetry technology [24,25] to counterbalance the argument against routine use in cardiac surgical patients. Large-scale multicenter clinical outcomes studies will be required in order to make a solid recommendation for the widespread use of cerebral oximetry in cardiac surgical patients or other specific subgroups of patients.

F. **CPP.** It represents the difference between driving pressure, or MAP, and downstream pressure, or intracranial pressure. During CPB, direct measure of intracranial pressure is not available; thus, CVP is often used as a surrogate. In the presence of impaired drainage from the SVC,

TABLE 24.6 Advantages and limitations of NIRS cerebral oximetry

Advantages
No interference from electrocautery
Ease of use
Measures balance of O_2 delivery and demand
Does not require pulsatile blood flow
Monitors watershed zone at the border of anterior and middle cerebral arteries
Limitations
Variable amount of extracerebral contamination (5%–15%)
Approximately 70% venous weighted
Measures a small volume (1 cc) of cortical brain tissue

7 **TABLE 24.7** Evidence-based guidelines for best practice bypass

The clinical team should manage adult patients undergoing moderate hypothermic CPB with α-stat pH management (Class I, Level A).
Limiting arterial line temperature to 37°C may be useful for avoiding cerebral hyperthermia (Class IIa, Level B).
The clinical team should maintain perioperative blood glucose concentration within an institution's normal clinical range in all patients including nondiabetics (Class I, Level B).
Direct reinfusion to the cardiopulmonary bypass circuit of unprocessed blood exposed to pericardial and mediastinal surfaces should be avoided (Class I, Level B).
Blood cell processing and filtration may be considered to decrease the deleterious effects of reinfused shed blood (Class IIb, Level B).
In patients undergoing cardiopulmonary bypass at increased risk of adverse neurological events, strong consideration should be given to intraoperative TEE or epiaortic ultrasound scanning of the aorta:
I. To detect nonpalpable plaque (Class I, Level A)
II. For reduction of cerebral emboli (Class IIa, Level B)
Arterial line filters should be incorporated in the CPB circuit to minimize the embolic load delivered to the patient (Class I, Level A).
Efforts should be made to reduce hemodilution including reduction of prime volume in order to avoid subsequent allogenic blood transfusion (Class I, Level A).
Reduction of circuit surface area and the use of biocompatible surface modified circuits may be useful/effect at attenuating the systemic inflammatory response to cardiopulmonary bypass and improve outcomes (Class IIa, Level B).

From Shann KG, Likosky DS, Murkin JM, et al. An evidence-based review of the practice of cardiopulmonary bypass in adults: A focus on neurologic injury, glycemic control, hemodilution, and the inflammatory response. *J Thorac Cardiovasc Surg.* 2006; 132:283–290.

which may occur during dislocation of the heart (particularly with use of a single two-stage cannula), cerebral venous hypertension may occur. Because atrial drainage is unimpaired, CVP measured from the atrium will be low; hence, this condition may be unrecognized. If sustained, cerebral venous hypertension can lead to cerebral edema and substantially decreased CPP, despite apparently adequate MAP (see Fig. 24.6). NIRS cerebral oximetry has been demonstrated to rapidly detect such events when cerebral desaturation occurs. **During CPB, cerebral venous pressure should be monitored by a catheter placed proximally (usually pulmonary artery catheter introducer sheath) in the SVC and by visual inspection of the face.**

VI. Prevention of CNS injury. As discussed in detail below, Table 24.7 shows a series of evidence-based recommendations designed to limit the risk of perioperative cerebral injury in cardiac surgical patients [26]. Table 24.8 outlines specific interventions designed to limit or avoid particular risk factors.

A. Embolic load

1. Aortic instrumentation

a. Although still the standard of care, palpation of the aorta has not proven sensitive to detect aortic atherosclerosis. Direct EAS scan of ascending aorta is the most sensitive technique for assessment of atherosclerotic burden. Alternatively, initial TEE screening of descending aorta, followed by EAS if TEE detects descending aortic atherosclerosis, represents an acceptable screening strategy. With extensive aortic atherosclerosis, distal aortic arch or axillary artery cannulation should be considered.

b. Minimize the number of aortic clampings. Use of all arterial grafts (e.g., mammary, gastroepiploic) or sutureless proximal anastomotic devices eliminates the need for aortic side clamping for proximal anastomoses. In cases of severe atherosclerosis, "no touch" techniques (OPCAB with zero manipulation of the ascending aorta) have been shown to significantly decrease stroke rate [27].

B. Off-pump versus conventional CAB

In one of the most recent meta-analyses of risk of stroke in OPCAB versus conventional on-pump CAB (CCAB) surgery, analysis of 59 most recent randomized clinical trials involving 8,961 patients, of whom 4,461 patients underwent OPCAB and 4,500 were randomized to

TABLE 24.8 Perioperative strategies minimize CNS brain injury

Mechanism of brain injury	Favorable intervention
Embolism	Epiaortic ultrasound No-touch technique in severe aortic atherosclerosis Dispersion aortic cannula Intra-aortic filters Cell saver for shed blood Early postoperative DW-MRI in high-risk patients
Hypoperfusion	Preoperative carotid Doppler in high-risk patients High intraoperative arterial BP (emerging consensus to maintain MAP >70 mm Hg during normothermic and tepid CPB) Monitor SVP and MAP simultaneously (CPP) NIRS cerebral oximetry Early postoperative DW-MRI in high-risk patients
Inflammation	Minimal-volume CPB circuit Surface-modified CPB circuit Minimize allogeneic transfusion Perioperative statin administration
Aggravating factors	Labile perfusion pressures Rewarming and postoperative hyperthermia Hyperglycemia Postoperative atrial fibrillation

The interventions have been classified according to corresponding mechanisms of injury.
DW-MRI, diffusion-weighted magnetic resonance; SVP, superior vena cava pressure; BP, blood pressure; MAP, median systemic arterial pressure; CPB, cardiopulmonary bypass; CPP, cerebral perfusion pressure; NIRS, near-infrared spectroscopy.

CCAB, determined a significant difference in composite stroke incidence of 1.4% in OPCAB versus 2.1% in CCAB groups [28]. Not inconsistent with this result, no studies have reported a higher stroke risk with OPCAB but have shown either no effect or a trend for decreased stroke rate associated with OPCAB. Accordingly, selective use of OPCAB for patients at increased risk of stroke related to aortic atherosclerosis would appear to be an important strategy to minimize early stroke risk.

1. **Perfusion equipment and techniques**
   - **a.** Precirculation of CPB circuit for a minimum of 30 min with a 5 μm filter before usage removes plasticizers and other manufacturing microdebris.
   - **b.** Incorporation of a micropore (20 to 40 μm) filter into the cardiotomy return line keeps tissue and other particulate debris from the surgical field out of the CPB circuit.
   - **c.** Retransfusion of cardiotomy suction blood after processing using cell saver. Of note, while this may decrease embolic load it has not been consistently shown to improve early postoperative cognitive outcomes but has been associated with increased transfusion requirements.
   - **d.** Use of a 40 μm filter on the arterial inflow line decreases delivery of emboli into the arterial circulation.
   - **e.** To minimize gas bubble formation due to decreased solubility with rewarming, the temperature gradient between the arterial inflow blood and the patient must be less than 10°C, particularly with use of a bubble oxygenator.
   - **f.** During rewarming, arterial blood inflow temperature must not exceed 37°C.
   - **g.** Be aware of the possibility of air entrainment from cardiac vents in the surgical field, and ensure meticulous deairing of CPB venous cannulae and syringes for injection into the CPB circuitry to decrease arterial gas embolization.
2. **Open-chamber deairing techniques**
   - **a.** Before ventricular ejection, needle aspiration of the LV and LA, combined with manual agitation of the heart, to dislodge air entrapped in trabeculae. This process should be

combined with concomitant manual ventilation of the lungs to mobilize residual air within the pulmonary veins.

b. Use of TEE to detect residual intracavitary air and to direct needle aspirations.

c. Tilting the patient's head down. This procedure achieves a dependent position of the great vessels of the head and is thought to minimize cerebral embolization although evidence for its efficacy is lacking.

d. Transient bilateral carotid compression during defibrillation and initial filling and commencement of heart ejection. This maneuver should be reserved for instances where the risk of intracavitary air remains high and there is no suspicion of carotid atherosclerosis.

C. Cerebral perfusion. In normal individuals during moderate hypothermia, relative hypotension is well tolerated because cerebral autoregulation is preserved down to CPP 20 mm Hg with α-stat blood gas management. However, in elderly patients or those with cerebrovascular disease, higher pressure should be maintained as the lower autoregulatory threshold has been shown to vary markedly in such patients [12,14]. As assessed by NPT, the brain rewarms rapidly; therefore, hypotension (MAP less than 50 mm Hg) should be avoided after commencement of rewarming in all patients. Inadvertent compromise of CPP should also be avoided by monitoring proximal SVC pressure to detect cerebral venous hypertension. Diabetics and patients with previous CVA have impaired cerebral autoregulation and CBF is directly dependent on MAP. Such patients, as well as those with chronic hypertension, may benefit from close CNS monitoring (see previous discussion) and maintenance of higher perfusion pressures.

D. Euglycemia. There is considerable evidence from experimental models and from patients with CVA that hyperglycemia increases the magnitude and extent of neurologic injury during ischemia. Hyperglycemia should be avoided as a basic approach. **Glucose-free infusions and a glucose-free prime should be used for CPB circuit**, because insulin resistance develops during CPB (partially as a result of increased endogenous catecholamines), producing glucose intolerance and increasing the tendency for refractory hyperglycemia. A structured approach to maintain normal values of blood glucose is considered favorable to patients' outcomes and is a recognized element of best practice CPB guidelines as shown in Table 24.7 [26].

E. Mild hypothermia. There is increasing evidence showing that EAAs are pivotal in the genesis of ischemic neurologic injury (see preceding discussion). Since EAA synthesis and release are critically temperature dependent and are significantly inhibited below 35°C [20], brain temperature (NPT) should be monitored continuously during rewarming, **hyperthermia (NPT greater than 37°C) must be avoided**, and brain temperature should be maintained less than 37°C until after separating from CPB and decannulation [26].

F. Best practice CPB. Recommendations from an **evidence-based review** for conducting safe, patient-centered CPB as based on a structured MEDLINE search coupled with a critical review of scientific literature and debates stemming from presentations at regional and national conferences, with the level of evidence and **finding**s graded using criteria promulgated by the American Heart Association and American College of Cardiology Task Force on Practice Guidelines, are shown in Table 24.7 [26].

VII. Pharmacologic cerebral protection

Despite a profound and ongoing increase in the understanding of the mechanisms involved in ischemic neuronal injury and the development of new classes of drugs, currently none represent a standard of practice; but these or related compounds may become part of the therapeutic armamentarium in the near future.

A. Metabolic suppression

1. Rationale and limitations. Metabolic activity is temperature dependent, and hypothermia produces an exponential decrease in CMR. Unlike pharmacologic metabolic suppressants, hypothermia decreases metabolic activity related both to functional activity (e.g., EEG activity) and basal activity (e.g., ion pumps). Hypothermia prolongs the tolerance for global ischemia (Fig. 24.9) and is undertaken particularly for circulatory arrest (see following discussion). During cardiac surgery, however, greatest risk for cerebral emboli occurs during normothermia with cannulation and decannulation; hence, pharmacologic metabolic suppressants have been investigated. While there was previously some interest

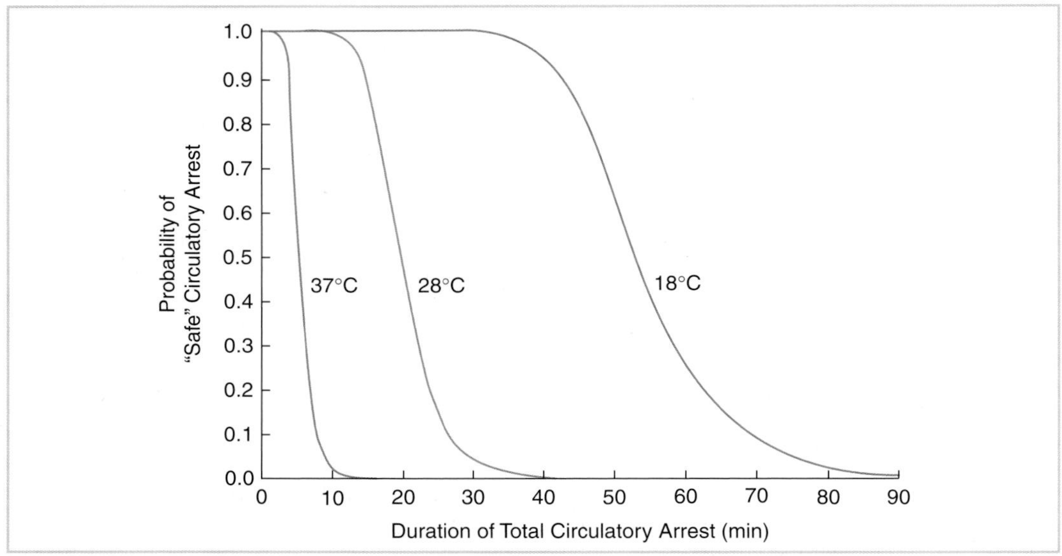

FIGURE 24.9 Nomogram of probability of "safe" total circulatory arrest according to duration of total arrest time as NPTs of 37°C, 28°C, and 18°C, defined as the duration of total arrest after which no structural or functional damage has occurred. (From Kirklin JK, Kirklin JW, Pacifico AD. Deep hypothermia and total circulatory arrest. In: Arciniegas E, ed. *Pediatric Cardiac Surgery.* Chicago, IL: Year Book; 1985:79–85, with permission.)

in high-dose thiopental, no consistent clinical benefit was demonstrated likely since any potential benefit resulting from such therapy was derived from the suppression of CMR associated with suppression of synaptic activity which would likely result only in prolongation of ischemia tolerance of a very few minutes.

2. **Agents.** As shown in Figure 24.10, various anesthetics have the ability to produce EEG burst suppression and result in profound decreases in CMR to approximately 50% of awake $CMRO_2$, averaging 25 mL/(100 g·min).
   a. **Thiopental.** A dosage of 5 to 8 mg/kg results in 5 min of EEG suppression at normothermia. Proportional decreases in both CBF and $CMRO_2$ are produced. An infusion at 0.5 to 1 mg/(kg·min) is required for prolonged EEG suppression, results in prolonged recovery and extubation times, and may increase the need for inotropic support because of myocardial depression.
   b. **Propofol.** Transient EEG burst suppression is obtained at dosages of 2 to 3 mg/kg and results in proportional decreases in CBF and $CMRo_2$. Infusion at 0.1 to 0.3 mg/(kg·min) produces sustained EEG suppression and is rapidly metabolized; therefore, it does not prolong recovery and extubation times. Hypotension from systemic vasodilation may require administration of phenylephrine or other such vasoconstrictor.
   c. **Sevoflurane and Deflurane.** At inspired concentrations of 1.5 to 2 MAC, burst suppression is produced. Unlike the intravenous agents, EEG suppression with inhalational agents is not accomplished by any decrease in CBF, although $CMRo_2$ is significantly reduced. Rapid elimination is characteristic of volatile anesthetics. Of particular interest is the evidence of ischemic preconditioning and neuroprotection associated with administration of volatile anesthetics which have been variously demonstrated to decrease glutamate release, modulate calcium flux, and inhibit generation of free radicals as well as modulate apoptosis [29]. Large-scale clinical studies are currently lacking but it does appear as though usage of volatile anesthetics does not increase and may have a salutary effect on postoperative CNS dysfunction.

B. **Calcium-channel blockers.** Massive calcium influx is likely the final common pathway of ischemic neuronal injury (see preceding comments). In clinical trials, calcium-channel

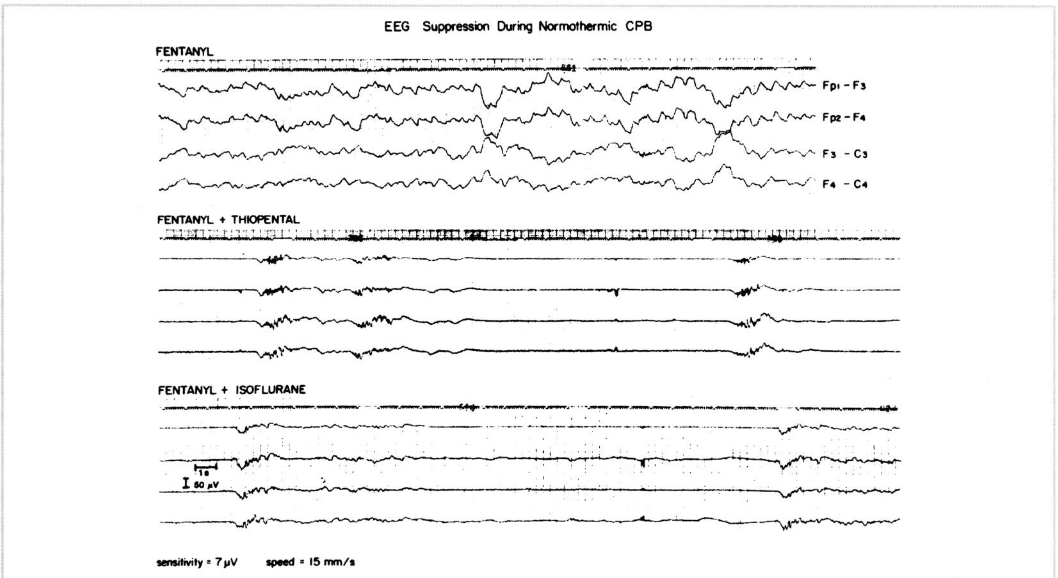

FIGURE 24.10 EEG tracings from three patients during normothermic CPB. The *top tracing* demonstrates characteristic low-voltage activity occurring during high-dose fentanyl anesthesia. The *middle tracing* shows the burst-suppression pattern resulting from thiopental administration. The *lower pattern* demonstrates burst suppression occurring during isoflurane administration. (From Woodcock TE, Murkin JM, Gentile PS, et al. Pharmacologic EEG suppression during cardiopulmonary bypass: Cerebral hemodynamic and metabolic effects of thiopental or isoflurane during hypothermia and normothermia. *Anesthesiology.* 1987;67:218–224, with permission.)

antagonists (nimodipine) have demonstrated efficacy in decreasing vasospasm after subarachnoid hemorrhage; however, nimodipine also has been associated with increased bleeding and higher mortality in cardiac surgical patients.

C. **Glutamate antagonists.** Since excitotoxicity is recognized as central to ischemic neuronal injury (see previous discussion), EAA receptor antagonists are being actively investigated. NMDA and AMPA receptor antagonists have been found to be neuroprotective following cardiac arrest but clinical studies in cardiac surgical patients remain inconclusive [30].

D. **Lidocaine.** Given its ability to decrease ischemia-mediated neuronal membrane depolarization and attendant excitotoxic cascades, two small clinical trials of lidocaine versus placebo have demonstrated lowered incidences of cognitive dysfunction in cardiac surgical patients. However, preliminary results from a larger clinical trial have been unable to confirm these results.

E. **Statins:** An increasingly promising line of investigation is the role of perioperative statin therapy, either alone or in combination with other medications. Evidence is accruing that when administered prior to CAB surgery, statins reduce the risk of perioperative mortality, stroke, and atrial fibrillation, and when combined with β-blocker administration there is suggestive evidence that statins may result in a significantly decreased risk of perioperative stroke in CAB patients [21]. Whether these results will be borne out in large-scale prospective studies is currently unclear but current evidence suggests that benefits seem to outweigh the risks associated with their use, both in the preoperative and postoperative period.

VIII. DHCA

A. **Clinical indications.** DHCA sometimes is used for major surgical procedures because it provides a motionless, cannula-free, bloodless field. By allowing unobstructed surgical access, DHCA facilitates repair of complex congenital anomalies in neonates and infants. In adults, DHCA allows temporary interruption of cerebral perfusion, primarily for aortic arch reconstruction or for resection of giant cerebral aneurysms.

B. Technique

1. **Core and external cooling.** In most North American centers, active external cooling (e.g., ice baths) has been eliminated but packing the head in ice is still recommended to inhibit secondary rewarming prior to onset of reperfusion. Core cooling using CPB allows efficient and controlled onset of hypothermia, and cooling persists until core temperature (bladder, rectal) is stable at 15 to 20°C. Cooling must be continued until stable brain temperature (e.g., NPT, jugular thermistry) has been achieved. Some centers use development of isoelectric EEG as the endpoint for cooling, necessitating careful selection and titration of anesthetic agents.
2. **Decannulation.** Before circulatory arrest, administration of long-acting muscle relaxants is essential to ensure profound paralysis in order to minimize systemic O_2 consumption. With cessation of perfusion, venous cannulas are unclamped, allowing passive exsanguinations into the CPB circuit and decreasing distention of the heart and bleeding into the surgical site. For pediatric surgery, venous cannulas are usually removed to facilitate surgical exposure. Often passive circulation of blood within the CPB circuit is continued ex vivo to avoid stasis and setting of blood with platelet clumping.

C. Brain protection

1. **Temperature.** Hypothermia is the primary component of brain protection during circulatory arrest. The temperature coefficient (Q_{10}), which is the ratio of metabolic rates at temperatures 10°C apart, has been shown to be 2.3 for human brain such that CMR is still 17% of baseline at 15°C [31]. A 20°C (37 to 17°C) decrease in brain temperature enhances cerebral tolerance for ischemia (see Fig. 24.9). Cooling the patient to a temperature of 10 to 15°C seems to offer the best protection to the brain. Minimizing rewarming of the brain is essential; therefore, external heat sources (e.g., overhead lights, ambient room temperature) should be minimized. Application of external ice packs to the head has been shown experimentally to delay brain rewarming and increase ischemic tolerance. Thiopental and/or steroids are administered before circulatory arrest in some centers, although any beneficial effect is unproven.
2. **Anterograde and retrograde perfusion.** Because of cerebral autoregulation with preferential shunting of blood to the brain, even low perfusion rates (e.g., 10 to 25 mL·kg·min) during deep hypothermia have been shown to significantly improve cerebral ischemic tolerance in comparison to total circulatory arrest. A prospective randomized study has shown that continuous low-flow perfusion (0.71/min·m^2) at 18°C for pediatric patients younger than 3 months undergoing arterial switch operations results in significantly lower incidences of clinical seizures and brain creatinine kinase isoenzyme versus HCA and is now the standard of care.

   For aortic arch procedures in which arterial inflow is restricted, selective cerebral perfusion (SCP) via brachiocephalic or carotid perfusion is employed in many centers. Since these techniques assume adequacy of circle of Willis, there is increasing clinical interest in bihemispheric NIRS cerebral oximetry to assess adequacy of unilateral SCP. NIRS cerebral oximetry has been reported to detect catheter kinking or inadequacy of flow in a number of cases. Retrograde cerebral perfusion does not provide sufficient substrate supply to maintain brain metabolic demand but may prevent rewarming and decrease cerebral embolization. In a recent case report, RCP with pressure-augmented perfusion guided by cNIRS was felt to provide enhanced cerebral perfusion and was not associated with neurologic deficit despite prolonged duration of perfusion [32]. There is general clinical consensus that cerebral oximetry monitoring is beneficial when SCP or RCP is employed.
3. **pH management.** Although in a large randomized clinical trial, use of α-stat versus pH-stat acid–base management strategy during reparative infant cardiac operations with deep hypothermic CPB was not consistently related to either improved or impaired early neurodevelopmental outcomes, experimental and clinical studies have demonstrated more homogeneous brain cooling with pH-stat. Conversely, pH-stat impairs cerebral autoregulation and potentially increases cerebral embolization; therefore, a considered approach is to employ pH-stat during cooling and α-stat during rewarming.

TABLE 24.9 Summary of deep hypothermic circulatory arrest (DHCA)

1. Administer muscle relaxants prior to DHCA.
2. Cool until stable core (NPT) is achieved.
3. Eliminate glucose from solutions and pump prime.
4. Minimize ambient room temperature.
5. Place external ice packs around head.
6. Continuously monitor NPT during DHCA.
7. Use intermittent- or low-flow perfusion when possible.
8. Minimize duration of DHCA.
9. Ensure adequate anticoagulation prior to DHCA.
10. pH-stat during cooling, α-stat during rewarming
11. Cerebral oximetry with use of RCP or SCP

D. Summary (Table 24.9)

IX. Cardiac surgery in patients with cerebrovascular disease

A. Incidence. Coronary atherosclerosis increases the likelihood of coexisting carotid arteriopathy. Presence or absence of carotid bruits is a poor predictor of carotid stenosis or the risks of perioperative stroke. In a survey of patients undergoing CABG, 5.5% showed significant unilateral carotid stenosis, 2.2% had bilateral stenoses, and 1.5% of patients had unilateral or bilateral carotid occlusion. Another study of over 200 CABG patients demonstrated a 54% incidence of significant cerebrovascular (carotid or intracranial) atherosclerosis preoperatively [19]. In general, however, noninvasive (ultrasonography) and invasive (contrast arteriography) investigations are usually reserved for patients who have had overt symptoms of cerebrovascular insufficiency (e.g., transient ischemic attacks or stroke) during the previous 3 to 6 months [33]. In part, this reflects the clinical recognition that carotid endarterectomy (CEA) does not appreciably reduce risk of perioperative CVA in cardiac surgical patients (see later) [33].

B. Morbidity. Neurologic injury associated with cardiovascular surgery is a consequence of both cerebral emboli and hypoperfusion. Carotid disease is an important etiologic factor in the pathophysiology of post-CAB stroke but is probably only responsible for, at most, about 50% of all strokes [1,33]. Carotid stenosis is associated with a greater incidence of aortic atherosclerosis and concomitant cerebrovascular disease. The presence of combined carotid and cardiac disease suggests more advanced and severe atherosclerosis and a higher risk of embolization and/or hypoperfusion during cardiac surgery and emphasizes the role of adequate intraoperative management (e.g., neuromonitoring and avoidance of hypoperfusion) in susceptible patients.

C. Combined carotid and cardiac procedures

1. **Rationale.** Indications for CEA and CAB should be considered independently. There is no compelling evidence that, in the absence of significant symptomatology, CEA decreases perioperative stroke risk [1,33]. The role of carotid stenting is promising and remains to be defined. Approximately 9% to 11% of patients undergoing either staged or synchronous procedures will die or suffer a nonfatal stroke/MI in the perioperative period. Prospective community-based studies have reported the worst outcomes [1,33].
2. **Morbidity.** In asymptomatic patients CEA does not decrease perioperative stroke risk. The reported combined risk of death, CVA, and MI for synchronous procedures (CEA + CAB) is 11.5%, and for staged procedures (CEA then CAB) it is 10.2%, suggesting that institutional experience is of primary importance. Because of the paucity of natural history data, there is no systematic evidence that staged or synchronous operations confer any benefit over isolated CAB surgery [1,33].

   As such, while there is a strong correlation between risk of perioperative stroke and presence of carotid stenosis, it is not clear that CEA in any way mitigates this risk. In a meta-analysis of 11 studies in which 760 CAB patients underwent either staged or synchronous CAB plus CEA, it was noted that 87% of the patients were neurologically asymptomatic and 82% had unilateral carotid disease [34]. Overall, the 30-day risk of death or stroke was

9.1% and while it was observed that staged CAB then CEA was considered less invasive, the authors concluded that "it remains questionable whether the observed 9% risks of CEA can be justified in any **asymptomatic** patient with unilateral carotid disease" [34].

X. Summary

There is an evidence-based rationale in support of a number of procedural and technical modifications that have been shown to decrease perioperative CNS complications. Avoidance of instrumentation of ascending aortic atheroma by enhanced screening techniques (e.g., preoperative MRI, intraoperative EAS) and selective use of OPCAB and no-touch techniques for patients with significant aortic atherosclerosis, more judicious use of cerebral monitoring and NIRS for assessing adequacy of cerebral perfusion during CPB, avoidance of cerebral hyperthermia during rewarming on CPB and postoperatively, attenuation of perioperative and CPB-related inflammatory responses, enhanced usage of techniques to decrease postoperative atrial fibrillation, as well as administration of aspirin and statins throughout the perioperative period have all been shown as efficacious in decreasing perioperative CNS complications. The challenge is to better understand which patients are at increased risk and to encourage more widespread assessment and adoption of these various strategies.

REFERENCES

1. Serruys PW, Morice MC, Kappetein AP, et al; SYNTAX Investigators. Percutaneous coronary intervention versus coronary-artery bypass grafting for severe coronary artery disease. *N Engl J Med.* 2009;360:961–972.
2. Bronster DJ. Neurologic complications of cardiac surgery: Current concepts and recent advances. *Curr Cardiol Rep.* 2006;8:9–16.
3. Arrowsmith JE, Grocott H, Reves JG, et al. Central nervous system complications of cardiac surgery. *Br J Anaesth.* 2000;84:378–393.
4. Nishiyama K, Horiguchi M, Shizuta S, et al. Temporal pattern of strokes after on-pump and off-pump coronary artery bypass graft surgery. *Ann Thorac Surg.* 2009;87:1839–1844.
5. Hedberg M, Boivie P, Engström KG. Early and delayed stroke after coronary surgery - An analysis of risk factors and the impact on short- and long-term survival. *Eur J Cardiothorac Surg.* 2011;40:379–387.
6. Dacey LJ, Likosky DS, Leavitt BJ, et al. Perioperative stroke and long-term survival after coronary bypass graft surgery. *Ann Thorac Surg.* 2005;79:532–536.
7. Newman MF, Kirchner JL, Phillips-Bute B, et al. Neurological Outcome Research Group and the Cardiothoracic Anesthesiology Research Endeavors Investigators. Longitudinal assessment of neurocognitive function after coronary-artery bypass surgery. *N Engl J Med.* 2001;344:395–402.
8. Selnes OA, Grega MA, Bailey MM, et al. Do management strategies for coronary artery disease influence 6-year cognitive outcomes? *Ann Thorac Surg.* 2009;88:445–454.
9. Sellke FW, DiMaio JM, Caplan LR, et al. Comparing on-pump and off-pump coronary artery bypass grafting: Numerous studies but few conclusions: A scientific statement from the American Heart Association council on cardiovascular surgery and anesthesia in collaboration with the interdisciplinary working group on quality of care and outcomes research. *Circulation.* 2005;111:2858–2864.
10. Barber PA, Hach S, Tippett LJ, et al. Cerebral ischemic lesions on diffusion-weighted imaging are associated with neurocognitive decline after cardiac surgery. *Stroke.* 2008;39:1427–1433.
11. Grigore AM, Grocott HP, Mathew JP, et al. The rewarming rate and increased peak temperature alter neurocognitive outcome after cardiac surgery. *Anesth Analg.* 2002;94:4–10.
12. Brady K, Joshi B, Zweifel C, et al. Real-time continuous monitoring of cerebral blood flow autoregulation using near-infrared spectroscopy in patients undergoing cardiopulmonary bypass. *Stroke.* 2010;41:1951–1956.
13. Joshi B, Brady K, Lee J, et al. Impaired autoregulation of cerebral blood flow during rewarming from hypothermic cardiopulmonary bypass and its potential association with stroke. *Anesth Analg.* 2010;110:321–328.
14. Murkin JM, Martzke JS, Buchan AM, et al. A randomized study of the influence of perfusion technique and pH management strategy in 316 patients undergoing coronary artery bypass surgery. II. Neurologic and cognitive outcomes. *J Thorac Cardiovasc Surg.* 1995;110:349–362.
15. Ryu KH, Hindman BJ, Reasoner DK, et al. Heparin reduces neurological impairment after cerebral arterial air embolism in the rabbit. *Stroke.* 1996;27:303–309.
16. Ura M, Sakata R, Nakayama Y, et al. Ultrasonographic demonstration of manipulation-related aortic injuries after cardiac surgery. *J Am Coll Cardiol.* 2000;35:1303–1310.
17. Murkin JM, Baird DL, Martzke JS, et al. Cognitive dysfunction after ventricular fibrillation during implantable cardiovertor/defibrillator procedures is related to duration of the reperfusion interval. *Anesth Analg.* 1997;84:1186–1192.
18. Yoon BW, Bae HJ, Kang DW, et al. Intracranial cerebral artery disease as a risk factor for central nervous system complications of coronary artery bypass graft surgery. *Stroke.* 2001;32:94–99.
19. Auriel E, Bornstein NM. Neuroprotection in acute ischemic stroke–current status. *J Cell Mol Med.* 2010;14:2200–2202.
20. Grau AJ, Boddy AW, Dukovic DA, et al; CAPRIE Investigators. Leukocyte count as an independent predictor of recurrent ischemic events. 2004;35:1147–1152.
21. Albert AA, Beller CJ, Walter JA, et al. Preoperative high leukocyte count: A novel risk factor for stroke after cardiac surgery. *Ann Thorac Surg.* 2003;75:1550–1557.

22. Murkin JM, Adams SJ, Novick RJ, et al. Monitoring brain oxygen saturation during coronary bypass surgery: A randomized, prospective study. *Anesth Analg.* 2007;104(1):51–58.
23. Heringlake M, Garbers C, Käbler JH, et al. Preoperative cerebral oxygen saturation and clinical outcomes in cardiac surgery. *Anesthesiology.* 2011;114:58–69.
24. Murkin JM, Arango M. Near-infrared spectroscopy as an index of brain and tissue oxygenation. *Br J Anaesth.* 2009;103(suppl 1): i3–i13.
25. Highton D, Elwell C, Smith M. Noninvasive cerebral oximetry: Is there light at the end of the tunnel? *Curr Opin Anaesthesiol.* 2010;23(5):576–581.
26. Shann KG, Likosky DS, Murkin JM, et al. An evidence-based review of the practice of cardiopulmonary bypass in adults: A focus on neurologic injury, glycemic control, hemodilution, and the inflammatory response. *J Thorac Cardiovasc Surg.* 2006;132:283–290.
27. Bergman P, Hadjinikolaou L, Dellgren G, et al. A policy to reduce stroke in patients with extensive atherosclerosis of the ascending aorta undergoing coronary surgery. *Interact Cardiovasc Thorac Surg.* 2004;3:28–32.
28. Afilalo J, Rasti M, Ohayon SM, et al. Off-pump vs. on-pump coronary artery bypass surgery: An updated meta-analysis and meta-regression of randomized trials. *Eur Heart J.* 2011 Oct 10. [Epub ahead of print]
29. Yu Q, Wang H, Chen J, et al. Neuroprotections and mechanisms of inhalational anesthetics against brain ischemia. *Front Biosci (Elite Ed).* 2010;2:1275–1298.
30. Bhutta AT, Schmitz ML, Swearingen C, et al. Ketamine as a neuroprotective and anti-inflammatory agent in children undergoing surgery on cardiopulmonary bypass: A pilot randomized, double-blind, placebo-controlled trial. *Pediatr Crit Care Med.* 2011 Sep 15. [Epub ahead of print]
31. Bouchard D, Carrier M, Demers P, et al. Statin in combination with β-blocker therapy reduces postoperative stroke after coronary artery bypass graft surgery. *Ann Thorac Surg.* 2011;91:654–659.
32. Murkin JM. Pathophysiological basis of CNS injury in cardiac surgical patients: Detection and prevention. *Perfusion.* 2006;21:203–208.
33. Kubota H, Tonari K, Endo H, et al. Total aortic arch replacement under intermittent pressure-augmented retrograde cerebral perfusion. *J Cardiothorac Surg.* 2010;5:97.
34. Naylor AR, Bown MJ. Stroke after cardiac surgery and its association with asymptomatic carotid disease: An updated systematic review and meta-analysis. *Eur J Vasc Endovasc Surg.* 2011;41:607–624.
35. Naylor AR, Mehta Z, Rothwell PM. A systematic review and meta-analysis of 30-day outcomes following staged carotid artery stenting. *Eur J Vasc Endovasc Surg.* 2009;37:379–387.

V THORACIC ANESTHESIA AND PAIN MANAGEMENT

25 Anesthetic Management for Thoracic Aortic Aneurysms and Dissections

Amanda A. Fox and John R. Cooper, Jr.

KEY POINTS

1. An aortic dissection usually occurs when blood penetrates the aortic intima, forming either an expanding hematoma within the aortic wall or simply a false channel for blood flow between the medial layer.
2. An aortic aneurysm involves dilation of all three layers of the aortic wall.
3. The term dissecting aneurysm, although commonly used, is often a misnomer because the aorta may not be dilated.
4. Nitroprusside, a potent arterial dilator, and a β-blocker to decrease LV ejection velocity are critical to prevent further propagation of aortic dissection, rupture of a torn aorta, or leaking thoracic aortic aneurysm.
5. Aortic valve repair or replacement is often needed with repair of aortic dissections or aneurysms. Which procedure is used depends on involvement of the sinus of Valsalva and the aortic annulus.

(*continued*)

6. Management of left heart bypass (LHB) can be very challenging for the cardiac anesthesiologist while repairing descending thoracic aneurysms or aortic tears (see Table 25.12). TEE is very useful to guide volume management, as native cardiac output must be preserved to provide adequate blood flow to the brain.
7. Cerebral spinal drainage has been shown to significantly decrease postoperative paraplegia and paraparesis in a randomized controlled trial in patients undergoing descending thoracic surgery.

ANESTHESIOLOGISTS CARING FOR THORACIC AORTIC surgical patients encounter considerable variation between patients with regard to the cause and location of aortic disease. It is vital that anesthesiologists understand the implications of and the challenges related to these variations in providing optimal perioperative care. Members of both the American Society of Anesthesiologists and the Society of Cardiovascular Anesthesiologists were involved in the multidisciplinary development of the 2010 ACCF/AHA/AATS/ACR/ASA/SCA/SCAI/SIR/STS/SVM Guidelines for the Diagnosis and Management of Patients with Thoracic Aortic Disease [1]. This chapter gives a concise overview of the pathophysiology of thoracic aortic surgery, a review of its surgical approaches and results, and a rational approach to managing patients undergoing thoracic aortic surgery. Surgery on the thoracic aorta and, in particular, the descending and thoracoabdominal aorta may obviously involve complicated surgical and anesthetic management. Therefore, each team member must have a clear understanding of what is being planned. Often, all that is required is a brief preoperative conversation between the surgeon and the anesthesiologist as to the exact requirements for a particular procedure.

I. Classification and natural history

1 **A. Dissections.** An **aortic dissection** usually occurs when blood penetrates the aortic intima, forming either an expanding hematoma within the aortic wall or simply a false channel for flow between the medial layers. (This expanding hematoma may be called a dissecting hematoma.) The true lumen of the dissecting aorta is generally not dilated; rather, it is often compressed by the dissection. Because the dissection does not necessarily involve the entire circumference of the aorta, branching vessels may be not affected, they may be occluded, or they may arise
2 from the false lumen. In contrast, an **aortic aneurysm** involves dilation of all three layers of the aortic wall and has different pathophysiology and management concerns. The term **dissecting**
3 **aneurysm**, although commonly used, is often a misnomer because the aorta may not be dilated.

1. Incidence and pathophysiology

a. Incidence. The incidence of dissection in the United States is unclear mainly because of under-reporting; however, European studies have reported an incidence of 3.2 dissections per 100,000 autopsies, with increasing numbers over time. Also, dissections resulted in more deaths than did aneurysm rupture [2].

b. Predisposing conditions. The medical conditions predisposing to aortic dissection are listed in Table 25.1 in their order of importance. Interestingly, **atherosclerosis** by itself may not contribute to the risk of subsequent aortic dissection.

c. Inciting event. The onset of aortic dissections has been associated with increased physical activity or emotional stress. Dissections also have been associated with blunt trauma

TABLE 25.1 Conditions predisposing to aortic dissections

History of hypertension	Present in ~90% of patients
Advanced age	>60 yrs
Sex	Male preponderance age <60 yrs
Arachnodactyly (Marfan syndrome)	Also other connective tissue diseases
Congenital heart disease	Coarctation of aorta, bicuspid aortic valve
Pregnancy	Uncommon
Other causes	Toxins and diet

TABLE 25.2 Sites of primary intimal tears in acute dissections of the aorta (398 autopsy cases)

Site	Percent incidence
Ascending	61
Descending	24
Isthmus	16
Other	8
Arch	9
Abdominal	3
Other	1

Modified from Hirst AE Jr, Johns VJ Jr, Kime W Jr. Dissecting aneurysm of the aorta: A review of 505 cases. *Medicine.* 1958;37:243.

to the chest; however, the temporal relationship of blunt trauma and subsequent dissections has not been well established. Dissections can occur without any physical activity. They may also occur during cannulation for cardiopulmonary bypass (CPB), either antegrade from the ascending aorta or retrograde from the femoral artery.

d. **Mechanism of aortic tear.** An intimal tear is the initial event in aortic dissection. The intimal tear of aortic dissections usually occurs in the presence of a weakened aortic wall, predominantly involving the middle and outer layers of the media. In this area of weakening, the aortic wall is more susceptible to shear forces produced by pulsatile blood flow in the aorta. The most frequent locations of intimal tears are the areas experiencing the greatest mechanical shear forces, as listed in Table 25.2. The ascending and isthmic (just distal to the left subclavian artery) segments of the aorta are relatively fixed and thus subject the aortic wall to the greatest amount of mechanical shear stress. This explains the high incidence of intimal tears in these areas.

   In large autopsy series, however, up to 4% of dissections had no identifiable intimal disruption. In these cases, rupture of the **vasa vasorum**, the vessels that supply blood to the aortic wall, has been implicated as an alternative cause of dissections. The thin-walled vasa vasorum are located in the outer third of the aortic wall, and their rupture would cause the formation of a medial hematoma and propagation of a dissection in the presence of an already diseased vessel, without formation of an intimal tear.

e. **Propagation.** Propagation of an aortic dissection can occur within seconds. The factors that contribute to propagation are the hemodynamic forces inherent in pulsatile flow: pulse pressure and ejection velocity of blood.

f. **Exit points.** Exit points of dissections are found in a relatively small percentage of cases. Exit point tears usually occur distal to the intimal tear and represent points at which blood from the false lumen re-enters the true lumen. The presence or absence of an exit point does not appear to have an impact on the clinical course.

g. **Involvement of arterial branches.** The origins of the major branches of the aorta, including the coronary arteries, may be involved in aortic dissections. Their involvement ranges from branch vessel occlusion via mechanical compression by the false lumen or from propagation of the dissecting hematoma into the arterial branch. The incidence of involvement of arterial branches gathered from a large autopsy series is listed in Table 25.3 [3].

2. **DeBakey classification of dissections** (Fig. 25.1). This classification consists of three different types based upon the location of the intimal tear and which section of the aorta is involved.

   a. **Type I.** The intimal tear is located in the ascending portion, but the dissection involves all portions (ascending, arch, and descending) of the thoracic aorta.

   b. **Type II.** The intimal tear is in the ascending aorta, but the dissection involves the ascending aorta only, stopping before the takeoff of the innominate artery.

TABLE 25.3 Involvement of major arterial branches in aortic dissections

Artery	Percent incidence
Iliac	25.2
Common carotid	14.5
Innominate	12.9
Renal (either)	12.0
Left subclavian	10.9
Mesenteric	8.2
Coronary (either)	7.5
Intercostal	4.0
Celiac	3.2
Lumbar	1.6

Modified from Hirst AE Jr, Johns VJ Jr, Kime W Jr. Dissecting aneurysm of the aorta: A review of 505 cases. *Medicine.* 1958;37:243.

c. **Type III.** The intimal tear is located in the descending segment. If the dissection involves the descending portion of the thoracic aorta only, starting distal to the origin of the left subclavian artery and ending above the diaphragm, it is a Type III A. If the dissection propagates below the diaphragm, it is a Type III B. By definition, Type III dissections can extend proximally into the arch, but this is rare.

3. **Stanford (Daily) classification of dissections** (Fig. 25.2). This classification is simpler than DeBakey's and has more clinical relevance.
   a. **Type A.** Type A dissections are those that have any involvement of the ascending aorta, regardless of where the intimal tear is located and regardless of how far the dissection propagates. Clinically, Type A dissections run a more virulent course and are generally considered urgent or emergent cases.
   b. **Type B.** Type B dissections are those that involve the aorta distal to the origin of the left subclavian artery.

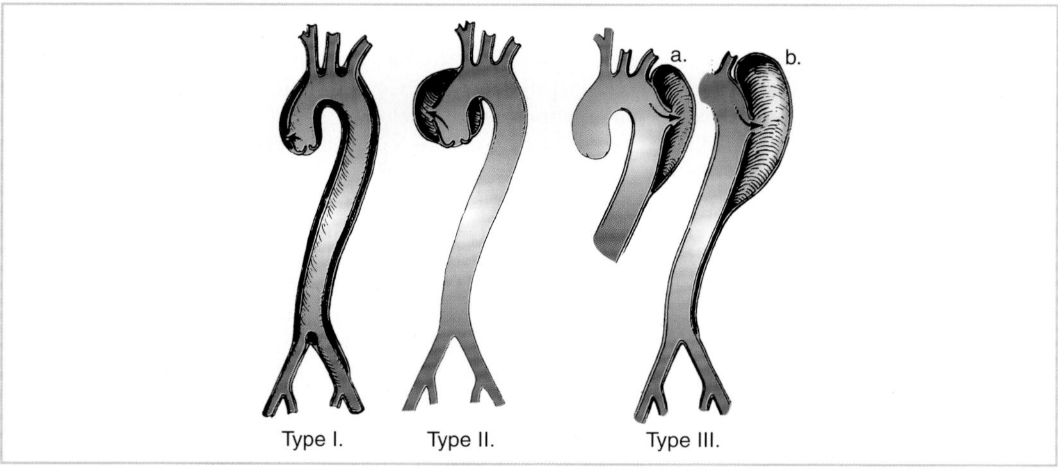

FIGURE 25.1 DeBakey classification of aortic dissections by location: Type I, with intimal tear in the ascending portion and dissection extending to descending aorta; Type II, ascending intimal tear and dissection limited to ascending aorta; Type III, intimal tear distal to left subclavian, but dissection extending for a variable distance, either to the diaphragm (a) or to the iliac artery (b). (From DeBakey ME, Henly WS, Cooley DA, et al. Surgical management of dissecting aneurysms of the aorta. *J Thorac Cardiovasc Surg.* 1965;49:131, with permission.)

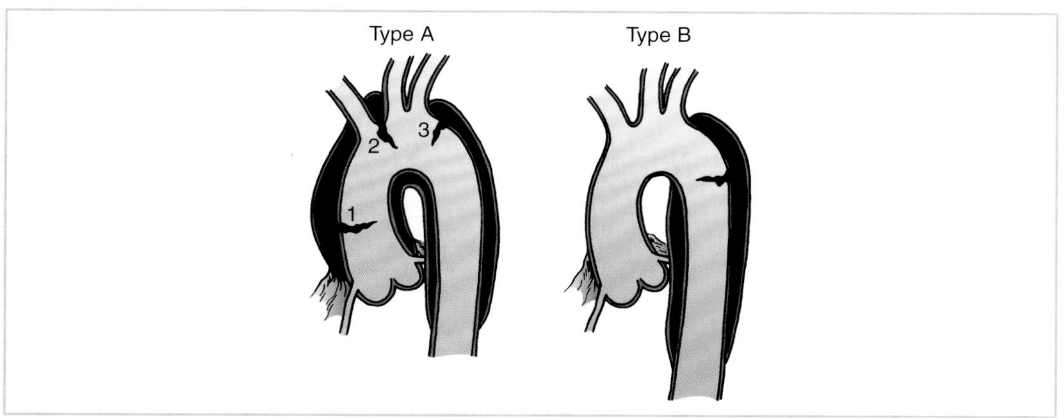

FIGURE 25.2 Stanford (Daily) classification of aortic dissections. Type A describes a dissection involving the ascending aorta regardless of site of intimal tear (*1,* ascending; *2,* arch; *3,* descending). In Type B, both the intimal tear and the extension are distal to the left subclavian. (From Miller DC, Stinson EB, Oyer PE, et al. Operative treatment of aortic dissections. Experience with 125 patients over a sixteen-year period. *J Thorac Cardiovasc Surg.* 1979;78:367, with permission.)

4. **Natural history**
   a. **Mortality—untreated.** The survival rate of untreated patients with ascending aortic dissections is dismal, with a 2-day mortality of up to 50% in some series and 3-month mortality approaching 90% [3]. The usual cause of death is rupture of the false lumen into the pleural space or pericardium. Mortality is lower with DeBakey Type III or Stanford B dissections. Other causes of death include progressive cardiac failure (aortic valve involvement), myocardial infarction (coronary artery involvement), stroke (occlusion of cerebral vessels), and bowel gangrene (mesenteric artery occlusion).
   b. **Surgical mortality.** Overall mortality ranges from 3% to 24% and varies with the section of aorta that is affected. Dissections involving the aortic arch carry the highest mortality, while those confined to the descending thoracic aorta carry the lowest [2].

B. **Aneurysms**
1. **Incidence.** The European studies cited above report an incidence of thoracic aneurysms in approximately 460 autopsies per 100,000. In one study, 45% of thoracic aneurysms involved the ascending aorta, 10% the arch, 35% the descending aorta, and 10% the thoracoabdominal aorta [4].
2. **Classification by location and cause.** In general, the causes and pathophysiology of aortic aneurysms are site dependent. Most commonly, medial degeneration affects the ascending aorta, while degenerative conditions associated with atherosclerosis affect the descending and thoracoabdominal portions of the aorta. Other causes are listed in Table 25.4.
3. **Classification by shape**
   a. **Fusiform.** Fusiform aneurysmal dilation involves the entire circumference of the aortic wall.
   b. **Saccular.** Saccular aneurysms involve only part of the circumference of the aortic wall. Isolated **aortic arch aneurysms** are commonly saccular.
4. **Natural history.** The natural history of aortic aneurysms is one of progressive dilation, with more than half of aortic aneurysms eventually rupturing. The untreated, 5-yr rate of survival for patients with thoracic aortic aneurysms ranges from 13% to 39% [2]. Other complications of thoracic aortic aneurysms include mycotic infection, atheroembolism to peripheral vessels, and dissection. This last complication is rare, probably occurring in fewer than 10% of cases. Some predictors of poor prognosis are large size (greater than 10 cm maximum transverse diameter), presence of symptoms, and associated cardiovascular disease, especially coronary artery disease, myocardial infarction, or cerebrovascular accident.

TABLE 25.4 Causes of aneurysms based on location in the aorta

Ascending	
Medial necrosis	Accumulation of mucoid material between elastic elements in the outer third of aortic wall, eventually involving the entire media
Syphilis	Major cause before 1950, distinguished by invasion of the aortic wall by *Treponema pallidum*
Congenital	Secondary to inborn errors in metabolism (Marfan syndrome, Ehlers–Danlos syndrome) leading to generalized defect of connective tissue
Poststenotic dilation	Secondary to long-standing aortic stenosis
Atherosclerosis	Not a major cause in ascending pathology
Arch	
Isolated	Atherosclerosis
Associated with ascending disease	Same causes as for disease in ascending aorta
Descending	
Atherosclerosis	Begins as intimal disease; major cause of thoracoabdominal and abdominal aneurysms
Congenital	See under Ascending, above
Trauma	Causal relationship difficult to prove; history of blunt trauma may be distant
Infection	Syphilis, *Salmonella,* tuberculosis

Causes are listed in order of frequency.

C. Thoracic aortic rupture (tear)

1. **Etiology.** The overwhelming majority of thoracic aortic ruptures occur after trauma and almost always involve a **deceleration injury** from a motor vehicle accident. Sudden deceleration places large mechanical shear stress on points of the aortic wall that are relatively immobile. While aortic rupture leads to immediate exsanguination and death in many patients, approximately 10% to 15% of these patients maintain integrity of the adventitial covering of the aortic lumen and survive to emergency care. Surgical treatment of these survivors is often successful.
2. **Location.** Most thoracic aortic ruptures occur just distal to the origin of the left subclavian artery (isthmus) because of the relative fixation of the aorta at this point by the ligamentum arteriosum (Fig. 25.3). The second most common site of aortic rupture is in the ascending aorta, just distal to the aortic valve.

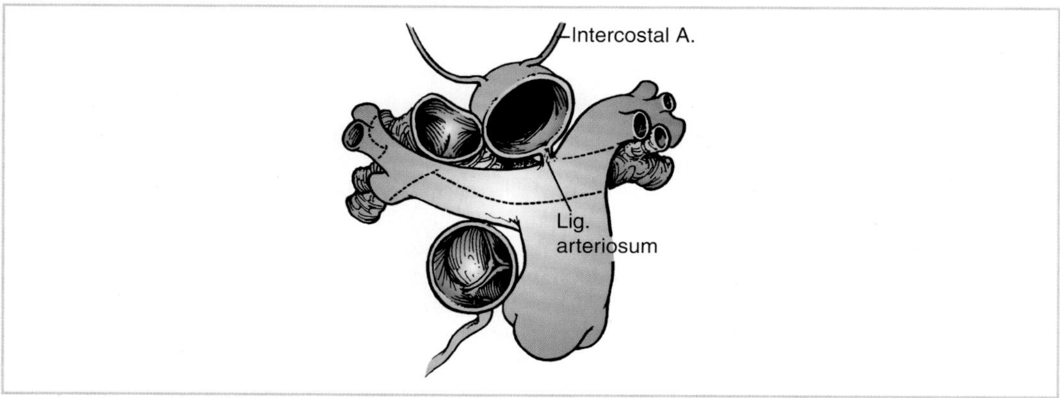

FIGURE 25.3 The heart and great vessels are relatively mobile in the pericardium, whereas the descending aorta is relatively fixed by its anatomic relations. The attachment of the ligamentum arteriosum enhances this immobility and increases the risk of aortic tear due to deceleration injury. (From Cooley DA, ed. *Surgical Treatment of Aortic Aneurysms.* Philadelphia, PA: WB Saunders; 1986:186, with permission.)

II. Diagnosis

A. Clinical signs and symptoms (Table 25.5)

1. **Dissections.** Aortic dissections usually present with a dramatic onset and a fulminant course. Clinical presentation of Stanford Types A and B are listed in Table 25.5.
2. **Aneurysms.** Aneurysms of the ascending, arch, or descending thoracic aorta are often asymptomatic until late in their course. In many circumstances, the presence of an aneurysm is not diagnosed until medical evaluation is conducted for an unrelated problem or for a problem related to a complication of the aneurysm.
3. **Traumatic rupture.** Ruptures most commonly occur just distal to the left subclavian artery. If the patient survives the initial trauma, signs and symptoms are similar to those seen with aneurysms of the descending thoracic aorta.

B. Diagnostic tests

1. **Electrocardiogram (ECG).** Many patients with aortic disease will have evidence of **left ventricular (LV) hypertrophy on ECG**, secondary to the high incidence of hypertension in these patients. In the setting of aortic dissection, the ECG may show ischemic changes caused by coronary artery involvement or evidence of pericarditis from hemopericardium.
2. **Chest X-ray film.** A **widened mediastinum** is a classic X-ray finding with thoracic aortic pathology. Widening of the aortic knob is often seen, with **disparate ascending-to-descending aortic diameter.** A double shadow has been described in the setting of aortic dissection, secondary to visualization of the false lumen.
3. **Serum laboratories.** There are no laboratory findings specifically found with asymptomatic aortic aneurysms. Aortic dissections or ruptures will decrease hemoglobin. Dissections may cause elevated cardiac enzymes from coronary artery occlusion, may increase blood urea nitrogen and creatine from renal artery involvement, and may lead to metabolic acidosis from low cardiac output or ischemic bowel. Fibrinogen may decrease in patients experiencing associated disseminated intravascular coagulation.
4. **Computed tomographic (CT) scans and magnetic resonance imaging.** CT is a useful tool for ascertaining aneurysm size and location and has replaced angiography in many instances. It is also useful for following the progression of aortic disease. Digital images can be manipulated into a three-dimensional form, which may make it easier to assess the lesion and plan repair. Magnetic resonance imaging is extremely sensitive and specific in identifying the entry tear location, presence of false lumen, aortic regurgitation, and pericardial effusion accompanying aortic dissections [5].
5. **Angiography.** This technique remains useful for determining the severity and extent of aortic aneurysms and dissections. With dissections it can be used to locate the site of an intimal tear, to assess aortic valve integrity, and to identify the distal and proximal spread. It can especially delineate involvement of the coronary arteries, as well as the presence of significant coronary artery disease in patients with ascending aortic pathology. Patients with disease of the thoracic aorta often have concurrent coronary artery disease, and bypassing significant lesions helps prevent perioperative myocardial infarction and improves ventricular function when weaning from CPB. Aortography can also determine if other major branch arteries off the aorta are involved. Unfortunately, aortography only rarely identifies those intercostal vessels that are critical for providing blood supply to the spinal cord (see Section **IV.G**).
6. **Transesophageal echocardiography (TEE).** TEE has been found to be highly sensitive and specific for diagnosing aortic dissection. In many cases, pulsed-wave and color-flow Doppler imaging can aid in defining the presence, extent, and type of dissection. Identification of a mobile intimal flap provides a prompt bedside diagnosis that can be lifesaving. In addition, entry and re-entry tears can be defined; aortic regurgitation can be identified and quantified; assessment of LV function and wall motion abnormalities can be made; presence of pericardial effusion with possible associated cardiac tamponade can be identified; and follow-up studies of the false lumen can be made after therapeutic intervention.

TABLE 25.5 Presenting clinical signs and symptoms by location and type of aortic pathology

	Aneurysm	Dissection	Aortic tear
General presentation	Chronic symptoms, but leaking or ruptured aneurysm can lead to fulminant course (see aortic tear for symptoms and signs)	Dramatic onset and fulminant course; symptoms depend on location (Type A or Type B) Patient presents in shock, anxious, diaphoretic	History of deceleration injury; usually fulminant course (good chance of survival if patient gets to treatment center); patient can present in hypovolemic shock
Symptoms and signs			
Ascending and arch		**Type A dissection**[a]	
Location of pain	Anterior chest pain secondary to compression of the following: I. Coronary arteries II. Sensory mediastinal nerves	Anterior chest pain secondary to the following: I. Extension of dissection (ripping or tearing sensation) II. Angina, from dissection of coronaries	Chest pain secondary to compression of structures by enlarging adventitia (the only structure maintaining aortic integrity)
Cardiovascular	CHF symptoms secondary to aortic annular enlargement include the following: I. Widened pulse pressure II. Diastolic murmur Facial and upper trunk venous congestion secondary to superior vena cava compression Blood pressure usually elevated chronically	CHF symptoms include the following: I. Murmur of aortic valve insufficiency II. Narrowing of true-lumen (increased afterload) systolic ejection murmur Blood pressure changes include the following: I. Hypotension secondary to rupture into the retroperitoneal, intra-abdominal, intrathoracic, or pericardial spaces II. Hypertension secondary to pain, anxiety Asymmetry of pulses, or pulseless extremity	Blood pressure changes include the following: I. Hypotension from hypovolemia II. Hypertension from pain
Respiratory	Hoarseness secondary to compression of recurrent laryngeal nerve Dyspnea or stridor due to tracheal compression Hemoptysis due to erosion into trachea Rales secondary to CHF	Hoarseness secondary to compression of recurrent laryngeal nerve Dyspnea and stridor due to tracheal compression Hemoptysis due to erosion into trachea (chronic) Rales secondary to CHF	Lung contusion if chest trauma is significant
Gastrointestinal	Not usually affected	See under Descending	Not usually affected
Renal	Not usually affected	See under Descending	Decreased function secondary to hypotension
Neurologic	Possible due to emboli to carotid artery from aortic valve or aneurysmal segment (see Dissection, at right)	Hemiparesis or hemiplegia secondary to involvement of single carotid artery Reversible or progressive coma	Symptoms related to hypoperfusion

TABLE 25.5 Presenting clinical signs and symptoms by location and type of aortic pathology (*continued*)

	Aneurysm	Dissection	Aortic tear
Descending		**Type B dissection**	
Location of pain	Chronic back pain may occur	Located in back, midscapular region	Located in midscapular region
Cardiovascular	Blood pressure usually normal or elevated (chronic hypertension)	Blood pressure changes include the following: I. Elevated secondary to pain (common) II. Hypotension if rupture of dissection has occurred	Blood pressure changes include the following: I. Elevated secondary to pain (especially with other injuries from trauma) II. Hypotension if hypovolemic
Respiratory	Dyspnea from left main stem bronchial obstruction Hemoptysis due to erosion into left bronchus Hemorrhagic pleural effusion	Dyspnea due to left main stem bronchial obstruction Hemorrhagic pleural effusion	Sequelae of lung contusion or rib fracture
Gastrointestinal	Usually normal	Mimics an acute abdomen, as follows: I. Pain, rigid abdomen, nausea, and vomiting II. Gastrointestinal bleeding Bowel ischemia secondary to compression or dissection of mesenteric or celiac artery	Usually normal
Renal	Renal insufficiency or renovascular hypertension if occlusive aortic disease develops	Ischemia due to involvement of renal arteries in dissection, as follows: I. Infarction and renal failure II. Renal insufficiency	Renal hypofunction from hypoperfusion or hypovolemia
Neurologic	Usually not affected	Paraparesis or paraplegia possible secondary to occlusion of critical spinal cord blood flow	Paraplegia possible

[a]Type A dissections may involve the entire aorta; therefore, symptoms of both ascending and descending pathology may be present. CHF, congestive heart failure.

TEE can also be used to assess many thoracic aortic aneurysms. For ascending or descending thoracic aortic aneurysms in particular, the location, diameter, and extent of the aneurysm, as well as whether the aneurysm contains significant atheroma, can often be well described. TEE can also be used to determine if the aneurysm is saccular or fusiform in shape. TEE can be rarely used to define definitive aneurysmal involvement of the aortic arch and distal ascending aorta. This is because the trachea obscures the latter section from transesophageal ultrasound imaging and the entire arch is not usually visible on TEE. If the surgeon desires detailed preoperative imaging of the aortic arch, he or she should confer with a radiologist about magnetic resonance or CT imaging.

Because traumatic aortic transection generally occurs just distal to the left subclavian takeoff, it is often easily and rapidly identified by TEE imaging. In addition, aortic transection operations are usually emergencies, so TEE imaging is advantageous because it can be conducted quickly and in most locations.

7. **Recommendation for diagnostic strategies.** In hemodynamically stable patients, Nienaber and colleagues recommend diagnosis of thoracic aortic dissection noninvasively

via magnetic resonance imaging because of its high degree of sensitivity (98.3%) and specificity (97.8%) [6]. For patients too unstable for this rather lengthy procedure (40 to 45 min), TEE, which has an average duration of about 15 min and a sensitivity and specificity of 97.7% and 76.9%, respectively, is recommended. Because of its general inability to provide additional information to that provided by more noninvasive methods and its higher incidence of complications, aortography is only useful in very select cases.

C. Indications for surgical correction

1. Ascending aorta

a. Dissections. Acute Type A dissections should be surgically corrected, given their virulent course and high mortality if not surgically treated.

b. Aneurysms. Indications for surgical resection include the following:

(1) Presence of persistent pain despite a small aneurysm

(2) Aortic valve involvement producing aortic insufficiency

(3) Presence of angina from LV strain secondary to aortic valve involvement or from coronary artery involvement by the aneurysm

(4) Rapidly expanding aneurysm or an aneurysm greater than 5 to 5.5 cm in diameter, because the chance of aortic rupture increases as the aneurysm's size increases

2. Aortic arch

a. Dissections. Acute dissection limited to the aortic arch is rare but is an indication for surgery.

b. Aneurysms. Since even elective surgical treatment of arch aneurysms is more difficult than surgery for other aortic aneurysms and is associated with a higher morbidity and mortality, management may be more conservative. However, arch involvement is often seen with ascending aneurysms (less so with descending aneurysms) and is dealt with during surgical repair of these lesions. Surgical indications include the following:

(1) Persistent symptoms

(2) Aneurysm greater than 5.5 to 6 cm in transverse diameter

(3) Progressive aneurysmal expansion

3. Descending aorta

a. Dissection. Some controversy remains concerning the best treatment for an acute Type B dissection. Because of similar in-hospital mortality statistics for medical versus surgical interventions [7], Type B dissections are often treated medically in the acute phase, especially if the patient's comorbidities make the chance of surgical mortality prohibitively high. However, patients with Type B dissections who have the following complications are treated surgically:

(1) Failure to control hypertension medically

(2) Continued pain (indicating progression of the dissection)

(3) Enlargement on chest X-ray film, CT scan, or angiogram

(4) Development of a neurologic deficit

(5) Evidence of renal or gastrointestinal ischemia

(6) Development of aortic insufficiency

Note, as shown in Table 25.6, that the 10-yr survival of patients receiving medical management only for Type B dissections is slightly better than the combined survival of patients treated surgically for Type A and B dissections [7].

TABLE 25.6 Surgical versus medical therapy for aortic dissections

	Hospital mortality (%)	
	Surgical	**Medical**
Type A	32	72
Type B	32	27
10-yr survival	20–25 (A and B)	33 (B only)

Modified from Miller DC, Stinson EB, Oyer PE, et al. Operative treatment of aortic dissection. *J Thorac Cardiovasc Surg.* 1979;78:365.

b. **Aneurysm.** Indications for surgical repair of descending thoracic aneurysms include the following:

(1) Aneurysm greater than 5 to 6 cm in diameter

(2) Aneurysm expanding

(3) Aneurysm leaking (more fulminant symptoms)

(4) Chronic aneurysm causing persistent pain or other symptoms

III. Preoperative management of patients requiring surgery of the thoracic aorta. Emergency preoperative management of **aortic dissections** is discussed below. However, emergency preoperative management is similar for a **leaking thoracic aortic aneurysm** or a **contained thoracic aortic rupture**.

A. **Prioritizing: Making the diagnosis versus controlling blood pressure (BP).** In the setting of a suspected aortic dissection, aortic tear, or leaking aortic aneurysm, the first priority is always to control the BP and ventricular ejection velocity, as these propagate aortic dissection or rupture. **If dissection is strongly suspected, making a definitive diagnosis with radiographic studies should occur after proper monitoring, intravenous (IV) access, hemodynamic stability, and heart rate and BP control have been established (if possible).** During diagnostic procedures, the patient should be monitored closely, with a physician present as clinically indicated. An anesthesiologist should become involved as early as possible, if needed, to lend expertise in monitoring and airway and hemodynamic management in cases where clinical deterioration occurs before the patient reaches the operating room. Rapid diagnosis using TEE may save critical minutes in initiating definitive surgical treatment in patients with suspected thoracic aortic dissection or rupture.

4 B. **Achieving hemodynamic stability and control.** The ideal drug to control BP is administered by IV and is rapidly acting with a short half-life and few, if any, side effects. Systolic and diastolic BPs and LV ejection velocity should be reduced, because all these factors can propagate aortic dissection.

1. **Monitoring.** Patients must have an ECG for detection of ischemia and dysrhythmias, two large-bore IV catheters for volume resuscitation, an arterial line in the appropriate location (discussed below), and, if time permits, a central venous catheter or pulmonary artery (PA) catheter for monitoring filling pressures and infusing drugs centrally.

2. **BP-lowering agents**

a. **Vasodilators**

(1) **Nitroprusside** has emerged as a useful agent for controlling BP in patients with critical aortic lesions, because its rapid onset and offset make it quickly effective and easily regulated. A vasodilator that relaxes both arterial and venous smooth muscle, it is given as an IV infusion, and while central administration is probably optimal, it can be administered through a peripheral vein with good effect. The usual starting dose is 0.5 to 1 μg/kg/min, titrated to effect. Doses of 8 to 10 μg/kg/min have been associated with cyanide toxicity (see Chapter 2).

(2) **Nitroglycerin** is a less potent vasodilator than sodium nitroprusside, and it causes more venous than arterial dilation. It can be useful in settings where ascending aortic pathology is coupled with myocardial ischemia, as it can improve coronary blood flow via coronary artery vasodilation. Infusion dosage usually ranges from 1 to 4 μg/kg/min.

(3) **Fenoldopam** is a rapidly acting vasodilator that is a selective D_1 dopamine receptor agonist. It has little affinity for the D_2, α_1, or β adrenoreceptors. Fenoldopam causes vasodilation in many vascular beds, but it increases renal blood flow to a significant degree. Therefore, it may have some renal protective effects while also being used to treat acute hypertension. Dosing starts at 0.05 to 0.1 μg/kg/min and can be increased incrementally to a maximum dose of 0.8 μg/kg/min.

(4) **Nicardipine** is a calcium-channel blocker that inhibits calcium influx into vascular smooth muscle and the myocardium. It may be used as a single 0.5 to 2 mg IV "push" or as a 5 to 15 mg/hr infusion titrated to the desired effect.

b. β_1-antagonists

Decreasing LV ejection velocity is important for decreasing risk of propagating aortic dissection. Medications to lower heart rate may be particularly useful for attenuating reflex tachycardia and increased ventricular contractility that can occur with use of sodium nitroprusside. Nitroprusside can increase LV ejection velocity by increasing dP/dt and heart rate. For this reason, β-adrenergic blockade should be used with nitroprusside to decrease both tachycardia and contractility (see Chapter 2).

(1) Propranolol, a nonselective β-antagonist, has been used for many years as first-line therapy for this role and can be administered as an IV bolus of 1 mg, but doses of 4 to 8 mg may be required for adequate heart rate control. Propranolol has been somewhat supplanted by selective β_1-antagonists.

(2) Labetalol is a combined α- and β-blocker and offers an alternative to the nitroprusside–propranolol combination. It should be given initially as a 5 to 10 mg loading bolus; once the effect has been assessed, the dose is doubled, allowing a few minutes for onset of effect. This process should be repeated until target BP or a total dose of 300 mg is reached. Once target BP and heart rate are achieved via the loading dose, a continuous infusion may be started at 1 mg/min, or a small bolus dose can be repeated every 10 to 30 min to maintain BP control.

(3) Esmolol is a β-blocking agent with a short half-life that may be useful in this setting. It is administered as a bolus loading dose of 500 μg/kg over 1 min and then continued as an infusion starting at 50 μg/kg/min and titrated to effect to a maximum dose of 300 μg/kg/min. This drug is particularly useful in patients with obstructive lung disease because it is β_1 selective and its action can be terminated quickly if β_2-mediated respiratory symptoms ensue.

(4) Metoprolol, another β_1-selective agent, is used in doses of 2.5 to 5 mg titrated to effect over a few minutes to a maximum dose of 15 to 20 mg. It provides a longer effect, which may be useful.

3. **Desired endpoints.** In order to decrease the chance of propagating aortic dissection or rupture, systolic BP should usually be lowered to approximately 100 to 120 mm Hg or to a mean pressure of 70 to 90 mm Hg. Heart rate should be 60 to 80 beats/min. If a PA catheter is in place, the cardiac index may be lowered to a range of 2 to 2.5 L/min/m^2 to reduce ejection velocity from a hyperdynamic LV.

C. Bleeding and transfusion. Coagulopathy is frequently encountered in the thoracic aortic surgical patient. Many of these patients require left heart or full CPB during surgery to help maintain sufficient end-organ perfusion during aortic repair; thus, they also require heparinization. CPB may cause a consumptive coagulopathy and enhanced fibrinolysis, thus increasing blood loss [8,9]. Patients requiring deep hypothermic circulatory arrest (DHCA) for aortic arch surgery also may experience substantial platelet dysfunction secondary to extreme hypothermia. Platelet consumption has also been noted in the abdominal aortic surgical population [10]. In patients undergoing thoracoabdominal aortic aneurysm repairs, "back-bleeding" through intercostal vessels increases blood loss, and very large losses necessitating transfusion of multiple units of blood products can occur [11].

1. A total of 8 to 10 units of packed red blood cells should be typed and cross-matched before surgery.
2. Use of blood scavenging/reprocessing devices decreases the amount of banked blood transfused, but extensive bleeding and the logistics of effectively scavenging autologous blood during these operations may frequently require transfusion of packed cells and procoagulant blood products.
3. Antifibrinolytic therapy during aortic surgery is controversial but commonly used. Few adequately powered trials have examined this surgical population, so it is unclear if significant benefit is derived from antifibrinolytics, particularly in patients in whom left heart bypass (LHB) is used and full heparinization is unnecessary [12].

a. Tranexamic acid or ϵ-aminocaproic acid. A retrospective study of 72 patients who underwent descending thoracic aortic surgery with LHB and tranexamic acid or

ϵ-aminocaproic acid infusion versus no antifibrinolytic therapy found no difference in incidence of transfusion or chest tube output; however, all of these patients also received intraoperative methylprednisolone and platelet-rich plasmapheresis before aortic repair [12]. These authors did find that intraoperative hypothermia independently predicted chest tube output and that preoperative hemoglobin, older age, and duration of cross-clamp time independently predicted transfusion. Casati and colleagues conducted a single-institution, double-blind, randomized, controlled study of 60 consecutive elective thoracic aortic surgical patients, half of whom received perioperative tranexamic acid and the other half received a normal saline placebo [13]. This study found that the tranexamic acid recipients required significantly fewer packed red blood cell transfusions, as well as overall allogeneic transfusions, than the placebo recipients. No differences in perioperative thrombotic complications were noted between the tranexamic acid intervention group and the placebo group. However, this was a small study that was not statistically powered to evaluate the occurrence of adverse perioperative thrombotic events. Larger prospective randomized studies are needed to determine whether tranexamic acid or ϵ-aminocaproic acid effectively reduce bleeding and do not cause thrombotic complications in thoracic aortic operations, because there are no other data regarding the risk/benefit of these agents in thoracoabdominal aortic surgical patients.

b. On the basis of available data, the authors can neither recommend nor advise against the use of antifibrinolytic therapies in thoracic aortic surgery. Potential thrombotic risks, including neurocognitive and renal dysfunction, are of concern, and the clinician should weigh these risks against the benefits of potential decreases in transfusion.

D. Assessment of other organ systems

1. **Neurologic.** Preoperatively the patient should be monitored closely for change in neurologic status, as this is an indication for immediate surgical intervention. Involvement of the artery of Adamkiewicz may lead to lower extremity paralysis, while propagation of a dissection into a cerebral vessel may lead to a change in mental status or stroke symptoms.
2. **Renal function.** Urine output should be monitored, as development of anuria or oliguria in the euvolemic setting is an indication for immediate surgical intervention.
3. **Gastrointestinal.** Serial abdominal examinations should be performed, and blood gas analysis should be done routinely to assess changes in acid–base status. Ischemic bowel can cause significant metabolic acidosis.

E. Use of pain medications. Patients with aortic dissections may be anxious and in severe pain. Not only is pain relief important for patient comfort, but it is beneficial in controlling BP and heart rate. Oversedation should be avoided so that ongoing patient assessments may occur. In addition to neurologic or abdominal symptoms, worsening of back pain may indicate aneurysm expansion or further aortic dissection and is regarded by many surgeons as an emergent situation.

IV. Surgical and anesthetic considerations

A. Goal of surgical therapy (for aortic dissections, aneurysms, or rupture). The foremost goal in treating acute aortic disruption is to control hemorrhage. Once control is achieved, the objectives of management of both acute and chronic lesions are to repair the diseased aorta and restore its relationships with major arterial branches.

Thoracic aortic aneurysm repair is usually conducted by replacing the diseased segment of the aorta with a synthetic graft and then reimplanting major arterial branches into the graft. In contrast, when repairing an aortic dissection the goal is to resect the segment of the aorta that contains the intimal tear. When this segment is removed, it may be possible to obliterate the false lumen and interpose graft material. It is usually not possible or necessary to replace the entire dissection portion of aorta, because, if the origin of dissection is controlled, re-expansion of the true lumen usually compresses and obliterates the false lumen. With contained aortic rupture, the objective is to resect the area of the aorta that ruptured and either reanastomose the natural aorta to itself in an end-to-end fashion or interpose graft material for the repair.

TABLE 25.7 Incidence of coexisting diseases in patients with aortic pathology who present for surgery

Coronary artery disease	66%
Hypertension	42%
Chronic obstructive pulmonary disease	23%
Peripheral vascular disease	22%
Cerebrovascular disease	14%
Diabetes mellitus	8%
Other aneurysms	4%
Chronic renal disease	3%

Modified from Romagnoli A, Cooper JR Jr. Anesthesia for aortic operations. *Cleve Clinic Q.* 1981; 48:147–152.

B. Overview of intraoperative anesthetic management (for aortic dissections, aneurysms, or rupture)

1. **Key principles**
   a. **Managing BP.** BP control should be sought during the transition from the preoperative to the intraoperative period. Such control is important in light of the surgical and anesthetic manipulations that will profoundly affect BP.
   b. **Monitoring of organ ischemia.** If possible, the central nervous system, heart, kidneys, and lungs should be monitored for adequacy of perfusion. The liver and gut cannot be monitored continuously, but their metabolic functions can be checked periodically.
   c. **Treating coexisting disease.** Patients with aortic pathology often have associated cardiovascular and systemic diseases, as outlined in Table 25.7.
   d. **Controlling bleeding.** Patients undergoing aortic surgery often experience an inflammatory response to foreign graft material and cardiopulmonary or LHB. This inflammation can interact with the coagulation cascade and lead to significant perioperative coagulopathy. Furthermore, patients with acute dissection and lower fibrinogen and platelet counts may already have a consumptive process from the clotting that often occurs in the false lumen. The challenges of coagulation abnormalities and their treatment are discussed in Chapter 19.
2. **Induction and anesthetic agents.** Many thoracic aortic operations are emergent procedures that require aspiration precautions when securing the airway. However, rapid sequence induction and intubation typically done for patients with full stomachs may not be appropriate for the patient with thoracic aortic pathology, as wide swings in hemodynamics may occur. A compromise in this situation is a smooth, controlled IV induction, with gentle manual ventilations and cricoid pressures held. This "modified" rapid sequence induction allows not only some airway protection but also titration of anesthetic induction drugs that control BP with laryngoscopy. Use of nonparticulate antacids, H_2-blockers, and metoclopramide should be considered before induction of anesthesia. Other anesthetic considerations and agents are described more fully in Section **IV.D**. Despite precautions, marked changes in hemodynamics are common when securing the patient's airway, and vasoactive drugs (nitroglycerin, esmolol, or others) should be available to immediately treat an undesirable hemodynamic response to intubation [14].
3. **Importance of site of lesion** (Table 25.8). Although the principles of anesthetic induction and maintenance are similar for all aortic lesions, the location of the thoracic aortic lesion is also important for intraoperative management.

C. Ascending aortic surgery

1. **Surgical approach.** Ascending aortic surgery is conducted through a midline sternotomy.
2. **CPB.** CPB is required because of proximal aortic involvement.
   a. If the aneurysm ends in the proximal portion or midportion of the ascending aorta, the arterial cannula for CPB can be placed in the upper ascending aorta or proximal arch.

TABLE 25.8 Anesthetic and surgical management for thoracic aortic surgery

	Surgical site		
	Ascending	**Arch**	**Descending**
Surgical approach	Median sternotomy	Median sternotomy	Left thoracotomy
Perfusion	CPB—aortic cannula distal to lesion, or in femoral or right axillary artery	CPB—femoral artery cannula or right axillary artery cannula	Simple cross-clamp Heparinized Gott shunt ECC with LHB or CPB (femoral–femoral)
Involvement of the following:			
Aortic valve	Sometimes	Sometimes	No
Coronary arteries	Sometimes	Sometimes	No
Pericardium	Sometimes	Sometimes	No
Invasive monitoring	Left radial or femoral arterial catheter PA catheter[a]	Arterial catheter—either arm or femoral[b] PA catheter[a]	Proximal arterial (right radial or brachial) Distal arterial (femoral)[a] PA catheter[a]
Special techniques	Renal preservation EEG	DHCA Cerebral protection (DHCA, DHCA with RCP, or anterograde cerebral perfusion) Renal preservation EEG	Motor-evoked potentials[a] One-lung ventilation Renal preservation CSF drainage[a]
Common complications	Bleeding Cardiac dysfunction	Bleeding Hypotension from cerebral protective doses of thiopental Neurologic deficits	Bleeding Paralysis Renal failure Cardiac dysfunction

[a]Optional, depending on physician's preferences.
[b]Depends on whether the left subclavian or innominate arteries are involved in the pathologic process or whether axillary arterial cannulation is used. If there is uncertainty preoperatively, use a femoral artery catheter.
CPB, cardiopulmonary bypass; ECC, extracorporeal circulation; LHB, left heart bypass; PA, pulmonary artery; EEG, electroencephalogram; DHCA, deep hypothermic circulatory arrest; CSF, cerebrospinal fluid; RCP, retrograde cerebral perfusion.

b. If the entire ascending aorta is involved, the femoral artery may be cannulated, because an **aortic cannula cannot be placed distal to the lesion without jeopardizing perfusion to the great vessels. Arterial flow on CPB in this case is retrograde from the femoral artery toward the great vessels. Another, newer approach is to cannulate the right axillary, the innominate, or occasionally the right carotid artery, allowing retrograde perfusion into the innominate artery and then into the aorta in an antegrade manner.**

c. Venous cannulation is usually through the right atrium; however, femoral venous cannulation may be necessary if the aneurysm is very large and obscures the atrium.

3. **Aortic valve involvement.** Aortic valvuloplasty or valve replacement is often needed with repair of ascending aortic dissections or aneurysms. Which procedure is used depends on the degree of involvement of the sinus of Valsalva and the aortic annulus.

5

4. **Coronary artery involvement.** Ascending aortic dissections or aneurysms may involve the coronary arteries. Aortic dissections may cause coronary occlusion by compression of the coronary ostia by an expanding false lumen; such occlusion will require surgical coronary artery bypass grafting to restore myocardial blood flow. Displacement of the coronary arteries from their normal position distal to the aortic annulus with proximal aortic aneurysms usually requires coronary artery reimplantation into the reconstructed aortic tube graft or coronary artery bypass grafting.

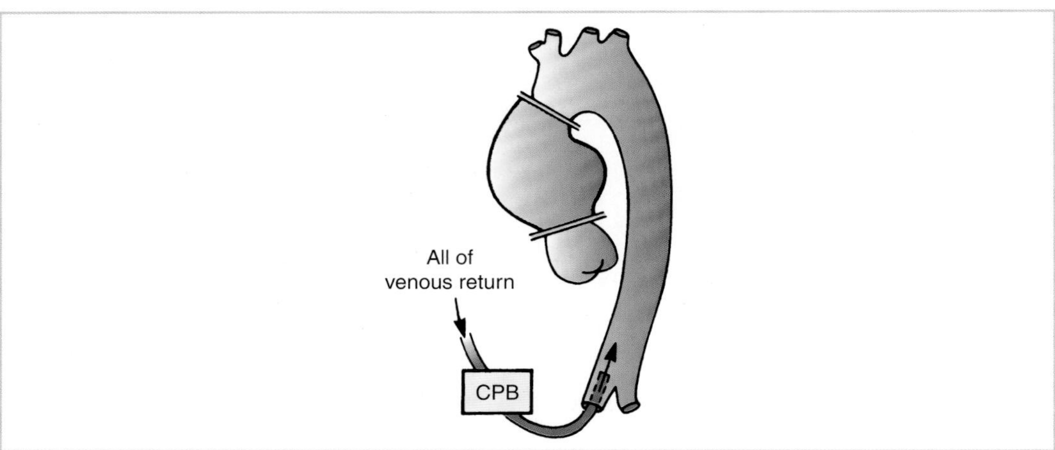

FIGURE 25.4 Circulatory support and clamp placement for surgery of the ascending aorta if femoral arterial cannulation is used; the distal clamp must be distal to the diseased segment. This may be the only clamp required. CPB, cardiopulmonary bypass. (From Benumof JL. Intraoperative considerations for special thoracic surgery cases. In: Benumof JL, ed. *Anesthesia for Thoracic Surgery*. Philadelphia, PA: WB Saunders; 1987:384, with permission.)

5. **Surgical techniques.** An example of the usual cross-clamp placement used in surgery of the ascending aorta is shown in Figure 25.4. Note that placement of the distal clamp is more distal than when cross-clamping for coronary artery bypass surgery and might include a part of the innominate artery. If aortic insufficiency is present, a large portion of the cardioplegic solution infused into the aortic root will flow through the incompetent aortic valve and into the LV instead of the coronary arteries. This can cause distention of the LV with increased myocardial oxygen utilization and diminished myocardial protection from reduced distribution of cardioplegia. For these reasons, an immediate aortotomy is often performed after aortic cross-clamping with direct infusion of cardioplegia into individual coronary arteries. Many centers also use retrograde coronary perfusion for cardioplegia administration as an alternative or in addition to an antegrade technique.

   If the aortic valve and annulus are both normal size and unaffected by concurrent ascending aortic pathology, surgery is limited to replacing the diseased section of the aorta with graft material. If the annulus is normal size, but the aortic valve is incompetent, the valve may be resuspended or replaced. If both aortic insufficiency and annular dilation are present, either a composite graft (i.e., a tube graft with an integral artificial valve) or an aortic valve replacement with a graft sewn to the native annulus can be used. The coronary arteries must be reimplanted into the wall of a composite graft, but they may not need to be reimplanted if separate aortic valve replacement and aortic tube grafts are used for the repair and the native sinus of Valsalva can be left in place (Fig. 25.5) [15]. The posterior wall of the native aneurysm can be wrapped around the graft material and sewn in place to help with hemostasis.

   In patients with ascending dissections, the aortic root is opened and the site of the intimal tear is located. The section of the aorta that includes the intimal tear is excised, and the edges of the true and false lumens are sewn together. Graft is used to replace the excised portion of the aorta.

6. **Complications.** Complications include any that can occur with an operation involving CPB and an open ventricle:
   a. Air emboli
   b. Atheromatous or clot emboli
   c. LV dysfunction secondary to difficult myocardial protection during aortic cross-clamping

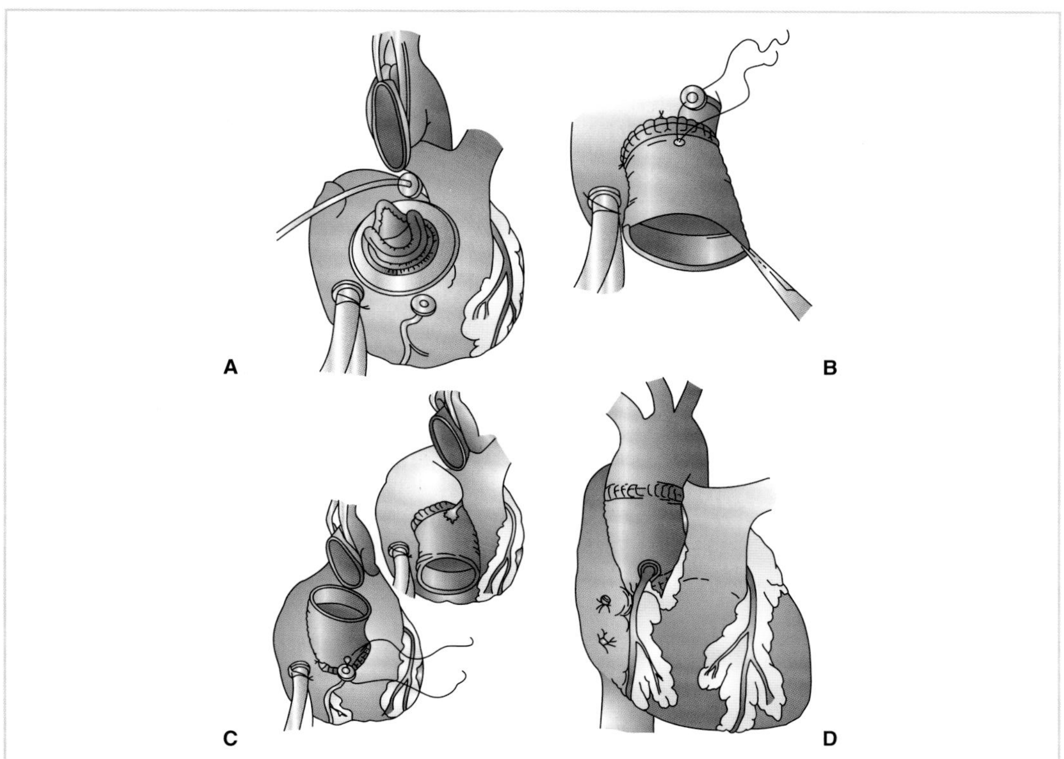

FIGURE 25.5 Surgical repair of ascending aortic aneurysm or dissection. **A:** Aortic valve has been replaced and the aorta is transected at native annulus, leaving "buttons" of aortic wall around coronary ostia. **B:** Graft material anastomosed to the annulus, with left coronary reimplantation. **C:** Completion of left and beginning of right coronary reimplantation. **D:** Completion of distal graft anastomosis. (From Miller DC, Stinson EB, Oyer PE, et al. Concomitant resection of ascending aortic aneurysm and replacement of the aortic valve—operative results and long-term results with "conventional" techniques in ninety patients. *J Thorac Cardiovasc Surg.* 1980;79:394, with permission.)

d. Myocardial infarction or myocardial ischemia secondary to technical problems with reimplantation of the coronaries
e. Renal or respiratory failure
f. Coagulopathy
g. Hemorrhage, especially from suture lines, which can be especially difficult to control

D. Anesthetic considerations for ascending aortic surgery

1. Monitoring

a. **Arterial line placement.** The ascending aortic lesion or procedures for its repair may involve the innominate artery, so a left radial or femoral arterial line is inserted for direct BP monitoring. Also, if right axillary cannulation is used, arterial pressure measurements will be falsely elevated because of increased flow (see below).

b. **ECG.** Five-lead, calibrated ECG should be used to monitor both leads II and V_5 for ischemic changes.

c. **PA catheter.** Because of the advanced age of many of these patients and the presence of severe systemic disease that may lead to pulmonary hypertension or low cardiac output, a PA catheter may be useful in selected patients in the perioperative period.

d. **TEE.** In addition to its preoperative diagnostic importance, TEE is a useful adjunct for the intraoperative management of these patients. Hypovolemia, hypocontractility,

TABLE 25.9 Anesthetic considerations and choice of anesthetic agent for surgery of the aorta

Patient variables	Opioids[a]	Volatile agent[b]	Other intravenous agents
Full stomach	Rapid acting (especially sufentanil, alfentanil)	Prolonged induction	Rapid acting if tolerated
Hemodynamic instability	Minimal myocardial depression Potent analgesics useful for treating intraoperative hypertension	Dose-dependent myocardial depression Indicated if hypertensive with adequate cardiac output	T, P: Myocardial depression M, E: Minimal myocardial depression K: Worsens hypertension
Ventricular function (VF)	Indicated with poor VF	Use in patients with good VF	M, E, and K maintain VF Avoid T, P if VF is poor
Neurologic function	Decrease $CMRo_2$	Decrease $CMRo_2$, especially isoflurane; unclear in vivo protective effects	T, P decrease $CMRo_2$, probably protective, used with hypothermic arrest or open ventricle
Myocardial ischemia (coronary involvement)	Oxygen balance: Increases supply/demand ratio and therefore will have adverse effects in the presence of hypertension	Decrease supply/demand ratio but will have negative effect in the presence of hypotension	T, P: Adversely affects supply secondary to hypotension K: Increases oxygen demand; decreases supply (secondary to tachycardia)

[a]Refers to fentanyl, sufentanil, and alfentanil.
[b]Halothane, sevoflurane, desflurane, and isoflurane.
T, thiopental; P, propofol; M, midazolam; E, etomidate; K, ketamine; VF, ventricular function; $CMRo_2$, cerebral metabolic rate of oxygen consumption.

myocardial ischemia, intracardiac air, the location of an intimal tear, and the presence and extent of valvular dysfunction can all be detected with TEE. Caution should be exercised when placing this probe in the presence of a large ascending aortic aneurysm because of theoretical risk of rupture.

e. **Neuromonitoring**

(1) **Electroencephalogram (EEG).** Either raw or processed EEG data may be helpful for judging the adequacy of cerebral perfusion during CPB. Monitoring the bispectral index might help to assess the depth of anesthesia during these procedures, but the benefits of such monitoring are unproven.

(2) **Temperature.** When correctly placed at the back of the oropharynx, a nasopharyngeal or oropharyngeal temperature probe probably gives the anesthesiologist the best overall approximation of brain temperature.

f. **Renal monitoring.** As with all cases involving CPB, urine output should be monitored.

2. **Induction and anesthetic agents.** See Table 25.9.
3. **Cooling and rewarming.** Hypothermic CPB is used in most cases of ascending aneurysms. DHCA is needed if the proximal arch is involved. If femoral cannulation is used and the femoral artery is small, a smaller cannula may be needed. This may delay cooling and rewarming, because lower blood flows on CPB will have to be used to avoid excessive arterial line pressures between the roller pump and the arterial cannula.

E. **Aortic arch surgery**

1. **Surgical approach.** The arch is exposed through a median sternotomy.
2. **CPB.** In most cases, CPB with femoral or right axillary arterial and right atrial venous cannulation is required.
3. **Technique.** Typical aortic clamp placement for this procedure is shown in Figure 25.6. Note that blood flow to the innominate, left carotid, and left subclavian arteries will

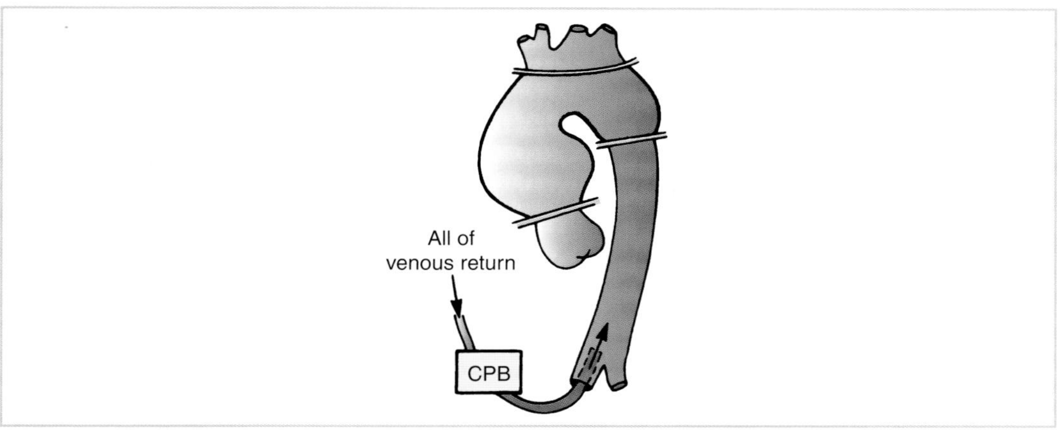

FIGURE 25.6 Representation of cannula and clamp placement for surgery of the aortic arch if femoral bypass is used. Proximal clamp is placed to arrest the heart. Distal clamp isolates the arch so that the distal anastomosis can be performed. Middle clamp on major branches isolates the head vessels so that en bloc attachment to graft is possible. The distal and arch anastomoses may be performed without clamps by using circulatory arrest. CPB, cardiopulmonary bypass. (From Benumof JL. Intraoperative considerations for special thoracic surgery cases. In: Benumof JL, ed. *Anesthesia for Thoracic Surgery.* Philadelphia, PA: WB Saunders; 1987:384, with permission.)

cease during resection of the aneurysmal or dissected section of the aortic arch, thus necessitating DHCA.

The attachments of the arch vessels are usually excised en bloc so that all three vessels are located on one "button" of tissue, as shown in Figure 25.7 [16]. This facilitates rapid reimplantation and re-establishment of blood flow through the arch vessels. Once the distal arch anastomosis is completed, the surgeon sutures the aortic button containing the arch vessels to the graft that is replacing the diseased aortic arch. The aortic cross-clamp can then be placed on the graft proximal to the arch vessels, after which the arch portion of the aortic graft is deaired, and blood flow is re-established to the cerebral vessels via the arterial CPB cannula. The proximal aortic arch anastomosis is then completed.

4. **Cerebral protection.** As discussed above, resection of the aortic arch requires interruption or alteration of cerebral blood flow, which may contribute to postoperative stroke and neurocognitive dysfunction—both significant causes of morbidity and mortality in patients undergoing aortic arch surgery. Although various surgical approaches are used to reduce cerebral ischemia, all include lowering patient temperature with CPB in order to decrease the cerebral metabolic rate, the corresponding oxygen demand, and the production of toxic metabolites.
   a. DHCA is used for arch surgery, because blood flow through the aorta to the brain can be stopped and surgical exposure is maximized. DHCA requires cooling the patient's core temperature to 15 to 22°C, depending on the anticipated complexity and duration of the procedure and the adjunctive technique used (antegrade cerebral perfusion [ACP] or retrograde cerebral perfusion [RCP]). Turning off CPB and partially draining the patient's blood volume into the venous reservoir provides a bloodless surgical field, with effective protection of the brain and other organs, such as the kidneys, for 40 min [17], or perhaps longer. DHCA has improved outcomes for aortic arch surgery but is associated with longer CPB times to adequately cool and rewarm the patient. Animal studies suggest that it is important to rewarm patients relatively slowly after DHCA, and also not to rewarm the brain above 37°C, because this may cause increased cerebral injury [18]. Because of the limited time that patients can undergo DHCA before suffering cerebral injury, some surgeons use either selective retrograde perfusion or ACP as an adjunct to DHCA to prolong the "safe time" allowed for complicated reconstruction

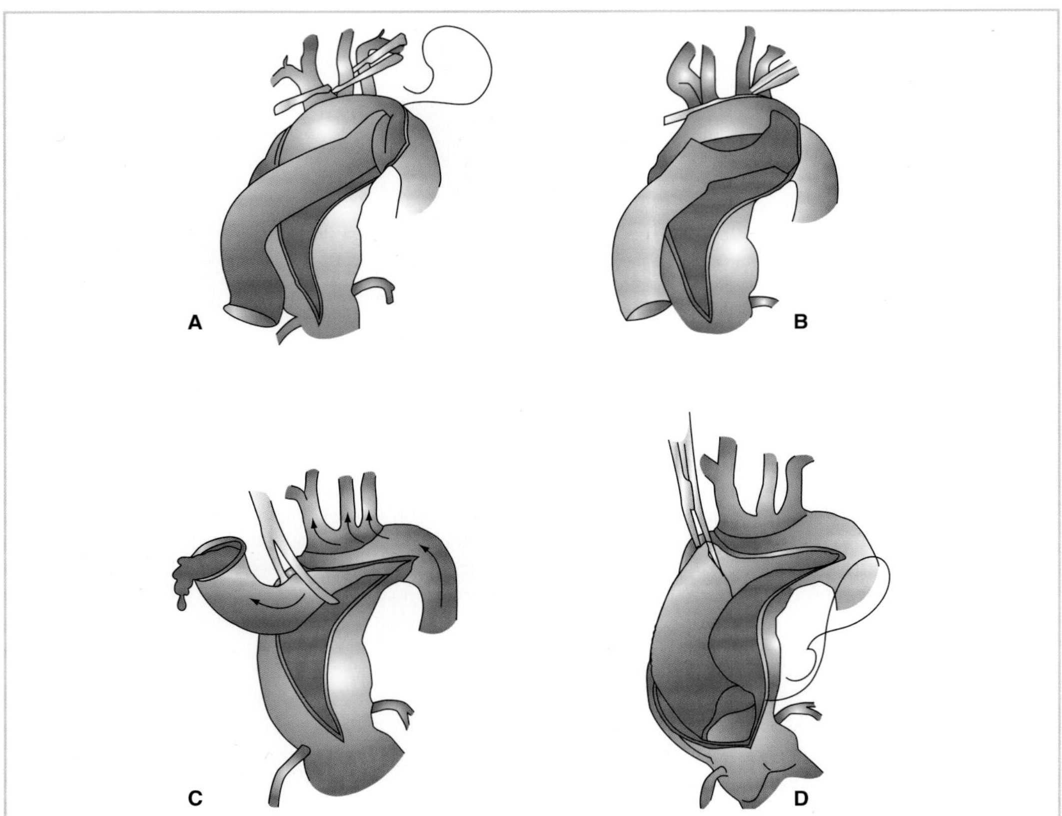

FIGURE 25.7 Aortic arch replacement. **A:** The distal suture line is completed first, followed by **(B)** reattachment of the arch vessels. **C:** Flow is re-established to these vessels by moving the clamp more proximally. **D:** The proximal suture line is completed. (From Crawford ES, Saleh SA. Transverse aortic arch aneurysm—improved results of treatment employing new modifications of aortic reconstruction and hypokalemic cerebral circulatory arrest. *Ann Surg.* 1981;194:186, with permission.)

of the aortic arch and its branch vessels while circulation to the rest of the body is stopped.

b. **RCP does necessitate individual caval cannulation.** At circulatory arrest, the arterial line of the CPB circuit is connected to the superior vena cava cannula and low flows are directed through the cannula to maintain a central venous pressure (CVP) of around 20 mm Hg [19], although this pressure is not necessarily associated with improved outcomes. Advantages of RCP include relative simplicity, uniform cerebral cooling, efficient deairing of the cerebral vessels (thus reducing the risk of embolism), and provision of oxygen and energy substrates. Outcome studies have identified the following risk factors for mortality and morbidity in RCP during DHCA: time on CPB, urgency of surgery, and patient age [20]. Controversy exists as to how much flow is actually directed to the brain and how much flow courses through the extracranial vessels.

c. **ACP.** With this technique, the brain is selectively perfused via the innominate or carotid arteries [19]. As shown in Figure 25.8, one method for administering ACP is to take blood from the CPB circuit's oxygenator and to deliver it via arterial access to the brain by using a separate roller pump from the one used for CPB [21]. Many centers use this same technique to deliver antegrade or retrograde cardioplegia.

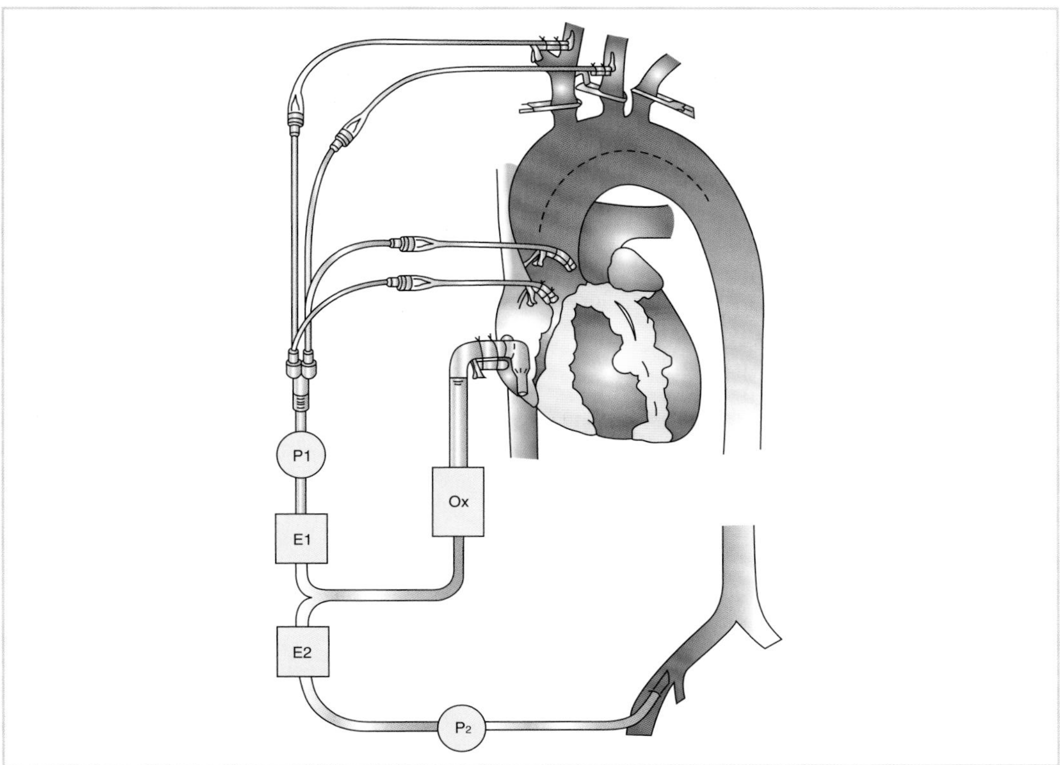

FIGURE 25.8 Perfusion circuit for anterograde cerebral perfusion for aortic arch surgery. Venous blood from the right atrium drains to the oxygenator (*Ox*) and is cooled to 28°C by heat exchange (*E2*) before passing via the main roller pump (*P2*) to a femoral artery. A second circuit derived from the oxygenator with a separate heat-exchanger (*E1*) and roller pump (*P1*) provides blood at 6 to 12°C to the brachiocephalic and coronary arteries. (From Bachet J, Guilmet D, Goudot B, et al. Antegrade cerebral perfusion with cold blood: A 13-year experience. *Ann Thorac Surg.* 1999;67:1875, with permission.)

Figure 25.8 [21] depicts direct cannulation of both carotid arteries for ACP, but this technique has been simplified in many practices by cannulating the right axillary artery or other arteries, as discussed above, for placement of the arterial line from the CPB circuit instead of using the femoral artery. This is usually done by anastomosing (side-to-end) a tube graft to the axillary artery and attaching the arterial line from the pump to the graft. After the patient is placed on CPB and cooled, at the time of circulatory arrest the base of the innominate artery is clamped and ACP is delivered at lower flow rates (e.g., 10 mL/kg/min) through the axillary artery cannula and thus up the right carotid artery (Fig. 25.9) [22]. This allows bilateral cerebral perfusion, assuming that the circle of Willis is intact. If there is uncertainty about the integrity of collateral blood flow to the left cerebral hemisphere, the left common carotid also can be cannulated directly through the surgical field, as shown. Pressure during this method of ACP can be monitored via a right radial arterial line, but monitoring pressure and maintaining a certain pressure is not known to improve outcome.

Cannulating the right axillary artery instead of the femoral artery to provide CPB before and after circulatory arrest reduces the risk of systemic atheroembolism. This is because right axillary artery cannulation provides antegrade aortic flow, whereas femoral artery cannulation produces retrograde flow through an often atherosclerotic descending aorta [23].

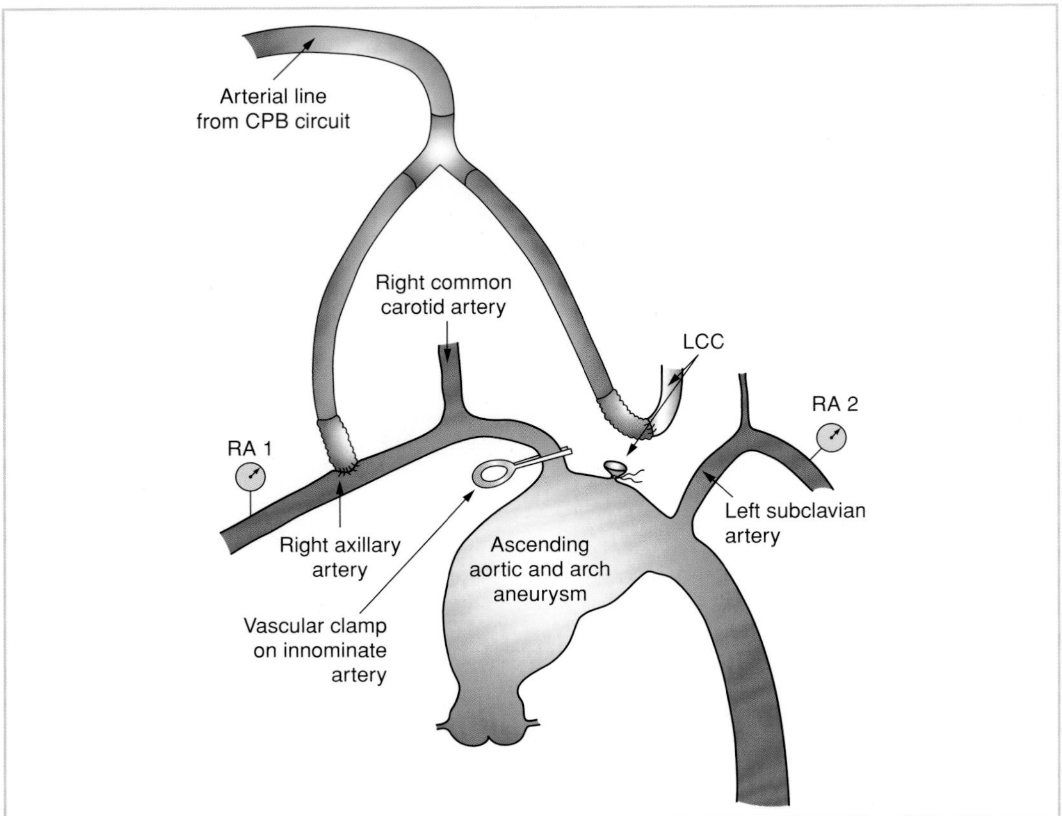

FIGURE 25.9 ACP via right axillary artery cannulation. Figure demonstrates routes of cannulation and monitoring of arterial pressures for extensive arch reconstruction. RA 1, right radial arterial line; RA 2, left radial arterial line. Thick lines indicate native arterial vessels. Thin lines indicate CPB circuit tubing and connectors. Hatched areas indicate Dacron grafts. (From Cook R, Min G, Macnab A, et al. Aortic arch reconstruction: Safety of moderate hypothermia and antegrade cerebral perfusion during systemic circulatory arrest. *J Card Surg.* 2006;21:159, with permission of Blackwell Publishing.)

Additionally, DHCA is required only for completion of the distal and arch anastomoses. Then the aortic graft may be clamped proximally and full CPB perfusion reinitiated to the rest of the body while the proximal anastomosis is performed.

Many groups accept ACP as the safest method of brain protection during arch surgery [21]. Antegrade perfusion may take advantage of autoregulation of cerebral blood flow, which is thought to remain intact even at low temperatures when α-stat blood gas management is used. With intact autoregulation, physiologic protection against ischemia of hyperperfusion will be active. However, proponents of pH-stat blood gas management argue that the cerebral vasodilation that accompanies elevated pCO_2 will produce more uniform cooling and perfusion of the brain (see Chapters 21 and 24).

5. **Complications.** Complications from aortic arch surgery include those of any procedure in which CPB is used. Irreversible cerebral ischemia is a distinct possibility with this type of surgery. Hemostatic difficulties may be increased secondary to the multiple suture lines, long CPB times, and prolonged periods of intraoperative hypothermia.

F. **Anesthetic considerations for aortic arch surgery**

1. **Monitoring**

   a. **Arterial BP.** An intra-arterial catheter can be placed in either the right or left radial artery, depending on which of the head and neck arteries that extend off of the aortic arch are involved. If both the right- and left-sided arteries are involved, the femoral artery may need to be catheterized. As noted earlier, if the right axillary artery is cannulated for CPB, right radial arterial line BPs will not accurately reflect systemic BP during CPB. If the right axillary artery is used for CPB, and DHCA with ACP is planned, some surgeons may ask that the patient have a right radial arterial line placed for monitoring arterial pressures during ACP. Also, with profound hypothermia, many have found that the radial artery does not provide accurate pressures for a period during rewarming, and they electively and pre-emptively insert a femoral arterial catheter.

   b. **Neurologic monitors**

      (1) EEG is often used to ensure that the patient has been cooled sufficiently such that the EEG is isoelectric before DHCA. Thiopental or propofol is given by many anesthesiologists to achieve or extend this isoelectric state [24].

      (2) Nasal or oropharyngeal temperature can be used to monitor brain cooling.

      (3) **Near-infrared regional spectroscopy (NIRS).** This relatively new technology measures frontal cerebral oxygenation through light transmittance. Although the technology is complex, it is easily applied and seems to be most useful as a trend monitor during ascending aortic and arch surgery, particularly when ACP is employed. Significant reductions in left-sided sensor values compared with right-sided ones may indicate an incomplete circle of Willis. We have found that these values are usually restored when separate left carotid perfusion begins. However, clear outcome data are not yet available. Longer periods of lower cerebral oxygenation during DHCA, as indicated by NIRS, have been associated with longer postoperative hospital stays, but large, well-designed prospective studies are needed to validate the efficacy of these approaches [25,26].

   c. **TEE.** It provides useful information similar to that for ascending aortic surgery (see Section **IV.D.1**), but care should be taken when placing the probe, because patients undergoing aortic arch surgery are even more prone to developing perioperative coagulopathy.

2. **Choice of anesthetic agents.** See Table 25.9.

3. **Management of hypothermic circulatory arrest.** The technique involves core cooling to 15 to 20°C, packing the head in ice, using pharmacologic adjuncts to aid in cerebral protection, avoiding glucose-containing solutions, and using appropriate monitoring for selective cerebral perfusion. More details are provided in Chapter 24.

4. **Complications.** Complications related directly to anesthesia for aortic arch surgery are uncommon. One potential complication could be myocardial depression secondary to the use of thiopental for cerebral protection; inotropic agents are often needed during weaning from CPB, probably to counter the effects of prolonged myocardial ischemia during DHCA.

G. **Descending thoracic and thoracoabdominal aortic surgery**

1. **Surgical approach.** Aneurysms of the descending thoracic aorta frequently extend into the abdominal cavity and involve the entire aorta. They are often classified according to Crawford's classification (Fig. 25.10). Exposure of the affected segment of aorta may be accomplished through a left thoracotomy incision alone or through a thoracoabdominal incision. Extent IV aneurysms involve the supraceliac abdominal aorta but still require thoracic aortic clamping. The patient is placed in a full right lateral decubitus position with the hips rolled slightly to the left to allow access for potential cannulation of the femoral vessels for left heart or CPB. When positioning the patient, it is important to protect pressure points via measures such as using an axillary roll, placing pillows between

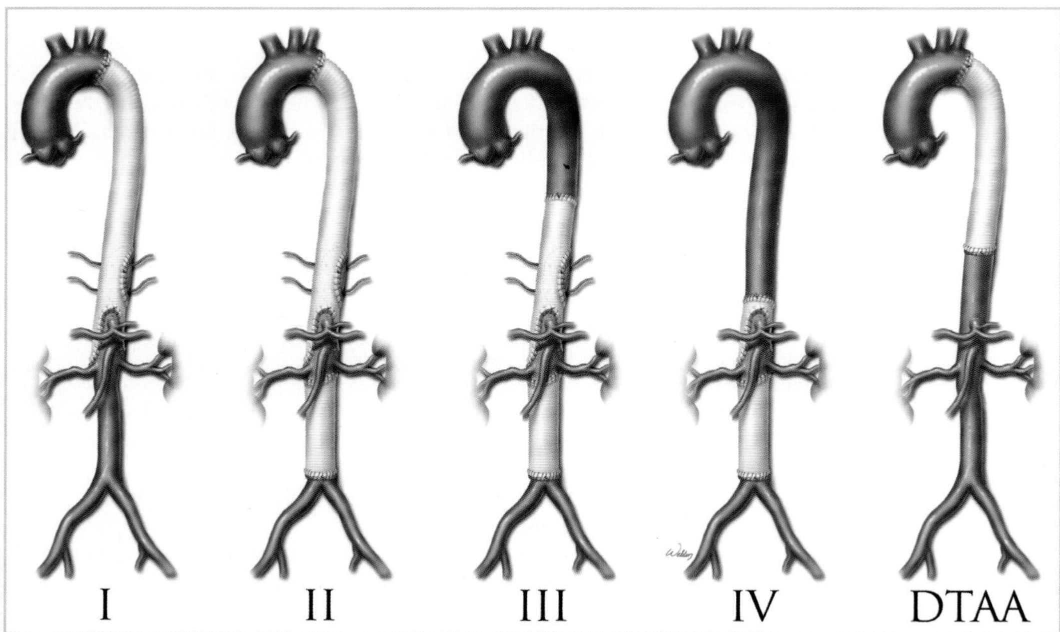

FIGURE 25.10 The Crawford classification of repair for thoracoabdominal aortic aneurysm surgery, with a descending thoracic aortic repair for comparison. The descending aortic repair does not extend beyond the diaphragm, whereas all the others do. Extent I aneurysms involve an area that begins just distal to the left subclavian artery and extends to most or all of the abdominal visceral vessels but not the infrarenal aorta. Extent II aneurysms also begin distal to the left subclavian and involve most of the aorta above the abdominal bifurcation. Extent III lesions begin in the mid-thoracic aorta and involve various lengths of the abdominal aorta. Finally, Extent IV lesions originate above the celiac axis and end below the renal arteries; these aneurysms necessitate a thoracoabdominal approach for proximal aortic cross-clamping. (Reproduced with permission from Baylor College of Medicine.)

the knees, and padding the head and elbows. It is also important to maintain the occiput in line with the thoracic spine to prevent traction on the brachial plexus.

2. **Surgical techniques.** Regardless of whether a patient has a descending thoracic aortic aneurysm, a thoracoabdominal aneurysm, a dissection, or aortic rupture, surgical repair usually involves placing aortic cross-clamps both above and below the affected region of the aorta and then opening the aorta and replacing the diseased segment with a graft.
   a. **Simple cross-clamping.** Some groups report success with cross-clamping the aorta above and below the lesion without using additional measures to provide perfusion distal to the aortic lesion. This technique has the advantage of simplifying the operation and reducing the amount of heparin needed (Fig. 25.11) because more heparin is required when using bypass circuits. However, there is the obvious disadvantage of potentially compromising flow to the distal aorta and its perfused organs when the simple cross-clamp technique is used.

      Clamping the descending thoracic aorta generally produces marked hemodynamic changes, with profound **hypertension** in the proximal aorta and **hypotension** distal to the cross-clamp. The increase in afterload that occurs when the majority of the cardiac output goes only to the arteries perfusing the head and upper extremities can cause acutely elevated LV filling pressures and a corresponding progressive drop in cardiac output. Presumably, LV failure may result if this increased afterload is maintained for a significant length of time. Furthermore, hypertension

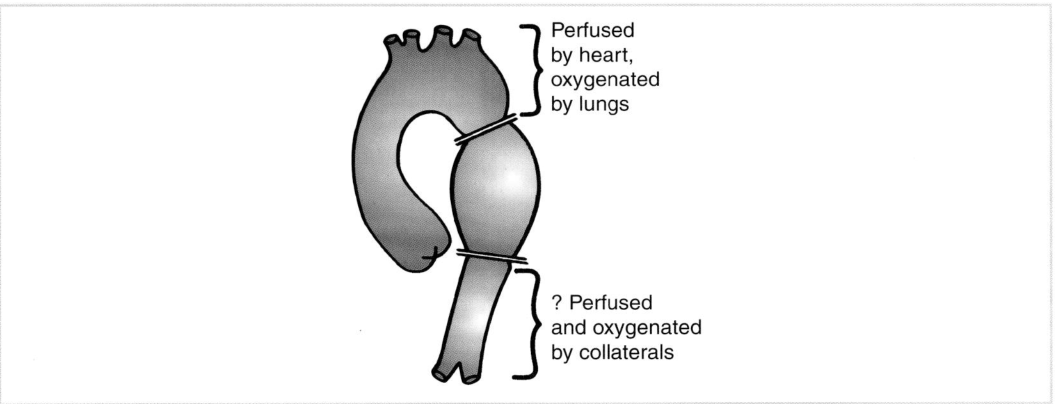

FIGURE 25.11 Illustration of simple cross-clamp placement for repair of descending aortic aneurysm or dissection. Distal clamp placement dictates that flow to the spinal cord and major organs proceeds through collateral vessels. (From Benumof JL. Intraoperative considerations for special thoracic surgery cases. In: Benumof JL, ed. *Anesthesia for Thoracic Surgery.* Philadelphia, PA: WB Saunders; 1987:384, with permission.)

in the proximal aorta could precipitate a catastrophic cerebral event, particularly in patients with unidentified cerebral aneurysms. Mean arterial pressure (MAP) distal to the aortic cross-clamp may decrease to less than 10% to 20% of the patient's baseline BP. This decrease will cause a decrease in renal perfusion and, perhaps, spinal cord perfusion. The physiology of aortic cross-clamping can change depending on the actual site of the clamp and is influenced by many factors, a discussion of which is beyond the scope of this chapter. Gelman's review of the subject remains an excellent reference [27].

The presence of chronic obstruction to distal aortic blood flow such as that which occurs with aortic coarctations generally results in well-developed collateral flow and will lessen the hemodynamic changes usually encountered when a cross-clamp is placed on the descending thoracic aorta. This is illustrated by BPs taken proximal and distal to the aortic cross-clamp in a series of patients with aortic coarctations versus descending thoracic aortic aneurysms (Table 25.10) [28].

TABLE 25.10 Proximal versus distal blood pressure in simple aortic clamping

	Proximal systolic/diastolic; mean (mm Hg)	Distal mean (mm Hg)
Coarctation	160/85; 110	23
	145/80; 102	54
	150/85; 107	18
	155/80; 105	36
Average	152/82; 106	33
Thoracic aneurysm	260/160; 194	12
	240/135; 170	8
	245/150; 182	24
	235/140; 172	4
	240/155; 184	10
	255/160; 192	6
Average	245/150; 182	10

Modified from Romagnoli A, Cooper JR Jr. Anesthesia for aortic operations. *Cleve Clinic Q.* 1981;48:147–152.

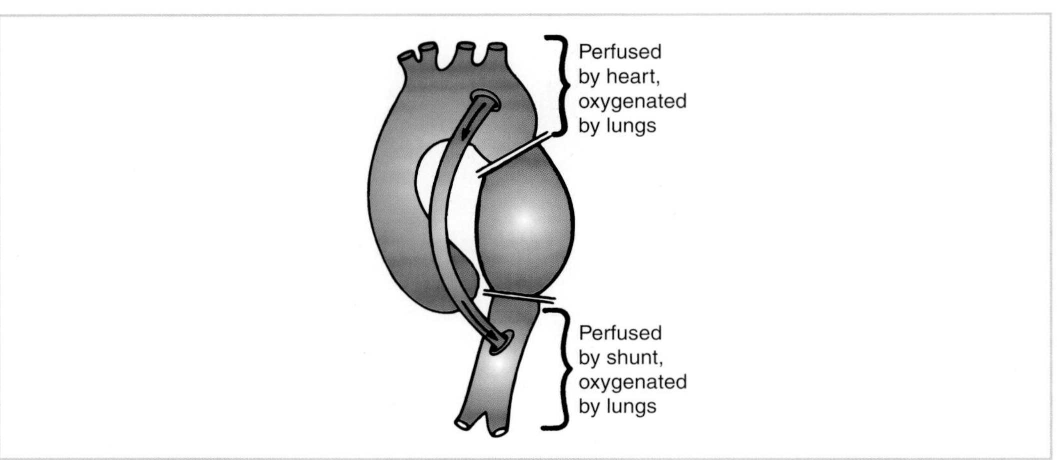

FIGURE 25.12 Placement of a heparin-coated vascular shunt from proximal to distal aorta during repair of descending aneurysm or dissection. (From Benumof JL. Intraoperative considerations for special thoracic surgery cases. In: Benumof JL, ed. *Anesthesia for Thoracic Surgery*. Philadelphia, PA: WB Saunders; 1987:384, with permission.)

Another method of simple aortic cross-clamping is use of an "open" technique, in which no cross-clamp is used distal to the aortic pathology. This technique allows direct inspection of the distal aorta for debris such as thrombus and atheroma, and graft material can be anastomosed in an oblique fashion that reincorporates the maximal number of intercostal arteries.

b. **Shunts.** A method that provides decompression of the proximal aorta and perfusion to the distal aorta involves placement of a heparin-bonded (Gott) extracorporeal shunt from the LV, aortic arch, or left subclavian artery to the femoral artery (Fig. 25.12). Systemic heparinization is usually not required. The advantage of this technique is that distal aortic perfusion and proximal aortic decompression are achieved. However, there may be problems related to technical difficulties with placement and kinking of the shunt, which result in inadequate distal flows. Furthermore, only two sizes of these shunts are available: 7 mm (5-mm inner diameter) and 9 mm (6-mm inner diameter). These relatively small diameters may limit blood flow and, thereby, limit the amount of proximal LV decompression and augmentation of distal aortic perfusion that can be accomplished.

c. **Extracorporeal circulation (ECC).** Historically, the first method used for distal aortic perfusion and proximal decompression in the repair of descending thoracic aortic lesions was ECC. There are several ways to perform ECC, but all involve removal of blood from the patient, passage into an extracorporeal pump, and reinfusion into the femoral artery to provide perfusion distal to the aortic cross-clamp (Fig. 25.13). An alternative technique is to perfuse the body of the aneurysm with ECC while the proximal anastomosis is being performed and then open the aneurysm and perfuse the major visceral vessels individually until they can be incorporated into the anastomosis.

Blood can be drained from the patient into the extracorporeal pump from the femoral vein, which is technically the easiest site to access for surgery on the descending thoracic aorta. However, using a venous drainage site necessitates placing an oxygenator in the ECC circuit to provide oxygenated blood for systemic reinfusion. This form of CPB in conjunction with DHCA arrest may be necessary to repair descending thoracic aortic aneurysms that involve the aortic arch.

Alternatively, LHB may be used. The left atrium, LV apex, or left axillary artery may be cannulated to carry oxygenated patient blood to the ECC pump; this blood is then returned to the distal aorta or femoral artery. This technique does not require an oxygenator in the LHB circuit (Fig. 25.14).

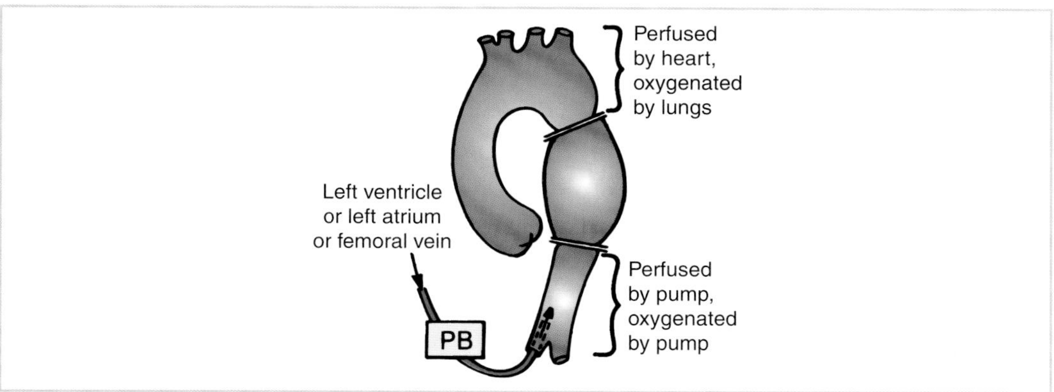

FIGURE 25.13 Partial bypass (*PB*) (or extracorporeal circulation [ECC]) method for maintaining distal perfusion pressure and preventing proximal hypertension. Oxygenated blood can be taken directly from the LV or atrium (or aortic arch) and pumped either by roller head or centrifugal pump into the femoral artery. Alternatively, unoxygenated blood can be taken from the femoral vein, passed through a separate oxygenator, and pumped into the femoral artery. Use of an oxygenator dictates the use of a full heparinizing dose. (From Benumof JL. Intraoperative considerations for special thoracic surgery cases. In: Benumof JL, ed. *Anesthesia for Thoracic Surgery*. Philadelphia, PA: WB Saunders; 1987:384, with permission.)

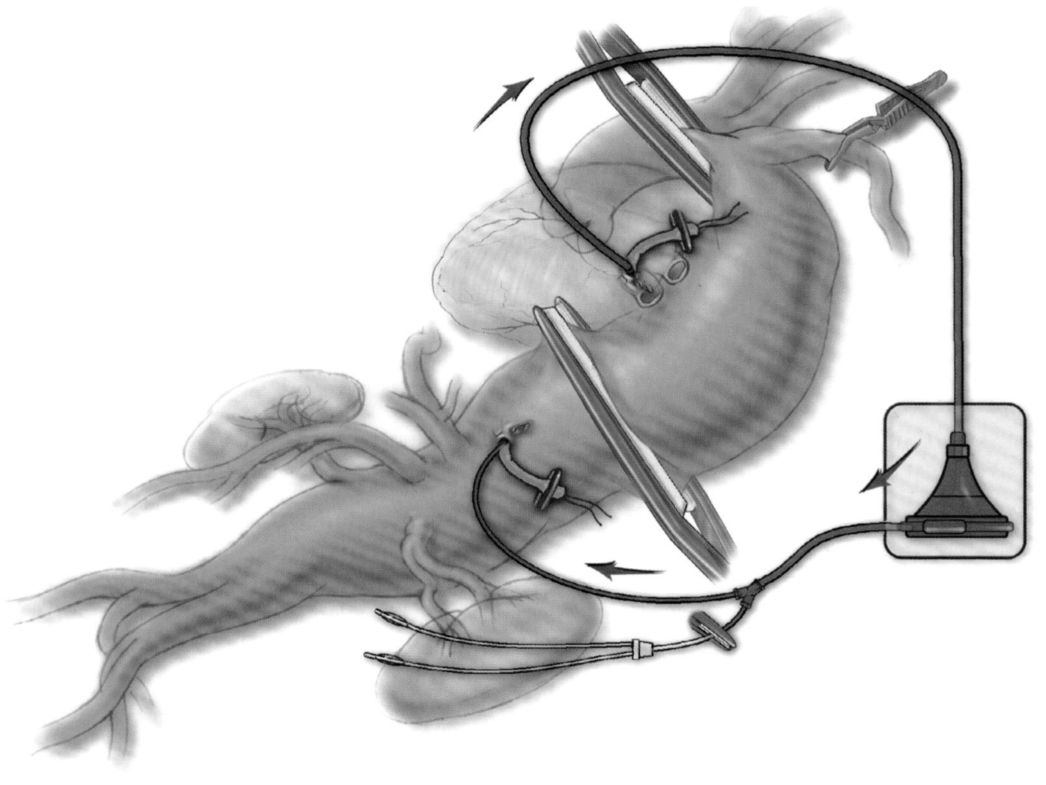

FIGURE 25.14 Left heart bypass. Perfusing the aneurysm allows completion of the proximal anastomosis while distal perfusion is maintained. After the aneurysm is opened, perfusion of the celiac, superior mesenteric, and renal arteries may be performed by individual cannulation before these arteries are attached to the graft. (From Coselli JS, LeMaire SA. Tips for successful outcomes for descending thoracic and thoracoabdominal aortic aneurysm procedures. *Semin Vasc Surg.* 2008;21:13–20, with permission.)

TABLE 25.11 Options for increasing distal perfusion in descending aortic surgery

Blood removed from	Blood infused into	Heparinized shunt	Perfusion apparatus		Extracorporeal bypass	
			Roller	Centrifugal	Oxygenator	Heparin (ACT)[a]
LV, AoA, LSA	FA, DAo	Yes	No	No	No	None (nl)
FV	FA, DAo	No	Either		Yes	Full (>480)
LA, AoA, LSA, LV	FA, DAo	No	No	Yes	No	Minimum (nl–250)[b]

[a]Refers to the activated clotting time (in seconds); if used, optimum ACT is controversial.
[b]Some groups will not use heparin when using a centrifugal pump.
AoA, aortic arch; DAo, descending aorta; FA, femoral artery; FV, femoral vein; LA, left atrium; nl, normal; LSA, left subclavian artery; LV, left ventricle.

Both of these ECC techniques have disadvantages. Use of an oxygenator requires complete systemic heparinization, which is associated with an increased incidence of hemorrhage, especially into the left lung. Left atrial or ventricular cannulation for LHB without an oxygenator may allow the use of less heparin, but this approach increases the risk for systemic air embolism. Also, in the venous-to-arterial–circulation CPB technique, a heat exchanger is included in the ECC circuit, which helps to avoid significant perioperative hypothermia and corresponding coagulopathy. When LHB is used, a heat exchanger is often not added to the ECC circuit. Table 25.11 summarizes the possible cannulation sites and the major differences between heparinized shunts and ECC for perfusion distal to the aortic cross-clamp.

3. **Complications of descending thoracic aortic repairs**
   a. **Cardiac.** Major cardiac morbidity and mortality was approximately 12% in one large series of thoracoabdominal aneurysm repairs [29].
   b. **Hemorrhage.** Significant perioperative bleeding is a common complication.
   c. **Renal failure.** The incidence of renal failure in large case series ranges from 13% to 18% [29,30]. The mortality rate is substantially higher in those patients experiencing postoperative renal failure [29]. The cause is presumed to be a decrease in renal blood flow during aortic cross-clamping. However, renal failure may still occur in the presence of apparently adequate perfusion (heparinized shunt or ECC). Pre-existing renal dysfunction increases a patient's likelihood of developing postoperative renal failure.
   d. **Paraplegia.** The reported incidence of paraplegia with open surgical repair of aneurysms of the descending thoracic or thoracoabdominal aorta ranges from 0.5% to 38% [29–32]. The cause is either complete interruption of blood supply or prolonged hypoperfusion (more than 30 min) [32] of the spinal cord via the anterior spinal artery. The anterior spinal artery is formed by fusion of the vertebral arteries and is the major blood supply to the anterior spinal cord. As the anterior spinal artery traverses the spinal cord from cephalad to caudad, it receives collateral blood supply from radicular branches of the intercostal arteries (Fig. 25.15). In most patients, one radicular arterial branch, known as the **great radicular artery** (**of Adamkiewicz**), provides a major portion of the blood supply to the midportion of the spinal cord. It may arise anywhere from T_5 to below L_1. Unfortunately, this vessel is difficult to identify by angiography or by inspection during surgery. Interruption of flow may lead to paraplegia, depending on the contribution of other collateral arteries to spinal cord perfusion. With anterior spinal artery hypoperfusion, an **anterior spinal syndrome** can result, in which motor function is usually completely lost (anterior horns) but some sensation may remain intact (posterior columns).
   e. **Miscellaneous.** Other significant complications may arise during surgery of the descending thoracic aorta. Some of these are specific to the type of aortic pathology being addressed. For example, death from multiorgan trauma and failure is a major entity in patients who initially survive traumatic aortic rupture. Furthermore, thoracic

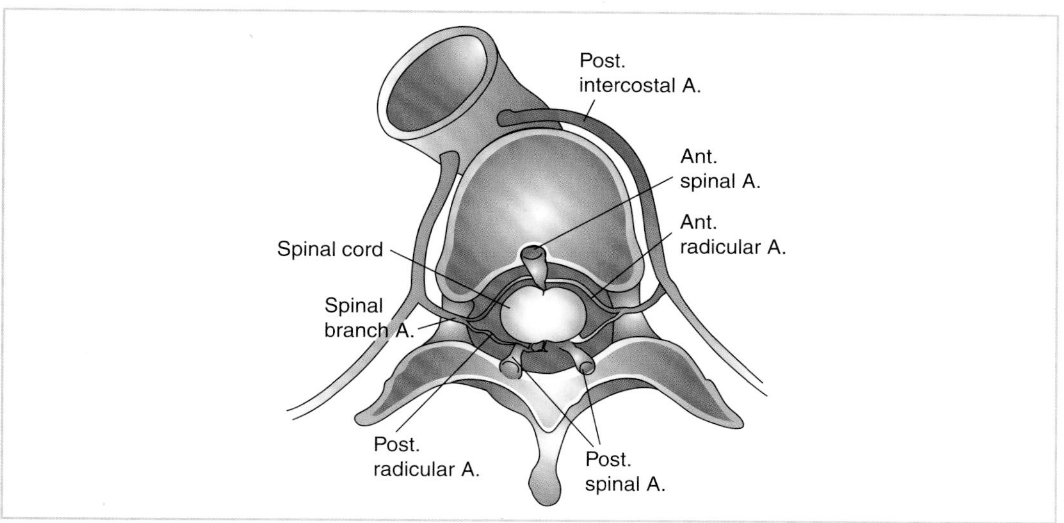

FIGURE 25.15 Anatomic drawing of the contribution of the radicular arteries to spinal cord blood flow. If the posterior intercostal artery is involved in a dissection or is sacrificed to facilitate repair of aortic pathology, critical blood supply may be lost, causing spinal cord ischemia. (From Cooley DA, ed. *Surgical Treatment of Aortic Aneurysms.* Philadelphia, PA: WB Saunders; 1986:92, with permission.)

aortic surgical patients are more likely to succumb to respiratory failure or multiorgan failure than patients with isolated abdominal aortic disease. Patients who undergo thoracoabdominal aortic repair may develop postoperative diaphragmatic dysfunction. Cerebrovascular accidents are seen in a small number of thoracic aortic surgical patients. Also, left vocal cord paralysis due to recurrent laryngeal nerve damage commonly occurs during descending thoracic aortic surgery because of the proximity of the nerve to the site of the aneurysm. All descending thoracic and thoracoabdominal aneurysms may be associated with major complications, but Crawford extent II lesions involve more potential hazards because more of the aorta is affected.

H. Anesthetic considerations in descending thoracic aortic surgery

1. **General considerations.** Providing anesthesia for descending thoracic aortic surgery can be extremely demanding because of profound hemodynamic changes and compromised perfusion of organs distal to the aortic cross-clamp. Anesthesia for descending thoracic aortic surgery is summarized in several good reviews [33,34].
2. **Monitoring**
   a. **Arterial BP.** A right radial or brachial arterial catheter is needed to monitor pressures above the proximal clamp because the left subclavian artery may be occluded with the application of the aortic cross-clamp. To assess perfusion distal to the lower aortic cross-clamp, many centers place a femoral artery catheter in addition to the right radial or brachial catheter in order to monitor pressure below the distal clamp. Should the LHB technique of ECC be used, the left femoral artery is typically cannulated for distal perfusion of the aorta, and the right femoral artery can be used for monitoring BP.
   b. **Ventricular function.** Some operative teams monitor LV function during proximal aortic cross-clamping. A TEE can be useful for directly assessing LV function and volume, but, occasionally, the TEE probe in the esophagus can interfere with the surgical placement of retractors or clamps. In those cases, TEE cannot be used. A PA catheter allows for indirect assessment of LV filling and cardiac output, presuming that the right heart and tricuspid valve function well and the patient does not have pulmonary hypertension. However, a PA catheter is not as helpful as TEE for intraoperative real-time patient monitoring.

c. **Other monitors.** ECG lead V_5 cannot be used because of the surgical approach, which limits the assessment of anterior myocardial ischemia. However, TEE should allow good assessment of anterior LV wall motion.

3. **One-lung anesthesia.** In order to provide good surgical access, double-lumen endobronchial tubes allow deflation of the left lung during surgery on the descending thoracic and thoracoabdominal aorta. This not only improves surgical exposure but also protects the left lung from trauma associated with surgical manipulation. Furthermore, if trauma to the left lung leads to hemorrhage into the airway, the double-lumen tube can protect the right lung from blood spillage. A left-sided double-lumen endotracheal tube may generally be easier for the anesthesiologist to place and is often used for operations on the descending thoracic aorta. However, in some patients, the aortic aneurysm distorts the trachea or left main stem bronchus to the degree that placing a left-sided double-lumen tube is impossible. Patients with aortic rupture may also have a distorted left main stem bronchus. Right-sided double-lumen endobronchial tubes may be used, but proper alignment with the right upper lobe bronchus should be checked with a fiberoptic bronchoscope. Alternatively, use of a single-lumen endotracheal tube with an endobronchial blocker can be considered when a double-lumen tube cannot be placed, or when changing a double-lumen tube over to a single-lumen endotracheal tube is anticipated to be challenging (i.e., the patient has a difficult intubation before undergoing an operation that involves major transfusion and fluid resuscitation). For a detailed description of double-lumen and endobronchial blocker tube placement and single-lung ventilation, see Chapter 26.

4. **Anesthetic management before and during aortic cross-clamping.** Before the aorta is cross-clamped, mannitol (0.5 g/kg) is often administered to try to provide some renal protection during aortic cross-clamping, when the kidneys may experience low perfusion. Even when shunting or ECC is used, changes in the distribution of renal blood flow may make efforts at renal protection prudent.

   After the aortic cross-clamp is applied, it is important to closely monitor acid–base status with serial arterial blood gas measurements, as it is common for metabolic acidosis to develop because of hypoperfusion of critical organ beds. Acidosis should be treated aggressively with sodium bicarbonate and with attempts to increase distal aortic perfusion pressure if LHB or shunting is used (particularly if the patient is normothermic). If simple aortic cross-clamping without shunting or ECC is used, proximal hypertension should be controlled, again realizing that distal organ flow may be diminished. In treating proximal hypertension, regional blood flow studies have shown that infusing nitroprusside may decrease renal and spinal cord blood flow in a dose-related fashion. Ideally, aortic cross-clamp time (regardless of technique) should be less than 30 min, because the incidence of complications, especially paraplegia, starts to increase substantially beyond this time [32].

   If a heparinized shunt is used and proximal **hypertension** cannot be treated without producing subsequent distal **hypotension** (less than 60 mm Hg), the surgeon should be made aware that there could be a technical problem with the shunt's placement. If LHB is used, pump speed can be increased such that proximal hypertension can be reduced by moving blood volume from the proximal to the distal aorta. This also simultaneously increases lower-body perfusion. Usually, little or no pharmacologic intervention is needed during LHB, because changing the pump speed allows for rapid control of proximal and distal aortic pressures. Table 25.12 lists the treatment options for several clinical scenarios when using ECC.

   Before the surgeon removes the aortic cross-clamp, the patient should be adequately volume resuscitated, and a vasopressor should be available in case substantial hypotension occurs after the aorta is unclamped. The anesthesiologist must be constantly aware of the stage of the operation so that major events such as clamping and unclamping of the aorta are anticipated.

5. **Declamping shock.** When **simple cross-clamping** of the aorta is used, subsequent unclamping can lead to serious and even life-threatening consequences, usually from

6 **TABLE 25.12** Management of extracorporeal circulation for surgery of the descending aorta

Proximal arterial pressure	Distal arterial pressure	Pulmonary wedge pressure	Treatment
↑	↓	↓	Volume; increase pump flow
↑	↓	↑	Increase pump flow
↑	↑	↓	Volume; vasodilator
↑	↑	↑	Vasodilator; diuretic; maintain pump flow, hold volume in pump reservoir (if in use)
↓	↓	↓	Volume; look for partial occlusion of arterial outflow cannula (if reservoir in use)
↓	↓	↑	Increase pump flow; inotrope
↓	↑	↑	Decrease pump flow; inotrope; diuretic
↓	↑	↓	Decrease pump flow; may need volume

severe hypotension or myocardial depression. There are several theoretical causes of declamping syndrome, including washout of acid metabolites, vasodilator substances, sequestration of blood in the gut or lower extremities, and reactive hyperemia. The usual cause, however, is relative or absolute hypovolemia. Anesthesiologists may be fooled into under-resuscitating patients while the aortic cross-clamp is on because of high proximal arterial pressures. To attenuate the effects of clamp removal, the patient's volume should be optimized, particularly in the 10 to 15 min before unclamping. This includes elevating filling pressures by infusing blood products, colloid, or crystalloids. Some advocate prophylactic bicarbonate administration just before clamp removal to minimize myocardial depression from "washout acidosis." It is advisable for the surgeon to release the cross-clamp slowly over a period of 1 to 2 min to allow enough time for compensatory hemodynamic changes to occur and for the anesthesiologist to assess whether further volume resuscitation is indicated.

Vasopressors may be needed to compensate for hypotension after the aortic cross-clamp is removed, but the anesthesiologist should take care not to "overshoot" target BP, as even transient hypertension may result in significant bleeding from the aortic suture lines. With a volume-resuscitated patient and a slow cross-clamp release, any significant post-clamp hypotension is usually short lived and well tolerated. If hypotension is severe, the easiest intervention is reapplication of the clamp and further volume infusion.

If shunts or ECC are used, declamping hypotension is usually mild, as the vascular bed below the clamp is less "empty," and there will be less proximal-to-distal aortic volume shifting after the aortic cross-clamp is released. If a volume reservoir is used in the bypass circuit, ECC also provides a means for rapid volume infusion after the aortic cross-clamp is removed.

6. **Fluid therapy and transfusion.** Even patients undergoing elective repair of a descending thoracic aneurysm versus aortic rupture or dissection may be relatively hypovolemic. Fluid therapy should have the following aims: correcting the patient's starting fluid deficit, providing maintenance fluids, compensating for evaporative and "third space" losses, decreasing red cell loss by mild hemodilution, and replacing blood loss as needed.

   Despite proximal and distal control of portions of the aorta undergoing surgical repair, blood loss can be considerable in these cases because of back-bleeding from the intercostal arteries, which are often ligated when the aorta is opened. Use of intraoperative cell-scavenging devices has become common and has reduced the need for banked blood transfusions. However, large-volume blood loss can occur rapidly in these operations, and banked blood transfusions are often needed. As long as liver perfusion is adequate, even with a large blood loss, citrate toxicity is usually not a problem because of rapid "first pass" metabolism in the liver. Repair of a thoracic aneurysm, particularly with simple clamping, however, presents a unique situation because hepatic arterial blood flow to the liver is compromised for an extended period of time. In this circumstance, transfusion of large amounts of banked blood may rapidly produce citrate toxicity, resulting in myocardial depression that requires vigilant calcium chloride infusion.

7. **Spinal cord protection.** In addition to the use of ECC, shunts, and expeditious surgery, several other methods have been promoted to protect the spinal cord during aortic cross-clamping [35].
   a. **Maintaining perfusion pressure.** Some groups prefer to maintain perfusion pressure of the distal aorta in the range of 40 to 60 mm Hg to increase blood flow to the middle and lower spinal cord. This practice should be regarded as controversial because at present, few data exist regarding outcome. **No method used to maintain blood flow to the distal aorta (i.e., shunt or partial bypass) guarantees that spinal cord blood flow, and therefore function, will be preserved.** Proximal and distal clamp placement to isolate the diseased aortic segment may include critical intercostal vessels that provide blood flow to the spinal cord and whose loss is not compensated for by distal aortic perfusion. In addition, distal perfusion may be hindered by the presence of atherosclerotic disease in the abdominal aorta, a condition that may also compromise blood flow to the kidneys and spinal cord. Finally, these crucial arterial vessels may be disrupted in gaining surgical exposure. The largest studies have shown no difference in the incidence of paraplegia, regardless of the type of surgical adjunct used.
   b. **Somatosensory-evoked potentials (SEPs).** SEPs have been promoted as a means of assessing the functional status of the spinal cord during periods of possible ischemia [35]. Briefly, SEPs monitor spinal cord function by stimulating a peripheral nerve and monitoring the response in the brainstem and cerebral cortex. Normal SEPs seem to ensure the integrity of the posterior (sensory) columns. However, SEPs have several shortcomings. First, during aortic surgery, the **anterior** (motor) horns are more at risk. Perhaps for this reason, there have been reports of patients having normal SEPs during cross-clamping but subsequently being found to have paraplegia. Second, it must be remembered that many anesthetics, including all of the halogenated drugs, nitrous oxide, and several IV drugs (e.g., thiopental and propofol), will alter the amplitude and latency of the evoked potential. Ongoing dialogue should therefore occur between the anesthesiologist and the individual(s) performing and evaluating the neuromonitoring during the operation in order to create an anesthetic plan that will be compatible with effective SEP monitoring (i.e., one-half minimum alveolar concentration of volatile anesthetic, etc.). In addition, if simple cross-clamping is used, ischemia of the peripheral nerves will interfere with SEPs interpretation.

      Other than being used as an intraoperative tool to help identify intercostal arteries that should be reimplanted to preserve spinal cord perfusion, SEPs monitoring has not been shown to decrease the incidence of paraplegia.
   c. **Motor-evoked potentials (MEPs).** Because of the noted deficiencies in SEPs monitoring, the use of MEPs has been advocated as a potentially superior method of monitoring for spinal cord ischemia, because MEP monitoring can accurately assess the integrity of the anterior horn of the spinal cord. However, because access to the central nerve roots for direct stimulation is not possible in thoracic surgery, transcranial stimulation over the motor cortex is used. In addition to being cumbersome, this method has been reported to trigger seizures in susceptible patients. However, some groups have successfully used MEPs, particularly as an adjunct to SEPs, to detect spinal cord injury in patients undergoing thoracic and thoracoabdominal aortic aneurysm repairs. Although studies have shown these neuromonitoring techniques to be helpful for predicting spinal cord injury during operations on the thoracic aorta, these monitoring methods cannot definitively rule out intraoperative spinal cord injury that will result in paraplegia. Therefore, these methods should be used as an addition to, and not a replacement for, intraoperative spinal cord protection strategies such as cerebrospinal fluid (CSF) drainage and other efforts to maintain arterial perfusion of the spinal cord

[36–38]. As with SEP monitoring, MEP monitoring requires good communication between the anesthesiologist and the neuromonitoring personnel, particularly because neuromuscular blockade cannot be used during intervals where MEP assessments are needed.

d. Hypothermia. Allowing the core body temperature to passively drift down to 32 to 34°C during surgery will lower the metabolic rate of the spinal cord tissue, possibly providing some protection from reduced or interrupted blood flow. Adequate temperature reduction can be usually accomplished by exposing the patient to a cool operating room. Other methods, such as topical cooling (cooling blankets, bags of crushed ice) and cold saline gastric lavage, also may be used. Precise control of temperature is difficult, though. At temperatures below 32°C, the myocardium may become more prone to ventricular arrhythmias, and there is increased risk of coagulopathy with hypothermia. Despite these potential problems, using vigorous methods to rewarm the patient is ill advised because of the risk of rapidly warming neural tissue that may be ischemic.

e. CSF drainage. Spinal cord damage may also be mediated by the increases in cerebrospinal fluid pressure (CSFP) that often accompany aortic cross-clamping. CSFP may increase to levels as high as the mean distal **aortic** pressure. Spinal cord perfusion pressure (SCPP) is proportional to the patient's MAP minus the CSFP or CVP—whichever is highest. SCPP may be reduced to zero during aortic cross-clamping. One approach to improving perfusion is placement of a lumbar spinal drain, which not only allows for measurement of the CSFP, but also, by removal of CSF, reduces CSFP and increases SCPP, with an apparent reduction in risk of paraplegia [39]. CSF drainage has been shown to significantly decrease postoperative paraplegia and paraparesis in a randomized controlled trial of 145 patients undergoing surgical repair of extent I or II thoracoabdominal aneurysms, with 13% and 2.6% of patients experiencing postoperative paraplegia or paraparesis in the control group versus the spinal drain group, respectively [31].

7

(1) Potential complications of spinal drain placement. Removal of CSF in the presence of an elevated intraspinal pressure can provide a gradient for herniation of cerebral structures. Also, CSF drainage, particularly more rapid CSF drainage to lower CSFPs, may cause intracranial bleeding from traction of the brain on the meninges, torn bridging veins, and the formation of subdural hematomas [40–42]. Risk of intracranial bleeding may be decreased by maintaining CSFP above at least 10 cm H_2O (7.4 mm Hg) during CSF drainage [41]. To reduce the incidence of intracranial hemorrhage and subdural hematoma, some centers have recently changed their practice regarding perioperative CSF drainage in patients with no indications of spinal cord injury (e.g., changes on intraoperative SEP or MEP monitoring, postoperative paraplegia). For these patients, CSF drainage is now targeted to less aggressive minimum CSFP thresholds, such as 10 to 15 mm Hg, and hourly CSF drainage is not to exceed 15 mL/h even if CSFP is above the minimum CSFP. If the patients develop paraplegia, CSF drainage is then liberalized to try to provoke resolution of the paralysis [40]. If a patient develops a subdural hematoma and CSF is still leaking from the insertion site after drain removal, an epidural blood patch may be warranted at the site [41]. In addition, placement of a spinal drain followed by systemic heparinization could lead to the formation of an epidural hematoma at the insertion site [42]. This is of more concern in patients who are undergoing concurrent aortic arch and descending thoracic aortic repairs that involve CPB with full heparinization and DHCA and who are, thus, at increased risk of bleeding. Another risk of drain placement is catheter fracture in the subarachnoid space.

(2) Technique for inserting and monitoring spinal drains. There are a variety of commercially available spinal drain catheters, but the insertion technique is similar for all. Spinal drain catheters are generally placed using anatomic landmarks through a 14 G (or smaller) Touhy needle that has been inserted into the subarachnoid space at a lumbar interspace (usually L_3 to L_4 or L_4 to L_5). Once the catheter

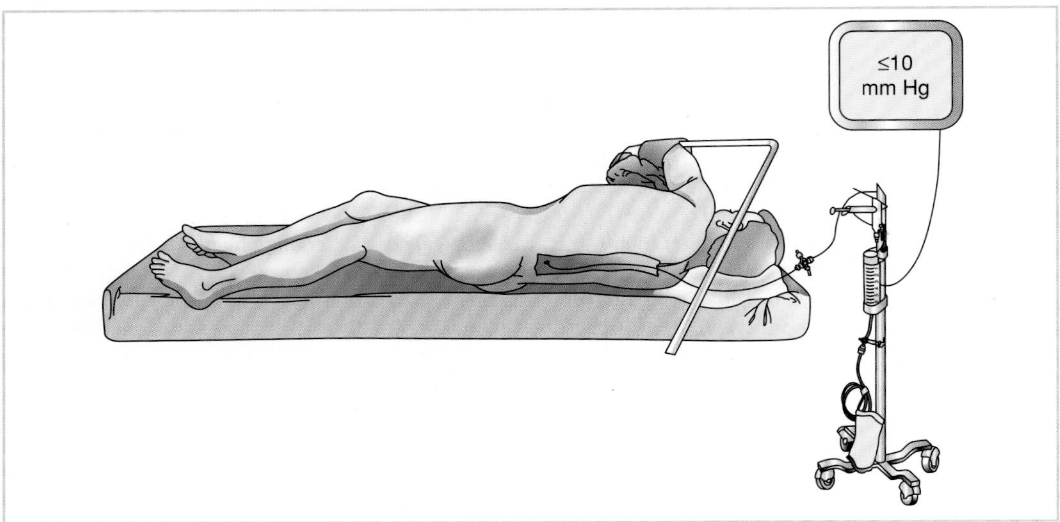

FIGURE 25.16 Intraoperative CSF drainage during thoracoabdominal aortic repair. (From Safi HJ, Miller CC III, Huynh TT, et al. Distal aortic perfusion and cerebrospinal fluid drainage for thoracoabdominal and descending thoracic aortic repair: Ten years of organ protection. *Ann Surg.* 2003;238:372–380, with permission.)

is threaded into the subarachnoid space and the needle is removed, the drain is attached to a stopcock that allows toggling between measurement of CSFP and a collection bag for drainage (Fig. 25.16) [43]. Some practitioners remove CSF intermittently to reduce CSFP, while others prefer to allow continuous drainage whenever the CSFP exceeds a predetermined set point. Although many try maintaining CSFP at 8 to 10 mm Hg in order to balance the benefit of increasing SCPP against the risk of supratentorial bleeding with a lower CSFP, there is no consensus in the literature regarding what the optimal target CSFP should be or how much CSF may be removed over a set time period.

(3) Postoperative spinal drain management. There is also no consensus regarding when spinal drains should be removed, and this is of concern considering that 30% or more of all neurologic deficits are delayed in onset [43,44]. Spinal drains are commonly left in for 48 to 72 h postoperatively [31,40] and are replaced if neurologic deficits occur after the drain is removed. In addition to maintaining CSFP between 10 to 15 mm Hg in the postoperative setting, efforts must be made to avoid systemic hypotension and associated decreased spinal cord perfusion. If delayed-onset paraparesis or paraplegia evolves, systemic hypotension should be treated and the CSF drained. This combination of measures can result in some recovery of neurologic function [43]. As with any patient with a dural puncture, headaches related to residual CSF leaks may be expected, and some will require therapy with epidural blood patches. Reviewing our own experience, we recently found that the incidence of post-dural puncture headaches and need for an epidural blood patch were elevated in patients with connective tissue diseases such as Marfan syndrome (Youngblood S, Tolpin D, LeMaire SA, et al., unpublished data; presented at the Annual Meeting of the American Society of Anesthesiologists, Chicago, Illinois, October 2011).

(4) Other methods of spinal cord protection. Additional "protective" measures, such as IV steroids, pharmacologic suppression of spinal cord function through IV or intrathecal drug administration, local hypothermia, and free radical scavengers, are not widely used or are considered experimental.

8. **Pain relief.** Thoracic and thoracoabdominal aortic surgical patients may be given IV opioid and oral analgesics for relief of postoperative pain. However, anesthesiologists may also consider using thoracic epidural anesthesia as an adjunctive perioperative pain-control measure, although, depending upon the length of the surgical incision, analgesic coverage may not be complete. Whereas thoracic epidural analgesia may potentially enhance perioperative pain control, the risk of additional significant complications associated with thoracic epidural placement should also be considered. In a patient who will undergo partial or even full heparinization and who may have significant intraoperative and early postoperative coagulopathy, instrumenting the epidural space may increase the chance of an epidural hematoma (just as placing a spinal drain does). This possibility is particularly worrisome because these patients already have a primary risk of significant neurologic complications. Additionally, it has been reported that use of a thoracic epidural may mask neurologic complications related to the removal of a CSF drainage catheter [45]. Thoracic epidural use may delay the diagnosis and treatment of spinal cord ischemia, such as when a patient cannot move his or her legs postoperatively, and the presence of epidural hematoma or motor blockade related to local anesthesia must also be considered.
9. **Prevention of renal failure.** Many patients who require thoracoabdominal aortic repair also present with renal dysfunction. It is therefore important to try to prevent the development of acute or chronic renal failure during the perioperative period. The cause of renal failure is thought to be ischemia from the interruption of blood flow during clamping, although embolism remains another possibility. Use of CPB or a shunt may be protective, but superior outcome data are lacking, and renal failure still occurs despite these surgical adjuncts. Adequate volume loading is probably important for renal protection, and some clinicians also use mannitol. In some centers, cold crystalloid or cold blood renal perfusion is administered during thoracoabdominal aneurysm repair. If the renal arteries can be surgically exposed during periods of the operation when renal arterial blood flow is interrupted, perfusate can be administered with a roller-head pump into perfusion catheters that are inserted into the renal arteries [46]. In a randomized controlled trial, intermittent cold crystalloid renal perfusion prevented postoperative renal dysfunction more effectively than renal perfusion with isothermic blood [47]. Another randomized, controlled trial indicated that cold crystalloid and cold blood renal perfusion produced comparable renal outcomes [48].

I. **Endovascular (EV) graft repair of the thoracic aorta.** Successful EV graft abdominal aortic aneurysm repair was first reported in 1991 [49]. Since then, EV graft design has improved to allow reliable deployment in the higher pulse pressure zones of the thoracic aorta, permitting repair of thoracic aortic aneurysms and dissections that were previously only reparable with open procedures. Initially, EV grafting of the descending thoracic aorta was only possible in relatively straight sections of the aorta with good "landing zones" for the proximal and distal portions of the EV graft and no major branches of the aorta in that region. Surgeons are now performing **carotid-to-subclavian** or **aorta-to-visceral** bypass operations before EV graft placement to permit placement of these devices where they would otherwise occlude the origin of a critical vessel. This has led to EV therapy of more complex aortic arch and descending thoracic aortic lesions.

1. **Surgical approach.** Placing EV grafts in the thoracic aorta generally requires femoral arterial access through which fluoroscopically guided wires and catheters may be passed to allow optimal EV graft positioning. The femoral artery is exposed and isolated via a small groin incision, but, if the femoral artery is too small or stenotic to accommodate the relatively large thoracic EV graft delivery system, a retroperitoneal dissection may be required to attain access to the iliac artery. There have been reports of EV grafts placed into the descending thoracic aorta via alternative arterial access sites such as the axillary arteries, but the femoral artery remains the typical access site for EV graft delivery [50]. The delivery system is positioned fluoroscopically at the desired implantation site, and when the delivery device is withdrawn, the endograft expands at this final aortic position.

After EV graft deployment, fluoroscopy and TEE are generally used to reassess for blood leakage around the graft [51]. Patients are positioned supine on the fluoroscopy table throughout the procedure.

2. **Surgical techniques**
   a. Patients must be systemically anticoagulated, usually with heparin, during the procedure.
   b. It is important that patients do not move during angiography, particularly during EV graft deployment. Sometimes the interventionalist will ask the anesthesiologist to hold respirations during the procedure so that they may more closely assess the portion of the aorta in which the EV graft will be deployed. This is one reason why EV graft placement into the descending thoracic aorta is usually performed with general anesthesia.
   c. EV grafts are designed to withstand continuous forward and pulsatile forces of blood flow in the aorta. Advances have led to the development of self-expanding stents that reliably adhere to the aortic wall after deployment and do not require temporarily occlusive balloon inflation within the aorta. This removes the risks of proximal hypertension associated with aortic occlusion within the thoracic aorta.
   d. EV graft design is evolving rapidly, and therefore, the number of patients ineligible for EV grafts is decreasing. However, there remain limitations regarding who can receive an EV graft in the descending thoracic aorta. The patient's aortic pathology must have a proximal "landing zone" of at least 10 to 15 mm in length and a diameter not greater than the diameter of the largest available EV graft [52]. Many descending thoracic aneurysms and dissections involve the distal aortic arch, including the take-off of the left subclavian artery. EV stent grafts are now placed that cover the ostia of the left subclavian artery, but prophylactic preprocedural left subclavian artery transposition or left subclavian-to-left common carotid artery bypass is frequently performed for the purpose of trying to prevent post-EV graft complications, including left arm ischemia, stroke, and spinal cord ischemia [53,54]. These complications can occur because the left subclavian artery not only is the main source of blood flow to the left arm, but branches into the vertebral artery (which contributes to the blood flow to the posterior portion of the Circle of Willis), the left internal mammary artery, and costocervical trunk [54]. Myocardial ischemia in patients who have a patent left internal mammary arterial bypass graft is also possible when the left subclavian arterial takeoff is covered by an EV graft [54]. It is important to note that stroke can also occur as a complication of left subclavian artery transposition or left subclavian-to-left common carotid artery bypass, so patients' cerebral blood flow anatomy and institutional comfort with performance should be considered before left subclavian arterial revascularization is performed [54]. The distal site for EV graft attachment needs to be nonaneurysmal and also of sufficient length. Furthermore, fenestrated stents are being developed to accommodate aortic side branches, but the location of aortic side branches still must be carefully evaluated and considered when one is selecting and placing EV grafts. Aortic tortuosity, calcification, and atheromatous disease are also considerations in determining whether a patient is an appropriate candidate for EV graft placement.
3. **Advantages of EV graft repair**
   a. **Reduced mortality.** Randomized controlled trials have shown significantly decreased mortality in patients undergoing EV repair of abdominal aortic aneurysms [55,56]. Nonrandomized studies of descending thoracic aorta repair have associated EV grafting with significantly lower 30-day mortality than open surgical repair; however, this mortality benefit may not persist at 1 yr after thoracic aortic repair [57]. The randomized controlled INvestigation of STEnt-grafts in Aortic Dissection (INSTEAD) trial reported no significant 2-yr mortality advantage for EV stenting versus medical therapy alone in patients with uncomplicated Type B dissections [58].

b. **Reduced morbidity.** Patients experience substantially less blood loss with EV procedures and are spared the prolonged recovery and pulmonary complications that often occur with large thoracoabdominal incisions. EV procedures also allow for increased hemodynamic stability and decreased ischemic risk to the heart and other organs when compared with open repairs. Patients with pulmonary and cardiac comorbidities that would eliminate them as candidates for open repair are often acceptable candidates for thoracic aortic EV graft placement. A recent meta-analysis of 42 nonrandomized studies that included 5,888 patients with aneurysm, trauma, or dissection of the descending thoracic aorta revealed that patients who underwent EV repair versus open surgical repair had significantly less perioperative paraplegia, cardiac complications, transfusions, reoperation for bleeding, renal dysfunction, and pneumonia, and they had a shorter hospital length of stay [57]. In addition, many patients who undergo EV repair require substantially shorter intensive care unit (ICU) stays [52,59,60].

4. **Complications of EV repair**

a. **Need for emergency conversion to open repair** may occur if the aorta is ruptured or dissected during manipulations to place the EV graft or if the EV graft becomes malpositioned such that it presents substantial risk for visceral ischemia.

b. **Bleeding.** Although blood loss during EV repair of the thoracic aorta is markedly lower (approximately 500 mL) [59] than blood loss with open surgery, bleeding does occur from the femoral artery introducer when it is traversed by wires and catheters during the interventional procedure. Because many patients with thoracic aortic disease have comorbidities that make anemia unfavorable, bleeding may be significant enough to warrant periprocedural blood transfusion. Large-volume blood loss may also occur if the internal iliac artery is damaged during removal of what is generally a large-diameter graft deployment device. Massive blood loss should be anticipated in the setting of aortic rupture.

c. **Endoleak.** Endoleak occurs when blood continues to flow into the aneurysmal sac after EV graft placement. It confers continued risk of aortic rupture and thus requires early identification and intervention. If identified, responses range from observation over several months to see if the leak resolves spontaneously to another EV procedure to occlude the source of the leak to, in some cases, an open surgical repair. The degree of intervention depends upon the type of leak identified [52]. Type I endoleaks occur with an inadequate seal between the EV graft and the wall of the aorta at either the proximal or the distal attachment site, such that there is persistent flow into the native aneurysm. A Type II endoleak occurs when the portion of the aorta that was to be excluded by the graft fills in a retrograde fashion from back-bleeding collateral vessels, such as the lumbar or inferior mesenteric arteries. There is no definitive approach for addressing Type II endoleak: Both observation and side-branch embolization are used. A Type III endoleak occurs from failure within the EV graft itself and requires conversion to an open repair so that the EV graft does not dislodge.

d. **Stroke.** The incidence of periprocedural stroke is ~5% [57] and appears to be higher in patients who undergo EV graft placement in the region of the distal arch that includes the take-off of the left subclavian artery. Among patients who undergo EV graft placement across the left subclavian artery, stroke risk may be lower in those who undergo a staged carotid-to-subclavian-artery bypass procedure first, as this may prevent vertebrobasilar arterial insufficiency and potential ensuing posterior cerebral infarction [54]. Stroke risk is increased in patients with a history of stroke, patients whose CT scans reveal severe atheromatous disease of the aortic arch, and patients in whom EV grafting involves the distal aortic arch [61]. For these reasons, it seems likely that stroke is secondary to embolic events that result from intra-aortic or carotid arterial manipulation during positioning and deployment of the EV graft.

e. **Paraplegia.** Although some data suggest that the risk of lower-extremity paraparesis or paralysis is reduced in patients undergoing EV graft versus open thoracic aortic repair, its incidence is still 3% to 4% [57,59,62]. Many surgeons and interventional radiologists, therefore, prefer that a lumbar spinal drain be placed before the procedure and that CSF drainage be conducted in the same manner as described in this chapter for open thoracoabdominal operations.

f. **Contrast nephropathy (CN).** Although patients undergoing open aortic surgical repairs are susceptible to postoperative acute renal failure from ischemia during aortic cross-clamping, patients undergoing EV graft repairs are susceptible to CN. Patients with pre-existing renal insufficiency, especially those with diabetic nephropathy, are particularly susceptible to CN [63]. Older age, hypertension, repeat contrast exposure within a short time, use of high osmolality contrast, and preprocedural medications such as nonsteroidal anti-inflammatory drugs and ACE inhibitors also put patients at increased risk for CN [63]. Although the pathogenesis of CN is not completely understood, it appears to be related to decreased renal medullary perfusion and associated ischemia, as well as a direct toxic effect of contrast on the renal epithelial cells. We refer the reader to two excellent reviews of CN for a more detailed discussion [63,64].

J. **Anesthetic considerations for patients undergoing EV stent graft repair of the thoracic aorta**

1. **General considerations**

a. Although thoracic aortic EV graft placement is a minimally invasive procedure, the possibility of aortic rupture, dissection, or malposition of the EV graft should be considered when the location for the procedure is selected and the anesthetic planned, as any of these complications would require urgent or emergent conversion to an open procedure. If the procedure cannot be conducted in an operating room because it lacks appropriate angiographic equipment, the entire care team involved with the procedure in a radiology suite must be familiar with resuscitation plans and with transport plans to the operating room. If a cardiac or vascular surgeon is not performing the EV graft procedure, he or she should be immediately available if conversion to open surgery is necessary.

b. Although there have been reports of placing thoracic aortic EV grafts under regional anesthesia, this approach has several disadvantages in comparison to general anesthesia.

(1) In the event that there needs to be an emergency conversion to open aortic repair, this conversion will be slowed by the need for airway control before positioning the patient for the operation.

(2) If the patient is intubated at the start of the procedure and the surgeon feels that the patient is at reasonably high risk for open conversion, the anesthesiologist can place a bronchial blocker in the left main stem bronchus without inflating it. The bronchial blocker can then be quickly inflated in the setting of emergency conversion to provide single-lung ventilation.

(3) Many of the thoracic aortic EV graft procedures are too lengthy for regional anesthesia.

(4) General anesthesia with endotracheal intubation allows the anesthesiologist or cardiologist to conduct TEE evaluation throughout the procedure. This has been found to be particularly useful in assessing for endoleaks and for differentiating slow blood flow associated with the porosity of the EV stent graft from true high-velocity peri-stent endoleaks [51,52,65]. In patients undergoing EV stent graft placement for complicated Type B dissections, TEE can also be helpful for repositioning the guidewire from the false to the true lumen and for detecting new intimal tears in the thoracic aorta after EV stent placement [65]. Such new distal aortic tears might require additional EV stents to be placed.

2. **Monitoring.** All patients should have standard ASA monitors and a radial arterial line for BP monitoring to help in maintaining hemodynamic stability. The majority of patients presenting for thoracic aortic EV grafts have significant cardiovascular comorbidities that warrant tight hemodynamic control. Furthermore, surgeons may request transient,

mild hypotension during stent deployment to help prevent graft migration. In the event that emergent conversion to open surgery is needed, an arterial line will be extremely useful in guiding volume resuscitation and possible cardiopulmonary resuscitation. The location of arterial access for stent delivery should be discussed with the surgical team, because, if the femoroiliac vasculature is not adequate for the procedure, they may guide stent placement via a brachial artery. Typically, a right radial arterial line is ideal for hemodynamic monitoring because it allows monitoring of arterial pressure proximal to the distal aortic arch. Central venous access for monitoring right atrial pressure and for effective administration of vasoactive drugs is reasonable for most patients. Some centers monitor SEPs and/or MEPs, as well as CSFP, during placement of thoracic aortic EV grafts. Urine output should be monitored to help assess adequacy of fluid administration during what can often be long procedures. A fluid warmer and warming blanket should be used if possible to help prevent hypothermia, and oropharyngeal temperature should be monitored.

3. **Fluid therapy and transfusion**
   a. Large-bore IV access should be placed in case of the need for rapid volume resuscitation.
   b. Cross-matched, packed red blood cells should be available.
   c. A system for rapid infusion of blood products and other fluids should be immediately available in cases where volume resuscitation is needed.
4. **CSF drainage.** Risk for paraplegia or paraparesis after EV graft placement remains approximately 3% to 4%, as noted above, particularly if long segments of the descending thoracic aorta are involved in EV graft placement or if the patient has previously undergone abdominal aortic aneurysm repair [52,66,67]. Therefore, many surgeons, interventionalists, and anesthesiologists prefer to place and manage lumbar spinal drains for EV graft procedures in the manner described above. IV hydration and vasopressor drugs should be administered to maintain higher MAPs. As with patients who undergo open surgical repairs of the descending thoracic aorta, delayed-onset paraparesis or paraplegia also occurs in patients who receive EV stent grafts [66,67], so patients should undergo frequent post-procedural neurologic examinations, and if signs of spinal cord ischemia/injury are detected, aggressive efforts should be made to increase MAPs and to drain more CSF.
5. **CN.** Because EV grafting of the thoracic aorta is often a long procedure that involves a substantial volume of IV contrast, the anesthesiologist should consider strategies to attenuate risk for CN, particularly in patients presenting with renal insufficiency.
   a. **Hydration.** Studies suggest that preprocedural hydration with 0.9% normal saline is beneficial in mitigating the risk of developing CN [63]. There is no consensus regarding the duration of IV 0.9% normal saline infusion before or after the procedure, but avoiding hypovolemia in these patients during the procedure is advisable [64].
   b. **N-acetylcysteine (NAC).** NAC has antioxidant and vasodilatory effects. Some studies have shown a benefit in pretreating patients with NAC for 24 h before procedures requiring IV contrast, while other studies have shown that there is no benefit [63,64].
   c. **Diuretics.** Diuretic use does not seem to prevent CN. Some advocate that, if possible, diuretics be withdrawn for the 24 h before procedures requiring contrast [63] because of concern that they may increase the risk of CN.
   d. **Dopamine and fenoldopam.** Neither of these drugs has been found to prevent CN in human studies [63].

K. **Future trends.** Just as the past several decades of treatment of aortic diseases have been marked by innovation and the refinement of surgical and anesthetic techniques, so also will future years. The most promising recent developments have been made in the area of EV stenting of aneurysmal, dissected, or traumatically transected segments of the thoracoabdominal aorta. EV stent graft technology will probably continue to advance, with the industry focusing on newer fenestrated grafts that will not obstruct blood flow to important aortic side branches and other grafts that are able to adhere to curved portions of the aorta, such as the aortic arch. There will also probably be innovations regarding alternate arterial access points for inserting

EV stent-deployment devices. Hopefully, greater strides will also be made toward even better protection strategies for organs (i.e., spinal cord, gut, and kidneys), including novel approaches to mitigating end-organ ischemia-reperfusion injury. Anesthetic developments will focus on refining understanding of the physiology of organ preservation and the pharmacology needed to achieve this. Such advances should continue to improve the survival of patients with thoracic aortic disease.

REFERENCES

1. Hiratzka LF, Bakris GL, Beckman JA, et al. 2010 ACCF/AHA/AATS/ACR/ASA/SCA/SCAI/SIR/STS/SVM guidelines for the diagnosis and management of patients with thoracic aortic disease: A report of the American College of Cardiology Foundation/American Heart Association Task Force on Practice Guidelines, American Association for Thoracic Surgery, American College of Radiology, American Stroke Association, Society of Cardiovascular Anesthesiologists, Society for Cardiovascular Angiography and Interventions, Society of Interventional Radiology, Society of Thoracic Surgeons, and Society for Vascular Medicine. *Circulation.* 2010;121:e266–e369.
2. Kouchoukos NT, Dougenis D. Surgery of the thoracic aorta. *N Engl J Med.* 1997;336:1876–1888.
3. Hirst AE Jr, Johns VJ Jr, Kime SW Jr. Dissecting aneurysm of the aorta: A review of 505 cases. *Medicine (Baltimore).* 1958;37:217–279.
4. Bickerstaff LK, Pairolero PC, Hollier LH, et al. Thoracic aortic aneurysms: A population-based study. *Surgery.* 1982;92:1103–1108.
5. Hartnell GG. Imaging of aortic aneurysms and dissection: CT and MRI. *J Thorac Imaging.* 2001;16:35–46.
6. Nienaber CA, von Kodolitsch Y, Nicolas V, et al. The diagnosis of thoracic aortic dissection by noninvasive imaging procedures. *N Engl J Med.* 1993;328:1–9.
7. Miller DC, Stinson EB, Oyer PE, et al. Operative treatment of aortic dissections. Experience with 125 patients over a sixteen-year period. *J Thorac Cardiovasc Surg.* 1979;78:365–382.
8. Gertler JP, Cambria RP, Brewster DC, et al. Coagulation changes during thoracoabdominal aneurysm repair. *J Vasc Surg.* 1996;24:936–943; discussion 43–45.
9. Schneiderman J, Bordin GM, Engelberg I, et al. Expression of fibrinolytic genes in atherosclerotic abdominal aortic aneurysm wall. A possible mechanism for aneurysm expansion. *J Clin Invest.* 1995;96:639–645.
10. Balduini CL, Salvini M, Montani N, et al. Activation of the hemostatic process in patients with unruptured aortic aneurysm before and in the first week after surgical repair. *Haematologica.* 1997;82:581–583.
11. Cina CS, Clase CM. Coagulation disorders and blood product use in patients undergoing thoracoabdominal aortic aneurysm repair. *Transfus Med Rev.* 2005;19:143–154.
12. Shore-Lesserson L, Bodian C, Vela-Cantos F, et al. Antifibrinolytic use and bleeding during surgery on the descending thoracic aorta: A multivariate analysis. *J Cardiothorac Vasc Anesth.* 2005;19:453–458.
13. Casati V, Sandrelli L, Speziali G, et al. Hemostatic effects of tranexamic acid in elective thoracic aortic surgery: A prospective, randomized, double-blind, placebo-controlled study. *J Thorac Cardiovasc Surg.* 2002;123:1084–1091.
14. Cooper JR Jr, Skeehan TM, Cooley DA. Case 4—1991. A 57-year-old man requires complex management for surgery on a dissecting thoracic aortic aneurysm. *J Cardiothorac Vasc Anesth.* 1991;5:390–398.
15. Miller DC, Stinson EB, Oyer PE, et al. Concomitant resection of ascending aortic aneurysm and replacement of the aortic valve: Operative and long-term results with "conventional" techniques in ninety patients. *J Thorac Cardiovasc Surg.* 1980;79:388–401.
16. Crawford ES, Saleh SA. Transverse aortic arch aneurysm: Improved results of treatment employing new modifications of aortic reconstruction and hypothermic cerebral circulatory arrest. *Ann Surg.* 1981;194:180–188.
17. Svensson LG, Crawford ES, Hess KR, et al. Deep hypothermia with circulatory arrest. Determinants of stroke and early mortality in 656 patients. *J Thorac Cardiovasc Surg.* 1993;106:19–28; discussion 31.
18. Shum-Tim D, Nagashima M, Shinoka T, et al. Postischemic hyperthermia exacerbates neurologic injury after deep hypothermic circulatory arrest. *J Thorac Cardiovasc Surg.* 1998;116:780–792.
19. Ehrlich MP, Wolner E. Neuroprotection in aortic surgery. *Thorac Cardiovasc Surg.* 2001;49:247–250.
20. Ueda Y, Okita Y, Aomi S, et al. Retrograde cerebral perfusion for aortic arch surgery: Analysis of risk factors. *Ann Thorac Surg.* 1999;67:1879–1882; discussion 91–94.
21. Bachet J, Guilmet D, Goudot B, et al. Antegrade cerebral perfusion with cold blood: A 13-year experience. *Ann Thorac Surg.* 1999;67:1874–1878; discussion 91–94.
22. Cook RC, Gao M, Macnab AJ, et al. Aortic arch reconstruction: Safety of moderate hypothermia and antegrade cerebral perfusion during systemic circulatory arrest. *J Card Surg.* 2006;21:158–164.
23. Strauch JT, Spielvogel D, Lauten A, et al. Axillary artery cannulation: Routine use in ascending aorta and aortic arch replacement. *Ann Thorac Surg.* 2004;78:103–108; discussion 8.
24. Dewhurst AT, Moore SJ, Liban JB. Pharmacological agents as cerebral protectants during deep hypothermic circulatory arrest in adult thoracic aortic surgery. A survey of current practice. *Anaesthesia.* 2002;57:1016–1021.
25. Murkin JM, Arango M. Near-infrared spectroscopy as an index of brain and tissue oxygenation. *Br J Anaesth.* 2009;103(suppl 1):i3–i13.
26. Harrer M, Waldenberger FR, Weiss G, et al. Aortic arch surgery using bilateral antegrade selective cerebral perfusion in combination with near-infrared spectroscopy. *Eur J Cardiothorac Surg.* 2010;38:561–567.
27. Gelman S. The pathophysiology of aortic cross-clamping and unclamping. *Anesthesiology.* 1995;82:1026–1060.
28. Romagnoli A, Cooper JR Jr. Anesthesia for aortic operations. *Cleve Clin Q.* 1981;48:147–152.

29. Cambria RP, Clouse WD, Davison JK, et al. Thoracoabdominal aneurysm repair: Results with 337 operations performed over a 15-year interval. *Ann Surg.* 2002;236:471–479; discussion 9.
30. Svensson LG, Crawford ES, Hess KR, et al. Experience with 1509 patients undergoing thoracoabdominal aortic operations. *J Vasc Surg.* 1993;17:357–368; discussion 68–70.
31. Coselli JS, LeMaire SA, Köksoy C, et al. Cerebrospinal fluid drainage reduces paraplegia after thoracoabdominal aortic aneurysm repair: Results of a randomized clinical trial. *J Vasc Surg.* 2002;35:631–639.
32. Shenaq SA, Svensson LG. Paraplegia following aortic surgery. *J Cardiothorac Vasc Anesth.* 1993;7:81–94.
33. O'Connor CJ, Rothenberg DM. Anesthetic considerations for descending thoracic aortic surgery: Part 1. *J Cardiothorac Vasc Anesth.* 1995;9:581–588.
34. O'Connor CJ, Rothenberg DM. Anesthetic considerations for descending thoracic aortic surgery: Part II. *J Cardiothorac Vasc Anesth.* 1995;9:734–747.
35. Robertazzi RR, Cunningham JN Jr. Intraoperative adjuncts of spinal cord protection. *Semin Thorac Cardiovasc Surg.* 1998;10:29–34.
36. Horiuchi T, Kawaguchi M, Inoue S, et al. Assessment of intraoperative motor evoked potentials for predicting postoperative paraplegia in thoracic and thoracoabdominal aortic aneurysm repair. *J Anesth.* 2011;25:18–28.
37. Min HK, Sung K, Yang JH, et al. Can intraoperative motor-evoked potentials predict all the spinal cord ischemia during moderate hypothermic beating heart descending thoracic or thoraco-abdominal aortic surgery? *J Card Surg.* 2010;25:542–547.
38. Keyhani K, Miller CC 3rd, Estrera AL, et al. Analysis of motor and somatosensory evoked potentials during thoracic and thoracoabdominal aortic aneurysm repair. *J Vasc Surg.* 2009;49:36–41.
39. Ling E, Arellano R. Systematic overview of the evidence supporting the use of cerebrospinal fluid drainage in thoracoabdominal aneurysm surgery for prevention of paraplegia. *Anesthesiology.* 2000;93:1115–1122.
40. Estrera AL, Sheinbaum R, Miller CC, et al. Cerebrospinal fluid drainage during thoracic aortic repair: Safety and current management. *Ann Thorac Surg.* 2009;88:9–15; discussion 15.
41. Dardik A, Perler BA, Roseborough GS, et al. Subdural hematoma after thoracoabdominal aortic aneurysm repair: An underreported complication of spinal fluid drainage? *J Vasc Surg.* 2002;36:47–50.
42. Murakami H, Yoshida K, Hino Y, et al. Complications of cerebrospinal fluid drainage in thoracoabdominal aortic aneurysm repair. *J Vasc Surg.* 2004;39:243–245.
43. Safi HJ, Miller CC 3rd, Huynh TT, et al. Distal aortic perfusion and cerebrospinal fluid drainage for thoracoabdominal and descending thoracic aortic repair: Ten years of organ protection. *Ann Surg.* 2003;238:372–380; discussion 80–81.
44. Wong DR, Coselli JS, Amerman K, et al. Delayed spinal cord deficits after thoracoabdominal aortic aneurysm repair. *Ann Thorac Surg.* 2007;83:1345–1355; discussion 55.
45. Heller LB, Chaney MA. Paraplegia immediately following removal of a cerebrospinal fluid drainage catheter in a patient after thoracoabdominal aortic aneurysm surgery. *Anesthesiology.* 2001;95:1285–1287.
46. Coselli JS. Strategies for renal and visceral protection in thoracoabdominal aortic surgery. *J Thorac Cardiovasc Surg.* 2010;140:S147–S149; discussion S85–S90.
47. Köksoy C, LeMaire SA, Curling PE, et al. Renal perfusion during thoracoabdominal aortic operations: Cold crystalloid is superior to normothermic blood. *Ann Thorac Surg.* 2002;73:730–738.
48. LeMaire SA, Jones MM, Conklin LD, et al. Randomized comparison of cold blood and cold crystalloid renal perfusion for renal protection during thoracoabdominal aortic aneurysm repair. *J Vasc Surg.* 2009;49:11–19; discussion 9.
49. Parodi JC, Palmaz JC, Barone HD. Transfemoral intraluminal graft implantation for abdominal aortic aneurysms. *Ann Vasc Surg.* 1991;5:491–499.
50. Saadi EK, Dussin LH, Moura L, et al. The axillary artery—a new approach for endovascular treatment of thoracic aortic diseases. *Interact Cardiovasc Thorac Surg.* 2010;11:617–619.
51. Swaminathan M, Lineberger CK, McCann RL, et al. The importance of intraoperative transesophageal echocardiography in endovascular repair of thoracic aortic aneurysms. *Anesth Analg.* 2003;97:1566–1572.
52. Kahn RA, Moskowitz DM, Marin M, et al. Anesthetic considerations for endovascular aortic repair. *Mt Sinai J Med.* 2002;69:57–67.
53. Weigang E, Parker JA, Czerny M, et al. Should intentional endovascular stent-graft coverage of the left subclavian artery be preceded by prophylactic revascularisation? *Eur J Cardiothorac Surg.* 2011;40:858–868.
54. Rehman SM, Vecht JA, Perera R, et al. How to manage the left subclavian artery during endovascular stenting of the thoracic aorta. *Eur J Cardiothorac Surg.* 2011;39:507–518.
55. Greenhalgh RM, Brown LC, Kwong GP, et al. Comparison of endovascular aneurysm repair with open repair in patients with abdominal aortic aneurysm (EVAR trial 1), 30-day operative mortality results: Randomised controlled trial. *Lancet.* 2004;364:843–848.
56. Prinssen M, Verhoeven EL, Buth J, et al. A randomized trial comparing conventional and endovascular repair of abdominal aortic aneurysms. *N Engl J Med.* 2004;351:1607–1618.
57. Cheng D, Martin J, Shennib H, et al. Endovascular aortic repair versus open surgical repair for descending thoracic aortic disease: A systematic review and meta-analysis of comparative studies. *J Am Coll Cardiol.* 2010;55:986–1001.
58. Nienaber CA, Rousseau H, Eggebrecht H, et al. Randomized comparison of strategies for type B aortic dissection: The INvestigation of STEnt Grafts in Aortic Dissection (INSTEAD) trial. *Circulation.* 2009;120:2519–2528.
59. Makaroun MS, Dillavou ED, Kee ST, et al. Endovascular treatment of thoracic aortic aneurysms: Results of the phase II multicenter trial of the GORE TAG thoracic endoprosthesis. *J Vasc Surg.* 2005;41:1–9.
60. Gopaldas RR, Huh J, Dao TK, et al. Superior nationwide outcomes of endovascular versus open repair for isolated descending thoracic aortic aneurysm in 11,669 patients. *J Thorac Cardiovasc Surg.* 2010;140:1001–1010.
61. Gutsche JT, Cheung AT, McGarvey ML, et al. Risk factors for perioperative stroke after thoracic endovascular aortic repair. *Ann Thorac Surg.* 2007;84:1195–1200; discussion 200.

62. Leurs LJ, Bell R, Degrieck Y, et al. Endovascular treatment of thoracic aortic diseases: Combined experience from the EUROSTAR and United Kingdom Thoracic Endograft registries. *J Vasc Surg.* 2004;40:670–679; discussion 9–80.
63. Maeder M, Klein M, Fehr T, et al. Contrast nephropathy: Review focusing on prevention. *J Am Coll Cardiol.* 2004;44:1763–1771.
64. Barrett BJ, Parfrey PS. Clinical practice. Preventing nephropathy induced by contrast medium. *N Engl J Med.* 2006;354:379–386.
65. Rocchi G, Lofiego C, Biagini E, et al. Transesophageal echocardiography-guided algorithm for stent-graft implantation in aortic dissection. *J Vasc Surg.* 2004;40:880–885.
66. Baril DT, Carroccio A, Ellozy SH, et al. Endovascular thoracic aortic repair and previous or concomitant abdominal aortic repair: Is the increased risk of spinal cord ischemia real? *Ann Vasc Surg.* 2006;20:188–194.
67. Gravereaux EC, Faries PL, Burks JA, et al. Risk of spinal cord ischemia after endograft repair of thoracic aortic aneurysms. *J Vasc Surg.* 2001;34:997–1003.

26 Anesthetic Management for Surgery of the Lungs and Mediastinum

Peter Slinger and Erin A. Sullivan

KEY POINTS

1. Preoperatively respiratory function should be assessed in three related but independent areas: Respiratory mechanics, gas exchange, and cardiopulmonary interaction.
2. The most useful preoperative predictor of difficult endobronchial intubation is the chest film.
3. The most important predictor of $P_{a}O_2$ during one-lung ventilation is the $P_{a}O_2$ during two-lung ventilation in the lateral position before one-lung ventilation.
4. Absolute indications for lung isolation include purulent secretions, massive pulmonary hemorrhage, bronchopleural fistula, blebs, and bullae (blood, pus, and air).
5. Iatrogenic injury has been estimated to occur in 0.5 to 2 per 1,000 cases using double-lumen tubes.
6. The rapidity of the fall in $P_{a}O_2$ after the onset of one-lung ventilation is an indicator of the risk of subsequent desaturation.
7. Because of the risk of increased shunt and pulmonary edema in the dependent lung, no volume should be given for theoretical third-space losses during thoracotomy.
8. Desaturation during bilateral lung procedures is particularly a problem during the second period of one-lung ventilation.
9. The postoperative mortality following pneumonectomy is 17% in patients who develop arrhythmias versus 2% in those without this complication.
10. During induction of general anesthesia in patients with an anterior mediastinal mass, airway obstruction is the most common and feared complication.
11. Hemoptysis in a patient with a PA catheter must be assumed to be caused by perforation of a pulmonary vessel by the catheter until proven otherwise. The mortality rate may exceed 50%.
12. In a patient with pulmonary hypertension, abrupt cessation of treatment with a prostacyclin analog can result in potentially catastrophic rebound pulmonary hypertension.
13. For transplantation of CMV-negative donors and recipients, leukocyte-poor filters should be used to reduce exposure to CMV during transfusion of blood and blood products. Likewise, to avoid human leukocyte antigen alloimmunization, leukocyte-poor blood is necessary for transplant candidates.
14. There may be an increase in the dose of nondepolarizing neuromuscular blocking agents required in posttransplantation patients receiving azathioprine.

I. Preoperative assessment

A. Overview. Advances in anesthetic management, surgical techniques, and perioperative care have expanded the envelope of patients now considered to be operable. The principles described apply to all types of pulmonary resections and other chest surgery. In patients with malignancy, the risk/benefit ratio of canceling or delaying surgery pending other investigation/therapy is always complicated by the risk of further spread of cancer during any interval before resection.

A patient with a "resectable" lung cancer has a disease that is still local or locoregional in scope and can be encompassed in a plausible surgical procedure. An "operable" patient is one who can tolerate the proposed resection with acceptable risk.

1. **Risk assessment.** It is the anesthesiologist's responsibility to use the preoperative assessment to identify patients at elevated risk and then to use that risk assessment to stratify perioperative management and focus resources on the high-risk patients to improve their outcome. This is the primary function of the preanesthetic assessment.
2. **Initial and final assessments.** Commonly, the patient is initially assessed in a clinic and often not by the member of the anesthesia staff who will administer the anesthesia. The actual contact with the responsible anesthesiologist may be only 10 to 15 min before induction. It is necessary to organize and standardize the approach to preoperative evaluation for these patients into two temporally disjoint phases: The initial (clinic) assessment and the final (day-of-admission) assessment.
3. **"Lung-sparing" surgery.** Postoperative preservation of respiratory function has been shown to be proportional to the amount of functioning lung parenchyma preserved. To

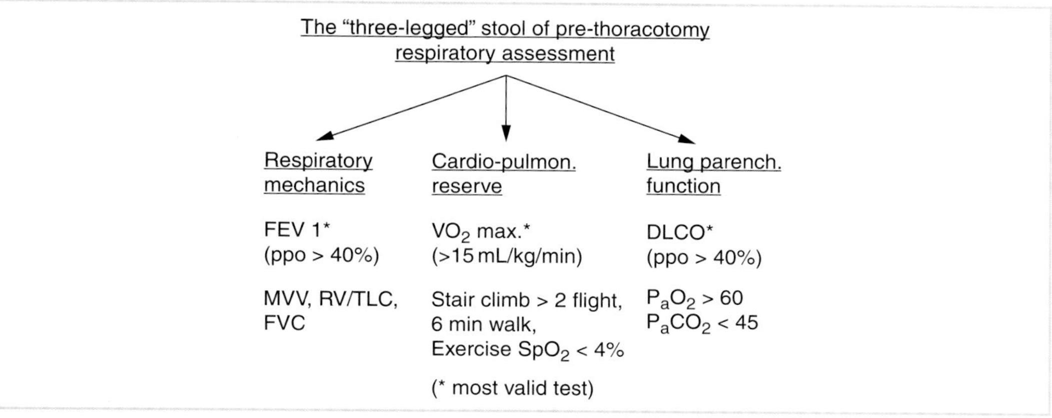

FIGURE 26.1 "Three-legged" stool of prethoracotomy respiratory assessment. ppo, predicted postoperative; FEV 1, Forced expiratory volume in one second; MVV, Maximum voluntary ventilation; RV/TLC, Residual volume/Total lung capacity; FVC, Forced vital capacity; VO_2 max, Maximum Oxygen consumption; SpO_2, Oxygen saturation by pulse oximetry; DLCO, Diffusing capacity for carbon monoxide; P_aO_2, Arterial partial pressure of oxygen; P_aCO_2, Arterial partial pressure of carbon dioxide.

assess patients with limited pulmonary function, the anesthesiologist must understand these surgical options in addition to conventional lobectomy and pneumonectomy.

Prethoracotomy assessment naturally involves all of the factors of a complete anesthetic assessment: Past history, allergies, medications, and upper airway. The major cause of perioperative morbidity and mortality in the thoracic surgical population is respiratory complications. Atelectasis, pneumonia, and respiratory failure occur in 15% to 20% of patients. Cardiac complications, such as arrhythmia and ischemia, occur in 10% to 15% of the thoracic population.

B. Risk stratification

1. **Assessment of respiratory function.** The best assessment of respiratory function comes from a history of the patient's quality of life. An asymptomatic American Society of Anesthesiologists (ASA) Class I or II patient with full exercise capacity does not need screening
1 cardiorespiratory testing. Assess respiratory function in three related but independent areas: Respiratory mechanics, gas exchange, and cardiopulmonary interaction. These three factors give the "three-legged stool" of prethoracotomy respiratory assessment (Fig. 26.1).

   a. **Lung mechanics.** The most valid single test [1] for post-thoracotomy respiratory complications is the predicted postoperative forced expiratory volume in 1 s ($ppoFEV_1\%$), which is calculated as follows:

$$\mathbf{ppoFEV_1\% = preop.\ FEV_1\% \times (1\text{-}\%\ functional\ lung\ tissue\ removed/100)}$$

   Consider the right upper and middle lobes combined as approximately equivalent to each of the other three lobes and the right lung 10% larger than the left lung.

   Low risk = $ppoFEV_1$ > 40% predicted.
   Moderate risk = $ppoFEV_1$ 30% to 40% predicted.
   High risk = $ppoFEV_1$ < 30% predicted.

   b. **Pulmonary parenchymal function.** Traditionally, arterial blood gas (ABG) data such as P_aO_2 less than 60 mm Hg or P_aCO_2 greater than 45 mm Hg have been used as cutoff values for pulmonary resection. Cancer resections now have been successfully done or even combined with volume reduction in patients who do not meet these criteria, although they remain useful as warning indicators of increased risk. The most useful test of the gas exchange capacity of the lung is the diffusing capacity for carbon monoxide (DLCO). DLCO correlates with the total functioning surface area of alveolar–capillary interface. A ppoDLCO less than 40% correlates with both increased respiratory and cardiac complications [2].

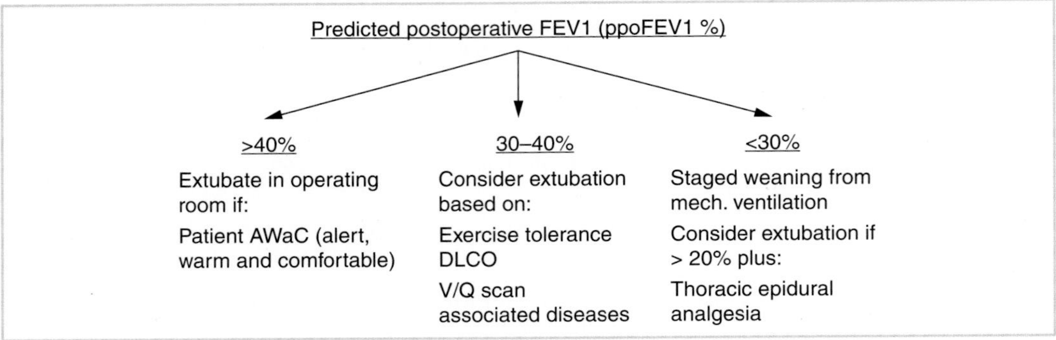

FIGURE 26.2 Post-thoracotomy anesthetic management. FEV1, Forced expiratory volume in 1 second; ppo, Predicted postoperative; DLCO, Diffusing capacity for carbon monoxide; V/Q, Ventilation/Perfusion.

c. **Cardiopulmonary interaction.** The traditional test in ambulatory patients is stair climbing. The ability to climb three flights or more is associated with decreased mortality. Formal laboratory exercise testing is currently the "gold standard" for assessment of cardiopulmonary function. The maximal oxygen consumption Vo_2 max is the most valid exercise predictor of post-thoracotomy outcome. An estimate of Vo_2 max can be made by dividing the distance walked in meters in 6 min (6MWT) by 30 (i.e., 450 m/30 = 15 mL/kg/min):

Low risk = Vo_2 max > 20 mL/kg/min.
Moderate risk = Vo_2 max = 15 to 20 mL/kg/min.
High risk = Vo_2 max < 15 mL/kg/min.

d. **Ventilation–perfusion scintigraphy** is particularly useful in pneumonectomy patients and should be considered for any patient who has $ppoFEV_1$ less than 40%. Assessments of $ppoFEV_1$, DLCO, and Vo_2 max can be upgraded if the lung region to be resected is nonfunctioning.

e. **Split-lung function studies.** These tests have not shown sufficient predictive validity for universal adoption in potential lung resection patients.

f. **Combination of tests** (Fig. 26.2). If a patient has $ppoFEV_1$ greater than 40%, it should be possible for the patient to be extubated in the operating room at the conclusion of surgery, assuming the patient is alert, warm, and comfortable ("AWaC"). If $ppoFEV_1$ is greater than 30% and exercise tolerance and lung parenchymal function exceed the increased risk thresholds, then extubation in the operating room should be possible depending on the status of associated diseases. Patients with $ppoFEV_1$ 20% to 30% and favorable predicted cardiorespiratory and parenchymal function can be considered for early extubation if thoracic epidural analgesia is used.

2. **Intercurrent medical conditions**

a. **Age.** For patients older than 80 yrs, the rate of respiratory complications (40%) is double that expected in a younger population, and the rate of cardiac complications (40%), particularly arrhythmias, is nearly triple. The mortality from pneumonectomy (22% in patients older than 70 yrs), particularly right pneumonectomy, is excessive.

b. **Cardiac disease**

(1) **Ischemia.** Pulmonary resection is generally regarded as an intermediate-risk procedure for perioperative ischemia. Beyond the standard history, physical examination, and electrocardiogram, routine screening testing for cardiac disease does not appear to be cost effective for all prethoracotomy patients. Noninvasive testing is indicated in patients with active cardiac conditions (unstable ischemia, recent infarction, decompensated heart failure, severe valvular disease, significant arrhythmia), multiple clinical predictors of cardiac risk (stable angina, remote infarction, previous congestive failure, diabetes, renal insufficiency, or cerebrovascular

disease), or in the elderly. Timing of lung resection surgery after a myocardial infarction is always a difficult decision. Limiting the delay to 4 to 6 wks in a medically stable and fully investigated and optimized patient seems acceptable.

(2) **Arrhythmia.** Atrial fibrillation is a common complication (10% to 15%) of pulmonary resection surgery. Factors correlating with an increased incidence of arrhythmia are the amount of lung tissue resected, age, intraoperative blood loss, and intrapericardial dissection. Prophylactic digoxin does not prevent these arrhythmias, but diltiazem may.

c. **Chronic obstructive pulmonary disease (COPD).** Assessment of the severity of COPD is based on FEV_1% predicted, as follows—Stage I: Greater than 50%; Stage II: 35% to 50%; and Stage III: Less than 35%. The following factors in COPD need to be considered.

Respiratory drive. Many Stage II or III COPD patients have an elevated P_aCO_2 at rest. It is not possible to differentiate "CO_2 retainers" from nonretainers on the basis of history, physical examination, or spirometry. These patients need an ABG preoperatively. Supplemental oxygen causes the P_aCO_2 to increase in CO_2 retainers by a combination of decreased respiratory drive and increased dead space.

Nocturnal hypoxemia. COPD patients desaturate more frequently and severely than normal patients during sleep. This is due to the rapid/shallow breathing pattern that occurs during rapid eye movement sleep.

Right ventricular (RV) dysfunction. Cor pulmonale occurs in 40% of adult COPD patients with FEV_1 less than 1 L and in 70% with FEV_1 less than 0.6 L. COPD patients who have resting P_aO_2 less than 55 mm Hg and those who desaturate to less than 44 mm Hg with exercise should receive supplemental home oxygen. The goal of supplemental oxygen is to maintain P_aO_2 at 60 to 65 mm Hg. Pneumonectomy candidates with ppoFEV_1 less than 40% should have transthoracic echocardiography to assess right heart function. Elevation of right heart pressures places these patients in a very high-risk group.

3. **Preoperative therapy of COPD.** The four treatable complications of COPD that must be actively sought and therapy begun at the initial prethoracotomy assessment are atelectasis, bronchospasm, chest infection, and pulmonary edema. Patients with COPD have fewer postoperative pulmonary complications when a perioperative program of chest physiotherapy is initiated preoperatively. Pulmonary complications are decreased in thoracic surgical patients who are not smoking versus those who continue to smoke up until the time of surgery.
4. **Lung cancer considerations.** At the time of initial assessment, cancer patients should be assessed for the "4 M's" associated with malignancy: **M**ass effects, **M**etabolic abnormalities, **M**etastases, and **M**edications. Prior use of medications that can exacerbate oxygen-induced pulmonary toxicity, such as bleomycin, should be considered (Table 26.1).
5. **Postoperative analgesia.** The risks and benefits of the various forms of post-thoracotomy analgesia should be explained to the patient at the time of initial preanesthetic assessment. Potential contraindications to specific methods of analgesia should be determined, such as coagulation problems, sepsis, and neurologic disorders. If the patient is to receive prophylactic anticoagulants and it is elected to use epidural analgesia, appropriate timing of anticoagulant administration and neuraxial catheter placement need to be arranged.

TABLE 26.1 Anesthetic considerations in lung cancer patients (the "4 M's")

I. **Mass effects:** Obstructive pneumonia, superior vena cava syndrome, tracheobronchial distortion, Pancoast syndrome, recurrent laryngeal nerve or phrenic nerve paresis
II. **Metabolic effects:** Lambert–Eaton syndrome, hypercalcemia, hyponatremia, Cushing syndrome
III. **Metastases:** Particularly to brain, bone, liver, and adrenal
IV. **Medications:** Chemotherapy agents, pulmonary toxicity (bleomycin, mitomycin), cardiac toxicity (doxorubicin), renal toxicity (cis-platinum)

TABLE 26.2 Summary of preanesthetic assessment

Initial preanesthetic assessment for pulmonary resection
I. All patients: Exercise tolerance, ppoFEV_1%, discuss postoperative analgesia, D/C smoking
II. Patients with ppoFEV_1 <40%: DLCO, V/Q scan, Vo_2 max
III. Cancer patients: The "4 M's": Mass effects, metabolic effects, metastases, medications
IV. COPD patients: ABG, physiotherapy, bronchodilators
Final preanesthetic assessment for pulmonary resection
I. Review initial assessment and test results
II. Assess difficulty of lung isolation: Chest x-ray film, computed tomographic scan
III. Assess risk of hypoxemia during OLV

D/C, discontinue; DLCO, diffusing capacity for carbon monoxide; ppoFEV_1, predicted postoperative forced expiratory volume in 1 s; V/Q, ventilation/perfusion; VO_2 max, Maximum oxygen consumption; COPD, chronic obstructive pulmonary disease; ABG, arterial blood gas; OLV, one-lung ventilation.

American Society of Regional Anesthesia guidelines suggest an interval of 2 to 4 h before or 1 h after catheter placement for prophylactic heparin administration. Low-molecular-weight heparin precautions are less clear, but an interval of 24 h before catheter placement is recommended.

6. **Premedication.** Avoid inadvertent withdrawal of drugs that are being taken for concurrent medical conditions (bronchodilators, antihypertensives, β-blockers). For esophageal reflux surgery, oral antacid and H_2-blockers are routinely ordered preoperatively. Mild sedation, such as an intravenous (IV) short-acting benzodiazepine, is often given immediately before placement of invasive monitoring lines and catheters. In patients with copious secretions, an anti-sialagogue (e.g., glycopyrrolate 0.2 mg) is useful to facilitate fiberoptic bronchoscopy (FOB) for positioning of a double-lumen tube (DLT) or bronchial blocker (BB).
7. **Final preoperative assessment.** The final preoperative anesthetic assessment is made immediately before the patient is brought to the operating room. Review the data from the initial prethoracotomy assessment (Table 26.2) and the results of tests ordered at that time. Two other concerns for thoracic anesthesia need to be assessed: (i) The potential for difficult lung isolation and (ii) the risk of desaturation during one-lung ventilation (OLV).
    a. **Assessment of difficult endobronchial intubation.** The most useful predictor of dif-
    2 ficult endobronchial intubation is the chest x-ray film. Clinically important tracheal or bronchial distortions or compression from tumors or previous surgery can be usually detected on plain chest films. Distal airway problems not detectable on the plain x-ray film may be visualized on chest computed tomographic (CT) scans. These abnormalities often will not be mentioned in a written or verbal report from the radiologist or surgeon. The anesthesiologist must examine the chest image before placing a DLT or BB.
    b. **Prediction of desaturation during OLV.** It is possible to determine patients who are most at risk for desaturation during OLV for thoracic surgery [3]. The factors that correlate with desaturation during OLV are listed in Table 26.3. The most important
    3 predictor of P_aO_2 during OLV is the P_aO_2 during two-lung ventilation in the lateral position before OLV. The proportion of perfusion or ventilation to the non-operated lung on preoperative ventilation/perfusion (V/Q) scans also correlates with the P_aO_2 during OLV. The side of the thoracotomy has an effect on P_aO_2 during OLV. With the left lung being 10% smaller than the right lung, there is less shunt when the left lung is collapsed. The degree of obstructive lung disease correlates in an inverse fashion with P_aO_2 during

TABLE 26.3 Factors that correlate with an increased risk of desaturation during one-lung ventilation

I. High percentage of ventilation (V) or perfusion (Q) to the operative lung on preoperative V/Q scan
II. Poor P_aO_2 during two-lung ventilation, particularly in the lateral position intraoperatively
III. Right-sided surgery
IV. Good preoperative spirometry (FEV_1 or FVC)

V/Q, ventilation/perfusion; FEV_1, forced expiratory volume in 1 s; FVC, forced vital capacity.

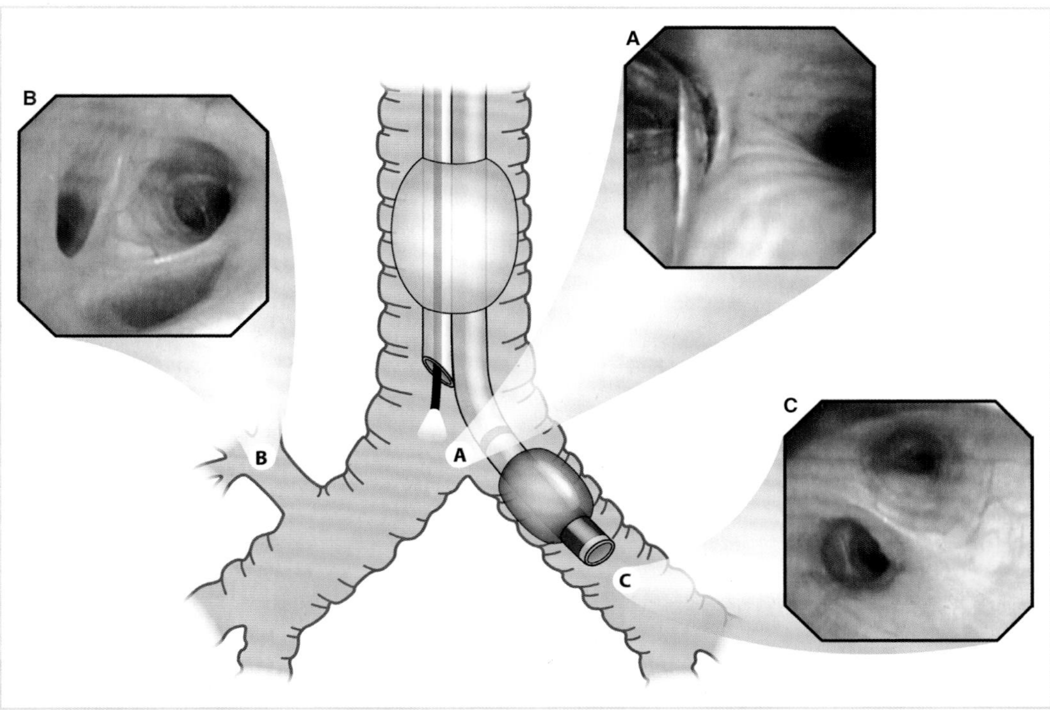

FIGURE 26.3 The optimal position of a left-sided double lumen endotracheal tube. **A:** Unobstructed view of the entrance of the right mainstem bronchus as seen from the tracheal lumen. **B:** Take-off of the right-upper lobe bronchus with the three segments. **C:** Unobstructed view of the left-upper and left-lower bronchus as seen from the bronchial lumen. (Reproduced from Campos J. Lung isolation. In: Slinger P, ed. *Principles and Practice of Thoracic Anesthesia.* New York, NY: Springer; 2011, with kind permission of Springer Science + Business Media.)

OLV. Patients with more severe airflow limitation on preoperative spirometry tend to have a better P_aO_2 during OLV. This is related to the development of auto positive end-expiratory pressure (PEEP) during OLV in the obstructed patients.

Stratifying the perioperative risks allows the anesthesiologist to develop a systematic focused approach to these patients at the time of initial contact and immediately before induction, which can be used to guide anesthetic management (Fig. 26.2).

II. Intraoperative management

A. Lung separation. There are three basic options for lung separation: Single-lumen endobronchial tubes (EBTs), DLTs (left- or right-sided) (see Figs. 26.3 and 26.4), and BBs. The second half of the twentieth century has seen refinements of the DLT from that of Carlens to a tube specifically designed for intraoperative use (Robertshaw) with larger, D-shaped lumens and without a carinal hook. Current disposable polyvinyl chloride DLTs have incorporated high-volume/low-pressure tracheal and bronchial cuffs. Recently, there has been a revival of interest in BBs due to several factors: New blocker designs (see Figs. 26.5 and 26.6) [4] and greater familiarity of anesthesiologists with fiberoptic placement of BBs (see Fig. 26.7).

1. **Indications for lung separation.** Absolute indications for lung isolation include purulent secretions, massive pulmonary hemorrhage, and bronchopleural fistula, blebs, and bullae
4 (blood, pus, and air). More commonly, lung separation is provided intraoperatively to facilitate surgical exposure.
2. **Techniques of lung separation.** The optimal methods for lung isolation are listed in Table 26.4. Because it is impossible to describe one technique as best in all indications for OLV, the various indications are considered separately.

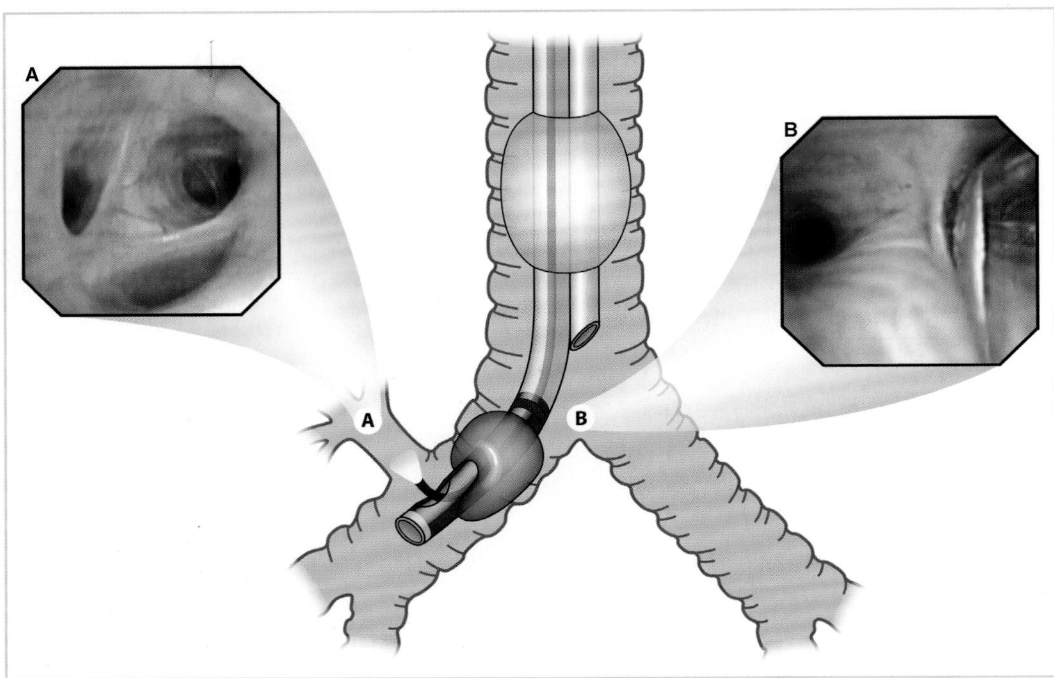

FIGURE 26.4 Optimal position of a right-sided double lumen endotracheal tube as seen with a fiberoptic bronchoscope. **A:** View of the right upper lobe bronchus seen through the ventilating side slot of the bronchial lumen. **B:** View of the carina showing the left mainstem bronchus and the bronchial lumen in the right mainstem bronchus seen from the tracheal lumen. (Reproduced from Campos J. Lung isolation. In: Slinger P, ed. *Principles and Practice of Thoracic Anesthesia.* New York, NY: Springer; 2011, with permission of Springer Science + Business Media.)

TABLE 26.4 Selection of airway device for lung isolation

Surgery	Primary choice[a]	Secondary options (in order of preference)
Pulmonary resection, right sided	Left DLT	BB, EBT
Pulmonary resection, left sided, not pneumonectomy	Left DLT	BB, right DLT
Pulmonary resection, left sided pneumonectomy/ left main bronchial surgery	Right DLT	BB, left DLT
Thoracoscopy	Left DLT	Right DLT, BB, EBT
Pulmonary hemorrhage	DLT/BB/EBT	
Bronchopleural fistula/abscess	Left DLT	Right DLT, BB, EBT
Esophageal, thoracic aortic, transthoracic vertebral surgery	Left DLT/BB	Right DLT, EBT
Lung transplantation, bilateral/right single	Left DLT	EBT, BB
Lung transplantation, left single	Right DLT	BB, left DLT
Abnormal upper airway, left thoracotomy	BB	Right DLT/left DLT, EBT
Abnormal upper airway, right thoracotomy	EBT/BB	Left DLT/right DLT

[a]Options separated by a slash (/) are equivalent choices.
BB, bronchial blocker ipsilateral to side of surgery; EBT, single-lumen tube placed endobronchial contralateral to surgery; left DLT, left-sided double-lumen tube; right DLT, right-sided double-lumen tube.

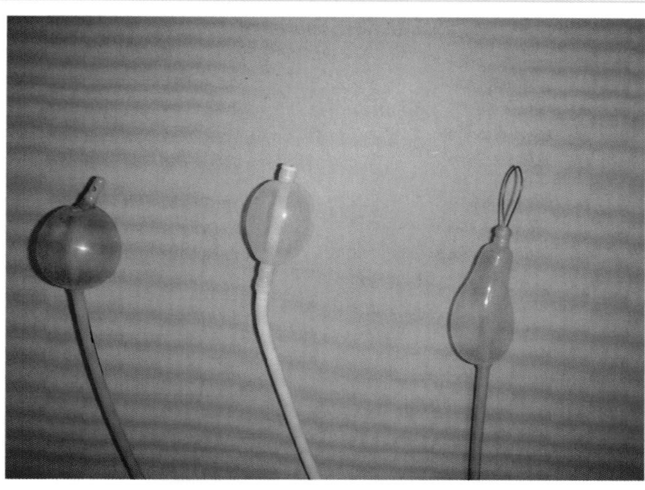

FIGURE 26.5 Three independent endobronchial blockers currently available in North America. **Left:** The Cohen® tip-deflecting endobronchial blocker (Cook Critical Care, Bloomington, IN, USA), which allows anesthesiologists to establish one lung ventilation by directing its flexible tip left or right into the desired bronchus using a control wheel device on the proximal end of the blocker in combination with fiberoptic bronchoscopic (FOB) guidance. **Middle:** The Fuji Uniblocker® (Fuji Corp., Tokyo, Japan). It has a fixed distal curve that allows it to be rotated for manipulation into position with FOB guidance. Unlike its predecessor, the Univent blocker, the Uniblocker is used with a standard endotracheal tube. **Right:** The wire-guided endobronchial blocker (Arndt® bronchial blocker; Cook Critical Care) introduced in 1999. It contains a wire loop in the inner lumen; when used as a snare with a fiberoptic bronchoscope, it allows directed placement. The snare is then removed, and the 1.4 mm lumen may be used as a suction channel or for oxygen insufflation. (Reproduced from Campos J. Lung isolation. In: Slinger P, ed. *Principles and Practice of Thoracic Anesthesia.* New York, NY: Springer; 2011, with kind permission of Springer Science + Business Media.)

a. **Elective pulmonary resection, right-sided.** The first choice is a left DLT. The widest margin of safety in positioning is with left DLTs. With blind positioning, the incidence of malposition can exceed 20% but is correctable in virtually all cases by fiberoptic adjustment. There is continuous access to the nonventilated lung for suctioning, fiberoptic monitoring of position, and continuous positive airway pressure (CPAP). There are two possible alternatives. (i) Single-lumen EBT: A standard 7.5 mm diameter, 32 cm long endotracheal tube (ETT) can be advanced over an FOB into the left main stem bronchus. (ii) Univent tube or BB: The BB can be placed external to or intraluminally with an ETT.

b. **Elective pulmonary resection, left-sided**
   (1) **Not pneumonectomy.** There is no obvious best choice between a BB and a left DLT. Use of a left DLT for a left thoracotomy can be associated with obstruction of the tracheal lumen by the lateral tracheal wall and subsequent problems with gas exchange in the ventilated lung. A right DLT is an alternate choice.
   (2) **Left pneumonectomy.** When a pneumonectomy is foreseen, a right DLT is the best choice. A right DLT will permit the surgeon to palpate the left hilum during OLV without interference from a tube or blocker in the left main stem bronchus. The disposable right DLTs currently available in North America vary greatly in design, depending on the manufacturer (Mallinckrodt, Rusch, Kendall). The Mallinckrodt design, currently, is the most reliable. All three designs include a ventilating side slot in the distal bronchial lumen for right upper lobe ventilation. If left lung isolation is impossible despite extremely high pressures in the right DLT bronchial cuff, a Fogarty catheter can be passed into the left main bronchus as a BB. As an alternative, there is no clear preference between a left DLT or BB. These all require repositioning before clamping the left main stem bronchus.

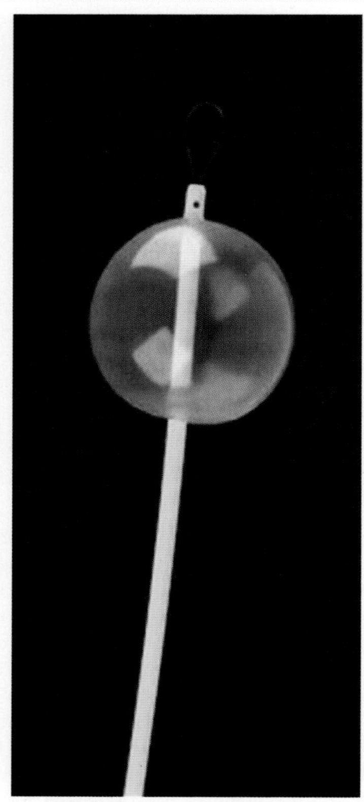

FIGURE 26.6 The recently introduced Arndt® spherical endobronchial blocker cuff (Cook Critical Care, Bloomington, IN, USA). Some clinicians prefer to use the spherical cuff for right-sided surgery versus the original elliptical cuff because of the short length of the right mainstem bronchus. (Reproduced from Campos J. Lung isolation. In: Slinger P, ed. *Principles and Practice of Thoracic Anesthesia.* New York, NY: Springer; 2011, with kind permission of Springer Science + Business Media.)

c. **Thoracoscopy.** Lung biopsies, wedge resection, bleb/bullae resections, and some lobectomies can be done using video-assisted thoracoscopic surgery (VATS). During open thoracotomy, the lung can be compressed by the surgeon to facilitate collapse before inflation of a BB. A left DLT is preferred for thoracoscopy of either hemithorax because it gives more rapid deflation of the nonventilated lung.

d. **Pulmonary hemorrhage.** Instances of life-threatening pulmonary hemorrhage can occur due to a wide variety of causes, such as aspergillosis, tuberculosis, and pulmonary artery (PA) catheter trauma. The primary risk for these patients is asphyxiation, and first-line treatment is lung isolation and suctioning the lower airways. Lung isolation can be with a DLT, BB, or single-lumen EBT, depending on availability and the clinical circumstances (see Section 24 III-M). Tracheobronchial hemorrhage from blunt chest trauma usually resolves with suctioning; only rarely is lung isolation necessary.

e. **Bronchopleural fistula.** The anesthesiologist is faced with the triple problem of avoiding tension pneumothorax, ensuring adequate ventilation, and protecting the healthy lung from the fluid collection in the involved hemithorax. Management depends on the site of the fistula and the urgency of the clinical situation. For a peripheral bronchopleural fistula in a stable patient, a BB may be acceptable. For a large central fistula and in urgent situations, the most rapid and reliable method of securing one-lung isolation and ventilation is a DLT. In life-threatening situations, a DLT can be placed in awake patients with direct FOB guidance.

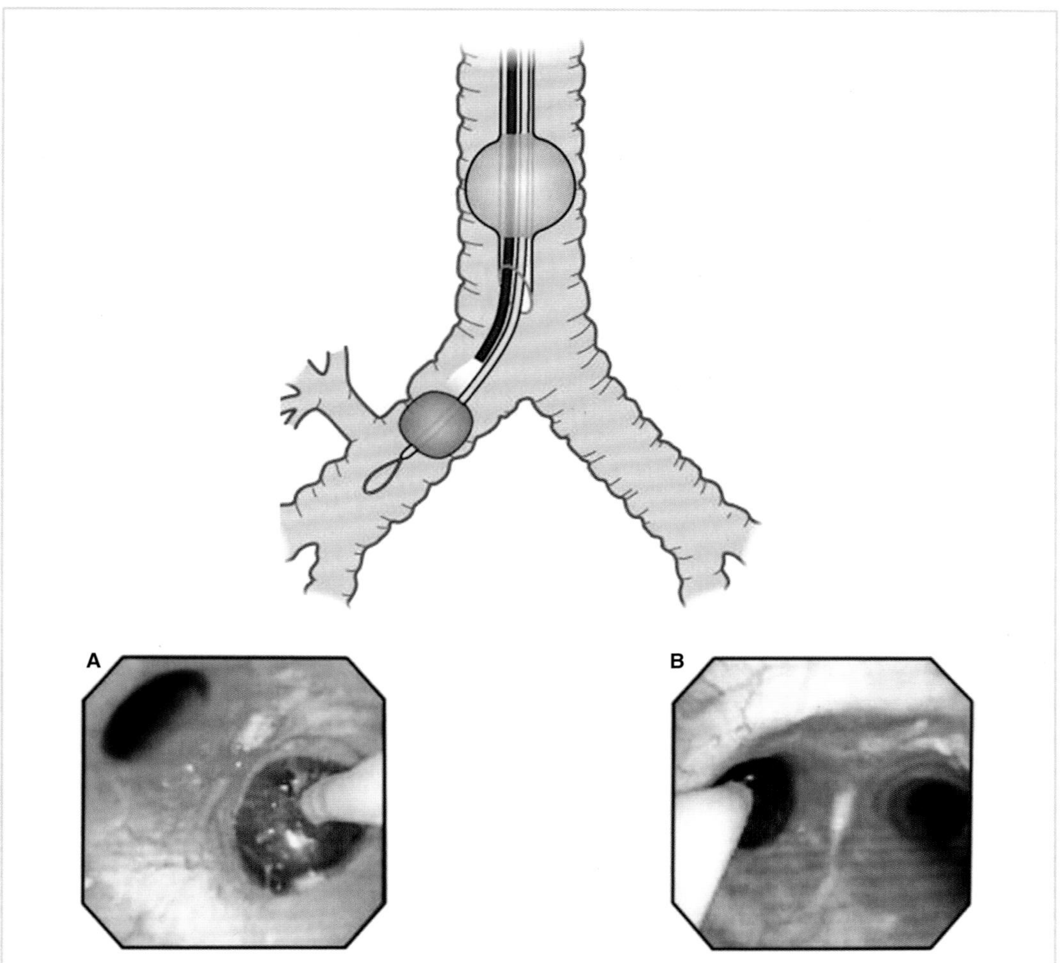

FIGURE 26.7 Diagram **(top):** Placement of an Arndt® blocker through a single-lumen endotracheal tube in the right mainstem bronchus with the fiberoptic bronchoscope. Photographs **(bottom):** Optimal position of an endobronchial blocker in the right **(A)** or left **(B)** mainstem bronchus as seen through a fiberoptic bronchoscope. (Reproduced from Campos J. Lung isolation. In: Slinger P, ed. *Principles and Practice of Thoracic Anesthesia.* New York, NY: Springer; 2011, with kind permission of Springer Science + Business Media.)

f. **Purulent secretions** (lung abscess, hydatid cysts). Lobar or segmental blockade is ideal. Loss of lung isolation in these cases is not merely a surgical inconvenience but may be life threatening. Univent tubes can be used for lobar blockade. A secure technique in these cases is the combined use of a BB and a DLT.
g. **Nonpulmonary thoracic surgery.** Thoracic aortic and esophageal surgeries require OLV. Because there is no risk of ventilated-lung contamination, a left DLT and a BB are equivalent choices.
h. **Bronchial surgery.** An intrabronchial tumor, bronchial trauma, or bronchial sleeve resection during a lobectomy requires that the surgeon have intraluminal access to the ipsilateral main stem bronchus. Either a single-lumen EBT or a DLT in the ventilated lung is preferred.
i. Unilateral lung lavage, independent lung ventilation, and lung transplantation are all best accomplished with a left DLT.

3. **Upper airway abnormalities.** It is occasionally necessary to provide OLV in patients who have abnormal upper airways due to previous surgery or trauma or in patients who are known for unanticipated difficult intubations. There are four basic options for these patients: (i) Fiberoptic-guided intubation with a DLT; (ii) secure the airway with an ETT and then use a "tube exchanger" to place a DLT; (iii) use a BB; and (iv) use an uncut single-lumen tube as an EBT.

   The optimal choice will depend on the patient and the operation. At all times it is best to maintain spontaneous ventilation and to do nothing blindly in the presence of blood or pus. Awake FOB intubation with a DLT requires thorough topical anesthesia of the airway. It is important when using a tube exchanger to have a second person perform a direct laryngoscopy to expose as much of the glottis as possible during the tube change. Direct laryngoscopy decreases the angles between the oropharynx and trachea and reduces the chance of trauma to the airway from the DLT. The video-laryngoscopes (e.g., glidescope) are useful for this.

   BBs are often the best choice for some of these patients. If the ET tube is too narrow to easily accommodate both a bronchoscope and a BB, the BB can be introduced through the glottis independently external to the ET tube with fiberoptic guidance. Bilateral BBs can be used for bilateral resections or the same blocker can be manipulated from side to side. Bilateral single-lumen EBTs or BBs can be used for lung isolation in patients with tracheal fistulas, trauma, or other abnormalities in the region of the carina. Smaller DLTs (32, 28, and 26 Fr) are available, but they will not permit passage of an FOB of the diameter commonly available to monitor positioning (3.5 to 4.0 mm). An ETT designed for microlaryngoscopy (5 to 6 mm inner diameter [ID] and greater than 30 cm long) can be used as an EBT, with FOB positioning. If the patient's trachea can accept a 7.0 mm ETT, a Fogarty catheter (8 Fr venous thrombectomy catheter with a 10 mL balloon) can be passed through the ETT via an FOB adapter for use as a BB.

4. **Chest trauma.** It is common in both open and closed chest trauma to have some hemoptysis from alveolar hemorrhage. The majority of these cases can be managed without lung isolation after bronchoscopy and suction. The majority of the deaths in these patients are due to their other injuries and not from airway hemorrhage or air embolus. Lung isolation may be helpful in some of these cases, but if resources and time are limited the priority must be the resuscitation of the patient.

5

5. **Avoiding iatrogenic airway injury.** Iatrogenic injury has been estimated to occur in 0.5 to 2 per 1,000 cases with DLTs.
   a. **Examine the chest x-ray film or CT scan**, which can help predict the majority of difficult endobronchial intubations.
   b. **Use an appropriate size tube.** Too small tube will make lung isolation difficult. Too large a tube is more likely to cause trauma. Useful guidelines for DLT sizes in adults are as follows:
      (1) **Females' height < 1.6 m (63 inch): 35 Fr (possibly 32 Fr if <1.5 m).**
      (2) **Females >1.6 m: 37 Fr.**
      (3) **Males <1.7 m (67 inch): 39 Fr (possibly 37 Fr if <1.6 m).**
      (4) **Males >1.7 m: 41 Fr.**
   c. **Depth of insertion of DLT.** Tracheobronchial dimensions correlate with height. The average depth at insertion, from the teeth, for a left DLT is 29 cm in an adult and varies ±1 cm for each 10 cm of patient height above/below 170 cm.
   d. **Avoid nitrous oxide.** Nitrous oxide 70% can increase the bronchial cuff volume from 5 to 16 mL intraoperatively.
   e. **Inflate the bronchial cuff/blocker only to the minimal volume required for lung isolation and for the minimal time.** This volume is usually less than 3 mL. Inflating the bronchial cuff does not stabilize the DLT position when the patient is turned to the lateral position.
      (1) Endobronchial intubation must be done gently and with fiberoptic guidance if resistance is met. A significant number of case reports are from cases of esophageal surgery, where the elastic supporting tissue may be weakened and predisposed to rupture from DLT placement.

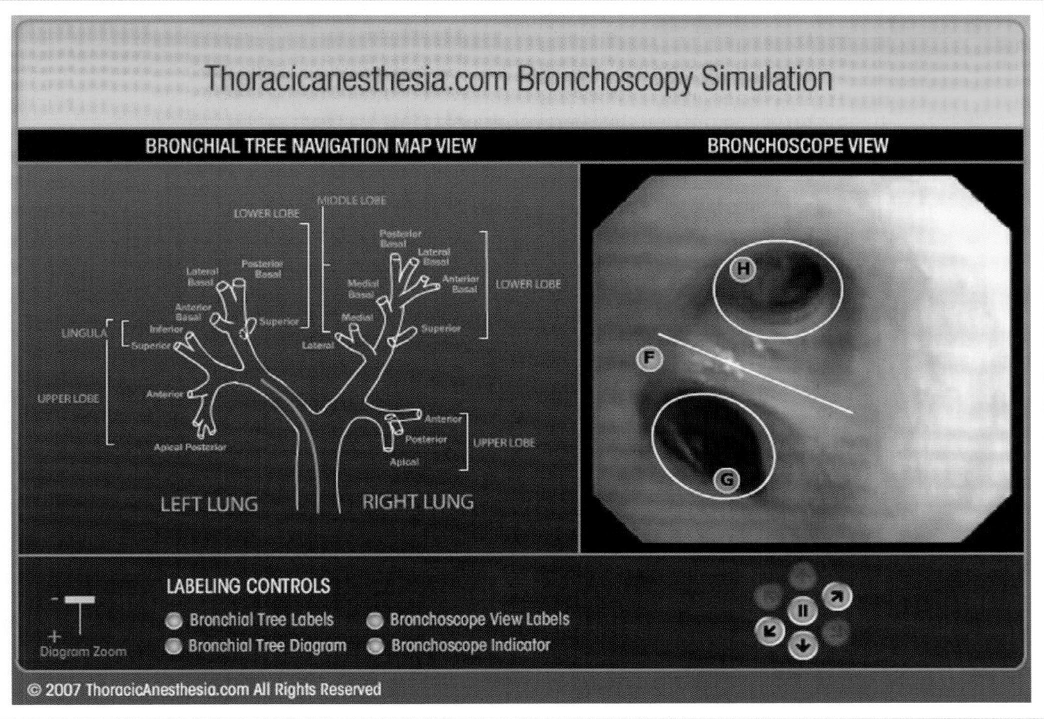

FIGURE 26.8 The free online bronchoscopy simulator at www.thoracicanesthesia.com. The user can navigate the tracheobronchial tree using real-time video by clicking on the lighted directional arrows under the "Bronchoscopic view" **(right)**. Clicking on the labels on the "Bronchoscopic view" gives details of the anatomy seen. The process is aided by the "Bronchial Tree Navigational Map" **(left)**, which shows the simultaneous location of the bronchoscope as the orange line in the airway. (Reproduced from Campos J. Lung isolation. In: Slinger P, ed. *Principles and Practice of Thoracic Anesthesia.* New York, NY: Springer; 2011, with kind permission of Springer Science + Business Media.)

6. **Other complications of lung separation**
   a. **Malpositioning.** Initial malpositioning of DLTs with blind placement can occur in greater than 30% of cases. Verification and adjustment with FOB immediately before initiating OLV is mandatory because these tubes will migrate during patient positioning. Malpositioning after the start of OLV due to dislodgment is more of a problem with BBs than DLTs.
   b. **Airway resistance.** The resistance from a 37 F DLT exceeds that of a no. 9 Univent by less than 10% over the range of airflows seen with spontaneous ventilation. These flow resistances both are less than that of an 8.0 mm ID ETT but exceed that of a 9.0 mm ETT. For short periods of postoperative ventilation and weaning, airflow resistance is not a problem with a DLT.
7. The **ABC**s of lung separation will always apply:
   a. Know the tracheobronchial **a**natomy [5].
   b. Use the fiberoptic **b**ronchoscope (see Fig. 26.8) [6].
   c. Look at the **c**hest x-ray film and **CT** scan in advance.

B. **Positioning.** The majority of thoracic procedures are performed with the patient in the lateral position, but, depending on the surgical technique, a semisupine or semiprone lateral position may be used. It is awkward to induce anesthesia in the lateral position; thus, monitors will be placed and anesthesia will be usually induced in the supine position and the anesthetized patient will then be repositioned for surgery. It is possible to induce anesthesia in the lateral position. This may rarely be indicated with unilateral lung diseases, such as bronchiectasis or hemoptysis, until lung isolation can be achieved. However, even these patients will have to be repositioned and the diseased lung turned to the nondependent side. Due to the loss of venous vascular tone in the anesthetized patient, it is not uncommon to see hypotension when the patient is turned to or from the lateral position.

All lines and monitors will have to be secured during position change and their function reassessed after repositioning. The anesthesiologist should take responsibility for the head, neck, and airway during position change and must be in charge of the operating team to direct repositioning. It is useful to make an initial "head-to-toe" survey of the patient after induction and intubation, checking oxygenation, ventilation, hemodynamics, lines, monitors, and potential nerve injuries. This survey must be repeated after repositioning. It is nearly impossible to avoid some movement of a DLT or BB during repositioning. The patient's head, neck, and EBT should be turned en bloc with the patient's thoracolumbar spine. The margin of error in positioning EBTs or blockers is often so narrow that even small movements can have significant clinical implications. EBT/blocker position and adequacy of ventilation must be rechecked by auscultation and FOB after patient repositioning.

1. **Neurovascular complications.** The brachial plexus is the site of the majority of intraoperative nerve injuries related to the lateral position. The brachial plexus is fixed at two points: Proximally by the transverse process of the cervical vertebrae and distally by the axillary fascia. This two-point fixation plus the extreme mobility of neighboring skeletal and muscular structures make the brachial plexus extremely liable to injury. The patient should be positioned with padding under the dependent thorax to keep the weight of the upper body off the dependent arm brachial plexus. This padding will exacerbate the pressure on the brachial plexus if it migrates superiorly into the axilla. It is useful to survey the patient from the side of the table immediately after the patient is turned to ensure that the entire vertebral column is aligned properly.

   The dependent leg should be slightly flexed with padding under the knee to protect the peroneal nerve lateral to the proximal head of the fibula. The nondependent leg is placed in a neutral extended position and padding placed between it and the dependent leg. The dependent leg must be observed for vascular compression. Excessively tight strapping at the hip level can compress the sciatic nerve of the nondependent leg. A "head-to-toe" protocol to monitor for possible neurovascular injuries related to the lateral decubitus position is given in Table 26.5.

2. **Physiologic changes in the lateral position**

   a. **Ventilation.** Significant changes in ventilation develop between the lungs when the patient is placed in the lateral position. The compliance curves of the two lungs are different because of their difference in sizes. The lateral position, anesthesia, paralysis, and opening the thorax all combine to magnify these differences between the lungs.

      In a spontaneously breathing patient, the ventilation of the dependent lung will increase approximately 10% when the patient is turned to the lateral position. Once the patient is anesthetized and paralyzed, the ventilation of the dependent lung will

TABLE 26.5 Avoiding neurovascular injuries specific to the lateral position

Routine "head-to-toe" survey
I. Dependent eye
II. Dependent ear pinna
III. Cervical spine alignment
IV. Dependent arm: (i) Brachial plexus, (ii) circulation
V. Nondependent arm[a]: (i) Brachial plexus, (ii) circulation
VI. Nondependent leg sciatic nerve
VII. Dependent leg: (i) Peroneal nerve, (ii) circulation

[a]Neurovascular injuries of the nondependent arm are more likely to occur if the arm is suspended or held in an independently positioned armrest.

TABLE 26.6 Intraoperative complications that occur with increased frequency during thoracotomy

Complication	Etiology
I. Hypoxemia	Intrapulmonary shunt during one lung ventilation
II. Sudden severe hypotension	Surgical compression of the heart or great vessels
III. Sudden changes in ventilating pressure or volume	Movement of endobronchial tube/blocker, air leak
IV. Arrhythmias	Direct mechanical irritation of the heart
V. Bronchospasm	Direct airway stimulation, increased frequency of reactive airways disease
VI. Massive hemorrhage	Surgical blood loss from great vessels or inflamed pleura
VII. Hypothermia	Heat loss from the open hemithorax

decrease 15%. The compliance of the entire respiratory system will increase once the nondependent hemithorax is open.

Applying PEEP to both lungs in the lateral position, PEEP preferentially goes to the most compliant lung regions and hyperinflates the nondependent lung without causing any improvement in gas exchange. In the lateral position, atelectasis will develop in a mean of 5% of lung volume, all in the dependent lung.

b. **Perfusion.** Turning the patient to the lateral position decreases the blood flow of the nondependent lung due to gravity by approximately 10% of the total pulmonary blood flow.

The matching of ventilation and perfusion will usually decrease in the lateral position compared to the supine position. Pulmonary arteriovenous shunt usually increases from approximately 5% in the supine position to 10% to 15% in the lateral position.

C. **Intraoperative monitoring**

1. **General to all pulmonary resections.** The majority are major operative procedures of moderate duration (2 to 4 h) and performed in the lateral position with the hemithorax open. Consideration for monitoring and maintenance of body temperature and fluid volume should be given to all of these cases. All cases should have standard ASA monitoring. Additional monitoring is guided by a knowledge of which complications are likely to occur (Table 26.6).
2. **Specific to certain types of resection.** There are complications that are more prone to occur with certain resections, such as hemorrhage from an extrapleural pneumonectomy, contralateral lung soiling with resection of a cyst or bronchiectasis, air leak hypoventilation, or tension pneumothorax with a bronchopleural fistula.
3. **Oxygenation.** Significant arterial oxygen desaturation (less than 90%) during OLV occurs in approximately 1% of the surgical population with a high F_{IO_2} of 1.0. Pulse oximetry (S_pO_2) has not negated the need for direct measurement of arterial P_aO_2 via intermittent blood gases in the majority of thoracotomy patients. P_aO_2 offers a more useful estimate of the margin of safety above desaturation than S_pO_2. The rapidity of the fall in P_aO_2 after the onset of OLV is an indicator of the risk of subsequent desaturation. Measure P_aO_2 by ABG before OLV and 20 min after the start of OLV.
4. **Capnometry.** End-tidal CO_2 ($P_{et}CO_2$) is a less reliable indicator of the P_aCO_2 during OLV than during two-lung ventilation and the $P_{a\text{-}et}CO_2$ gradient increases during OLV. As the patient is turned to the lateral position, the $P_{et}CO_2$ of the nondependent lung falls relative to the dependent lung because of increased perfusion of the dependent lung and increased dead space of the nondependent lung. At the onset of OLV, the $P_{et}CO_2$ of the dependent lung usually falls transiently as all the minute ventilation is transferred to this lung. The $P_{et}CO_2$ then rises as the fractional perfusion is increased to this dependent lung by collapse and pulmonary vasoconstriction of the nonventilated lung. If there is no correction of minute ventilation, the net result will be increased baseline P_aCO_2 and $P_{et}CO_2$ with an increased gradient. Severe (greater than 5 mm Hg) or prolonged falls in $P_{et}CO_2$ indicate a maldistribution of perfusion between ventilated and nonventilated lungs and may be an early warning of a patient who will desaturate during OLV.

5. **Invasive hemodynamic monitoring**
   a. **Arterial line.** There is a significant incidence of transient severe hypotension from surgical compression of the heart or great vessels during intrathoracic procedures. For this reason, plus the utility of intermittent ABG sampling, it is useful to have beat-to-beat assessment of systemic blood pressure during the majority of thoracic surgery cases. Exceptions are limited procedures such as thoracoscopic resections in younger/healthier patients. For most thoracotomies, placement of a radial artery catheter can be in either the dependent or nondependent arm.
   b. **Central venous pressures (CVPs).** CVP readings obtained intraoperatively with the chest open are not completely reliable. It is our practice to routinely place CVP lines in pneumonectomy patients but not for lesser resections unless there is significant other concurrent illness. Our choice is to use a high anterior approach to the right internal jugular vein with ultrasound guidance to minimize the risk of pneumothorax for CVP access unless there is a contraindication.
   c. **PA catheters.** The risk/benefit ratio for the routine use of PA catheters for pulmonary resection surgery favors their use only in certain specific cases, such as patients with life-threatening coexisting disease and/or patients undergoing particularly extensive procedures. Several recently developed systems of noninvasive cardiac output monitoring may prove equally as useful for this purpose (e.g., Flowtrac®, Edwards Lifesciences, Irvine, CA, USA).
6. **FOB.** Significant malpositions of left-sided or right-sided DLTs that can lead to desaturation during OLV are often not detected by auscultation or other traditional methods of confirming placement. Positioning of DLTs or BBs should be confirmed after placing the patient in the surgical position because a large number of the tubes/blockers migrate during repositioning of the patient.
7. **Continuous spirometry.** Side-stream spirometry monitors inspiratory and expiratory pressures, volume, and flow interactions during anesthesia. The adequacy of lung isolation can be monitored by breath-to-breath comparison of inspiratory and expiratory tidal volumes. This also gives a sense of the magnitude of air leaks from the ventilated lung. Changes in the position of a DLT can be detected by changes in the pressure–volume loops.

D. **Anesthetic technique.** Any anesthetic technique that provides safe and stable general anesthesia for major surgery can and has been used for lung resection. Many centers use combined thoracic epidural and general anesthesia for thoracic surgery.

1. **IV fluids.** Because of hydrostatic effects, excessive administration of IV fluids can cause increased shunt and lead to pulmonary edema of the dependent lung. Because the 7 dependent lung is the lung that must carry on gas exchange during OLV, it is best to be as judicious as possible with fluid administration. IV fluids are administered to replace volume deficits and for maintenance only during lung resection anesthesia. No volume is given for theoretical third-space losses during thoracotomy (Table 26.7).
2. **Nitrous oxide.** Nitrous oxide/oxygen mixtures are more prone to cause atelectasis in poorly ventilated lung regions than oxygen by itself. The optimal method to prevent dependent lung atelectasis is the use of air/oxygen mixtures during both two-lung ventilation and OLV, titrating the F_{IO_2} to avoid hypoxemia. Nitrous oxide also tends to increase PA pressures in patients who have pulmonary hypertension.

TABLE 26.7 Fluid management for pulmonary resection surgery

I. Total positive fluid balance in the first 24 h perioperatively should not exceed 20 mL/kg.
II. For an average adult patient, crystalloid administration should be limited to <3 L in the first 24 h.
III. No fluid administration for "third-space" fluid losses during pulmonary resection
IV. Urine output >0.5 mL/kg/h is unnecessary.
V. If increased tissue perfusion is needed postoperatively, it is preferable to use invasive monitoring and inotropes rather than to cause fluid overload.

3. **Temperature.** Maintenance of body temperature can be a problem during thoracic surgery because of heat loss from the open hemithorax. This is particularly a problem at the extremes of the age spectrum. Most of the body's physiologic functions, including hypoxic pulmonary vasoconstriction (HPV), are inhibited during hypothermia. Increasing the ambient room temperature and using a lower-limb forced-air patient warmer are the best methods to prevent inadvertent intraoperative hypothermia.
4. **Prevention of bronchospasm.** Due to the high incidence of coexisting reactive airways disease in the thoracic surgical population it is generally advisable to use an anesthetic technique that decreases bronchial irritability. This is particularly important because the added airway manipulation caused by placement of a DLT or BB is a potent trigger for bronchoconstriction. Avoid manipulation of the airway in a lightly anesthetized patient, use bronchodilating anesthetics, and avoid drugs which release histamine.

   For IV induction of anesthesia, either propofol or ketamine diminish bronchospasm. For maintenance of anesthesia, propofol and/or any of the volatile anesthetics will diminish bronchial reactivity. Sevoflurane may be the most potent bronchodilator of the volatile anesthetics.
5. **Coronary artery disease.** Since the lung resection population is largely composed of elderly patients and smokers there is a high coincidence of coronary artery disease. This consideration will be a major factor in the choice of the anesthetic technique for most thoracic patients. The anesthetic technique should optimize the myocardial oxygen supply/demand ratio by maintaining arterial oxygenation and diastolic blood pressure while avoiding unnecessary increases in cardiac output and heart rate. Thoracic epidural anesthesia (TEA)/analgesia may help to achieve these goals.

E. Management of one-lung ventilation

1. **Hypoxemia.** There is an incidence of <4% of hypoxemia (arterial saturation <90%) during OLV for thoracic surgery. Hypoxemia is more likely to occur when OLV is in the supine position.
2. **HPV.** HPV is thought to decrease the blood flow to the nonventilated lung by 50%. The stimulus for HPV is primarily the alveolar oxygen tension (P_aO_2), which stimulates precapillary vasoconstriction redistributing pulmonary blood flow away from hypoxemic lung regions via a pathway involving nitric oxide (NO) and/or cyclo-oxygenase synthesis inhibition. All of the volatile anesthetics inhibit HPV. This inhibition is dose dependent. Isoflurane, sevoflurane, and desflurane cause less inhibition than other volatiles [7]. No clinical benefit has been shown for total IV anesthesia beyond that seen with isoflurane 1 MAC (minimum alveolar concentration) or less. HPV is decreased by all vasodilators such as nitroglycerin and nitroprusside. In general, vasodilators can be expected to cause a deterioration in P_aO_2 during OLV.
3. **Cardiac output.** The net effects of an increase in cardiac output during OLV tend to favor an increase in P_aO_2. However, elevation of cardiac output beyond physiologic needs tends to oppose HPV and may cause P_aO_2 to fall.
4. **Ventilation during one-lung anesthesia.** It is possible to improve gas exchange for selected individual patients by altering the ventilatory variables that are under the control of the anesthesiologist: Tidal volume, rate, inspiratory/expiratory ratio, P_aCO_2, peak and plateau airway pressures, and PEEP (Table 26.8).
   a. **Respiratory acid–base status.** The overall efficacy of HPV is optimal with normal pH and P_aCO_2.
   b. **Tidal volume.** 5–6 mL/kg ideal body weight for OLV is a reasonable starting point. The tidal volume should be adjusted during OLV to keep the airway peak pressure less than 35 cm H_2O and the plateau airway pressure less than 25 cm H_2O.
   c. **PEEP.** Most patients with either normal or supra-normal (restrictive lung disease) lung elastic recoil will benefit from low levels (5 cm H_2O) of PEEP during OLV. A recruitment maneuver (e.g., static inflation to 20 cm H_2O for 20 s, observing for hypotension) to the ventilated lung is useful at the start of OLV. Auto-PEEP is prone to occur in patients with decreased lung elastic recoil, such as those with emphysema. Auto-PEEP

TABLE 26.8 Ventilation parameters for one-lung ventilation

Parameter	Suggested	Note
I. Tidal volume	5–6 mL/kg (ideal body weight)	Maintain Peak airway pressure <35 cm H_2O Plateau airway pressure <25 cm H_2O
II. PEEP	5 cm H_2O (recruitment maneuver at start of OLV and prn)	Avoid added PEEP in patients with moderate–severe COPD who have auto-PEEP
III. Respiratory rate	12/min	$P_{a\text{-}et}CO_2$ gradient usually will increase 1–3 mm Hg during OLV. Mild hypercapnia (P_aCO_2 50–55 mm Hg) OK
IV. Mode	Volume or pressure control	Patients at risk for lung injury (pneumonectomy, lung transplantation, bullae) pressure-control ventilation preferred
V. FiO_2	0.8–1.0 initially	Add air to decrease FiO_2 guided by oxygen saturation after 20 min of stable OLV

PEEP, positive end-expiratory pressure; OLV, one-lung ventilation; COPD, chronic obstructive pulmonary disease; $P_{a\text{-}et}CO_2$, Arterial-end tidal CO_2 partial pressure; P_aCO_2, Arterial partial pressure of CO_2; FiO_2, Inspired oxygen concentration.

is difficult to detect using currently available anesthetic ventilators. Applied PEEP combines with auto-PEEP in an unpredictable fashion.

d. **Volume control versus pressure control.** Pressure-control OLV is useful in patients with severe obstructive disease and to limit airway pressure in patients with blebs, bullae, or fresh resections in the lung, and also in patients at risk of acute lung injury (pneumonectonies, lung transplantation).

e. **FIO_2.** The FIO_2 should be increased at the start of OLV to 80% to 100% and then can be decreased as tolerated over the next 20 min.

5. **Treatment of hypoxemia during OLV (see Table 26.9)**

In cases of severe and/or acute desaturation resume two-lung ventilation immediately, deflate the bronchial cuff or blocker, and then check the position of the DLT or BB. In cases of desaturation that have not become life-threatening:

a. **Increase FIO_2.** The first-line therapy is to increase the FIO_2, which is an option in essentially all patients except those who received bleomycin or similar therapy that potentiates pulmonary oxygen toxicity.

TABLE 26.9 Treatment options for hypoxemia during one-lung ventilation

Severe/acute: Resume two-lung ventilation
Gradual desaturation:

- **I.** Assure $FiO_2 = 1.0$
- **II.** Check position of DLT/BB with FOB
- **III.** Optimize cardiac output
- **IV.** Recruitment maneuver of ventilated lung
- **V.** Apply PEEP 5 cm H_2O to ventilated lung (except COPD)
- **VI.** Apply CPAP 1–2 cm H_2O to nonventilated lung (recruitment maneuver first)
- **VII.** Intermittent reinflation of nonventilated lung
- **VIII.** Partial ventilation of nonventilated lung:
  - **A.** Segmental oxygen insufflation via FOB
  - **B.** Lobar reinflation
  - **C.** Lobar collapse
  - **D.** Oxygen insufflation
  - **E.** High-frequency ventilation
- **IX.** Mechanical restriction of nonventilated lung pulmonary blood flow

FiO_2, Inspired oxygen concentration; DLT, double-lumen tube; BB, bronchial blocker; FOB, fiberoptic bronchoscopy; PEEP, positive end-expiratory pressure; COPD, chronic obstructive pulmonary disease; CPAP, continuous positive airway pressure.

b. **PEEP.** PEEP to the ventilated dependent lung will improve oxygenation in patients with normal lung mechanics and those with increased elastic recoil due to restrictive lung diseases. Apply a recruitment maneuver to the ventilated lung before application of PEEP.

c. **Pharmacologic manipulations.** Increasing cardiac output will result in a small but clinically useful increase in both $P_{v}O_2$ and $P_{a}O_2$ if cardiac output has decreased. Eliminating potent vasodilators, such as nitroglycerin and halothane, will improve oxygenation during OLV. Selective pulmonary vasodilators such as NO have not yet proven to be reliable.

d. **CPAP.** It must be applied to a fully inflated or re-inflated lung for optimal effect. When CPAP is applied to a fully inflated lung, as little as 2 to 3 cm H_2O can be used. All that is required is a CPAP valve and an oxygen source. Ideally the circuit should permit variation of the CPAP level and should include a reservoir bag to allow easy reinflation of the nonventilated lung and a manometer to measure the actual CPAP supplied. Such circuits are commercially available or can be readily constructed. When the bronchus of the operative lung is obstructed or open to atmosphere, CPAP will not improve oxygenation. During thoracoscopic surgery, CPAP can significantly interfere with surgery.

e. **Alternative ventilation methods.** Several alternative methods of OLV, all of which involve partial ventilation of the nonventilated lung, have been described and improve oxygenation during OLV. These techniques are useful in patients who are particularly at risk for desaturation, such as those with previous pulmonary resections of the contralateral lung.

(1) Oxygen insufflation (5 L/min) for brief periods via the suction channel of an FOB to partially recruit a segment of the nonventilated lung remote from the site of surgery (e.g., a basilar segment of the lower lobe for upper lobe surgery). This is particularly useful in VATS surgery [8].

(2) Selective lobar collapse of only the operative lobe in the open hemithorax by placement of a blocker in the appropriate lobar bronchus of the ipsilateral operative lung.

(3) Differential lung ventilation by only partially occluding the lumen of the DLT to the operative lung.

(4) Intermittent reinflation of the nonventilated lung by regular re-expansion of the operative lung via an attached CPAP circuit.

(5) Conventional OLV of the nonoperative lung and high-frequency jet ventilation of the operative lung

f. **Mechanical restriction of pulmonary blood flow.** It is possible for the surgeon to directly compress or clamp the blood flow to the nonventilated lung. This can be done temporarily in emergency desaturation situations or definitively in cases of pneumonectomy or lung transplantation. Another technique is inflation of a PA catheter balloon in the main PA of the operative lung.

6. **Prevention of hypoxemia.** The treatments outlined as therapy for hypoxemia can be used prophylactically to prevent hypoxemia in patients who are at high risk for desaturation during OLV. Desaturation during bilateral lung procedures is particularly a problem during the second period of OLV. It is advisable to operate first on the lung that has better gas exchange. For the majority of patients this means operating on the right side first.

III. Specific procedures

A. Thoracotomy

1. Operations

a. **Lobectomy.** Lobectomy is the most common pulmonary resection for lung cancer. Early functional loss exceeds the amount of lung tissue resected, but function recovers over a period of 6 wks so that the final net loss of respiratory function is equivalent to the amount of functioning lung tissue excised. The recovery of pulmonary function after thoracotomy is unique because it shows a plateau with no early recovery during the first 72 h postoperatively. This period coincides with the occurrence of the majority of post-thoracotomy respiratory complications (atelectasis, pneumonia), which are the major causes of mortality after pulmonary resection. These complications are particularly associated with lobectomy and its variations, probably due to the transient dysfunction that occurs in the remaining lobe(s). The right middle lobe is particularly at risk for these complications after a right upper lobectomy and can develop torsion about its broncho-vascular pedicle or lobar bronchial kinking as it expands into the apex of the right hemithorax.

b. **Sleeve lobectomy.** A sleeve lobectomy is the excision of a lobe plus the adjacent segment of mainstem bronchus with bronchoplastic repair of the bronchus by end-to-end anastomosis to preserve the distal functioning pulmonary parenchyma. It is done to preserve functioning lung tissue when the tumor encroaches to less than 2 cm from the lobar bronchial orifices, precluding simple lobectomy. This procedure is usually done for right upper lobe tumors but can be used for other lobes. The anesthetic implications of this procedure are that no airway catheter (single-lumen or DLT) or BB can be placed in the ipsilateral main stem bronchus. Mucus clearance across the bronchial anastomosis may be impaired after sleeve resection, and local tumor recurrence is a problem.

c. **Bi-lobectomy.** In the right lung, a bi-lobectomy may be used to conserve either a functioning upper or lower lobe when the tumor extends across the lobar fissure or for malignancies involving the bronchus intermedius (the portion of the right main stem bronchus distal to the right upper lobe orifice). The complication rate is slightly higher than for a simple lobectomy but is less than for a pneumonectomy. The incidence of cardiac dysrhythmias increases postoperatively versus lobectomy, whereas the incidence of respiratory complications remains the same. The residual lobe cannot completely fill the hemithorax, and all patients will have a degree of pneumothorax that can be expected to resolve gradually.

d. **Pneumonectomy.** Complete removal of the lung is required when a lobectomy or its modifications is not adequate to remove the local disease and/or ipsilateral lymph node metastases. Atelectasis and pneumonia occur after pneumonectomy as they do after lobectomy but may be less of a problem because of the absence of residual parenchymal dysfunction on the operative side. The mortality rate after pneumonectomy exceeds that for lobectomy because of complications that are more likely with pneumonectomy.

   (1) **Postpneumonectomy pulmonary edema.** The syndrome presents clinically with dyspnea and an increased alveolar–arterial oxygen gradient on the second or third postoperative day [9]. Radiologic changes precede clinical symptoms by approximately 24 h. The factors that are known about this syndrome are listed in Table 26.10. This syndrome has such a high case of fatality rate (greater than 50%) that it represents a large portion of mortality after lung resection. Excessive perioperative administration of IV crystalloids or colloids can exacerbate this syndrome. There is no evidence that judicious amounts of fluids cause this problem. The residual nonoperated lung has an increased pulmonary capillary permeability after pneumonectomy that is not seen in the nonoperated lung after lobectomy. The cause of this increased permeability may be related to surgical lymphatic damage, capillary stress injury from increased flow, or increased airway pressure and hyperinflation

TABLE 26.10 Postpneumonectomy pulmonary edema

Incidence 2–4% of pneumonectomies
Case fatality >50%
Incidence right > left pneumonectomy (3–4:1)
Clinical onset 2–3 days postoperatively
Associated with increased pulmonary capillary permeability
Not associated with increased PA pressures
Exacerbation by fluid overload

PA, pulmonary artery.

of the ventilated lung during OLV. The majority of lobectomies have the potential to become a pneumonectomy, so caution is needed with fluids in most thoracic cases.

(2) **Atrial fibrillation.** Up to 50% of postpneumonectomy patients will develop supraventricular arrhythmias in the first week postoperatively and the majority of these are atrial fibrillation. The perioperative mortality is 17% in patients who develop arrhythmias versus 2% in those without this complication. The etiology of these arrhythmias seems to depend on two factors: RV strain and increased sympathetic nervous activity. Similar arrhythmias occur after lesser pulmonary resections with a lower incidence. Prophylactic digoxin is not effective in preventing these arrhythmias. Diltiazem 10 mg IV every 8 h is of some benefit [10].

(3) **Mechanical effects.** A variety of potentially lethal intrathoracic mechanical derangements of cardiorespiratory function can occur after pneumonectomy. The most important of these is cardiac herniation through an incompletely closed pericardium. This is particularly a risk after right pneumonectomy and presents with acute severe hypotension in the immediate postoperative period. The only useful therapy is immediate re-operation to return the heart into the pericardium. A subacute form of cardiac herniation can occur after a left pneumonectomy and presents with a picture of myocardial ischemia as the apex of the heart herniates through the pericardial defect and compresses the coronary blood flow. Less acute presentations of cardiovascular or respiratory symptoms may develop related to shifts of the mediastinum that can compress the great vessels or airways after pneumonectomy.

e. **Sleeve pneumonectomy.** Tumors involving the most proximal portions of the main stem bronchus and the carina may require a sleeve pneumonectomy. These are performed most commonly for right-sided tumors and usually can be performed without cardiopulmonary bypass (CPB) via a right thoracotomy. A long single-lumen EBT can be advanced into the left main stem bronchus during the period of anastomosis, or the lung can be ventilated via a separate sterile ETT and circuit that is passed into the operating field and used for temporary intubation of the open distal bronchus. High frequency positive pressure ventilation (HFPPV) also has been used for this procedure.

Because the carina is surgically more accessible from the right side, left sleeve pneumonectomies are commonly performed as a two-stage operation, first a left thoracotomy and pneumonectomy, and then a right thoracotomy for the carinal excision. The complication rate and mortality are higher and the 5-yr survival significantly lower than for other pulmonary resections.

f. **Lesser resections (segmentectomy, wedge).** These procedures are commonly performed in the elderly or in patients with limited cardiopulmonary reserves to preserve functioning pulmonary parenchyma. These lesser resections are associated with a lower 5-yr survival rate compared to lobectomy due to loco-regional recurrence of cancer. The decrease of pulmonary function (FEV_1) for lesser resections is in proportion to the amount of lung tissue removed. Lesser resections are acceptable therapy for nonmalignant lung lesions.

g. **Extended resections.** Portions of the chest wall, diaphragm, pericardium, left atrium, vena cava, brachial plexus, or vertebral body may be excised with adjacent lung tumor. Resection of any of these structures has important anesthetic implications for choice and placement of intraoperative monitors and lines and for postoperative management.

h. **Subsequent pulmonary resections.** Lung resection surgery after previous lung resection is increasingly frequent. These operations can be performed for either benign or malignant disease. Ten percent of lung cancer patients can be expected to develop a second primary tumor. Prediction of postoperative lung function for these patients is accurate based on the assessment of preoperative function (lung mechanics, gas exchange, and cardiopulmonary reserve) and estimation of the amount of functional lung tissue removed at surgery (Fig. 26.1). Lobectomy after pneumonectomy can be performed safely if the patient meets minimal standards for predicted postoperative pulmonary function. Intraoperative collapse of the ipsilateral lung is not possible, but surgery can be facilitated by selective lobar or segment bronchial blockade or the use of HFPPV.

Completion pneumonectomy after a previous ipsilateral resection for cancer has a greater than 40% 5-yr survival rate. Intraoperative hemorrhage is the specific anesthetic concern with this procedure, and more than 50% of patients experience blood loss of greater than 1,000 mL. Hemorrhage is particularly a problem in completion pneumonectomy for nonmalignant lung disease (lung abscess, bronchiectasis, tuberculosis). Inflammatory lung disease tends to destroy the tissue planes around the hilum and makes the surgical dissection more difficult, with an attendant increase in perioperative mortality.

i. **Incomplete resections.** In general, a lung cancer patient's prognosis is not improved from an incomplete resection. There are several exceptions. Incompletely resected tumors with direct mediastinal invasion or tumors of the superior sulcus may benefit if the resection is combined with adjuvant brachytherapy or external irradiation. Also, if the residual tumor is limited to microscopic involvement of the cut mucosal margin of the bronchus, 5-yr survival is increased beyond that seen without surgery. Incomplete resections may be indicated for palliation in cases of airway obstruction or hemoptysis if these are not amenable to endoscopic or radiologic procedures.

j. **Adjuvant and neoadjuvant therapy.** The benefits of pre- and/or postoperative prophylactic chemotherapy and/or radiotherapy are unclear for lung cancer patients who have undergone complete resections. Thoracic irradiation is usually given to patients with resected N_2 node involvement disease. Chemotherapy may be of some benefit after resection of advanced adenocarcinoma. Neoadjuvant cisplatin-based regimens for marginally resectable Stage IIIa or IIIb disease are currently under investigation. Preoperative radiotherapy does not appear to offer any survival benefits and makes the surgery technically more difficult.

2. **Surgical approaches.** Any given pulmonary resection can be accomplished by a variety of different surgical approaches. The approach used in an individual case depends on the interaction of several factors, which include the site and pathology of the lesion(s) and the training and experience of the surgical team. Each approach has specific anesthetic implications. Common thoracic surgical approaches and their generally accepted advantages and disadvantages are listed in Table 26.11.

TABLE 26.11 Surgical approaches for pulmonary resections

Incision	Pro	Con
Posterolateral thoracotomy	Excellent exposure to entire operative hemithorax	Postoperative pain; ±respiration dysfunction (short and long term)
Lateral muscle-sparing thoracotomy	Decreased postoperative pain	Increased incidence of wound seromas
Anterolateral thoracotomy	Better access for laparotomy, resuscitation, or contralateral thoracotomy, especially in trauma	Limited access to posterior thorax
Axillary thoracotomy	Decreased pain; adequate access for first rib resection, sympathectomy, apical blebs, or bullae.	Limited exposure
Sternotomy	Decreased pain; bilateral access	Decreased exposure of posterior structures
Trans-sternal bilateral ("clamshell")	Good exposure for bilateral lung transplantation	Postoperative pain and chest wall dysfunction
Video-assisted thoracoscopic/robotic surgery	Less postoperative pain and respiratory dysfunction	Technically difficult with lung adhesions

a. **Posterolateral thoracotomy.** This is the traditional incision in thoracic surgery. The patient is placed in the lateral decubitus position. Chest access is usually via the fifth or sixth intercostal space. The left seventh or eighth space may be used for access to the esophageal hiatus. The serratus anterior, latissimus dorsi, and trapezius muscles all will be partially divided during incision, with subsequent postoperative pain and disability. Chest access may be obtained directly through an intercostal space or by excision of a rib. Exposure to all ipsilateral intrathoracic structures is excellent.

b. **Muscle-sparing lateral thoracotomy.** The lateral muscle-sparing thoracotomy has been advocated to reduce the pain and disability associated with a standard posterolateral thoracotomy. The skin incision is basically the same, but an extensive subcutaneous dissection is required to mobilize the latissimus and serratus muscles.

c. **Anterolateral thoracotomy.** This is a particularly useful incision in trauma because it allows complete access to the patient for ongoing resuscitation and does not require repositioning for laparotomy or exploration of the contralateral chest. Exposure to the posterior hemithorax is limited in comparison to a posterolateral incision. Because this approach requires incision of only the pectoralis muscles, pain and shoulder disability may be less than with a standard thoracotomy.

d. **Axillary thoracotomy.** The transaxillary approach provides limited access, only to the apical areas of the hemithorax. The ipsilateral arm must be draped free or suspended and access to this arm will be limited intraoperatively. Thus, it is preferable for vascular access and monitoring to use the contralateral arm. Postoperative pain and disability are less than with a standard thoracotomy. This is an adequate incision for first rib resection, resection of apical bullae/blebs, or thoracic sympathectomy.

e. **Median sternotomy.** This incision, which is the standard for cardiac surgery, has potential benefits for certain thoracic procedures. Bilateral excisions for metastases and bullae are best performed via this incision. It has been demonstrated that postoperative spirometry is superior and pain is less after median sternotomy than thoracotomy. Most pulmonary resections can be performed via a median sternotomy, which obviates the need for a separate incision in cases of combined cardiac and thoracic surgery (see Section **III.J**). Certain procedures are more difficult via a median sternotomy, including procedures performed for superior sulcus tumors, tumors with posterior chest wall extension, and left lower lobe tumors. OLV is more of a necessity for surgical exposure than for lateral thoracotomies because of the limited surgical access and desaturation is more common with OLV in the supine than the lateral position.

f. **Trans-sternal bilateral thoracotomy (the "clamshell" incision).** This is the common incision for bilateral lung transplantation. Because of increased pain and postoperative chest wall dysfunction, it is not commonly used for other intrathoracic procedures. It has been used for resection of bilateral metastases, pericardiectomy, resection of a posterior ventricular aneurysm, and cardiac surgery in a patient with a tracheotomy.

B. **Video-assisted thoracoscopic (VATS) and robotic surgery.** Essentially any surgical procedure that is performed via thoracotomy has been attempted by VATS. VATS has been advocated for pulmonary resection of lung cancer in patients with limited respiratory reserves because of decreased postoperative pain and loss of early postoperative spirometric respiratory function that is only approximately half of that seen when the same operation is performed by thoracotomy. VATS is the procedure of choice for resection of nonmalignant pulmonary lesions (blebs, bullae, granulomas). VATS will probably become the commonest procedure for the majority of cancer resections. Also, VATS is used for sympathectomy for palmar hyperhidrosis and for the intrathoracic portion of esophagogastrectomy. Bilateral VATS can be performed in the supine position for apical lesions, but for most operations bilateral VATS requires change from one lateral position to the other intraoperatively. Robotic thoracic surgery is being used increasingly for minimally invasive procedures due to better visualization.

Some procedures are attempted by VATS initially with conversion to thoracotomy if the surgery proves impractical. OLV with complete collapse of the operative lung is more of a priority than for open thoracotomy, and application of CPAP to the nonventilated lung is more detrimental to surgery than in open thoracotomy. To aid collapse of the lung, particularly in patients with COPD and poor lung elastic recoil, it is best to ventilate with oxygen instead of air/oxygen mixtures during the period of two-lung ventilation before lung collapse and to apply suction (−20 cm H_2O) to the nonventilated lung after the start of OLV until collapse is complete. Postoperative management is essentially the same as for thoracotomy, and most patients initially will have chest drains. The amount of postoperative pain after VATS varies greatly depending on the surgical procedure performed. Simple wedge excisions will have only the pain of several small intercostal incisions and the chest drain(s), and this can usually be easily managed with oral medications. Pleural abrasions or instillation of pleural sclerosing agents, which are often done for recurrent pneumothoraces or effusions, are extremely painful and may require full postoperative analgesic management, up to and including thoracic epidural analgesia, in patients with limited pulmonary function.

C. **Bronchopleural fistula.** A persistent communication between the airway and the interpleural space can develop after medical conditions, such as rupture of a bleb or bulla, infection, or malignancy. Bronchopleural fistula can develop as a postoperative complication after lung surgery. The large majority of persistent lung air leaks will heal with drainage and conservative management.

Surgical intervention is indicated when conservative therapy is unable to permit adequate gas exchange (this is more likely to occur in the immediate postoperative period, particularly after pneumonectomy) or when conventional chest tube drainage and suction are unable to re-expand the ipsilateral lung, or for a second ipsilateral or first contralateral pneumothorax.

There are three specific **anesthetic goals** in all patients with a bronchopleural fistula:

1. Healthy lung regions must be protected from soiling by extrapleural fluid from the affected hemithorax.
2. The ventilation technique must avoid development of a tension pneumothorax in the affected hemithorax.
3. The anesthetic technique must ensure adequate alveolar gas exchange in the presence of a low-resistance air leak.

To achieve these goals there are two **management principles** that should be used in essentially all cases:

1. A functioning chest drain should be placed before the induction of anesthesia and connected to an underwater seal without suction.
2. A method of lung separation should be placed so that the fistula can be isolated as necessary intraoperatively.

After placement of a chest drain there are three **options for induction** of anesthesia [11]:

1. A single-lumen or double-lumen EBT or blocker can be placed in an awake patient with topical anesthesia and its position checked fiberoptically before induction. This is often not the best choice in a patient with severely compromised gas exchange because maintaining adequate oxygenation in an already hypoxemic patient can be a problem during awake intubation.
2. Induction of anesthesia maintaining spontaneous ventilation until lung isolation is secured. A spontaneous-ventilation induction may not be desirable if there is a risk of aspiration and in patients with compromised hemodynamics.
3. IV induction of general anesthesia and muscle relaxation after meticulous preoxygenation and manual ventilation using small tidal volumes and low airway pressures until the lung isolation is confirmed. The efficiency of this technique can be improved by using a bronchoscope to guide DLT placement during intubation.

   The air leak through a bronchopleural fistula is dependent on the pressure gradient between the mean airway pressure at the site of the fistula and the interpleural space. High-frequency ventilation, with and without lung or lobar blockade, has been used in certain cases. High-frequency techniques may permit relatively lower proximal mean airway pressures than conventional mechanical ventilation and may be more useful in large central air leaks.

D. **Bullae and blebs.** Whenever positive-pressure ventilation is applied to the airway of a patient with a bulla or bleb, there is the risk of lesion rupture and development of a tension pneumothorax that will require drainage and may progress to a bronchopleural fistula. The anesthetic considerations are similar to those for a patient with a bronchopleural fistula, except that it is best not to place a chest drain prophylactically because the chest tube may enter the bulla and create a fistula and there is not the risk of soiling healthy lung regions from extrapleural fluid that exists with fistulas. For induction of anesthesia it is usually optimal to maintain spontaneous ventilation until the lung or lobe with the bulla or bleb is isolated. When there is a risk of aspiration or it is believed that the patient's gas exchange or hemodynamics may not permit spontaneous ventilation for induction, the anesthesiologist will need to use small tidal volumes and low airway pressures during positive-pressure ventilation until the airway is isolated. Nitrous oxide will diffuse into a bleb or bulla, causing it to enlarge, and must be avoided.

E. **Abscesses, bronchiectasis, cysts, and empyema.** As with bronchopleural fistulas, there is the risk of soiling healthy lung regions by uncontrolled spillage from these lesions. Lung isolation is a primary requirement for anesthesia and the anesthetic principles and management are similar to those described for fistulas. When an intrathoracic space-occupying lesion is removed, there is the potential for re-expansion pulmonary edema to develop after reinflation of the ipsilateral lung. A slow and gradual reinflation may decrease the severity of this complication.

F. **Mediastinoscopy.** Cervical mediastinoscopy is a diagnostic sampling of the mediastinal nodes to assess if a pulmonary resection will improve outcome. Basically, it is an attempt to differentiate between Stage I or II and Stage III lung cancer because the benefits of surgery vary tremendously between these stages. Mediastinoscopy can avoid some but not all unnecessary exploratory thoracotomies. Mediastinoscopy is often omitted from the cancer staging if the CT scan of the mediastinum is negative (mediastinal nodes less than 1 cm in the short axis). Because there are a significant number of false-positive results on cancer staging with CT scan, all patients with positive mediastinal nodes on CT should have a mediastinoscopy.

Mediastinoscopy can be done at a separate anesthetic before pulmonary resection, often as an outpatient, or immediately after induction as part of the same procedure before the pulmonary resection. Apart from the specific anesthetic considerations of mediastinoscopy itself, the anesthetic implication of starting the case with these diagnostic procedures is that the resection may be aborted based on the initial mediastinoscopy findings. Consider avoiding the use of long-acting nondepolarizing muscle relaxants until the biopsy results indicate that the resection will proceed. The likelihood of not proceeding to thoracotomy must enter into each individual assessment of risk/benefit when considering placing an epidural catheter before induction.

Mediastinoscopy is most commonly done via a cervical approach with an incision in the suprasternal notch. Any structure in the upper chest can be injured during the procedure, including great vessels, pleura (pneumothorax), nerves (recurrent laryngeal), and airways.

Hemorrhage is the most frequent major complication, particularly due to inadvertent PA biopsy, and this must always be considered with respect to vascular access, monitoring, and the availability of means for resuscitation. Fortunately, significant hemorrhage during mediastinoscopy can usually be tamponaded temporarily by the surgeon when resuscitation is required. In only a minority of mediastinoscopy hemorrhages it is necessary to proceed to thoracotomy for surgical control of bleeding.

A frequent complication of cervical mediastinoscopy is transient compression of the brachiocephalic (innominate) artery by the mediastinoscope. The surgeon is usually unaware that this is occurring, and it is part of the anesthetic considerations to always continuously monitor the pulse in the right arm (pulse oximetry or arterial line or palpation) so that the surgeon can be notified and avoid the risk of cerebral ischemia in patients who may not have good collateral cerebral circulation.

Because of the different pattern of lymphatic drainage of the left upper lobe, patients with left upper lobe tumors often will have an anterior left parasternal mediastinoscopy or median sternotomy instead of or in addition to a cervical mediastinoscopy. The serious complications associated with cervical mediastinoscopy are not as frequent with parasternal mediastinoscopy.

Endobronchial ultrasound (EBUS)-guided mediastinal nodal biopsies via an FOB are increasingly used as an alternative to traditional mediastinoscopy as a lung cancer staging procedure. These can be performed awake with topical anesthesia of the airway or under general anesthesia.

TABLE 26.12 Grading scale for symptoms in patients with an anterior mediastinal mass

Asymptomatic
Mild: Can lie supine with some cough/pressure sensation
Moderate: Can lie supine for short periods but not indefinitely
Severe: Cannot tolerate supine position

G. Anterior mediastinal mass. Patients with anterior mediastinal masses present unique problems to the anesthesiologist. A large number of such patients require anesthesia for biopsy of these masses by mediastinoscopy or VATS, or they may require definitive resection via sternotomy or thoracotomy. Tumors of the anterior mediastinum include thymoma, teratoma, lymphoma, cystic hygroma, bronchogenic cyst, and thyroid tumors. Anterior mediastinal masses may cause obstruction of major airways, main pulmonary arteries, atria, and superior vena cava. Any one of these complications can be life threatening. During induction of general
10 anesthesia in patients with an anterior mediastinal mass, airway obstruction is the most common and feared complication.

It is important to note that the point of tracheal compression usually occurs distal to the ETT. A history of supine dyspnea or cough should alert the clinician to the possibility of airway obstruction upon induction of anesthesia. Life-threatening complications may occur in the absence of symptoms. The other major complication is cardiovascular collapse secondary to compression of the heart or major vessels. Symptoms of supine syncope suggest vascular compression. Death upon induction of general anesthesia in patients with an anterior mediastinal mass is always a risk. Anesthetic deaths have mainly been reported in children. These deaths may be the result of the more compressible cartilaginous structure of the airway in children or because of the difficulty in obtaining a history of positional symptoms in children.

The most important diagnostic test in the patient with an anterior mediastinal mass is the CT scan of the trachea and chest. Children with tracheobronchial compression greater than 50% on CT cannot be safely given general anesthesia [12]. Flow–volume loops, specifically exacerbation of a variable intrathoracic obstruction pattern (expiratory plateau) when supine, are unreliable for predicting which patients will have intraoperative airway complications. Echocardiography is indicated for patients with vascular compressive symptoms.

Management. General anesthesia will exacerbate extrinsic intrathoracic airway compression in at least three ways. First, reduced lung volume occurs during general anesthesia; second, bronchial smooth muscle relaxes during general anesthesia allowing greater compressibility of large airways; and third, paralysis eliminates the caudal movement of the diaphragm seen during spontaneous ventilation. This eliminates the normal trans-pleural pressure gradient that dilates the airways during inspiration and minimizes the effects of extrinsic intrathoracic airway compression.

Management of these patients is guided by their symptoms (Tables 26.12–26.14) and the CT scan. All of these patients requiring general anesthesia need a step-by-step induction of anesthesia with continuous monitoring of gas exchange and hemodynamics. This **"NPIC"**

TABLE 26.13 Stratification of patients regarding safety for "NPIC" general anesthesia

A. Safe	(I) Asymptomatic adult
	(II) CT minimum tracheal/bronchial diameter >50% of normal
B. Unsafe	(I) Severely symptomatic adult or child
	(II) Children with CT tracheal/bronchial diameter <50% of normal
C. Uncertain	(I) Mild/moderate symptomatic adult
	(II) Asymptomatic adult with CT tracheal/bronchial diameter <50% of normal
	(III) Mild/moderate symptomatic child with CT tracheal/bronchial diameter >50% of normal
	(IV) Adult or child unable to give history

CT, computed tomography. "NPIC" (Noli Pontes Ignii Consumere; i.e., Don't burn your bridges).

TABLE 26.14 Management for all "uncertain" patients for "NPIC" general anesthesia

I. Secure airway beyond stenosis awake if feasible
II. Rigid bronchoscope and surgeon available at induction
III. Laryngeal mask airway available
IV. Determine optimal positioning of patient
V. Monitor for airway compromise postoperatively "NPIC" (Noli Pontes Ignii Consumere; i.e., Don't burn your bridges)

(Noli Pontes Ignii Consumere, i.e., don't burn your bridges) anesthetic induction can be an inhalation induction with a volatile agent such as sevoflurane or IV titration of propofol with or without ketamine, which maintains spontaneous ventilation until either the airway is definitively secured or the procedure is completed [13]. Awake intubation of the trachea before induction is a possibility in some adult patients if the CT scan shows an area of noncompressed distal trachea to which the ETT can be advanced before induction. If muscle relaxants are required, ventilation should first be gradually taken over manually to assure that positive-pressure ventilation is possible and only then can a short-acting muscle relaxant be administered. Development of airway or vascular compression requires that the patient be awakened as rapidly as possible and then other options for the surgery to be explored. Intraoperative life-threatening airway compression has usually responded to one of two therapies: Either **repositioning** of the patient (which should be determined before induction if there is one side or position that causes less compression) or **rigid bronchoscopy** and ventilation distal to the obstruction (this means that an experienced bronchoscopist and equipment must always be immediately available in the operating room with these cases).

Femoro-femoral CPB before induction of anesthesia is a possibility for some patients who are considered "unsafe" for "NPIC" general anesthesia. The concept of CPB "standby" during attempted induction of anesthesia is fraught with danger because there is not enough time after a sudden airway collapse to establish CPB before hypoxic cerebral injury occurs [14]. Other options for "unsafe" patients include local anesthetic biopsy of the mediastinal mass or biopsy of another node (e.g., supraclavicular), preoperative radiotherapy with a nonradiated "window" for subsequent biopsy, preoperative chemotherapy or short-course steroids, and CT-guided biopsy of mass or drainage of a cyst.

H. **Tracheal and bronchial stenting.** Regional narrowing of the trachea or bronchi can be treated temporarily or definitively by placement of tracheal or bronchial stents [15]. The only previous options for these lesions were dilation, laser excision, or surgical excision. Airway stenting is an option for palliation of patients with mediastinal masses pending other therapy. There are two major varieties of stent: Metallic and Silastic (Dumon). Both are commonly placed during rigid bronchoscopy, although there is an option to place the self-expanding metallic stents with flexible FOB. The metallic stents are more stable and more resistant to dislocation in the airway but are difficult (often impossible) to remove once placed. Thus, metallic stents are commonly only used for palliation in malignant airway obstructions.

Anesthetic management for tracheal stenting is similar to management of patients with mediastinal masses. General anesthesia with muscle relaxation is optimal, but in patients with severe symptoms of airway obstruction, induction of anesthesia should follow a step-by-step "NPIC" protocol as discussed above.

I. **Tracheal resection.** Anatomically, the trachea has a necessary structural rigidity and a segmental blood supply that complicate its resection and repair. Many different prosthetic designs and materials have been evaluated as tracheal substitutes. Because of unresolved problems with anatomic disruption, poor healing, and infection, end-to-end anastomosis of the trachea remains the ideal method of repair.

Endotracheal intubation and resulting strictures were the primary cause of the need for tracheal resection, but using less irritating ETT materials and limiting the duration of prolonged endotracheal intubation have decreased this complication. Benign and malignant tumors (e.g., adenocarcinomas and cylindromas) constitute the remaining indications for tracheal resection.

For a controlled and methodical operation on the trachea, full control of the airway must be maintained at all times. Cooperation between the surgeon and anesthesiologist is of utmost importance. Both should visualize the lesion preoperatively (CT and bronchoscopy). With preoperative planning and discussions, they can avoid unnecessary hasty procedures that might compromise the end result or worse. Benign lesions can be dilated preoperatively to allow the passage of a small ETT through the lesion. Operatively, the area below the lesion is addressed first. If the degree of obstruction increases, a sterile ETT can be placed directly. The patient should be spontaneously ventilating at the end of the case to allow for extubation. Some surgeons will temporarily place a Montgomery "T" tube distal to the anastomosis with the side arm of the "T" brought out anteriorly through the neck incision to ensure gas exchange in case of proximal tracheoglottic obstruction or edema. Some surgeons will leave a temporary "chin retention" suture for several days postoperatively. This heavy suture between the chin and the sternum restricts head extension and limits traction on the fresh tracheal anastomosis. CPB greatly complicates the conduct of the operation and has largely been unnecessary.

J. **Combined pulmonary resection and cardiac surgery.** Potentially, most cardiac operations (aorto-coronary bypass, valve repair/replacement, congenital defects) can be combined with thoracic procedures for either malignant or benign disease (pneumonectomy, lobectomy, wedge resection). There is no agreement about the surgical management of patients found to have both cardiac and thoracic surgical lesions.

The one-stage combined procedure avoids a second anesthetic and incision and may reduce hospital stay. The two-stage procedure may be associated with less blood loss than with pulmonary resection in heparinized patients and may allow better operative exposure and staging of mediastinal nodes for malignant lung lesions. Patients with combined surgical lesions present in one of three patterns:

1. An asymptomatic lung lesion is discovered during evaluation for cardiac surgery.
2. A patient being investigated for lung pathology is found to have significant cardiac disease.
3. A previously undetected lung lesion is discovered intraoperatively after sternotomy.

In the first or second scenario, adequate pulmonary assessment can be arranged preoperatively to guide perioperative anesthetic management. When a lesion is discovered intraoperatively, anesthetic management will be more *ad hoc.* Many of these "surprise" lesions are benign (granulomas) and require only simple wedge resection without intraoperative lung isolation or loss of postoperative pulmonary function.

Due to the difficulty assessing subcarinal nodes for staging via a sternotomy, all known lung cancer patients should have a mediastinoscopy as the first step of a combined procedure. For cardiac valvular surgery, because of the risk of contamination of the operative field from an open bronchus, it is recommended to complete the cardiac procedure, wean from CPB, and close the pericardium before the pulmonary resection. Lung isolation and OLV are necessary for lung resection in these cases. A double-lumen EBT placed at induction is the preferred airway management.

For aorto-coronary bypass, lung isolation and OLV may not be necessary. It is optimal to perform the pulmonary resection at the end of CPB after the aortic cross-clamp is removed. It is important to examine and suction the airway with FOB after the pulmonary resection is completed and before weaning from CPB since there can be significant concealed bleeding into the airway in these cases. For cases where difficult weaning from CPB is anticipated (poor ventricular function, prolonged CPB, redo), the preferred management is to wean from CPB and stabilize the patient, then perform the pulmonary resection. Lung isolation will aid in these cases. Because problems weaning from CPB are not always predictable, a BB may be useful in these cases. Because of the increased incidence of phrenic nerve injury and diaphragmatic paralysis associated with topical cooling (slush) of the heart during CPB, topical cooling is not advised during combined cardiac and thoracic procedures.

K. **Combined cancer and emphysema surgery.** The combination of lung volume reduction surgery (LVRS) or bullectomy in addition to lung cancer surgery has been reported in emphysematous patients who previously would not have met minimal criteria for pulmonary resection because of their concurrent lung disease. Although the numbers of patients reported are small, the expected improvements in postoperative pulmonary function have been seen and the outcomes are encouraging. This offers an extension of the standard indications for surgery in a small, well-selected number of patients.

L. **Combined pulmonary resection and thoracic spine surgery.** Patients with extension of lung tumors to the thoracic spine may be candidates for combined resection of the lung and involved portions of the spine. These procedures may be done in one or two stages. The preferred practice at my (PS) institution is the two-stage procedure with an initial operation using a posterior approach to the thoracic spine for placement of stabilization devices. This is followed after a brief period of recovery (1 wk) with a lateral thoracotomy for lung resection and anterior approach to the spine. This second-stage operation is usually a long procedure (6 to 10 h) requiring a prolonged period of **OLV**. In addition to the usual considerations for long surgery (temperature, positioning, fluid status, etc.), considerations for prolonged **OLV** include minimizing atelectasis in the dependent lung using air–oxygen mixtures and PEEP and avoiding over-hydration. It may be possible for the surgeon to place a catheter in the epidural space intraoperatively under direct vision for postoperative analgesia.

M. **Pulmonary hemorrhage.** Massive hemoptysis is defined as expectoration of >200 mL of blood in 24 to 48 h. The commonest causes are carcinoma, bronchiectasis, and trauma (blunt, penetrating, or secondary to a PA catheter). Death can occur quickly due to asphyxia. Management requires four sequential steps: Lung isolation, resuscitation, diagnosis, and definitive treatment. The anesthesiologist is often called to deal with these cases outside of the operating room. There is no consensus on the best method of lung isolation for these cases. The initial method for lung isolation will depend on the availability of appropriate equipment and an assessment of the patient's airway. All three basic methods of lung isolation have been used: DLTs, single-lumen EBTs, and BBs. FOB is usually not helpful to position EBTs or blockers in the presence of torrential pulmonary hemorrhage and lung isolation must be guided by clinical signs (primarily auscultation). DLTs will achieve rapid and secure lung isolation. Even if a left-sided tube enters the right mainstem bronchus, only the right upper lobe will be obstructed. However, suctioning large amounts of blood or clots is difficult through the narrow lumens of a DLT. An option is initial placement of a single-lumen tube for oxygenation and suctioning and then replacement with a DLT either by laryngoscopy or with an appropriate tube exchanger. An uncut single-lumen ETT can be advanced directly into the right mainstem bronchus or rotated 90° counterclockwise for advancement into the left mainstem bronchus. A BB will normally pass easily into the right mainstem bronchus and is useful for right-sided hemorrhage (90% of PA-catheter–induced hemorrhages are right-sided). After lung isolation and resuscitation have been achieved, both diagnosis and definitive therapy are now most commonly performed by radiology [16] (except for blunt and penetrating trauma).

   1. **PA-catheter–induced hemorrhage.** Hemoptysis in a patient with a PA catheter must be
11
   assumed to be caused by perforation of a pulmonary vessel by the catheter until proven otherwise. The mortality rate may exceed 50%. This complication seems to be occurring less than previously, possibly related to stricter indications for the use of PA catheters and more appropriate management of PA catheters with less reliance on wedge measurements. Therapy for PA-catheter–induced hemorrhage should follow an organized protocol with some variation depending on the severity of the hemorrhage (see Table 26.15).

TABLE 26.15 Management of the patient with a PA-catheter–induced pulmonary hemorrhage

I.	Initially position the patient with the bleeding lung dependent.
II.	Endotracheal intubation, oxygenation, airway toilet
III.	Lung isolation. Endobronchial double- or single-lumen tube or BB
IV.	Withdraw the PA catheter several centimeters, leaving it in the main PA. Do not inflate the balloon (except with fluoroscopic guidance).
V.	Position the patient with the isolated bleeding lung nondependent. PEEP to the bleeding lung if possible
VI.	Transport to medical imaging for diagnosis and embolization if feasible.

BB, bronchial blocker; PA, pulmonary artery; PEEP, positive end-expiratory pressure.

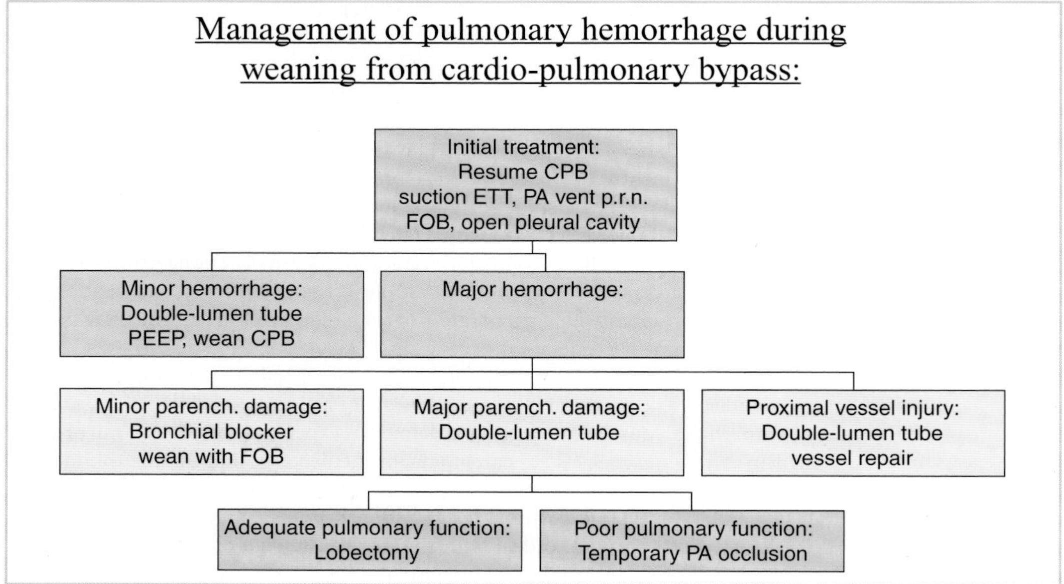

FIGURE 26.9 Management of pulmonary hemorrhage during weaning from cardio-pulmonary bypass. CPB, cardio-pulmonary bypass; ETT, endotracheal tube; PA, pulmonary artery; FOB, fiberoptic bronchoscopy; PEEP, positive end expiratory pressure; Parenc., lung parenchyma.

2. **During weaning from CPB:** Weaning from CPB is one of the times when PA-catheter–induced hemorrhage is most likely to occur. Management of the PA catheter during CPB by withdrawal from a potential wedge depth and observing the PA pressure waveform to avoid wedging during CPB may decrease the risk of this complication. When hemoptysis does occur in this situation there are several management options available (see Fig. 26.9). The anesthesiologist should resist the temptation to rapidly reverse the anticoagulation in order to quickly get off CPB since this can lead to disaster. Resumption of full CPB ensures oxygenation while the tracheobronchial tree is suctioned and then visualized with FOB. The use of a PA vent may be required to decrease the pulmonary blood flow sufficiently to define the bleeding site (usually the right lower lobe). The pleural cavity should be opened to assess the lung parenchymal damage. Conservative management with lung isolation, avoiding lung resection, is optimal therapy, if possible. In patients with persistent hemorrhage who are not candidates for lung resection, temporary lobar PA occlusion with a vascular loop may be an option.

N. **Post-tracheostomy hemorrhage.** Hemorrhage in the immediate postoperative period following a tracheostomy is usually from local vessels such as the anterior jugular or inferior thyroid veins. Massive hemorrhage 1 to 6 wks postoperatively is most commonly due to tracheo-innominate artery fistula [17]. A small sentinel bleed occurs in most patients before a massive bleed. The management protocol for tracheo-innominate artery fistula is outlined in Table 26.16.

TABLE 26.16 Management of tracheo-innominate artery fistula hemorrhage

1. Overinflate the tracheostomy cuff to tamponade the hemorrhage. If this fails:
2. Replace the tracheostomy tube with an oral ETT. Position the cuff with FOB guidance just above the carina.
3. Digital compression of the innominate artery against the posterior sternum using a finger passed through the tracheostomy stoma. If this fails:
4. Slow withdrawal of the ETT and overinflation of the cuff to tamponade
5. Then proceed with definitive therapy: Sternotomy and ligation of the innominate artery.

ETT, endotracheal tube; FOB, fiberoptic bronchoscopy.

IV. Pulmonary thromboendarterectomy

A. Overview. PTE, a complete endarterectomy of the pulmonary vascular tree, is the definitive treatment for chronic thromboembolic pulmonary hypertension (CTEPH). Pulmonary embolism (PE) is a relatively common cardiovascular event, and in a small percentage of cases it leads to a chronic condition in which repeated microemboli as well as ongoing inflammatory response lead to accumulation of connective and elastic tissue on the surface of the pulmonary vessels with resultant end-stage lung disease due to pulmonary hypertension [18]. The only potentially curative options are lung transplantation and PTE, with PTE preferred because of its favorable long-term morbidity and mortality profile. Surgical mortality rates vary in the range of 3% to 6% [19].

No clear etiology has been defined for the development of CTEPH in most cases, although hypercoagulability is certainly a risk. Lupus anticoagulant, Factor V Leiden, elevated plasma levels of Factor VIII, previous splenectomy, permanent IV catheters, ventriculo-atrial shunts, and chronic inflammatory conditions have been associated with CETPH.

The most common symptom of CTEPH, as with pulmonary hypertension in general, is exertional dyspnea. This dyspnea is out of proportion to abnormalities found on clinical examination. Other symptoms may include chest tightness, hemoptysis, peripheral edema, and early satiety.

Investigation includes chest radiograph (CXR), pulmonary function testing, right heart catheterization with pulmonary angiography, high-resolution magnetic resonance imaging, ABG analysis, ventilation/perfusion scanning, and echocardiography. Diffusing capacity (DLCO) is often reduced and may be the only abnormality on pulmonary function testing. Pulmonary arterial pressures are elevated (mean >25 mm Hg), sometimes supra-systemic. Resting cardiac output is often low. Many patients exhibit hypoxia, particularly with exercise. CO_2 tension is often slightly reduced, although dead space ventilation is increased. Ventilation–perfusion studies show moderate mismatch, but correlate poorly with the degree of pulmonary vascular obstruction.

Transthoracic echocardiography is often the first study to provide clear evidence of pulmonary hypertension. An estimate of PA systolic pressure is often provided by Doppler of the tricuspid regurgitant envelope. Echocardiographic findings vary depending on the stage of the disease and include RV enlargement, leftward displacement of the interventricular septum, and encroachment of the enlarged right ventricle on the left ventricular cavity with abnormal systolic and diastolic functions of the left ventricle. Many of these abnormalities resolve after successful PTE.

Pulmonary angiography is the gold standard for defining pulmonary vascular anatomy and is performed to confirm the diagnosis and to determine the location and surgical accessibility of thromboembolic disease. Many CTEPH patients receive medical pulmonary vasodilator therapy. This therapy may consist of phosphodiesterase 5 inhibition (e.g., sildenafil), endothelin-1 inhibition (e.g., bosentan), and prostacyclin analogs (e.g., iloprost, flolan, remodulin). It is prudent to continue these medications preoperatively and to consider their use postoperatively if the surgical result is suboptimal. Abrupt cessation of a prostacyclin analog can result in
12 potentially catastrophic rebound pulmonary hypertension. If a patient presents with an epoprostenol (Flolan™) infusion, this infusion is continued in the pre-CPB period, discontinued during CPB, and restarted after CPB if needed.

B. Surgical procedure. PTE, being an endarterectomy of the entire pulmonary vascular tree, is performed through a midline sternotomy, and requires CPB with deep hypothermic circulatory arrest (DHCA) in most centers. Details of anesthetic and CPB management at the Toronto General Hospital are presented in Tables 26.17 and 26.18. Following median sternotomy, CPB is established with cannulation of the ascending aorta and the inferior and superior vena cava. Cooling is instituted immediately. A gradient of not more than 10°C is maintained between the CPB waterbath temperature and the bladder/rectal temperature. This helps to prevent release of gas bubbles into the circulation upon rewarming. Circulatory arrest is limited to 20-min epochs. An experienced surgeon can usually accomplish the entire unilateral endarterectomy within this time period. If additional arrest time is necessary, reperfusion is carried out at 18°C core temperature for a minimum of 10 min. At the completion of the endarterectomy, perfusion is re-established while the PA incision is closed. Any additional procedures such as closure of a PFO or coronary artery bypass grafting can be performed during the rewarming period.

TABLE 26.17 Pulmonary thromboendarterectomy anesthesia, key points

I. Pre-induction Cooling/warming blanket below patient, supine back-head elevated position Peripheral large-bore venous access, arterial line (radial + femoral post-induction) Right internal jugular access, oximetric PA catheter, in vitro calibration Baseline ABG, activated clotting time (ACT), SVO_2, CI, and PVR, defibrillation pads
II. Induction of anesthesia[a] Intubation with single-lumen ETT Urinary catheter with temperature probe Forced air warming blanket on legs (not connected) Triple-lumen CVP post-induction for postoperative access (subclavian preferred site) Naso- or oropharyngeal probe for temperature Neuromonitoring as per institutional protocol for other CPB cases[a] Drugs Midazolam + fentanyl (or sufentanil) + ketamine (or etomidate) Propofol infusion ± volatile anesthetic Methylprednisolone 1 g on induction (30 mg/kg in some centers) Cephalosporine 1 g if <80 kg, 2 g if >80 kg (repeat q4h), or vancomycin 1 g Tranexamic acid 30 mg/kg loading dose plus infusion of 16 mg/kg/h on CPB Heparin 400 U/kg to raise and maintain ACT >480 s
III. TEE Assess RV/LV function, PFO, intracardiac and PA thrombi Assess aortic and mitral valve functions Monitor intracardiac air emboli during weaning Reassess post-CPB
IV. Post-CPB Pressure control ventilation, VT 6–7 mL/kg, PEEP 5 cm, decrease FiO_2 as tolerated Minimal doses of furosemide (5–10 mg) if indicated (to avoid excessive diuresis once patient is warmed) aim for urine output greater than 1 L while on CPB, total 1.5–2 L at the end of the procedure Norepinephrine to wean off CPB, limit maximum cardiac index to 2.0–2.5 L/min/M^2 to decrease pulmonary reperfusion injury Dopamine/epinephrine if indicated to raise CI, aim at SVO_2 greater than 60% Protamine to reverse heparin, platelets, and clotting factors only for indication (these patients usually have a thrombophilia). Bleeding post-CPB is not common despite long CPB times. NG tube after TEE probe removed, FOB at end of case

[a]In patients with very high PA pressures: Risk of hemodynamic collapse on induction, induction after urinary catheter, patient prepped and draped.
PA, pulmonary artery; ABG, arterial blood gas; PVR, pulmonary vascular resistance; ETT, endotracheal tube; CVP, central venous pressure; CPB, cardiopulmonary bypass; PEEP, positive end-expiratory pressure; TEE, transesophageal echocardiography; ACT, activated clotting time; SVO_2, mixed venous oxygen saturation; RV/LV, right ventricular/left ventricular; PFO, patent foramen ovale; CI, cardiac index; NG, naso-gastric; FOB, fiberoptic bronshoscopy.

C. **Anesthetic management.** A typical anesthetic for a pulmonary endarterectomy is similar to most cases of cardiac surgery with DHCA. However, the majority of lines and monitors are placed pre-induction due to the risk of hemodynamic collapse on induction.

Because of the high right-sided pressures, the coronary blood supply to right ventricle is at risk. Maintenance of adequate mean systemic blood pressure, systemic vascular resistance (SVR), inotropic state, and normal sinus rhythm is critical. Elevated PA systolic >2/3 systemic, RVEDP (>14 mm Hg), severe tricuspid regurgitation, and preoperative pulmonary vascular resistance (PVR) >1000 dyne s cm^{-5} are signs of impending decompensation. Vasopressor (norepinephrine) support is begun prior to induction with addition of inotropic support (e.g., dopamine or epinephrine) as indicated. Generally, patients with CTEPH have fixed PVR because of mechanical obstruction. However, high PVR can still be exacerbated by factors that increase PVR (e.g., hypoxia, hypercarbia, acidosis, pain, and anxiety). Thus, these stressors should be minimized during induction and immediate pre-CPB period. Attempts to lower the PVR pharmacologically (e.g., nitroglycerin, nitroprusside) should be avoided as they have minimal efficacy in treating CTEPH and can dangerously jeopardize the coronary perfusion pressure to

TABLE 26.18 Pulmonary thromboendarterectomy cardiopulmonary bypass (CPB)

Key points
Initiation
Standard CPB prime, retrograde autologous prime if hemodynamically stable
Hemodilution to a hematocrit of 28–30% during cooling
Perfusion index: 2.4–2.5 L/min/m^2, and about 1.7 L/m^2 during hypothermia
Aim for mean BP of 70 to 90 mm Hg during CPB if possible
Thiopental 10 mg/kg (if available) in CPB circuit just before aortic cross-clamp
Cardioplegia every 30–45 min
Start cooling to 18–20°C (rectal) once on full bypass
Head and neck packed in ice or cooling blanket, eyes protected
Circulatory arrest when PA back-bleeding from bronchial arteries obstructs surgical view
All anesthesia monitoring/access lines closed to the patient prior to circulatory arrest
Lung recruitment maneuver as pump turned off
Two episodes of circulatory arrest of maximum 20 min each
Rewarming
Start slow warming to 37°C, warming rate <1°C/q3min (CPB waterbath-rectal temp. grad. <8°C)
Unclamp LV and PA vent
Ventilation with PEEP 5 cm H_2O, pressure control ventilation, tidal volume 6 mL/kg, F_IO_2 21%, and respiratory rate of 15/min
Weaning
Once 37°C reached
Slowly wean CPB
Aim for cardiac index of 2.0–2.5 maximum
Aim for SVO_2 of greater than 60%
Aim for hematocrit of 30% by the end of the rewarming period
Aim for total urine output of 1.5–2 L at the end of the procedure

CPB, cardiopulmonary bypass; PA, pulmonary artery; PEEP, positive end-expiratory pressure; BP, blood pressure; LV, left ventricular; SVO_2, mixed venous oxygen saturation.

the RV myocardium. Direct pulmonary vasodilators such as nitric oxide and prostaglandins, which may be useful in the medical management of patients with other types of pulmonary hypertension, generally show limited benefit for pulmonary endarterectomy patients in the perioperative period.

End-tidal carbon dioxide ($ETCO_2$) is a poor measure of ventilation adequacy in these patients both pre- and post-CPB, since dead space ventilation is an integral part of the disease process. Transesophageal echocardiography (TEE) is valuable in monitoring and assessing cardiac function and filling during PTE. If a PFO is present, it is repaired, since, postoperatively, some patients may experience high right-sided pressures. Such pressures, in the presence of a PFO, could lead to right-to-left shunt and hypoxemia. During the periods of DHCA, all monitoring lines are turned off to the patient, decreasing the risk of entraining air into the vasculature during exsanguination.

The process of separation from CPB is similar to other surgeries involving CPB. Modest vasopressor/inotropic support (e.g., Nor-epinephrine 0.01 to 0.05 μg/kg/min) is often necessary initially because of the long hypothermic period and long aortic cross-clamp time. In patients with poor left ventricular function, epinephrine or dopamine is added. If the surgery has only been partially successful because of small-vessel disease, pulmonary vasodilators such as inhaled prostacyclin or nitric oxide are considered. If the surgery has been successful, the TEE reveals immediate improvements in the left- and right-sided geometry. The distention of the right ventricle and tricuspid regurgitation is decreased. Improvement in the cardiac index is usually seen with a dramatic decrease in PA pressures and a drop in the PVR.

D. **Post-CPB.** Frothy sputum, if present, likely indicates the onset of reperfusion pulmonary edema. In this case, the ETT is suctioned, FOB is used to evaluate the source of bleeding, and increasing amounts of PEEP are applied beginning with 5 cm H_2O. If frank blood is emanating from the ETT, surgical bleeding is possible. PEEP is increased and aggressive suctioning of the blood is undertaken. If severe bleeding persists and is predominantly unilateral, lung isolation (double-lumen EBT) and independent lung ventilation are considered. Topical vasopressors such as vasopressin and epinephrine, administered via the ETT, may also be useful.

After heparin reversal, a bleeding diathesis is rare, and transfusion requirements are usually minimal. Prophylactic antifibrinolytics are not given in some centers. PTE patients are usually awakened within 1 to 2 h after surgery, and a brief neurologic examination is performed. The patient is then sedated with a propofol infusion and analgesics. They remain intubated over night, since the onset of reperfusion pulmonary edema may be delayed with the use of vasopressors to limit the cardiac index. If pulmonary, cardiac, and neurologic functions are good, and there is no bleeding diathesis, extubation occurs the following morning. Discharge from the intensive care unit typically occurs on the second or third postoperative day.

V. Lung transplantation. End-stage pulmonary disease (ESPD) is one of the five leading causes of mortality and morbidity in adults in the United States. ESPD results from destruction of the pulmonary parenchyma and vasculature. Lung transplantation is the definitive treatment for these patients. Depending on the patient's pathophysiology, there are several surgical options: Single-lung transplantation (SLT), bilateral sequential lung transplantation (BSLT), *en bloc* double-lung transplantation (DbLT), heart–lung transplantation (HLT), and living-related lobar transplantation (LRT). Due to a severe shortage of suitable donor lungs, other therapeutic options were developed that may offer alternatives to those patients who otherwise might succumb to their disease while awaiting lung transplantation. Several improvements in the management of a highly selected group of patients with emphysema via LVRS, patients with cystic fibrosis (CF) via newer antibiotic agents, and patients with pulmonary hypertension via long-term prostacyclin therapy have been reported as viable options.

A. Epidemiology

1. **Total candidates.** There are in excess of one million potential lung transplant recipients among those suffering from ESPD.
2. **Survival of candidates.** Because the number of lung transplant recipients far exceeds the number of suitable lung donors, up to one-third of recipients die while awaiting transplantation. Recently, improvements to the method for allocation of lungs have served to decrease recipient waiting time for transplantation. In May 2005, the lung allocation score (LAS) was adopted in the United States [20]. This system is based on the severity of the recipient's disease and coupled with medical urgency for transplantation. The LAS attempts to balance the risk of death while awaiting transplantation with posttransplant survival. Since the LAS has been implemented, the total number of recipients on the waiting list has decreased by 50% and the total waiting time has also decreased from a median of 792 days in 2004 to 200 days or less during the time period of 2005 to 2008 [21]. Statistics from November 2011 indicate that there are 1,716 lung recipients and 69 heart–lung recipients awaiting transplantation (United Network Organ Sharing Critical Data, *http://www.unos.org*).
3. **Total procedures.** According to the most recent data supplied by the International Society of Heart and Lung Transplant (ISHLT) Registry, a total of 38,119 lung transplants and 4,248 HLT have been performed through June 30, 2010 [22].

B. Pathophysiology of end-stage pulmonary disease

1. **Parenchymal ESPD** is classified as obstructive, restrictive, or infectious.
   a. **Obstructive diseases** are characterized by elevation of airway resistance, diminished expiratory flow rates, severe V/Q mismatching, and pronounced air trapping. The most common cause is smoking-induced emphysema; however, other causes include asthma and several comparatively rare congenital disorders. Among these, α_1-antitrypsin deficiency is associated with severe bullous emphysema that manifests in the fourth or fifth decade of life.
   b. **Restrictive diseases** are characterized by interstitial fibrosis that results in a loss of lung elasticity and compliance. Most fibrotic processes are idiopathic in nature but they may also be caused by an immune mechanism or inhalation injury. Interstitial lung diseases may affect the pulmonary vasculature as well; therefore, pulmonary

hypertension is frequently present. Functionally, diseases in this category are associated with diminished lung volumes and diffusion capacities, albeit with preserved airflow rates. Respiratory muscle strength is usually adequate because of the increased work of breathing experienced by this patient population.

c. The common **infectious etiologic factors** are associated with CF and bronchiectasis.

(1) CF produces mucous plugging of peripheral airways leading to the development of pneumonia, chronic bronchitis, and bronchiectasis. The incidence of CF is 0.2% of live births in the United States.

(2) Smoking, α_1-antitrypsin deficiency, and environmental exposures may lead to the development of bronchiectasis.

2. **Etiologic factors of end-stage pulmonary vascular diseases** are (a) diffuse arteriovenous malformations, (b) congenital heart disease with Eisenmenger syndrome, or (c) pulmonary arterial hypertension (PAH). PAH is rare and most frequently idiopathic. It is characterized by marked elevation of PVR secondary to hyperplasia of the muscular pulmonary arteries combined with fibrosis and obliteration of the smallest arterioles.

C. **Recipient selection criteria: Indications and contraindications**

1. **Recipient selection criteria and indications** for lung transplantation are listed in Table 26.19 [23]. Referral and listing of potential candidates are based on the progression of the patient's disease along with their risk of death on the waiting list balanced with the likelihood

TABLE 26.19 Indications and contraindications for lung transplantation[a]

Indications
Untreatable end-stage pulmonary, parenchymal, and/or vascular disease
Absence of other major medical illnesses
Substantial limitation of daily activities
Projected life expectancy <50% 2–3 yrs predicted survival
NYHA Class III or IV functional level
Rehabilitation potential
Satisfactory psychosocial profile and emotional support system
Acceptable nutritional status
Disease-specific mortality exceeding transplant-specific mortality over 1–2 yrs
Relative contraindications
Age >65 yrs
Critical or unstable clinical conditions (e.g., shock, mechanical ventilation, or ECMO)
Severely limited functional status with poor rehabilitation potential
Colonization with highly resistant or virulent bacteria, fungi, or mycobacteria
Severe obesity defined as a BMI >30 kg/m^2
Severe or symptomatic osteoporosis
Other medical conditions not resulting in end-organ damage (e.g., diabetes mellitus, systemic hypertension, peripheral vascular disease, gastroesophageal reflux, patients with coronary artery disease s/p coronary artery stenting, or PTCA)
Absolute contraindications
Untreatable advanced dysfunction of another major organ system (e.g., heart, liver, or kidney)
Active malignancy within the previous 2 yrs
Noncurable chronic extrapulmonary infection
Chronic active viral hepatitis B, hepatitis C, and HIV
Significant chest wall/spinal deformity
Documented nonadherence or inability to follow through with medical therapy, office follow-up, or both
Untreatable psychiatric or psychologic condition associated with inability to cooperate or comply with medical therapy
Absence of a consistent or reliable social support system
Substance addiction (e.g., alcohol, tobacco, or narcotics) that is either active or within the previous 6 months

NYHA, New York Heart Association; ECMO, extra-corporeal membrane oxygenation; BMI, body mass index; PTCA, percutaneous transluminal coronary angioplasty; HIV, human immunodeficiency virus.

[a]Orens JB, Estenne M, Arcasoy P, et al. International Guidelines for the Selection of Lung Transplant Candidates: 2006 Update-A Consensus Report from the Pulmonary Scientific Council of the International Society for Heart and Lung Transplantation. *J Heart Lung.* 2006;25:145–155.

of survival after transplantation; however, each patient must be considered on an individual basis and subject to standardized selection criteria.

2. **Relative and absolute contraindications** to lung transplantation are listed in Table 26.19. Although candidates for organ transplantation frequently have abnormal physical or laboratory findings, such information must be distinguished from concurrent primary organ failure or a systemic disease that otherwise might disqualify candidacy. The relative contraindications to lung transplant have changed as improvements in the medical management of potential recipients have evolved. For example, coronary artery disease and corticosteroid usage, once absolute contraindications, are now not prohibitive, particularly if left ventricular function is preserved and corticosteroid doses are moderate [24]. Another highly controversial and debated issue is the transplantation of patients with multiple or pan-resistant bacteria, in particular, patients with CF who concurrently have been diagnosed with *Burkholderia cepacia* [25]. Although the international guidelines do not regard the presence of *B. cepacia* as an absolute contraindication to lung transplantation, there are multiple transplant centers that limit organ allocation and treatment to these patients. It has been reported in the literature that triple antimicrobial therapy can be bacteriocidal toward multiresistant *B. cepacia* [26]. The decision to ultimately transplant CF patients with this microbe rests with each transplant center because the previous data indicate a much higher incidence of preoperative and postoperative morbidity and mortality in this population.

D. **Medical evaluation of lung transplant candidates.** All candidates are systematically evaluated by history, physical examination, and the laboratory studies discussed previously in Section **I.B.** Additionally, evaluation includes chest radiographs, ABG values, spirometric and respiratory flow studies, ventilation and perfusion scanning, and right heart catheterization. On the basis of studies of the natural history of ESPD, specific laboratory criteria for referral to most lung transplantation programs have been developed and depend on the specific underlying disease (e.g., cardiac index less than 2 L/min/m^2 in patients with PAH and FEV_1 less than 30% predicted in patients with COPD or CF). Most centers provide documentation of the evaluation results on a summary sheet that is readily available to the anesthesiology team on short notice.

E. **Choice of lung transplant procedure** is based upon (a) the consequences of leaving a native lung in situ; (b) the procedure most likely to yield the best functional outcome for a given pathophysiologic process; and (c) the relative incidence of perioperative complications associated with a particular procedure.

1. **SLT**

   a. SLT is commonly selected for transplant recipients with nonseptic lung pathophysiology. SLT is a frequent option for older patients with end-stage pulmonary fibrosis or emphysema; however, in patients with severe bullous emphysema, SLT may exacerbate native lung hyperinflation and result in severe acute and/or chronic allograft compromise secondary to compression atelectasis. Preoperative measurement of the recipient static lung compliance has been suggested as a screening technique to determine whether SLT alone, SLT plus LVRS, or BSLT is most beneficial.

   b. SLT offers several advantages over the less frequently used *en bloc* DbLT: (a) allograft availability is optimized to the lung transplant recipient population; (b) SLT is feasible in many patients without the use of CPB, so complications arising from coagulopathic states are less frequent; and (c) bronchial anastomoses used in SLT show a decreased rate of dehiscence compared to tracheal anastomosis used for *en bloc* DbLT.

   c. SLT can be used to treat PPH and postoperative survival is similar when compared to DbLT and BSLT [22]. Because of the hemodynamic instability of these patients, CPB is often used during SLT, DbLT, or BSLT. In this setting, SLT frequently results in severe reperfusion injury to the allograft secondary to its increased pulmonary compliance. There are some data suggesting that early intervention with extracorporeal membrane oxygenation and NO administration intraoperatively and postoperatively may attenuate the effects of reperfusion injury.

   d. SLT involves pneumonectomy and implantation of the lung allograft. The choice of the native lung to be extracted is determined preoperatively. The lung with the poorest pulmonary function as delineated by V/Q scanning is generally chosen for replacement by the allograft. If the native lungs are equally impaired and pleural scarring is absent, the left lung is chosen for relative technical simplicity.

(1) The native left pulmonary veins are more accessible than those on the right.

(2) The left hemithorax can more easily accommodate an oversized donor lung.

(3) The recipient's left main stem bronchus is longer.

2. **DbLT**
   - **a.** Since 1996, there has been a proportional increase in adult BSLT for every major indication for lung transplantation except for CF (which remains essentially a 100% indication for BSLT) and in 2009 it accounted for 72% of lung transplant procedures.
   - **b.** While SLT is still performed frequently for end-stage IPF and emphysema in older recipients (>65 yrs of age), BSLT is also increasingly utilized for these conditions. Between 1996 and 2009, the share of BSLT for these conditions almost doubled [22].
   - **c.** BSLT is the procedure of choice for septic lung disease (e.g., generalized bronchiectasis), CF, young patients with COPD, and PAH. In contrast to *en* bloc DbLT, the BSLT procedure offers several advantages: (a) It permits two lungs to be implanted without CPB; (b) it decreases the incidence of bronchial anastomotic complications; and (c) it is less technically difficult.
   - **d.** In some instances, BSLT may lead to better functional outcomes in the treatment of end-stage pulmonary hypertension.
3. **HLT**
   - **a.** The indications for HLT are diminishing as experience with isolated lung transplantation evolves. The latter operation will suffice in most cases when it is performed before irreversible heart failure occurs or in concert with intracardiac repair of simple congenital defects. The total number of centers performing HLT has increased from 37 in 2003 to 114 in 2009 due to the addition of reporting centers to the Registry. Participating centers reported a total of 87 adult and pediatric HTL for calendar year 2009 [22].
   - **b.** HLT is **indicated** for patients with ESPD complicated by irreversible heart failure or end-stage congenital heart disease with secondary pulmonary vascular involvement (Eisenmenger syndrome). Specific pathologic diagnoses in recipients include idiopathic PAH, COPD/emphysema, acquired heart disease, CF, and fibrotic and granulomatous diseases of the lung. Congenital heart disease, PAH, and CF remain the main indications for adult HLT [22].
4. **Living-related donor lobar transplantation**
   - **a.** As of May 2006, 243 living-donor lobar transplants have been performed in the United States. Although outcomes in adult recipients are similar to cadaveric transplants, results in the pediatric recipient population are reported to be superior to those who receive cadaveric allografts [27,28]. Improved function and a decrease in the incidence of bronchiolitis obliterans have been noted. Despite these findings, LRT is rarely performed.
   - **b.** Although lobar donation is considered to be a relatively safe procedure, one group noted a 61% postoperative complication rate in the living donors. Complications included pleural effusions, bronchial stump fistulas, phrenic nerve injury, and bronchial strictures.

F. Selection criteria for donor lungs

1. Suitable lung allografts are characterized by **P_aO_2 greater than 300 mm Hg during mechanical ventilation with FIO_2 of 1.0 and PEEP of 5 cm H_2O.**
2. Unilateral pneumonia or trauma does not preclude use of the contralateral lung. In general, the donor **ideally should be younger than 60 yrs with a smoking history of no more than 20 to 30 pack-years.** Smoking criteria for donor lungs have been liberalized in some incidences, particularly if there is strong evidence indicating that a recipient's death is imminent should there be a prolonged waiting period. Outcomes have been similar when the more liberal smoking criteria have been used for donor lung selection [29,30].
3. In an attempt to provide a larger pool of suitable lung donors, the lungs from **non–heart-beating donors** have been transplanted and reported to produce a successful recipient outcome [31].

4. As experience in the field of genetic therapy continues to grow, **cytokine profiling** has come to represent a significant method to identify organs suitable for donation and transplantation. Fisher et al. [32] reported that elevated levels of interleukin-8 in donor lungs were associated with early graft failure and decreased recipient survival. These data suggest that cytokine profiles could be an early indicator of recipient outcome.
5. **Harvesting procedure.** Because both the heart and lungs are often harvested from the same donor for different recipients, a method has been developed to perform cardiectomy and reduce the risk of lung injury. During cardiectomy, a residual atrial cuff is left attached to the donor lungs. The trachea is stapled and divided at its midpoint, and the lungs are removed *en bloc.* Subsequently, the pulmonary vasculature is flushed and immersed in a hypothermic preservative (most commonly Euro-Collins or University of Wisconsin solution ± Prostaglandin $E_{1[PGE1]}$).
6. **Lung allograft preservation**
   a. There are several relevant issues surrounding donor lung preservation; however, all focus on methods to provide ready sources of energy and cryoprotection and to prevent vasospasm, cellular swelling, and accumulation of toxic metabolites. For example, free radical scavengers such as superoxide dismutase and catalase can be added to prevent oxygen-derived free radicals from damaging key intracellular constituents after reperfusion, and PGE_1 can be added to promote even cooling and distribution of preservative solutions.
   b. **Standard preservation techniques allow a reported maximum allograft ischemic time of 6 to 8 h.**
   c. Normothermic ex vivo lung perfusion (EVLP) is a newer preservation technique aimed at reconditioning and improving the function of marginal donor lungs. The harvested donor lung is perfused in an ex vivo circuit using an acellular normothermic perfusate while they are ventilated at body temperature to mimic physiologic conditions. Cypel et al. demonstrated that transplantation of high-risk donor lungs that were physiologically stable during 4 h of EVLP had a lower incidence of primary graft dysfunction 72 h posttransplant compared with controls [33].
7. **Clinical immunology of organ matching.** ABO matching is essential before transplantation because the donor-specific major blood group iso-agglutinins have been implicated as a cause of allograft hyperacute rejection. Once procured, the practical matter of a 6- to 8-h donor lung ischemic time limit severely restricts prospective matching of histocompatibility antigens, percentage of reactive antibody screens, and the geography of organ donation. One study suggests that the total ischemic time alone is not predictive of a poor outcome after transplantation. Rather, the additive effects of increased donor age (older than 55 yrs) plus increased ischemic allograft time (more than 6 to 7 h) are a more reliable indicator of poor posttransplantation survival [34].

G. **Preanesthetic considerations**

1. Because of a chronic shortage of suitable lungs available for transplantation, many patients experience long waiting periods ranging from several months to several years. **Interval changes** may occur since completion of the initial medical evaluation (see Section **IV.D**). Specifically, reduction in exercise tolerance; new drug regimens or requirements for oxygen and steroids; appearance of purulent sputum; signs or symptoms indicative of right heart failure (e.g., hepatomegaly, peripheral edema); or presence of fever are among the most common occurrences that should be explored in the immediate preoperative period.
2. Lung transplants are always performed as emergency procedures because of the relatively short, safe ischemic time for allografts. As is customary for any emergent surgical procedure, the time of **last oral intake** should be ascertained before induction of general anesthesia.
3. Patients undergoing lung transplantation may exhibit signs and symptoms of anxiety. They usually have not received the benefit of anxiolytic **premedication** before their arrival in the operating room. One should be vigilant when administering anxiolytic agents to these patients so that their impaired respiratory drive is not further compromised.

4. Insertion of a **thoracic epidural catheter** for both intraoperative and postoperative analgesia may be performed before induction of general anesthesia. The catheter should be inserted at a spinal level that provides appropriate anesthesia and analgesia in concordance with the surgical incision site (e.g., T-4 to T-5 or T-5 to T-6) [35]. Alternatively, bilateral paravertebral catheters may be inserted. Placement of a thoracic epidural catheter or bilateral paravertebral catheters when anticoagulation is anticipated for CPB remains controversial.
5. Chronically cyanotic patients are frequently severely polycythemic (hematocrit greater than 60%) and may manifest clotting abnormalities. In these instances, phlebotomy and hemodilution may be beneficial in minimizing the occurrence of end-organ infarction.
6. **Size matching** between donor and recipient is facilitated by comparing the vertical and transverse radiologic chest dimensions of the donor and recipient. Organs are also matched on the basis of ABO compatibility, because the value of histocompatibility matching is still unknown and requires time in excess of the tolerable ischemic time for the lung allograft.
7. Some **transfusion practices** are specific for transplantation. For example, cytomegalovirus (CMV) seronegative blood products must be available for seronegative recipients if CMV sepsis is to be avoided. When transplantation of CMV-negative donors and recipients occurs, leukocyte-poor filters are used to reduce exposure to CMV during transfusion of blood and blood products. Likewise, if human leukocyte antigen alloimmunization is to be avoided, leukocyte-poor blood is necessary for transplant candidates, particularly if they require transfusion before organ transplantation.
8. Close **coordination and effective communication** between the transplant team and the organ harvesting team is vital so that excess allograft ischemic time is avoided.
9. Arrangements should be made for intraoperative availability of a multimodality ventilator for patients with the most severe forms of lung disease. Useful **ventilator settings** include the ability to deliver minute volumes greater than 15 L/min (especially helpful if airway leaks are present); adjustable inflation pressure "pop-offs" (to allow high inflation pressures to be delivered to noncompliant lungs); adjustable respiratory cycle waveforms; and availability of high levels of PEEP (e.g., 15 to 20 cm H_2O during reperfusion pulmonary edema).
10. NO and inhaled nebulized prostacyclin have been shown to be effective therapies for treatment of pulmonary hypertension and early reperfusion injury in some patients.

13

H. Induction and maintenance of anesthesia

1. **Preoperative laboratory studies.** These studies are useful to predict difficulties during the induction of general anesthesia. For example, air trapping and diminished expiratory flow rates may exacerbate hypercapnia and lead to hemodynamic instability during mask ventilation and after endotracheal intubation. Elevated PA pressures may indicate the likelihood that CPB may be necessary.
2. **Intraoperative monitoring**
   a. Both **systemic and PA pressure monitoring** are essential during lung transplant procedures. Dyspnea, arrhythmias, RV dilation, and pulmonary hypertension may complicate PA catheter insertion before induction of general anesthesia. Oximetric PA catheters are useful in this setting to evaluate tissue oxygen delivery in patients who are subject to sudden cardiac instability. Some suggest that RV ejection fraction catheters may be useful for the diagnosis of right heart failure. Radial arterial cannulation with or without femoral artery cannulation is appropriate for monitoring of systemic arterial blood pressure. Femoral arterial catheters may interfere with groin cannulation for CPB.
   b. **Pulse oximetry** is useful for continuous monitoring of S_pO_2 during stressful intervals, such as the onset of OLV or cross-clamping of the PA.
   c. TEE is perhaps the most useful monitor available. TEE allows for (a) direct visualization of RV and left ventricular wall motion and function as well as assessment of intracardiac valvular function; (b) assessment of PA and pulmonary vein anastomoses and blood flow; (c) assessment of the elimination of intracardiac air that occurs during pulmonary venous anastomosis; and (d) calculation of PA pressure as measured by color Doppler flow velocity.

3. **IV access.** Large-caliber IV catheters inserted peripherally and centrally (e.g., 14-gauge peripheral IV; 8.5 to 9.0 Fr central venous introducer), supplemented by a rapid infusion device, are essential for lung transplant operations where massive transfusion requirements are anticipated (e.g., HLT for congenital heart disease with Eisenmenger syndrome; BSLT for CF with pleural scarring). When the clamshell incision is used for BSLT, placement of IV catheters in the antecubital fossae should be avoided.
4. **Positioning.** Full lateral decubitus position is typically used during SLT, even when CPB is anticipated (e.g., SLT for PPH). One groin is usually prepped into the field to allow for the option of femoral cannula insertion for CPB. General considerations for the thoracotomy position are reviewed in Section **II.B.** The supine position is used for BSLT, facilitating either median sternotomy, the clamshell incision, or bilateral anterior thoracotomy incision.
5. **"Pump standby."** This safeguard is prudent for patients with pulmonary hypertension or borderline ABG values, even when SLT is planned.
6. **Selection of anesthetic agents**
   a. Agents that promote hemodynamic homeostasis are preferred for induction of general anesthesia. One example is etomidate and a nondepolarizing neuromuscular blocking agent such as rocuronium, which may be used during a modified rapid sequence induction technique. Modest amounts of fentanyl (5 to 10 μg/kg) administered IV may be used if indicated to control cardiovascular responses to endotracheal intubation.
   b. For **maintenance** using conventional anesthetic agents, moderate-to-high doses of opioids (e.g., fentanyl 20 to 75 μg/kg) supplemented with low doses of a potent inhaled agent (e.g., isoflurane, 0.2% to 0.6%) and a long-acting neuromuscular blocking agent are recommended. **TEA**, in addition to providing excellent postoperative analgesia, may be used to enhance general anesthesia intraoperatively. Continuous infusion of a local anesthetic, such as 0.2% to 0.5% ropivacaine, provides ideal surgical anesthesia and analgesia and allow for reduced doses of both IV opioids and inhaled agents.
   c. **Nitrous oxide** is generally avoided for the following reasons: (a) 100% oxygen is almost always required to maintain an acceptable arterial saturation during OLV; (b) bullae may expand and compress the residual normal lung parenchyma, thus exacerbating V/Q mismatching; and (c) occult pneumothoraces may occur.
7. **Securing the airway.** Lung isolation is required for optimal surgical exposure. Both double-lumen EBTs and BBs are useful for this purpose. A general discussion of these choices is given in Section **II.A**.
   a. Advantages of double-lumen EBTs in the setting of lung transplantation include the following:
      (1) Facilitation of lung isolation
      (2) Ability to suction the nonventilated lung
      (3) Ability to apply CPAP to the nonventilated lung
      (4) Provision for postoperative independent lung ventilation
   b. Left-sided EBTs (Robertshaw) are recommended for both right and left SLTs as well as for BSLT (right-sided DLTs are used for left SLT in some centers). There is a higher incidence of right upper lobe obstruction when right-sided double-lumen EBTs are used because the right upper lobe orifice is relatively close to the right main stem bronchus.
   c. **Selecting the correct size of EBT** was discussed in Section **II.A.5.B**. In general, the largest sized EBT that can be placed without causing airway trauma is preferred to facilitate therapeutic flexible bronchoscopy both intraoperatively and postoperatively.
   d. Many lung transplant recipients have limited pulmonary reserve, and desaturation during intubation may occur rapidly. Therefore, **initial EBT positioning** can be accomplished quickly and accurately with the aid of a flexible FOB. A complete discussion of bronchoscopic placement is given in Section **II.A**.
8. **Management of ventilation**
   a. **Lateral decubitus positioning** may be associated with significant alterations in oxygenation and ventilation, depending on the underlying pulmonary pathophysiology.

Positional improvement or deterioration in blood gas values is sometimes predictable on the basis of the patient's preoperative V/Q scan.

b. General strategies for supporting oxygenation during OLV (i.e., during SLT and BSLT) are discussed in Section **II.E.5**.

c. Alteration of the inspired to expired ratios during mechanical ventilation may be useful during SLT of patients with emphysema. Increasing the expiratory time during each respiratory cycle allows for adequate exhalation, thus reducing the possibility of overinflation of the native lung and subsequent compromise of the allograft.

d. Similarly, **independent or differential ventilation** is often used during SLT for emphysema recipients, particularly those with gross V/Q mismatching.

e. After allograft implantation, **the lowest possible** $\mathbf{F_{IO_2}}$ to maintain adequate oxygenation is used in concert with **5 to 10 cm** $\mathbf{H_2O}$ **PEEP**. In patients with emphysema, independent lung ventilation allows PEEP to be selectively delivered to the allograft and avoid air trapping and overinflation of the native lung.

f. Frequent **suctioning and lavage** via **flexible FOB** is helpful to maintain airway patency during BSLT for CF or whenever airway bleeding and secretions are sufficient to cause obstruction and impair gas exchange.

I. **Surgical procedures and anesthesia-related interventions**

1. **Surgical dissection** is complicated by extensive pleural adhesions, vascular anomalies, vascular collaterals, or previous cardiac or thoracic surgery.
2. **OLV** is almost always used during lung transplantation to facilitate dissection. The relevant physiology was reviewed in Sections **II.A** and **II.E**. With the onset of OLV, acute deterioration in gas exchange and hemodynamics must be anticipated. Strategies for improving oxygenation under these circumstances include the following:
   a. PEEP applied to the dependent (ventilated) lung provided that bullous disease or emphysema is absent
   b. CPAP or high-frequency jet ventilation in the nondependent (nonventilated) lung
   c. Ligation of the branch PA of the operative lung
3. **Clamping the branch PA** when PA pressures are low is usually well tolerated and improves V/Q matching and ABG values. If elevated PA pressures exacerbate right heart failure, vasodilators and inotropes may improve systemic hemodynamics; however, gas exchange may be further impaired, depending on the agents that are selected (e.g., nitroprusside may worsen V/Q mismatching). Should the patient's condition deteriorate despite pharmacologic intervention, implementation of CPB should be considered.
4. Immediately before implantation of the donor lung, the donor hilar structures are trimmed to match the size of the recipient bronchus, branch PA, and atrial cuff containing the pulmonary venous orifices. While the allograft is kept scrupulously cold, the atrial PA and bronchial anastomoses are completed in sequence.
5. The **ischemic interval** ends with the removal of vascular clamps, but until ventilation is restored, systemic arterial saturation remains unchanged. Immediately before vascular unclamping, **methylprednisolone** (500 to 1,000 mg) is administered IV to minimize the potential for hyperacute allograft rejection.
6. **Reinflation of the allograft** follows, sometimes with the aid of a flexible FOB to clear airway secretions. This procedure allows for direct viewing of the airway anastomosis to ensure patency.
7. After SLT for emphysema, independent lung ventilation can be instituted if indicated using the anesthesia ventilator for the native lung (increased expiratory time, low tidal volume, no PEEP) and an intensive-care-unit–quality ventilator for the allograft (increased respiratory rates, low tidal volumes, 5 to 10 cm H_2O PEEP).
8. **Reperfusion injury**, characterized by increasing alveolar–arterial gradients, deteriorating compliance, and gross pulmonary edema, may follow allograft reperfusion within minutes to hours. The most effective treatments are PEEP and strict limitation of volume infusion, both crystalloid and colloid. Rarely, reperfusion injury may be accompanied by pulmonary hypertension. Inhaled NO (40 to 80 ppm) has been the agent of choice in this instance;

however, inhaled prostacyclin has also been effective in decreasing PA pressure [36]. If evidence of right heart failure occurs, continuous IV infusion of norepinephrine (0.05 to 0.2 μg/kg/min), milrinone (0.375 to 0.5 μg/kg/min), or a combination of the two may prove efficacious.

9. At the conclusion of surgery, the EBT can be exchanged for a standard single-lumen ETT or retained for independent lung ventilation in the intensive care unit.
10. **BSLT** is used to treat the same spectrum of patients as those treated by the *en bloc* DbLT procedure. BSLT is the preferred technique in many centers. BSLT can often be accomplished without the use of CPB. Its major disadvantage is that serial implantation prolongs the ischemic time for the second allograft lung.

J. **Postoperative management and complications**

1. The immediate priorities are acute, intensive **respiratory and cardiovascular support**.
   a. Early **respiratory insufficiency** is usually due to reperfusion injury, which is characterized by large alveolar–arterial O_2 gradients, poor pulmonary compliance, and parenchymal infiltrates despite low cardiac filling pressures. Mechanical ventilation with PEEP is essential, but inflation pressures are kept to a minimum in consideration of the new airway anastomoses.
   b. FIO_2 is maintained at the lowest levels compatible with an acceptable arterial oxygen saturation.
   c. Fifteen percent of lung transplant recipients may develop severe lung injury secondary to reperfusion injury and lymphatic disruption during the surgical procedure. This pattern of lung injury can be treated with extracorporeal membrane oxygenation, NO, or selective lung ventilation if indicated.
   d. Acute allograft dysfunction can occur and is associated with a mortality rate of up to 60%.
   e. **Cardiovascular deterioration** may be secondary to hemorrhage, PA or pulmonary venous anastomotic obstruction, tension pneumothorax, or pneumopericardium. TEE may be a useful diagnostic tool in the setting of vascular obstructive lesions. Hemorrhage most frequently occurs after HLT or *en bloc* DbLT, particularly in patients with pleural disease and Eisenmenger syndrome. Tension pneumothorax occurs more frequently in patients with concomitant end-stage emphysema.
2. **Immunosuppression drug regimens** have been developed to control the recipient's immune response and prevent allograft rejection [37]. Clinical immunosuppression for lung transplant can be considered in several different contexts: (1) Induction therapy, (2) maintenance therapy, and (3) anti-rejection therapy. Most centers use a triple-drug regimen that includes steroids, cyclosporine, and azathioprine. Although these regimens may adequately control acute rejection, chronic rejection still accounts for a majority of long-term morbidity and mortality.
   a. **Cyclosporine** is a cyclic polypeptide derived from a soil fungus. Its major actions are to inhibit macrophage and T-cell production of interleukins and to block activation of helper T cells.
   b. **Azathioprine blocks** de novo purine biosynthesis, which is important to both DNA and RNA production, thus inhibiting both T- and B-cell proliferation.
   c. **Prednisone** is an anti-inflammatory drug that suppresses helper T-cell proliferation and interleukin production by T cells.
   d. **FK506 (tacrolimus)** is a macrolide antibiotic with immunosuppressant properties that blocks interleukin production and proliferation of T lymphocytes. It is used as a substitute for cyclosporine in the setting of acute allograft rejection. FK506, in comparison to cyclosporine, has been associated with a lower rate of rejection, similar infection rates, and increased incidence of new-onset diabetes mellitus. It is effective in slowing progression of bronchiolitis obliterans. Some suggest using FK506 as a primary immunosuppressive agent for these reasons.
   e. **Antibodies** include antithymocyte globulin, a polyclonal immunoglobulin G antibody that rapidly reduces circulating T lymphocytes and promotes formation of suppressor T cells. OKT3 is a murine monoclonal antibody directed against the CD3 surface antigen

on mature T lymphocytes that blocks the recognition of MHC antigens on foreign cells and the subsequent immune response.

3. The rate of **postoperative infectious complications** is higher in lung transplant patients compared with other solid organ transplant recipients. Therefore, one must be able to differentiate **infection versus allograft rejection**.
   a. Several factors increase the susceptibility of transplanted lungs to infection: (a) Exposure to the external environment; (b) pulmonary lymphatic disruption; (c) impairment of mucociliary function; (d) prolonged mechanical ventilation predisposing the patient to nosocomial infection and airway colonization; and (e) presence of airway foreign bodies (e.g., sutures).
   b. Proper diagnosis is crucial to successful outcome and is usually performed via a transbronchial biopsy using flexible FOB. Occasionally, open lung biopsy is necessary.
   c. During the initial 2 postoperative months, nosocomial gram-negative bacteria are the most frequent **causes of pneumonia**. Thereafter, CMV pneumonitis becomes more common and is associated with progression to a state of chronic allograft rejection.
4. The **vagus, phrenic, and recurrent laryngeal nerves** are jeopardized during lung transplantation. Their injury complicates weaning from mechanical ventilation.
5. **Tracheal anastomotic leaks** often lead to fatal mediastinitis. In contrast, **bronchial fistulas** lead to the development of strictures that are treated by placing silicone stents and repeated airway dilation procedures. Airway complications have decreased as experience with successful lung transplants has increased. Although telescoping of the donor bronchus into the recipient has decreased the incidence of anastomotic dehiscence, the occurrence of anastomotic stenosis remains and varies with the surgical technique used at each center.

K. **Outcome**

1. **Survival.** Recent reports from the ISHLT Registry indicate that the unadjusted benchmark survival rate was 88% at 3 months, 79% at 1 yr, 64% at 3 yrs, 53% at 5 yrs, and 30% at 10 yrs for the time period of January 1994 through 2010 [22]. These rates are the same or slightly higher than previously reported.
   a. Independent predictors of an adverse outcome at 1 yr after transplantation are (a) pre-transplant ventilator requirement, (b) retransplant, (c) pre-transplant diagnosis other than emphysema, and (d) recipient age.
   b. Post–lung-transplant morbidity factors include (a) hypertension, (b) renal dysfunction, (c) hyperlipidemia, (d) diabetes mellitus, (e) bronchiolitis obliterans, and (f) development of malignancy (predominantly skin and lymphatics).
   c. Donor age and total allograft ischemic time appear to be significant risk factors for development of bronchiolitis obliterans.
2. **Exercise tolerance has** been shown to improve after lung transplantation, as has the quality-of-life factors for survivors.

L. **Special considerations for pediatric lung transplantation**

1. **Epidemiology**
   a. Since 1986, there have been 1,664 lung transplant procedures reported in children 17 yrs old and younger [38]. During the interval from January 1994 to June 2010, 105 retransplant procedures were performed.
   b. CF, idiopathic PAH, IPF, congenital heart disease, and surfactant protein B deficiency account for almost all diagnoses in pediatric lung recipients. DbLT/BSLT is the most frequent procedure.
2. **Outcome.** One-year survival is currently comparable with that reported for adults [38].
3. **Pathophysiology.** In children with severe developmental anomalies of the lung (e.g., congenital diaphragmatic hernia with pulmonary hypoplasia, and cystadenomatous malformations), isolated lung transplantation may offer the only chance for survival. Rarely, HLT may be indicated during childhood for PPH, CF, or Eisenmenger syndrome.
4. **Donor lungs.** Size considerations place additional limitations on organ matching for pediatric recipients and thereby exacerbate shortages. The scarcity of suitable donor organs

has propagated living-related lung lobe donation; however, the success of this approach is somewhat uncertain. In addition, donor and recipient morbidity and mortality inherent for this operation have sparked considerable controversy.

5. **Intubation.** In smaller children, using DLTs is not feasible; instead, **selective endobronchial intubation** with a conventional cuffed single-lumen tube is the most frequent choice.

M. **Anesthesia for the post–lung-transplant patient.** In addition to certain specific considerations, several general principles apply to all patients who have undergone successful lung transplantation, including the toxicity of immunosuppressants, potential for infectious and malignant complications, and interactions between immunosuppressants and other pharmacologic agents (including anesthetics).

1. **Cardiac denervation** may result after *en bloc* DbLT because extensive retrocardiac dissection is often necessary.
2. Airway anastomoses may be associated with chronic strictures and **inadequate clearance of secretions.**
3. **Toxic systemic effects of immunosuppressants**
   a. **Cyclosporine** is a potent nephrotoxin. Blood urea nitrogen and creatinine levels increase and most patients develop systemic hypertension. Cyclosporine can produce hepatocellular injury, hyperuricemia, gingival hypertrophy, hirsutism, and tremors or seizures (at high serum levels).
   b. **Azathioprine** suppresses all formed elements in the bone marrow. Anemia, thrombocytopenia, and occasionally aplastic anemia may result. Azathioprine is associated with hepatocellular and pancreatic impairment, alopecia, and gastrointestinal distress.
14 There may be an increased requirement in the dosage of nondepolarizing neuromuscular blocking agents in this patient population.
   c. **Prednisone** produces adrenal suppression, glucose intolerance, peptic ulceration, aseptic osteonecrosis, and integument fragility. Controversy surrounds the need to administer intraoperative "stress doses" of glucocorticoids to patients with chronic adrenal suppression.
   d. **FK506 (tacrolimus)** exhibits a spectrum of toxicities including nephrotoxicity similar to cyclosporine.
   e. **Antithymocyte globulin and OKT3** use may be accompanied by fever and other mild systemic symptoms, and rarely by pulmonary edema or aseptic meningitis.
4. **Infections**
   a. Early posttransplantation bacterial infections are typically related to **pneumonia** (*Streptococcus pneumoniae;* gram-negative bacilli), **wound infection** (*Staphylococcus aureus*), and use of **urinary catheters** (*Escherichia coli*). Because of the particular susceptibility of pneumonia, early extubation of the trachea after general anesthesia is highly recommended.
   b. CMV is the most frequent viral pathogen in lung transplant recipients and results either from primary infection (after contaminated allograft implantation or blood transfusion in seronegative recipients) or secondary to reactivated infection in a seropositive patient.
   c. After the first few months of immunosuppression, vulnerability to **opportunistic pathogens** increases (CMV, *Pneumocystis carinii,* herpes zoster). If diagnosis is rapid and treatment decisive, survival prevails. Prophylactic antibiotic regimens are available and have been successful in reducing the prevalence of some of these infections (e.g., trimethoprim-sulfamethoxazole for *P. carinii*).
5. **Posttransplant lymphoproliferative disorders** are more likely to develop in immunosuppressed patients. Posttransplant lymphoproliferative disorder is the third leading cause of death outside the perioperative period, with an incidence ranging from 1.8% to 20%. Other neoplasms have been associated with immunosuppression, including (a) non-Hodgkin lymphoma; (b) squamous cell carcinoma of the skin and lip; (c) Kaposi sarcoma; and (d) carcinoma of the vulva, perineum, kidney, and hepatobiliary tree.

6. **Drug interactions**
   a. Both cyclosporine and prednisone are metabolized by the cytochrome P450 enzyme system in hepatocytes. Drugs that inhibit those enzymes (e.g., calcium channel blockers) may increase their serum concentrations and promote toxic side effects.
   b. Other drugs (e.g., barbiturates and phenytoin) may induce the P450 enzymes and decrease cyclosporine levels below therapeutic range.

N. **The future of lung transplantation.** Lung transplantation has been a viable therapeutic option for many patients with ESPD. Obstacles with regard to graft availability, allograft function, and prolongation of patient survival remain to be overcome. New therapies, such as LVRS and nebulized prostacyclin for patients with end-stage pulmonary hypertension, may eliminate the need for transplantation altogether in a small select group of patients [39]. Gene therapy for transplant-related injuries shows much promise. Refinements of current methods for organ harvest and preservation, along with the development of improved techniques to evaluate donor organs, are important obstacles that are currently being addressed. Ultimately, further technologic advances may lead to the success of xenotransplantation and the development of pulmonary organogenesis, providing a solution to the ongoing shortage of suitable organs available for transplantation. In the longer term, fully implantable artificial lung technology will require evolution of ECMO to a self-renewing biologic interface propagated on new bronchocompatible materials.

VI. Lung volume reduction surgery.

Approximately 13.5 million persons in the United States are afflicted with COPD, and 3.1 million of these patients have emphysema (Cure Research™.com, http://www.cureresearch.com). Airflow obstruction associated with chronic bronchitis or emphysema occurs due to a loss of the elastic recoil properties of the lung and chest wall. As the disease progresses, patients become increasingly debilitated. Patients exhibit symptoms of severe dyspnea, require supplemental oxygen, and display poor exercise tolerance. LVRS offers a select group of patients the possibility of improved exercise tolerance, reduction in dyspnea, improved quality of life, and extended life span. It has been suggested that LVRS may provide these patients with a benefit that otherwise cannot be achieved by any means other than lung transplantation.

A. **History of lung volume reduction surgery**
   1. In 1957, Otto Brantigan, M.D., described a surgical technique for patients with end-stage emphysema that was designed to alleviate symptoms of severe dyspnea and exercise intolerance. It was Brantigan's intent to remove functionally useless areas of the lung in order to restore pulmonary elastic recoil, thus increasing the outward traction on small airways and subsequently improve airflow. Brantigan believed that this technique could restore diaphragmatic and thoracic contours that would improve respiratory excursion. Additionally, he reasoned that by excising the nonfunctional lung tissue, the compressive effects exerted on normal lung tissue could be relieved and result in improved V/Q matching. Unfortunately, the operative mortality was significant and no objective measures of benefit could be documented. Thus, early LVRS was abandoned as a viable therapy for patients with end-stage emphysema until 1993.
   2. In 1996, Joel Cooper, M.D., authored an editorial advocating the technique of LVRS as a "logical, physiologically sound procedure of demonstrable benefit for a selected group of patients with no alternative therapy [40]." He further stated that the successful application of LVRS was "made possible through an improved understanding of pulmonary physiology, improved anesthetic and surgical techniques, and lessons learned from experience with lung transplantation." Although Dr. Cooper touted the benefits of LVRS for certain patients, he did not minimize the surgical risk and suggested that this was not a procedure to be performed in all healthcare centers across the country. He made the following proposal: (1) Healthcare providers should restrict the application of this (LVRS) procedure to a limited number of centers of excellence; (2) such centers should be required to document and report specified information regarding morbidity, mortality, and objective measures of outcome; and (3) these data should be periodically reviewed and evaluated by a scientific panel before approval to continue performing the procedure is obtained.

      Additionally, he advocated that the patients who would otherwise qualify for lung transplantation should be simultaneously evaluated for LVRS so that they would receive the procedure proving to be most appropriate. Although Dr. Cooper did not necessarily advocate a long-term prospective randomized trial to validate the benefit of LVRS, his proposals led to the design and implementation of the National Emphysema Treatment Trial (NETT).

B. **The NETT** was conducted from January 1998 and July 2002. It was a prospective, randomized, multicenter trial sponsored by the National Heart, Lung, and Blood Institute in conjunction with Health Care Financing Administration (now known as Center for Medicare and Medicaid Services [CMS]). 3,777 patients were evaluated and 1,218 patients were ultimately randomized to receive either LVRS or medical therapy.
   1. The **primary objective** of the NETT was to determine if the addition of LVRS to medical therapy improves patient survival and increases exercise capacity.
   2. **Secondary objectives** included defining the profile of patients likely to benefit from LVRS and determining if LVRS improves quality of life, reduces debilitating symptoms, and improves overall pulmonary function.
   3. Patients were randomized to either medical therapy alone ($N = 610$) or medical therapy plus surgery ($N = 608$). Surgical patients were further randomized to intervention via either **median sternotomy** or **bilateral thoracoscopy**.
   4. A successful procedure was defined as a **60% to 70% increase in FEV_1 by 3 months postoperatively that is sustained for at least 1 yr; decreased total lung capacity and residual volume; improved exercise tolerance; and significant reduction in supplemental oxygen requirement.**

C. **Results.** The final results of the NETT were published in the May 22, 2003 issue of the New England Journal of Medicine [41]. Of the 608 patients assigned to LVRS, 580 underwent surgery (406 via median sternotomy; 174 VATS). Among the 610 patients assigned to medical therapy alone, 33 underwent LVRS outside the study and 15 received lung transplantation. Overall mortality was 0.11 deaths per person-year in both treatment groups. After 24 months, exercise capacity improved more than 10 W in 15% of patients in the surgery group compared with 3% in the medical-therapy-alone group. After exclusion of 140 patients at high risk for death from surgery [38] according to an interim analysis, overall mortality in the surgery group was 0.09 deaths per person-year versus 0.10 in the medical group. Among patients with predominantly upper-lobe emphysema and low baseline exercise capacity, mortality was lower in the surgery group than in the medical-therapy-alone group.

D. **Conclusions.** The data from the trial suggested that, overall, LVRS increased the chance of improved exercise capacity but did not demonstrate a survival advantage as compared with medical therapy alone. There was a survival advantage demonstrated for those patients with both predominantly upper-lobe emphysema and low baseline exercise capacity. Patients reported in the interim analysis [42] and those with non–upper-lobe emphysema and high baseline exercise capacity were found to be poor candidates for LVRS because of the increase in mortality and negligible functional gain.

E. **Anesthetic management for lung volume reduction surgery.** Anesthesiologists and their expertise are essential to the continued successful outcomes for patients undergoing LVRS. Our expertise in cardiopulmonary physiology, pharmacology, and pain management allows us to minimize complications in the postoperative period.
   1. **Preoperative assessment.** All patients scheduled for LVRS receive the following preoperative physiologic studies: (a) Standard pulmonary function studies; (b) plethysmographic measurement of lung volumes; (c) standardized 6-min walk test; (d) ABG values; (e) quantitative nuclear lung perfusion scans; and (f) radionuclide cardiac ventriculogram and/or dobutamine stress echocardiogram.
   2. **Preoperative pulmonary rehabilitation program.** After the initial preoperative evaluation, all patients are enrolled into a pulmonary rehabilitation program for a minimum of 6 wks before surgical intervention.
   3. **Monitors.** In addition to the standard monitors, large-bore IV access and an arterial line are recommended. The use of central venous catheters and PA catheters should be considered on an individual patient basis.

4. The judicious use of **TEA**, both intraoperatively and postoperatively, affords advantages as follows: (a) Preserved ability to cough and clear secretions, thus decreasing atelectasis and possibly reducing pulmonary infection; (b) decreased airway resistance; (c) improved phrenic nerve function; (d) stabilization of coronary endothelial function; (e) improved myocardial perfusion; (f) earlier return of bowel function; (g) preservation of immunocompetence; and (h) decreased cost of perioperative care through reduction of perioperative complications. Best results are obtained with catheters placed at the T-4 to T-5 or T-5 to T-6 spinal level.
   a. **Intraoperative TEA.** TEA can be used as an adjunct to general anesthesia. Local anesthetics, such as 2% lidocaine or 0.5% ropivacaine, provide optimal surgical conditions. The local anesthetics can be delivered via intermittent bolus or as continuous infusion.
      (1) Because persistent air leaks may be a problem in the postoperative period and may be exacerbated by positive-pressure ventilation, it is optimal to extubate the patients either at the conclusion of surgery or as soon as possible thereafter.
      (2) Caution must be exercised if opioids are added to the infusate because they have the potential to severely depress the patient's respiratory efforts.
   b. **Postoperative TEA.** TEA provides superior postoperative analgesia for both median sternotomy and bilateral thoracoscopic surgical procedures. A reduced concentration of local anesthetic plus a small dose of opioids delivered by continuous infusion is suggested (e.g., 0.2% ropivacaine plus 0.01 mg/mL hydromorphone).
   c. **Paravertebral nerve blocks** (PVN) may be used as an alternative to TEA. They may be performed either by multiple injections or by inserting a catheter into the paravertebral space for use with a continuous infusion of local anesthetic. This technique requires the use of a multimodal analgesic regimen including IV opioids and nonsteroidal anti-inflammatory agents. The effect of PVN on morbidity and mortality following thoracic surgery, in particular LVRS, has yet to be determined.
5. A **left-sided double-lumen EBT** should be used to secure the patient's airway.
6. **General anesthesia.** Induction of general anesthesia can be conducted with agents that promote hemodynamic homeostasis. An example is etomidate 0.2 mg/kg plus an easily reversible nondepolarizing neuromuscular blocking agent such as rocuronium. Maintenance anesthesia may consist of low doses of a volatile agent (e.g., 0.2% to 0.4% isoflurane) and oxygen in addition to TEA. The anesthetic plan for each patient should be individualized appropriately.
7. **Postoperative management.** Problems that should be anticipated in the postoperative period include (a) oversedation, (b) accumulation of airway secretions, (c) pneumothorax, (d) bronchospasm, (e) PE, (f) pneumonia, (g) persistent air leaks, (h) arrhythmias, (i) myocardial infarction, and (j) PE. Re-intubation and mechanical ventilation are associated with high morbidity and mortality. Several measures can be taken to minimize these adverse side effects:
   a. Judicious pulmonary toilet
   b. Bronchodilators
   c. Effective analgesia with TEA or PVN/multimodal analgesia
   d. Avoidance of systemic corticosteroids

F. **Endobronchial valves and blockers for lung volume reduction.** Although LVRS has been shown to benefit patients with a heterogeneous pattern of emphysema, this constitutes only about 20% of patients who are eligible candidates for this treatment. Procedures for bronchoscopic LVRS have been developed to treat patients with heterogeneous and homogeneous patterns of emphysema. The rationale for this minimally invasive approach is that by endobronchially obstructing the emphysematous segments of the lung, collapse of these areas should occur, thereby reducing hyperinflation and alleviating symptoms without the need for surgery. Currently available bronchoscopic techniques include endobronchial blockers/valves, biologic glues, and airway bypass. Although there are significant improvements achieved with endobronchial valves/blockers, the results have not been as substantial as those obtained with surgical LVRS.

G. Conclusions. LVRS is a viable option for a select group of emphysema patients and endobronchial valves and blockers that are undergoing clinical trials in the United States hold much promise as a treatment alternative for all emphysema patients. Regardless of the selection of treatment modality, the goals remain the same: Improvements in dyspnea, exercise tolerance, quality of life, and prolonged patient survival.

The anesthesiologist must be actively engaged in the perioperative management of these patients. Patient history and preoperative status as well as the results obtained from the evaluation of chest radiographs, high-resolution CT scans, and right heart catheterizations should be carefully weighed when planning for the patient's care.

REFERENCES

1. Poonyagariyagorn H, Mazzone PJ. Lung cancer: Preoperative pulmonary evaluation of the lung resection candidate. *Semin Respir Crit Care Med.* 2008;29:271.
2. Slinger PD, Darling G. Preanesthetic assessment for thoracic surgery. In: Slinger P, ed. *Principles and Practice of Anesthesia for Thoracic Surgery.* New York, NY: Springer; 2011:11–34.
3. Slinger P, Suissa S, Triolet W. Predicting arterial oxygenation during one-lung ventilation. *Can J Anaesth.* 1992;39:1030–1035.
4. Campos JH. An update on bronchial blockers during lung separation techniques in adults. *Anesth Analg.* 2005;97:1266.
5. Campos JH, Hallam E, Van Natta T, et al. Devices for lung isolation used by anesthesiologists with limited thoracic experience: Comparison of double-lumen endotracheal tube, Univent(R) torque control blocker, and Arndt wire-guided endobronchial blocker(R). *Anesthesiology.* 2006;104:261–266.
6. Slinger P. Fiberoptic bronchoscopic positioning of double lumen tubes. *J Cardiothorac Anesth.* 1989;3:486–496. For photographs see "Bronchoscopic positioning of Double-Lumen Tubes" in the Living Library section at the web site *www.thoracicanesthesia.com.*
7. Karzai W, Schwarzkopf K. Hypoxemia during one-lung ventilation. *Anesthesiology.* 2009;110:1402.
8. Ku C-M, Slinger P, Waddell T. A novel method of treating hypoxemia during one-lung ventilation for thoracoscopic surgery. *J Cardiothorac Vasc Anesth.* 2009;23:850.
9. Slinger P. Postpneumonectomy pulmonary edema: Good news, bad news. *Anesthesiology.* 2006;105:2–5.
10. Amar D, Roistacher N, Burt ME, et al. Effects of diltiazem versus digoxin on dysrhythmias and cardiac function after pneumonectomy. *Ann Thorac Surg.* 1997;63:1374.
11. Riley RH, Wood BM. Induction of anesthesia in a patient with a bronchopleural fistula. *Anaesth Intensive Care.* 1994;22:625.
12. Shamberger RC, Hozman RS, Griscom NT, et al. Prospective evaluation by computed tomography and pulmonary function tests of children with mediastinal masses. *Surgery.* 1995;118:468.
13. Frawley G, Low J, Brown TCK. Anaesthesia for an anterior mediastinal mass with ketamine and midazolam infusion. *Anaesth Intensive Care.* 1995;23:610–612.
14. Turkoz A, Gulcan O, Tercan F. Hemodynamic collapse caused by a large unruptured aneurysm of the ascending aorta in an 18 year old. *Anesth Analg.* 2006;102:1040–1042.
15. Licker M, Schweizer A, Nicolet G, et al. Anesthesia of a patient with an obstructing tracheal mass: A new way to manage the airway. *Acta Anaesthesiol Scand.* 1997;41:84–86.
16. Fortin M, Turcotte R, Gleeton O, et al. Catheter induced pulmonary artery rupture; using balloon occlusion to avoid lung isolation. *J Cardiothorac Vasc Anesth.* 2006;20:376–378.
17. Grant CA, Dempsey G, Harrison J, et al. Tracheo-innominate artery fistula after percutaneous tracheostomy: Three case reports and a clinical review. *Br J Anaesth.* 2006;96:127.
18. Manecke G, Banks D, Madani M, et al. Pulmonary thrombo-endarterectomy. In: Slinger P, ed. *Principles and Practice of Anesthesia for Thoracic Surgery.* New York, NY: Springer; 2011.
19. de Perrot M, McRae K, Shargall Y, et al. Early postoperative pulmonary vascular compliance predicts outcome after pulmonary endarterectomy for chronic thromboembolic pulmonary hypertension. *Chest.* 2011;140:34.
20. Egan TM, Murray S, Bustami RT, et al. Development of the new lung allocation system in the United States. *Am J Transplant.* 2006;6:1212–1227.
21. Yusen RD, Shearon TH, Quian Y, et al. Lung transplantation in the United States 1999–2008. *Am J Transplant.* 2010;10:1047–1068.
22. Christie JD, Edwards LB, Kucheryavaya AY, et al. The Registry of the International Society for Heart and Lung Transplantation: Twenty-eighth Adult Lung and Heart-Lung Transplant Report—2011. *J Heart Lung Transplant.* 2011;30:1104–1122.
23. Orens JB, Estenne M, Arcasoy S, et al. International guidelines for the selection of lung transplant candidates: 2006 update-a consensus report from the Pulmonary Scientific Council of the International Society for Heart and Lung Transplantation. *J Heart Lung Transplant.* 2006;25:745–755.
24. Snell GI, Richardson M, Griffiths AP, et al. Coronary artery disease in potential lung transplant recipients greater than 50 years old: The role of coronary intervention. *Chest.* 1999;116:874.
25. DeSoyza A, Corris PA. Lung transplantation and the *Burkholderia cepacia* complex. *J Heart Lung Transplant.* 2003;22:954–958.
26. Aris RM, Gilligan PH, Neuringer IP, et al. The effects of pan-resistant bacteria in cystic fibrosis patients on lung transplant outcome. *Am J Respir Crit Care Med.* 1997;155:1699.

27. Starnes VA, Woo MS, MacLaughlin EF, et al. Comparison of outcomes between living donor and cadaveric lung transplantation in children. *Ann Thorac Surg.* 1999;68:2279.
28. Bowdish ME, Barr ML, Schenkel FA, et al. A decade of living lobar lung transplantation: Perioperative complications after 253 donor lobectomies. *Am J Transplant.* 2004;4:1283–1288.
29. Reyes KG, Mason DP, Thuita L, et al. Guidelines for donor lung selection: Time for revision? *Ann Thorac Surg.* 2010;89:1756–1764.
30. Bhorade SM, Vigneswaran W, McCabe MA, et al. Liberalization of donor criteria may expand the donor pool without adverse consequence in lung transplantation. *J Heart Lung Transplant.* 2000;19:1199.
31. Snell GI, Levvy BJ, Oto T, et al. Early lung transplantation success utilizing controlled donation after cardiac death. *Am J Transplant.* 2008;8:1282–1289.
32. Fisher AJ, Donnelly SC, Hirani N, et al. Elevated levels of interleukin-8 in donor lungs is associated with early graft failure after lung transplantation. *Am J Respir Crit Care Med.* 2001;163:259.
33. Cypel M, Yeung JC, Liu M, et al. Normothermic ex vivo lung perfusion in clinical lung transplantation. *N Engl J Med.* 2011;364:1431–1440.
34. Novik RJ, Bennett LE, Meyer DM, et al. Influence of graft ischemic time and donor age on survival after lung transplantation. *J Heart Lung Transplant.* 1999;18:425.
35. Feltracco P, Barbieri S, Milefoy M, et al. Thoracic epidural analgesia in lung transplantation. *Transplant Proc.* 2010;42:1265–1269.
36. Khan TA, Schnickel G, Ross D, et al. A prospective, randomized, cross-over study of inhaled NO versus inhaled prostacyclin in heart transplant and lung transplant recipients. *J Thorac Cardiovasc Surg.* 2009;138:1417–1424.
37. Allan JS. Immunosuppression for lung transplantation. *Semin Thorac Cardiovasc Surg.* 2004;16:333–341.
38. Benden C, Aurora P, Edwards LB, et al. The Registry of the International Society for Heart and Lung Transplantation: Fourteenth Pediatric Lung and Heart-Lung Transplantation Report-2011. *J Heart Lung Transplant.* 2011;30:1123–1132.
39. Meyers BF, Yusen RD, Guthrie TJ, et al. Outcome of bilateral lung volume reduction in patients with emphysema potentially eligible for lung transplantation. *J Thorac Cardiovasc Surg.* 2001;122:10–17.
40. Cooper JD, Lefrak SS. Is volume reduction surgery appropriate in the treatment of emphysema? Yes. *Am J Respir Crit Care Med.* 1996;153:1201–1204.
41. National Emphysema Treatment Trial Research Group. A randomized trial comparing lung-volume-reduction surgery with medical therapy for severe emphysema. *N Engl J Med.* 2003;348:2059–2073.
42. National Emphysema Treatment Trial Research Group. Patients at high risk of death after lung-volume-reduction surgery. *N Engl J Med.* 2001;345:1075–1082.

27 Pain Management for Cardiothoracic Procedures

Mark Stafford-Smith and Thomas M. McLoughlin, Jr.

KEY POINTS

1. Chronic pain due to intercostal nerve injury develops in approximately 50% of postthoracotomy patients, and in 5% this pain becomes severe and disabling.
2. Thoracic epidural analgesia for cardiac surgery is associated with reduced supraventricular arrhythmias and postoperative pulmonary complications relative to standard approaches.
3. Highly lipophilic drugs, such as fentanyl, are best used with catheters placed near the involved dermatomes. Hydrophilic drugs, such as morphine, are most useful for remote catheters such as those positioned in the lumbar region.
4. Epidural opioids should generally not be administered unless postoperative observation and monitoring for delayed respiratory depression are planned.

5. Patients with severe lung disease have the most to gain in terms of improved outcome from optimal postoperative analgesia such as continuous thoracic epidural.
6. The risk of nephrotoxicity appears to be low (1:1,000 to 1:10,000) with perioperative ketorolac administration.
7. Respiratory depression requiring naloxone administration is reported to occur in 0.2% to 1% of patients receiving epidural narcotics.
8. Pending additional contributions to our understanding of the risk of peridural bleeding, the trend in expert opinion has recently shifted to argue for caution, particularly regarding thoracic epidural catheter placement prior to "full" heparinization for cardiac surgery.

I. Introduction

A. Incidence and severity of pain after cardiothoracic procedures. Pain is an unpleasant sensation occurring in varying degrees of severity as a consequence of injury or disease. Chest surgery, via sternotomy and especially via thoracotomy, is among the most debilitating for patients due to pain and consequent respiratory dysfunction. Important sources of postoperative discomfort after cardiothoracic surgery, in addition to incisional pain, include indwelling thoracostomy tubes, rib or sternal fractures, and costovertebral joint pain due to sternal retrac-
1 tion. Chronic pain due to intercostal nerve injury develops in approximately 50% of postthoracotomy patients, and in 5% this pain becomes severe and disabling. Despite the early belief that minimally invasive thoracic and cardiac surgical procedures involving smaller incisions would reduce the incidence and severity of postoperative pain compared to traditional cardiac surgery, clinical experience has not borne out this assumption for most patients. No single thoracotomy technique has been shown to reduce the incidence of chronic postthoracotomy pain, and patients should be warned in advance of this potential postoperative complication.

B. Transmission pathways for nociception. An understanding of the anatomy and physiology of pain pathways underpins the logical choice of analgesic strategies during and after cardiothoracic surgery. Multimodal approaches take advantage of numerous therapeutic targets in the signaling chain to optimize pain control while minimizing side effects [1].

In the thoracic region, pain signals are relayed through myelinated $A\delta$ and unmyelinated C fibers in peripheral intercostal nerves. The ventral, posterior, and visceral branches of each intercostal nerve innervate the anterior chest wall, posterior chest wall, and visceral aspects of the chest, respectively. These branches join together just before entering the paravertebral space and then pass through the intervertebral foramina in the spinal canal. Sensory intercostal nerve fibers form a dorsal root that fuses with the spinal cord dorsal horn to enter the central nervous system (CNS). Somatic pain is mediated predominantly through myelinated $A\delta$ fibers in the ventral and posterior branches. Sympathetic (visceral) pain is mediated by unmyelinated C fibers in all three branches. Sympathetic afferent pain signals are directed from intercostal nerve branches through the sympathetic trunk (a paravertebral structure found just beneath the parietal pleura in the thorax) and then pass back into the peripheral nerves to enter the CNS from T-1 to L-2. In addition, the vagus nerve provides parasympathetic visceral innervation of the thorax. This cranial nerve enters the CNS through the medulla oblongata and, therefore, is not normally affected by epidural or intrathecal (IT) methods of pain control.

The spinal cord and spinal canal are considerably different in length, and consequently spinal cord dermatomal segments do not typically lie at the level of their respective vertebrae. Thus, knowledge of spinal anatomy is essential if regional analgesia techniques are to be successful. This is particularly true with the use of lipid-soluble epidural opioids because the targeted dorsal horn often is significantly cephalad relative to the associated intervertebral foramen and nerve.

Most spinal pain signals are transmitted to the brain after crossing from the dorsal horn to contralateral spinal cord structures (e.g., spinothalamic tract). Distribution of nociceptive messages occurs to numerous locations in the brain resulting in cognitive, affective, and autonomic responses to noxious stimuli.

Endogenous modification of pain signals begins at the site of tissue trauma and includes hyperalgesia related to inflammation and other CNS-mediated phenomena such as "windup." The substantia gelatinosa of the dorsal horn is an important location for pain signal modulation, including effects that are mediated through opioid, adrenergic, and N-methyl-D-aspartate (NMDA) receptor systems.

C. **Analgesia considerations: The procedure, patient, and process.** The degree and location of surgical trauma, particularly in relation to the site of skin incision and route of bony access to the chest, are particularly important in anticipating analgesic requirements after cardiothoracic surgery. Notably, minimally invasive procedures that reduce total surgical tissue disruption but relocate it to more pain-sensitive regions may not translate into reduced postoperative pain (e.g., minithoracotomy vs. sternotomy). Analgesic strategies are best individualized, particularly for high-risk patients in whom outcome benefits may be the greatest. This includes not only appropriate postoperative analgesia delivery but also preoperative education regarding pain reporting, procedures, and devices to provide analgesia, and expectations for postoperative transition to oral medications and home administration.

D. **Adverse consequences of pain.** In addition to unpleasant emotional aspects of pain, nociceptive signals have several other effects that can be harmful and delay patient recovery. These include activation of neuroendocrine reflexes constituting the surgical stress response (including inflammation and elevated circulating catecholamines), a catabolic state associated with high levels of several other humoral substances (e.g., cortisol, vasopressin, renin, angiotensin), decreased vagal tone, and increased oxygen consumption. Spinal reflex responses to pain include localized muscle spasm and activation of the sympathetic nervous system.

Pathophysiologic consequences of the neuroendocrine local and systemic responses to pain include respiratory complications related to diaphragmatic dysfunction, myocardial ischemia, ileus, urinary retention and oliguria, thromboembolism, and immune impairment [2].

E. **Outcome benefits of good analgesia for cardiothoracic procedures.** A primary benefit of effective pain control is patient satisfaction. Studies have documented additional advantages of optimizing analgesia, especially in recovery from thoracotomy. Belief that the pain of median sternotomy is less severe and inconsequential to outcome leads many institutions to employ conventional analgesia protocols involving fixed dosing of analgesics on a timed schedule. However, after coronary bypass grafting, attention to profound analgesia in the early postoperative period may decrease the incidence and severity of myocardial ischemia. A meta-
2 analysis of 28 randomized studies suggests that thoracic epidural analgesia for cardiac surgery is associated with reduced supraventricular arrhythmias and postoperative pulmonary complications relative to standard approaches [3].

Evidence supporting reductions in perioperative complications related to pain relief are reported for many different analgesia techniques and may be related to their effectiveness in blocking the surgical stress response and nociceptive spinal reflexes. In this regard, neuraxial and regional analgesia are most often reported as being effective. Nonetheless, beyond reduced pain, any outcome benefits related to the incidence of major morbidities and mortality of specific analgesia techniques remain difficult to prove, possibly due to the insufficient numbers of patients studied and the low frequency of these events, as is well summarized in a review by Liu et al. [4]. In general, reported benefits of good analgesia rely on reporting of surrogate markers that correlate with major adverse outcomes (e.g., arterial oxygen saturation) that imply attenuation of the adverse consequences of pain outlined in Section I.D. For example, in the setting of thoracic surgery, thoracic epidural analgesia provides superior pain relief compared to systemic opioids and decreases the incidence of atelectasis, pulmonary infections, hypoxemia, and other pulmonary complications [5]. In addition, effective analgesia established before surgery in some circumstances may provide pre-emptive protection against the development of chronic pain syndromes. Aggressive pain control in the early postoperative period was associated with a greater than 50% reduction in the number of patients continuing to experience chronic pain 1 year after thoracotomy in one study [6]. Unfortunately, in cardiac surgery, reports of neuraxial techniques generally involve small numbers and fail to demonstrate clinical outcome benefit, although benefits in hospital length of stay and cost avoidance have been commonly shown [7].

TABLE 27.1 Opioid receptors

Type	Mediated effects
μ_1	Analgesia
μ_2	Respiratory depression, euphoria, physical dependence, pruritus, nausea and vomiting
K	Spinal analgesia, sedation, miosis, dieresis
Σ	Dysphoria, hypertonia
Δ	Spinal analgesia, μ-receptor modulation

Outcome benefit following cardiac surgery with central neuraxial analgesia was not demonstrated in a meta-analysis published in 2004 nor in a randomized trial published in 2011 [8,9].

II. Pain management pharmacology

A. Opioid analgesics

1. **Mechanisms.** Opioid analgesics are a broad group of compounds that include naturally occurring extracts of opium (e.g., morphine, codeine), synthetic substances (e.g., fentanyl, hydromorphone), and endogenous peptides (e.g., endorphins, enkephalins). The analgesic effects of these drugs are all linked to their interaction with opioid receptors; however, individual agents may function as agonists, antagonists, or partial agonists at different receptor subtype populations. Opioid receptors are widely distributed throughout the body, but they are particularly concentrated within the substantia gelatinosa of the dorsal horn of the spinal cord, as well as regions of the brain including the rostral ventral medulla, locus ceruleus, and midbrain periaqueductal gray area. Stimulation of opioid receptors inhibits the enzyme adenyl cyclase, closes voltage-dependent calcium channels, and opens calcium-dependent inwardly rectifying potassium channels, resulting in inhibitory effects characterized by neuronal hyperpolarization and decreased excitability. Opioid receptor subtypes have been sequenced and cloned, and they belong to the growing list of G-protein-coupled receptors. The effects of agonist binding at different opioid receptor subtypes are summarized in Table 27.1.
2. **Perioperative use.** Opioids are commonly administered throughout the perioperative period for cardiothoracic procedures. Preoperatively, they can be given orally, intramuscularly (IM), or intravenously (IV) alone or as part of a sedative cocktail to provide anxiolysis and analgesia for transport and placement of intravascular catheters. Intraoperatively, they are given IV most commonly as part of a balanced anesthetic technique that includes potent inhaled anesthetics, benzodiazepines, and other agents. Finally, they can be injected directly into the thecal sac or included as a component of epidural infusions to provide intraoperative and postoperative analgesia. Opioids administered epidurally have varying spread and analgesic potency based in part on their water solubility and are best matched with analgesic requirements with knowledge of the position of the epidural catheter relative to the dermatomes affected by pain and the relative lipophilicity of the drug. Highly lipophilic drugs, such as fentanyl, are best used with catheters placed near the involved dermatomes. Hydrophilic drugs, such as morphine, are most useful for remote catheters such as those positioned in the lumbar region. Drugs with intermediate lipophilicity, such as hydromorphone, are considered ideal by most and can be used for more balanced spread.

3

3. **Side effects and cautions**
   - **a.** Respiratory depression (increased risk with higher dosing, coadministration of other sedatives, opioid-naive patients, advanced age, central neuraxial administration of hydrophilic opioid agents)
   - **b.** Sedation
   - **c.** Pruritus
   - **d.** Nausea
   - **e.** Urinary retention, especially common in the elderly and in males receiving spinal opioids

f. Inhibition of intestinal peristalsis/constipation
g. CNS excitation/hypertonia, much more notable with rapid IV administration of lipophilic agents
h. Miosis
i. Biliary spasm

All of the above effects can be reversed with administration of opioid antagonist drugs (e.g., naloxone). Opioid rotation, or changing the narcotic drug that a patient is receiving, may also be useful in reducing the incidence or severity of complicating side effects or also in enhancing the patient's experience of analgesia [10].

B. **Nonsteroidal anti-inflammatory drugs**

1. **Mechanisms.** Nonsteroidal anti-inflammatory drugs (NSAIDs) act principally through both central and peripheral inhibition of cyclo-oxygenase, resulting in decreased synthesis of prostaglandins from arachadonic acid, including prostacyclin and thromboxane. Prostaglandins are involved in the physiology of numerous signaling pathways, including those influencing renal perfusion, bronchial smooth muscle tone, hemostasis, the gastric mucosal secretions, and the inflammatory response. Prostaglandin E_2 is the eicosanoid produced in greatest quantity at sites of trauma and inflammation and is an important mediator of pain. The full therapeutic effects of NSAIDs are complex and likely involve mechanisms that are independent of prostaglandin effects. For example, prostaglandin synthesis is effectively inhibited with low doses of most NSAIDs; however, much higher doses are required to produce anti-inflammatory effects.
2. **Perioperative use.** NSAIDs are useful for postoperative analgesia. They are most commonly administered in cardiothoracic surgical patients as a complement to neuraxial techniques. Their principal advantage is the absence of respiratory depression and other opioid side effects. Many NSAIDs are available for oral or rectal administration. Ketorolac is a nonselective NSAID intended for short-term use (5 days or less) with preparations available for intravenous or intramuscular injection, in addition to tablets for ingestion.
3. **Side effects and cautions**
   a. Decreased renal blood flow/parenchymal ischemia
   b. Gastrointestinal mucosal irritation
   c. Impaired primary hemostasis
4. **COX-2 inhibitors**

   The effects of cyclo-oxygenase are mediated by two distinct isoenzymes termed COX-1 and COX-2. COX-1 is the constitutive form responsible for production of prostaglandins involved in homeostatic processes of the kidney, gut, endothelium, and platelets. COX-2 is predominantly an inducible isoform responsible for production of prostaglandins during inflammation. Highly selective COX-2 inhibitors have potent analgesic properties and, until recently, were used frequently to treat perioperative pain. Unfortunately, combined data from several large randomized double-blind trials [11] revealed an increased incidence of cardiovascular complications including myocardial infarction with agents in this drug class. Celecoxib is the only remaining COX-2 inhibitor widely available for prescription in the US. The difference between celecoxib and the other agents may be due to its relatively modest COX-2 versus COX-1 subtype selectivity compared to the other agents (30 : 1 vs. >300 : 1). However, celecoxib use remains largely limited to treatment of severe arthritis, rheumatoid arthritis, and ankylosis spondylitis in circumstances where treatment of these conditions with several other NSAIDs has failed. Prothrombotic effects from COX-2 inhibition are likely due to reduced prostacyclin generation. In addition, COX-2 inhibitors lack the antiplatelet effects of aspirin and even favor vasoconstrictive effects. Thus, use of these agents for perioperative pain relief is not recommended.

C. **Acetaminophen (paracetamol)**

1. **Mechanism**

   Acetaminophen is a synthetic, non-opiate, analgesic drug that is distinct from most other NSAIDs in that it is a weak inhibitor of the synthesis of prostaglandins and of COX-1 and COX-2. Its mechanisms appear to be primarily central, resulting in analgesia and antipyresis, with only minimal anti-inflammation. COX-3, a splice variant of COX-1, has been suggested to be the site of action. Other proposed actions include activation of descending serotonergic pathways and/or inhibition of the nitric oxide pathway mediated by a variety of neurotransmitter receptors including NMDA and substance P. Although the exact site and mechanism of analgesic action is not clearly defined, acetaminophen appears to produce analgesia by elevation of the pain threshold.

2. **Perioperative use and cautions**
Until recently, acetaminophen was only available for oral and rectal administration and thus infrequently used in the immediate perioperative period. In 2010, the FDA approved an intravenous form of the drug for relieving pain or fever in surgical patients, approved for use in adults and children aged 2 and older. It has been shown useful in the treatment of moderate to severe post-surgical pain, demonstrating an opioid-sparing effect with good patient acceptance and few adverse effects, especially in orthopedic surgical populations [12]. A modest opioid-sparing effect, with no reduction in the incidence of nausea and vomiting, was shown when intravenous acetaminophen was compared to oral acetaminophen in a postoperative population of coronary artery bypass surgical patients [13].
The primary risk of acetominaphen is hepatotoxicity secondary to overdose. Acetaminophen toxicity is the leading cause of acute liver failure in the United States. A typical intravenous adult dosing schedule involves administration of 650 to 1,000 mg every 6 hrs, with infusion of the drug timed to occur over at least 15 min.

D. **Local anesthetics**

1. **Mechanisms.** Local anesthetics interrupt neural conduction thus disrupting transmission of pain and other nerve impulses through blockade of neuronal voltage-gated sodium channels. This blockade does not change the resting potential of the nerve. However, altered sodium ion channel permeability slows depolarization such that, in the presence of a sufficient concentration of local anesthetic, threshold for propagation of an action potential cannot be reached.
2. **Perioperative use.** Local anesthetics are used throughout the perioperative period for topical, infiltration, peripheral nerve, or central neuraxial anesthesia. Their advantage lies in the capacity to provide profound analgesia without the undesired side effects seen with opioids or NSAIDs. Effective regional anesthesia is the best technique to most completely attenuate the neurohumoral stress response to pain. Thoracic epidural analgesia is particularly useful in treating pain, both somatic and visceral, for patients with occlusive coronary artery disease.
3. **Side effects and cautions**
   a. Not surprisingly, side effects from sodium channel blockade due to local anesthetic toxicity resemble those observed with severe hyponatremia. Excessive local anesthetic blood concentrations, reached through absorption or inadvertent intravascular injection, predictably result in toxic effects on the CNS (seizures, coma) and the heart (negative inotropy, conduction disturbances, arrhythmias). Table 27.2 lists commonly accepted maximum local anesthetic dosing for infiltration anesthesia.

TABLE 27.2 Maximum recommended dosing of local anesthetic agents for local infiltration

	Maximum dose for 70 kg adult (mg)	
Drug	**Plain solution**	**Containing epinephrine (1:200,000)**
Chloroprocaine	600–800	1,000
Lidocaine	300	500
Mepivacaine	300	500
Bupivacaine	175	225
Ropivacaine	200	250

Dose may be increased modestly for use in compartments where absorption will be delayed (e.g., brachial plexus) and decreased for use in more vascular regions (e.g., epidural space, intercostal).

b. Caution must be exercised in the performance of any invasive regional anesthesia procedure in the setting of ongoing or proposed anticoagulation or thrombolysis.

Although regional anesthesia can be initiated without an apparent increase in the risk of bleeding in patients taking only aspirin or NSAIDs, The American Society of Regional Anesthesia and Pain Medicine (ASRA; www.ASRA.com) has recently updated their consensus recommendations for regional anesthesia in patients receiving antithrombotic therapy [14]. The group recommends holding the antiplatelet agents clopidogrel (Plavix) for 7 days, ticlopidine (Ticlid) for 14 days, and GP IIb/IIIa antagonists for 4 to 48 hrs before neuraxial block. ASRA also recommends holding the anticoagulant warfarin for 4 to 5 days, low molecular weight heparins for 12 to 24 hrs depending on drug and dose, and unfractionated heparin for 8 to 12 hrs depending on dosing interval, before neuraxial block placement. It should be noted that these same guidelines are recommended for consideration of deep plexus or peripheral nerve blockade in the setting of drug-altered hemostasis.

c. Allergic reactions are not uncommon, particularly to the para-aminobenzoic acid metabolites of ester local anesthetics or to preservative materials in commercial local anesthetic preparations. True allergic reactions to preservative-free amide local anesthetics (e.g., lidocaine) are rare, and suspected cases are often attributed in retrospect to inadvertent intravascular injection of epinephrine-containing solutions.

d. Concentration-dependent neurotoxicity of local anesthetics (e.g., cauda equina syndrome following IT local anesthetic injection) is now well described.

E. α_2-Adrenergic agonists

Clonidine is the prototypical drug in this class, although dexmedetomidine is also approved for clinical use. Both drugs produce analgesia through agonism at central α_2-receptors in the substantia gelatinosa of the spinal cord and sedation through receptors in the locus coeruleus in the brainstem. They also may act at peripheral α_2-receptors located on sympathetic nerve terminals to decrease norepinephrine output in sympathetically mediated pain. The analgesic effect of these drugs is distinct and complementary to that of opioids when used in combination. Clonidine may be administered orally to provide sedation and analgesia as a premedication. Preservative-free clonidine may be included as a component of epidural infusions or IT injections. Although these agents have limited respiratory depressant properties, hypotension, sedation, and dry mouth are common side effects from analgesic doses.

F. Ketamine. Ketamine has complex interactions with a variety of receptors but is thought to act primarily through blockade of the excitatory effects of the neurotransmitter, glutamic acid, at the NMDA receptor in the CNS. It can be administered orally or parenterally to provide sedation, potent analgesia, and "dissociative anesthesia." The principal advantages of ketamine stem from its sympathomimetic properties and lack of ventilatory depression. Cautions include increased secretions and dysphoric reactions. Ketamine administered by low-dose intravenous infusion as an adjunct to a post-sternotomy analgesic regimen may increase patient satisfaction and provide an opioid-sparing effect [15]. Ketamine may also be added as an adjunctive medication to epidural infusions, including thoracic epidural infusions for acute post-thoracotomy pain [16].

G. Nonpharmacologic analgesia

1. **Cryoablation.** A cryoprobe can be introduced into the intercostal space and used to produce transient (1 to 4 days) numbness in the distribution of the intercostal nerve. A cryoprobe circulates extremely cold gas on the order of −80°C. When applied for two to three treatments of approximately 2 min each, it temporarily disrupts neural function. Cryoablation has been shown to reduce pain and the need for systemic analgesics after lateral thoracotomy for cardiac surgery [17].
2. **Nursing care.** Empathic nursing care and nursing-guided relaxation techniques are important components to patient comfort throughout the perioperative period and should not be overlooked [17].

III. Pain management strategies

A. Oral. Gastrointestinal ileus is rarely a concern after routine cardiothoracic surgical procedures; therefore, transition to oral administration of analgesics should be considered as soon as pain management goals are likely to be effectively achieved by this route. This is particularly important because oral agents are currently the simplest, cheapest, and most reliable way to continue effective analgesia after hospital discharge, and they should be used as the mainstay of any "fast track" analgesia protocol.

B. **Subcutaneous/intramuscular.** Subcutaneous (SC) and (IM) injections remain effective and inexpensive alternate parenteral routes to intravenous (IV) administration for delivery of potent systemic analgesia using opioids (e.g., morphine, hydromorphone, meperidine). SC or IM injection results in slower onset of analgesia than the IV route and, therefore, is more suitable for scheduled dosing (e.g., every 3 to 6 hrs) rather than "as needed." A notable disadvantage of the SC route is injection-related discomfort, which can be largely avoided by slow injection through an indwelling SC butterfly needle.

C. **Intravenous.** In the absence of neuraxial analgesia, IV opioid analgesia is generally the primary tool to provide effective pain relief for the early postoperative patient. The advantages of this route include rapid onset and ease of titration to effect. In addition, for the awake patient, patient-controlled IV delivery of opioids (i.e., patient-controlled analgesia [PCA]) has become widely available. PCA units combine options for baseline continuous infusion of drug with patient-administered bolus doses after programmed lockout periods to minimize risk of overdose and maximize the patient's sense of "control" over their pain. Patient satisfaction using PCA analgesia rivals that with neuraxial analgesia.

Analgesic agents that have traditionally been available only for oral administration are becoming available for parenteral usage. IV ketorolac and acetominophen have gained widespread acceptance as analgesic alternatives for thoracic surgical patients that are devoid of respiratory depressant effects.

D. **Interpleural.** Interpleural analgesia involves placement of a catheter between the visceral and parietal pleura and subsequent instillation of local anesthetic solution. Ensuing pain relief is believed to be the result of blockade of intercostal nerves in addition to local actions on the pleura. Disadvantages of this technique include the requirement for relatively high doses of local anesthetic with relatively enhanced vascular uptake, poor effectiveness, and possible impairment of ipsilateral diaphragmatic function. For these reasons, interpleural analgesia has been largely abandoned as a strategy for pain control in cardiothoracic surgery patients.

E. **Intercostal.** Sequential intercostal blocks (e.g., T-4 to T-10) can contribute to unilateral postoperative chest wall analgesia for thoracic surgery. Bilateral intercostal nerve blocks (ICB) may be used for pain relief after median sternotomy [18]. ICB requires depositing local anesthetic (e.g., 4 mL of 0.5% bupivacaine per nerve) at the inferior border of the associated rib near the proximal intercostal nerve. ICBs are generally performed through the skin before surgery or by the surgeon under direct vision within the chest. ICBs contribute to analgesia for up to 12 hrs, but in general they do not include blockade of the posterior and visceral rami of the intercostal nerve; therefore, they often require additional NSAID or parenteral analgesia to be effective.

F. **Paravertebral.** Paravertebral blocks (PVBs) can provide unilateral chest wall analgesia for thoracic surgery. Sequential thoracic PVB injections (e.g., T-4 to T-10, 4 mL of 0.5% ropivacaine per level) may be combined with "light" general anesthesia for thoracotomy procedures and provide analgesia for several hours postoperatively. Anticipated chest tube insertion sites usually dictate the lowest PVB level required. Although use of PVBs reduces intraoperative opioid requirement, NSAID and/or opioid supplementation is often required after thoracotomy to achieve adequate comfort. "Emergence" from PVB-mediated analgesia may occur on the day after surgery, often after transfer from an intensive care environment; therefore, it is important that other analgesia alternatives be immediately available at this time. Advantages of PVBs and ICBs relative to neuraxial techniques include the avoidance of opioid side effects, risk of spinal hematoma, and hypotension related to bilateral sympathetic block. Nonetheless, disadvantages of ICB and PVB analgesia include that they are less reliable than thoracic epidural analgesia and can themselves be complicated by epidural spread of local anesthetic. Notably, compared to PVBs, ICBs do not affect the posterior and visceral ramus of the intercostal nerve and recede more rapidly. The paravertebral space, where peripheral nerves exit from the spinal canal, is limited superiorly and inferiorly by the heads of associated ribs, anteriorly by the parietal pleura, and posteriorly by the superior costotransverse ligament.

G. **Intrathecal.** IT opioid analgesia is a suitable treatment for major pain after median sternotomy or thoracotomy [19]. The benefits and risks of a spinal procedure should always be carefully weighed before using this technique, particularly with regard to the risk of spinal hematoma in patients with abnormal hemostasis. Small-caliber noncutting spinal needles (e.g., 27-gauge Whitacre needle) are often selected for lumbar spinal injection of preservative-free morphine. Age rather than weight predicts proper IT opioid dosing in adults; 10 μg/kg IT morphine dosing is effective for cardiothoracic surgery in most adults, usually administered before induction of general anesthesia. Smaller doses (e.g., 0.3 to 0.5 mg, total dose) are required to reduce the likelihood of respiratory depression in elderly patients (older than 75 yrs). It is prudent to avoid the use of IT morphine in patients 85 years or older. Since rare patients will develop significant delayed respiratory depression, hourly monitoring of respiratory rate and consciousness for 18 to 24 hrs is mandatory with this technique. Reduced doses of sedative and hypnotic agents during general anesthesia are required to avoid excessive postoperative somnolence. Onset of thoracic analgesia is approximately 1 to 2 hrs after injection, lasting up to 24 hrs. Postoperative NSAID therapy complements IT morphine analgesia without sedative effects. IT clonidine (1 μg/kg) combined with IT morphine produces superior analgesia compared to either drug administered alone [20]. IV or oral analgesia must be immediately available in anticipation of the resolution of IT morphine analgesia approximately 24 hrs after injection because significant pain may develop rapidly. IT administration of other drugs for cardiac and thoracic surgery, such as local anesthetic agents or short-acting opioids (e.g., sufentanil), is mainly limited to the intraoperative period.

H. **Epidural.** Epidural anesthesia is ideal for thoracic surgery and is the most widely studied and used form of regional analgesia for this purpose [5]. Although epidural catheter placement for use during and after cardiac surgery is reported to have benefits [21], this approach has not gained a similar level of acceptance.

Thoracic epidural catheter location (T-4 to T-10) is generally preferred over lumbar for thoracic surgery. Proponents of thoracic catheter placement cite the reduced local anesthetic dosing requirements, closer proximity to thoracic segment dorsal horns, and reduced likelihood of dislodgement postoperatively. Concern regarding increased risk of spinal cord injury using a thoracic compared to a lumbar approach for epidural catheter placement has not been borne out; however, it is commonly recommended that thoracic epidural catheter placement occur while the patient is sufficiently alert to reliably report paresthesias or other complaints during the procedure. Selection of the thoracic interspace should be dictated by surgical site. The epidural catheter should be placed 4 to 6 cm into the epidural space and securely taped.

Intraoperative use of an epidural catheter enhances the benefits of regional anesthesia for thoracotomy surgery by permitting a "light general" anesthetic technique with reduced residual respiratory depressant effects. Epidural local anesthetic block should be preceded by a "test dose" of epinephrine-containing local anesthetic to rule out intravascular or IT catheter placement. Epidural block can then proceed prior to incision, and administration of preincision
4 epidural opioids may contribute to a pre-emptive analgesic effect. Epidural opioids should generally not be administered unless postoperative observation and monitoring for delayed respiratory depression is planned. To minimize postoperative somnolence and the risk of respiratory depression, administration of potent IV sedatives and opioids should be reduced or avoided during surgery, and agents used to maintain general anesthesia should be easily reversible (e.g., volatile anesthetic agents). Monitoring inhaled volatile anesthetic concentrations or using a bispectral analysis monitor to assess the level of consciousness may permit guided and reduced dosing of these sedative agents. A popular mixture for postoperative epidural analgesia is dilute local anesthetic (e.g., 0.125% bupivacaine) containing an opioid with intermediate lipid solubility properties (e.g., hydromorphone, 10 μg/mL); this is administered by continuous infusion at a starting rate of 4 to 7 mL/hr, ideally starting at least 15 min before the end of surgery and titrated to clinical effect. Since early titration of epidural analgesic infusions is often required and pain is not effectively reported by the awakening patient, an initial analgesic dose of hydromorphone and local anesthetic agent should be administered to the patient (e.g., a 200 μg IT hydromorphone bolus and 3 mL preservative-free 2% lidocaine) before emergence.

IV ketorolac or acetominophen can also be administered at this time when indicated. Ketorolac is often especially effective in helping to manage shoulder discomfort secondary to indwelling thoracostomy tubes, since this complaint often persists in the setting of good incisional pain control with epidural analgesia alone. Titration of epidural analgesia to comfort should be completed in the postoperative recovery area where transfer of care to the acute pain care team should occur.

IV. Pain management regimens for specific cardiothoracic procedures

A. Conventional coronary artery bypass and open chamber procedures. Over the past three decades, anesthetic design for cardiac surgery has commonly included large doses of potent opioids (e.g., fentanyl, sufentanil), thus assuring intraoperative hemodynamic stability and excellent analgesia but often requiring considerable periods of postoperative ventilation. Although this remains a useful approach for the management of selected high-risk patients, it has been recognized that most procedures are suitable for analgesia regimens compatible with more rapid recovery. Standard regimens for cardiac surgery currently include more modest intraoperative opioid dosing than in the past, with postoperative bedside availability of parenteral opioids as required in the first 12 to 24 hrs, either patient-controlled or administered by a nurse. Transition to oral agents is encouraged as soon as food is tolerated.

The move away from traditional high-dose opioid anesthesia has increased interest in different approaches to analgesia after cardiac surgery. Routine NSAID therapy for uncomplicated patients is a safe and cost-effective way to complement opioid analgesia. Preoperative IT morphine has gained popularity in some centers. In experienced hands, imaginative combinations such as preoperative IT morphine and intraoperative IV remifentanil infusion provide reproducible excellent analgesia, with tracheal extubation often possible in the operating room [18].

B. Off-pump (sternotomy) cardiac procedures. One interpretation of "minimally invasive" cardiac surgery involves the avoidance of cardiopulmonary bypass (CPB). Whether outcomes from off-pump are equivalent, superior, or inferior to on-pump surgery for coronary artery disease remains to be answered; however, these procedures are common. Theoretically, avoidance of CPB with off-pump procedures may reduce the systemic inflammatory response associated with surgery and ironically *increase* the perception of pain. Practically, with the introduction of a "fast track" approach that has accompanied off-pump cardiac surgery, standard analgesia regimens are challenged, and inadequate pain relief has become a more common reason for delayed hospital discharge than in the past. Interest in analgesic approaches other than parenteral opioids has paralleled that for the patients undergoing traditional cardiac surgery with CPB, as outlined above (see Section **IV.A**). Because reduced heparin administration and avoidance of CPB-related impairment of hemostasis are part of off-pump surgery, IT morphine, oral NSAID therapy, and even interpleural local anesthetic regimens are being tried as analgesia strategies, and new approaches may ultimately gain approval in this patient group.

C. Minimally invasive (minithoracotomy/para- or partial sternotomy/robotic) cardiac procedures. In contrast to off-pump procedures, a second interpretation of "minimally invasive" cardiac surgery involves port-access catheter-based CPB employing very small incisions to achieve surgical goals. Although early hopes were that port-access procedures would be associated with less pain, this has not been proven to be true, most likely because of the relocation of the smaller incisions to more pain-sensitive areas (e.g., minithoracotomy). In addition to the alternate analgesic approaches outlined for patients undergoing traditional cardiac surgery with CPB (see Section **IV.A**), the possibility of using novel approaches to minithoracotomy analgesia including ICBs, one-shot PVBs, and PVB by continuous infusion exists but has not been explored sufficiently to recommend these approaches.

D. Thoracotomy/thoracoscopy procedures (noncardiac). An increasing number of the patients presenting for lung surgery have end-stage lung disease and would not have been considered eligible for an operative procedure several years ago [22]. In part, these changes in eligible candidates for lung resection are due in part to the introduction of less invasive techniques including minimally invasive video-assisted thoracic surgical (VATS) procedures. Patients with severe lung disease have the most to gain in terms of improved outcome from optimal postoperative analgesia (e.g., continuous thoracic epidural) [22]. As the potential of VATS is being realized, more physiologically invasive procedures (e.g., lobectomy) are now routinely performed using

VATS approaches. Finally, some procedures (e.g., pneumonectomy) still require the traditional and more painful thoracotomy incision.

"Light" general anesthesia with regional blockade of the chest wall is a particularly suitable anesthetic approach for lung and other chest surgery. Sedatives (e.g., midazolam) should be used sparingly throughout; often a small dose of midazolam (e.g., 0.5 mg) will extend the actions of shorter-acting sedatives such as propofol (e.g., 10 mg) for line placement. Using this technique, residual sedative/hypnotic effects can be minimized, early tracheal extubation reliably achieved, and the transition to postoperative pain management facilitated.

Analgesia for VATS and thoracotomy procedures in the intraoperative and postoperative period is often achieved through a multimodal approach including parenteral opioids, NSAIDs, and regional anesthesia. A spectrum of regional anesthesia procedures are available including thoracic epidural, spinal, paravertebral, intercostal, and interpleural blocks. These can be performed transcutaneously by the anesthesiologists or in some cases from within the rib cage during surgery by the surgeon. Options include one-shot injections or catheters tunneled under the parietal pleura that can be left in place for infusions of local anesthetic and/or opioid. Selection of a regional analgesia approach should include a plan for transition to oral medication and be matched to the expected hospital discharge timing; neuraxial opioids may delay discharge if given inappropriately. Many patients with normal pulmonary function having a minor surgical procedure will have good analgesia with IV PCA morphine or fentanyl alone.

Selection of regional blockade technique is best made after evaluation of both patient status and the demands of the surgery. American Society of Anesthesiologists class I to II patients anticipating postoperative hospital stays up to 48 hrs may benefit from single-shot local anesthetic blocks (e.g., PVBs and ICBs); however, anxious patients in this group should not be overly pressured to undergo a regional procedure. In contrast, patients who are deconditioned or undergoing more extensive procedures are more likely to benefit from regional anesthesia and placement of a thoracic epidural catheter unless contraindicated. Routine postoperative NSAID or acetominophen therapy should be considered, since these agents are devoid of sedation and are particularly effective analgesics in combination with regional analgesia. Local anesthetic/opioid mixtures are popular analgesic regimens for use as continuous epidural infusions (see Section III.H). However, in high-risk cases (e.g., lung volume reduction or lung transplant surgery) where avoidance of all respiratory depressants is desirable, analgesia can be achieved using a dilute local anesthetic agent alone. Tachyphylaxis is a common problem with any local anesthetic-alone technique requiring frequent rate readjustments. Removal of an epidural catheter subjects a patient to all the same risks as insertion. When transfer from epidural to oral analgesia is being considered, thromboprophylaxis protocols should be coordinated with epidural catheter removal to minimize the risk of epidural hematoma. If the patient is taking warfarin, the international normalized ratio at the time of catheter removal should be <1.5 to minimize the risk of bleeding.

E. Open and closed (total endovascular aortic repair [TEVAR]) descending thoracic aortic procedures. Major surgical procedures to treat the disease of the descending thoracic aorta often require both an extensive left thoracotomy incision and a long midline abdominal incision. Unfortunately, serious complications are common with these procedures and include high incidences of bleeding/coagulopathy due to the extensive surgery, paraplegia from spinal cord ischemia, and acute kidney injury. Despite the extent and pain associated with these incisions, analgesia is often relegated to a secondary concern. In addition, increased risks of renal and spinal cord injury are relative contraindications to some of the most useful agents of a multimodal approach to severe postoperative pain. However, some creative approaches to analgesia are being considered. In addition to standard intravenous opioid techniques, a tunneled catheter under the left parietal pleura can be placed to extend cephalad over several dermatomes of the chest wall and deliver dilute local anesthetic. Unfortunately, there is little research in this area to guide clinicians. Some anesthesiologists and surgical teams even feel that the benefits of thoracic epidural analgesia merit placement of a thoracic epidural catheter either preoperatively or after surgery. Finally, it is likely that more patients will present for descending thoracic aortic procedures in the future as endovascular stent-grafting techniques improve. Fortunately, these latter procedures are minimally invasive, rarely involve more than groin incisions for access to the femoral vessels and should not be associated with severe pain.

V. Approach to specific complications and side effects of analgesic strategies

A. Complications of nonsteroidal anti-inflammatory drugs

1. **Renal toxicity.** Normal patients exhibit a low rate of prostaglandin synthesis in the renal vasculature, such that cyclo-oxygenase inhibition has little effect. However, vasodilatory prostaglandins may play an important role in preservation of renal perfusion in disease states. Nephrotoxicity, secondary to vasoconstriction of both afferent and efferent renal arterioles leading to reduced glomerular filtration rate, is commonly seen with NSAID administration in patients with dehydration, sepsis, congestive heart failure, or other causes of renal hypoperfusion. Avoiding NSAID-induced renal toxicity is best accomplished by limiting or avoiding their use in patients with decreased renal reserve and in those at risk
6 for hypoperfusion. Risk appears to be low with perioperative ketorolac administration (1 : 1,000 to 1 : 10,000) [23]. NSAID-induced nephrotoxicity is usually reversible with discontinuation of the drug.
2. **Gastrointestinal mucosal irritation.** Gastrointestinal mucosal irritation is the most common NSAID side effect. It can occur regardless of route of administration. It may result in erosion and severe gastrointestinal bleeding. Prostaglandins are involved in multiple aspects of gastric mucosal protection, including mucosal blood flow, epithelial cell growth, and surface mucus and bicarbonate production. Prophylaxis may involve administration of histamine (H_2) receptor antagonists, proton pump inhibitors (omeprazole), protective agents (sucralfate), or prostaglandin analogs (misoprostol). Each of these treatments appears to be effective in decreasing ulceration with NSAID treatment.
3. **Impaired primary hemostasis.** Nonspecific cyclo-oxygenase inhibition leads to impaired platelet aggregation. It may increase intraoperative or postoperative bleeding. Duration of effect is highly variable depending on individual drug (reversible vs. irreversible enzymatic inhibition). The only effective prophylaxis or treatment is to discontinue NSAIDs for a sufficient duration preoperatively (ibuprofen more than 3 days, aspirin more than 7 to 10 days).

B. Nausea and vomiting.

B. Nausea and vomiting. Nausea and vomiting as a consequence of analgesia is most commonly associated with opioids. Opioids cause nausea primarily through activation of the chemoreceptor trigger zone of the brainstem in the floor of the fourth ventricle. A vestibular component is also postulated because it is clear that motion increases the incidence of nausea. Finally, the inhibitory effects of opioids on gastrointestinal motility may contribute. Nausea can accompany opioid therapy regardless of the route of administration. It occurs in roughly 25% to 35% of patients treated with spinal opioids and is more frequent with spinal use of hydrophilic drugs (e.g., morphine) secondary to enhanced rostral spread of these agents [24].

Treatment can include traditional antiemetic drugs such as prochlorperazine, chlorpromazine, promethazine, metoclopramide, or dexamethasone. However, many of these treatments can be complicated by excessive sedation and/or extrapyramidal side effects secondary to central dopamine receptor antagonism. In contrast, serotonin (5-HT) receptor type 3 antagonists are effective antiemetics with fewer side effects. A range of 5-HT_3 antagonists with differing half-lives are available or being studied, including ondansetron (4 to 6 hrs), granisetron (5 to 8 hrs), dolasetron (7 hrs), and palonosetron (40 hrs). Scopolamine, administered via transdermal patch to deliver 0.5 mg/day, is an effective antiemetic for spinal opioids. IV naloxone in doses up to 5 μg/kg/hr is extremely effective in reversing nausea from spinal opioids, without apparent antagonism of analgesia. Often, however, such symptomatic treatment is effective in reducing, but not eliminating, nausea.

C. Pruritus. Pruritus is a common side effect of opioids administered by any route, but it can be particularly problematic after central neuraxial administration. The mechanism is unclear and likely complex, but pruritis is not likely caused solely by either preservatives within the opioid preparation or histamine release. Pruritus often improves as the duration of opioid treatment lengthens. Pruritus is most effectively treated with antihistamines, mixed agonist–antagonist opioids such as nalbuphine, or by naloxone infusion as outlined above.

D. **Respiratory depression.** Hypoventilation is a potentially life-threatening complication of opioids. It can occur early after administration by any route, but it is particularly feared as a delayed complication of neuraxial opioid administration. Whatever the method of administration, opioid-related hypoventilation occurs secondary to elevated cerebrospinal fluid drug levels with depression of the medullary respiratory center, either from systemic absorption or
7 rostral spread of neuraxially administered drug. Respiratory depression requiring naloxone administration is reported to occur in 0.2% to 1% of patients receiving epidural narcotics [25], but the incidence is likely higher in opioid-naive patients being treated for acute pain. Other factors that may increase the risk include advanced age, poor overall medical condition, higher narcotic dosing (particularly of hydrophilic drugs), increased intrathoracic or intra-abdominal pressure (as may occur during mechanical ventilation), and coincident administration of other CNS depressants. Patients who have received spinal narcotics in the prior 18 to 24 hrs or in whom continuous infusions are being administered should have their ventilatory rate and level of alertness confirmed at least hourly. Caretakers should be aware that deteriorating levels of consciousness might portend severe respiratory depression even if ventilatory rates appear preserved. Arterial blood gas analysis should be used early in the investigation of decreased alertness. Modest doses of naloxone (0.04 to 0.1 mg IV) are usually sufficient to temporarily reverse respiratory depression if discovered before it has become severe.

E. **Neurologic complications.** Although neurologic complications from analgesic procedures are extremely rare, when these occur they can be catastrophic, and appropriate management is key to minimizing adverse consequences. Nerve injury may be heralded by an acute discomfort with nerve trauma during a procedure but may only be apparent when local anesthetic effects recede. Therefore, it is essential that this diagnosis is not overlooked in the evaluation of a prolonged block. In particular, if a spinal cord hematoma is being considered, it should be remembered that the promptness of surgical decompression of a spinal hematoma is the most important predictor of recovery of neurologic function [26]. Eighty-eight percent of neurologic deficits related to spinal hematoma will resolve if surgical decompression occurs within 12 hrs of symptom onset, whereas only 40% will have improvement when surgery occurs beyond 24 hrs. A key aspect in evaluation of a possible nerve injury is the involvement of a neurologist in consultation. Most nerve injuries are transient and recover over several days, but the opinion of a specialist in this area will assure that effective acute treatments are not delayed.

VI. Risk versus benefit: Epidural/intrathecal analgesia for cardiac surgical procedures requiring systemic anticoagulation

Controversy has surrounded the subject of whether the risks of neuraxial blockade (principally, epidural hematoma or other spinal bleeding) outweigh the potential benefits (principally, reduced postoperative myocardial ischemia and infarction) in patients undergoing cardiac surgery requiring systemic anticoagulation. Clearly, extensive clinical experience and literature support the safety of neuraxial procedures in the setting of heparin anticoagulation accompanying major vascular surgery; but, in these cases, heparin is typically administered in doses smaller than for cardiac surgery, and its anticoagulant effects are not compounded by the consumptive coagulopathy, inflammatory response, and fibrinolysis that sometimes accompany CPB. For some time, the pro/con debate seemed to favor the safety of neuraxial blockade, provided that commonly recommended precautions are followed. These precautions include avoiding such procedures in patients with any pre-existing hemostatic disorder, postponing cardiac surgery for at least 24 hrs in the event of a traumatic ("bloody") tap at the time of needle or catheter insertion, and delaying heparin administration for at least 60 min after performance of an uncomplicated neuraxial procedure. These beliefs were supported by an oft-cited mathematical analysis published in 2000 suggesting that the risk of spinal bleeding was likely acceptable given the postulated benefits [27]. Up until this time, there were no published reports of epidural hematoma complicating thoracic epidural anesthesia/analgesia for cardiac surgery. The ASRA consensus guidelines only indicate that "insufficient data and experience are available to determine if the risk of neuraxial hematoma is increased when combining neuraxial techniques with the full anticoagulation of cardiac surgery" [14].

Since 2000, however, a body of literature has assembled that does not support the belief that central neuraxial analgesia improves important clinical outcome [8]. Outcome after cardiac surgery rests on many factors, and it may well be that influences such as quality of the surgical intervention and the extent of major organ dysfunction after surgery (factors largely outside the anesthesiologist's control) outweigh the importance of quality analgesia on major morbidity or mortality. Also, in 2004, the first published report of epidural hematoma complicating thoracic epidural placement for cardiac surgery appeared [28], and several other such bleeding complications have occurred in the United States since 2000. It is still true that no reports exist of spinal bleeding complicating single-shot IT drug placement prior to cardiac surgery, and the risk for epidural cathether insertion prior to cardiac surgery has been assessed to be equivalent to that for obstetric anesthesia [29].

Despite widespread belief in the salutatory effects of excellent analgesia, the principal patient-related benefit of central neuraxial analgesia for cardiac surgery is patient satisfaction. Additional benefits of epidural or IT analgesia are not supported by the literature. Pending additional contributions to our understanding, the trend in expert opinion has recently shifted to argue for caution, particularly regarding thoracic epidural catheter placement prior to "full" heparinization for cardiac surgery.

VII. Considerations in facilitating transitions of care

Reliable postoperative analgesia is a key component in facilitating prompt tracheal extubation (within 6 hrs) after cardiac surgery. Such "fast tracking" of low-risk cardiac surgery patients appears to be safe and has been adopted by many centers throughout the world as a process to decrease intensive care unit and hospital lengths of stay. Patients may receive additional benefits such as improved cardiac function and reduced rates of respiratory infections and complications. Attention to reducing risk and to institutional resource utilization has expanded the scale of attention for speeding and improving transitions of care to all cardiothoracic surgical patients, not just those deemed "low risk" in advance. Similarly, the role of the anesthesiologist in care pathway design has expanded well beyond facilitating early extubation and early postoperative analgesia, toward greater preoperative and postoperative integration as a key perioperative physician [30].

IT morphine is used in many centers for eligible cardiac surgery patients to provide analgesia and mild sedation in the early postoperative period. However, some studies have failed to demonstrate a beneficial effect of IT morphine either in improving early analgesia or in facilitating early extubation. NSAIDs complement opioid analgesia regardless of how the opioid is administered. Indomethacin, administered rectally as 100-mg suppositories, is a common component of fast-tracking protocols for cardiac surgery aimed at reducing pain and early postoperative narcotic use. Some NSAIDs may antagonize opioid-induced respiratory depression [31]. Intraoperative and postoperative continuous infusions of remifentanil or alfentanil (with or without supplemental propofol infusion) are used in some centers to allow controlled analgesia and "scheduled extubation." Both a high-dose narcotic technique using the ultra-short-acting narcotic remifentanil [18] or an anesthetic incorporating high thoracic epidural conduction block [21] have been suggested as good methods that may improve outcome through inhibition of perioperative stress response while facilitating early extubation and fast tracking.

Postoperative analgesia strategy for thoracic surgery patients often influences disposition when continuous epidural infusions are used, since the care team must be equipped and trained to intervene when potentially serious complications of postoperative analgesia occur such as hypotension from local anesthetic-mediated reductions in sympathetic tone and delayed respiratory depression due to cephalad spread of neuraxial opioids. In formulating an analgesia plan for thoracic surgery, considerable respect must be paid to failure to achieve tracheal extubation—a serious complication of emergence whose occurrence is partly under the influence of the anesthesiologist. This is particularly important since major pulmonary complications of lung resection surgery are more than twice as likely in the setting of postoperative respiratory failure and highly associated with other markers of adverse outcome, including postoperative mortality. Contributors to the heightened risk of respiratory failure after lung resection include "variable" factors amenable to optimization such as inadequate respiratory mechanics from pain-related chest wall splinting, poor positioning, and residual paralysis.

Since pain at emergence from anesthesia for lung resection is extremely difficult to treat without increasing the risk of acute respiratory depression and interfering with efforts to extubate the patient, the anesthesiologist must be confident that analgesia is established pre-emergence. If a thoracic epidural catheter has been placed, a common practice 10 to 15 min prior to emergence is to supplement existing analgesia with an additional 2 mL bolus of 2% preservative-free lidocaine for an average adult male; this represents a modest investment in protection from emergence pain that rarely causes block-mediated hypotension but allows tracheal extubation before more pain management interventions are needed. Fortunately, difficult emergence sequences are relatively infrequent, but the patient with limited respiratory reserve likely has the most to gain from an experienced anesthesia team to avoid a prolonged episode of postoperative mechanical ventilation. Rarely, sequential blood gas determinations immediately following tracheal extubation (e.g., every 3 min) identify the marginal patient whose CO_2 levels are rising despite optimal analgesia, a concerning finding that requires further prompt intervention and optimization to avert respiratory failure and tracheal reintubation.

REFERENCES

1. Lui F, Ng KF. Adjuvant analgesics in acute pain. *Expert Opin Pharmacother.* 2011;12(suppl 3):363–385.
2. Brame AL, Singer M. Stressing the obvious? An allostatic look at critical illness. *Crit Care Med.* 2010;38(suppl 10):S600–S607.
3. Svircevic V, van Dijk D, Nierich AP, et al. Meta-analysis of thoracic epidural anesthesia versus general anesthesia for cardiac surgery. *Anesthesiology.* 2011;114(suppl 2):271–282.
4. Liu SS, Wu CL. Effect of postoperative analgesia on major postoperative complications: a systematic update of the evidence. *Anesth Analg.* 2007;104(suppl 3):689–702.
5. Manion SC, Brennan TJ. Thoracic epidural analgesia and acute pain management. *Anesthesiology.* 2011;115(suppl 1):181–188.
6. Gottschalk A, Cohen SP, Yang S, et al. Preventing and treating pain after thoracic surgery. *Anesthesiology.* 2006;104(suppl 3): 594–600.
7. Dowling R, Thielmeier K, Ghaly A, et al. Improved pain control after cardiac surgery: results of a randomized, double-blind, clinical trial. *J Thorac Cardiovasc Surg.* 2003;126(suppl 5):1271–1278.
8. Liu SS, Block BM, Wu CL. Effects of perioperative central neuraxial analgesia on outcome after coronary artery bypass surgery: a meta-analysis. *Anesthesiology.* 2004;101(suppl 1):153–161.
9. Svircevic V, Nierich AP, Moons KG, et al. Thoracic epidural anesthesia for cardiac surgery: a randomized trial. *Anesthesiology.* 2011;114(suppl 2):262–270.
10. Inturrisi CE. Clinical pharmacology of opioids for pain. *Clin J Pain.* 2002;18(suppl 4):S3–S13.
11. Nussmeier NA, Whelton AA, Brown MT, et al. Complications of the COX-2 inhibitors parecoxib and valdecoxib after cardiac surgery. *N Engl J Med.* 2005;352(suppl 11):1081–1091.
12. Sinatra RS, Jahr JS, Reynolds LW, et al. Efficacy and safety of single and repeated administration of 1 gram intravenous acetaminophen injection (paracetamol) for pain management after major orthopedic surgery. *Anesthesiology.* 2005;102(suppl 4):822–831.
13. Pettersson PH, Jakobsson J, Owall A. Intravenous acetaminophen reduced the use of opioids compared with oral administration after coronary artery bypass grafting. *J Cardiothorac Vasc Anesth.* 2005;19(suppl 3):306–309.
14. Horlocker TT, Wedel DJ, Rowlingson JC, et al. Regional anesthesia in the patient receiving antithrombotic or thrombolytic therapy: American Society of Regional Anesthesia and Pain Medicine Evidence-Based Guidelines (Third Edition). *Reg Anesth Pain Med.* 2010;35(suppl 1):64–101.
15. Lahtinen P, Kokki H, Hakala T, et al. S(+)-ketamine as an analgesic adjunct reduces opioid consumption after cardiac surgery. *Anesth Analg.* 2004;99(suppl 5):1295–1301; table of contents.
16. Ryu HG, Lee CJ, Kim YT, et al. Preemptive low-dose epidural ketamine for preventing chronic postthoracotomy pain: a prospective, double-blinded, randomized, clinical trial. *Clin J Pain.* 2011;27(suppl 4):304–308.
17. Oates HB. Non-pharmacologic pain control for the CABG patient. *Dimens Crit Care Nurs.* 1993;12(suppl 6):296–304.
18. Zarate E, Latham P, White PF, et al. Fast-track cardiac anesthesia: use of remifentanil combined with intrathecal morphine as an alternative to sufentanil during desflurane anesthesia. *Anesth Analg.* 2000;91(suppl 2):283–287.
19. Rathmell JP, Lair TR, Nauman B. The role of intrathecal drugs in the treatment of acute pain. *Anesth Analg.* 2005;101(suppl 5): S30–S43.
20. Lena P, Balarac N, Arnulf JJ, et al. Intrathecal morphine and clonidine for coronary artery bypass grafting. *Br J Anaesth.* 2003;90(suppl 3):300–303.
21. Scott NB, Turfrey DJ, Ray DA, et al. A prospective randomized study of the potential benefits of thoracic epidural anesthesia and analgesia in patients undergoing coronary artery bypass grafting. *Anesth Analg.* 2001;93(suppl 3):528–535.
22. Licker MJ, Widikker I, Robert J, et al. Operative mortality and respiratory complications after lung resection for cancer: impact of chronic obstructive pulmonary disease and time trends. *Ann Thorac Surg.* 2006;81(suppl 5):1830–1837.
23. Myles PS, Power I. Does ketorolac cause postoperative renal failure: how do we assess the evidence? *Br J Anaesth.* 1998;80(suppl 4): 420–421.
24. Carr DB, Cousins MJ. Spinal route of analgesia: opioids and future options for spinal analgesic chemo therapy. In: Cousins MJ, Carr DB, Horlocker TT, Bridenbaugh P, eds. *Cousins & Bridenbaugh's Neural Blockade in Clinical Anesthesia and Pain Medicine.* 4th ed. Philadelphia, PA: Lippincott Williams & Wilkins; 2008:899.

25. Ready L. Regional anesthesia with intraspinal opioids. In: Loeser J, ed. *Bonica's Management of Pain.* Philadelphia, PA: Lippincott, Williams & Wilkins; 2001:1953–1966.
26. Kunz U. Spinal hematoma: a literature survey with meta-analysis of 613 patients. *Neurosurg Rev.* 2003;26(suppl 1):52.
27. Ho AM, Chung DC, Joynt GM. Neuraxial blockade and hematoma in cardiac surgery: estimating the risk of a rare adverse event that has not (yet) occurred. *Chest.* 2000;117(suppl 2):551–555.
28. Rosen DA, Hawkinberry DW 2nd, Rosen KR, et al. An epidural hematoma in an adolescent patient after cardiac surgery. *Anesth Analg.* 2004;98(suppl 4):966–969.
29. Bracco D, Hemmerling T. Epidural analgesia in cardiac surgery: an updated risk assessment. *Heart Surg Forum.* 2007;10(suppl 4): E334–E337.
30. White PF, Kehlet H, Neal JM, et al. The role of the anesthesiologist in fast-track surgery: from multimodal analgesia to perioperative medical care. *Anesth Analg.* 2007;104(suppl 6):1380–1396, table of contents.
31. Moren J, Francois T, Blanloeil Y, et al. The effects of a nonsteroidal antiinflammatory drug (ketoprofen) on morphine respiratory depression: a double-blind, randomized study in volunteers. *Anesth Analg.* 1997;85(suppl 2):400–405.

Index

Note: Page number followed by *f* and *t* indicates figure and table respectively.

D

J

K

L

M

P

T

W

X

Z